Cardiovascular Catheterization and Intervention

A Textbook of Coronary, Peripheral, and Structural Heart Disease

Second Edition

T0321016

Cardiovascular Catheterization and Intervention

A Textbook of Coronary, Peripheral, and Structural Heart Disease

Second Edition

Edited by

Debabrata Mukherjee

Eric R. Bates

Marco Roffi

Richard A. Lange

David J. Moliterno

Managing Editor

Nadia M. Whitehead

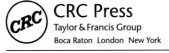

CRC Press
Taylor & Francis Group
Boca Raton London New York

CRC Press is an imprint of the
Taylor & Francis Group, an **informa** business

CRC Press
Taylor & Francis Group
6000 Broken Sound Parkway NW, Suite 300
Boca Raton, FL 33487-2742

First issued in paperback 2020

ISBN 13: 978-0-367-57293-8 (pbk)
ISBN 13: 978-1-4987-5019-6 (hbk)

Library of Congress Cataloging-in-Publication Data

Names: Mukherjee, Debabrata, editor. | Bates, Eric R., editor. | Roffi,
Marco, editor. | Lange, Richard A., editor. | Moliterno, David J., editor.
Title: Cardiovascular catheterization and intervention / [edited by]
Debabrata Mukherjee, Eric R. Bates, Marco Roffi, Richard Lange, David J. Moliterno.
Other titles: Cardiovascular catheterization and intervention (Mukherjee)
Description: Second edition. | Boca Raton, FL : CRC Press/Taylor & Francis
Group, 2018. | Includes bibliographical references and index.
Identifiers: LCCN 2017006001| ISBN 9781498750196 (pack-hardback and ebook :
alk. paper) | ISBN 9781498750264 (ebook) | ISBN 9781498752169 (ebook) |
ISBN 9781498752671 (ebook)
Subjects: | MESH: Cardiac Catheterization--methods | Cardiovascular
Diseases--diagnosis | Cardiovascular Diseases--therapy | Catheterization,
Peripheral--methods | Coronary Angiography--methods
Classification: LCC RC683.5.C25 | NLM WG 141.5.C2 | DDC 616.1/20754--dc23
LC record available at https://lccn.loc.gov/2017006001

Visit the Taylor & Francis Web site at
http://www.taylorandfrancis.com

and the CRC Press Web site at
http://www.crcpress.com

Printed and bound in Great Britain by TJ Books Limited, Padstow, Cornwall

Dedication

To all the cardiology fellows who enrich my academic experience every day, to my parents who continue to inspire me, to wonderful Suchandra for her love, friendship, and support, and to my beloved nephew, Rohin Hegde.

Debabrata Mukherjee

I would like to thank my wife, Nancy, and children, Andrew, Lyndsay, Alexis, and Evan, for all their love and support during the writing of this book.

Eric R. Bates

To my spouse, Muriel, and our children, Emma, Thomas, Giulia, and Edouard, with love and gratitude.

Marco Roffi

The truly important matters of the heart have been imparted to me by my parents, my lovely wife, Bobette, and our three sons—David, Jonathan, and Brian. My dedication is to them, as my love and admiration for them is ineffable.

Richard A. Lange

To my loving wife, Judith, and our sons, Nathaniel and Benjamin, of whom I am forever proud.

David J. Moliterno

Contents

Preface

The field of interventional cardiovascular medicine continues to rapidly evolve in both the diagnostic and therapeutic arenas. Over the past decade, substantial advances have been made on many fronts, including the development and utilization of techniques and devices for intravascular and intracardiac imaging, percutaneous hemodynamic support, newer drug-eluting stents, drug-coated balloons, and percutaneous valve repair and replacement. The evolution of newer drugs and devices challenges the cardiologist to stay abreast of cutting-edge pharmacological and mechanical strategies for optimal patient care. The second edition of *Cardiovascular Catheterization and Intervention: A Textbook of Coronary, Peripheral, and Structural Heart Disease* aims to provide clinicians with comprehensive guidance on the preprocedural, procedural, and postprocedural aspects of coronary, peripheral, and structural heart disease interventions. The text features evidence-based discussions on patient selection, vascular access, general principles of interventional cardiology, and postprocedure management of these patients; it also serves as a comprehensive, easily accessible reference for busy practitioners and cardiovascular trainees.

Of foremost importance, the topic areas covered are relevant to the daily practice of interventional cardiology. The book begins with several chapters dedicated to key concepts associated with cardiac catheterization and interventional cardiovascular medicine. The subsequent chapters focus on hemodynamic assessment and coronary angiography in general and in specific situations, such as those in pediatric patients and in adults with congenital heart disease. The bulk of the text addresses coronary and noncoronary interventions, including structural heart disease interventions. Finally, we have included dedicated chapters on credentialing and organizing prehospital and hospital systems that focus on cardiovascular care. A large number of high-quality illustrations make this textbook particularly attractive to the practitioner.

Essential to the quality and appropriateness of the text is the expertise of the chapter authors. We are fortunate to have assembled a stellar roster of interventional cardiovascular experts to create this book. The contributing authors from leading medical centers around the world have collectively performed hundreds of thousands of procedures and have published thousands of peer-reviewed manuscripts. We are greatly indebted to them. The practice of interventional cardiovascular medicine is exciting, rewarding, and a privilege that each of us enjoys. Likewise, it has been our personal honor to work with these superb contributors, our colleagues in interventional cardiology, as well as the editorial team at CRC Press. It is our hope that you will enjoy this book and that it will be a valuable resource to you in providing the highest quality of care to your patients.

Debabrata Mukherjee
Texas Tech University Health Sciences Center El Paso

Eric R. Bates,
University of Michigan

Marco Roffi
University Hospital of Geneva, Switzerland

Richard A. Lange
Texas Tech University Health Sciences Center El Paso

David J. Moliterno
University of Kentucky

Editors

Debabrata Mukherjee, MD, is a Professor and Chair of Internal Medicine and Chief of Cardiovascular Medicine at Texas Tech University Health Sciences Center El Paso (TTUHSC El Paso) in El Paso, Texas.

Eric R. Bates, MD, is a Professor of Internal Medicine at the University of Michigan, Ann Arbor.

Marco Roffi, MD, is a Professor of Medicine, Vice-Chariman of Cardiology, and Director of the Interventional Cardiology Unit at the University Hospital of Geneva, Switzerland.

Richard A. Lange, MD, MBA, is President of TTUHSC El Paso and Dean of the Paul L. Foster School of Medicine at TTUHSC El Paso in El Paso, Texas.

David J. Moliterno, MD, is a Professor and Chair of Internal Medicine at the University of Kentucky, Lexington.

Contributors

Aamer Abbas MD
Heart and Vascular Center at Titus, Titus Regional Medical Center, Mount Pleasant, Texas, USA

J. Dawn Abbott MD
Cardiovascular Institute, Rhode Island Hospital, Warren Alpert Medical School, Brown University, Providence, Rhode Island, USA

Shikhar Agarwal MD MPH
Interventional Cardiology and Structural Interventions, Geisinger Medical Center, Danville, Pennsylvania, USA

Jorge R. Alegria MD
Sanger Heart & Vascular Institute, Carolinas HealthCare System, Charlotte, North Carolina, USA

Syed Sohail Ali MD
Toledo Cardiology Consultants, Toledo, Ohio, USA

Basil Alkhatib MD
College of Medicine, The University of Arizona, Phoenix, Arizona, USA

Guilherme F. Attizzani MD
Cardiovascular Imaging Core Laboratory, Cardiac Catheterization Laboratory, University Hospitals Cleveland Medical Center, Case Western Reserve University School of Medicine, Cleveland, Ohio, USA

Sawsan Mokhtar M. Awad MD MSc
Rush University Medical Center, Rush Center for Congenital and Structural Heart Disease, Chicago, Illinois, USA

Steven R. Bailey MD
Janey and Dolph Briscoe Division of Cardiology, Long School of Medicine, University of Texas Health Science Center at San Antonio, San Antonio, Texas, USA

Sumit Baral MD
Icahn School of Medicine at Mount Sinai, Mount Sinai Hospital, New York, New York, USA

Thomas M. Bashore MD
Division of Cardiology, Duke University Medical Center, Durham, North Carolina, USA

Chirag Bavishi MD MPH
Department of Cardiology, Mount Sinai St Luke's, New York, New York, USA

Jeroen J. Bax MD PhD
Department of Cardiology, Leiden University Medical Center, Leiden, The Netherlands

Martin R. Bennett MD PhD
Division of Cardiovascular Medicine, University of Cambridge, Cambridge, United Kingdom

Hiram G. Bezerra MD PhD
Cardiovascular Imaging Core Laboratory, Cardiac Catheterization Laboratory, University Hospitals Cleveland Medical Center, Case Western Reserve University School of Medicine, Cleveland, Ohio, USA

Ion Botnaru MD
Olympia Multi-specialty Clinic, Olympia, Washington, USA

Adam J. Brown MD PhD
Division of Cardiovascular Medicine, University of Cambridge, Cambridge, United Kingdom

Adriano Caixeta MD PhD
Hospital Israelita Albert Einstein, Escola Paulista de Medicina, Universidade Federal de São Paulo, São Paulo, Brazil

Qi-Ling Cao MD
Echo and Research Lab, Sidra Cardia Program, Department of Pediatrics, Sidra Medical and Research Center, Doha, Qatar

Blase A. Carabello MD
East Carolina Heart Institute, Brody School of Medicine, East Carolina University, Greenville, North Carolina, USA

John D. Carroll MD
Division of Cardiology, School of Medicine, University of Colorado, Aurora, Colorado, USA

Joseph P. Carrozza Jr. MD
Tufts University School of Medicine,
St. Elizabeth's Medical Center,
and
Steward Health Care Cardiovascular Network, Boston, Massachusetts, USA

Saurav Chatterjee MD
Interventional Cardiology, Temple University Hospital, Philadelphia, Pennsylvania, USA

Jack P. Chen MD
Northside Heart and Vascular Institute, Northside
Hospital, Atlanta, Georgia, USA

Leslie Cho MD
Women's Cardiovascular Center, Preventive Cardiology
& Rehabilitation, Cleveland Clinic Foundation, Cleveland,
Ohio, USA

Marco A. Costa MD PhD
Harrington Heart & Vascular Institute, Interventional
Cardiovascular Center, University Hospitals Cleveland
Medical Center, Case Western Reserve University School
of Medicine, Cleveland, Ohio, USA

Charis Costopoulos MD MPhil
Division of Cardiovascular Medicine, University of
Cambridge, Cambridge, United Kingdom

Fernando Cura MD
Cardiology Clinic, Cardiovascular Institute of Buenos
Aires, Anchorena Hospital, Buenos Aires, Argentina

Charles J. Davidson MD
Division of Cardiology, Department of Medicine, Bluhm
Cardiovascular Institute, Northwestern University
Feinberg School of Medicine, Chicago, Illinois, USA

Laura Davidson MD
Division of Cardiology, Department of Medicine, Bluhm
Cardiovascular Institute, Northwestern University
Feinberg School of Medicine, Chicago, Illinois, USA

Gregory J. Dehmer MD
Division of Cardiology, Baylor Scott & White Health, Texas
A&M College of Medicine, Temple, Texas, USA

Victoria Delgado MD PhD
Department of Cardiology, Leiden University Medical
Center, Leiden, The Netherlands

José G. Díez MD
Interventional Cardiology, Baylor College of Medicine,
Texas Heart Institute, Houston, Texas, USA

Steven P. Dunn PharmD
Heart and Vascular Center, University of Virginia Health
System, University of Virginia School of Medicine,
Charlottesville, Virginia, USA

Franz R. Eberli MD
Division of Cardiology, Triemli Hospital Zurich, Zurich,
Switzerland

John P. Erwin MD
Division of Cardiology, Baylor Scott & White Health, Texas
A&M College of Medicine, Temple, Texas, USA

Amir-Ali Fassa MD
Department of Cardiology, La Tour Hospital, Geneva,
Switzerland

Stefano Galli MD
Centro Cardiologico Monzino, Milan, Italy

Joel A. Garcia Fernandez MD
Orlando Health Heart Institute, Orlando, Florida, USA

Irakli Gogorishvili MD
Jo Ann Medical Centre, T'bilisi, Georgia

Mario Gössl MD PhD
Minneapolis Heart Institute, Abbott Northwestern
Hospital, Minneapolis, Minnesota, USA

Matthias Greutmann MD
Department of Cardiology, University Heart Center,
University Hospital Zurich, Zurich, Switzerland

Paul Michael Grossman MD
Frankel Cardiovascular Center, University of Michigan,
Ann Arbor, Michigan, USA

Christiane Gruner MD
Department of Cardiology, University Heart Center,
University Hospital Zurich, Zurich, Switzerland

Evan L. Hardegree MD
Division of Cardiology, Baylor Scott & White Health,
Temple, Texas, USA

Ziyad M. Hijazi MD MPH
Weil Cornell Medical College, Cornell University,
and
Department of Pediatrics, Sidra Medical and Research
Center, Doha, Qatar

John W. Hirshfeld Jr. MD
Penn Heart and Vascular Center, Perelman School of
Medicine, University of Pennsylvania, Philadelphia,
Pennsylvania, USA

Claudia P. Hochberg MD
The Cardiovascular Center, Boston Medical Center,
Boston, Massachusetts, USA

Eric Horlick MDCM
Peter Munk Cardiac Centre, Toronto General Hospital,
University Health Network, Toronto, Canada

Nay Htyte MD
NYU Cardiac Catheterization Associates, New York
University, Langone Medical Center, New York,
New York, USA

Arif Jivan MD
Division of Cardiology, Feinberg School of Medicine,
Northwestern University, Chicago, Illinois, USA

Brinder Kanda MD
Minneapolis Heart Institute, Abbott Northwestern
Hospital, Minneapolis, Minnesota, USA

David E. Kandzari MD
Piedmont Heart Institute, Piedmont Healthcare, Atlanta,
Georgia, USA

Samir R. Kapadia MD
Department of Cardiovascular Medicine, Cleveland Clinic
Foundation, Cleveland, Ohio, USA

Subrata Kar DO
Department of Internal Medicine, Paul L. Foster School of
Medicine, Texas Tech University Health Sciences Center El
Paso, El Paso, Texas, USA

Morton J. Kern MD
Division of Cardiology, Veterans Affairs Long Beach
Healthcare System, Long Beach, California, USA
and
University of California, Irvine Medical Center, Orange,
California, USA

Spencer B. King, III MD
Emory University School of Medicine, Atlanta, Georgia, USA

Nicholas Kipshidze MD PhD
New York Cardiovascular Research
New York, New York, USA

Amartya Kundu MD
Department of Medicine, University of Massachusetts
Medical School, Worcester, Massachusetts, USA

Rony Lahoud MD MPH
Heart and Vascular Institute, Cleveland Clinic Foundation,
Cleveland, Ohio, USA

Richard A. Lange MD MBA
Paul L. Foster School of Medicine, Texas Tech University
Health Sciences Center El Paso, El Paso, Texas, USA

Michael J. Lim MD
Center for Comprehensive Cardiovascular Care, School of
Medicine, Saint Louis University
St. Louis, Missouri, USA

Robert A. Lookstein MD
Division of Vascular and Interventional Radiology, Icahn
School of Medicine at Mount Sinai, New York, New York, USA

Tracy E. Macaulay PharmD
College of Pharmacy, University of Kentucky, Lexington,
Kentucky, USA

Akiko Maehara MD
Columbia University Medical Center, Cardiovascular
Research Foundation, New York, New York, USA

Alberto Maud MD
Department of Neurology, Paul L. Foster School of
Medicine, Texas Tech University Health Sciences Center El
Paso, El Paso, Texas, USA

Vallerie V. McLaughlin MD
Frankel Cardiovascular Center, University of Michigan,
Ann Arbor, Michigan, USA

Bernhard Meier MD
Department of Cardiology, University Hospital of Bern,
Bern, Switzerland

Mellita Mezody MD
Peter Munk Cardiac Centre, Toronto Western Hospital,
University Health Network, Toronto, Canada

Gary S. Mintz MD
Cardiovascular Research Foundation, New York,
New York, USA

David J. Moliterno MD
Gill Heart and Vascular Institute, University of Kentucky,
Lexington, Kentucky, USA

Piero Montorsi MD
Department of Clinical Sciences and Community Health,
University of Milan, Centro Cardiologico Monzino, Milan, Italy

Motaz Moussa MD
Marietta Memorial Hospital, Memorial Health System,
Marietta, Ohio, USA

Debabrata Mukherjee MD
Department of Internal Medicine, Paul L. Foster School of
Medicine, Texas Tech University Health Sciences Center
El Paso, El Paso, Texas, USA

David W. M. Muller MBBS MD
Department of Cardiology, St. Vincent's Hospital, St.
Vincent's Clinical School, University of New South Wales,
Sydney, New South Wales, Australia

Srihari S. Naidu MD
Hypertophic Cardiomyopathy Program, Westchester
Heart and Vascular Institute, Westchester Medical Center
Health Network, New York Medical College, Hawthorne,
New York, USA

Jose Andrés Navarro MD
Cardiovascular Institute of Buenos Aires,
Buenos Aires, Argentina

Fabian Nietlispach MD PhD
University Heart Center, University Hospital Zurich, Zurich,
Switzerland

Stéphane Noble MD
Division of Cardiology, University Hospital of Geneva,
Geneva, Switzerland

Theophilus Owan MD
Division of Cardiovascular Medicine, Department of Internal
Medicine, The University of Utah, Salt Lake City, Utah, USA

Akhil Parashar MD
Department of Internal Medicine, Cleveland Clinic
Foundation, Cleveland, Ohio, USA

Myung H. Park MD
Houston Methodist DeBakey Heart & Vascular Center,
Houston Methodist Hospital, Houston, Texas, USA

Gabriel Tensol Rodrigues Pereira MD
Cardiovascular Imaging Core Laboratory, Harrington
Heart & Vascular Institute, University Hospitals Cleveland
Medical Center, Cleveland, Ohio, USA

Raffaele Piccolo MD
Department of Cardiology, University Hospital of Bern,
Bern, Switzerland

Mark J. Ricciardi MD
Cardiac Catheterization Labs and Interventional
Cardiology, Northwestern Bluhm Cardiovascular Institute,
Northwestern University Feinberg School of Medicine,
Chicago, Illinois, USA

Albert P. Rocchini MD
Department of Pediatrics, University of Michigan, C.S.
Mott Children's Hospital, Ann Arbor, Michigan, USA

Gustavo J. Rodriguez MD
Department of Neurology, Paul L. Foster School of
Medicine, Texas Tech University Health Sciences Center El
Paso, El Paso, Texas, USA

Marco Roffi MD
Division of Cardiology, University Hospital of Geneva,
Geneva, Switzerland

Robert J. Rosen MD
Lenox Hill Heart and Vascular Institute, New York,
New York, USA

Gregg F. Rosner MD
Division of Cardiovascular Medicine, Columbia University
Medical Center, New York, New York, USA

John H. Rundback MD
Interventional Institute, Holy Name Medical Center,
Advanced Interventional Radiology Svcs LLP, Teaneck,
New Jersey, USA

Fadi A. Saab MD
Michigan State University,
and
Pulmonary Embolism and DVT Program, Department of
Cardiovascular Medicine, University of Michigan Health,
Grand Rapids, Michigan, USA

Robert D. Safian MD
Center for Innovation and Research in Cardiovascular
Diseases, Department of Cardiovascular Medicine,
Beaumont Health, Royal Oak, Michigan, USA

M. Rizwan Sardar MD
Division of Cardiology, Warren Alpert Medical School,
Brown University, Providence, Rhode Island, USA

Partha Sardar MD
Division of Cardiovascular Medicine, The University of
Utah, Salt Lake City, Utah, USA

Arnold H. Seto MD
Division of Cardiology, Veterans Affairs Long Beach
Healthcare System, Long Beach, California, USA
and
University of California, Irvine Medical Center, Orange,
California, USA

Richard W. Smalling MD PhD
Division of Cardiovascular Medicine, McGovern Medical
School, University of Texas Health Science Center at
Houston,
and
Memorial Hermann Heart and Vascular Institute, Houston,
Texas, USA

Athanasios Smyrlis MD
South Nassau Cardiac Care, South Nassau Communities
Hospital, Oceanside, New York, USA

Amirreza Solhpour MD
Division of Cardiovascular Medicine, McGovern Medical
School, University of Texas Health Science Center at Houston
and
Memorial Hermann Heart and Vascular Institute, Houston,
Texas, USA

Paul Sorajja MD
Center for Valve and Structural Heart Disease,
Minneapolis Heart Institute, Abbott Northwestern
Hospital, Minneapolis, Minnesota, USA

Mohamad Soud MD
Cardiovascular Imaging Core Laboratory, Harrington
Heart & Vascular Institute, University Hospitals Cleveland
Medical Center, Cleveland, Ohio, USA

Roberto Spina MBBS MS
Department of Cardiology, St. Vincent's Hospital, Sydney,
New South Wales, Australia

Garrick C. Stewart MD MPH
Division of Cardiovascular Medicine, Brigham and
Women's Hospital, Boston, Massachusetts, USA

Saad Hussain Syed MD
Department of Internal Medicine, Paul L. Foster School of
Medicine, Texas Tech University Health Sciences Center El
Paso, El Paso, Texas, USA

James E. Tcheng MD
Division of Cardiology, Duke University School of
Medicine, Duke University Health System, Durham, North
Carolina, USA

Carl L. Tommaso MD
Cardiac Catheterization Laboratory, NorthShore
University HealthSystem, Rush Medical School
Evanston, Illinois, USA

Laurens F. Tops MD PhD
Department of Cardiology, Leiden University Medical
Center, Leiden, The Netherlands

E. Murat Tuzcu MD
Department of Cardiovascular Medicine, Cleveland Clinic
Abu Dhabi, Abu Dhabi, United Arab Emirates

Zoltan G. Turi MD
Seton Hall University School of Medicine, Structural
Heart Program and Cardiac Catheterization Laboratory,
Hackensack University Medical Center, New Brunswick,
New Jersey, USA

Dennis W. den Uijl MD PhD
Department of Cardiology, Leiden University Medical
Center, Leiden, The Netherlands

Michele Doughty Voeltz MD
Henry Ford Health System, Detroit, Michigan, USA

Peter Wenaweser MD
Department of Cardiology, University Hospital of Bern,
Cardiovascular Center Zurich, Hirslanden Clinic in the
Park, Bern and Zurich, Switzerland

Christopher J. White MD
Department of Cardiology, Ochsner Medical Center, New
Orleans, Louisiana, USA

David O. Williams MD
Harvard Medical School, Cardiovascular Division, Brigham
and Women's Hospital, Boston, Massachusetts, USA

James M. Wilson MD
Interventional Cardiology, Houston, Texas, USA

Stephan Windecker MD
Department of Cardiology, University Hospital of Bern,
Bern, Switzerland

Hong Jun Yun MD
Frankel Cardiovascular Center, University of Michigan,
Ann Arbor, Michigan, USA

PART 1

General Concepts

Introduction to cardiac catheterization

RICHARD A. LANGE AND STEVEN R. BAILEY

INTRODUCTION

Cardiac catheterization is one of the most frequently performed procedures in the United States. Over the past 25 years, the number of procedures has increased 3.5-fold because of expanded indications and improvements in techniques and equipment.[1] In 2005, an estimated 1,322,000 inpatient left heart diagnostic catheterizations and 1,271,000 inpatient percutaneous coronary interventional (PCI) procedures were performed in the United States.[1] According to the most recent American Hospital Association survey, 36% of the 4,836 hospitals in the United States have adult diagnostic catheterization laboratories. Of the 1,728 hospital-centered adult diagnostic laboratories, 78% are PCI capable.[2]

Historical perspective

THE EARLY YEARS OF CATHETERIZATION: ANIMAL AND CADAVERIC STUDIES (1711–1927)

The earliest known cardiac catheterization of an animal was performed in 1710 by Reverend Stephen Hales, an English physiologist and parson, who "bled a sheep to death and then led a gun barrel from the neck vessels into the still beating heart. Through this, he filled the hollow chambers with molten wax and then measured from the resultant cast the volume of the heartbeat and the minute-volume of the heart, which he calculated from the pulse beat."[3,4] In addition, Hales was the first to determine systemic arterial pressure, when, in 1727, he measured the rise in a column of blood in a long glass tube secured in an artery (Figure 1.1). Brass pipes placed in the carotid artery and jugular vein of a horse were connected to an 11-ft-high glass tube for pressure measurements, with the trachea of a goose used as a flexible connector. Hales astutely noted that the pressure was different in arteries and veins (blood from the carotid artery rose to a height of more than 8 ft in the glass tube, whereas blood from the jugular vein rose less than 1 ft) and between contractions and relaxations of the heart.

In 1844, the term *cardiac catheterization* was coined by Claude Bernard, a French physiologist who inserted long glass thermometers into a horse's right and left ventricles from its jugular vein and carotid artery, respectively. By demonstrating that blood temperature was higher in the right ventricle than in the left, he established that "chemical reactions" (i.e., metabolism) occurred in the body rather than the lungs. Subsequently, he used this technique to acquire blood samples from various arterial and venous sites for metabolic studies, and he performed intracardiac pressure recordings in dogs and sheep to study the regulation of systemic arterial pressure by the nervous system. He was the first to describe right and left heart catheterization via the femoral vein and artery.[5,6] Although Bernard was not the first to perform catheterization, his careful application of scientific methods to the study of cardiac physiology demonstrated the potential importance of cardiac catheterization and initiated an era of cardiovascular physiologic investigation.

In 1861, Etienne Jules Marey, another French physiologist, in collaboration with Jean Baptiste Auguste Chauveau, a veterinarian, elucidated the nature of the apex beat by simultaneously recording its movement and the right atrial and right ventricular pressures of a conscious horse.[7] Their observation that the apical impulse was caused by early forceful ventricular contraction remains a milestone as the first graphic recording of intracardiac events in a conscious animal (Figure 1.2).[8] Gaining access to the left ventricle via the carotid artery, they studied left ventricular pressure waveforms and characterized various phases of the cardiac cycle, and they were the first to obtain simultaneous recordings of left ventricular and aortic pressures. In addition,

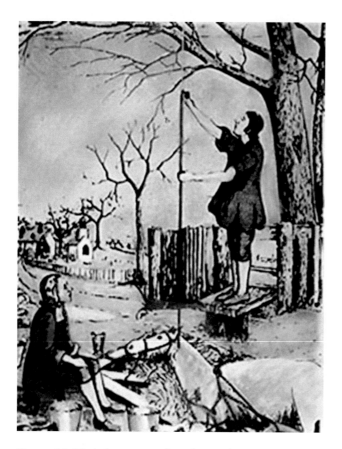

Figure 1.1 First documented cardiac catheterization performed by Hales in 1711. (Courtesy of the Bettmann Archives.)

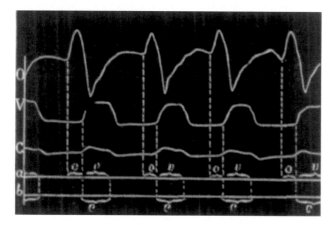

Figure 1.2 First published records of pressure pulses in a cardiac chamber obtained by catheterization of the right atrium (O) and ventricle (V) via the jugular vein in an unanesthetized horse. The third tracing (C) is from an intrathoracic balloon catheter placed to detect the cardiac impulse. (From Chaveau, A., and Marey, É. J., *Circulation Research*, 22, 96, 1968. With permission.)

Marey and Chaveau invented the double-lumen catheter, with which they simultaneously measured pressures in contiguous cardiac chambers in horses and dogs. Decades later, André Cournand (see following text) utilized this catheter design to perform similar studies in humans.

In 1870, Adolph Fick (Figure 1.3), a German physicist and physiologist, proposed a direct method of measuring cardiac output. In a commentary to his local medical society that resulted in a publication less than one page long (the Fick principle, 1870), Fick proposed that the cardiac output could be measured by dividing the oxygen uptake by the corresponding arteriovenous oxygen content difference.[9] Interestingly, in 1873 Fick published the results of right and left heart catheterizations that he performed in animals, but he did not utilize or validate his method.[10] Only two decades later did physiologists begin to apply the Fick principle in animals. Although Grehant and Quinquand published a brief report describing use of the technique in dogs in 1886, it was not until 1898, when Zuntz and Hageman made a detailed study of cardiac output in the horse at rest and during exercise, that the Fick method was established as reliable and reproducible.[11] Application of the Fick principle in humans was hindered by the difficulty of obtaining samples of mixed venous blood. Invasive catheterization was thought to be too dangerous to be applied to human subjects because of excessive blood loss and the risk of infection. Furthermore, radiography was not yet available, so attempts to obtain samples of mixed venous blood were made by such avant-garde interventions as direct transthoracic needle puncture of the right ventricle.[12]

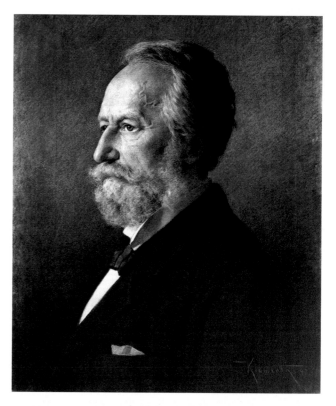

Figure 1.3 Adolph Fick (1829–1901), a mathematician, physicist, and physiologist. His major research interest was in the physiology of muscular contraction. He described the calculation of cardiac output as an outgrowth of his mathematical approach to physiologic events.

With the discovery of X-rays in 1895 by William Roentgen, radiographic equipment was quickly introduced into laboratories in universities and medical schools throughout Europe and North America.[13] Within a month of the publication of Roentgen's paper, two European physicians published the first arteriogram, which was obtained by injecting chalk into the brachial artery of a cadaver and observing the arterial supply of the hand with a roentgenogram.[14] In October 1896, Francis Williams, a radiologist at Boston City Hospital, published his observations on the use of the fluoroscope to evaluate the beating heart.[15] A decade later, Friedrich Jamin and Hermann Merkel, German physicians, published the first roentgenographic atlas of human coronary arteries.[16] In their 1907 description of 29 excised hearts, coronary arteries were injected with a suspension of red lead in gelatin, after which stereoscopic roentgenograms were obtained (Figure 1.4).[13] In some of the specimens, coronary arterial obstructions and collateral blood vessels were noted, which helped form the basis of James Herrick's seminal 1912 paper, titled "Certain Clinical Features of Sudden Obstruction of the Coronary Arteries." His observations served to advance our understanding of the pathophysiology of coronary artery disease, angina pectoris, and myocardial infarction (MI).[17,18]

For angiography to be safe and practical in a living human subject, several developments were necessary, including the availability of a nontoxic radiopaque material that could be safely injected intravascularly. In this regard, an important advance occurred in 1921 with the introduction of lipiodol, a 40% solution of iodine in poppy oil.[19] The injection of lipiodol into an antecubital vein permitted roentgenographic visualization of the pulmonary circulation. Sodium iodide, originally introduced as a urographic contrast agent in 1918, was first administered intravascularly by Osborne et al. at the Mayo Clinic in 1923.[20] The following year, Barney Brooks, a vascular surgeon at Washington University, described the intraarterial injection of sodium iodide in patients with suspected peripheral vascular disease.[21] The application of vascular roentgenography to the coronary arteries did not take place in the 1920s, in large part because the technique for human heart catheterization had not yet been described.

CARDIAC CATHETERIZATION PERFORMED IN HUMANS (1928–1929)

In 1929, Werner Forssmann (Figure 1.5) first reported the passage of a catheter into the heart of a living subject: himself.[22] As a medical student, Forssmann learned of the work of Bernard, Chauveau, and Marey, and became interested in using catheterization for the intracardiac

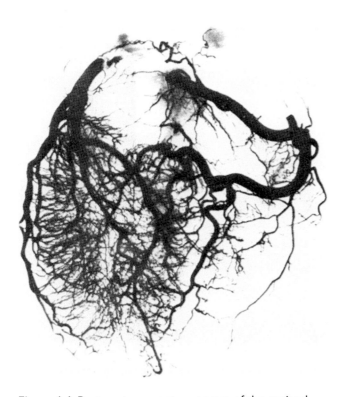

Figure 1.4 Postmortem roentgenogram of the excised heart of a 20-year-old man who died of pneumonitis. The coronary arteries were injected with a mixture of red lead and gelatin.

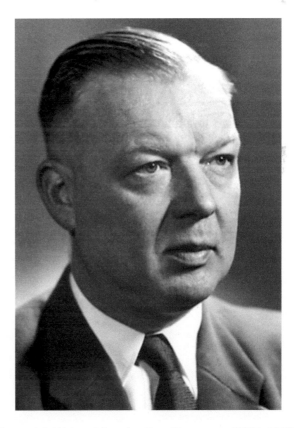

Figure 1.5 Werner Theodor Otto Forssmann (1904–1979). In 1929, interested in direct injections into the heart for resuscitation, he demonstrated on himself the feasibility of cardiac catheterization. In 1956, he shared the Nobel Prize in Physiology or Medicine with André Cournand and Dickinson Richards. From 1950 onward, he practiced as a urologist.

administration of drugs for attempted cardiac resuscitation.[4] Believing that catheterization could be applied as safely in humans as in animals, he performed the self-catheterization during his surgical residency at the Auguste-Viktoria Hospital in Eberswalde, Germany (Figure 1.6). According to Forssmann's daughter,[23]

> [H]e inserted the [ureteral] catheter through a vena sectio of the left cubital vein and pushed it up to about 65 cm—the estimated distance to the right heart. He experienced a sensation of warmth on the wall of the vein when he moved the catheter and a slight cough, which he attributed to stimulating the vagus nerve. With the catheter in his heart, he walked from the operating room downstairs to the X-ray room. He took X rays [Figure 1.7] while moving the catheter with the help of a nurse. This nurse held a mirror in front of Forssmann so that he could observe the position of the catheter and take X rays when the tip of the catheter passed the axilla and entered the right atrium, respectively. He could not continue to move the catheter forward into the right ventricle because the catheter was not long enough.

Forssmann's successful procedure was performed under inauspicious circumstances. He had discussed his ideas about heart catheterization with the chief of surgery, who forbade him from performing studies in humans without preliminary research in experimental animals to demonstrate the procedure's safety. To procure the surgical instruments for the vena sectio, Forssmann assuaged the scrub nurse's concerns about the procedure's safety by agreeing to allow her to be the subject, as she had requested.[24] He had her lie down on the operating table and then strapped her arms and legs. While distracting her by applying iodine to

her elbow, he anesthetized his own arm, performed a cutdown of the antecubital vein, and inserted a ureteral catheter into it. At that point, he released her and enlisted her help in assisting him down the stairs to the X-ray room to perform fluoroscopy. When word of Forssmann's self-catheterization reached the chief of surgery, Forssmann was reprimanded for his disobedience and promptly fired. When his work was published the following year (1929), it was acclaimed by the popular press but ridiculed and vilified by the medical community.[22] He was immediately dismissed from his new position at a Berlin hospital and informed that "he could lecture in a circus, but never in a respectable German university."[23] Before being dismissed, he performed experiments in animals to demonstrate the value of contrast angiography as a diagnostic tool. He used rabbits in his first experiments and later confessed that "if he had started experimenting with rabbits, he would never have experimented on himself. When the tip of catheter touched the rabbit's endocardium, the electrocardiogram showed temporary cardiac arrest."[23]

Forssmann ultimately continued his studies in dogs at another institution and reported in 1931 that angiography was a safe and useful diagnostic procedure.[25] During this time period, he catheterized himself nine more times in an attempt to obtain a publishable angiogram of his heart, but he was unsuccessful. "The response of the academic community ranged from laughter and disbelief to admiration."[23] He left academic medicine in 1932 to practice urology, remaining in obscurity until he, André Cournand, and Dickinson Richards were awarded the 1956 Nobel Prize in Physiology or Medicine, he for pioneering the procedure

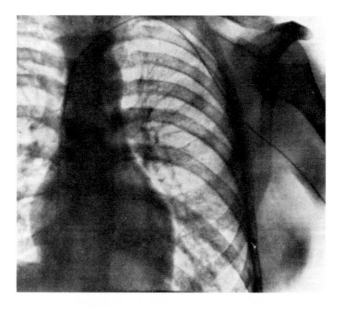

Figure 1.7 First documented human cardiac catheterization. As a 25-year-old surgical resident, Forssmann passed a ureteral catheter via a left basilic vein cutdown into his right atrium and then took this roentgenogram. (From Forssmann, W., *Klinische Wochenschrift*, 8, 2085–2087, 1929. With permission.)

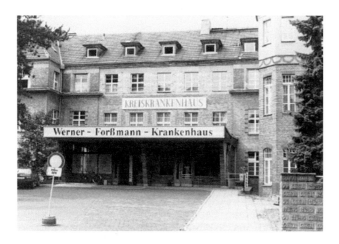

Figure 1.6 The hospital in Eberswalde where Forssmann performed the first catheterization. (From Forssmann-Falck, R., *American Journal of Cardiology*, 79(5), 651–660, 1997. With permission.)

and the others for developing its application. Although Forssmann is credited with being the first to report heart catheterization in human subjects, Otto Klein, in fact, should be recognized for performing the first diagnostic right heart catheterizations. In 1929, Klein performed 11 successful right heart catheterizations, including passage of a catheter into the right atrium and right ventricle, and he estimated the cardiac output in his human subjects using the Fick principle.[26]

THE ERA OF HEMODYNAMIC CARDIAC STUDIES (1930–1940s)

Although isolated reports of pulmonary[27,28] and right heart angiography via right atrial injection[29] appeared soon after Forssmann's publication, cardiac catheterization progressed slowly in the 1930s because of the poor quality of the radiographic images and concerns about safety. In a 1932 book on the measurement of cardiac output, Forssmann's technique was considered "not only dangerous to the subject, but useless as far as cardiac output determinations are concerned... This method must thus be considered merely a clinical curiosity."[30] In addition, progress in the field was hindered by the events leading to World War II that interrupted biomedical research in Europe. However, in the Western Hemisphere, Castellano (in Cuba) and Rob and Steinberg (in New York) obtained high-quality images of all four cardiac chambers and the great vessels using a rapid intravenous injection of radiographic contrast material.[31,32]

As Forssmann noted in his Nobel Prize acceptance speech in 1956, "A turning point in the history of cardiology is the year 1941, when Cournand and Ranges made known their first experiments with the heart catheter as a clinical method of investigation."[4] They showed that "consistent values for blood gases could be obtained from the right atrium, that with this, cardiac output could be reliably and fairly accurately determined by the Fick principle, and

furthermore that the catheter could be left in place for considerable periods without harm."[33] Prior to their published studies, cardiac catheterization was not routinely considered "a safe and sound procedure to study cardiac physiology,"[34] so their article served as a breakthrough.

The development of pressure manometers and the double-lumen catheter, through which simultaneous pressures in two contiguous heart chambers and large vessels could be recorded, served as important advances that allowed Cournand et al. to obtain the first tracings of pressures recorded simultaneously from the right ventricle and pulmonary artery (Figure 1.8).[35] Their "tracing holds a unique place, since it is the first demonstration that the tip of a catheter was placed in the pulmonary artery of man in order to record pressure pulses."[35] Cournand and his colleague Dickinson W. Richards developed the technique of heart catheterization for safe and widespread use "not only to normal man but to patients even in the most severe and acute stages of decompensation."[33] As a result of their efforts, cardiopulmonary physiologic investigation accelerated rapidly. As noted previously, their seminal work was acknowledged when they (along with Werner Forssmann) received the 1956 Nobel Prize in Physiology or Medicine (Figure 1.9).

While Cournand and Richards used right heart and pulmonary arterial catheterization primarily to study the pulmonary circulation, Lewis Dexter refined its use in patients with heart disease. In 1946, he described the placement of a stiff catheter in the pulmonary capillary "wedge" position, where he obtained blood samples for determination of oxygen saturation; the following year, he reported hemodynamic and oximetric data from normal subjects and those with congenital heart disease.[36,37]

The development of new synthetic catheter material in the 1940s (including polyethylene, nylon, woven Dacron, polyurethane, and metal braiding) facilitated heart catheterization, which was previously performed with modified

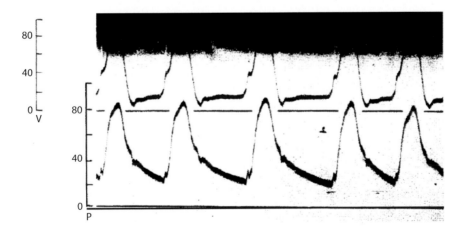

Figure 1.8 The first published pressure recordings from the pulmonary artery of man. The simultaneous tracings in the pulmonary artery and the right ventricle were obtained with a double-lumen catheter in a patient with severe pulmonary hypertension. (Note: the scale is in mmHg.) (From Cournand, A., in *Nobel Lectures, Physiology or Medicine 1942–1962,* Elsevier Publishing Company, Stockholm, 1956. With permission from the ©The Nobel Foundation, 1956/Andre F. Cournand.)

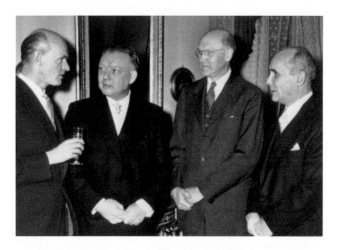

Figure 1.9 Nobel Prize Ceremony, Stockholm, Sweden, December, 1956. From left to right: Professor Sten Friberg of the Karolinska Institute chatting with Nobel Laureates Werner Forssmann, Dickinson W. Richards and André Cournand. (From Forssmann-Falck, R., *American Journal of Cardiology*, 79(5), 651–660, 1997. With permission.)

rubber urologic catheters. In part, the development of such synthetic material resulted from the difficulty of obtaining rubber during World War II. Concomitantly, improvements in radiographic equipment and techniques (e.g., rapid series "cut films," image intensifiers, cineangiography, etc.) paved the way for the subsequent development of diagnostic and therapeutic left heart catheterization and coronary angiography. Finally, safer and more widely applicable techniques with which to gain access to the aorta were developed during this time. Direct needle access of the aorta was abandoned in favor of retrograde catheterization of the femoral, brachial, or radial arteries via cutdown or percutaneous puncture.[6] Although aortography had been performed in the late 1940s, the passage of a catheter in a retrograde fashion across the aortic valve into the left ventricle was considered to be excessively dangerous. Instead, left ventriculography was performed via direct left ventricular transthoracic needle puncture.[6]

LEFT HEART CATHETERIZATION AND CORONARY ANGIOGRAPHY (1950–1960s)

Retrograde left heart catheterization was initially reported in 1950 by Zimmerman, who performed "pull-back" pressure measurements in a patient with aortic regurgitation.[38] Although enthusiasm for left heart catheterization escalated, the lack of safe and reliable access to the arterial system tempered its use. In 1953, Sven-Ivar Seldinger, a Swedish radiologist, developed a technique of introducing catheters into the arterial circulation. "A needle is introduced, a guidewire is pushed into it, and the needle is removed. The catheter then is guided in over the wire, which also is removed."[39,40] This technique, which bears his name (the "Seldinger technique"), continues to be used in virtually all catheterization procedures.

A new era in cardiovascular medicine began in 1958 when selective coronary angiography was performed in a patient undergoing left heart catheterization. Previously, visualization of the coronary arterial system was obtained nonselectively by a variety of techniques, including the following:

1. Balloon occlusion of the ascending aorta during aortic root injection of contrast material[41]
2. Aortic root injection of contrast material enhanced by acetylcholine-induced ventricular arrest[42]
3. Phasic injections of contrast material timed to occur during ventricular diastole[43]
4. Use of various catheters designed to opacify the coronary sinuses while directing jets of contrast material toward the coronary arterial ostia[44]

Selective coronary angiography was not attempted because of concerns that it would cause myocardial hypoxia, which might lead to an electrical imbalance and a resultant fatal ventricular arrhythmia. In support of these concerns, Nobel Laureate André Cournand reported "his personal experience of a 100% fatality rate when contrast was selectively injected in the coronary arteries of dogs."[45]

On October 30, 1958, Mason Sones, a pediatric cardiologist, inadvertently performed the first selective coronary angiogram in a 26-year-old patient with aortic regurgitation.[46] After performing left ventriculography, Sones reported[47]:

I asked my associate to withdraw the catheter tip across the aortic valve into the ascending aorta so that we could complete the procedure by performing an aortogram with the catheter tip in the ascending aorta. My associate complied and we relied on the pressure change from the left ventricle to the ascending aorta without sliding the table top back under the 5 inch amplifier to confirm the exact location of the tip. I didn't think this was necessary because I was quite certain that the catheter tip lay in the ascending aorta just above the aortic valve. My associate, Dr. Royston Lewis, made an injection of 40 cc of 90% Hypaque through the catheter. About one second before the injection was initiated, I had the switch to initiate a cine run. When the injection began, I was horrified to see the right coronary artery become heavily opacified and realized the catheter tip was actually inside the orifice of the dominant right coronary artery. I shouted, "Pull it out." Our combined reaction times to accomplish withdrawal of the catheter consumed from 3–4 seconds which meant that approximately 30 cc of 90% Hypaque had been delivered into the right coronary artery. I was of course horrified because I was certain the patient would develop ventricular fibrillation. At that time we did not have direct current defibrillators and knew nothing about the application of closed chest cardiac massage. I climbed out of the hole and ran around the table looking for a scalpel to open his chest in order to defibrillate him by direct application of the paddles of an alternating current defibrillator. I looked at the oscilloscope tracing of his electrocardiogram and it was evident that he was in asystole rather than in ventricular fibrillation. I knew that an explosive cough could produce a very effective pressure pulse in the aorta and hoped that this might push the contrast media through his myocardial capillary bed. Fortunately, he was still conscious and responded to my demand that he cough repeatedly. After three to four explosive coughs, his heart began to beat again with initially a sinus bradycardia which accelerated into a sinus tachycardia within 15 to 20 seconds. He then made a perfectly uneventful recovery with no neurological deficit or other sequelae.

The failure of ventricular arrhythmias to materialize during this inadvertent selective coronary arterial opacification convinced Sones that the human coronary circulation was different from that of dogs, so he continued to perform selective coronary angiography in patients, with access to the arterial system obtained via a brachial artery cutdown. Sones' seminal discovery eventually opened the door to coronary artery bypass surgery and interventional cardiology. The development of preformed coronary catheters by Judkins, Amplatz, Schoonmaker, and others;[6,48–50] a percutaneous femoral arterial approach;[51] and sheaths with a hemostatic valve[52] further refined the technique, which has become standard in thousands of catheterization laboratories around the world.

Shortly after selective coronary angiography was adopted, quantitation of left ventricular function and correlation with coronary anatomy transpired. In 1960, Dodge and coworkers reported methods to determine left ventricular volumes via "angiocardiography" and to quantitate global function by introducing the concept of ejection fraction.[53] Subsequently, their work provided the basis for the quantitative assessment of regional wall motion.

Concomitant with the development of selective coronary angiography and quantitative ventriculography, the early foundations for coronary intervention were laid by Charles Dotter, a radiologist in Portland, Oregon. In 1963, he inadvertently recanalized an occluded right iliac artery by passing a catheter through the site of occlusion.[54] The following year, Dotter and his trainee, Melvin Judkins, performed the first intentional percutaneous transluminal angioplasty on the popliteal artery of an 82-year-old woman with gangrene who refused amputation. The site of severe obstruction was dilated with rigid catheters of increasing diameter, the patient's leg was salvaged, and angiography 2 years later demonstrated a patent vessel.[54] The "Dotter technique" was not widely embraced in the United States because it was considered to be crude, technically cumbersome, and associated with a high incidence of failure and complications. However, it was widely employed in Germany, where

Andreas Gruentzig, a young German angiology fellow, learned the technique in 1969 and conceived of adding a balloon to the Dotter catheter so that it could be applied to other arterial systems.

THE AGE OF PERCUTANEOUS CORONARY REVASCULARIZATION (1970–1980s)

Attempts to improve on Dotter's techniques by adding a balloon to the dilatation catheter were met with limited success, in large part because the balloon material was too fragile or too compliant for dilatation of rigid plaques. Gruentzig set out to develop a suitable catheter with a nondistensible balloon for use in narrowed coronary arteries. He chose polyvinyl chloride at the suggestion of a professor emeritus of chemistry who was working across the street from Gruentzig's institution, the University Hospital of Zurich.[55] Using heat molding and compressed air, he manufactured balloon catheters in his kitchen at night and on weekends with the help of his wife and friends.[6] After testing these balloon catheters in animals, he performed the first of several hundred successful percutaneous balloon angioplasties of peripheral arteries in human subjects in February 1974.[56] Subsequently, he refined and miniaturized his balloon catheters so that they could be used in the coronary arterial circulation. Although he conducted extensive studies in animals and human cadavers (Figure 1.10), skepticism concerning the utility of coronary balloon angioplasty was widespread. After successful coronary angioplasty in a dog,[57]

the pathologist wrote in his report that Gruentzig should stop doing whatever he was doing and certainly never come close to a human being with this terrible balloon instrument because the canine heart and coronary arteries looked terrible.

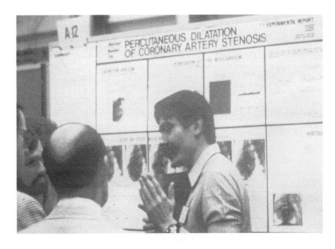

Figure 1.10 Andreas R. Gruentzig standing in front of his poster describing percutaneous dilatation of a canine coronary arterial stenosis at the American Heart Association meeting in Miami, Florida, in November 1976. (From King, S. B. 3rd, and Meier, B., *Circulation*, 102(20 Suppl 4), IV81–IV86, 2000. With permission.)

Despite widespread skepticism, Gruentzig performed the first successful percutaneous transluminal coronary angioplasty (PTCA) in a human subject in Zurich, Switzerland, on September 16, 1977. The patient, a 38-year-old man, had unstable angina and a discrete stenosis in his proximal left anterior descending coronary artery. Following two balloon dilatations, he became free of angina, and when he underwent catheterization at Emory University on September 16, 1987—precisely 10 years after his original procedure—his left anterior descending coronary artery was widely patent. In 2000, repeat catheterization performed for chest pain thought to be atypical for angina showed that "the dilated area was pristine" (Figure 1.11).[55]

PTCA was first performed in the United States on March 1, 1978, simultaneously by Richard Myler in San Francisco and Simon Stertzer in New York.[6] It was rapidly adopted by American cardiologists, but in Europe it was received with skepticism. Gruentzig encountered obstacles that prevented him from developing the technique in Zurich, so in 1980 he moved to Emory University in Atlanta, Georgia, where he continued to refine the procedure until his untimely death in 1985 in an airplane crash. Several technical developments led to the widespread use of PTCA, the most important of which was the introduction of steerable guidewires, which allowed the application of PTCA to distal coronary arterial stenoses and tortuous vessels. At the same time, softer, smaller diameter guiding catheters and lower profile, more flexible

balloons were manufactured. Altogether, these technologic advances resulted in higher rates of success and lower rates of complications, even though PTCA was being used in patients with more technically difficult stenoses and in those with multivessel coronary artery disease.

Throughout the 1980s, the balloon catheter remained the primary device for performing angioplasty, but by the late 1980s, new equipment began to emerge. The first addition, the directional atherectomy device developed by John Simpson, was based on the idea that removal of atherosclerotic tissue would be superior to simple dilation of the artery. Peripheral arterial atherectomy was first reported in 1985,[58] and the following year the device was successfully applied to coronary arteries.[59] Although higher procedural success rates were noted with atherectomy than with balloon angioplasty in randomized comparisons, atherectomy was not widely adopted, since it was more tedious and expensive and was associated with a higher rate of non–Q wave MIs. Subsequently, other atherectomy (extraction, rotational, thermal, laser) and thrombectomy devices were developed. In randomized comparisons with balloon angioplasty or stenting (see following text), many of the atherectomy devices were associated with higher acute complication rates without improving late results. Therefore, their use is currently restricted to coronary arterial stenoses that are not thought to be amenable to balloon angioplasty or stenting.

THE STENT ERA (1990s–2000s)

The derivation of the term *stent* is attributed to Dr. Charles Stent (1807–1885) (Figure 1.12), who developed a material that enabled him to secure better dental molds.[60] The concept of endovascular stents is attributed to Alexis Carrel, 1912 Nobel laureate and vascular surgeon, who implanted glass and metal tubes into the aorta of dogs.[61] Fifty years later, Charles Dotter developed "sleeve" graft devices and metallic coils, which he used in experimental animals, but he never implanted them in patients.[6] The recognition that PTCA resulted in acute vessel closure in ~5% of patients and restenosis in >30% in those in whom it was attempted, accelerated the development of an endoprosthetic device (e.g., stent) to enhance procedural results, avert vessel closure, and prevent restenosis. The first implantation of coronary arterial stents in humans occurred in 1986 in Europe, with insertion of the spring-loaded, self-expanding Wallstent.[6] The following year, a balloon-mounted, wire coil stent designed by Cesar Gianturco was implanted at Emory University Hospital in Atlanta, Georgia, and a slotted tube stent designed by Julio Palmaz was inserted in a patient in São Paulo, Brazil. The Gianturco-Roubin stent was approved for use by the U.S. Food and Drug Administration (FDA) in 1993 in subjects with abrupt and threatened arterial closure (Figure 1.13). In 1994, the Palmaz-Schatz stent was approved by the FDA.[62]

Initially, intensive anticoagulation and antiplatelet therapy were administered to patients in whom intracoronary stents were deployed to prevent acute (in-hospital) and

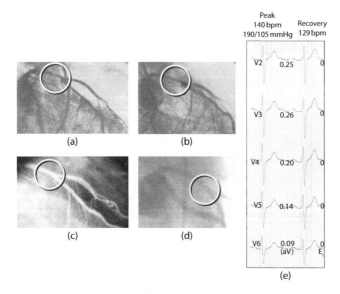

Peak
140 bpm
190/105 mmHg

Recovery
129 bpm

V2 0.25 0

V3 0.26 0

V4 0.20 0

V5 0.14 0

V6 0.09 0
(aV) E,

(e)

Figure 1.11 Stenosis **(a)** before, **(b)** immediately after, **(c)** 10 years after, and **(d)** 23 years after the world's first coronary balloon angioplasty in a human subject, performed by Andreas Gruentzig in Zurich, Switzerland, on September 16, 1977. The functional long-term success is documented by normal stress tolerance and a normal exercise ECG **(e)** of the 61-year-old patient, who underwent the intervention at the age of 38 years. (From King, S. B. 3rd, and Meier, B., *Circulation*, 102(20 Suppl 4), IV81–IV86, 2000. With permission.)

subacute (within 30 days of implantation) stent thrombosis. As a result, bleeding complications at the peripheral arterial puncture site were common. Two major developments advanced the use of stents. First, the abandonment of warfarin in favor of dual antiplatelet therapy (aspirin and ticlopidine) substantially reduced the incidence of the aforementioned bleeding complications. Second, the discovery (with intravascular ultrasound) that stents were often not fully expanded and in poor apposition against the coronary

arterial wall led to the use of high-pressure balloon inflations to achieve more complete stent expansion. Both advances improved the acute and chronic success rates of stents.

Soon after coronary stents were introduced, it was recognized that in-stent restenosis from neointimal hyperplasia occurs in ~20% to 25% of patients with discrete, short de novo stenoses, and in as many as 60% of those with small caliber vessels, long lesions, bifurcation lesions, or diabetes mellitus. Furthermore, in contradistinction to the discrete restenotic lesions that sometimes occurred following balloon angioplasty, in-stent restenosis was noted often to be a much more diffuse lesion that was not readily amenable to repeat dilatation or atherectomy. Extensive research was performed in the late 1990s to seek a solution to the problem of in-stent restenosis. Numerous immunosuppressive and antiplatelet regimens were evaluated but were unsuccessful in reducing its incidence. In 2001, intracoronary radiation (i.e., brachytherapy) after balloon dilatation was reported to be moderately successful in treating in-stent restenosis, but its drawbacks, including late thrombosis, limited applicability, high cost, and the required presence of a radiation oncologist during the procedure, rendered it unsuitable for widespread, routine clinical practice.

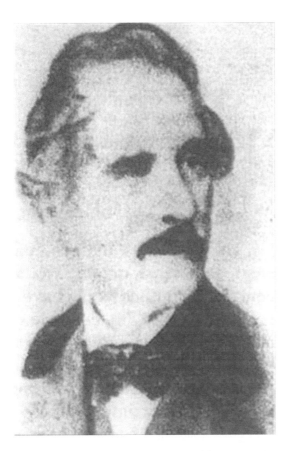

Figure 1.12 Charles Stent, an English dentist, formulated a stable dental mold. In 1916 a plastic surgeon who utilized the material for facial reconstruction was the first to use the term *stent* when he noted, "The dental composition for this purpose is that put forward by Stent and a mold composed of it is known as a 'Stent.'"

In early 2000, stents that eluted antiproliferative pharmacologic agents directly into the vessel wall were developed. The antiproliferative drug was bound to the stent via a polymer coating, which permitted controlled release of the drug for days, weeks, or months after stent implantation. A sirolimus-coated (CYPHER, Cordis Corp: a Johnson & Johnson Company, Miami, FL) stent was approved for clinical use in Europe in April 2002, and in the United States in May 2003, following randomized studies that demonstrated a marked reduction in restenosis when compared with uncoated (bare-metal) stents.[63] A paclitaxel-coated stent (TAXUS, Boston Scientific, Natick, MA) was approved for use in Europe in January 2003, and in the United States in March 2004, following studies that demonstrated that it too was accompanied by a lower incidence of restenosis in comparison with bare-metal stents. Subsequently, additional drug-eluting stents (DESs) have been developed, each varying in its delivery platform, polymer coating, and antiproliferative agent. At present, DESs are utilized for the majority of patients undergoing

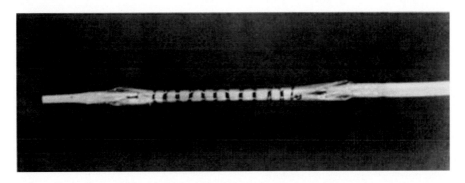

Figure 1.13 Historic image of a balloon-expandable flexible coil stent (Gianturco-Roubin Fslex-Stent, Cook, Inc., Bloomington, IN). (Courtesy of Cook Medical, Bloomington, IN.)

stent implantation for coronary artery disease because of their expected very low incidence of in-stent restenosis. In October 2014, the first drug-coated angioplasty balloon catheter (LUTONIX DCB, C.R. Bard Inc., Tempe, AZ) was approved for use to treat peripheral vascular disease. The balloon is coated on its outer surface with the paclitaxel to prevent restenosis following balloon dilatation.

At the same time, devices were developed to improve the evaluation of arteries, selection of therapies, and success of the procedures described above. Intravascular ultrasound was developed in the late 1980s but did not achieve widespread use until the 1990s. Although it had long been known to provide an image of the arterial wall that was not available with angiography, its use became commonplace with the development of atherectomy devices and intracoronary stenting, with which operators needed to evaluate vessel characteristics, including lumen size, extent and location of plaque, and presence and distribution of calcium deposits within the arterial wall. For patients with coronary luminal narrowings of indeterminate hemodynamic significance, methods to assess the physiology of coronary flow were developed, including (1) the Doppler flow wire, which can record the velocity of blood flow in the coronary artery and thereby determine if a stenosis is impeding flow, and (2) the pressure wire, which can be used to assess the presence or absence of a pressure decline across a coronary stenosis at rest or after the administration of a vasodilator.

INDICATIONS AND CONTRAINDICATIONS

During its early years, cardiac catheterization was performed sparingly and with substantial risk. As time has elapsed, considerable advances have occurred, and the associated morbidity and mortality have fallen precipitously. Today, diagnostic cardiac catheterization is performed with minimal risk, and therapeutic catheterization (i.e., PCI and valvuloplasty) is performed without incident in most patients. Cardiac catheterization now plays a central role in the diagnostic evaluation of the patient with suspected or known cardiac disease, and it offers percutaneous therapeutic possibilities in many individuals.

Diagnostic cardiac catheterization is appropriate in several circumstances. First, it is indicated to confirm or to exclude the presence of a condition already suspected from the history, physical examination, and/or noninvasive evaluation. In such a circumstance, it allows physicians to both establish the presence and to assess the severity of cardiac disease. Second, catheterization is indicated to clarify a confusing or obscure clinical picture in a patient whose clinical findings and noninvasive data are inconclusive. Third, it is performed in some patients for whom corrective cardiac surgery is contemplated to confirm the suspected abnormality and to exclude associated abnormalities that might require the surgeon's attention. Fourth, catheterization occasionally is performed purely as a research procedure.

Therapeutic catheterization is appropriate in several circumstances. Percutaneous coronary revascularization (e.g., angioplasty, rotational atherectomy, or endovascular stenting) may be indicated in the patient with symptomatic atherosclerotic coronary artery disease whose coronary anatomy is suitable for the procedure. Valvuloplasty is indicated in the subject with symptomatic isolated pulmonic stenosis, and it is an acceptable alternative to surgery in the patient with mitral stenosis or aortic stenosis in whom valvular anatomy is suitable and surgery is believed to offer an unfavorable risk-to-benefit ratio due, for example, to advanced age or comorbid medical conditions (i.e., chronic pulmonary, hepatic, or renal disease or an underlying malignancy).

Catheterization is absolutely contraindicated if a mentally competent individual does not consent. It is relatively contraindicated if an intercurrent condition exists that, if corrected, would improve the safety of the procedure.

RISKS AND COMPLICATIONS

As cardiac catheterization has been more frequently performed, the incidence of complications has diminished (Table 1.1). However, even in skilled hands, the procedure is not without risk. The overall incidence of in-hospital mortality is 0.09% for diagnostic catheterization and 0.8% for PCI.[1] Such deaths may be caused by perforation of the heart or great vessels, cardiac arrhythmias, acute MI, or anaphylaxis to radiographic contrast material. Individuals with an increased risk of death include those with (1) advanced (>70 years old) or very young (<1 year old) age, (2) marked functional impairment (class IV angina or heart failure), (3) severe left ventricular dysfunction or coronary artery disease (particularly left main disease), (4) severe valvular disease, (5) severe comorbid medical conditions (i.e., renal, hepatic, or pulmonary disease), or (6) history of an allergy to radiographic contrast material. Patients with significant narrowing of the left main coronary artery have a substantially greater risk of periprocedural death (2.8%) compared with those without left main stenosis (0.1%).[64]

Table 1.1 Complications associated with diagnostic cardiac catheterization

Complication	Percent
Major	
Death	<0.1
Cerebrovascular accident	0.07
Myocardial infarction	0.07
Arrhythmia (life threatening)	0.5
Vascular compromise	0.5–1.5
Anaphylaxis (to contrast material)	0.007
Minor	
Hives	2.0–3.0
Nausea/vomiting	~5.0
Vasovagal reaction	3.0

Major complications (allergic reaction to radiographic contrast media, cardiogenic shock, cerebrovascular accident, congestive heart failure, cardiac tamponade, and renal failure) occurring during or within 24 hours of diagnostic catheterization or PCI occur in 1.3% of patients undergoing a diagnostic study and in 2.3% of those undergoing PCI.[1] MI during or immediately following diagnostic catheterization occurs in about 0.07% of patients, but most are small and uncomplicated. Cerebrovascular accidents in the pericatheterization period may be (1) embolic (from the arterial catheter, guidewire, left ventricular or atrial thrombus, or dislodged atherosclerotic plaque) or (2) ischemic (i.e., existence of extensive cerebrovascular disease that, in association with the hemodynamic alterations induced by angiography, leads to inadequate cerebral perfusion).

Catheterization may result in vascular complications, such as bleeding at the entry site, retroperitoneal bleeding, vascular access occlusion at the entry site, peripheral embolization, vascular dissection, pseudoaneurysm, and arteriovenous fistula. The incidence of vascular complications in patients undergoing diagnostic catheterization is <0.5%, and in those undergoing PCI, it is 2.1%,[1,65] with the latter being higher because of the use of intensive antiplatelet and anticoagulant therapy and larger lumen catheters than those used in diagnostic catheterization.

Numerous minor complications may cause morbidity but exert no effect on mortality. Local vascular complications occur in 0.5% to 2.0% of patients. The incidence is similar for the brachial and femoral approaches and somewhat higher for the radial approach. Following arterial catheterization by the brachial or radial approach, thrombosis, dissection, intimal flap formation, or subintimal hemorrhage may compromise blood flow to the hand or arm, and the patient may require thrombectomy or surgical exploration after catheterization. With the percutaneous femoral approach, hemorrhage and/or hematoma formation at the arterial puncture site are the most common problems and, if severe, may require limited surgical exploration. Arteriovenous fistulae or pseudoaneurysm formation may occur, especially if protracted bleeding at the puncture site occurs after sheath removal, as may result from inadequate compression of the femoral vessel, insertion of large sheaths, severe systemic arterial hypertension, prolonged heparinization, or administration of thrombolytic or antiplatelet agents. Less commonly, femoral arterial thrombosis occurs, which requires immediate thrombectomy. Compression by a large hematoma or groin clamp may cause local nerve damage. Local infection may occur at the site of catheter insertion and manipulation, but this can usually be treated with meticulous wound care and antibiotics.

The administration of radiographic contrast material may cause nausea and vomiting as well as a transient fall in systemic arterial pressure. Occasionally, such injections are associated with allergic reactions of varying severity, and a rare individual has anaphylaxis. Interestingly, only 15% of individuals with a previous allergic reaction to contrast material have another adverse reaction with repeat administration, and most of these are minor (urticaria, nausea, vomiting).[66] In most patients with a history of contrast allergy, angiography can be performed safely; however, premedication with glucocorticosteroids and antihistamines, as well as use of a different contrast agent are usually recommended. The endocardial injection of contrast material during ventriculography (so-called, *endocardial staining*) may cause ventricular irritability. Finally, use of excessive quantities of radiographic contrast material may cause renal insufficiency, which is usually transient. This is particularly likely to occur in patients with preexisting renal dysfunction and diabetes mellitus, and its occurrence can be minimized by (1) limiting the amount of contrast material used during catheterization on the basis of the patient's weight and serum creatinine,[67] (2) administering sufficient oral and intravenous fluids during and after the procedure to ensure that the osmotic diuresis caused by the hyperosmolar contrast material does not induce intravascular volume depletion, and (3) avoiding other nephrotoxic agents before the procedure.[68]

CARDIAC CATHETERIZATION SETTINGS

Cardiac catheterization procedures were originally only performed on inpatients. Nowadays, however, most elective diagnostic catheterizations are performed on outpatients in laboratories based at a hospital with available cardiovascular surgery. These laboratories may be fixed or mobile, with the latter being located on the hospital premises. Outpatient catheterization is widely accepted because of its excellent safety record when performed in properly selected patients (see following text). In 16 studies reporting the results of 20,129 individuals who underwent diagnostic catheterization at a hospital outpatient laboratory, mortality rates ranged from 0 to 0.3%, MI rates from 0 to 0.7%, the rate of stroke or transient ischemic attack from 0 to 0.4%, the incidence of vascular complications from 0 to 2%, and the rate of bleeding or hematoma from 0 to 7%.[69] These complication rates are similar to those reported in a very large multicenter registry of 222,553 patients who had inpatient diagnostic catheterization.[70]

For patients considered to be at low risk of suffering a complication or having extensive coronary artery disease, the procedure may be performed at a community hospital without cardiovascular surgical capability or in a freestanding catheterization facility, which may be a fixed structure or a mobile unit. Since a freestanding laboratory is not physically attached to a hospital, quick transportation of a patient by stretcher to a hospital is usually not possible. The most recent Society of Cardiac Angiography and Intervention survey of cardiac catheterization laboratories (published in 2007) identified 75 non-hospital-based laboratories in the United States, up from 58 in a 1999 survey.[71]

Some freestanding catheterization laboratories are privately owned by physicians. Regardless of who owns and operates them, all freestanding laboratories should have a clearly defined working relationship with one or more nearby hospitals to facilitate emergency transfer of patients when required. Such freestanding facilities must be able to stabilize the occasional patient who has a complication, and they must have the equipment required for endotracheal intubation and ventilator support. The physicians using such facilities should be facile in performing endotracheal intubation (since on-site anesthesiologists are not available) and intra-aortic balloon insertion. Quality assurance and quality improvement programs should be in place and reviewed regularly by an outside consultant. Currently, only diagnostic procedures (i.e., left or right heart catheterization, ventriculography, and coronary angiography) are performed in freestanding laboratories; performance of PCI is restricted by state edict only to hospital-based laboratories.

By providing a setting exclusively for low-risk diagnostic procedures, freestanding facilities can eliminate the long waiting periods that sometimes occur with inpatient facilities. In addition, cost savings are touted as one of the advantages of such freestanding facilities.[69] In many circumstances, however, the growth of freestanding laboratories has been driven by a desire to "capture market share" rather than to improve patient access to expert catheterization. Since most of these facilities are physician owned, the potential exists for financial incentives that inappropriately influence the decision to perform the procedure at such a facility. Other concerns associated with freestanding facilities include the ability to perform an adequate caseload to maintain the operators' skills, limited experience with recognition and management of complications, inadequate regulation and quality control, and the time required to transfer patients to nearby hospitals in the event of an emergency.

The authors of the American College of Cardiology/ Society for Cardiac Angiography and Interventions (ACC/ SCAI) Clinical Expert Consensus Document on Cardiac Catheterization Laboratory Standards[72] recommended patient selection criteria for individuals deemed suitable for consideration of diagnostic catheterization in an outpatient facility. They recommended the following exclusion criteria for adult patients:

1. Age >75 years
2. New York Heart Association (NYHA) class III or IV heart failure
3. Acute intermediate- or high-risk ischemic syndromes
4. Recent MI with postinfarction ischemia
5. Pulmonary edema thought to be caused by ischemia
6. Markedly abnormal noninvasive test indicating a high likelihood of left main or severe multivessel coronary artery disease
7. Known left main coronary artery disease
8. Severe valvular dysfunction, especially in the setting of depressed left ventricular systolic performance
9. Patients at increased risk for vascular complications
10. Complex adult congenital heart disease

Patients with any of these exclusion criteria would not be candidates for catheterization in a freestanding facility, nor would any patients considered to be at high risk because of the presence of comorbid conditions, including the need for anticoagulation therapy, poorly controlled hypertension or diabetes mellitus, allergy to radiographic contrast material, or renal insufficiency.

Although several case series have reported the rate of complications of diagnostic catheterization in freestanding facilities, no randomized trials have compared the complication rates in freestanding facilities with those in hospital-based laboratories. The rates of mortality, MI, stroke, and vascular complications in these case series are comparable to those observed in hospital outpatient facilities.[69] In recent years, diagnostic catheterization procedures have been combined with PCI if the diagnostic study indicates a need for intervention. Combining the two procedures may lower the overall cost. Patients who undergo diagnostic catheterization at a freestanding facility or a diagnostic-only hospital do not have the option of a combined procedure if PCI is deemed appropriate; for these individuals, the PCI must be performed at a different institution at a separate time. Approximately 30% of patients who undergo diagnostic catheterization in an outpatient setting are referred for subsequent PCI.[69]

REFERENCES

1. Rosamond W, et al. Heart disease and stroke statistics—2008 update: A report from the American Heart Association Statistics Committee and Stroke Statistics Subcommittee. *Circulation* 2008;117(4):e25–e146.
2. American Hospital Association. *Facilities and services*: Health Forum LLC, 2008.
3. Burchell HB. Editorial Stephen Hales, September 17, 1677–January 4, 1761. *Circulation* 1961;23:1–6.
4. Forssmann W. The role of heart catheterization and angiocardiography in the development of modern medicine. In: Nobel lectures, *physiology or medicine 1942–1962*. Amsterdam, The Netherlands: Elsevier Publishing Company, 1964.
5. Bernard C, et al. *Notes of M. Bernard's lectures on the blood; with an appendix*. Philadelphia: Lippincott, Grambo & Co, 1854.
6. Mueller RL, Sanborn TA. The history of interventional cardiology: Cardiac catheterization, angioplasty, and related interventions. *Am Heart J* 1995;129(1):146–172.
7. Luderitz B. Etienne Jules Marey (1830–1904). *J Interv Card Electrophysiol* 2005;12(1):91–92.
8. A. Chaveau and É.J. Marey. Classic pages. *Circ Res* 1968;22:96.
9. Fick A. Uber die Messung des Blutquantums in den Herzventrikeln. *Phys-Med Ges Wurzburg*, 1870.
10. Fick A. Ueber die schwankungen des blutdruckes in verschmdenen abschnitten des gefass-systems (zum theil nach versuchen von D Naceff aus Belgrad un Rumanien) Vorhandl der Wurzburg Physlol Med Gesellsch 1873;4:223.
11. Zuntz N, Hagemann O. Untersuchungen iiber den Stoffwechsel des Pferdes bei Ruhe und Arbeit. *Landwirtschaftliche Jahrbucher* 1898;27:1–438.
12. Fishman AP. A century of pulmonary hemodynamics. *Am J Respir Crit Care Med* 2004;170(2):109–113.
13. Fye WB. Coronary arteriography—it took a long time! *Circulation* 1984;70(5):781–787.

14. Haschek ELO. Ein beitrag zur praktischen verwerthung der photographie nach Roentgen. *Wiener Klin Wochenschr* 1896;9:63–64.

15. Williams F. A method for more fully determining the outline of the heart by means of the fluoroscope together with other uses of this instrument in medicine. *Boston Med Surg J* 1896;135(14):335.

16. Jamin F, Merkel H. Die Koronararterien des menschlichen Herzens unter normalen und pathologischen Verhiiltnissen Jena, 1907.

17. Herrick JB. Certain clinical features of sudden obstruction of the coronary arteries. *J Am Med Assoc* 1912;59(23):1757–1762.

18. Herrick JB. Landmark article (JAMA 1912). Clinical features of sudden obstruction of the coronary arteries. By James B. Herrick. *JAMA* 1983;250(13):1757–1765.

19. Sicard JA, Forestier J. Methode radiographique d'exploration de la cavite epidurale par la lipiodol. *Rev Neurol* 1921;37:1264–1266.

20. Osborne ED, et al. Landmark article Feb 10, 1923: Roentgenography of urinary tract during excretion of sodium iodid. By Earl D. Osborne, Charles G. Sutherland, Albert J. Scholl Jr. and Leonard G. Rowntree. *JAMA* 1983;250(20):2848–2853.

21. Brooks B. Intra-arterial injection of sodium iodid preliminary report. *J Am Med Assoc* 1924;82:1016–1019.

22. Forssmann W. Sondierung des rechten Herzens. *Klin Wochenschr* 1929;8:2085–2087.

23. Forssmann-Falck R. Werner Forssmann: A pioneer of cardiology. *Am J Cardiol* 1997;79(5):651–660.

24. King SB 3rd. The development of interventional cardiology. *J Am Coll Cardiol* 1998;31(4 Suppl B):64B–88B.

25. Forssmann W. Ueber kontrastdarstellung der hohlen des lebenden rechten herzens und der lungenschlagader. *Munch Med Wochenschr* 1931;78:489–492.

26. Klein O. Zur Bestimmung des zirkulatorischen Minutenvolumens nach dem Fickschen Prinzip. *Munchener Medizinische Wochenschrift* 1930;77:1311–1312.

27. Moniz E, et al. La visibilite des vaisseaux pulmonaires aus rayons X par injection dans l'oreillette droite de fortes solutions d'Iodure de sodium. *Bull Acad Med Paris* 1931;105:627–629.

28. Perez Ara A. El sondage del corazon derechia su tecnica y aplicationes. *Rev Med Cir Habana* 1931;36:491–508.

29. Moniz E, et al. Angiopneumographie. *J Radiol d'Electrol* 1932;16:469–472.

30. Grollman A. *The Cardiac Output of Man in Health and Disease.* Baltimore: C.C. Thomas, 1932.

31. Castellanos A, et al. La angiocardiografia radioopaca. *Arch Estud Clin Habana* 1937;31:523–527.

32. Robb GP, Steinberg I. A practical method of visualization of the chambers of the heart, the pulmonary circulation, and the great blood vessels in man. *J Clin Invest* 1938;17:507 (abstr).

33. Richards DW. The contributions of right heart catheterization to physiology and medicine, with some observations on the physiopathology of pulmonary heart disease. In: Nobel Lectures, Physiology of Medicine 1942–1962. Amsterdam, The Netherlands: Elsevier Publishing Company, 1964.

34. Cournand A, Ranges HA. Catheterization of the right auricle in man. *Proc Soc Exp Biol Med* 1941;46:462–466.

35. Cournand A. Control of the pulmonary circulation in man with some remarks on methodology. In: *Nobel Lectures, Physiology or Medicine 1942–1962.* Amsterdam, The Netherlands: Elsevier Publishing Company, 1964.

36. Dexter L, et al. Oxygen content of pulmonary "capillary" blood in unanesthetized human beings. *J Clin Invest* 1946;25:913 (abstr).

37. Dexter L, et al. Studies of congenital heart disease: II. The pressure and oxygen content of blood in the right auricle, right ventricle, and pulmonary artery in control patients, with observations on the oxygen saturation and source of pulmonary 'capillary' blood. *J Clin Invest* 1947;26(3):554–560.

38. Zimmerman HA, et al. Catheterization of the left side of the heart in man. *Circulation* 1950;1(3):357–359.

39. Doby T. A tribute to Sven-Ivar Seldinger. *AJR Am J Roentgenol* 1984;142(1):1–4.

40. Seldinger SI. Catheter replacement of the needle in percutaneous arteriography:A new technique. *Acta Radiol* 1953;39(5):368–376.

41. Dotter CT, Frische LH. Visualization of the coronary circulation by occlusion aortography: A practical method. *Radiology* 1958;71(4):502–524.

42. Arnulf G. L'arteriographie methodique des arteres coronaires grace a l'utilisation de l'acetylcholine; donnees experimentales et cliniques. *Bull Acad Natl Med* 1958;142:661–672.

43. Richards LS, Thal AP. Phasic dye injection control system for coronary arteriography in the human. *Surg Gynecol Obstet* 1958;107(6):739–743.

44. Bellman S, et al. Coronary arteriography.I. Differential opacification of the aortic stream by catheters of special design–experimental development. *N Engl J Med* 1960;262:325–328.

45. Ryan TJ. The coronary angiogram and its seminal contributions to cardiovascular medicine over five decades. *Circulation* 2002;106(6):752–756.

46. Fye WB. *American Cardiology. The History of a Specialty and Its College.* Baltimore, Md: The Johns Hopkins University Press; 1996:175.

47. Hurst JW. History of cardiac catheterization. In: King SB III, Douglas JS Jr., eds. *Coronary arteriography and angioplasty.* New York: McGraw-Hill, 1985, pp. 1–9.

48. Judkins MP. Selective coronary arteriography. I. A percutaneous transfemoral technic. *Radiology* 1967;89(5):815–824.

49. Schoonmaker FW, King SB III. Coronary arteriography by the single catheter percutaneous femoral technique. Experience in 6,800 cases. *Circulation* 1974;50(4):735–740.

50. Wilson WJ, et al. Biplane selective coronary arteriography via percutaneous transfemoral approach. *Am J Roentgenol Radium Ther Nucl Med* 1967;100(2):332–340.

51. Ricketts HJ, Abrams HL. Percutaneous selective coronary cine arteriography. *JAMA* 1962;181:620–624.

52. Hillis LD. Percutaneous left heart catheterization and coronary arteriography using a femoral artery sheath. *Cathet Cardiovasc Diagn* 1979;5(4):393–399.

53. Dodge HT, et al. The use of biplane angiocardiography for the measurement of left ventricular volume in man. *Am Heart J* 1960;60:762–776.

54. Dotter CT. Transluminal angioplasty: A long view. *Radiology* 1980;135(3):561–564.

55. King SB 3rd, Meier B. Interventional treatment of coronary heart disease and peripheral vascular disease. *Circulation* 2000;102(20 Suppl 4):IV81–IV86.

56. Gruentzig A. Perkutane rekanalisation chronischer arterieller verschlusse mit einem neuen dilatationskatheter modifikation der Dotter technik. *Deutsch Med Wochenschr* 1974;99:2502–2510.

57. Meier B, Gruentzig, the father of balloon angioplasty—I was there! Interview with Dr. George A. Beller. ESC Congress, Rapid News Summaries, Cardiosource, 2003.

58. Simpson JB, et al. Transluminal atherectomy: A new approach to the treatment of atherosclerotic vascular disease. *Circulation* 1985;72:146 (abstr).

59. Simpson JB, et al. Transluminal atherectomy: Initial clinical results in 27 patients. *Circulation* 1986;74:203 (abstr).

60. Ring ME. How a dentist's name became a synonym for a life-saving device: The story of Dr. Charles Stent. *J Hist Dent* 2001;49:77–80.

61. Akerman J. Award Ceremony Speech. In: Nobel Lectures, Physiology or Medicine 1901–1921. Amsterdam, The Netherlands: Elsevier Publishing Company, 1967.

62. Schatz RA. A view of vascular stents. *Circulation* 1989;79(2):445–457.

63. Morice MC, et al. A randomized comparison of a sirolimus-eluting stent with a standard stent for coronary revascularization. *N Engl J Med* 2002;346(23):1773–1780.

64. Boehrer JD, et al. Markedly increased periprocedure mortality of cardiac catheterization in patients with severe narrowing of the left main coronary artery. *Am J Cardiol* 1992;70(18):1388–1390.

65. Applegate RJ, et al. Trends in vascular complications after diagnostic cardiac catheterization and percutaneous coronary intervention via the femoral artery, 1988 to 2007. *JACC Cardiovasc Interv* 2008;1(3):317–326.

66. Brogan WC III, et al. Contrast agents for cardiac catheterization: Conceptions and misconceptions. *Am Heart J* 1991;122(4 Pt 1):1129–1135.

67. Cigarroa RG, et al. Dosing of contrast material to prevent contrast nephropathy in patients with renal disease. *Am J Med* 1989;86(6 Pt 1):649–652.

68. Marenzi G, et al. N-acetylcysteine and contrast-induced nephropathy in primary angioplasty. *N Engl J Med* 2006;354(26):2773–2782.

69. Agency for Healthcare Research and Quality (AHRQ). *Cardiac catheterization in freestanding clinics: A review.* Rockville, MD: Department of Health and Human Services;2005, pp. 1–120.

70. Johnson LW, et al. Coronary arteriography 1984–1987: A report of the Registry of the Society for Cardiac Angiography and Interventions. I. Results and complications. *Cathet Cardiovasc Diagn* 1989;17(1):5–10.

71. Dehmer GJ, et al. The current status and future direction of percutaneous coronary intervention without on-site surgical backup: An expert consensus document from the Society for Cardiovascular Angiography and Interventions. *Catheter Cardiovasc Interv* 2007;69(4):471–478.

72. Bashore TM, et al. American College of Cardiology/Society for Cardiac Angiography and Interventions clinical expert consensus document on cardiac catheterization laboratory standards: Summary of a report of the American College of Cardiology Task Force on clinical expert consensus documents. Catheter *Cardiovasc Interv* 2001;53:281–286.

2

Setting up a catheterization laboratory: Organizational, architectural, and equipment considerations

JOHN W. HIRSHFELD, JR.

OVERVIEW

A cardiac catheterization laboratory is a complex facility that integrates multiple pieces of equipment and multiple groups of clinical personnel with differing skill sets and responsibilities. This hospital component serves different roles in different institutions with different missions and, consequently, has varying degrees of complexity. The laboratory relates to multiple facilities within the greater hospital system. Thus, how the facility is designed architecturally and organized administratively can have a major influence on its operational efficiency and smoothness.

The multidimensional missions of current cardiac catheterization laboratories raise complex issues related to physical location (in relation to other related cardiovascular facilities), architectural design, and administrative organization.

Currently, cardiac catheterization laboratories fulfill a variety of missions, from what would be considered minor outpatient surgery to urgent and emergent treatment of acutely ill patients. They are also used for establishing circulatory support in critically ill patients and for complex therapeutic procedures that require infrastructure and capabilities ordinarily thought of as cardiac surgical procedures. In addition, many hospitals operate clinical electrophysiology laboratories that have many similar qualities and procedures but have major differences in the types of procedures and operational equipment.

Depending on the nature of its particular program, the cardiac catheterization laboratory has the potential to be a large cost center with respect to fixed capital costs and ongoing personnel and supply costs. Consequently, it is important that the facility be properly organized to operate efficiently. This requires careful thought and planning in developing its architectural design, determining its operational scale, selecting and integrating its equipment, and developing its operating procedures and protocols.

Clinical electrophysiology laboratories are similar to cardiac catheterization laboratories in that both are built around X-ray fluoroscopic equipment. Consequently, there is pressure to combine both functions into a single procedure room, particularly for laboratories with low utilization levels. This pressure should be resisted. The equipment used and procedures performed in the two types of facilities are very different. Converting from a catheterization function to a clinical electrophysiology function can be complex. Thus, while catheterization and clinical electrophysiology labs can be located in a common suite and share support space, it is ideal to have separate procedure rooms for each function.

Many of the issues and considerations discussed in this chapter have been reviewed in depth in an expert consensus document published by the American College of Cardiology (ACC) and Society for Cardiovascular Angiography and Interventions (SCAI).[1]

General considerations

A cardiac catheterization laboratory suite is an integrated facility that provides care to a variety of patients as discussed above. These patients range from stable outpatients undergoing diagnostic procedures to critically ill patients presenting to the emergency room with a ST-segment elevation myocardial infarction (STEMI) requiring emergent interventional procedures. This lab is also equipped to treat patients with circulatory failure requiring mechanical circulatory support and patients undergoing complex elective interventional procedures that may potentially require full cardiac surgical collaboration. This complement of services requires that the facility be architecturally configured to accommodate a broad range of patients.

Location

The architectural placement of a cardiac catheterization suite within a health care institution requires balancing many competing requirements. For clinical, operational, and administrative purposes, it is ideal to have the entire cardiac catheterization facility in a single contiguous space. Because the cardiac catheterization facility serves stable outpatients, critically ill inpatients, emergency room patients, and patients undergoing complex structural and hybrid cardiac surgical procedures alike, the facility ideally will be located in close proximity to the following hospital facilities:

1. The cardiac medical critical care unit
2. The cardiac surgery critical care unit
3. The hospital emergency department
4. Cardiac operating rooms
5. Outpatient surgery facilities

There are three basic reasons why these architectural relationships are important:

1. Patients are frequently transported between these facilities. Many of these patients are critically ill and medically unstable. Short transportation distances and minimal elevator rides are important safety considerations.
2. Patients who have recently undergone invasive diagnostic and therapeutic procedures are frequently cared for in critical care units. In the event that they develop a postprocedure problem, the cardiac catheterization laboratory staff can check on them promptly and efficiently if the patients are located in close proximity to the cardiac catheterization suite.
3. Support staff needed to respond to emergencies occurring in the cardiac catheterization suite, such as anesthesiologists and respiratory therapists, frequently congregate in operating rooms and critical care units. Being in close proximity to the cardiac catheterization laboratory suite allows these support personnel to respond promptly.

Physical facilities and space requirements

Securing a location with sufficient space that is also accessible from the aforementioned facilities would be an administrative and architectural tour de force that would be virtually impossible to achieve in most existing health care facilities, and challenging to achieve even in a new, clean-sheet construction. Despite these challenges, planners should strive to optimize the arrangement to include as many of the ideal components as possible.

Facilities required in a cardiac catheterization suite include the following:

1. Procedure rooms with attached control rooms and X-ray equipment electronics rooms
2. Patient pre- and postprocedural care areas, including patient changing areas and lockers
3. Equipment and supply storage areas
4. A patient registration and waiting area for families
5. An area for data review and report generating
6. An office space for administrative personnel

The design of a cardiac catheterization suite begins with developing programmatic requirements to determine the scale of the facility. This includes the number of procedure rooms and the space allotted to the nonprocedural room functions. An additional architectural challenge is arranging the components of the suite so that they relate well to each other and provide for efficient circulation of staff and patients.

The cardiac catheterization suite also interacts closely with other hospital facilities. These include critical care units, the emergency department, and cardiac operating rooms. Ideal architectural design places the cardiac catheterization suite in close proximity to these facilities.

Since outpatients constitute an increasing fraction of cardiac catheterization laboratory patients, the facility must include the space requisite for intake and registration, pre- and postprocedural care, and waiting facilities for patients' family members. These functions can be combined with outpatient surgery programs in order to use space and facilities efficiently, provided that the intake and recovery spaces are conveniently accessible to the procedure rooms, and that the clinical personnel who provide aftercare are highly experienced in the management of catheterization patients.

Procedure room design

Since the procedure room is the core of the facility, its design should not be compromised by competing architectural considerations. The first consideration is to provide adequate floor space. Many state department health codes specify minimum floor areas. In addition, X-ray equipment manufacturers specify minimum room sizes and minimum clearances between equipment and adjacent walls. However, irrespective of whatever code requirements exist, procedure rooms should be a minimum of 500 square feet; however, 600 square feet is ideal. Biplane X-ray systems require additional space. If a laboratory is to function as a hybrid operating room, 800 square feet is required to contain all the necessary equipment and provide sufficient space for circulation.

In laying out the procedure room, particular attention should be paid to circulation, sightlines, and relationships to supporting utilities.

Patient entry points and circulation space around the procedure table should be designed to facilitate ease of patient entry and transfer to and from the procedure table. With respect to circulation, planners should consider the most demanding scenarios, such as transferring a patient who is in an oversized hospital bed on mechanical ventilation, as well as providing adequate circulatory support in and out of the procedure room.

Sightline considerations are also important to facilitate communications and interactions between the procedure room staff and the control room staff. These considerations include the location of the control room, its window to the procedure room, and audio communication between the control room and the procedure room.

The X-ray imaging system has four groups of components:

1. The X-ray gantry supporting the X-ray tube, the imaging system, and the patient procedure table.
2. The X-ray video monitors mounted on a ceiling-suspended monitor boom in the procedure room.
3. The X-ray system's supporting electronic equipment, which should be housed in a separate, climate-controlled room adjacent to the procedure room.
4. The X-ray control system, which is housed in the control room, along with a duplicate set of video monitors.

The procedure room, control room, and X-ray electronics equipment room should be designed with adequate space, with attention to physical relationships and sightlines to optimize the positioning and configuration of the X-ray system.

The procedure room also needs to be able to accommodate portable ancillary equipment. This requires that there be sufficient floor space for the portable equipment and appropriate utility connections. Examples include portable imaging equipment (e.g., external ultrasound systems, intravascular and intracardiac ultrasound systems), portable physiologic monitoring equipment (e.g., pressure wire and flow wire consoles), and circulatory support equipment (e.g., intra-aortic balloon pump [IABP], Impella, and various extracorporeal circulatory support devices, such as full extracorporeal membrane oxygenator [ECMO] systems).

Each of these units requires space when in use and utility connections. Some require connections to dedicated monitors located on the X-ray imaging monitor boom; some require connections to the laboratory's physiologic monitoring system in order to send and receive signals (e.g., electrocardiographic [ECG] signals for IABP and ultrasound machines). Each of these utility and monitor connections should be specified at the time the procedure room is designed so that the appropriate connectors and cabling are allocated to the room at the time of construction.

Since the procedure room is a source of diagnostic radiation, its walls must be shielded. Construction codes from the state departments of health specify the type and extent of shielding required, as well as X-ray signage requirements.

Design considerations for X-ray equipment room

The supporting electronics for current X-ray equipment have progressively decreased in size compared to systems of one to two decades ago. Now, less space needs to be reserved for this equipment. However, much of the current equipment is high-capacity computing equipment that has demanding environmental requirements. It is not feasible or appropriate to place this equipment in the procedure room. Consequently, a separate equipment room to house supporting electronics should be located adjacent to the procedure room, and a door should be provided connecting the two rooms to facilitate equipment servicing. This room should have a high-efficiency air conditioning system. The amount of space required varies, but is generally on the order of 150 square feet for a single-plane X-ray system, or 250 square feet for a biplane system. The majority of the system's network connection hardware is also ideally located in this space.

Control room design

The design and layout of the control room are among the most complex and frequently overlooked tasks when designing a cardiac catheterization laboratory suite. The challenge is to arrange all of the equipment needed in the control room (frequently provided by different manufacturers) with appropriate cabling and ergonomic arrangement to facilitate control room operations. The design should also provide for future changes in equipment configuration. The control room requires a seating area for the staff monitoring the procedure with adequate sightlines to the procedure room and to the physiologic monitoring and X-ray equipment. Wall-mounted video monitors that display the X-ray system's live and roadmap images should be furnished.

The numerous computer cases and monitors associated with these functions need to be arranged and cabled appropriately. Cabling includes dedicated signal cables from the procedure room and the X-ray equipment control room, as well as hospital network connections and electrical power connections. In addition, the room design needs to provide the flexibility to accommodate future changes in X-ray imaging or physiologic monitoring equipment.

Numerous cables transmit signals between the control room, the procedure table pedestal, the X-ray system supporting electronics in the equipment room, and the procedure room monitors. In planning the room, it is important to provide adequate wireways under the floor between these locations. These wireways should be designed for ready access to cabling and with sufficient capacity to accommodate additional cables.

Design of pre- and postprocedure care areas

The pre- and postprocedure care area provides all of the functions of an outpatient surgery facility. It must provide comfortable, private areas for individual patients with appropriate staff access and monitoring capabilities. The overall purpose and functions provided by these units influence design considerations. At a minimum, these units provide a facility for the preprocedure intake of patients, and for their short-term aftercare. Some units also function as 23-hour stay facilities for patients undergoing interventional procedures. Thus, the particulars of design and capabilities of the unit will vary depending on its intended functionalities. Anticipated utilization levels will determine the total capacity designed into the unit.

While there may be an operational incentive to combine this function with other hospital short-stay and day surgery functions, it is important to emphasize that the clinical and nursing care issues of catheterization patients are different from most day surgery patients. The principal challenge for catheterization patients involves managing vascular access sites. This requires a unique clinical care knowledge base not generally held by outpatient surgery staff; thus, a dedicated unit with dedicated staff is preferred.

Supply storage

A cardiac catheterization facility must maintain a large inventory of devices readily accessible on-site, as it is not possible to anticipate and procure all of the devices that may be required to complete a given procedure in advance. Thus, the facility needs to have a supply storage area located in close proximity to the procedure room(s) so that devices can be obtained promptly as the need arises. The laboratory's overall scale of operation determines the size of this facility.

Storage of ancillary equipment

Cardiac catheterization suites acquire numerous small portable equipment items, including ultrasound imaging machines, pressure and flow wire consoles, and circulatory assistance machines. While it is tempting to keep these portable units in the procedure room, they take up space and add to clutter when not in use. Consequently, these machines should be stored in a designated area in a suite outside of general circulation (not in the procedure rooms or in the corridors) where they can be appropriately supported (connected to an electrical power line, if necessary to maintain battery charge) and readily available when needed. The size of this facility is determined by the amount and type of equipment stored.

The IABP console is an exception to the principle of keeping unused, portable equipment out of the room. It is a comparatively small unit and one of the more frequently used devices that should be promptly applied when needed.

HOSPITAL NETWORK CONSIDERATIONS

General considerations

Cardiac catheterization laboratories transmit and receive large volumes of computer network traffic. X-ray images, as well as data from the physiological monitoring and report-generating systems, are transmitted to and from the laboratory's archive server. The laboratory's X-ray and monitoring systems read ADT (admissions, discharge, transfer), demographic, and accounting data from the hospital information system and post accounting data from completed procedures to the hospital information system. Ideally, the laboratory also makes its reports available throughout the hospital network for access by physicians and clinical staff caring for the patient. The catheterization laboratory information system is becoming increasingly integrated with the hospital electronic medical record (EMR) system. Both the X-ray and physiological monitoring systems require maintenance and troubleshooting. This is frequently accomplished by vendor service personnel connecting remotely via network connections to the equipment in the procedure rooms.

As described above, a cardiac catheterization laboratory's computer network demands are substantial. These demands must be considered in the design of the system's network backbone. The network must have sufficient bandwidth to support real-time communications between the core systems in the procedure rooms, the archive servers, and the client terminals used to access images and procedure data outside of the procedure rooms. Much of the data transmitted is high-resolution video that requires substantial bandwidth to transmit in real-time. The bandwidth issue is particularly important given that hospital information networks experience large fluctuations in traffic volume. Consequently, a network design that is adequate for low-traffic periods may choke during high-traffic periods. One solution is to isolate the core network that connects the procedure rooms and the related archive servers from the hospital network so that the local area network (LAN) performance between procedure rooms and archive servers is not affected by traffic elsewhere.

Network security is also a vital attribute. While the ability to achieve secure transmission of confidential patient information within the institution's network is axiomatic, it is also important for the protection of the network and the facility's equipment from unwanted malware intrusions. The network must also be sufficiently secure to protect against the intrusion of viruses and other computer malware into the core system components. Many X-ray and physiological monitoring systems run under a Windows operating environment using open-source hardware and are vulnerable to viruses and other malware. Systems should be configured to prohibit installation of unauthorized applications on any hardware. Ideally, the systems should have neither a web browser nor an e-mail client installed; they should be isolated from the Internet. However, because Internet-based connections are needed for remote monitoring and servicing of the system, Internet access is needed. Thus, the challenge is to configure firewalls to provide remote monitoring and servicing access while excluding potentially harmful Internet traffic.

Equipment considerations and system integration

A cardiac catheterization laboratory has two major equipment systems that work together: the X-ray cinefluorographic unit and the physiological monitoring system.

The majority of current physiological monitoring systems provide both physiologic signal conditioning and display functions for monitoring and recording purposes; they also generate reports and data archives. The X-ray and physiological monitoring systems need to communicate with each other in order to link angiographic and physiological data into a single procedure file and report.

Many X-ray system vendors also furnish physiological monitoring systems and archiving systems. A single vendor providing all capabilities (X-ray, physiological monitoring, and image/data archiving systems) has operational advantages. With a single vendor, the communication protocols needed to import X-ray system variables into the clinical information system are built in and should operate seamlessly.

However, there are considerable differences between X-ray systems and catheterization information systems furnished by different vendors. In addition, there are catheterization information systems in the marketplace from companies that do not furnish X-ray systems. Consequently, after evaluating competing products, a catheterization facility's clinical leadership may prefer one vendor's X-ray system, but a different vendor's information system. In making these equipment and system selections, it is important to verify that the systems selected can establish communications with each other in order to transfer patient and procedure identifier data, as well as angiographic image data, if they are included in the system's capabilities. This requirement also extends to communication with the hospital information system and the institution's EMRs. Compatibility and communications between systems must be ensured to avoid operational problems.

As discussed above, when selecting equipment, it is important to confirm that working communication links can be established between X-ray and physiological monitoring systems, and within the hospital information system to enable transmission of registration, accounting data, and publication of completed procedure reports. These capabilities should be specified contractually at the time the systems are ordered.

X-ray cinefluorographic unit

GENERAL IMAGING CONSIDERATIONS

The X-ray cinefluorographic unit is the core equipment around which the entire laboratory facility is based.

The technology of these units has matured, and all of the vendors currently in the marketplace offer systems that are capable of generating excellent fluorographic images. X-ray generator and X-ray tube design have now become relatively uniform across vendors. Imaging chains have now migrated almost completely from X-ray image intensifier/video camera systems to integrated, flat panel detector systems.

A major advantage of the migration to flat panel detector imaging chains is detector uniformity, making the quest for "the best possible image intensifier" a thing of the past. X-ray system manufacturers frequently make claims that flat panel detectors require smaller X-ray input doses. However, in practice, this turns out not to be the case.

With current systems, X-ray image quality is influenced more by the interaction of X-ray input dose and image processing software than by the actual hardware components. Consequently, any quality system in the current marketplace should be capable of generating high-quality images if its X-ray-generating system, dose-modulating system, and image processing algorithms are optimally calibrated. If a system is generating poor images, the fault is likely with calibration rather than with defective components in the imaging chain.

The impact of current image processing algorithms on image characteristics cannot be overstated. In fact, many qualitative differences in default image characteristics between different X-ray manufacturers are attributable to philosophical choices of the characteristics of an optimal image. While the raw initial image data generated by different X-ray vendors are quite similar, the final image displayed on the monitor is strongly influenced by image processing choices, such as contrast ratio, white compression, and edge enhancement algorithms. Thus, the end user should collaborate with the X-ray system manufacturer's imaging specialists to achieve optimal image quality in the opinion of the end-user physician.

It is important that the end-user physician keep in mind the trade-off between X-ray input dose and image quality. It is easy for an X-ray vendor, in response to a request for better image quality, to increase the X-ray input dose. While this can reduce image noise, it also increases radiation exposure for both the patient and laboratory clinical personnel. Consequently, it is important that the hospital's radiology physicist and radiation safety officer oversee the calibration of the X-ray system to ensure that optimal image quality is being generated at the lowest input doses possible.

The excellent image quality that current X-ray systems generate can exceed the image quality needed for certain basic catheterization laboratory procedures. This offers the opportunity to reduce X-ray dose to the patient (and secondarily to operating personnel) by choosing to decrease the X-ray dose and accepting a lower quality image or a slower image framing rate. Ideal X-ray systems have table-side dose and framing rate controls that enable operators to readily select dose and framing rates, providing the optimal balance between image quality and radiation dose.

UNIT CONFIGURATION ISSUES

A number of issues need to be considered when specifying the configuration of an X-ray unit. These include detector size, image processing capabilities, procedure table capabilities, and biplane configurations.

Detector size

X-ray image detectors suitable for cardiovascular imaging come in two sizes: 20 × 20 cm and 40 × 30 cm. The 20 cm detectors are square and have 1024 × 1024 pixel matrices. The 40 cm detectors are rectangular and have 2048 × 1536 pixel matrices. It is important to point out that flat panel detectors provide multiple image magnification (zoom) modes. However, as these are digital devices, a magnified image (e.g., a 20 cm detector, which generally offers three image sizes) is achieved by using only the detector's central pixels and stretching their display to a larger size, thereby magnifying the image. This stretching of pixels is accompanied by a commensurate increase in X-ray input dose, maintaining a constant dose-area product, in order to reduce image noise that would otherwise become evident in response to pixel magnification. The 40 cm detectors generate rectangular images in the 40 cm mode, but change to square images in magnified modes.

Selection of detector size is an important consideration, and should be based on the unit's anticipated usage pattern. The 40 cm detectors offer the ability to achieve a larger image field of view, but do so at the cost of greater bulk, which impairs the ability to achieve extreme degrees of cranial and caudal skew. The 40 cm detector is ideal for imaging large areas of the peripheral vasculature and substantially enlarged hearts (e.g., the left atrium [LA] and left ventricle [LV]) in a patient with severe enlargement of both chambers due to chronic mitral regurgitation, or the LV and thoracic aorta in a patient with severe left ventricular enlargement due to severe aortic regurgitation secondary to a thoracic aortic aneurysm). Therefore, a 20 cm detector is ideal for a laboratory that will be doing mostly coronary imaging in patients with normal-sized or only moderately enlarged hearts. A 40 cm detector will prove to be more cumbersome for coronary imaging and may actually preclude achieving certain highly skewed projections but is ideal for imaging enlarged hearts with valvular disease and patients with peripheral vascular disease.

Digital subtraction and table-stepping

Peripheral angiography is facilitated by two capabilities in addition to detector size: digital subtraction and table-stepping. Digital subtraction is very valuable when imaging below the diaphragm or in the neck. It frequently permits acquisition of diagnostic-quality images with smaller contrast (but not X-ray) doses. Thus, it is a valuable adjunct for peripheral vascular work. Table-stepping is useful primarily for following a contrast bolus injection below the inguinal ligament to the feet. Thus, it is of value for assessing infrainguinal arterial anatomy.

Rotational three-dimensional imaging

Another capability of current digital X-ray units is rotational three-dimensional (3D) angiography. This technique rotates the gantry rapidly through a 180° arc during a coronary injection, acquiring images of the opacified coronary artery in multiple projections. Computed tomography (CT)–type reconstruction algorithms can be applied to the image dataset to enable a 3D reconstruction of the coronary anatomy. The potential of this technique is to enable a comprehensive anatomic assessment of a coronary artery with a single contrast agent injection.

Biplane configurations

Biplane configurations have attributes that are of value in three circumstances:

1. It minimizes contrast agent dose in patients with renal insufficiency. In such patients, if an operator is skilled and experienced at performing biplane coronary angiography, a biplane X-ray unit offers the potential for substantial contrast agent dose reduction. It is possible that, in the future, 3D rotational angiography may supercede this particular indication for biplane angiography.
2. Patients with complex congenital heart disease who require multiple contrast injections with images acquired in multiple projections can also benefit from studies conducted on a biplane unit.
3. On occasion, biplane fluoroscopy is an adjunct when performing interventional cardiovascular procedures as it enables rapid switching between fluoroscopic views, which is sometimes helpful when conducting a complex interventional procedure.

A biplane X-ray unit costs nearly twice the price of a single plane unit. As mentioned above, it also requires a larger procedure room. The investment is wasted if the lateral imaging plane sits unused in the corner of the procedure room. Thus, the choice to specify a biplane unit should be made carefully considering the uses intended for the particular laboratory. Many multiple-procedure room facilities will equip one room with a biplane unit, scheduling patients with the above-cited conditions in it while equipping other rooms with single plane units. Similarly, a multi-room facility may have a mixture of detector sizes in its different rooms, using the rooms with large detectors for patients with severe cardiac enlargement and for peripheral vascular procedures, while doing straightforward coronary work in rooms with 20 cm detectors.

DISPLAY MONITOR CONFIGURATION

The configuration of monitor displays is an important ergonomic feature of procedure room design. The ceiling suspended monitor system should facilitate positioning the monitors where they can be easily viewed from all possible catheter entry site locations. In addition, the monitor configuration will include the physiological recorder/monitor system for monitoring the patient during the procedure. Given the increasingly frequent use of adjunctive imaging systems, such as ultrasound and optical coherence tomography (OCT), monitors are incorporated to display these images.

Historically, ceiling suspended monitor support systems were designed to support up to eight individual monitors. Basic design criteria were to provide two video monitors (live and roadmap) for each X-ray plane. Naturally, these display mounts became bulky and somewhat unwieldy.

Video monitors were historically monochrome cathode ray tube units. Subsequently, monochrome flat panel monitors superseded cathode ray tube units as these units were progressively refined.

The ideal monitor system is currently the single, ceiling-suspended large format (typically 50 in or 60 in diagonal) color flat panel screen. Flat panel color displays have been refined to the degree that they can display monochrome images with quality comparable to a monochrome display. In addition, the principal value of the large format monitor is that it can be divided into individual display areas for each of the functions: X-ray video display, physiologic monitor display, and ancillary equipment display. The color display capability makes a single unit capable of providing displays from all equipment.

PHYSIOLOGICAL MONITOR, RECORDER, AND DATABASE

In the past decade, the physiologic monitor and recorder system have undergone a major evolution. This component, which descended from a multichannel oscillograph with analog signal conditioning preamplifiers and an optical strip chart recorder, has evolved into a comprehensive cardiac catheterization laboratory information system. These systems now function as digital recorders and monitors that also incorporate procedure logging (preprocedure, intraprocedure, and postprocedure), inventory management, report-generating, and database capabilities. The addition of these capabilities is the logical development of the progressive application of computer technology to what was originally an analog device. These systems now interface with hospital information systems and EMRs providing a single solution to establishing a comprehensive record and report of the entire cardiac catheterization procedure from initial preprocedure intake to discharge from the cardiac recovery unit.

For intraprocedure monitoring and data acquisition, the current system typically incorporates basic pressure, ECG, and other signal acquisition, display, and recording capabilities. The system has logic to measure digital values that characterize intracardiac and intravascular pressure waveforms as well as calculate valve pressure gradients, cardiac output, vascular resistance, valve orifice areas, and intracardiac shunt flows. In addition, the unit, through its user interface, records a time-stamped procedure log of all procedure events and tabulates devices used for reporting and for inventory maintenance purposes. The recorder system archives the physiologic data from the procedure, including all of the physiologic signal data obtained during the procedure. In addition, the system has the ability either to generate a clinical procedure report using its recorded data or to export its data to another report-generating application. These functions, combined with physician interpretation of the angiographic image data, form the basis of the system's clinical procedure report.

The physiologic recorder/database interfaces with the procedure room X-ray system to establish links between the procedure's physiologic data and its angiographic images. Some systems are comprehensive physiologic data and image archiving systems, while others do not archive the angiographic data. If the latter type of system is employed, a separate angiographic archive is needed.

Particular attention should be paid to the ability of the physiologic recorder/database to interface with and communicate with the X-ray system. The X-ray vendors supply physiologic recorder/database systems that are specifically designed to interface with their X-ray systems. In addition, third-party vendors offer physiologic recorder/database systems and compete with X-ray vendors on feature complement. A given cardiac catheterization suite may contain X-ray equipment from more than one vendor, but should have a single physiologic recorder/database system if it intends to use the system for reporting. Thus, there is the potential, depending on the supplier of the physiologic recorder/database system, to need to interface one X-ray manufacturer's physiologic recording system with another X-ray manufacturer's X-ray unit. Given the potential for conflict, considerable planning must be conducted to configure a blended manufacturer system. This should include contractual guarantees to achieve full interoperability of all linked systems.

There is not currently a common architecture for catheterization laboratory information systems database structures. Consequently, the file structure of a given catheterization laboratory information system is not compatible with others. This creates a major issue if a facility decides to change cardiac catheterization laboratory information systems. Migrating archived information from one information system to another is challenging at best, and likely not fully achievable. As a consequence, there is considerable inertia opposing a change of information system applications. Laboratory leadership should be fully cognizant of this issue when selecting an information system, as should one subsequently desire to change systems, there will be considerable operational forces opposing such a change.

DATABASE SERVERS

The heart of the laboratory information system is its database server(s). Depending on vendors used and configurations, the laboratory may have a single archive server that stores both angiographic image data and physiologic monitoring and report-generation data. Alternatively, depending on the particulars of equipment configuration and vendors supplying the systems, these functions may be supported by different servers. In addition, it is also feasible to use the hospital radiology department's image archiving server for this purpose, provided that it is configured to archive cineangiographic images. It is important to point out that these servers do not need to be located physically in the laboratory suite provided and that they have connections with sufficient bandwidth as discussed above. In fact, it is likely preferable that these servers be located in the hospital's larger computer facility where they can be maintained by dedicated computer support staff rather than be an item that requires periodic attention from the laboratory's clinical staff (who are less likely to be adept at these functions). The same considerations regarding Internet connections described for the X-ray systems and monitoring systems apply to the database servers.

Database server capacity is an important consideration with financial implications. The server system is generally a combination of three units. The server itself with an associated RAID (redundant array of independent disks) storage system provides immediate online storage. A server "juke box," which contains an array of mountable, removable media data storage units, provides near-line storage generally available automatically within several minutes of a request. Offline storage is removable media not stored in a "juke box" that must be physically mounted by an operator in a server drive in response to a request. Data in offline storage units require variable amounts of time for retrieval. When specifying a database server configuration, there is an obvious financial trade-off between the amount of online and near-line capacity and the cost of the system. These are functionality considerations that should be made at that time of system specification.

Ancillary diagnostic equipment: Provision, integration

ULTRASOUND

A cardiac catheterization laboratory may utilize a variety of ultrasound equipment. This will entail portable consoles that drive transducers used for a variety of purposes.

A small duplex ultrasound machine is very useful for assisting with vascular access, particularly internal jugular access in which anatomy can be very variable with respect to external landmarks. This unit is also of value in assessing vascular access sites following catheter removal in case there is concern about vascular integrity.

Intravascular and intracardiac ultrasound imaging and OCT imaging are valuable adjuncts to a variety of invasive and interventional procedures. Since this imaging is used to support intracardiac catheter and device manipulation, these machines are ideally interfaced with the monitor mounted on the main monitor boom so that the operators have ready access to both ultrasound and fluoroscopic images in the same location.

GUIDEWIRE PRESSURE AND FLOW VELOCITY TRANSDUCERS

These devices are used for assessment of intracoronary pressure and flow for measuring fractional flow reserve and coronary vasodilator reserve. The devices are driven by portable consoles that need to be interfaced with the physiological recording system. This constitutes one of the requirements for procedure table pedestal input and output connections, other than the standard pressure transducer input connections. These connection capabilities must be designed into the table pedestal and cabled appropriately at the time of construction and installation.

REFERENCES

1. Bashore TM, et al. 2012 America College of Cardiology Foundation/Society for Cardiovascular Angiography and Interventions expert consensus document on cardiac catheterization laboratory standards update: A report of the America College of Cardiology Foundation Task Force on Expert Consensus documents developed in collaboration with the Society of Thoracic Surgeons and Society for Vascular Medicine. *J Am Coll Cardiol* 2012;59(24):2221–2305.

3

Radiation safety

THOMAS M. BASHORE

INTRODUCTION

According to a National Council on Radiation Protection and Measurements report,[1] Americans were exposed to seven times as much ionizing radiation in 2006 than in the early 1980s. While much of this increase is the result of computed tomography (CT) and nuclear imaging, procedures performed in the cardiac catheterization laboratory also are responsible for this increased exposure to radiation. The public has become increasingly aware of the potential hazards of ionizing radiation,[2] as have governmental agencies.[3] As a consequence, the use of as-low-as-reasonably-achievable (ALARA) radiation has become a mantra for health-care providers to more carefully examine the use of medical radiation. A review from the American Heart Association Science Advisory committee[4] and editorials[5-7] have emphasized the importance of considering radiation effects in cardiac imaging. In general, the effects of ionizing radiation have been a greater focus for radiologists than cardiologists. This overview will discuss the manner in which X-ray images are created to better understand the means by which a reduction in radiation dose may be accomplished. The radiobiology of ionizing radiation will also be addressed to provide insight into the consequences of X-rays on biologic tissue and how these adverse effects can be minimized.

FUNDAMENTALS OF THE X-RAY IMAGING SYSTEM IN THE CARDIAC CATHETERIZATION LABORATORY

Figure 3.1 outlines the basic operation of flat panel X-ray systems used in the cardiac catheterization laboratory. In the generator, electrons are pushed to the X-ray tube where they are converted into a beam of X-rays. This conversion is inefficient with most of the energy converted to heat. Indeed, the focal spot on the rotating anode within the X-ray tube can reach temperatures of up to 4,300°F. The beam of X-rays produced starts from the focal spot and quickly diverges once out of the X-ray tube. This beam then passes upward through the patient and toward the image receptor. The shape of the beam from the X-ray tube can be altered by movable collimators at the exit site. The beam is filtered by passing through copper and aluminum plates that remove lower-energy X-rays that do not contribute useful information to the final image. The X-rays that pass through the patient (i.e., are not absorbed or scattered) are further filtered by use of a movable grid attached to the front of the flat panel receptor. This grid helps eliminate stray or scattered X-rays before they strike the face of the image detector.

When X-rays strike the cesium iodide (CsI) crystal on the face of the flat panel, they are converted to light photons

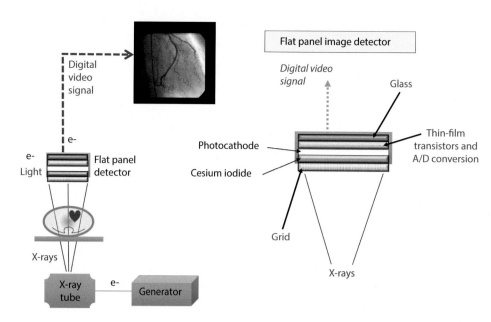

Figure 3.1 Basic operation of the flat panel X-ray system. On the left side is the overview of the imaging system, and on the right side is an expanded image of the flat panel image intensifier. X-rays are formed in the X-ray tube utilizing electrons from the generator. The generator produces both a potential gradient across the X-ray tube (kVp) and electrons that are converted in the X-ray tube (mA). The X-rays then diverge as they leave the X-ray tube, pass through the patient, and are detected on the image detector. There is a grid on the face of the image detector that filters out stray X-rays. The X-rays then strike a cesium iodide (CsI) crystal that converts them briefly to light, and then a photocathode converts the light back to electrons. These electrons hit the thin-film transistor that records their intensity and position and produces the video signal.

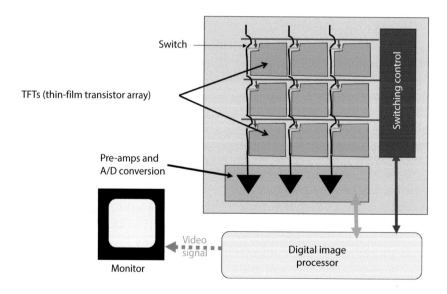

Figure 3.2 Thin-film transistors (TFTs) array inside the image detector. As shown in the figure, there is an array of TFTs within the image detector that correlate with the pixel array on the monitor. Each TFT records the intensity of the original X-ray and its location from the face of the image detector. This information produces the video signal that is then digitized (A/D converted) and sent to the monitor for display.

that strike a silicon photocathode that converts the light photons back to electrons. These electrons are then passed on to a thin-film transistor (TFT) that is part of an array of TFTs (Figure 3.2). Active matrix array sizes are available up to 43 × 43 cm with more than 9 million pixels. Each TFT then generates a current that is proportional to the number of electrons it received for each frame of the procedure. That generated current is called the video signal, and it reflects the amount of energy that struck each TFT and the location of that TFT on the sheet of transistors. This video signal is then digitized (converted from analog to digital) on the flat panel and sent directly to the computer monitor for display by recreating the "image" detected on the face of the image intensifier. By converting each pixel to light again, an image can be visually observed on the monitor screen. Direct image receptor imaging systems, primarily using amorphous selenium rather than CsI, are now being investigated where the electrical charge produced by each TFT in the active matrix can be produced directly by the X-ray interaction, rather than having to go through all the steps described.

Several features of the X-ray system are particularly relevant in order to understand how to minimize radiation exposure to both the operator and the patient. The most important is the functioning of the automatic exposure control (AEC). This control samples the middle of the image being generated and ensures that the maximal voltage across the X-ray tube (kVp) and the number of X-rays generated (a function of the mA) are optimal for the image being produced. It samples the image in every frame, and if at any time the X-ray dose needs adjustment, the AEC signals the generator to appropriately increase or decrease the number of X-rays produced.

Magnification always results in an increase in the number of X-rays required to produce an optimal image. Magnification occurs in two ways (Figure 3.3). First, because of the divergence of X-rays leaving the X-ray tube toward the detector, the farther the detector is from the source (source-to-image distance [SID]), the fewer the number of X-rays that will strike the face of the detector because some simply miss the detector altogether. This means the total X-ray dose must increase to satisfy the exposure requirement (mA times kVp times pulse width). Only displaying the middle section of the image on the monitor can also produce magnification. This is, in effect, digital magnification, and with it comes a loss in spatial resolution and an increase in

signal-to-noise that can only be overcome by increasing the X-ray dose. So it is important to keep the SID as narrow as possible and to use the fewest number of magnified images in order to minimize the X-ray dose. Other factors that increase the dose requirement per frame include panning over a dense structure like bones (compared to a less dense structure like the lungs) and imaging larger patients. Other issues related to the X-ray dose and satisfying the exposure requirement are presented below.

X-RAYS AND X-RAY SCATTER

X-rays are at the high end of the energy spectrum and have short wavelengths (from 10^{-8} to 10^{-9} m). X-rays differ from gamma rays in that their origin is from the outer shell of the atom while gamma rays originate from the nucleus. Both can be absorbed and attenuated (resulting in the image we are seeking) or result in X-ray scatter. Scattered X-rays provide no useful information and can result in loss of image contrast. Scatter is also a major source of radiation hazard for both the patient and the operator. Scatter mechanisms include (1) coherent or classical scattering, where the X-rays interact with atoms and change direction, (2) Compton scatter, where the X-ray knocks out an electron that travels in another direction, and (3) photoelectric scatter, where the X-ray is absorbed in the atom and another electron is ejected in another direction.

RADIOBIOLOGY

X-rays are harmful to tissue, resulting in ionization of atoms or deposition of energy into the tissue. Deposited energy can result in molecular changes. Ionization changes the chemical bonding properties of the atom and can result in

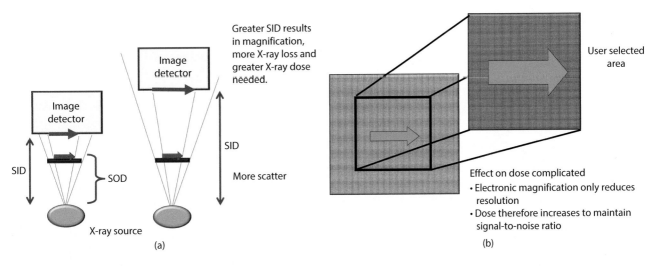

Figure 3.3 Magnification and the effect on X-ray dose. **(a)** Magnification occurs due to the divergence of the X-rays leaving the X-ray tube and striking the object, with the source-to-object distance (SOD) displayed. The greater the source-to-image distance (SID), the wider the spray of X-rays and the fewer usable X-rays strike the face of the image detector. In order to compensate the X-ray, dose must increase. **(b)** Magnification in the image detector occurs by selecting only the middle portion of the TFT data to display. This reduces the quality of the image, and a greater X-ray dose is required to restore an adequate signal-to-noise ratio.

the molecule breaking up or the atom relocating within the molecule. When this occurs, molecular and cellular function may be impaired, leading to cell death or mutation.

The radiosensitive molecule of greatest concern is DNA, although other moieties may also be altered. The cell is most susceptible to radiation damage during mitosis (i.e., cell division). Accordingly, organs most susceptible to radiation injury are those with frequently dividing cells.[8] These tend to be bone marrow cells, lymphoid tissue, and gonads. Stem cells are more radiosensitive than mature cells. Of interest, radiation has little effect during the first 2 weeks of the embryonic stage where loss of a pluripotent cell still allows other cells to continue normal development. Tissue with the highest metabolic rate or with a high proliferation rate is the most radiosensitive. Tissue is also more sensitive when irradiated in the oxygenated or aerobic state; hyperbaric conditions have been used in radiation oncology to take advantage of this.

DNA injury from radiation can be either direct or indirect (Figure 3.4). Direct damage to the DNA backbone of alternating sugar-phosphate molecules occurs when there is ionization of a backbone molecule and a break in the DNA backbone occurs. Indirect injury to DNA occurs when the X-ray interacts with cellular water, producing an electrically charged ion radical that decays to form a free radical by interacting with another water molecule. These free hydroxyl radicals are highly reactive and can result in DNA injury. Around two-thirds of DNA injury from radiation is by free radical injury and about one-third by the direct impact from X-rays.

When a DNA strand break does occur, it tends to be rapidly repaired using the opposite strand as a template. If the repair is deficient, a mutation may result, which predisposes to carcinogenesis.

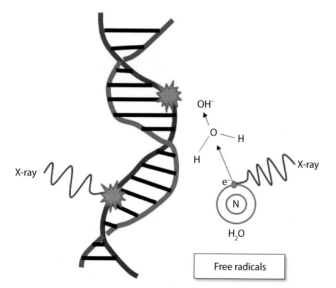

Figure 3.4 DNA injury. Radiation results in injury to the DNA backbone by either a direct hit or by first creating free radicals from contact with water within the cell. See text for further explanation.

From the DNA injury, one of two clinical scenarios may emerge. A *deterministic* radiation injury is present when a certain number of cells of an organ die following radiation injury. The classic example is a skin burn. These types of injuries are dose dependent, and there is a threshold when the effects become obvious. A *stochastic* radiation injury is evident when the cell lives but has mutated. This can result in either cancers or genetic defects. Stochastic injury, therefore, has no threshold dose (one X-ray can cause it), though the risk increases linearly with the amount of radiation exposure.

MEASURING RADIATION DOSAGES

The *radiation absorbed dose* (rad) is a measure of the energy absorbed per unit mass by an organ. It is expressed in units of milliGray (mGy). The *effective dose* (rem) strives to reflect the overall result of being exposed to ionizing radiation. It is an attempt to represent the amount of whole-body radiation that occurs when there is radiation of only a portion of the body, such as in the catheterization laboratory. It is expressed in milliSieverts (mSv). The effective dose is derived from simulations of radiation exposure using mathematical models plus radiation weighting factors.

Table 3.1 outlines the estimated effective dose for a variety of cardiovascular imaging procedures. In addition to man-made sources, individuals are routinely exposed to other sources of radiation (Figure 3.5), the bulk (55%) of which is from earth radon (an alpha particle). The average total background radiation exposure in the United States is 3.6 mSv. If a routine posteroanterior (PA) chest X-ray results in 0.04 mSv of exposure, we receive the equivalent of about 90 chest X-rays per year from inherent background radiation. Patient exposure in the cardiac catheterization laboratory amounts to about 7 mSv (range 2–20 mSv) for a diagnostic catheterization (twice that of background radiation) and approximately twice that (range 5–57 mSv) for a coronary interventional procedure.

To gauge how much radiation exposure the operator receives outside the lead apron, a radiosensitive badge is used—nowadays usually an optical simulated luminescent (OSL) badge. The OSL badge contains an aluminum oxide activated with carbon that releases light in proportion to the X-rays absorbed when the badge is later struck with a laser. Differing filters on the badge mimic the attenuation one might expect for shallow, eye lens, or deep exposure. To achieve proper use of the radiation badge, it should be worn on the thyroid collar.

Radiation dose to the patient can also be semi-quantitated (Figure 3.6). It is estimated using the dose-area-product (DAP) and/or the air kerma (kinetic energy released in matter). These data are now required as part of the cardiac catheterization report.[9] The DAP is calculated using data derived from an ionization chamber that is placed at the output of the X-ray tube. It is the absorbed radiation dose multiplied by the area radiated and is expressed in

Table 3.1 Typical effective radiation doses for cardiac procedures

Modality	Protocol	Typical dose (mSv)
X-ray (Fluoro)	Diagnostic coronary angiography	2–20
X-ray (Fluoro)	Percutaneous coronary intervention	5–57
X-ray (Fluoro)	TAVR (transfemoral)	33–100
X-ray (Fluoro)	EP radiofrequency ablation	1–25
X-ray (Fluoro)	Permanent pacemaker implantation	0.2–8
X-ray (MDCT)	Coronary CT, triggered axial	0.5–7
X-ray (MDCT)	CT angiography, high-pitch helical	<0.5–3
X-ray (MDCT)	Calcium score	1–5
Gamma (SPECT)	Tc-99m sestamibi rest/stress	11–18
Gamma (SPECT)	Tc-99m tetrofosmin rest/stress	14
Gamma (SPECT)	Thallium-201 rest/stress	15
Gamma (SPECT)	Dual isotope (thallium-201; Tc-99m sestamibi)	22–23
Positron (PET)	Rb-82; rest/stress	4
Positron (PET)	F-18 FDG	8

Source: Modified from Einstein, A.J., et al., *J. Am. Coll. Cardiol.*, 63(15), 1480–1489, 2014.
Note: CT, computed tomography; EP, electrophysiology; FDG, fluorodeoxyglucose; Fluoro, fluoroscopy; MDCT, multi-detector computed tomography; PET, positron emission tomography; Rb, rubidium; SPECT, single-photon emission computed tomography; TAVR, transcatheter aortic valve replacement; Tc, technetium.

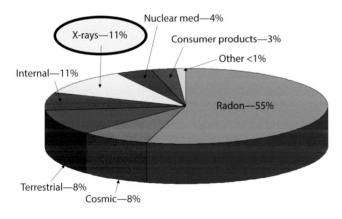

Figure 3.5 Sources of background radiation.

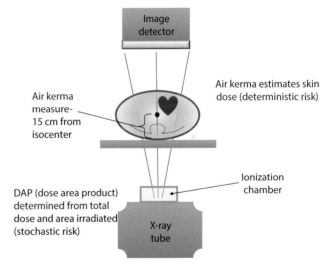

Figure 3.6 Dose-area-product (DAP) and air kerma definitions (kinetic energy released in matter). The DAP (or air kerma product) is derived from the total radiation that is detected from the ionization chamber on the output of the X-ray tube and the area of patient radiated. It is expressed in Gy/cm² and correlates with stochastic injury. An estimation of skin exposure (deterministic injury) is provided by the air kerma value. It estimates the radiation dose 15 cm from isocenter (and assumes this is the location of the skin). This point is sometimes called the interventional reference point. See text for further explanation.

Gy/cm². The DAP is a measure of the total X-ray dose that exited the X-ray tube during the procedure. It does not provide information on where the radiation went, but rather only defines how much radiation was emitted. For example, a 5 × 5 cm X-ray field with an entry dose of 1 mGy will result in a DAP value of 25 mGy/cm². The DAP has been shown to correlate with the risk of stochastic injury.[10] The air kerma value reported is an attempt to express how much radiation dose was delivered to the patient's skin. It is measured in Gray (Gy) units. It is sometimes referred to as the interventional reference point and is determined by assuming the patient's skin is about 15 cm from this isocenter.[11,12] Using the data from the ionizing chamber, and the data regarding location of the patient table, X-ray tube, and flat panel detector, a mathematical estimate of skin exposure can be derived. Thus, the air kerma value provides a semi-quantitative estimate of the risk for deterministic injury (for the skin

in particular) in much the same manner as the DAP provides data for estimating potential stochastic injury. Since the two measures require similar data from the ionizing chamber, the DAP is also referred to in some publications as the air kerma product.

Operators are exposed to less radiation than patients during their procedure, but they are exposed repeatedly over a lifetime. The effective dose becomes important in this situation, and operator limits are expressed in mSv.

Obtaining real-time radiation dosage data is a limitation in many cardiac catheterization laboratories, although devices are now available that provide real-time auditory or visual feedback during the catheterization procedure.[13] As these devices become more widespread and the technology matures, they may become powerful tools in alerting the operator of high levels of exposure and provide an opportunity to alter the procedure accordingly.

DEFINING THE RISKS FROM IONIZING RADIATION

The health effects from radiation have been the subject of much debate. The Committee on the Biological Effects of Ionizing Radiation (BEIR), an arm of the National Academy of Sciences, published the seventh in a series of reports on the issue (BEIR VII).[14] In it, they support the concept of a "linear-no-threshold" model for cancer risk. This assumes that even the smallest dose of ionizing radiation carries a potential risk. The committee pointed out that risk is a function of age at exposure (with younger patients more at risk), the gap between exposure and manifestation of disease, and whether the response was absolute or relative. There is a latent period (e.g., years) after radiation exposure before the risk of cancer is manifest. The magnitude of this risk is strikingly low, however, and for most occupational radiation exposures, the chances of dying from radiation exposure are about equivalent to the risk of dying from air travel.

Using data from the Japanese atomic bomb survivors, about 60% of survivors were exposed to less than 100 mSv. On average, assuming a sex and age distribution similar to the U.S. population, 1 in 100 persons would be expected to develop cancer from radiation exposure of 100 mSv, while 42 in 100 would be expected to develop cancer from other causes. The BEIR VII committee concluded that the risk of cancer from doses less than 100 mSv is extremely low and should drop linearly with no threshold value.[14]

Deterministic risks occur at known thresholds with skin erythema at about 2 Gy and permanent skin injury at about 5 Gy. Cataract risks may occur from acute exposure as low as 0.1 Gy and chronic exposure at 5 Gy.[15]

SPECIFIC PATIENT RISKS

The patient's skin takes the greatest risk from radiation (deterministic injury), with the amount of damage being dose dependent. Table 3.2 outlines the accepted threshold doses for the appearance of skin injury and the timing when this injury becomes evident after exposure. Note there is often a delay when the injury pattern is evident. Certain diseases appear to predispose the patient to skin injury from

Table 3.2 Threshold for skin entry doses that result in skin injury

Dose (Gy)	Effect	Onset
2 (2000 mSv)	Erythema	1 h
4–6	Late erythema	10 days to 10 weeks
7	Hair loss	3 weeks
10	Atrophy and fibrosis	14 weeks to 1 year
6–18	Necrosis	10 weeks to 1 year
Unknown	Skin cancer	>5 years

Source: Modified from Hirshfeld, J.W. Jr., et al., *Circulation*, 111(4), 511–532, 2005; Wagner, L.K., et al., *Radiology*, 213(3), 773–776, 1999.

radiation, including collagen vascular disease, diabetes mellitus, hyperthyroidism, ataxia telangiectasia, and prior exposure to radiation.[11,16,17]

The risk of a skin stochastic effect (cancer) is difficult to estimate, but a relative risk of 4:1 has been reported from exposure of 5–20 Gy, 14:1 from 40 to 60 Gy, and 27:1 from 60 to 100 Gy.[8] As opposed to deterministic effects, stochastic effects are cumulative, though it is very unlikely patients would receive doses of this magnitude from the low-radiation procedures performed in the cardiac catheterization laboratory.

The risk of stochastic effects to other organs in the patient is not completely known, but there may be a small but detectable increase in solid tumors at doses as low as 100 mSv.[18] The general risk of a fatal cancer has been estimated from 0.004% to 0.12% for each 10 mSv of radiation exposure.[11] Newborns are estimated to be 10 to 30 times more sensitive to radiation than adults, and women appear more susceptible than men.[19]

There are a number of international organizations that have weighed in on the patient's right to know how much radiation they receive from medical procedures. The International Commission on Radiation Protection established a 5-year limit of 100 mSv whole-body effect dose and a 50 mSv limit in any year.[20] When these limits are exceeded, appropriate action should be taken to inform the patient and document it in the medical record. The Society of Interventional Radiology proposed patients be informed if they have received >5 Gy air kerma, >500 Gray/cm^2 DAP, or fluoroscopy time >60 minutes.[21] A patient who has received a dose greater than these thresholds should be given written instructions to alert the operator or a medical physicist if irritated skin is noted after the procedure, and a clinic appointment should be arranged if there is skin injury. In 2013, the NRCP issued report #168,[22] which provides additional suggestions as to when the patient should be directly notified (Table 3.3).

Because of the greater risk of ionizing radiation in the pediatric population, many efforts have been made to reduce their radiation exposure. A variety of recent articles have addressed dose reduction and the development of

Table 3.3 NCRP suggested patient threshold values for first and subsequent notification to the patient regarding radiation dose

Dose metric	First notification	Subsequent notification
Peak skin dose	2 Gy	0.5 Gy
Air kerma*	3 Gy	1.0 Gy
DAP	300 Gy/cm^2	100 Gy/cm^2
Fluoroscopic time	30 min	15 min

Source: Mahesh, M., *J. Am. Coll. Radiol.*, 10(7), 551–552, 2013, with permission.

* Assumes a 100-cm field at the patient's skin. Subsequent notification implies an incremental dose from first notification. DAP, dose–area product; NRCP, National Council on Radiation Protection & Measurements.

Table 3.4 Dose limits for occupational exposure from the International Commission on Radiological Protection

Dose measure	Occupational dose limit
Effective dose	20 mSv per year averaged over 5 years (100 mSv total in 5 years) and <50 mSv in a single year
Equivalent dose	
Lens of the eye	20 mSv per year averaged over 5 years (100 mSv total in 5 years) and <50 mSv in a single year
Skin	500 mSv in a year
Extremities	500 mSv in a year

Source: Modified from Duran A, et al., *Catheter Cardiovasc. Interv.*, 82(1), 29–42, 2013.

awareness programs in pediatric catheterization laboratories.[23–26] Since most pediatric catheterizations are interventional in nature, the radiations doses vary widely.[27] The long-term effects of cardiac catheterization radiation in pediatric patients are only now being investigated in the French-sponsored Coccinelle study.[28]

Pregnancy is another special situation. While there is little risk during the first 2 weeks of an embryo's life due to the ability of the pluripotent cells to continue normal development should one of the early cluster of cells die, fetal risk is otherwise greatest during the first trimester. The risk of leukemia has been estimated at 0.06% per 10 mSv exposure during this time. The risk of later adult cancer is currently unknown. Neurologic tissue injury appears to be the greatest fetal concern as mental retardation was observed in atomic bomb survivors. Pregnancy is not an absolute contraindication to cardiac catheterization, but efforts to minimize radiation exposure must always be considered. Shielding the fetus from direct X-ray exposure is relatively effective during cardiac procedures; less than 2% of the radiation dose scatters internally to the uterus.[11]

SPECIFIC OCCUPATIONAL RISKS

Occupational risks from radiation in the cardiac catheterization laboratory are poorly understood, but by all measures they appear to be low. A radiation worker can expect to lose only 12 days from his or her life span due to radiation, compared to actual heart disease that would result in 2,100 days lost.[18]

Despite such reassuring data, a recent consensus statement from societies of physicians who work in the interventional laboratory environment noted that the risk is simply not well defined.[29] Increased cancers, particularly of the brain[30] and bone marrow,[31] have been reported in interventionalists. Radiation exposure has been associated with neural tumors[32] and brain tumors on the left side of the head where more radiation exposure is evident.[33] There is some evidence that cataract formation may be a stochastic and not a deterministic effect, and that the upper limits currently advised may not protect eyesight. In one study, slit-lamp examination of the

eyes of interventional cardiologists and nurses matched to a control group revealed the prevalence of posterior lens opacities "likely related to radiation" at around 50% contrasting to 9% in the control group.[34]

Table 3.4 outlines the 2013 recommendations for maximal radiation exposure to operators from the International Commission on Radiation Protection.[22] This differs only slightly from the World Health Organization suggestion that the maximal *monthly* limit for an operator be an effective dose of 0.5 mSv, a lens equivalent dose of 5 mSv, or an extremity dose of 15 mSv. During the average interventional procedure, the operator receives anywhere from 0.07 to 1.31 mSv on the badge[35] (the equivalent dose of about 1.5 to 7 chest X-rays). Note, that the *annual* maximal dose (on the badge) is 50 mSv to avoid a stochastic effect and 150 mSv to prevent a deterministic effect. Since stochastic effects are cumulative, the maximal dose over a lifetime is considered to be 10 mSv times your age or a maximum of 500 mSv. Unfortunately, there are a variety (up to six) of different formulae being used to convert the data from the badge into the effective dose, and the method used can result in considerable variability in the estimated dose,[35] further adding to the uncertainty and the wide variations in reported radiation doses received by operators.

An operator or staff member who becomes pregnant may continue working in the cardiac catheterization laboratory if she so chooses. However, she is required to meet with a radiation safety officer and monitor radiation exposure with two badges (worn on the collar and under the apron). If in any month the sum of the radiation exposure is >0.5 mSv or the total for the pregnancy is >5 mSv, she should consider removing herself from the cardiac catheterization laboratory environment.[36] In the United Kingdom, the whole-body radiation exposure must not exceed >6 mSv for the calendar year, and once the pregnancy is declared, the fetus is treated as a member of the general public and the radiation dose must be limited to a maximum of 1 mSv.[37] Many women choose to remove themselves from invasive procedures, not only for the radiation concern, but also because of the burden of wearing a lead apron while pregnant.

REDUCING RADIATION EXPOSURE IN THE CARDIAC CATHETERIZATION LABORATORY

Every member of the cardiac catheterization team should promote efforts to reduce radiation exposure to both the patients and the operators. Everything that reduces patient dose also reduces operator exposure. Education is important, and there are data that doses recorded in 2006 were 7- to 14-fold lower than 15 years prior.[38] Fluoroscopic time and radiation exposure are higher during fellowship training or during the learning curve of a new procedure.[39,40] The DAP is lower with more experienced operators.[41] Table 3.5 outlines the factors that every cardiac catheterization laboratory can utilize to reduce radiation risk.

Be aware of the positioning of the X-ray tube and image detector

The location of the operator to the X-ray tube is one factor that can influence radiation exposure. The dose of radiation received diminishes via the inverse square law (1/distance²). More radiation is received by the operator's left side than the right because of the relationship of the operator to the X-ray tube and to the patient during most of the acquisition.[35] In a left anterior oblique (LAO) cranial view, the X-ray tube is closest to the operator and the dose received may be six times that from the 30° right anterior oblique (RAO) view where the X-ray tube is on the opposite side of the table.[42] Increasing angulation always increases dose during both fluoroscopy and acquisition, not only because of the greater SID, but also due to more patient attenuation in angulated views.[43] Radial cases often put the operator closer to the X-ray tube, and catheter manifold extension tubing may help reduce operator exposure in this situation.[44,45] Since panning over bony structures results in increasing the dose requirement, patient's extremities should be kept out of the field whenever possible.

The height of the patient table has a major impact on the patient dose and on the scatter the operator receives. The closer the patient is to the X-ray tube, the more radiation he or she receives. Accordingly, the patient should be placed at the maximal distance from the X-ray tube, and the image detector should be positioned as close to the patient as possible to reduce the SID distance (Figure 3.3).

One of the newest considerations to reduce operator exposure is the use of robotic systems.[46,47] These new systems still face a number of technical and cost-effective issues, but given the rapid development of robotics in general, they may become a viable option in the future.

Keep the X-ray dose to a minimum

X-ray time should be kept to a minimum. Even though on a frame-by-frame basis, fluoroscopy results in 10 to 20 times less radiation exposure than cineangiography, fluoroscopy radiation accounts for 40%–60% of the total dose during a catheterization.[48] Pulsed fluoroscopy at rates below

Table 3.5 Reducing radiation risks in the cardiac catheterization laboratory for both the patient and the operator

1. **Be aware of the positioning of the X-ray tube, patient, and operator**
   Minimize angulated views with their wide SID
   Be aware of the operator position in relationship to the X-ray tube itself
   Elevate the patient away from the X-ray tube as much as possible
   Keep the image detector as close to the patient as possible
   Keep boney structures out of field of view as much as possible
   Use methods to increase the distance between the operator and the patient

2. **Keep the X-ray dose to a minimum**
   Minimize fluoroscopic and cine time
   Use last image held when possible
   Keep high-quality fluoroscopic images rather than cine when feasible
   Minimize the number of acquired images
   Use collimation and filters
   Optimize the imaging chain
   Keep frame rates to a minimum (7.5 f/sec for fluoroscopy and 15 f/sec for cine)
   Keep magnified imaging to a minimum
   Possible benefit to three-dimensional rotational angiography
   Possible benefit to removal of grid on face of image detector (children only)
   Be aware of real-time DAP and air kerma

3. **Use shielding**
   Equipment-mounted shielding (table drapes)
   Ceiling-mounted shielding
   Floor shielding
   Radioabsorbent drapes
   Personal shielding (thyroid collar, lead apron, glasses, shielding caps)

4. **Develop an educational program for the laboratory**
   Develop a training program for all staff
   Wear radiation monitoring badges and keep staff informed of results
   Document fluoroscopy time, air kerma, and DAP on all reports
   Report excessive patient dosages to the medical record and referring physician and arrange follow-up clinically

Note: DAP, dose–area product; f/s, frames per second; SID, source-to-image distance.

25 pulses/sec reduces dosage.[49] Most fluoroscopy can be performed at 7.5 frames/second.[4,23] Operators should limit the number of cine images by storing fluoroscopic images when high image quality is not needed. Collimation should be used to shape the X-ray image, and filters should be

utilized to remove unnecessary low-energy X-rays. Proper collimation can reduce DAP,[20] and virtual collimation can reduce dose without the need for fluoroscopy to adjust the collimators.[50] Since magnified views increase dose, they should be used only when necessary. A few of the newer X-ray systems can now produce "virtual magnification" that provides acceptable images without increasing X-ray dose.[10] In some instances, removal of the grid of the image detector has been tried where lower resolution might be acceptable (especially in the electrophysiology [EP] lab); this allows more X-rays to reach the flat panel face (the trade-off being the acquisition of more scattered X-rays).[51] Three-dimensional rotational imaging techniques for angiography have also been reported to reduce radiation exposure,[52] as has image chain optimization.[53]

Implementation of dose-reduction protocols should be considered in every laboratory to ensure that all possible technical settings are considered to reduce X-ray exposure.[43,54] In one study, the increased use of spectral filters, a reduction in fluoroscopic and acquisition imaging time, a reduction in the fluoroscopic frame rate, and active behavior changes reportedly reduced the air kerma dose by 40%.[41]

Use shielding

As outlined in a recent review,[10] shielding efforts include architectural shielding, equipment-mounted shielding, and personal protection. Architectural shielding amounts to rolling stationary lead screens. Equipment-mounted shielding includes the table-suspended drapes, ceiling-suspended shields, and disposable radioabsorbent drapes. To be effective, the shields have to be utilized.[55] Disposable radioprotective drapes have been shown to be effective in reducing operator exposure, with a 29-fold drop noted.[56] The drapes should not be placed directly within the X-ray imaging field as this will result in increased patient dose.[57] Shield draping may also be applied that reduces radiation exposure to the operator.[58]

Personal protective equipment is evolving. The half-value layer is a standard expression of how much radiation is absorbed by the lead apron. At a kVp of 75, a lead apron of 0.5 cm thickness will absorb 95% of all the X-rays produced. Two-piece wrap-around aprons offer more protection than single-piece lead aprons and reduce musculoskeletal aches. It is important the lead apron is stored properly to prevent any cracks from forming. More recently a "weightless" apron has been promoted that hangs from the ceiling and may help reduce back injury.[59] It may have an additional advantage of reducing side and cranial radiation exposure. Radiation glasses are effective in protecting the eyes from radiation, and they should have side shielding.[60]

The Brain Radiation exposure and Attenuation during INvasive (BRAIN) cardiology procedures study reported that there is substantially more radiation to the left side of the operator's head versus the right side during catheterization procedures.[33] This has furthered the speculation of radiation injury as reports have emerged of brain tumors in interventional cardiologists that are more frequently left-sided.[30] A protective cap (either of bismuth or lead) is now available, and there are data that confirm it can reduce cranial radiation exposure.[61]

Efforts in the cardiac catheterization laboratory to train all personnel on ways to reduce radiation exposure—reducing radiation time, increasing distance from the radiation source, and utilizing barriers—have met with very encouraging positive results,[62,63] and such an overall program should be instituted in every cardiac catheterization laboratory.

CONCLUSION

It is important to remember that many patients will have multiple procedures using ionizing radiation, and that stochastic risks are cumulative. Adhering to the ALARA principles is encouraged: (1) assume there is no absolutely safe dose of ionizing radiation; (2) the smaller the radiation dose, the less risk of an adverse event; and (3) incremental radiation doses have a cumulative effect over time.

REFERENCES

1. Balter S. Radiation dose management for fluoroscopically-guided interventional medical procedures. Report No. 168 (2010). National Council on Radiation Protection and Measurement. www.ncrppublications.org/reports/168.
2. Lauer MS. Elements of danger—The case of medical imaging. *Minn Med* 2009;92(12):40–41.
3. Vano E, et al. Radiation risks and radiation protection training for healthcare professionals: ICRP and the Fukushima experience. *J Radiol Prot* 2011;31(3):285–287.
4. Gerber TC, et al. Ionizing radiation in cardiac imaging: A science advisory from the American Heart Association Committee on Cardiac Imaging of the Council on Clinical Cardiology and Committee on Cardiovascular Imaging and Intervention of the Council on Cardiovascular Radiology and Intervention. *Circulation* 2009;119(7):1056–1065.
5. Wexler L. Gaining perspective on the risks of ionizing radiation for cardiac imaging. *J Am Coll Cardiol* 2014;63(15):1490–1492.
6. Einstein AJ, Knuuti J. Cardiac imaging: Does radiation matter? *Eur Heart J* 2012;33(5):573–578.
7. Einstein AJ, et al. Patient-centered imaging: Shared decision making for cardiac imaging procedures with exposure to ionizing radiation. *J Am Coll Cardiol* 2014;63(15):1480–1489.
8. Bushong SC (ed.). *Radiologic science for technologists: Physics, biology and protection.* 9th ed. St. Louis, MO: Elsiever, 2008.
9. Fazel R, et al. Approaches to enhancing radiation safety in cardiovascular imaging: A scientific statement from the American Heart Association. *Circulation* 2014;130(19):1730–1748.
10. Christopoulos G, et al. Optimizing radiation safety in the cardiac catheterization laboratory: A practical approach. *Catheter Cardiovasc Interv* 2016;87(2):291–301.
11. Hirshfeld JW Jr., et al. ACCF/AHA/HRS/SCAI clinical competence statement on physician knowledge to optimize patient safety and image quality in fluoroscopically

guided invasive cardiovascular procedures: A report of the American College of Cardiology Foundation/American Heart Association/American College of Physicians Task Force on Clinical Competence and Training. *Circulation* 2005;111(4):511–532.

12. Chida K, et al. Evaluation of patient radiation dose during cardiac interventional procedures: What is the most effective method? *Acta Radiol* 2009;50(5):474–481.

13. Christopoulos G, et al. Effect of a real-time radiation monitoring device on operator radiation exposure during cardiac catheterization: The radiation reduction during cardiac catheterization using real-time monitoring study. *Circ Cardiovasc Interv* 2014;7(6):744–750.

14. Monson RR CJ, et al. *Committee to Assess Health Risks from Exposure to Low Levels of Ionizing Radiation. Beir VII: health risks from exposure to low levels of ionizing radiation.* Washington, DC: National Academy Press; 2006.

15. Abbott JD. Controlling radiation exposure in interventional cardiology. *Circ Cardiovasc Interv* 2014;7(4):425–428.

16. Wagner LK, et al. Potential biological effects following high X-ray dose interventional procedures. *J Vasc Interv Radiol* 1994;5(1):71–84.

17. Koenig TR, et al. Skin injuries from fluoroscopically guided procedures: Part 2, review of 73 cases and recommendations for minimizing dose delivered to patient. *AJR Am J Roentgenol* 2001;177(1):13–20.

18. Pierce DA, Preston DL. Radiation-related cancer risks at low doses among atomic bomb survivors. *Radiat Res* 2000;154(2):178–186.

19. Brenner DJ, et al. Estimates of the cancer risks from pediatric CT radiation are not merely theoretical: Comment on "point/counterpoint: in X-ray computed tomography, technique factors should be selected appropriate to patient size. Against the proposition". *Med Phys* 2001;28(11):2387–2388.

20. Chambers CE, et al. Radiation safety program for the cardiac catheterization laboratory. *Catheter Cardiovasc Interv* 2011;77(4):546–556.

21. Stecker MS, et al. Guidelines for patient radiation dose management. *J Vasc Interv Radiol* 2009;20(7 Suppl):S263–S273.

22. Mahesh M, National Council on Radiation P, Measurements. NCRP 168: Its significance to fluoroscopically guided interventional procedures. *J Am Coll Radiol* 2013;10(7):551–552.

23. Covi SH, et al. Pulse fluoroscopy radiation reduction in a pediatric cardiac catheterization laboratory. *Congenit Heart Dis* 2015;10(2):E43–E47.

24. Glatz AC, et al. Patient radiation exposure in a modern, large-volume, pediatric cardiac catheterization laboratory. *Pediatr Cardiol* 2014;35(5):870–878.

25. Osei FA, et al. Radiation dosage during pediatric diagnostic or interventional cardiac catheterizations using the "air gap technique" and an aggressive "as low as reasonably achievable" radiation reduction protocol in patients weighing <20 kg. *Ann Pediatr Cardiol* 2016;9(1):16–21.

26. Verghese GR, et al. Characterization of radiation exposure and effect of a radiation monitoring policy in a large volume pediatric cardiac catheterization lab. *Catheter Cardiovasc Interv* 2012;79(2):294–301.

27. Borik S, et al. Achievable radiation reduction during pediatric cardiac catheterization: How low can we go? *Catheter Cardiovasc Interv* 2015;86(5):841–848.

28. Baysson H, et al. Follow-up of children exposed to ionising radiation from cardiac catheterisation: The Coccinelle study. *Radiat Prot Dosimetry* 2015;165(1–4):13–16.

29. Klein LW, et al. Occupational health hazards of interventional cardiologists in the current decade: Results of the 2014 SCAI membership survey. *Catheter Cardiovasc Interv* 2015;86(5):913–924.

30. Roguin A, et al. Brain and neck tumors among physicians performing interventional procedures. *Am J Cardiol* 2013;111(9):1368–1372.

31. Matanoski GM, et al. The current mortality rates of radiologists and other physician specialists: Deaths from all causes and from cancer. *Am J Epidemiol* 1975;101(3):188–198.

32. Finkelstein MM. Is brain cancer an occupational disease of cardiologists? *Can J Cardiol* 1998;14(11):1385–1388.

33. Reeves RR, et al. Invasive cardiologists are exposed to greater left sided cranial radiation: The BRAIN study (brain radiation exposure and attenuation during invasive cardiology procedures). *JACC Cardiovasc Interv* 2015;8(9):1197–1206.

34. Ciraj-Bjelac O, et al. Radiation-induced eye lens changes and risk for cataract in interventional cardiology. *Cardiology* 2012;123(3):168–171.

35. Kim KP, et al. Occupational radiation doses to operators performing cardiac catheterization procedures. *Health Phys* 2008;94(3):211–227.

36. Dauer LT, et al. Occupational radiation protection of pregnant or potentially pregnant workers in IR: A joint guideline of the Society of Interventional Radiology and the Cardiovascular and Interventional Radiological Society of Europe. *J Vasc Interv Radiol* 2015;26(2):171–181.

37. Best PJ, et al. SCAI consensus document on occupational radiation exposure to the pregnant cardiologist and technical personnel. *Catheter Cardiovasc Interv* 2011;77(2):232–241.

38. Vano E, et al. Occupational radiation doses in interventional cardiology: A 15-year follow-up. *Br J Radiol* 2006;79(941):383–388.

39. Jolly SS, et al. Effect of radial versus femoral access on radiation dose and the importance of procedural volume: A substudy of the multicenter randomized RIVAL trial. *JACC Cardiovasc Interv* 2013;6(3):258–266.

40. Alaswad K, et al. Transradial approach for coronary chronic total occlusion interventions: Insights from a contemporary multicenter registry. *Catheter Cardiovasc Interv* 2015;85(7):1123–1129.

41. Fetterly KA, et al. Radiation dose reduction in the invasive cardiovascular laboratory: Implementing a culture and philosophy of radiation safety. *JACC Cardiovasc Interv* 2012;5(8):866–873.

42. Balter S. Stray radiation in the cardiac catheterisation laboratory. *Radiat Prot Dosimetry* 2001;94(1–2):183–188.

43. Wassef AW, et al. Radiation dose reduction in the cardiac catheterization laboratory utilizing a novel protocol. *JACC Cardiovasc Interv* 2014;7(5):550–557.

44. Delewi R, Piek JJ. Cardiac catheterisation: radiation for radialists. *Lancet* 2015;386(10009):2123–2124.

45. Politi L, et al. Reduction of scatter radiation during transradial percutaneous coronary angiography: A randomized trial using a lead-free radiation shield. *Catheter Cardiovasc Interv* 2012;79(1):97–102.

46. Granada JF, et al. First-in-human evaluation of a novel robotic-assisted coronary angioplasty system. *JACC Cardiovasc Interv* 2011;4(4):460–465.

47. Smilowitz NR, et al. Robotic-enhanced PCI compared to the traditional manual approach. *J Invasive Cardiol* 2014;26(7):318–321.

48. Jurado-Roman A, et al. Effectiveness of the implementation of a simple radiation reduction protocol in the catheterization laboratory. *Cardiovasc Revasc Med* 2016;17(5):328–332.

49. Chida K, et al. Effect of radiation monitoring method and formula differences on estimated physician dose during percutaneous coronary intervention. *Acta Radiol* 2009;50(2):170–173.

50. Duran A, et al. Recommendations for occupational radiation protection in interventional cardiology. *Catheter Cardiovasc Interv* 2013;82(1):29–42.

51. Smith IR, et al. Radiation risk reduction in cardiac electrophysiology through use of a gridless imaging technique. *Europace* 2016;18(1):121–130.

52. Eloot L, et al. Three-dimensional rotational X-ray acquisition technique is reducing patients' cancer risk in coronary angiography. *Catheter Cardiovasc Interv* 2013;82(4):E419–E427.

53. Eloot L, et al. Novel X-ray imaging technology enables significant patient dose reduction in interventional cardiology while maintaining diagnostic image quality. *Catheter Cardiovasc Interv* 2015;86(5):E205–E212.

54. Bracken JA, et al. A radiation dose reduction technology to improve patient safety during cardiac catheterization interventions. *J Interv Cardiol* 2015;28(5):493–497.

55. Balter S. Radiation shielding really works, when you use it. *Catheter Cardiovasc Interv* 2006;67(1):24.

56. Jones MA, et al. The benefits of using a bismuth-containing, radiation-absorbing drape in cardiac resynchronization implant procedures. *Pacing Clin Electrophysiol* 2014;37(7):828–833.

57. King JN, et al. Using a sterile disposable protective surgical drape for reduction of radiation exposure to interventionalists. *AJR Am J Roentgenol* 2002;178(1):153–157.

58. Gilligan P, et al. Assessment of clinical occupational dose reduction effect of a new interventional cardiology shield for radial access combined with a scatter reducing drape. *Catheter Cardiovasc Interv* 2015;86(5):935–940.

59. Fattal P, Goldstein JA. A novel complete radiation protection system eliminates physician radiation exposure and leaded aprons. *Catheter Cardiovasc Interv* 2013;82(1):11–16.

60. van Rooijen BD, et al. Efficacy of radiation safety glasses in interventional radiology. *Cardiovasc Intervent Radiol* 2014;37(5):1149–1155.

61. Karadag B, et al. Effectiveness of a lead cap in radiation protection of the head in the cardiac catheterisation laboratory. *EuroIntervention* 2013;9(6):754–756.

62. Kuon E, et al. Efficacy of a minicourse in radiation-reducing techniques in invasive cardiology: A multicenter field study. *JACC Cardiovasc Interv* 2014;7(4):382–390.

63. Georges JL, et al. Reduction of radiation delivered to patients undergoing invasive coronary procedures. Effect of a programme for dose reduction based on radiation-protection training. *Arch Cardiovasc Dis* 2009;102(12):821–827.

64. Wagner LK, et al. Severe skin reactions from interventional fluoroscopy: Case report and review of the literature. *Radiology* 1999;213(3):773–776.

4

Contrast media

LAURA DAVIDSON AND CHARLES J. DAVIDSON

INTRODUCTION

Iodinated contrast agents used in the cardiac catheterization laboratory are the mainstay of visualization of coronary and peripheral vasculature as well as cardiac anatomy. Low osmolar and iso-osmolar agents have been developed to mitigate adverse events while providing optimal imaging. This chapter discusses contrast agents and the evidence-based strategies to prevent adverse events.

FUNDAMENTALS

Types of contrast agents

Various formulations of contrast agents containing iodine have been developed. They differ in ionicity and the ratio of iodine to particles. This ratio directly affects their viscosity and osmolarity (Table 4.1 and Figure 4.1).

First-generation, high-osmolar contrast media (HOCM) are ionic monomers, which consist of a single, negatively charged tri-iodinated benzene ring attached to a cation. Iodine provides the radiopacity. Osmolarity is determined by the number of particles in a solution rather than particle size. The particles dissociate in solution, thus creating a 3:2 iodine-to-particle ratio. First-generation agents have a sodium concentration similar to blood but are hyperosmolar relative to blood. These agents have osmolarity that is typically >1400 mOsm/kg compared with the 290 mOsm/kg found in blood. This high osmolarity can cause repolarization changes and arrhythmias during coronary angiography.[1] Both the ionicity and hyperosmolarity of these agents contribute to significant volume shifts and to adverse cardiac and renal effects. These include bradycardia, atrioventricular (AV) block, ventricular fibrillation, and acute kidney injury. First-generation HOCM agents include diatrizoate (Hypaque, Angiovist, Renografin), metrizoate (Isopaque), and iothalamate (Conray).

Second-generation, low osmolar contrast media (LOCM) were designed to minimize side effects. Among the first such agents was the ionic dimer, ioxaglate (Hexabrix). Ioxaglate is a monoacidic, double benzene ring with six iodine molecules at the 2, 4, and 6 positions on each ring. Dissociation occurs in solution at carbon 1, creating a 6:2 iodine-to-particle ratio. This agent has an osmolarity of 600 mOsm/kg, which is less than half that of HOCM but still twice that of blood. Early studies confirmed that ioxaglate was associated with fewer cardiovascular and renal effects compared to HOCM.[2]

Table 4.1 Comparison of various contrast media

Generation	Class	Type of molecule	Examples	Iodine (mgI/mL)	Sodium (mEq/L)	Osm (mOsm/kg)	Viscosity at 37.8°C
First	High osmolar	Ionic monomer	Diatrizoate (Hypaque) Metrizoate (Isopaque) Iothalamate (Conray)	325–370	160	1797–2076	2.8–8.4
Second	Low osmolar	Ionic dimer Nonionic monomer	Ioxaglate (Hexabrix) Iopamidol (Isovue) Iohexol (Omnipaque) Iopromide (Ultravist) Ioxilan (Oxilan) Ioversol (Optiray)	320 350–370	150 2–5	600 695–844	7.5 8.1–10.4
Third	Iso-osmolar	Nonionic dimer	Iodixanol (Visipaque)	320	19	290	11.8

Source: Modified from Baim, D.S., ed., *Grossman's Cardiac Catheterization, Angiography, and Intervention*, 8th edn, Lippincott Williams & Wilkins, Philadelphia, PA, 2013.

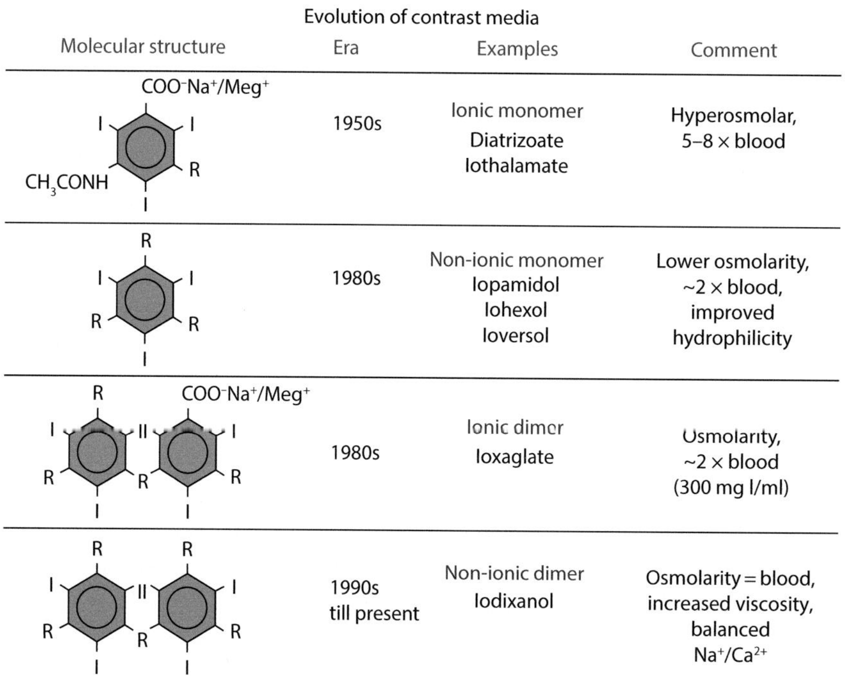

Figure 4.1 Chemical structures of various contrast media.

LOCM are also available as nonionic monomers. These are tri-iodinated with many hydrophilic hydroxyl groups. They possess a 3:1 iodine-to-particle ratio and have an osmolarity between 500 and 850 mOsm/kg. These include iopamidol (Isovue), iohexol (Omnipaque), iopromide (Ultravist), ioxilan (Oxilan), and ioversol (Optiray). The nonionic LOCM cause less ventricular irritability than their ionic predecessors but generally have a slightly higher viscosity. Nevertheless, there is no increased risk of thrombotic events compared to ionic agents.[3,4] Additionally, nonionic LOCM are associated with less nephrotoxicity and fewer allergic reactions compared to HOCM.[5]

There is some evidence that nonionic, iso-osmolar contrast media (IOCM) with an osmolarity similar to blood, may be safer than LOCM. Iodixanol (Visipaque) is a nonionic dimer that consists of two tri-iodinated benzene rings. It has a 6:1 iodine-to-particle ratio. IOCM have a higher viscosity than HOCM and LOCM, but have been shown in some studies to cause fewer allergic reactions and no increased adverse coronary events.[3,6] Iodixanol was initially thought to be associated with less acute kidney injury than ioxaglate.[7,8] However, recent larger randomized trials have not shown a reduced incidence of contrast-induced nephrotoxicity with iodixanol compared with other LOCM.[9,10] Multiple trials have shown a reduction in patient symptoms, allergic reactions, and organ toxicity with LOCM or IOCM compared to HOCM.

INDICATIONS

Contrast agents are used in the cardiac catheterization lab for coronary arteriography, ventriculography, aortography, and peripheral arterial assessment.

CLINICAL ASPECTS

Contrast reactions can be divided into two major categories: chemotoxic reactions and hypersensitivity reactions. Chemotoxic reactions are related to the chemical properties of the agents and are often dose- and rate-dependent. These include volume overload, vasovagal reactions, cardiotoxicity, and nephrotoxicity. Hypersensitivity reactions, or allergic reactions, are idiosyncratic and independent of rate or volume of contrast infusion.

CHEMOTOXIC REACTIONS

Volume overload

Most laboratories utilize LOCM contrast media that are hyperosmolar relative to blood. Since LOCM are two to three times the osmolarity of blood, rapid infusion of large amounts of contrast can result in large fluid shifts from the extravascular to the intravascular space. This causes elevated filling pressures or, in extreme cases, cardiogenic pulmonary edema. Minimization of contrast volume, use of IOCM, or deferral of angiography should be considered in patients with clinical evidence of acute heart failure or on measurement of left ventricular (LV) end-diastolic pressure or pulmonary capillary wedge pressure (PCWP).

Vasovagal reactions

It is common for patients to experience a sensation of flushing, warmth, or nausea with a large bolus injection of contrast media. Flushing is related to the osmolarity of the agent used. Therefore, it is more pronounced with administration of HOCM than with LOCM, and least with IOCM. Flushing is typically mild, transient, and self-limited. Rarely, this sensation can persist. If the reaction is severe, then transient hypotension may occur.

Bradycardia and vasovagal reactions from contrast administration can also occur. These reactions should be distinguished from hypersensitivity reactions and do not preclude further injection of contrast media. Decreasing the rate of injection may ameliorate further symptoms. If symptoms are prolonged, atropine (0.5–1 mg, bolus) should be administered intravenously.

Cardiotoxicity

Cardiotoxicity is less common with nonionic LOCM and IOCM compared to HOCM. The mechanism of direct cardiotoxicity is related to the hyperosmolarity of these agents or the calcium-chelation of anions, which dissociate from ionic contrast compounds. Observed electrocardiographic changes include sinus bradycardia, heart block, QRS widening, QT prolongation, ST segment changes, and giant T-wave inversions. Ventricular tachycardia and ventricular fibrillation may also rarely occur. This is often precipitated by injecting into a conus branch of the right coronary artery (RCA) or when the catheter is occlusive in the coronary ostium.

Transient LV systolic dysfunction and elevated LV end-diastolic pressure have also been observed after LV contrast injection and coronary angiography.

Nephrotoxicity

A common and important chemotoxic contrast reaction is contrast-induced acute kidney injury (CI-AKI). Although it is an infrequent event in unselected population-based studies, CI-AKI is the third leading cause of hospital-acquired renal failure.[11] There are many definitions of CI-AKI. It was traditionally accepted to be an increase in serum creatinine (SCr) that is 25% above baseline or an absolute increase of >0.5 mg/dL within 48 hours of contrast exposure. However, more recently, an alternative definition has been proposed by the Kidney Disease Improving Global Outcomes (KDIGO) guidelines.[14] This statement defines stage I CI-AKI as an SCr increase of ≥0.3 mg/dL within 48 hours of contrast exposure, an increase in SCr that is ≥1.5 times baseline, or a urine volume of less than 0.5 mL/kg/h for at least 6 hours. Stage II AKI is defined as an SCr that is 2–2.9 times baseline, or a urine volume of less than 0.5 mL/kg/h for ≥12 hours. Stage III AKI is defined as an SCr 3 or more times baseline, SCr ≥4 mg/dL, initiation of renal replacement therapy, urine output of less than 0.3 mL/kg/h for ≥24 hours, or anuria for ≥12 hours. The Valvular Academic Research Consortium (VARC)-2 initiative also utilizes this definition of AKI.[12] The European Renal Best Practice (ERBP) position statement on the KDIGO guidelines agrees with these definitions and expands upon them by stating that a baseline SCr should be determined prior to contrast administration and that high-risk patients have a repeat SCr performed 12–72 hours after contrast exposure.[13,14]

Epidemiology

The incidence of CI-AKI varies depending on the presence of risk factors, the type of contrast media, and the volume of contrast media administered. The incidence is 1.6% to 2.3% in patients undergoing diagnostic procedures.[15] This increases to 20% to 30% in patients with chronic kidney disease (CKD), diabetes, congestive heart failure (CHF), or advanced age.[2] In a registry of 7,586 patients undergoing percutaneous coronary intervention (PCI), the incidence of AKI (defined as a >0.5 mg/dL rise in SCr) was 3.3% overall and 22% in patients with a baseline SCr >2 mg/dL.[16] In a prospective evaluation of patients undergoing diagnostic cardiac catheterization, the incidence of AKI, defined as an SCr rise >0.5 mg/dL, was 6.4%.[17]

Pathophysiology

The pathophysiology of CI-AKI is unclear, although several potential mechanisms have been implicated. Animal models with renal biopsy have shown changes consistent with acute tubular necrosis.[18,19] However, since recovery from CI-AKI is faster than the 2 to 3 weeks expected after other types of acute tubular necrosis, this suggests less permanent or severe damage to tubular cells. In addition, the fractional excretion of sodium (FENa) observed in CI-AKI is often <1%, which suggests prerenal hypoperfusion as opposed to frank tubular necrosis. This potential mechanism highlights the need for adequate prehydration. *In vitro* studies have shown that contrast media causes apoptosis of renal tubular cells. Additionally, reactive oxygen species increase in a dose-dependent fashion when renal cells are exposed to contrast media in cell culture.[20]

Clinical features

CI-AKI typically begins in the first 12-24 hours following contrast exposure, peaks at 2–3 days, and resolves over 5–7 days. Renal failure is unusual with proper precautions (see below) and is typically nonoliguric. The need for dialysis is highly uncommon (<0.1%),[21] but when required it is associated with an in-hospital mortality rate of 36% (vs. 1% without hemodialysis) and a 2-year mortality of 81%.[22]

It is important to consider that other types of renal failure commonly occur after contrast exposure that are unrelated to the contrast exposure. These include (1) renal hypoperfusion due to hypotension or (2) acute tubular necrosis in the setting of CHF, volume depletion, sepsis, atheroemboli, interstitial nephritis, or obstructive uropathy.

Renal failure related to atheroemboli is most common in patients with peripheral arterial or abdominal aortic aneurysmal disease who undergo cardiac catheterization. Unlike CI-AKI, the onset is often delayed for days or even weeks after catheterization. Atheroemboli are associated with blue toes, livedo reticularis, fever, hypereosinophilia, hypocomplementemia, and ghost-like clefts on renal biopsy from

vacated cholesterol crystals that are dissolved during routine histologic preparation. Unlike CI-AKI, a high percentage of patients with atheroemboli-related kidney injury require hemodialysis, and recovery of renal function is minimal.[23]

Urinalysis in CI-AKI may reveal either low or elevated FENa depending on the degree of prerenal hypoperfusion versus actual tubular injury. Urine protein may be elevated for the first 24 hours after contrast media exposure.

Risk factors

Both modifiable and nonmodifiable risk factors predispose patients to CI-AKI (Table 4.2). The major nonmodifiable risk factor for CI-AKI is underlying CKD (SCr >1.5 mg/dL or a glomerular filtration rate [GFR] of <60 mL/min/1.73 m^2),[16,17,22] and this risk is increased further by the presence of diabetes. In adult patients with cardiovascular disease, it is recommended that the Modification of Diet in Renal Disease (MDRD) formula be utilized to calculate GFR (Table 4.3).

Age is an independent predictor of CI-AKI,[24] and this likely reflects the fact that elderly patients tend to have a lower GFR and more comorbid disease. In addition, the elderly are more likely to have multivessel coronary artery disease and revascularization with PCI, which translates to a higher volume of contrast media.

Inadequate renal perfusion in the setting of CHF or hemodynamic instability is also associated with increased risk for CI-AKI. This is particularly true in the setting of large myocardial infarction (MI) or the need for intra-aortic

Table 4.2 Risk factors for the development of contrast-induced acute kidney injury

Non-modifiable risk factors	Modifiable risk factors
Age	Recent contrast exposure
Baseline chronic kidney disease	Adequate hydration
Diabetes mellitus	Contrast volume
Shock	Other nephrotoxic drugs
Presence of intra-aortic balloon pump	
Anemia	
Acute decompensated heart failure	
Multiple myeloma	

Table 4.3 Estimating creatinine clearance (CrCl) and glomerular filtration rate (GFR[a])

Modification of diet in renal disease (MDRD):

(GFR mL/min/1.73 m^2) = $175 \times$ (serum creatinine [mg/dL])$^{-1.154} \times$ (Age)$^{-0.203} \times 0.742$ (if female) $\times 1.212$ (if African American)

Cockcroft – Gault: CrCl $= \dfrac{(140\text{-age}) \times \text{weight in kilograms} \times 0.85 \text{ (if female)}}{72 \times \text{serum creatinine (mg/dL)}}$

[a] MDRD GFR calculator available at: http://www.niddk.nih.gov/health-information/health-communication-programs/nkdep/lab-evaluation/gfr-calculators/adults-conventional-unit/Pages/adults-conventional-unit.aspx.

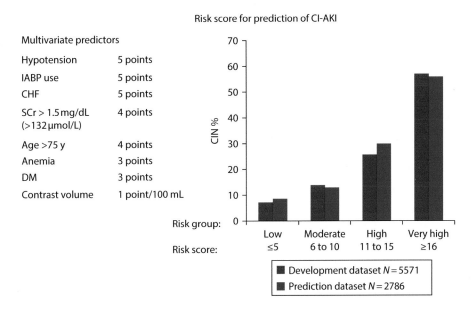

Figure 4.2 A risk score for predicting contrast-induced acute kidney injury following percutaneous coronary intervention. CHF, congestive heart failure; CI-AKI, chronic-induced acute kidney injury; CIN, contrast-induced nephropathy; DM, diabetes mellitus; IABP, intra-aortic balloon pump; SCr, serum creatinine. (From Mehran, R., et al., *J. Am. Coll. Cardiol.*, 44(7), 1393–1399, 2004. With permission.)

balloon counterpulsation.[24] Anemia has also been identified as an independent risk factor, perhaps related to decreased oxygen delivery to tubular cells.[25]

Diabetes is also a known risk factor for the development of CI-AKI.[22,24] One study demonstrated that while diabetes confers risk for CI-AKI (20% of patients), pre-diabetes is also associated with an increased risk (11.4%) compared to patients with a normal fasting glucose (5.5%).[26] Diabetic patients and preexisting CKD are additive risk factors, and together, the risk of CI-AKI is amplified.[27,28]

Multiple myeloma has been associated with an increased risk of CI-AKI, particularly with HOCM. The incidence is likely <1.5% with newer agents. Volume depletion, in particular, tends to cause tubular precipitation of myeloma proteins after contrast media exposure.[27]

Modifiable risk factors for CI-AKI include contrast volume, hydration status, recent contrast administration, and use of nephrotoxic drugs concomitantly. While there is no safe minimum volume of contrast that can be used to avoid CI-AKI, especially in high-risk patients, it has been suggested that using <30 mL for diagnostic studies and <100 mL for interventional procedures lessens the risk.[11] Often, multiple exposures to contrast media in patients may be necessary. If clinically possible, it is recommended that 10 days lapse between contrast exposures in individual patients.[28]

Nephrotoxic drugs can also increase the risk of CI-AKI. Nonsteroidal anti-inflammatory drugs (NSAIDs), aminoglycosides, and other nephrotoxins should be avoided if possible. The use of angiotensin-converting enzyme inhibitors is controversial, and studies examining whether these medications increase CI-AKI risk have had mixed results.[29,30]

Cumulative risk prediction models have been proposed to estimate the risk of CI-AKI in a given patient. One frequently utilized risk prediction score was developed in 2004 and includes baseline renal function, age, presence of intra-aortic balloon pump (IABP), CHF, anemia, hypotension, diabetes, and contrast media volume (Figure 4.2).[24]

HYPERSENSITIVITY REACTIONS

Unlike chemotoxic contrast reactions, hypersensitivity reactions are independent of the rate or volume of contrast infusion. Immediate hypersensitivity reactions typically occur within seconds to an hour after contrast exposure. Delayed hypersensitivity reactions can occur between 1 hour and 1 week, but these are much less common. Hypersensitivity reactions typically present with some combination of pruritus, urticaria, rash, angioedema, laryngospasm, bronchospasm, hypotension, syncope, shock, or even death. Most such reactions are mild, but they can (rarely) be fatal.

Epidemiology

The incidence of hypersensitivity reactions is up to 13% with HOCM, but much lower with LOCM and IOCM.[31,32,35] Overall, the incidence of mild reactions is approximately 9% and severe reactions is 0.2%.[33,34] The mortality due to hypersensitivity reactions is approximately 1/100,000 patients.[35]

Pathophysiology

The pathophysiology of hypersensitivity reactions is poorly understood. The clinical manifestations may be similar to those of a Type I hypersensitivity allergic reaction, but the vast majority of contrast hypersensitivity reactions are not immunoglobulin E (IgE)-mediated,[36,37] and one-third of anaphylactic reactions occur without prior exposure to the contrast agent.[38] However, serum tryptase levels are elevated in patients who react to contrast media, as is seen with anaphylactic reactions.[39] The most likely etiology is an anaphylactoid reaction involving direct mast cell activation and massive degranulation of histamine. Activation of the coagulation cascade and kinin, release of serotonin, and inhibition of platelets may also play a role.[39]

Risk factors

The type of contrast media used impacts the likelihood of a hypersensitivity reaction. Ionic HOCM causes mild, immediate reactions in as many as 13% of patients, compared to less than 3% with nonionic LOCM.[35] Severe reactions occur in 0.22% to 0.04% with ionic HOCM, compared to 0.04% to 0.004% with nonionic LOCM.[39] The incidence of hypersensitivity reactions may be even lower with the nonionic IOCM iodixanol.[31,32]

The most important risk factor for the development of an anaphylactoid reaction is a prior anaphylactoid reaction to contrast media, with a 21% to 60% risk of having another reaction with a subsequent exposure.[35] When a previous adverse reaction has occurred with an ionic contrast agent, the risk of a reaction with a nonionic agent is less. Patients with asthma have a sixfold increase in their risk of contrast-mediated reactions compared to those without asthma. Other risk factors include history of allergic disease, female gender, and beta-blocker exposure.[39,40]

A common misconception is that shellfish allergy confers an increased risk of contrast hypersensitivity due to iodine content.[41,42] This is likely not the case since the allergen in shellfish is the protein tropomyosin, not iodine. However, atopic individuals are commonly allergic to seafood and also tend to be at higher risk of a contrast reaction. Routine premedication for a history of shellfish allergy is not recommended prior to contrast. Patients with asthma and other food allergies should be treated with similar caution to those with a shellfish allergy.[43]

Clinical features

Hypersensitivity reactions are not related to the dose or the injection rate of contrast medium. Symptoms typically begin within minutes and up to 1 hour after contrast infusion. The severity of the reaction can be classified based on the grading system developed by Ring and Messmer (Table 4.4). Reactions that occur within seconds after contrast exposure may initially seem mild but can progress rapidly. Typical manifestations include pruritus and urticaria. More severe reactions may include angioedema, laryngospasm, bronchospasm, loss of consciousness, and even death. Danger signs are rapid progression of symptoms, respiratory distress, stridor, hypotension, arrhythmia, or chest pain.

It is important to distinguish an anaphylactoid reaction from other complications of contrast injection, such as vasovagal reactions or cardiogenic pulmonary edema. Like an anaphylactoid reaction, a vasovagal reaction can result in acute hypotension but typically involves bradycardia and nausea. Patients often will not have pruritus, urticaria, angioedema, stridor, or wheezing. Rapid volume expansion after contrast bolus can cause respiratory distress and wheezing from cardiogenic pulmonary edema. Likewise, this syndrome is not associated with pruritus, urticaria, or angioedema.

Lab testing for anaphylactoid reactions is not routinely performed as its utility remains unclear. However, postprocedure serum tryptase and serum histamine levels may help indicate that an anaphylactoid reaction has occurred if there

Table 4.4 Severity of immediate hypersensitivity reactions to iodinated contrast media

| Grade | Symptoms | | | |
	Skin	Abdomen	Respiratory tract	Circulation
I	Pruritus Flush Urticaria Angioedema			
II	Pruritus Flush (not obligatory) Urticaria Angioedema	Nausea Cramping	Rhinorrhea Hoarseness Dyspnea	Tachycardia ($\Delta > 20$ beats/min)
III	Pruritus Flush (not obligatory) Urticaria Angioedema	Vomiting Defecation Diarrhea	Laryngeal edema Bronchospasm Cyanosis	Hypotension ($\Delta > 20$ mmHg systolic) Arrhythmia Shock
IV	Pruritus Flush (not obligatory) Urticaria Angioedema	Vomiting Defecation Diarrhea	Respiratory arrest	Circulatory arrest

Source: Brockow, K., et al., Allergy, 60(2), 150–158, 2005. With permission.

is clinical uncertainty. Tryptase is a mast cell proteinase that is released in the setting of massive mast cell activation and degranulation such as anaphylaxis, anaphylactoid reactions, and systemic mastocytosis.[35,36] It has a 90-minute half-life and is only detectable for several hours after an anaphylactoid reaction. Serum levels obtained following an anaphylactoid reaction should be compared to baseline levels of serum tryptase 1–2 days following the reaction. Histamine has an even shorter half-life and can be detected within 1 hour of the reaction.[35]

Routine skin testing has not proven to be beneficial in predicting the recurrence of a hypersensitivity reaction to contrast media, although there may be a very small subset of patients with true IgE-mediated anaphylaxis who can be detected with skin testing.[37]

Treatment

The initial step in the treatment of a presumed anaphylactoid contrast reaction is to stop further administration of contrast (Table 4.5). Mild reactions, such as simple pruritus, may be treated with intravenous (IV) antihistamines (usually 25–50 mg diphenhydramine bolus) and observation. IV corticosteroids are also effective. However, it should be noted that mild reactions can quickly progress, and the clinician should anticipate and respond to a severe reaction when needed.

The first and most important active treatment of a severe anaphylactoid reaction is epinephrine. Other therapies are not as rapidly acting and may not be effective in reversing the underlying reaction. Intramuscular epinephrine 0.01 mg/kg (1:1000 dilution; 0.01 mL/kg), maximum of 0.3 mg, can be given and this can be repeated every 5–15 minutes with a maximum of 1 mg total.[44] Alternatively, if the patient has IV access, 0.01 mg/kg (1:10,000 dilution; 0.1 mL/kg), maximum of 0.3 mg, can be administered as an IV infusion and repeated every 5–15 minutes with a total of 1 mg dose. If there is evidence of impending airway obstruction from angioedema or stridor, immediate endotracheal intubation should take place. Delay may result in complete obstruction requiring cricothyroidotomy.

Adjunctive antihistamine therapy with 50 mg of diphenhydramine (IV or oral), an H1 blocker, may improve symptoms and prevent short-term recurrence. Glucocorticoids have little immediate benefit, but a 125 mg methylprednisolone IV bolus can be given to prevent a recurrent reaction several hours later.

SPECIAL ISSUES

Contrast-induced acute kidney injury prevention

The most effective therapy for CI-AKI is prevention, with recognition of patients at risk as the first step. Identification of risk factors and measurement of SCr with calculation of estimated GFR or creatinine clearance prior to contrast exposure is essential. When patients are deemed to be at high risk, the use of alternative diagnostic imaging of the cardiac chambers and valves, such as echocardiography or magnetic resonance imaging (MRI), should be considered. Nephrotoxic medications should be discontinued prior to the procedure when possible. In addition to these general measures, there are specific preprocedural and procedural approaches that are effective in minimizing the risk of CI-AKI (Table 4.6).

Hydration

There is no prospective randomized trial comparing hydration to no hydration, but there is universal consensus that hydration is beneficial. The mechanism by which hydration reduces the risk for CI-AKI is unknown; however, several mechanisms have been proposed. One hypothesis is that administration of saline dilutes contrast and reduces its

Table 4.5 Prophylaxis and treatment of contrast hypersensitivity reactions

Prophylaxis for a Known Contrast Allergy	Prednisone	50 mg PO, 13, 7, and 1 h before procedure
	OR hydrocortisone (for emergent procedures)	200 mg IV, prior to and every 4 h during procedure
	AND diphenhydramine	50 mg IV or PO, 1 h before procedure
	AND low-osmolar or iso-osmolar contrast	
Treatment for a Mild Contrast Reaction	Stop contrast injection	
	Diphenhydramine	50 mg IV or PO
	Observe for progression to severe reaction	
Treatment for a Severe Contrast Reaction	Stop contrast injection	
	Protect airway	Immediate intubation if stridor or angioedema with airway obstruction
	Epinephrine	0.01 mg/kg infusion IV or 0.3 mg IM; each repeated every 5–15 minutes with a maximum total of 1 mg
	Oxygen	6–10 L/min
	Normal saline	1 liter IV bolus

Note: IM, intramuscular; IV, intravenous; PO, oral.

Table 4.6 Prevention of contrast-induced acute kidney injury

Intervention	Dose	Mechanism	Proven efficacy?	Recommended?
0.9% saline	1 liter IV, 3 h prior to procedure; 100–150 mL/h postprocedure	Dilution/renal perfusion	Yes	Yes
Minimize contrast volume		Biplane, staged procedures	Yes	Yes
Use of low-osmolar or iso-osmolar contrast		Unclear	Yes	Yes
N-acetylcysteine	600 mg PO BID day prior and day of procedure	Antioxidant	No	Consider
Sodium bicarbonate	3 mL/h IV for 1 h prior and 1 mL/h IV for 6 h after procedure	Alkalinization	No	Consider
Fenoldopam, dopamine, theophylline		Increased renal artery perfusion	No	No
Statins		Modifying endothelial function	Controversial	Consider
Hemodialysis		Removal of contrast	No	No

Note: BID, twice daily; IV, intravenous; PO, oral.

tubular precipitation, thereby preventing obstruction of the tubule lumen. Another postulate is that normal saline delivered to the distal nephron decreases activation of the renin-angiotensin system, thereby allowing adequate renal blood flow to prevent tubular necrosis. In addition, there is evidence that hydration minimizes the reduction of nitric oxide in the renal circulation.[45]

The 2011 American College of Cardiology Foundation (ACCF)/American Heart Association (AHA)/Society for Cardiovascular Angiography and Interventions (SCAI) guidelines for PCI state that adequate preparatory hydration is a class I recommendation.[46] Furthermore, the ACCF/AHA–focused update of the guidelines for the management of patients with unstable angina/non-ST-segment elevation myocardial infarction (NSTEMI) has a class I recommendation for adequate preparatory hydration for patients undergoing cardiac catheterization.[47] Controversy remains as to the ideal regimen of hydration to best prevent CI-AKI. Early studies evaluated infusing 0.45% saline with mannitol, furosemide, and sodium bicarbonate to reduce the risk of CI-AKI.[45] Subsequently, Mueller et al. established that hydration with 0.9% saline reduced CI-AKI incidence by more than 50% compared with 0.45% saline (0.7% vs. 2%, respectively) in patients who received angioplasty.[48] Studies also established that IV saline was superior to oral hydration.[49]

The optimal dose of hydration is not determined, and regimens may need to be modified in patients with impaired LV function or evidence of preexisting volume overload. However, for those with normal LV function, it is generally recommended to administer at least 1 liter of isotonic saline IV at a rate of 100–150 mL/h beginning 3 hours before start of the procedure and continuing for 6–8 hours postprocedure.[11] One study suggested that overnight fluid infusion instead of a bolus trended toward a lower incidence of CI-AKI.[50]

Isotonic sodium bicarbonate has been proposed as an alternative form of hydration for the prevention of CI-AKI. The theory is that alkalinization may further protect from free radical–induced tubular injury or may decrease the viscosity of contrast agents passing through the vasa recta of the kidney. A reduction in CI-AKI (defined as a >25% increase in SCr) was found in a study of 119 patients randomized to isotonic sodium bicarbonate versus normal saline (1.7% vs. 13.6%, respectively).[51] Several subsequent trials demonstrated mixed results with sodium bicarbonate compared to saline hydration. The REMEDIAL trial of 326 patients with mild to moderate renal insufficiency (baseline SCr >2 mg/dL) showed a significant reduction in CI-AKI in those hydrated with isotonic sodium bicarbonate plus N-acetylcysteine (NAC) (1.9%), versus normal saline plus NAC (9.9%), or normal saline plus NAC and vitamin C (10.3%).[52] A subsequent trial of 356 high-risk patients, however, revealed no benefit of isotonic sodium bicarbonate compared with isotonic saline alone.[53] Two meta-analyses concluded that sodium bicarbonate probably does reduce the incidence of CI-AKI compared with saline alone, but the results may be exaggerated by publication bias.[54,55] Nevertheless, routine prophylactic use and superiority of sodium bicarbonate to normal saline for the prevention of CI-AKI remain unproven.

Type of contrast

Some LOCM have been shown to reduce the incidence of CI-AKI in patients with preexisting mild to moderate renal insufficiency when compared with HOCM.[2,3,5] A randomized trial of more than 1,100 patients referred for coronary angiography compared LOCM iohexol with the HOCM diatrizoate.[56] The incidence of acute nephrotoxicity (defined as a rise in SCr >0.5 mg/dL) was significantly lower with iohexol compared to diatrizoate (12.2% vs. 27%, respectively) in patients with baseline renal insufficiency.

The nonionic, IOCM iodixanol has been compared with various types of LOCM. Some randomized trials showed a reduced incidence of CI-AKI with iodixanol, while others did not.[7,9,57,58] A meta-analysis of 16 trials comparing iodixanol with LOCM concluded that iodixanol was less nephrotoxic, but many of the trials were not designed with CI-AKI as the primary endpoint, and thus the analysis may have suffered from ascertainment bias.[8] In addition, the difference was driven primarily by a large trial that compared iodixanol with the ionic LOCM ioxaglate, which may not be generalizable to nonionic LOCM contrast agents. A meta-analysis of 16 trials showed no difference in CI-AKI between iodixanol and various LOCM.[59] The most recent prospective randomized trial of patients at high risk for CI-AKI did not demonstrate superiority of CI-AKI prevention for iodixanol compared to LOCM.[10]

In the highest-risk patients, there is some experience with using gadolinium-containing contrast agents as a substitute for iodinated contrast.[60] Gadolinium has rarely been associated with nephrotoxicity, but it should be used with caution in patients with moderate to severe renal failure, given the increased risk of nephrogenic systemic fibrosis. Carbon dioxide angiography has also been used in the peripheral vasculature, but its use must be limited to below the diaphragm because of the potential risk of cerebral embolization, and digital subtraction radiography must be used.[61,62]

Volume of contrast

Volume of contrast administered is crucial to the development of CI-AKI, and minimization of contrast volume is of utmost importance in its prevention.[11] In order to decrease contrast volume used in patients at high risk of CI-AKI, it is recommended to use biplane or rotational coronary angiography, staged procedures if clinically feasible, and to not routinely perform left ventriculography.

Potential prophylactic therapy

Besides adequate hydration, contrast dose reduction, and staging of procedures, other therapies to prevent CI-AKI have been studied and are discussed below.

N-ACETYLCYSTEINE

Given the possibility of contrast-mediated oxidative kidney injury in CI-AKI, prophylactic use of the antioxidant NAC has been evaluated. An early, randomized trial showed a marked reduction in CI-AKI in 83 patients randomized to NAC 600 mg twice daily with saline hydration versus saline alone (2% vs. 21%, respectively).[63] Further studies suggest that 1200 mg twice daily may be superior to 600 mg twice daily, with a reported CI-AKI incidence of 8% versus 15%, respectively.[64] Trials have shown similar benefit with IV and oral NAC, but there is a risk of anaphylaxis with the IV form.[64,65]

However, since the promising original trials, several larger randomized prospective trials have shown no benefit for NAC compared with hydration alone.[15,66–68] Meta-analyses have demonstrated trends toward overall benefit, but the trials are heterogeneous, and the results are inconsistent.[45,69] Although generally well-tolerated, the 2011 ACCF/AHA/SCAI Guidelines for PCI considered use of NAC as a Class III recommendation, and it is therefore not recommended for routine use.[46]

STATINS

Statins have been evaluated for the prevention of CI-AKI by modifying endothelial function and inflammation. In a study of 410 patients with CKD when atorvastatin was given as pretreatment 24 hours prior to contrast exposure, there was a significant reduction in the rate of CI-AKI (4.5% vs. 17.8% of controls).[70] Similarly, in a retrospective analysis of 29,409 patients undergoing PCI, those on preprocedural statins had a lower incidence of CI-AKI (4.4% vs. 5.9%, $P < 0.001$) and a lower rate of requiring hemodialysis (0.32% vs. 0.49%, $P = 0.03$) than patients not on statin therapy.[71] Although further studies are needed, statins may favorably modify the risk of CI-AKI.

THEOPHYLLINE/AMINOPHYLLINE

Since adenosine is an intrarenal vasoconstrictor, adenosine antagonists are a plausible consideration for the reduction of CI-AKI. A meta-analysis published in 2004 demonstrated that theophylline or aminophylline given post-contrast administration protected against a decline in renal function.[72] However, this result has not been consistently demonstrated with these agents.[73] Thus, these medications cannot be recommended to provide protection from CI-AKI.

RENAL ARTERIOLAR VASODILATION

Fenoldopam is a selective dopamine A1 receptor agonist. Although it is an effective renal arterial vasodilator, systemic infusions of fenoldopam have failed to reduce CI-AKI compared with saline in two controlled studies.[74,75] Another renal arterial vasodilator, dopamine, has likewise been ineffective in reducing CI-AKI.[45] Overall, neither of these medications have adequate data to support their routine clinical use.

OTHER AGENTS

Furosemide and dual endothelin receptor antagonists are not beneficial, and in fact, can exacerbate CI-AKI. Similarly, vitamin C[52] and mannitol have no benefit in preventing CI-AKI.[45]

HEMODIALYSIS AND HEMOFILTRATION

Prophylactic hemodialysis does not diminish the incidence of CI-AKI in patients with preexisting renal insufficiency.[76] A meta-analysis of 412 patients from six studies with a baseline creatinine ranging from 2.5 to 4 mg/dL showed no benefit, with a suggestion of harm.[77]

Prophylactic continuous venovenous hemofiltration (CVVH) in moderate to severe renal insufficiency (mean SCr 3 mg/dL) resulted in a lower creatinine and lower mortality compared with standard of care, but the outcomes may have resulted from the fact that CVVH removes creatinine and was performed in the intensive care unit. The greater intensity of care CVVH patients received compared with the control patients may explain their improved survival.[78] A trial in patients with severe CKD (SCr = 4.9 mg/dL) referred for cardiac catheterization demonstrated a reduced incidence of long-term need for hemodialysis in those who received immediate hemodialysis compared to the control group (0% vs. 13%, respectively).[79] There may be a role for prophylactic hemodialysis in a subpopulation of patients who are at the highest risk of CI-AKI, but additional studies are warranted before routine use of this strategy can be recommended.

Hypersensitivity reaction prevention

As indicated earlier, the most significant risk factor for an allergic contrast reaction is a history of previous hypersensitivity. Premedication with a steroid and H1 blocker is crucial to minimize the risk of a repeat reaction. Additionally, the use of LOCM should be considered in high-risk patients.[40] Unless the procedure is urgent or emergent, premedication should be given 4–6 hours prior to contrast exposure. A validated protocol is 50mg prednisone by mouth at 13 hours, 7 hours, and 1 hour prior to the procedure.[44] In addition, 50mg diphenhydramine (IV or oral) should be given 1 hour prior to the procedure. Alternatively, 32 mg methylprednisolone can be administered orally 12 hours and 2 hours prior to exposure along with 50mg diphenhydramine (IV or oral) 1 hour prior to exposure (Table 4.5).

In an emergency procedure, a rapid premedication protocol may include 200 mg hydrocortisone IV or 40 mg methylprednisolone IV, and then every 4 hours until the procedure is complete, plus 50mg diphenhydramine IV 1 hour prior to contrast agent injection.

Less desirable, but used for patients with methylprednisolone, aspirin, or NSAID allergies, is 7.5 mg dexamethasone IV or 6 mg betamethasone IV every 4 hours until the study is performed. Diphenhydramine 50 mg IV is also given 1 hour prior to contrast agent injection.[35]

Use of LOCM reduces the chance of recurrent hypersensitivity reaction compared with HOCM. Use of the IOCM iodixanol may reduce this risk even further. The incidence of a repeat allergic contrast reaction using iodixanol was 0.7%, compared with 2% when using the ionic, LOCM ioxaglate.[4]

Gadolinium is even less likely to cause a repeat contrast reaction, with the incidence ranging from 1/100,000 to 1/500,000 cases, and essentially confined to rare case reports.[80] In addition, carbon dioxide angiography can be used for peripheral interventions below the diaphragm if digital subtraction radiography is available.

No routine empiric medications are recommended for prevention of first-time hypersensitivity reactions. However, in atopic individuals (e.g., asthma), one should consider using LOCM.

CONCLUSIONS

Iodinated contrast agents allow detailed visualization of the cardiac anatomy. Multiple formulations have been introduced in an attempt to minimize adverse effects. In general, LOCM and IOCM are similarly effective in minimizing adverse effects and are associated with less cardiac and renal toxicity than the HOCM. CKD is the primary risk factor for CI-AKI. Other risk factors include diabetes, advanced age, contrast dose, hypotension, multiple recent exposures to contrast, and anemia. Adequate hydration is mandatory to lessen the risk of CI-AKI. Many evidence-based methods have been developed to prevent anaphylactoid contrast reactions and CI-AKI. These strategies should be routinely utilized in patients predetermined to be at a higher risk for these complications.

REFERENCES

1. Zukerman LS, et al. Effect of calcium-binding additives on ventricular fibrillation and repolarization changes during coronary angiography. *J Am Coll of Cardiol* 1987;10(6):1249–1253.
2. Tepel M, et al. Contrast-induced nephropathy: A clinical and evidence-based approach. *Circulation* 2006;113(14):1799–1806.
3. Davidson CJ, et al. Randomized trial of contrast media utilization in high-risk PTCA: The COURT trial. *Circulation* 2000;101(18):2172–2177.
4. Davidson CJ, et al. Thrombotic and cardiovascular complications related to nonionic contrast media during cardiac catheterization: Analysis of 8,517 patients. *Am J Cardiol* 1990;65(22):1481–1484.
5. Barrett BJ, Carlisle EJ. Metaanalysis of the relative nephrotoxicity of high- and low-osmolality iodinated contrast media. *Radiology* 1993;188(1):171–178.
6. Sutton AG, et al. A randomized prospective trial of ioxaglate 320 (hexabrix) vs. iodixanol 320 (visipaque) in patients undergoing percutaneous coronary intervention. *Catheter Cardiovasc Interv* 2002;57(3):346–352.
7. Jo SH, et al. Renal toxicity evaluation and comparison between visipaque (iodixanol) and hexabrix (ioxaglate) in patients with renal insufficiency undergoing coronary angiography: The RECOVER study: A randomized controlled trial. *J Am Coll Cardiol* 2006;48(5):924–930.
8. McCullough PA, et al. A meta-analysis of the renal safety of isosmolar iodixanol compared with low-osmolar contrast media. *J Am Coll Cardiol* 2006;48(4):692–699.
9. Rudnick MR, et al. Nephrotoxicity of iodixanol versus ioversol in patients with chronic kidney disease: The Visipaque Angiography/Interventions with Laboratory Outcomes in Renal Insufficiency (VALOR) trial. *Am Heart J* 2008;156(4):776–782.

10. Laskey W, et al. Nephrotoxicity of iodixanol versus iopamidol in patients with chronic kidney disease and diabetes mellitus undergoing coronary angiographic procedures. *Am Heart J* 2009;158(5):822–828.e3.

11. Schweiger MJ, et al. Prevention of contrast induced nephropathy: Recommendations for the high risk patient undergoing cardiovascular procedures. *Catheter Cardiovasc Interv* 2007;69(1):135–140.

12. Kappetein AP, et al. Updated standardized endpoint definitions for transcatheter aortic valve implantation: The Valve Academic Research Consortium-2 consensus document. *EuroIntervention* 2012;8(7):782–795.

13. Ad-hoc working group of ERBP, et al. A European Renal Best Practice (ERBP) position statement on the Kidney Disease Improving Global Outcomes (KDIGO) clinical practice guidelines on acute kidney injury: Part 1: Definitions, conservative management and contrast-induced nephropathy. *Nephrol Dial Transplant* 2012;27(12):4263–4272.

14. Kidney Disease: Improving Global Outcomes (KDIGO) Acute Kidney Injury Work Group. KDIGO Clinical Practice Guideline for Acute Kidney Injury. *Kidney Int* Suppl 2012;2:1–138.

15. Pannu N, et al. Prophylaxis strategies for contrast-induced nephropathy. *JAMA* 2006;295(23):2765–2779.

16. Rihal CS, et al. Incidence and prognostic importance of acute renal failure after percutaneous coronary intervention. *Circulation* 2002;105(19):2259–2264.

17. Davidson CJ, et al. Cardiovascular and renal toxicity of a nonionic radiographic contrast agent after cardiac catheterization. A prospective trial. *An Intern Med* 1989;110(2):119–124.

18. Heyman SN, et al. Pathophysiology of radiocontrast nephropathy: A role for medullary hypoxia. *Invest Radiol* 1999;34(11):685–691.

19. Persson PB, et al. Pathophysiology of contrast medium-induced nephropathy. *Kidney Int* 2005;68(1):14–22.

20. Quintavalle C, et al. In vivo and in vitro assessment of pathways involved in contrast media-induced renal cells apoptosis. *Cell Death Dis* 2011;2:e155.

21. Liss P, et al. Renal failure in 57,925 patients undergoing coronary procedures using iso-osmolar or low-osmolar contrast media. *Kidney Int* 2006;70(10):1811–1817.

22. McCullough PA, et al. Acute renal failure after coronary intervention: Incidence, risk factors, and relationship to mortality. *Am J Med* 1997;103(5):368–375.

23. Modi KS, Rao VK. Atheroembolic renal disease. *J Am Soc of Nephrol* 2001;12(8):1781–1787.

24. Mehran R, et al. A simple risk score for prediction of contrast-induced nephropathy after percutaneous coronary intervention: Development and initial validation. *J Am Coll Cardiol* 2004;44(7):1393–1399.

25. Nikolsky E, et al. Low hematocrit predicts contrast-induced nephropathy after percutaneous coronary interventions. *Kidney Int* 2005;67(2):706–713.

26. Toprak O, et al. Impact of diabetic and pre-diabetic state on development of contrast-induced nephropathy in patients with chronic kidney disease. *Nephrol Dial Transplant* 2007;22(3):819–826.

27. Toprak O, Cirit M. Risk factors for contrast-induced nephropathy. *Kidney Blood Press Res* 2006;29(2):84–93.

28. McCullough PA. Contrast-induced acute kidney injury. *J Am Coll Cardiol* 2008;51(22):1419–1428.

29. Cirit M, et al. Angiotensin-converting enzyme inhibitors as a risk factor for contrast-induced nephropathy. *Nephron Clin Pract* 2006;104(1):c20–27.

30. Gupta RK, et al. Captopril for prevention of contrast-induced nephropathy in diabetic patients: A randomised study. *Indian Heart J* 1999;51(5):521–526.

31. Sutton AG, et al. Early and late reactions after the use of iopamidol 340, ioxaglate 320, and iodixanol 320 in cardiac catheterization. *Am Heart J* 2001;141(4):677–683.

32. Sutton AG, et al. Early and late reactions following the use of iopamidol 340, iomeprol 350 and iodixanol 320 in cardiac catheterization. *J Invasive Cardiol* 2003;15(3):133–138.

33. Thomsen HS, et al. Management of acute adverse reactions to contrast media. *Eur Radiol* 2004;14(3):476–481.

34. Tramer MR, et al. Pharmacological prevention of serious anaphylactic reactions due to iodinated contrast media: Systematic review. *BMJ* 2006;333(7570):675.

35. Brockow K, et al. Management of hypersensitivity reactions to iodinated contrast media. *Allergy* 2005;60(2):150–158.

36. Laroche D, et al. Mechanisms of severe, immediate reactions to iodinated contrast material. *Radiology* 1998;209(1):183–190.

37. Trcka J, et al. Anaphylaxis to iodinated contrast material: Nonallergic hypersensitivity or IgE-mediated allergy? *AJR Am J Roentgenol* 2008;190(3):666–670.

38. Kim MH, et al. Anaphylaxis to iodinated contrast media: Clinical characteristics related with development of anaphylactic shock. *PloS One* 2014;9(6):e100154.

39. Pasternak JJ, Williamson EE. Clinical pharmacology, uses, and adverse reactions of iodinated contrast agents: A primer for the non-radiologist. *Mayo Clin Proc* 2012;87(4):390–402.

40. Nayak KR, et al. Anaphylactoid reactions to radiocontrast agents: Prevention and treatment in the cardiac catheterization laboratory. *J Invasive Cardiol* 2009;21(10):548–551.

41. Huang SW. Seafood and iodine: An analysis of a medical myth. *Allergy Asthma Proc* 2005;26(6):468–469.

42. Beaty AD, et al. Seafood allergy and radiocontrast media: Are physicians propagating a myth? *Am J Med* 2008;121(2):158.e1–e4.

43. Rose TA Jr., Choi JW. Intravenous imaging contrast media complications: The basics that every clinician needs to know. *Am J Med* 2015;128(9):943–949.

44. ACR manual on contrast media, version 10.1. 2015. (Accessed March 15, 2016 at http://www.acr.org/Quality-Safety/Resources/Contrast-Manual.)

45. Stacul F, et al. Strategies to reduce the risk of contrast-induced nephropathy. *Am J Cardiol* 2006;98(6A):59K–77K.

46. Levine GN, et al. 2011 ACCF/AHA/SCAI Guideline for Percutaneous Coronary Intervention: Executive summary: A report of the American College of Cardiology Foundation/American Heart Association Task Force on Practice Guidelines and the Society for Cardiovascular Angiography and Interventions. *Circulation* 2011;124(23):2574–2609.

47. Wright RS, et al. 2011 ACCF/AHA Focused Update of the Guidelines for the Management of Patients With Unstable Angina/ Non-ST-Elevation Myocardial Infarction (updating the 2007 guideline): A report of the American College of Cardiology Foundation/American Heart Association Task Force on Practice Guidelines. *Circulation* 2011;123(18):2022–2060.

48. Mueller C, et al. Prevention of contrast media-associated nephropathy: Randomized comparison of 2 hydration regimens in 1620 patients undergoing coronary angioplasty. *Arch Intern Med* 2002;162(3):329–336.

49. Trivedi HS, et al. A randomized prospective trial to assess the role of saline hydration on the development of contrast nephrotoxicity. *Nephron Clin Pract* 2003;93(1):C29–C34.

50. Krasuski RA, et al. Optimal timing of hydration to erase contrast-associated nephropathy: The OTHER CAN study. *J Invasive Cardiol* 2003;15(12):699–702.

51. Merten GJ, et al. Prevention of contrast-induced nephropathy with sodium bicarbonate: A randomized controlled trial. *JAMA* 2004;291(19):2328–2334.

52. Briguori C, et al. Renal Insufficiency Following Contrast Media Administration Trial (REMEDIAL): A randomized comparison of 3 preventive strategies. *Circulation* 2007;115(10):1211–1217.

53. Brar SS, et al. Sodium bicarbonate vs sodium chloride for the prevention of contrast medium-induced nephropathy in patients undergoing coronary angiography: A randomized trial. *JAMA* 2008;300(9):1038–1046.

54. Hogan SE, et al. Current role of sodium bicarbonate-based preprocedural hydration for the prevention of contrast-induced acute kidney injury: A meta-analysis. *Am Heart J* 2008;156(3):414–421.

55. Meier P, et al. Sodium bicarbonate-based hydration prevents contrast-induced nephropathy: A meta-analysis. *BMC Med* 2009;7:23.

56. Rudnick MR, et al. Nephrotoxicity of ionic and nonionic contrast media in 1196 patients: A randomized trial. The Iohexol Cooperative Study. *Kidney Int* 1995;47(1):254–261.

57. Solomon RJ, et al. Cardiac Angiography in Renally Impaired Patients (CARE) study: A randomized double-blind trial of contrast-induced nephropathy in patients with chronic kidney disease. *Circulation* 2007;115(25):3189–3196.

58. Aspelin P, et al. Nephrotoxic effects in high-risk patients undergoing angiography. *N Engl J Med* 2003;348(6):491–499.

59. Reed M, et al. The relative renal safety of iodixanol compared with low-osmolar contrast media: A meta-analysis of randomized controlled trials. *JACC Cardiovasc Interv* 2009;2(7):645–654.

60. Boyden TF, Gurm HS. Does gadolinium-based angiography protect against contrast-induced nephropathy?: A systematic review of the literature. *Catheter Cardiovasc Interv* 2008;71(5):687–693.

61. Cho KJ. Carbon dioxide angiography: Scientific principles and practice. *Vasc Specialist Int* 2015;31(3):67–80.

62. Fujihara M, et al. Endovascular therapy by CO2 angiography to prevent contrast-induced nephropathy in patients with chronic kidney disease: A prospective multicenter trial of CO2 angiography registry. *Catheter Cardiovasc Interv* 2015;85(5):870–877.

63. Tepel M, et al. Prevention of radiographic-contrast-agent-induced reductions in renal function by acetylcysteine. *N Engl J Med* 2000;343(3):180–184.

64. Marenzi G, et al. N-acetylcysteine and contrast-induced nephropathy in primary angioplasty. *N Engl J Med* 2006;354(26):2773–2782.

65. Baker CS, et al. A rapid protocol for the prevention of contrast-induced renal dysfunction: The RAPPID study. *J Am Coll Cardiol* 2003;41(12):2114–2118.

66. Kay J, et al. Acetylcysteine for prevention of acute deterioration of renal function following elective coronary angiography and intervention: A randomized controlled trial. *JAMA* 2003;289(5):553–558.

67. Webb JG, et al. A randomized controlled trial of intravenous N-acetylcysteine for the prevention of contrast-induced nephropathy after cardiac catheterization: Lack of effect. *Am Heart J* 2004;148(3):422–429.

68. Azmus AD, et al. Effectiveness of acetylcysteine in prevention of contrast nephropathy. *J Invasive Cardiol* 2005;17(2):80–84.

69. Nallamothu BK, et al. Is acetylcysteine effective in preventing contrast-related nephropathy? A meta-analysis. *Am J Med* 2004;117(12):938–947.

70. Quintavalle C, et al. Impact of a high loading dose of atorvastatin on contrast-induced acute kidney injury. *Circulation* 2012;126(25):3008–3016.

71. Khanal S, et al. Statin therapy reduces contrast-induced nephropathy: An analysis of contemporary percutaneous interventions. *Am J Med* 2005;118(8):843–849.

72. Ix JH, et al. Theophylline for the prevention of radiocontrast nephropathy: A meta-analysis. *Nephrol Dial Transplant* 2004;19(11):2747–2753.

73. Shammas NW, et al. Aminophylline does not protect against radiocontrast nephropathy in patients undergoing percutaneous angiographic procedures. *J Invasive Cardiol* 2001;13(11):738–740.

74. Allaqaband S, et al. Prospective randomized study of N-acetylcysteine, fenoldopam, and saline for prevention of radiocontrast-induced nephropathy. *Catheter Cardiovasc Interv* 2002;57(3):279–283.

75. Stone GW, et al. Fenoldopam mesylate for the prevention of contrast-induced nephropathy: A randomized controlled trial. *JAMA* 2003;290(17):2284–2291.

76. Vogt B, et al. Prophylactic hemodialysis after radiocontrast media in patients with renal insufficiency is potentially harmful. *Am J Med* 2001;111(9):692–698.

77. Cruz DN, et al. Extracorporeal blood purification therapies for prevention of radiocontrast-induced nephropathy: A systematic review. *Am J Kidney Dis* 2006;48(3):361–371.

78. Marenzi G, et al. The prevention of radiocontrast-agent-induced nephropathy by hemofiltration. *N Engl J Med* 2003;349(14):1333–1340.

79. Lee PT, et al. Renal protection for coronary angiography in advanced renal failure patients by prophylactic hemodialysis. A randomized controlled trial. *J Am Coll Cardiol* 2007;50(11):1015–1020.

80. Dillman JR, et al. Allergic-like breakthrough reactions to gadolinium contrast agents after corticosteroid and antihistamine premedication. *AJR Am J Roentgenol* 2008;190(1):187–190.

5

Patient selection, preparation, risks, and informed consent

J. DAWN ABBOTT AND DAVID O. WILLIAMS

INTRODUCTION

Cardiac catheterization is one of the most common in-hospital procedures performed in the United States with an annual volume of over 1 million cases. The majority of procedures are performed for the evaluation and management of coronary artery disease (CAD). Trends in diagnostic catheterization and percutaneous coronary intervention (PCI) over the past decade show a decline in procedures from 2004 to 2008 with stabilization in 2009. During this time, there was a rapid uptake of drug-eluting stents (DES), an increase in the use of intravascular ultrasound (IVUS) and fractional flow reserve (FFR), and a steady reduction in coronary bypass surgery.[1] These trends support improved medical treatment and prevention of coronary disease and the effectiveness of DES. In the modern era, procedural capabilities have expanded to include the diagnosis and treatment of a wide range of structural and peripheral vascular diseases and more complex coronary interventions.

Independent of the type or complexity of the procedure, all share the common technique of insertion of catheters into the circulatory system guided by a combination of fluoroscopy, hemodynamic monitoring, and radiographic contrast. Paramount to patient safety is an experienced and competent catheterization lab team. The physician performing the procedure in each case is responsible for evaluating the potential risks and benefits of a given procedure based on both patient and technical factors. Proper patient selection and preparation can minimize the occurrence and severity of complications. The risks of angiography should be understood by all members of the catheterization lab team so that complications can be anticipated and responded to in a rapid, coordinated, and effective manner. Staff should receive continuing education on new devices or procedures introduced to the lab. An in-depth knowledge of the risks of each procedure is also required in order to obtain appropriate informed consent from the patient. The preprocedural aspects of cardiac catheterization deserve special review and are the basis for this chapter.

PATIENT SELECTION

Procedural indications

Before a decision to recommend cardiac catheterization is made, the indication for and alternatives to the procedure should be clear. Foremost, what clinical information is desired and how will the findings be used? An invasive study should only be performed when the value to the patient is incremental to a noninvasive approach. A thorough review of the patient's medical history, physical exam, electrocardiogram (ECG), and laboratory and cardiac testing results is required in order to determine the appropriateness of and type of procedure planned. Left heart catheterization is commonly performed for CAD and includes aortic and left ventricular pressures, coronary angiography, and, at times, left ventriculography and aortography. The practice guidelines for coronary angiography are detailed in a report from the American College of Cardiology (ACC) and American Heart Association (AHA) and are summarized in Table 5.1.[2]

In many clinical scenarios, such as valvular, myocardial, and congenital heart disease, one or more additional procedures, such as a right heart catheterization, exercise, or oximetry are required for a complete diagnostic study. The operator must, therefore, have the expertise to determine and perform the necessary procedural components. For patients who go on to require interventional procedures, including those detailed in the subsequent chapters of this book, clinical guidelines from the ACC/AHA exist for many diseases and procedures and can serve as a basis for clinical decisions.

Cardiac catheterization may be performed as part of a diagnostic or therapeutic research study, or solely for research purposes. In these circumstances, the protocol must be approved by the local institutional review board and the patient informed of the investigative nature of the study and consent obtained.

Procedural contraindications

As the field of interventional cardiology has evolved to routinely care for critically ill patients, such as those with myocardial infarction (MI) and cardiogenic shock, the number of absolute contraindications to cardiac catheterization has decreased. The majority of procedures are still done on an elective or urgent, nonemergent basis, and a number of relative contraindications to the procedure have been reported that can often be addressed beforehand to improve safety (Table 5.2). When possible, procedures should be delayed until all relative contraindications are evaluated and addressed.

The list of relative contraindications includes severe contrast allergy, which is uncommon but potentially life-threatening. Proper pretreatment, discussed below, can reduce the incidence and severity of recurrent reactions. Acute or chronic kidney disease (CKD) may alter the

Table 5.1 Indications for coronary angiography in patients with known or suspected coronary artery disease

Asymptomatic or stable angina	Unstable coronary syndromes
• High-risk criteria on noninvasive testing • Sudden cardiac death survivors • Sustained monomorphic or polymorphic ventricular tachycardia • Angina on medical treatment • Worsening abnormalities on serial noninvasive testing • Patients that cannot be adequately risk stratified by other means • Individuals whose occupation involves the safety of others and who have an abnormal stress test or high-risk clinical features • Abnormal but not high-risk stress test in a patient with high likelihood of disease • Ischemia demonstrated by noninvasive testing in a patient with a prior myocardial infarction • Postcardiac transplant evaluation • Preoperative organ transplant in individuals ≥40 years old • Patients with equivocal or abnormal non high-risk findings on noninvasive testing with recurrent hospitalizations for chest pain • Suspected in-stent restenosis or early bypass graft failure based on symptoms or noninvasive testing • Planned noncoronary cardiac surgery (valve surgery, hypertrophic cardiomyopathy, congenital heart disease) • Before surgery for aortic aneurysm or dissection • Unexplained systolic dysfunction • Suspicion for ischemia-mediated diastolic dysfunction • Prospective immediate cardiac transplant donor at risk for coronary disease • Kawasaki disease with coronary artery aneurysms detected noninvasively	• Unstable angina refractory to medical therapy • Unstable angina with intermediate-to-high short-term risk • Unstable angina with subsequent abnormal noninvasive testing • Suspected Prinzmetal variant angina • Suspected stent thrombosis • Patients with STEMI with the intent to perform primary or rescue percutaneous coronary intervention • Evaluation of non-STEMI • Cardiogenic shock • Postmyocardial infarction with angina, congestive heart failure, left ventricular ejection fraction <40%, or ventricular arrhythmia • Suspected or known mechanical complication post myocardial infarction • Myocardial infarction suspected to be from nonatherothrombotic cause (i.e., spontaneous dissection, arteritis) • Cardiac trauma

Note: STEMI, ST-segment elevation myocardial infarction.

Table 5.2 Relative contraindications to cardiac catheterization

Severe contrast allergy
Acute renal failure or advanced chronic kidney disease without the ability to perform hemodialysis
Uncontrolled ventricular arrhythmia
Metabolic derangements (electrolytes, acid–base abnormalities)
Drug toxicity (digoxin)
Malignant hypertension
Active noncardiac problems (bacteremia, bleeding, stroke)
Acute decompensated heart failure in the absence of ischemia
Coagulopathy or bleeding diathesis
Patient unable to cooperate with instructions

risk-benefit ratio of cardiac catheterization or may result in the requirement of hemodialysis. Measures such as ensuring adequate volume status, minimizing contrast volume administered, and consultation with a nephrologist may be required in such cases. Uncontrolled ventricular irritability may increase the incidence of ventricular tachycardia or fibrillation. Correction of electrolyte imbalances and diagnosis and treatment of potential drug toxicity should be sought, and medical therapy for ischemia should be optimized. Attention to control of hypertension can reduce the potential for ischemia, congestive heart failure, and bleeding related to angiography. Patients with decompensated congestive heart failure in the absence of acute myocardial ischemia or the need for hemodynamic support should be stabilized prior to catheterization when possible. Abnormal coagulation or blood counts should be corrected when feasible to reduce bleeding risk and ischemic complications. The presence of a febrile illness or bacteremia is an additional relative contraindication. Several of the relative contraindications will be determined and treatment optimized during patient preparation for cardiac catheterization.

Appropriateness criteria

Marked variability in the use of coronary angiography and revascularization in and outside the United States has led to concerns about the appropriate use of cardiovascular procedures.[3–5] In addition to regional variation in cost, both under and overuse of invasive procedures have the potential to adversely impact patient outcomes. Appropriateness criteria for diagnostic catheterization and coronary revascularization were therefore developed in an effort to optimize the quality of cardiovascular care and develop a tool that can be used to measure variability and utilization patterns. In determining whether diagnostic catheterization was appropriate, inappropriate, or uncertain, the following definition was used:

An appropriate diagnostic cardiac catheterization (left heart, right heart, ventriculography, and/or coronary angiography) is one in which the expected incremental information combined with clinical judgment exceeds the negative consequences by a sufficiently wide margin for a specific indication that the procedure is generally considered acceptable care and a reasonable approach for the indication.[6]

Indications for diagnostic catheterization were developed under the following assumptions: indications were evaluated on the basis of medical literature, recognition that published studies provide minimal information about the role of testing in clinical decision-making, determination of the risk-benefit tradeoff for the individual patient and indication, and that no circumstances preclude the performance of cardiac catheterization. The technical panel scored each indication on a scale from 1 to 9. Indications that were scored 7 to 9 by the panel were termed *appropriate*, meaning the test is generally acceptable. Indications with a score of 4 to 6 were termed *uncertain*, meaning the test may be acceptable and a reasonable approach but with uncertainty, signifying that more research and/or patient information was needed to further classify the indication. *Inappropriate* indications, scores of 1 to 3, were generally not acceptable.

Operators performing cardiac catheterization must be familiar with the appropriateness criteria. While the criteria are not meant to replace clinical judgment, they do provide guidance for decision-making and supplement practice guidelines developed by the ACC/AHA. Importantly, the criteria will certainly be used by health care facilities, third-party payers, and ultimately, patients.

PREPARATION

Patient preparation is one of the most important aspects of cardiac catheterization. Each patient has unique issues that must be addressed, for example, a history of contrast reaction, coumadin therapy, or diabetes mellitus. In addition to clinical factors, the physician must ensure that the patient is mentally prepared, understands instructions, and knows what to expect before, during, and after the procedure. A well-informed patient will be less anxious and more cooperative. The circumstances of the procedure will dictate the pace of preparation, but even in emergent situations, such as ST-elevation myocardial infarction (STEMI), patient safety cannot be compromised by inadequate preprocedural assessment. Patient preparation should follow an organized check-list of items to review prior to the official "time out" signifying that it is safe to proceed. At a minimum, the patient's name, intended procedure, confirmation of signed consent, review of allergies and lab values, and intended access site with marking if appropriate should be verbally reviewed in the presence of the entire team (American College of Cardiology Foundation [ACCF] and Society for Cardiovascular Angiography and Interventions [SCAI] catheterization lab standards update 2012).[7]

Preprocedural assessment

A detailed medical history, pertinent physical examination, and review of allergies and ancillary studies should be performed within 30 days and updated the day of the procedure. In patients with known or suspected CAD, assessment of compliance and ability to take dual antiplatelet therapy (DAPT) should be made. Any upcoming noncardiac procedures or surgeries should also be discussed with the patients. The ECG should be reviewed and available at the time of the procedure for comparison. In some individuals a chest X-ray may be warranted. Basic laboratories, including a complete blood count, glucose, electrolytes, blood urea nitrogen, and creatinine should be obtained in all patients to assess the status of chronic diseases or to identify clinically silent comorbidities such as kidney disease or anemia. Patients receiving anticoagulation or with a personal or family history of a bleeding diathesis should have coagulation studies. Abnormalities should be recorded and addressed if possible, such as correction of electrolytes. The procedure, if elective, should be delayed when problems are identified that could influence treatment strategies or complications, such as unexplained anemia. Abnormalities such as an elevated creatinine or thrombocytopenia may not alter plans for diagnostic cardiac catheterization but may require additional measures to reduce the risk of contrast nephropathy or bleeding, respectively.

For patients with prior cardiac catheterization, the approach, equipment, and findings, including a review of the images, should be reviewed whenever feasible. There is no use trying to engage the left coronary artery with a Judkins left 4 catheter when the previous operator was successful with a Judkins left 6, or to rediscover an anomalous coronary artery. For patients with prior coronary bypass surgery, the preoperative native coronary anatomy, operative report, and postoperative angiograms, if performed, should be reviewed. Every effort should be made to review the original operative report rather than rely on a summary of the graft anatomy, which may be misleading. Attention should be paid to the number and types of conduits and any special circumstances, such as use of a free versus *in situ* left internal mammary graft, use of uncommon conduits such as a gastroepiploic graft, or placement of a saphenous vein graft (SVG) off the descending aorta. When the operative report is unavailable and the procedure cannot be delayed, aortography and bilateral mammary injections should be considered to assist in locating grafts.

Access considerations

The femoral artery remains the most common site for arterial access in the United States. Radial artery access, however, is gaining momentum because of the lower risk of bleeding, vascular complications, and patient preference. In addition, transradial access may reduce mortality.[8] Importantly, there is a learning curve for transradial procedures that requires operators to obtain sufficient experience, generally 100 transradial PCIs, prior to performing transradial primary PCI for STEMI or high-risk anatomic subsets such as left main stenosis or chronic total occlusion (CTO).[9] With experience, access site crossover is uncommon, and radiation exposure is similar to the femoral approach. Radial artery occlusion is minimized with adequate procedural anticoagulation and patent hemostasis techniques. Access site options should be reviewed prior to catheterization to consider the risks and benefits of a femoral versus radial approach in an individual patient. Factors that may influence access site decisions are presented in Table 5.3. The brachial approach has the highest risk of complications and is rarely indicated.

While many operators and catheterization labs have a default strategy of using either the right radial or femoral artery, patient- and lesion-specific factors may obligate an alternative approach. A review of the patients' comorbidities, need for left versus right and left heart catheterization, and anticipated maximum sheath size can decrease the need for more than one access site. The femoral approach is often considered for procedures requiring a large sheath size, technical complexity, or simultaneous arterial and venous access.

Table 5.3 Arterial access considerations

Femoral approach	Radial approach
1. Operator inexperience with radial technique	1. Default strategy for proficient operators
2. Requirement of a large sheath size (≥8 Fr)	2. Aortic pathology (dissection, aneurysms, large atheroma)
3. Abnormal Allen test or Type D Barbeau	3. Peripheral arterial disease (aortic or iliac occlusions, iliac tortuosity)
4. Severe subclavian/innominate tortuosity or occlusive disease	4. Morbid obesity
5. CABG with bilateral internal mammary artery grafts	5. Difficulty with patient maintaining a supine position (back pain, lung disease)
6. ESRD with AV fistula	6. Anticoagulant use
	7. Coagulopathy

Note: AV, arteriovenous; CABG, coronary artery bypass grafting; ESRD, end-stage renal disease.

Vascular closure devices (VCDs) are commonly used with the femoral approach, but it should be acknowledged that transradial access is superior to transfemoral access combined with VCD with respect to bleeding and access site complications.[10] In addition, skilled radial operators can use sheathless radial guides with a 7.5-Fr internal diameter and brachial vein access for right heart catheterization or pacemaker access.[11]

Although there are no data on the predictive value of testing for dual radial artery circulation, most operators perform an assessment of the palmar arch prior to transradial catheterization.[9] In patients with an intact arch, extensive collaterals between the radial and ulnar arteries make radial artery occlusion, which occurs in approximately 5% of cases, clinically less relevant. Hand ischemia can occur with radial artery occlusion in patients who have incomplete palmar arches. The modified Allen test assesses the palmar arch and is one of the methods that can be used to assess hand circulation. The test is performed by compressing both the radial and ulnar arteries while the patient's hand is held high with the fist clenched. The hand is then lowered and opened and pressure over the ulnar artery released. If the superficial palmar arch is intact, color should return to the hand within 6 seconds, and ≥10 seconds is considered abnormal. Since the Allen test is subject to inaccuracy, many centers use pulse oximetry and plethysmography as a more direct assessment of blood flow, termed the Barbeau test.[12,13] Plethysmography is considered abnormal if during radial artery compression there is a loss of pulse tracing with no recovery during 2 minutes of observation. In 1,010 consecutive patients referred for cardiac catheterization, the modified Allen test was abnormal in 6.3% and plethysmography in 1.5%, but the clinical implications of using a particular method are not clear.[12]

An abnormal Allen test is observed in 6% to 27% of patients undergoing cardiac catheterization.[12,14] One small study of patients undergoing coronary angiography showed that patients with an abnormal Allen test had decreased thumb blood flow and increased capillary lactate after 30 minutes of radial artery occlusion compared to patients with a normal Allen test.[15] Given the potential risk of hand ischemia, the radial artery approach should not be used in patients with an abnormal Allen test unless the risks of alternative approaches are prohibitory.

Conditions requiring special preparations

ALLERGIES

A list of allergies should be recorded and patients should be specifically questioned regarding allergies to lidocaine, premedication (i.e., diazepam), and iodinated contrast. An alternative local anesthetic, bupivacaine (1mg/mL), can be used in patients with an allergy to lidocaine. Sedatives can be withheld or alternatives substituted for patients with prior reactions to benzodiazepines or narcotics.

The overall incidence of adverse reactions to intravascular contrast media is about 5%, but rates are higher in patients with a history of allergy, asthma, or prior contrast media reaction.[16,17] Reactions can be acute, which are non-IgE-mediated anaphylactoid reactions, or delayed. The latter can occur up to 48 hours postexposure, are IgE-mediated, and can be confused with drug reactions due to the presence of fever or rash.[18] Patients reporting contrast media reactions or a history of other life-threatening allergic reactions require premedication prior to cardiac catheterization. Premedication should also be considered in patients with severe asthma or prior anaphylaxis. An isolated history of shellfish allergy does not require premedication. Pretreatment with corticosteroids, when given at least 12 hours before the procedure, significantly decrease contrast reactions with the exception of hives, which have only a trend toward reduction. A single-dose regimen administered 2 hours prior to contrast exposure, however, does not reduce the incidence of reactions.[19] Based on the limited data available, nonemergent procedures should be delayed until adequate premedication can be administered to patients at risk of an allergic reaction. An acceptable regimen is oral prednisone 50 mg every 6 hours starting 13 hours preprocedure with the last dose 1 hour prior.[18] For emergent circumstances, 200 mg of intravenous (IV) hydrocortisone can be given despite the lack of known efficacy. In addition to steroids, 50 mg of oral or IV diphenhydramine and histamine-2 blockers can be given before the procedure. Compared to high-osmolar ionic contrast, there is a lower incidence of adverse reactions to the low-osmolar nonionic contrast agents primarily used today.[20]

ANTIPLATELETS AND ANTICOAGULANTS

Coronary angiography can generally be performed on patients receiving antiplatelet therapy. Patients should be instructed not to stop aspirin or to start it at least 24 hours prior to the procedure if not currently prescribed. If patients are on DAPT they can continue it. For patients undergoing elective PCI for stable CAD, pretreatment with clopidogrel is reasonable. Patients can be started on clopidogrel 75 mg daily for at least 5 days or receive a loading dose of 600 mg within 24 hours of PCI.

Patients on oral anticoagulant therapy should be assessed for the risk of bleeding associated with cardiac catheterization versus thrombotic or embolic events. When the risk of a subtherapeutic international normalized ratio (INR) is acceptable, coumadin can be held for several days in order to allow the INR optimally to drift down to less than 1.8 for femoral access. A higher INR, up to 2.1, is generally acceptable for radial access.[7] There are no studies to support a specific INR cut-off, and one small study suggested that catheterization can be performed safely without interruption of anticoagulation.[21] For high-risk clinical situations, such as recent pulmonary embolism, atrial fibrillation with prior embolic events, or mechanical mitral valve prosthesis, patients require periprocedural heparin to bridge the discontinuation of coumadin. Low molecular weight heparin can be administered on an outpatient basis or the patient can be admitted for IV unfractionated heparin (UFH).

In general, UFH is started 48 hours after discontinuation of coumadin or when the INR is less than 2. For pregnant patients, there is an increased risk of thrombosis due to the hypercoagulable state and a continuous infusion of dose-adjusted UFH is the preferred anticoagulant for bridging. In some circumstances catheterization must be performed while a patient is fully anticoagulated. For these cases, a radial approach may be preferable and vitamin K and fresh frozen plasma can be infused if bleeding complications occur.

Patients are increasingly being treated with novel oral anticoagulants (NOACs). A comprehensive guide to the use of these drugs in patients with nonvalvular atrial fibrillation was published by the European Heart Rhythm Association in 2013.[22] Temporary discontinuation of NOACs is indicated for patients undergoing cardiac catheterization. For patients with normal renal function, the NOAC should be discontinued 24 hours prior to the procedure. If CKD with a creatinine clearance <30 mL/min is present, then longer interruption, 48 hours, is recommended. The drug can be resumed postprocedure once access site hemostasis is achieved.

DIABETES MELLITUS

Patients with diabetes mellitus treated with oral agents or insulin require an adjustment in medication to prevent peri-procedural hypoglycemia while fasting. Patients taking subcutaneous insulin should be instructed to take half of their long-acting insulin preparation the morning of the procedure. Regular insulin should be held the day of the procedure and a blood glucose level checked by the catheterization lab staff for symptoms of hypo- or hyperglycemia. Oral agents should be held the morning of the procedure. Patients with diabetes, particularly those taking neutral protamine Hagedorn (NPH) insulin, have an increased sensitivity to protamine, an agent used to reverse systemic heparinization. Major reactions to protamine, including vasomotor collapse, occur 50-fold more frequently in NPH insulin-dependent diabetes patients than in patients who have never received NPH insulin; therefore, protamine should be used with caution in this patient subset.[23]

Patients on metformin require special instructions and monitoring due to rare cases of metformin-associated lactic acidosis reported in patients with diabetes and CKD.[24] Metformin is excreted in the urine, and 90% is eliminated within 24 hours; therefore, it is contraindicated in patients with elevated creatinine. Since radiographic contrast can induce acute renal failure, there is a small risk of lactic acidosis in metformin-treated patients receiving contrast agents. Nearly all the cases reported, however, were in individuals with preexistent renal impairment who were continued on metformin after contrast exposure.[25] Patients with a serum creatinine <1.5 mg/dL can undergo cardiac catheterization without discontinuing metformin until the morning of the procedure. Metformin should be held postprocedure and resumed in 48 hours in patients without signs of renal failure. In patients at high risk of renal failure due to concomitant mediation such as cyclosporine, volume depletion, or low cardiac output, the serum creatinine concentration should be measured prior to resuming metformin. In patients with an elevated serum creatinine, metformin should be discontinued 48 hours prior to an elective procedure. In emergent situations, metformin should be discontinued at the time of the procedure, hydration administered, and renal function monitored closely.[26]

RENAL DISEASE

CKD, diabetes mellitus, low cardiac output, hypovolemia, and contrast volume administration are risk factors for contrast-induced acute kidney injury (CI-AKI). CI-AKI is defined as either an increase in serum creatinine concentration of >0.5 mg/dL or a relative increase of >25%. The incidence of CI-AKI in contemporary PCI is 6.7% in patients with stable CAD and 12.2% in acute coronary syndromes, and is associated with an increased risk of all-cause mortality.[27] Patients at risk for CI-AKI should be adequately hydrated with IV saline for 12 hours preprocedure if possible.[28,29] Other strategies, such as pretreatment with oral N-acetylcysteine, are no longer recommended due to lack of supporting data. Additional measures, including minimizing contrast volume, staging procedures, and withholding diuretics and other nephrotoxins, such as nonsteroidal anti-inflammatory agents, should be considered.

RISKS

The risk of a complication from cardiac catheterization has decreased over time and is <1% in the majority of cases (Table 5.4). Even with experienced operators and modern equipment, however, complications will occur. Many factors, including patient demographics, comorbidities, cardiovascular anatomy, procedural type and circumstances, and operator and hospital volume, can influence the risk to an individual patient, and these should be weighed in each case.[30,31] The risks are lowest in stable patients undergoing elective procedures; diagnostic angiography in this setting has a <0.1% risk of a major adverse event such as death, MI, or stroke.[32–34] The risk can increase up to eightfold in patients with multivessel disease, congestive heart failure, and renal insufficiency.[35] To justify performance of the procedure, the expected benefits, in terms of diagnostic or therapeutic outcomes, should be greater than the potential risks. Physicians performing invasive procedures have to be knowledgeable about potential complications and capable of administering treatment. This way, every effort can be made to minimize the incidence and severity of complications, many of which are immediately life-threatening. The most common complications of cardiac catheterization will be reviewed here. Complications specific to PCI and noncoronary interventions are covered in other chapters.

Death

Despite an aging population and performance of coronary angiography in higher-risk individuals, the procedural

Table 5.4 Major complications of diagnostic left heart catheterization

Complication	Incidence (%)
Mortality[a]	0.08–0.14
Myocardial infarction	0.05–0.17
Stroke	0.18–0.4
Vascular-related requiring treatment	0.5
Ventricular tachycardia	0.4

[a] Increased risk in patients with left main disease (i.e., stenosis >50%), left ventricular ejection fraction <30%, New York Heart Association Class III or IV congestive heart failure, age over 60 years, three-vessel coronary artery disease, valvular heart disease, and renal disease.

mortality reported for 222,553 patients by the Registry of the Society for Cardiac Angiography and Interventions in 1989 was 0.098%, compared to 0.14% reported in 1982.[33,34] Procedure-related mortality in a subsequent multicenter registry of 58,332 patients in 1990 was 0.08%.[36] A later single-center study of 11,821 patients undergoing 7,953 diagnostic and 3,868 therapeutic procedures was congruent. The total mortality rate was 0.2%, with a fivefold higher rate for interventions compared to diagnostic procedures.[37] The cause of in-hospital death after PCI has been evaluated, and procedural complications accounted for about half of deaths with the remaining attributed to preexisting cardiac disease, predominantly low output failure.[38]

Several subgroups at higher risk of procedural mortality have been identified. In the initial registry, patients with left main disease (i.e., stenosis >50%), left ventricular ejection fraction <30%; New York Heart Association (NYHA) Class III or IV congestive heart failure, age over 60 years, or three-vessel disease were at increased risk of mortality from diagnostic cardiac catheterization.[39] Renal insufficiency, postprocedural renal function deterioration, and valvular heart disease are additional predictors of mortality.[40,41]

Myocardial infarction

Myocardial ischemia may occur during diagnostic angiography as a result of catheter engagement or contrast injection and more commonly during PCI with balloon inflations, but it is usually transient and self-limited. Development of anginal symptoms, ECG changes, or hemodynamic changes may indicate ischemia and should prompt an evaluation of the cause. Attention to catheter flushing and monitoring for pressure damping reduce the risk of ischemia due to technical-related factors, such as coronary embolization or vessel occlusion. Even with careful technique, removal of the catheter from the coronary ostium or administration of nitroglycerine may be required to reverse ischemia due to obstructive CAD or vasospasm.

During diagnostic catheterization, progression of ischemia to MI is uncommon. In the first, second, and third registries conducted by SCAI, the risk of MI was rare and

decreased over time, from 0.07% and 0.06% to 0.05%.[33,36,42] Patient-related factors such as the extent of CAD (0.06% for single-vessel disease, 0.08% for triple-vessel disease) and location (0.17% for left main disease) slightly increase the risk of MI.[33] Postprocedural MI is rare following an uncomplicated elective diagnostic catheterization, and the majority of patients can be discharged after several hours of observation.[43]

Cerebrovascular events

Stroke is an uncommon but potentially devastating complication of cardiac catheterization and PCI. In several large series involving over 43,000 patients, the rate of clinically diagnosed procedure-related stroke ranged from 0.18% to 0.4%.[44–48] Several patient and procedural factors are associated with an increased risk of stroke, including diabetes mellitus, prior stroke, longer procedure times, intra-aortic balloon pump placement, and treatment with thrombolytic therapy.[46,49] Stroke risk is independent of arterial access site. In a study examining 16,710 procedures from 2006 to 2012, the total incidence of stroke or transient ischemic attack was 0.16% and was not different in radial or femoral cases (0.165% vs. 0.160%, $P = 1$).[50] Patients that suffer from a periprocedural stroke have a poor prognosis with persistent neurologic deficits and a high in-hospital mortality rate of up to 32%.[44] In patients that have PCI, the incidence of stroke remains low. In the British Cardiovascular Society database from 2007 to 2012, the incidence of stroke was 0.13% among 426,046 patients.[51] In the Euro Heart Survey Programme, which included 46,888 procedures, the incidence was 0.3% in elective PCI and 0.6% in acute coronary syndrome cases.[52]

Cerebral microembolism is the primary mechanism of periprocedural ischemic stroke occurring with left heart catheterization. Manipulation of guidewires and catheters results in disruption of atheromatous plaques from the walls of the aorta. In more than 50% of PCIs, guiding catheter placement is associated with scraping debris from the aorta as indicated by retrieval of atheromatous material.[53] Transcranial Doppler and serial magnetic resonance imaging (MRI) studies of patients who underwent cardiac catheterization and PCI support embolization as the main cause of stroke, with asymptomatic microemboli detected in about 15% of patients.[54–56] Strokes can also result from embolization of air or thrombus or intracerebral hemorrhage. Stroke risk can be minimized, therefore, by meticulous procedural techniques, such as withdrawal of blood from and flushing of catheters with heparinized saline, and performing catheter exchanges over wires in the descending aorta. The optimal management of periprocedural stroke is unknown, but favorable results have been shown in a small series of patients treated with neurovascular intervention and intra-arterial thrombolytics.[57–59] The clinical situation should prompt an emergent response and multidisciplinary management with cardiology, neurology, and neurointerventional specialists.[60]

Vascular complications

Several complications can occur at the arterial site of catheter insertion that result in significant patient discomfort, and increased length of stay and health care costs. Vascular access site complications are not uncommon, but only about 0.5% of cases require specific intervention. The majority of these complications, including arterial thrombosis, dissection, uncontrolled or retroperitoneal bleeding, and hematoma formation, commonly occur during or within hours following catheterization. Development of a pseudoaneurysm or arteriovenous fistula (AVF), however, may not manifest for several days. In general, arterial thrombosis is more common with radial access, whereas all other vascular complications are more frequent with femoral or brachial approaches.[42,61] Radial artery occlusion is generally unassociated with symptoms in patients with an intact palmar arch and does not require treatment. However, over half of patients with radial artery occlusion are observed to have spontaneous recanalization 1 to 3 months postprocedure. If symptomatic from radial artery occlusion, treatment with enoxaparin or fondaparinux results in recanalization rates of 87% at 1 month.[62] Treatment of femoral vascular complications is often conservative for hematomas, but surgical or percutaneous intervention are required for arterial thrombosis, AVFs, large or expanding pseudoaneurysms, and retroperitoneal bleeds not responsive to supportive care.[63]

Hemostasis at the access site can be accomplished either by manual or device compression or with a closure device of which there are several types.[64-66] The approach chosen for hemostasis depends on the catheterization lab and patient-related factors, such as availability of trained staff for sheath removal, anticoagulation status, sheath size and location, presence of peripheral vascular disease, and patient comfort. In patients undergoing diagnostic procedures, collagen and suture-type arterial puncture closure devices shorten the time to ambulation and have comparable safety to manual compression.[65-67] In two large meta-analyses involving over 37,000 patients undergoing diagnostic and interventional procedures with numerous types of devices in 30 studies, closure devices had an increased risk of local complications.[67,68] The risk of complications, however, differed among the VCDs.[67]

The randomized Instrumental Sealing of Arterial Puncture Site-CLOSURE Device versus Manual Compression (ISAR-CLOSURE) Trial compared manual compression to two types of closure devices, intravascular and extravascular, in 4,524 patients undergoing diagnostic coronary angiography. The primary endpoint of access site–related vascular complications at 30 days occurred in 6.9% of VCDs and 7.9% of manual compression patients (*p* for noninferiority < 0.001). Time to hemostasis and closure device failure favored intravascular devices.[69] Overall, the data suggest that closure devices are an acceptable alternative to manual compression in appropriate patients.

Arrhythmias

Although predominantly benign and self-limited, a gamut of arrhythmias can occur during cardiac catheterization. Therefore, continuous ECG monitoring and a staff trained in arrhythmia treatment are necessary. The majority of arrhythmias can be induced solely by intracoronary contrast injection or right heart catheter manipulation. Ventricular tachycardia and fibrillation are rare but occurred in 0.4% of cases in the second registry of SCAI.[33] Bradycardia and conduction disturbances are also uncommon, with an incidence of approximately 1% in diagnostic catheterization and PCI. Bradycardia is generally responsive to forceful coughing and atropine administration; initiation of temporary pacing is rarely required (0.06% of diagnostic cases, 0.4% of PCI).[70] Vasovagal reactions occur more commonly, in up to 3% of patients, as a result of anxiety or pain. Patients generally respond to removal of painful stimuli, fluid administration, and atropine administration. These reactions, however, can be life-threatening in patients with severe valvular or ischemic disease and should be rapidly treated to prevent hemodynamic decompensation.

Perforation

The risk of perforation of the heart or blood vessels is exceedingly rare in diagnostic cardiac catheterization, but may occur with transseptal procedures, pacemaker placement, myocardial biopsy, or elective pericardiocentesis. Patients may demonstrate vagal reactions, hypotension, chest pain, or arrhythmia. Echocardiographic evaluation should be immediately available and anticoagulation should be reversed if possible. In a large single-center series, emergent pericardiocentesis relieved acute tamponade in 99% of patients and was the only therapy required in 82% of patients.[71]

Atheroembolism

Atheromatous debris can be dislodged from the arterial wall during catheter manipulation and exchanges and may result in systemic embolization. When systematically evaluated, approximately half of patients undergoing PCI had detectable atheromatous debris in blood removed after placement of the guiding catheter.[53] None of the patients, however, had clinical events, suggesting that operator technique is critical to the prevention of embolic events. The incidence of clinically evident atheroembolic events is reported to be 0.6% to 1.9%.[72] In a large prospective study, the incidence of cholesterol embolization syndrome, as defined by peripheral cutaneous involvement or renal dysfunction, was 1.4%. Forty-eight percent of patients had cutaneous involvement as defined by the presence of livedo reticularis, blue toe syndrome, or digital gangrene; 64% of patients had renal insufficiency. Eosinophil counts were significantly higher in patients suffering from atheroembolism both before and after catheterization, but the only independent predictor of cholesterol emboli syndrome was baseline serum C-reactive protein. Unadjusted mortality was 32-fold greater in patients with cholesterol emboli syndrome (16% vs. 0.5%) than in those without it. Unfortunately, there is no specific therapy, and care is supportive with hemodialysis and wound management as required.[73]

Infection

The risk of occupational exposure to communicable disease and procedure-related infections is fortunately rare. Nonetheless, attention to proper sterile techniques and donning of protective barrier gear is of paramount importance. Operators should wear hats, eyewear, masks, and shoe covers and follow proper hand washing techniques prior to placing on a sterile gown and gloves. Additional protection to lab staff comes from eyewear and proper handling and disposal of contaminated equipment. All personnel should receive vaccination for hepatitis B.[74] Immediate cleansing of needlestick injuries and prompt medical attention are required. Protocols should be in place to manage occupational exposure to blood or body fluids.

As cardiac catheterization is performed using sterile technique, the incidence of bacteremia or infection at the access site is rare, and routine use of prophylactic antibiotics is not recommended. Bacteremia related to PCI occurs in approximately 0.64% of patients and is generally transient. Septic endarteritis after catheterization via femoral access is extremely rare, but there have been 20 reported cases with manual compression hemostasis and 46 related to VCDs.[75] The SCAI infection control guidelines discuss techniques for minimizing risk to the patient and catheterization lab personnel.[76] The best practices for infection control are presented in Table 5.5.

Radiation exposure

Although the risk of radiation to patients and staff is an accepted consequence of cardiac catheterization, every effort should be made to minimize patient and staff radiation exposure.[77] All personnel working with fluoroscopy should be trained and competency monitored.[78,79] Radiation exposure is determined by multiple factors (Table 5.6).[80,81]

Cardiac catheterization lab systems should be equipped with the capability of monitoring cumulative radiation dose. The energy delivered to the air by the X-ray beam, or air kerma, is measured at a fixed reference point during a procedure to calculate the reference point dose. The reference point dose is the cumulative dose derived from fluoroscopy, cine, and dosimetric effects of patient size and is typically displayed as milligray (mGy).[77] Some systems use a kerma-area product meter, or dose-area product meter, to monitor dose.

The most common type of radiation injury to patients is skin burns. All patients receiving a skin dose of 5–10 Gy will have erythema. Obese patients and those with long fluoroscopy times are at highest risk. The rash is located at the radiation entry portal, which is usually on the back. When the institutional threshold for a significant dose is reached, a follow-up process should be initiated. Patients at risk should be instructed to survey their skin at 48 to 72 hours for early signs of transient erythema. Since reactions may be delayed, surveillance for skin changes should continue for 4–6 weeks following prolonged radiation exposure. The Joint Commission's sentinel event threshold is 15 Gy, and doses above this will result in deep tissue injury. The effect of radiation exposure on cancer risk is difficult to determine, but it should be recognized that diagnostic X-rays are the largest man-made source of radiation exposure and do contribute to cancer risk.[82]

INFORMED CONSENT

The process of obtaining informed consent is a critical aspect of cardiac catheterization intervention. Responsibility ultimately lies with the operating physician. While members of the catheterization lab team may take part in describing the flow of the day and aspects of the procedure, the physician should confirm that the risks, benefits, and alternative treatments to the planned procedure have been explained to the patient's satisfaction. A study observed that more than half of patients lack complete understanding of the risks of cardiac catheterization after verbal and written communication, and interactive computer-based information

Table 5.5 Patient preparation: Infection control recommendations

Procedure	Recommendation
Hair removal	Remove hair only at or around access site*
	Electric clippers or depilatory cream preferred over razor*
Skin Cleaning	Preferred: 2% chlorhexidine-based preparation*
	Alternatives: iodophor or 70% alcohol
Drapes	Material should resist liquid penetration*
Antibiotics	Not routinely indicated*
Arterial access	Percutaneous (avoid cut-down)
Closure device	Avoid placing in synthetic grafts, through infected skin, or with sheath dwell time >6 hours
Wound dressing	Use gauze or semipermeable dressing*
Staged procedure	Avoid re-puncture of femoral artery

* Centers for Disease Control recommendation.

Table 5.6 Factors that contribute to radiation exposure

Physician and patient

X-ray system

Body mass index/weight distribution of the patient

Duration of fluoroscopy

Cine usage

Table position (distance between patient and X-ray tube)

Technique selection (i.e., magnification, fluoroscopy, and cine modes [frames per second]) beam angulation)

Physician

Personal shielding (lead apron, thyroid shield, and glasses)

Use of table-mounted lead shielding and table skirts

Distance from the X-ray source

results in greater comprehension.[83] Sufficient details should be provided to adequately inform the patient without provoking undue fear. The patient or patient's legal representative should provide written consent, and documentation should be placed in the medical record. In rare circumstances when a patient is unable to provide consent and delay would compromise survival, such as with a cardiac arrest, medical justification for proceeding without consent should be documented in the medical record. Hospital personnel such as social workers can be of assistance in locating family members while care is being provided to the patient. The rationale for proceeding with emergent procedures should be explained to the patient and family as soon as feasible. Another special circumstance involving consent pertains to medical research. Research protocols that involve patients in the cardiac catheterization laboratory, such as studies involving drugs or devices, should be thoroughly explained to the patient prior to the initiation of the procedure. Patients must be given time to fully examine the research protocol consent form and must understand the protocol, including treatments, risks, and follow-up. Patients should not be pressured to consent to research protocols. Physicians should disclose their relationship to the study and any potential conflicts of interest. The ethical principles and guidelines for the protection of human subjects of research should be followed.[84,85]

CONCLUSIONS

In order to provide the highest level of care with the lowest risk, invasive and interventional cardiologists must ensure they have up-to-date, in-depth knowledge of procedural indications and risks, and meticulous technical skills. Appropriate patient selection and preparation require individualized care and attention to high-risk features. Procedural risk and patient stress can be minimized through the process of informed consent, patient preparation, and an experienced, trained catheterization lab staff.

REFERENCES

1. Riley RF, et al. Trends in coronary revascularization in the United States from 2001 to 2009: Recent declines in percutaneous coronary intervention volumes. *Circ Cardiovasc Qual Outcomes* 2011;4(2):193–197.
2. Scanlon PJ, et al. ACC/AHA guidelines for coronary angiography: Executive summary and recommendations. A report of the American College of Cardiology/American Heart Association Task Force on Practice Guidelines (Committee on Coronary Angiography) developed in collaboration with the Society for Cardiac Angiography and Interventions. *Circulation* 1999;99(17):2345–2357.
3. Guadagnoli E, et al. Impact of underuse, overuse, and discretionary use on geographic variation in the use of coronary angiography after acute myocardial infarction. *Med Care* 2001;39(5):446–458.
4. Hartford K, et al. Regional variation in angiography, coronary artery bypass surgery, and percutaneous transluminal coronary angioplasty in Manitoba, 1987 to 1992: The funnel effect. *Med Care* 1998;36(7):1022–1032.
5. Hannan EL, Kumar D. Geographic variation in the utilization and choice of procedures for treating coronary artery disease in New York State. Ischaemic Heart Disease Patient Outcomes Research Team (PORT). *J of Health Serv Res Policy* 1997;2(3):137–143.
6. Patel MR, et al. ACCF/SCAI/AATS/AHA/ASE/ASNC/HFSA/HRS/SCCM/SCCT/SCMR/STS 2012 appropriate use criteria for diagnostic catheterization: American College of Cardiology Foundation Appropriate Use Criteria Task Force Society for Cardiovascular Angiography and Interventions American Association for Thoracic Surgery American Heart Association, American Society of Echocardiography American Society of Nuclear Cardiology Heart Failure Society of America Heart Rhythm Society, Society of Critical Care Medicine Society of Cardiovascular Computed Tomography Society for Cardiovascular Magnetic Resonance Society of Thoracic Surgeons. *J Am Coll Cardiol* 2012;59(22):1995-2027.
7. Bashore TM, et al. 2012 American College of Cardiology Foundation/Society for Cardiovascular Angiography and Interventions expert consensus document on cardiac catheterization laboratory standards update: A report of the American College of Cardiology Foundation Task Force on Expert Consensus documents developed in collaboration with the Society of Thoracic Surgeons and Society for Vascular Medicine. *J Am Coll Cardiol* 2012;59(24):2221–2305.
8. Joyal D, et al. Meta-analysis of ten trials on the effectiveness of the radial versus the femoral approach in primary percutaneous coronary intervention. *Am J Cardiol* 2012;109(6):813–818.
9. Rao SV, et al. Best practices for transradial angiography and intervention: A consensus statement from the society for cardiovascular angiography and intervention's transradial working group. *Cath Cardiovasc Interv* 2014;83(2):228–236.
10. Ratib K, et al. Access site practice and procedural outcomes in relation to clinical presentation in 439,947 patients undergoing percutaneous coronary intervention in the United kingdom. *JACC Cardiovasc Interv* 2015;8 (1 Pt A):20–29.

11. Mamas M, et al. Use of the sheathless guide catheter during routine transradial percutaneous coronary intervention: A feasibility study. *Catheter Cardiovasc Interv* 2010;75(4):596–602.

12. Barbeau GR, et al. Evaluation of the ulnopalmar arterial arches with pulse oximetry and plethysmography: Comparison with the Allen's test in 1010 patients. *Am Heart J* 2004;147(3):489–493.

13. Hovagim AR, et al. Pulse oximetry for evaluation of radial and ulnar arterial blood flow. *J Cardiothorac Anesth* 1989;3(1):27–30.

14. Benit E, et al. Frequency of a positive modified Allen's test in 1,000 consecutive patients undergoing cardiac catheterization. *Cathet Cardiovasc Diagn* 1996;38(4):352–354.

15. Greenwood MJ, et al. Vascular communications of the hand in patients being considered for transradial coronary angiography: As the Allen's test accurate? *J Am Coll Cardiol* 2005;46(11):2013–2017.

16. Shehadi WH, Toniolo G. Adverse reactions to contrast media: A report from the Committee on Safety of Contrast Media of the International Society of Radiology. *Radiology* 1980;137(2):299–302.

17. Lang DM, et al. Increased risk for anaphylactoid reaction from contrast media in patients on beta-adrenergic blockers or with asthma. *Ann Intern Med* 1991;115(4):270–276.

18. Nayak KR, et al. Anaphylactoid reactions to radiocontrast agents: Prevention and treatment in the cardiac catheterization laboratory. *J Invasive Cardiol* 2009;21(10):548–551.

19. Lasser EC, et al. Pretreatment with corticosteroids to alleviate reactions to intravenous contrast material. *N Engl J Med* 1987;317(14):845–849.

20. Katayama H, et al. Adverse reactions to ionic and nonionic contrast media. A report from the Japanese Committee on the Safety of Contrast Media. *Radiology* 1990;175(3):621–628.

21. Ziakas AG, et al. Radial versus femoral access for orally anticoagulated patients. *Catheter Cardiovasc Interv* 2010;76(4):493–499.

22. Heidbuchel H, et al. European Heart Rhythm Association Practical Guide on the use of new oral anticoagulants in patients with non-valvular atrial fibrillation. *Europace* 2013;15(5):625–651.

23. Stewart WJ, et al. Increased risk of severe protamine reactions in NPH insulin-dependent diabetics undergoing cardiac catheterization. *Circulation* 1984;70(5):788–792.

24. Gan SC, et al. Biguanide-associated lactic acidosis. Case report and review of the literature. *Arch Intern Med* 1992;152(11):2333–2336.

25. Bailey CJ, Turner RC. Metformin. *N Engl J Med* 1996;334(9):574–579.

26. Heupler FA, Jr. Guidelines for performing angiography in patients taking metformin. Members of the Laboratory Performance Standards Committee of the Society for Cardiac Angiography and Interventions. *Cathet Cardiovasc Diagn* 1998;43(2):121–123.

27. Crimi G, et al. Incidence, prognostic impact, and optimal definition of contrast-induced acute kidney injury in consecutive patients with stable or unstable coronary artery disease undergoing percutaneous coronary intervention. Insights from the all-comer PRODIGY trial. *Catheter Cardiovasc Interv* 2015(1);86:E19–E27.

28. Trivedi HS, et al. A randomized prospective trial to assess the role of saline hydration on the development of contrast nephrotoxicity. *Nephron Clin Pract* 2003;93(1):C29–C34.

29. Mueller C, et al. Prevention of contrast media-associated nephropathy: Randomized comparison of 2 hydration regimens in 1620 patients undergoing coronary angioplasty. *Arch Intern Med* 2002;162(3):329–336.

30. Baim D, Grossman W. Complications of cardiac catheterization. In: Baim D, Grossman, W, ed. *Cardiac catheterization, angiography and intervention.* 6th ed. Baltimore, MD: Williams & Wilkins, 2000, pp. 35–65.

31. Hannan EL, et al. Volume-outcome relationships for percutaneous coronary interventions in the stent era. *Circulation* 2005;112(8):1171–1179.

32. Davis K, et al. Complications of coronary arteriography from the Collaborative Study of Coronary Artery Surgery (CASS). *Circulation* 1979;59(6):1105–1112.

33. Johnson LW, et al. Coronary arteriography 1984–1987: A report of the Registry of the Society for Cardiac Angiography and Interventions. I. Results and complications. *Cath Cardiovasc Diagn* 1989;17(1):5–10.

34. Lozner EC, et al. Coronary arteriography 1984–1987: A report of the Registry of the Society for Cardiac Angiography and Interventions. II. An analysis of 218 deaths related to coronary arteriography. *Cathet Cardiovasc Diagn* 1989;17(1):11–14.

35. Laskey W, et al. Multivariable model for prediction of risk of significant complication during diagnostic cardiac catheterization. The Registry Committee of the Society for Cardiac Angiography & Interventions. *Cathet Cardiovasc Diagn* 1993;30(3):185–190.

36. Noto TJ, Jr., et al. Cardiac catheterization 1990: A report of the Registry of the Society for Cardiac Angiography and Interventions (SCA&I). *Cathet Cardiovasc Diagn* 1991;24(2):75–83.

37. Chandrasekar B, et al. Complications of cardiac catheterization in the current era: A single-center experience. *Catheter Cardiovasc Interv* 2001;52(3):289–295.

38. Malenka DJ, et al. Cause of in-hospital death in 12,232 consecutive patients undergoing percutaneous transluminal coronary angioplasty. The Northern New England Cardiovascular Disease Study Group. *Am Heart J* 1999;137(4 Pt 1):632 638.

39. Kennedy JW, et al. Mortality related to cardiac catheterization and angiography. *Cathet Cardiovasc Diagn* 1982;8(4):323–340.

40. Gruberg L, et al. The prognostic implications of further renal function deterioration within 48 h of interventional coronary procedures in patients with pre-existent chronic renal insufficiency. *J Am Coll Cardiol* 2000;36(5):1542–1548.

41. Folland ED, et al. Complications of cardiac catheterization and angiography in patients with valvular heart disease. VA Cooperative Study on Valvular Heart Disease. *Cathet Cardiovasc Diagn* 1989;17(1):15–21.

42. Kennedy JW. Complications associated with cardiac catheterization and angiography. *Cathet Cardiovasc Diagn* 1982;8(1):5–11.

43. Mahrer PR, et al. Efficacy and safety of outpatient cardiac catheterization. *Cathet Cardiovasc Diagn* 1987;13(5):304–308.

44. Fuchs S, et al. Stroke complicating percutaneous coronary interventions: Incidence, predictors, and prognostic implications. *Circulation* 2002;106(1):86–91.

45. Lazar JM, et al. Predisposing risk factors and natural history of acute neurologic complications of left-sided cardiac catheterization. *Am J Cardiol* 1995;75(15):1056–1060.

46. Segal AZ, et al. Stroke as a complication of cardiac catheterization: Risk factors and clinical features. *Neurology* 2001;56(7):975–977.

47. Wong SC, et al. Neurological complications following percutaneous coronary interventions (a report from the 2000–2001 New York State Angioplasty Registry). *Am J Cardiol* 2005;96(9):1248–1250.

48. Dukkipati S, et al. Characteristics of cerebrovascular accidents after percutaneous coronary interventions. *J Am Coll Cardiol* 2004;43(7):1161–1167.

49. Sutton AGC, et al. A randomized trial of rescue angioplasty versus a conservative approach for failed fibrinolysis in ST-segment elevation myocardial infarction: The Middlesbrough Early Revascularization to Limit INfarction (MERLIN) trial. *J Am Coll Cardiol* 2004;44(2):287–296.

50. Raposo L, et al. Neurologic complications after transradial or transfemoral approach for diagnostic and interventional cardiac catheterization: A propensity score analysis of 16,710 cases from a single centre prospective registry. *Catheter Cardiovasc Interv* 2015;86(1):61–70.

51. Kwok CS, et al. Stroke following percutaneous coronary intervention: Type-specific incidence, outcomes and determinants seen by the British Cardiovascular Intervention Society 2007–12. *Eur Heart J* 2015;36(25):1618–1628.

52. Werner N, et al. Incidence and clinical impact of stroke complicating percutaneous coronary intervention: Results of the Euro heart survey percutaneous coronary interventions registry. *Circ Cardiovasc Interv* 2013;6(4):362–369.

53. Keeley EC, Grines CL. Scraping of aortic debris by coronary guiding catheters: A prospective evaluation of 1,000 cases. *J Am Coll Cardiol* 1998;32(7):1861–1865.

54. Hamon M, et al. Cerebral microembolism during cardiac catheterization and risk of acute brain injury: A prospective diffusion-weighted magnetic resonance imaging study. *Stroke* 2006;37(8):2035–2038.

55. Leclercq F, et al. Transcranial Doppler detection of cerebral microemboli during left heart catheterization. *Cerebrovasc Dis* 2001;12(1):59–65.

56. Busing KA, et al. Cerebral infarction: Incidence and risk factors after diagnostic and interventional cardiac catheterization—prospective evaluation at diffusion-weighted MR imaging. *Radiology* 2005;235(1):177–183.

57. Al-Mubarak N, et al. Immediate catheter-based neurovascular rescue for acute stroke complicating coronary procedures. *Am J Cardiol* 2002;90(2):173–176.

58. De Marco F, et al. Management of cerebrovascular accidents during cardiac catheterization: Immediate cerebral angiography versus early neuroimaging strategy. *Cath Cardiovasc Interv* 2007;70(4):560–568.

59. Khatri P, et al. The safety and efficacy of thrombolysis for strokes after cardiac catheterization. *J Am Coll Cardiol* 2008;51(9):906–911.

60. Hamon M, et al. Periprocedural stroke and cardiac catheterization. *Circulation* 2008;118(6):678–683.

61. Agostoni P, et al. Radial versus femoral approach for percutaneous coronary diagnostic and interventional procedures: Systematic overview and meta-analysis of randomized trials. *J Am Coll Cardiol* 2004;44(2):349–356.

62. Kotowycz MA, Dzavik V. Radial artery patency after transradial catheterization. *Circ Cardiovasc Interv* 2012;5(1):127–133.

63. Webber GW, et al. Contemporary management of postcatheterization pseudoaneurysms. *Circulation* 2007;115(20):2666–2674.

64. Pracyk JB, et al. A randomized trial of vascular hemostasis techniques to reduce femoral vascular complications after coronary intervention. *Am J Cardiol* 1998;81(8):970–976.

65. Ward SR, et al. Efficacy and safety of a hemostatic puncture closure device with early ambulation after coronary angiography. Angio-Seal Investigators. *Am J Cardiol* 1998;81(5):569–572.

66. Baim DS, Knopf WD, et al. Suture-mediated closure of the femoral access site after cardiac catheterization: Results of the suture to ambulate aNd discharge (STAND I and STAND II) trials. *Am J Cardiol* 2000;85(7):864–869.

67. Nikolsky E, et al. Vascular complications associated with arteriotomy closure devices in patients undergoing percutaneous coronary procedures: A meta-analysis. *J Am Coll Cardiol* 2004;44(6):1200–1209.

68. Koreny M, et al. Arterial puncture closing devices compared with standard manual compression after cardiac catheterization: Systematic review and meta-analysis. *JAMA* 2004;291(3):350–357.

69. Schulz-Schupke S, et al. Comparison of vascular closure devices vs manual compression after femoral artery puncture: The ISAR-CLOSURE randomized clinical trial. *JAMA* 2014;312(19):1981–1987.

70. Harvey JR, et al. Use of balloon flotation pacing catheters for prophylactic temporary pacing during diagnostic and therapeutic catheterization procedures. *Am J Cardiol* 1988;62(13):941–944.

71. Tsang TS, et al. Rescue echocardiographically guided pericardiocentesis for cardiac perforation complicating catheter-based procedures. The Mayo Clinic experience. *J Am Coll Cardiol* 1998;32(5):1345–1350.

72. Bashore TM, Gehrig T. Cholesterol emboli after invasive cardiac procedures. *J Am Coll Cardiol* 2003;42(2):217–218.

73. Fukumoto Y, et al. The incidence and risk factors of cholesterol embolization syndrome, a complication of cardiac catheterization: A prospective study. *J Am Coll Cardiol* 2003;42(2):211–216.

74. Heupler FA, Jr., et al. Infection prevention guidelines for cardiac catheterization laboratories. Society for Cardiac Angiography and Interventions Laboratory Performance Standards Committee. *Cathet Cardiovasc Diagn* 1992;25(3):260–263.

75. Franco J, et al. Infectious complications of percutaneous cardiac procedures. *Interv Cardiol* 2014;6(5):445–452.

76. Chambers CE, et al. Infection control guidelines for the cardiac catheterization laboratory: Society guidelines revisited. *Catheter Cardiovasc Interv* 2006;67(1):78–86.

77. Balter S, Moses J. Managing patient dose in interventional cardiology. *Catheter Cardiovasc Interv* 2007;70(2):244–249.

78. Hirshfeld JW, Jr., et al. ACCF/AHA/HRS/SCAI clinical competence statement on physician knowledge to optimize patient safety and image quality in fluoroscopically

guided invasive cardiovascular procedures. A report of the American College of Cardiology Foundation/American Heart Association/American College of Physicians Task Force on Clinical Competence and Training. *J Am Coll Cardiol* 2004;44(11):2259–2282.

79. Chambers CE, et al. Radiation safety program for the cardiac catheterization laboratory. *Catheter Cardiovasc Interv* 2011;77(4):546–556.

80. Laskey WK, et al. Variability in fluoroscopic X-ray exposure in contemporary cardiac catheterization laboratories. *J Am Coll Cardiol* 2006;48(7):1361–1364.

81. Cusma JT, et al. Real-time measurement of radiation exposure to patients during diagnostic coronary angiography and percutaneous interventional procedures. *J Am Coll Cardiol* 1999;33(2):427–435.

82. Berrington de Gonzalez A, Darby S. Risk of cancer from diagnostic X-rays: Estimates for the UK and 14 other countries. *Lancet* 2004;363(9406):345–351.

83. Tait AR, et al. Patient comprehension of an interactive, computer-based information program for cardiac catheterization: A comparison with standard information. *Arch Intern Med* 2009;169(20):1907–1914.

84. Code of Federal Regulations Regarding Protection of Human Subjects *(45 CFR 46)* (Accessed August 5, 2009, at http://ohsr.od.nih.gov/guidelines/45cfr46.html.)

85. The Belmont Report Ethical Principles and Guidelines for the protection of human subjects of research. (Accessed August 6, 2009, at http://ohsr.od.nih.gov/guidelines/belmont.html.)

6

Conscious sedation (local anesthetics, sedatives, and reversing agents)

STEVEN P. DUNN

INTRODUCTION

Conscious sedation, also known as moderate sedation, is the practice of choice during cardiac catheterization to relieve pain and anxiety, as recommended by the American College of Cardiology (ACC) and the Society for Cardiovascular Angiography and Interventions (SCAI).[1] The American Society of Anesthesiologists (ASA) has defined moderate sedation as a drug-induced depression of consciousness that continues to allow the patient to purposefully respond to commands and maintain airway, breathing, and circulation without mechanical or pharmacological support (Table 6.1).[2] This level of sedation is optimal for cardiac catheterization as patient symptoms can often be the first warning of a procedural complication. In addition, by allowing patients to maintain physiologic respiratory and cardiac function, postprocedure recovery time is significantly lessened. Whereas there are general recommendations regarding the most appropriate methods to achieve this level of sedation, significant variability in practice exists across different cardiac catheterization laboratories. The use of deep sedation or general anesthesia as an augment to complex interventional cases, or trans-catheter aortic valve replacement, are beyond the scope of this chapter and should require the use of anesthesia professionals.

FUNDAMENTALS

Preprocedure assessment

A preprocedure assessment is an important part of ensuring that safe and effective sedation therapy is applied to each patient situation, as many factors can put the patient at risk for adverse reaction to sedation (Table 6.2).[2] Ideally this would include an assessment of major organ systems functions, history of drug and alcohol abuse (including tobacco), date and time of last oral intake, and allergic history relative to local anesthesia and sedative drugs.

As sedative agents can affect airway reflexes, patients undergoing cardiac catheterization are at risk for aspiration of gastric contents. Therefore, patients undergoing this procedure electively should fast for an appropriate amount of time to allow for sufficient gastric emptying, generally 4 hours after a meal. Clear liquids may be permitted up to 2 hours prior to the procedure.[2] Medications, particularly antihypertensive and antiplatelet medications, should be ingested as ordered, unless proscribed by the invasive cardiologist.

A preprocedure assessment will include an evaluation of anatomic variables that may affect sedation or, if necessary, intubation and allow proactive planning. In planning for potential intubation, examination specific to the airway is recommended, including evaluation of

Table 6.1 Continuum of depth of sedation: Definition of general anesthesia and levels of sedation/analgesia

	Minimal sedation (anxiolysis)	Moderate sedation/analgesia (conscious sedation)	Deep sedation/ analgesia	General anesthesia
Responsiveness	Normal response to verbal stimulation	Purposeful[a] response to verbal or tactile stimulation	Purposeful[a] response after repeated or painful stimulation	Unarousable, even with painful stimulus
Airway	Unaffected	No intervention required	Intervention may be required	Intervention often required
Spontaneous ventilation	Unaffected	Adequate	May be inadequate	Frequently inadequate
Cardiovascular function	Unaffected	Usually maintained	Usually maintained	May be impaired

Source: American Society of Anesthesiologists Task Force on Sedation and Analgesia by Non-Anesthesiologists, *Anesthesiology*, 96(4), 1004–1017, 2002. With permission.

Note: Minimal Sedation (Anxiolysis) = a drug-induced state during which patients respond normally to verbal commands. Although cognitive function and coordination may be impaired, ventilatory and cardiovascular functions are unaffected.

Moderate Sedation/Analgesia (Conscious Sedation) = a drug-induced depression of consciousness during which patients respond purposefully[a] to verbal commands, either alone or accompanied by light tactile stimulation. No interventions are required to maintain a patent airway, and spontaneous ventilation is adequate. Cardiovascular function is usually maintained.

Deep Sedation/Analgesia = a drug-induced depression of consciousness during which patients cannot be easily aroused but respond purposefully[a] following repeated or painful stimulation. The ability to independently maintain ventilatory function may be impaired. Patients may require assistance in maintaining a patent airway, and spontaneous ventilation may be inadequate. Cardiovascular function is usually maintained.

General Anesthesia = a drug-induced loss of consciousness during which patients are not arousable, even by painful stimulation. The ability to independently maintain ventilatory function is often impaired. Patients often require assistance in maintaining a patent airway, and positive pressure ventilation may be required because of depressed spontaneous ventilation or drug-induced depression of neuromuscular function. Cardiovascular function may be impaired.

Because sedation is a continuum, it is not always possible to predict how an individual patient will respond. Hence, practitioners intending to produce a given level of sedation should be able to rescue patients whose level of sedation becomes deeper than initially intended. Individuals administering *Moderate Sedation/Analgesia (Conscious Sedation)* should be able to rescue patients who enter a state of *Deep Sedation/Analgesia*, while those administering *Deep Sedation/Analgesia* should be able to rescue patients who enter a state of general anesthesia.

Developed by the American Society of Anesthesiologists; approved by the ASA House of Delegates October 13, 1999.

[a] Reflex withdrawal from a painful stimulus is not considered a purposeful response.

Table 6.2 Preprocedure evaluation[2]

System	Rationale
Pre-existing cardiac or pulmonary disease	Sedative agents can cause cardiovascular or respiratory depression.
Pre-existing renal or hepatic disease	Abnormalities may impair how fast the drug is metabolized and excreted from the system, resulting in longer drug action and increased drug effect.
Time and type of last oral intake	Gag reflex suppression could result in aspiration
History of drug and alcohol abuse	The dose and action of sedative agents may be affected in patients that abuse drugs and alcohol. In addition, procedural agitation may be higher.
History of smoking	Patients who smoke are at increased risk of bronchospasm, airway problems, or coughing.
Previous experience with sedative agents	Any previous adverse reactions to sedation should be noted.

Source: Modified from the American Society of Anesthesiologists Task Force on Sedation and Analgesia by Non-Anesthesiologists, *Anesthesiology*, 96(4), 1004–1017, 2002.

the neck and dentition. The Mallampati Scale,[3] an objective anatomical assessment of the oral cavity that predicts ease of intubation, is also a useful examination tool (Table 6.3). In addition, a general physical assessment is warranted. This should include vital signs and auscultation of the heart and lungs.[2] Although many catheterization laboratories achieve adequate preprocedural sedation with the use of oral medications, intravenous (IV) access for medication administration is a necessity.

While there are many patient variables that affect the choice and the amount of sedation administered to achieve conscious sedation, a systematic approach to assessing the patient and selecting the therapeutic modality will ensure an optimal outcome.

Table 6.3 The Mallampati scale

	Anatomic findings	Difficulty of intubation
Class I	Soft palate, uvula, fauces, pillars available	No difficulty
Class II	Soft palate, uvula, fauces available	No difficulty
Class III	Soft palate, base of uvula available	Moderate difficulty
Class IV	Hard palate only visible	Severe difficulty

Source: Modified from Mallampati, S.R., et al., Can. Anaesth. Soc. J., 32(4), 429–434, 1985.

Monitoring of sedation

The ASA focuses on four key areas of monitoring for moderate sedation: level of consciousness, pulmonary ventilation, oxygenation, and hemodynamics.[2] Although the methods utilized to achieve moderate sedation may differ, universally accepted methods are used to assess whether appropriate sedation is achieved. Monitoring requires a combination of direct observation and assessment, along with various medical equipment as appropriate. Since respiratory depression is the principle concern with the use of moderate sedative modalities, monitoring of both ventilation and oxygenation is recommended.

The level of sedation can also be objectively assessed with the use of the Aldrete score (Table 6.4).[4] This score assigns a point value for activity, respiration, circulation, consciousness, and color.

LEVEL OF CONSCIOUSNESS

For moderate sedation, a level of consciousness where the patient purposefully responds to commands (physically or verbally) is appropriate. While there is little literature to suggest that monitoring level of consciousness improves clinical outcomes associated with procedural sedation, it is strongly felt that early intervention when the patient's level of sedation is supratherapeutic (e.g. no response, or response only to painful stimuli) will likely prevent adverse outcomes associated with oversedation such as respiratory or cardiac depression.

PULMONARY VENTILATION

One of the principle adverse effects from oversedation is drug-induced respiratory depression. Therefore, the ASA strongly recommends monitoring respiratory ventilation via observation or auscultation during moderate sedation. While there are noninvasive techniques to assess ventilation, such as impedance plethysmography, these are considered complementary to observation and auscultation and not substitutes.

In 2010, the ASA amended its standards for monitoring during moderate and deep sedation to include a requirement for the monitoring of exhaled carbon dioxide (end-tidal CO_2 monitoring [$EtCO_2$] using capnography) in addition to clinical monitoring.[5] Evidence for capnography during cardiac catheterization is limited, but a randomized, controlled study of capnography versus clinical monitoring only in patients receiving moderate sedation with propofol during colonoscopy demonstrated reduced oxygen desaturation and hypoxemia events with capnography.[6] However, other studies have failed to demonstrate benefit with capnography.[7] While the requirement for capnography has not been routinely mandated by various regulatory agencies due to limited evidence and the relatively high cost of implementation, $EtCO_2$ monitoring should be considered in areas where moderate sedation practices occur, including the cardiac catheterization lab.

OXYGENATION

Pulse oximetry has been shown to effectively monitor and prevent hypoxemia during moderate sedation and should be utilized in all patients undergoing cardiac catheterization. However, pulse oximetry is not singularly adequate for assessing respiratory function and should be combined with assessment of pulmonary ventilation, including patient observation and $EtCO_2$ monitoring where available.

Table 6.4 The Aldrete scoring system for sedation

Score[a]	Activity	Respiration	Circulation	Consciousness	Color
2	Able to move four extremities	Able to breathe deeply and cough	BP ± 20% of baseline	Fully alert and answers questions	Normal pink
1	Able to move two extremities	Limited respiratory effort (dyspnea)	BP ± 20–50% of baseline	Arousable	Pale, dusky, blotchy
0	Not able to control any extremities	No spontaneous respiratory effort	BP change >50% of baseline	Failure to elicit response	Frank cyanosis

Source: Reproduced from Dunn, S.P., Local anesthetics, sedatives, and reversing agents, In: Moliterno, D.J., et al., eds., CathSAP 3 (Cardiac Catheterization and Interventional Cardiology Self-Assessment Program), American College of Cardiology Foundation, Washington, DC, 2008, pp. 437–443. With permission. All rights reserved; Aldrete, J.A., Kroulik, D.A., Anesth. Analg., 49(6), 924–934, 1970.
Note: BP, blood pressure.
[a] A score is applied to each of the variables, with the sum of scores of <8 considered acceptable to indicate recovery from sedation.

HEMODYNAMICS

Pharmacologic agents used in moderate sedation have the potential to blunt autonomic responses to the procedure. Additionally, some local anesthetics and sedative agents may cause cardiac dysrhythmias, which may be more pronounced in patients with extensive cardiovascular disease. The ASA recommends monitoring vital signs at 5-minute intervals until adequate sedation is achieved. However, this monitoring may occur at more frequent or continuous intervals during cardiac catheterization. In addition, continuous electrocardiographic monitoring is warranted to monitor sedative adverse effects, although this is also generally part of standard monitoring independent of sedation practices.

EQUIPMENT

The ASA recommends a minimum level of emergency equipment in the event of pulmonary or cardiac arrest induced by procedural sedation and/or analgesia (Table 6.5). Also, given the high cardiovascular acuity of the patient undergoing cardiac catheterization and the potential for cardiac and/or pulmonary arrest independent of sedation use, the ACC/SCAI recommends a baseline level of emergency resuscitative equipment be immediately available.[1] In addition, cardiac catheterization lab personnel should possess a minimum level of training (basic life support), and advanced levels of training are highly recommended.

CLINICAL ASPECTS

Local anesthesia

Local anesthesia continues to be the preferred method to prevent discomfort associated with vascular access. Local anesthetics primarily act by competitive antagonism of the α-subunit of voltage-gated sodium channels in the nerve membrane. In addition, there are effects on G-protein-coupled receptors, calcium channels, and potassium channels, which complement the classically known effect on sodium channels.[8,9] Inhibition of these pathways essentially results in temporary cessation of nerve impulse conduction.

In general, local anesthetics are both safe and effective, although there are pharmacologic differences between agents (Table 6.6). Lidocaine (0.5%–2% concentration) is the local anesthetic of choice for cardiac catheterization due to its rapid onset, short duration of action, and minimal risk of cardiotoxicity. Cardiotoxicity induced by local anesthetics can be caused by several mechanisms,

Table 6.5 ASA recommended emergency equipment for moderate sedation

Airway management equipment	Compressed oxygen
	Endotracheal tubes
	Face masks
	Lubricant
	Stylets
	Suction
	Suction catheters
Intravenous equipment	Alcohol wipes
	Gloves
	Intravenous catheters
	Intravenous fluids
	Intravenous tubing
	Needles for drug administration, intramuscular, or intraosseous injection
	Sterile gauze pads
	Syringes
	Tape
	Tourniquets
Medications	Amiodarone
	Atropine
	Dextrose (50%)
	Diazepam or midazolam
	Diphenhydramine
	Epinephrine
	Hydrocortisone, methylprednisolone, or dexamethasone
	Lidocaine
	Nitroglycerin
	Vasopressin

Source: Modified from the American Society of Anesthesiologists Task Force on Sedation and Analgesia by Non-Anesthesiologists, *Anesthesiology*, 96(4), 1004–1017, 2002.

Table 6.6 Selected local anesthetic agents

Agent	Onset	Potency	Duration	Cardiotoxicity	Max. dose (mg/kg)	Max. dose with a vasoconstrictor (mg/kg)
Lidocaine	+++	++	++	+	5	7
Mepivicaine	+	++	++	+	5	7
Bupivacaine	+	+++	+++	+++	2	3
Ropivacaine	+	++	+++	++	2.5	4

Source: Reproduced from Dunn, S.P., Local anesthetics, sedatives, and reversing agents, In: Moliterno, D.J., et al., eds., *CathSAP 3 (Cardiac Catheterization and Interventional Cardiology Self-Assessment Program)*, American College of Cardiology Foundation, Washington, DC, 2008, pp. 437–443. With permission. All rights reserved.
Note: +, low; ++, intermediate; +++, high.

but classically is described as both direct and indirect (central nervous system [CNS] mediated) effects on the myocardium with conduction delays leading to a prolonged PR interval or a wide QRS complex.[10] In addition, many anesthetic agents can cause ventricular arrhythmias through this same mechanism by unidirectional block and re-entry,[8,9] the risk of which may be heightened by mechanical disturbance of myocyte electrophysiology during cardiac catheterization. Some agents also possess strong negative inotropic activity, which is generally not a desirable pharmacologic property for administration to a patient with significant structural heart disease.[11] Bupivacaine is widely regarded as the local anesthetic with the highest potential for cardiotoxicity and should be considered less preferable for use in cardiac catheterization.[10]

Since most anesthetics are vasodilators, a vasoconstrictor (typically epinephrine at 1:100,000 or 1:200,000) may be utilized in combination with a local anesthetic to minimize local bleeding and increase anesthetic duration. Use of a vasoconstrictor in this setting has not been shown to significantly affect hemodynamic parameters,[12,13] although few data exist establishing the safety of local vasoconstrictor use in the patient with high cardiovascular acuity. Of note, the administration of a vasoconstrictor in combination with a local anesthetic will reduce the potency of the anesthetic employed by reducing tissue diffusion, necessitating higher doses for equivalent effect. This also lowers the risk of local anesthetic toxicity by minimizing vascular uptake as a result of vasoconstriction of capillary beds.[14,15]

Sedation and analgesia

Cardiac catheterization is most often performed under the influence of agents with anxiolytic and amnestic properties in combination with an analgesic, if necessary. The most frequently used sedative agent is a benzodiazepine, which may also be combined with a sedating antihistamine. Opioid analgesics may also be utilized in combination with benzodiazepines to achieve adequate sedation. Literature suggests that combining a sedative with an opioid provides adequate moderate sedation,[16] but there are few data describing the superiority of the combination versus either agent alone. Furthermore, the combination of a sedative agent with an opioid increases the risk of adverse outcomes such as respiratory depression and hypoxemia.[17] Therefore, the combination of a benzodiazepine with an opioid may be utilized, but therapy should be individualized and the agents administered separately to determine the response of the patient and if the desired level of sedation can be achieved with minimal use of drug stacking. This also underscores the need for continuous monitoring of the patient, not only to achieve adequate sedation, but also to prevent adverse outcomes associated with the effort. Repeat dosing may be required with longer procedures.

ANTIHISTAMINES

Oral antihistamines, especially diphenhydramine, have been used since the early 1960s as sedative medication for cardiac catheterization.[18] They remain a popular preprocedural medication, typically in combination with an oral benzodiazepine, due to their sedative properties and because they blunt allergic reactions to contrast media. First-generation antihistamines exert sedative effects largely through a combination of anticholinergic properties and lipophilicity, allowing the drug to easily cross the blood–brain barrier and affect histamine-mediated neurologic function.[19] Diphenhydramine is most often used, and due to its strong anticholinergic effects, elderly individuals appear to have more pronounced and prolonged sedative effects.[20] In combination with diazepam, a drug that is also slowly metabolized by elderly patients, this may result in excessive and/or prolonged sedation.

BENZODIAZEPINES

The most commonly used agents for sedation for cardiac catheterization are the benzodiazepines, which act at the gamma-aminobutyric acid (GABA) complex in the CNS and produce hypnosis, anxiolysis, and an amnestic effect. Several methods of dosing are commonly utilized in the cardiac catheterization lab, including premedication with oral benzodiazepines (such as diazepam) and/or IV administration of rapid and short-acting benzodiazepines (such as midazolam). Drug properties of each benzodiazepine are listed in Table 6.7. Differences exist between agents in terms of onset and duration of action, with no data supporting the superiority of any benzodiazepine in terms of efficacy or safety for moderate sedation. Patients with altered clearance or significant drug–drug interactions will require either alternative benzodiazepines or lower doses. For example, patients who are elderly or those with significant liver disease will have prolonged clearance of diazepam due to slower hepatic oxidative activity and may experience a shorter recovery time with a drug that is conjugated without active metabolite formation (e.g. lorazepam).

Adverse effects of benzodiazepines in moderate sedation generally relate to respiratory depression as a result of oversedation. Hemodynamic effects are minimal, but hypotension can result with rapid administration of IV benzodiazepines containing propylene glycol (diazepam, lorazepam).

OPIATES

The opiates, such as morphine, fentanyl, and meperidine, are commonly used for analgesia in moderate sedation practice in combination with local anesthesia. Opiates are preferred in part due to their superior pharmacological profiles for procedural analgesia (quick onset and offset), but also due to their lack of interaction with the renal prostaglandin system (unlike nonsteroidal compounds), resulting in safer interactions with nephrotoxic contrast media. Unfortunately, opiates carry a greater risk of respiratory depression, particularly in combination with benzodiazepines, and their use should only occur with careful monitoring of the patient. Table 6.8

Table 6.7 Selected benzodiazepines for use in procedural sedation

	Dose		Peak effect	Duration of effect	Metabolic pathway	Active metabolite?	Protein binding (%)
Midazolam	IV: 0.5–2 mg Max: 5–10 mg		3–5 min	30–80 min	Oxidation	Yes	95
Diazepam	Oral: 5 mg	IV: 5–10 mg Max: 20 mg	Oral: 30 min IV: 8–10 min	2–4 h	Oxidation	Yes	80
Lorazepam	Oral: 4 mg	IV: 2 mg Max: 4 mg	Oral: 60–90 min IV: 15–20 min	6–8 h	Conjugation	No	85

Table 6.8 Selected opiates for use in procedural sedation

	Dose	Peak effect	Duration of effect	Active metabolite?	Cardiovascular effects	Protein binding (%)
Fentanyl	IV: 25–50 mcg Max: 3 mcg/kg	1 min	30–60 min	No	Low	80–86
Morphine	IV: 1–2 mg Max: 0.15 mg/kg	1–2 min	3–4 h	Yes	Moderate	20–30
Meperidine	IV: 10–20 mg Max: 1.5 mg/kg	1–2 min	2–3 h	Yes	Low	65–80

lists the various opiates that could be considered for use during cardiac catheterization. Of note, meperidine should not be used in patients with severe renal insufficiency as seizures may be provoked via active metabolite accumulation.

SPECIAL ISSUES

Local anesthetic allergies

While occasionally patients report a history of an allergic reaction to a local anesthetic, there is no documentation of a true IgE-mediated hypersensitivity reaction to amide anesthetics, which are the most commonly employed in vascular procedures.[21] In many cases, these reactions are misclassified adverse effects or allergic responses from preservatives (e.g., methylparaben) or other excipients contained within the anesthetic solution, such as bisulfate compounds designed to prevent oxidation of vasoconstrictors. There is some potential for certain local anesthetics containing ester compounds (i.e., prilocaine, tetracaine, or benzocaine), which are derivatives of para-aminobenzoic acid (PABA), to cause an allergic reaction because their structures contain a potentially immunogenic amine substitution. When confronted with a history consistent with an anesthetic-induced allergic reaction, the safest course of action without undergoing allergy testing would be to choose an amide anesthetic (i.e., lidocaine, mepivicaine, bupivacaine, or ropivacaine) in a preservative-free solution (typically denoted

as "MPF" or "methylparaben free") that does not contain a vasoconstrictor. The use of an amine anesthetic could be considered when faced with an uncertain history of allergy in a patient receiving preservative-free amide anesthetic.

Reversal of sedation and analgesia

Pharmacologic antagonists are available for both opiates and benzodiazepines (Table 6.9) and should be immediately accessible for use. Naloxone is a competitive antagonist at all receptors affected by opiates (mu, kappa, sigma) and possesses no agonist effects. Complete antagonism of analgesic response, although sometimes necessary, can result in severe onset of pain and physiological pain response (hypertension, tachycardia) by the patient and may require further intervention. Flumazenil is an antagonist of the benzodiazepine receptor and is beneficial in reversing the CNS-depressant effects of the benzodiazepines; reversal of benzodiazepine-induced respiratory depression is less clear, although some literature supports this.[22] Caution must be exercised in complete reversal in the patient receiving long-term benzodiazepine therapy, as this may provoke withdrawal symptoms, including seizures.[23] Of note, many benzodiazepines and opiates have longer elimination half-lives than their pharmacologic antagonists and may require additional doses. Successful reversal should be followed up with an appropriate duration of monitoring based on

Table 6.9 Pharmacological reversal of sedation and analgesia

	Dose	Peak effect	Duration of effect
Flumazenil (benzodiazepine antagonist)	IV: 0.2 mg initial Max (total): 1 mg	6–10 min	1–4 h
Naloxone (opioid antagonist)	IV: 0.4 mg initial Max (total): 2 mg	5–10 min	45 min–3 h

Source: Reproduced from Dunn, S.P., Local anesthetics, sedatives, and reversing agents, In: Moliterno, D.J., et al., eds., *CathSAP 3 (Cardiac Catheterization and Interventional Cardiology Self-Assessment Program)*, American College of Cardiology Foundation, Washington, DC, 2008, pp. 437–443. With permission. All rights reserved.
Note: IV, intravenous.

the elimination half-life of the offending agent and particularly close attention should be paid to patients with altered drug clearance.

FUTURE DIRECTIONS

While current methods to achieve moderate sedation are effective, there remains room for improvement in the efficacy and safety of sedation practice. An ideal agent would be a drug that has rapid onset and offset, minimal effects on respiratory function at maximal efficacy, and is not affected by altered organ function.

Literature exists for the use of ketamine as an alternative analgesic agent, which also produces a "dissociative" anesthetic effect.[24] Although the mechanism of action of ketamine is not entirely clear, it appears to act on a wide variety of CNS receptors, including n-methyl-d-aspartate (NMDA) opiate, serotonin, and norepinephrine receptors.[24] An advantage of ketamine in procedural sedation is that it has minimal effects on respiratory function, which may render it more desirable in situations where intensive analgesia is required.

Dexmedetomidine has also gained considerable interest as a central alpha-2 agonist that achieves adequate sedation without affecting respiratory function.[25] Although it is more selective for alpha-2 receptors than its structural relative clonidine,[25] significant decreases in blood pressure and heart rate have been noted with its use that may limit widespread applicability to patients with significant cardiovascular disease.

CONCLUSIONS

The preferred level of sedation during cardiac catheterization is defined as moderate sedation. Sedation requires constant monitoring to ensure adequate efficacy without oversedation. Short-acting benzodiazepines are the preferred pharmacologic agents to induce sedation in the catheterization lab and may be paired with opioid analgesia, with extreme care to avoid oversedation. While variability in individual sedation practice exists, a systematic approach to administering and monitoring conscious sedation aids in improving patient comfort during cardiac catheterization, while avoiding potential adverse effects.

REFERENCES

1. Bashore TM, et al. 2012 American College of Cardiology Foundation/Society for Cardiovascular Angiography and Interventions expert consensus document on cardiac catheterization laboratory standards update: A report of the American College of Cardiology Foundation Task Force on Expert Consensus documents developed in collaboration with the Society of Thoracic Surgeons and Society for Vascular Medicine. *J Am Coll Cardiol* 2012;59(24):2221–2305.
2. American Society of Anesthesiologists Task Force on Sedation and Analgesia by Non-Anesthesiologists. Practice Guidelines for sedation and analgesia by non-anesthesiologists. *Anesthesiology* 2002;96(4):1004–1017.
3. Mallampati SR, et al. A clinical sign to predict difficult tracheal intubation: A prospective study. *Can Anaesth Soc J* 1985;32(4):429–434.
4. Aldrete JA, Kroulik D. A postanesthetic recovery score. *Anesth Analg* 1970;49(6):924–934.
5. American Society of Anesthesiologists. *Standards for Basic Anesthetic Monitoring*. 2010. Available at: https://www.asahq.org/~/media/Sites/ASAHQ/Files/Public/Resources/standards-guidelines/standards-for-basic-anesthetic-monitoring.pdf. Accessed April 14, 2016.
6. Beitz A, et al. Capnographic monitoring reduces the incidence of arterial oxygen desaturation and hypoxemia during propofol sedation for colonoscopy: A randomized, controlled study (ColoCap Study). *Am J Gastroenterol* 2012;107(8):1205–1212.
7. Mehta PP, et al. Capnographic monitoring in routine EGD and colonoscopy with moderate sedation: A prospective, randomized, controlled trial. *Am J Gastroenterol* 2016;111(3):395–404.
8. Hollmann MW, et al. Local anesthetic inhibition of G protein-coupled receptor signaling by interference with Galpha(q) protein function. *Mol Pharmacol* 2001;59(2):294–301.
9. Xiong Z, et al. Local anesthetics inhibit the G protein-mediated modulation of K+ and Ca++ currents in anterior pituitary cells. *Mol Pharmacol* 1999;55(1):150–158.
10. Mather LE, Chang DH. Cardiotoxicity with modern local anaesthetics: Is there a safer choice? *Drugs* 2001;61(3):333–342.
11. David JS, et al. Effects of bupivacaine, levobupivacaine and ropivacaine on myocardial relaxation. *Can J Anaesth* 2007;54(3):208–217.
12. Niwa H, et al. Cardiovascular response to epinephrine-containing local anesthesia in patients with cardiovascular disease. *Oral Surg Oral Med Oral Pathol Oral Radiol Endod* 2001;92(6):610–616.

13. Rosenberg M. The cardiovascular response of oral and maxillofacial surgeons during administration of local and general anesthesia. *J Oral Maxillofac Surg* 1987;45(4):306–308.

14. Karmakar MK, et al. Arterial and venous pharmacokinetics of ropivacaine with and without epinephrine after thoracic paravertebral block. *Anesthesiology* 2005;103(4):704–711.

15. Yagiela JA. Intravascular lidocaine toxicity: Influence of epinephrine and route of administration. *Anesth Prog* 1985;32(2):57–61.

16. Kennedy PT, et al. Conscious sedation and analgesia for routine aortofemoral arteriography: A prospective evaluation. *Radiology* 2000;216(3):660–664.

17. Bailey PL, et al. Frequent hypoxemia and apnea after sedation with midazolam and fentanyl. *Anesthesiology* 1990;73(5):826–830.

18. Akdikmen SA, et al. Diphenhydramine hydrochloride in premedication for cardiac catheterization. *Anesth Analg* 1966;45(3):293–297.

19. Carruthers SG, et al. Correlation between plasma diphenhydramine level and sedative and antihistamine effects. *Clin Pharmacol Ther* 1978;23(4):375–382.

20. Agostini JV, et al. Cognitive and other adverse effects of diphenhydramine use in hospitalized older patients. *Arch Intern Med* 2001;161(17):2091–2097.

21. Becker DE, Reed KL. Essentials of local anesthetic pharmacology. *Anesth Prog* 2006 Fall;53(3):98–108.

22. Pitman V, et al. Flumazenil for reversal of respiratory depression. *Am J Hosp Pharm* 1994;51(2):235–236,239.

23. Penninga EI, et al. Adverse events associated with flumazenil treatment for the management of suspected benzodiazepine intoxication—A systematic review with meta-analyses of randomised trials. *Basic Clin Pharmacol Toxicol* 2016;118(1):37–44.

24. White PF, et al. Ketamine—Its pharmacology and therapeutic uses. *Anesthesiology* 1982;56(2):119–136.

25. Peden CJ, Prys-Roberts C. Dexmedetomidine—A powerful new adjunct to anaesthesia? *Br J Anaesth* 1992;68(2):123–125.

7

Vasopressors, vasodilators, and antithrombotics in the catheterization laboratory

TRACY E. MACAULAY AND DAVID J. MOLITERNO

INTRODUCTION

This chapter provides an overview of medications commonly used during cardiac catheterization and interventional procedures. It focuses on medications that provide hemodynamic optimization during procedures, as well as agents used to prevent thrombotic complications. Other chapters addressing specific clinical scenarios (e.g., ST-segment elevation myocardial infarction [STEMI]) may address individual treatments in more detail, while this chapter serves as a broad overview of pharmacology, therapeutic applications, monitoring, and safety of pharmacologic agents.

VASOACTIVE OVERVIEW

In critically ill patients, hemodynamic stability can be achieved using mechanical support with intra-aortic balloon pumps and mechanical assist devices. However, an initial pharmacologic approach is typically preferred. The main goal of using vasoactive medications is to maintain tissue perfusion and optimize oxygen delivery. Although hemodynamic goals vary depending on the situation, the overall goal of meeting metabolic demands and preventing multisystem organ dysfunction and death remains the same.[1,2] When considering the use of vasodilators, inotropes, and vasopressors, the aim is to provide adequate oxygen delivery while also maintaining adequate perfusion pressure. This approach limits myocardial oxygen demand and ischemia, as well as other deleterious effects associated with these agents.

ANATOMIC CONSIDERATIONS WITH VASOACTIVE AGENTS

Vasodilator therapy is most frequently used in the treatment of hypertension. It is also useful in patients with left ventricular systolic dysfunction (LVSD)—with or without pulmonary edema—in whom both acute and chronic therapy has demonstrated a mortality reduction.[3,4] In the catheterization laboratory, these medications can be given systemically to lower peripheral vascular resistance or locally as direct coronary arterial vasodilators. Some vasodilators may also be used in the characterization and treatment of pulmonary arterial hypertension.

Intravenous (IV) inotropic therapy is often necessary for the treatment of cardiogenic shock, particularly in patients with LVSD. In cardiogenic shock, a decrease in cardiac output results in a hypoperfusion state, thereby increasing adrenergic drive. The release of endogenous catecholamines may be temporarily effective; however, it may be necessary to stimulate beta-1 receptors or administer phosphodiesterase (PDE) inhibitors to augment cardiac output.[5] Use of inotropic agents such as dobutamine or milrinone to achieve an adequate cardiac index of 2.2 L/min/m^2 may provide necessary circulatory support, but they do not provide a mortality benefit.[6–8] Temporary increases in cardiac preload and afterload may also be required and can be achieved by increasing intravascular volume (blood or intravenous fluids) and/or stimulation of alpha-receptors in the periphery.

When treating patients with vasopressor therapy, targeting a minimal perfusion pressure or mean arterial pressure of approximately 65 mmHg is widely accepted.[9] Because blood pressure is not an isolated determinant of adequate oxygen delivery, advanced hemodynamic monitoring and individualized goals are appropriate. This will allow for selection of the appropriate vasoactive medication based on the clinical situation while limiting deleterious side effects.

PHARMACOLOGIC FUNDAMENTALS

Vasodilators

NITRIC OXIDE

Nitric oxide (NO) is a potent vasodilator that acts through stimulation of guanylate cyclase, which leads to the formation of cyclic guanosine monophosphate (cGMP). In turn, cGMP activates protein kinase G, leading to reuptake of calcium and opening of calcium-activated potassium channels. Ultimately, the fluctuation in calcium concentration ensures that myosin light-chain kinase can no longer be phosphorylated, leading to vascular smooth muscle cell relaxation. Within the cardiac catheterization laboratory, pharmacologically available inhaled NO is the gold standard for vasodilatory challenges.

NITROGLYCERIN

Nitroglycerin (NTG) provides an exogenous source of NO, which works by increasing vascular cGMP, resulting in smooth muscle relaxation (Table 7.1). NTG's major effect is in preload reduction, making it an ideal choice for the hypertensive patient with elevated pulmonary capillary wedge pressure (PCWP). For the same reason, caution should be used in administering it to patients who are preload-dependent, such as those with right ventricular failure (or acute infarction involving the right ventricle). NTG also causes endothelium-independent coronary artery dilation, antagonizes vasoconstriction and vasospasm, and increases collateral vessel blood flow. These effects make it useful in treatment of ischemic symptoms, although no mortality reduction has been demonstrated in large clinical trials of patients with myocardial infarction (MI).[10,11] Tachyphylaxis can develop within 24 hours of continuous NTG therapy, but can generally be overcome by increasing the dose or providing a nitrate-free interval.[5]

SODIUM NITROPRUSSIDE

Sodium nitroprusside is an endothelium-independent vasodilator like NTG, though it has greater arterial than venous vasodilating properties.[12] Unlike other vasodilators, nitroprusside causes only mild increases in heart rate. The molecular composition of sodium nitroprusside includes five cyanide ions, which can accumulate systemically as either cyanide or thiocyanate in patients with liver or renal failure, respectively. Patients receiving high doses (10 mcg/kg/min) of nitroprusside for a prolonged time (>2 days) are particularly at risk of cyanide or thiocyanate toxicity. Nitroprusside is the recommended intravenous antihypertensive for hypertensive emergency because of its remarkable effectiveness and rapid onset (and resolution) of action (Table 7.2).

ADENOSINE

Adenosine is a purine nucleoside involved in cellular metabolism. Exogenously administered adenosine decreases sinus

Table 7.1 Vasodilator overview

Generic (brand)	Starting dose	Maintenance and titration	Intracoronary dose	ADR	Precautions and CI	Uses
Nitroglycerin (nitrostat IV)	5 mcg/min	Increase every 3 min to maximum 200 mcg/min	50–250 mcg	Headache, tachyphylaxis	RV failure (preload-dependent patients)	Used to treat symptoms of ischemia at low doses, hypertension with or without pulmonary edema at higher doses
Nitroprusside (nipride)	0.5 mcg/kg/min	Increase every 5 min to maximum of 5–10 mcg/kg/min (ideally for <48 h)	25–100 mcg	With prolonged use (or high doses) cyanide toxicity and methemoglobinemia may develop	Severe renal or liver impairment, COPD	Cardiac failure due to increase afterload, ADHF, vasodilatory challenges (pulmonary HTN)

(Continued)

Table 7.1 (Continued) Vasodilator overview

Generic (brand)	Starting dose	Maintenance and titration	Intracoronary dose	ADR	Precautions and CI	Uses
Diltiazem (cardizem)	For arrhythmias 10 mg IVP (0.25 mg/kg)	5–20 mg/h continuous infusion. Consider rebolus with each uptitration		AV blockade	LVSD, AV blockade, sick sinus syndrome, WPW	AF/flutter, PSVT
Verapamil (isoptin)	For arrhythmias 2.5–5 mg IVP		100–200 mcg (up to 4 times)	AV blockade	LVSD, AV blockade, sick sinus syndrome, WPW	AF/flutter, PSVT
Nicardipine (cardene)		3–15 mg/h		Hypotension, tachycardia, headache, peripheral edema	Severe aortic stenosis, peripheral edema	Stability of more concentrated solution unknown, therefore infusion provides large volume of fluid
Adenosine			12–24 mcg			

Note: ADR, adverse drug reaction; ADHF, acute decompensated heart failure; AF, atrial flutter; AV, atrioventricular; CI, contraindications; COPD, chronic obstructive pulmonary disease; HTN, hypertension; IV, intravenous; IVP, intravenous push; LVSD, left ventricular systolic dysfunction; PSVT, paroxysmal supraventricular tachycardia; RV, right ventricular; WPW, Wolff-Parkinson-White syndrome.

Table 7.2 Comparison of intravenous vasodilators

	NTG	Nitroprusside	Diltiazem	Verapamil	Nicardipine	Clevidipine
MOA	Exogenous NO, cyclic guanosine monophosphate					
Overall hemodynamic effect	Venovasodilation	Arterial and venous dilator	Decrease heart rate and vasodilation	Decrease heart rate and vasodilation	Decrease blood pressure	Decrease blood pressure
Contractility	0	0	2	4	0	
Heart rate	0	1 (reflex)	0/1	0/1	1 (reflex)	
SA automaticity	0	0	4	4	0	
Atrioventricular conduction	0	0	4	5	0	
Vasodilation	2	4	3	4	5	

Note: 0 to 5, none to substantial; MOA, mechanism of action; NO, nitric oxide; NTG, nitroglycerin; SA, sinoatrial.

node automaticity and slows atrioventricular (AV) node conduction, interrupting reentry pathways; it can restore sinus rhythm in some dysrhythmias.[13,14] The most common therapeutic use for adenosine is treatment of AV nodal reentrant tachycardia. For this purpose, adenosine is given as a 6 mg IV rapid injection. After 2 minutes, if the 6 mg dose is not effective, a 12 mg bolus can be given and then repeated if needed (for a total dose of 30 mg). With this regimen, AV nodal reentrant tachycardia is terminated with a nearly 90% success rate. When administering adenosine, it is important to follow each dose with an intravenous flush to ensure rapid distribution, as the onset of action is immediate and the duration of effect is mere seconds. Importantly, when given through a central venous catheter, the aforementioned doses should be halved, as there are case reports of full-dose adenosine initiating atrial fibrillation. In cardiac catheterization, adenosine can be used to evaluate coronary flow reserve since it causes maximal coronary vasodilation. The benefit of its short half-life is that adverse effects (angina, dyspnea, AV nodal block, and flushing) are very transient.

CALCIUM CHANNEL BLOCKERS

Calcium channel blockers (CCBs) inhibit calcium from entering "slow channels" or voltage-sensitive areas of vascular smooth muscle, producing smooth muscle relaxation and vasodilation. CCBs are classified as dihydropyridine or non-dihydropyridine on the basis of differences in structure and pharmacologic effects. Diltiazem and verapamil are non-dihydropyridines and offer greater negative chronotropic effects than dihydropyridines. Both non-dihydropyridine agents slow AV nodal conduction and exert a negative inotropic effect. In the catheterization laboratory, these agents are most often used for treatment of rapid ventricular rate secondary to atrial fibrillation. Nifedipine is the prototypical dihydropyridine CCB, although newer second-generation agents are more often used in the acute setting. Dihydropyridines have selectivity for peripheral vasculature, resulting in extensive blood pressure lowering with little to no direct effect on heart rate. In fact, more often compensatory tachycardia is observed following administration of a dihydropyridine CCB. Use in the setting of an acute coronary syndrome (ACS) or among patients with heart failure is controversial, as they can result in fluid retention in addition to adrenergic activation.

INOTROPES

Inotropic agents are indicated for the treatment of low-output heart failure in patients with elevated left ventricular filling pressures.[14] Effects are either directly mediated through beta-1 adrenergic receptor agonism or indirectly through an increase in intracellular cyclic adenosine monophosphate (cAMP), increasing ventricular contractility and heart rate and thereby cardiac output (Table 7.3). All inotropes have arrhythmogenic properties, and, as such, should be reserved for acutely ill patients and used for the shortest duration necessary.

DOBUTAMINE AND ISOPROTERENOL

Dobutamine and isoproterenol primarily act as beta-1 adrenergic-receptor agonists, but dobutamine also exhibits mild beta-2 and alpha-adrenergic receptor effects (beta-1 >> beta-2 > alpha).[15] For inotropy in left ventricular heart failure, dobutamine infusion doses of 1 to 20 mcg/kg/min are used. Isoproterenol has more chronotropic effects than dobutamine and is used for treatment of bradycardia post cardiac transplantation and to prevent recurrence of torsades de pointes.[16] Inotropes are not indicated as monotherapy in shock as they provide little effect on blood pressure.

MILRINONE

Milrinone is a selective PDE inhibitor that increases vascular PDE III and intracellular cAMP in cardiac tissue.[8] Pharmacologic effects include positive inotropy (increasing cardiac output) and peripheral vasodilation (decreasing cardiac myocardial oxygen demands and PCWP). Additional benefits include both positive lusitropy (improved diastole) and pulmonary arterial vasodilation. Like dobutamine, milrinone is indicated for severe LVSD. Milrinone may be more beneficial than dobutamine in patients on chronic beta-blockade therapy (based on its nonadrenergic mechanism) and in those with normal to high blood pressure. Conversely, milrinone is eliminated via the kidneys and should be avoided or administered at a reduced dose in patients with severe renal dysfunction. No difference in clinical outcomes or arrhythmogenicity has been demonstrated in comparisons of dobutamine and milrinone among hospitalized patients awaiting cardiac transplantation.[17] In comparison to placebo, short-term use of milrinone for mild to moderate heart failure exacerbation did not decrease hospital length of stay and was associated with an increase in arrhythmias,[7] further supporting that inotropic agents should be reserved for use in patients with severe heart failure.

VASOPRESSORS

During cardiac catheterization, it may be necessary to provide temporary hemodynamic support for a patient in shock or experiencing severe hypotension. This sometimes requires use of vasopressors, most commonly dopamine,

Table 7.3 Inotrope overview

Generic name	Brand name	Starting dose	Maintenance and titration	PK properties	Adverse effects
Dobutamine	Dobutrex	1 mcg/kg/min	20 mcg/kg/min	Metabolized by methylation and conjugation, renal excretion of inactive metabolites, $t_{1/2}$ 2 min	Angina, hypertension, tachyarrhythmia, headache
Isoproterenol	Isuprel	0.01 mcg/kg/min	Increase every 5 min to maximum 0.3 mcg/kg/min	Hepatic metabolism, $t_{1/2}$ 3–5 min	Syncope, tachyarrhythmia, confusion, tremor
Milrinone	Primacor	0.25 mcg/kg/min	0.75 mcg/kg/min	Renal excretion (83% unchanged), $t_{1/2}$ 2.3 h (prolonged in renal failure)	Ventricular arrhythmias, hypotension, headache

Note: PK, pharmacokinetic.

Table 7.4 Vasopressor overview

Drug type and generic name	Brand name	Starting dose	Maintenance and titration
Dopamine	Intropin	3–10 mcg/kg/min	Up to 20 mcg/kg/min
Epinephrine	Adrenalin	1 mcg/min	10 mcg/min
Norepinephrine	Levophed	2 mcg/min	30 mcg/min
Phenylephrine	Neo-Synephrine	100 mcg/min	Decrease to maintenance of 40–60 mcg/min
Vasopressin	Pitressin	0.01 units/min	0.04 units/min

norepinephrine, epinephrine, or phenylephrine (Table 7.4). Administration of medications with vasoconstrictive properties requires use of a central venous catheter to avoid tissue ischemia that can occur with extravasation. If extravasation does occur, phentolamine, an alpha-adrenergic blocking agent, can be injected directly into the areas of ischemic tissue, and warm compresses should be applied.

DOPAMINE

Dopamine exhibits unique pharmacologic actions according to dosage. Low-dose infusion (<5 mcg/kg/min) primarily stimulates dopaminergic (DA) receptor activity, resulting in vasodilation, with resultant increases in renal, mesenteric, and coronary blood flow. Historically, low or "renal-dose" dopamine was thought to be renal protective and beneficial in preventing contrast-induced nephropathy. However, studies show no certain evidence of a renal-protective benefit with dopamine in patients.[18-20] Dopamine infusions of 3 to 10 mcg/kg/min stimulate beta-1 and beta-2-adrenergic receptors (beta-1 > beta-2), resulting in similar inotropic effects as dobutamine. At maximal infusion doses of 10 to 20 mcg/kg/min, alpha-adrenergic receptor agonism predominates, providing blood pressure support. Doses in this range can increase myocardial oxygen demand, resulting in myocardial ischemia, limiting its attractiveness in ACS. Pulmonary vein vasoconstriction can occur in patients receiving dopamine, therefore, rendering PCWP measurement less reliable as an estimate of left ventricular end-diastolic filling pressure.[9]

NOREPINEPHRINE AND EPINEPHRINE

Norepinephrine and epinephrine exhibit mixed receptor activity. Norepinephrine has potent beta-1 and alpha-adrenergic receptor activity, with less beta-2 activity. This translates clinically into more potent vasoconstrictive properties and less inotropic effects as compared with dopamine. For this reason, norepinephrine remains the initial catecholamine of choice for septic or vasodilatory shock. Epinephrine is the most potent agonist for the beta-1, beta-2, and alpha-adrenergic receptors. Adverse effects—including arrhythmias, ischemia, tachycardia, hyperglycemia, cerebral hemorrhage, pulmonary edema, and diminished splanchnic blood flow—limit use of continuous epinephrine infusion. As such, epinephrine should be reserved for patients who are unresponsive to dopamine or norepinephrine.[21]

Epinephrine has a role in treatment of pulseless ventricular tachycardia, ventricular fibrillation, asystole, and pulseless electrical activity. Epinephrine at doses of 0.5 to 1 mg intravenous bolus (0.1 to 0.5 mg intracardiac or 0.1 mg/kg given via endotracheal tube) remains the first-line medication for use in advanced cardiac life support and the most common reason for its use in cardiac catheterization procedures. Another emergent use is in anaphylactoid reactions to medications or, more commonly, contrast agents. For systemic anaphylactoid reactions (i.e., hypotension), epinephrine should be given as an intravenous bolus dose of 10 mcg. This dose should be repeated in 1-minute intervals until an intravenous infusion of epinephrine can be initiated or until the patient's hemodynamics have been adequately stabilized. A 10 mcg/mL syringe of epinephrine for this use can be rapidly prepared by diluting 0.1 mL of 1:1000 epinephrine to 1 mL with saline or (more easily) diluting 1 mL of 1:10,000 epinephrine to a total volume of 10 mL. For less severe reactions, epinephrine 0.3 to 0.5 mg (0.3–0.5 mL of 1:1000 solution) can be given subcutaneously or intramuscularly. Repeated doses are often necessary while steroids and other treatments take effect.

Vasopressin, given as a bolus of 40 units, can be used as an alternative to epinephrine in acute cardiac arrest.[22] The proposed mechanism of vasopressin activity is maintenance of vascular tone and modulation of cardiovascular homeostasis.[21,23] One potential advantage of vasopressin over epinephrine is in patients with acidosis, as catecholamine response is diminished in these patients. In patients with vasodilatory shock despite norepinephrine treatment, the addition of vasopressin infusion is recommended.

PHENYLEPHRINE

Phenylephrine is the drug of choice when a clinical situation calls for pure vasoconstriction. Phenylephrine is an alpha-adrenergic receptor agonist with no beta receptor activity. It is the preferred agent for treatment of anesthetic-induced hypotension or unopposed parasympathetic activity (i.e., spinal cord injuries). Dosing typically begins at 100 to 180 mcg/min infusion until blood pressure is stable, and then infusion is decreased to a maintenance dose of 40–60 mcg/min. The potent vasoconstrictor activity may cause a reflexive decrease in adrenergic drive. Therefore, caution should be exercised in administering it to patients

Table 7.5 Hemodynamic effects of vasopressors and inotropes[a]

Drug type, generic (brand)	HR	MAP	PAWP	SVRI	CO	Receptor activity
Vasopressors						
Dopamine (Inotropin)	2					
<3		0	0	0	0	$D > b_1$
3–10		1	1	0	1	$b_1 > b_2 > D$
>10		2	2	1	1	$a_1 > b_1 \gg b_2$
Epinephrine (Adrenalin)	3					
<0.05		0	0	0/1	3	$b_1 \gg b_2$
0.05–0.15		1	2	1	3	$b_1 > a_1 > b_2$
>0.15		2	2	3	2	$a_1 > b_1$
Norepinephrine (Levophed)	2	3	3	3.5	0	$a_1 \gg b_1$
Phenylephrine (Neo-Synephrine)	0	2	2	1	0	a_1
Vasopressin						
Inotropes						
Dobutamine (Dobutrex)	1					$b_1 > b_2 > a_1$
2–10		1	1	1	1	
10–20		0/1	1	0/1	2	
Isoproterenol (Isuprel)		2	2	3	3	$b_1 \gg b_2$
Amrinone (Inocor)	1	0	1	2	1	Phosphodiesterase inhibitor
Milrinone	1	2	1	2	2	Phosphodiesterase inhibitor

Note: a, alpha-adrenergic; b, beta-adrenergic; CO, cardiac output; D, dopamine, HR, heart rate; MAP, mean arterial pressure; PAWP, pulmonary artery pressure; SVR, systemic vascular resistance.

[a] All listed doses are in mcg/kg/min.

with myocardial ischemia or heart failure–induced shock where inotropy is needed. Table 7.5 details the hemodynamic effects of vasopressors and inotropes.

ANTITHROMBOTIC OVERVIEW

To prevent the two most frequent complications associated with percutaneous coronary intervention (PCI)—thrombosis and bleeding—it is important to achieve adequate protection from thrombosis without resultant hemorrhage. This balance is reached by using an optimal combination of anticoagulant and antiplatelet medications. The ideal extent of anticoagulation is the lowest possible, yet adequately effective, regimen. This section examines currently approved U.S. Food and Drug Administration (FDA) antithrombotic medications that are used to manage ACS and support cardiac catheterization.

ANATOMIC CONSIDERATIONS WITH ANTITHROMBOTIC AGENTS

Under normal circumstances, opposing mechanisms finely regulate the body's hemostatic system. Prostacyclin, NO, tissue plasminogen activator, thrombomodulin, protein C, and protein S protect against coagulation in individuals with intact endothelium. In cases of vascular damage, life-threatening hemorrhage may be prevented by thrombus formation. However, the same thrombotic mechanisms are activated when coronary endothelial damage occurs (as in ACS), and this can result in deleterious effects. Exposure of circulating blood to the thrombogenic subendothelial surface results in platelet activation and aggregation, release of vasoconstriction substances and fibrin formation, which further stimulates platelet activity. Once formed, a thrombus may be degraded by endogenous or therapeutic thrombolysis, or mechanically via balloon angioplasty, which may promote further platelet activation and thrombosis.

Two types of agents discussed in this chapter act on different aspects of the thrombotic process. Antiplatelet medications prevent platelet aggregation, while anticoagulants limit fibrin formation. These differing mechanisms of action allow for additive, or potentially synergistic, effects resulting in greater efficacy with combination (antiplatelet and antithrombin) therapy. Unfortunately, combination therapy also increases bleeding risk

PHARMACOLOGIC FUNDAMENTALS

Antiplatelet agents

Currently available antiplatelet medications target various aspects of platelet function (Figure 7.1). Antiplatelet medications can protect against platelet activation,

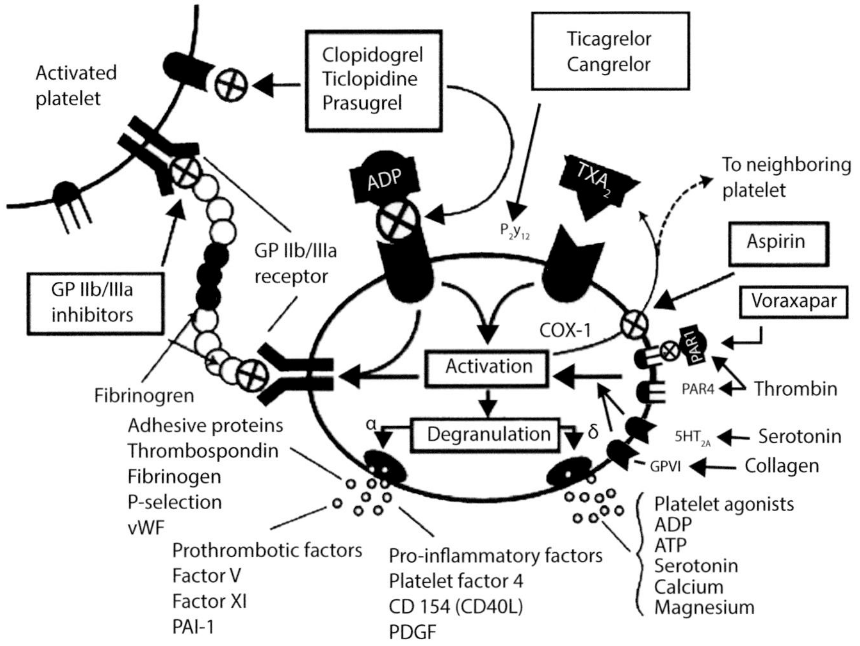

Figure 7.1 Platelet activation is an important early step in the pathophysiology of atherothrombosis. Platelet activation involves (1) a shape change in which the platelet membrane surface area is greatly increased; (2) the release of proinflammatory, prothrombotic, vasoconstrictor, and chemotactic mediators; and (3) activation of the GP IIb/IIIa receptor. Multiple agonists, including thromboxane A2, adenosine diphosphate, thrombin, serotonin, epinephrine, and collagen, can activate the platelet and thus contribute toward establishing the environmental conditions necessary for platelet aggregation. Aspirin inhibits the production of thromboxane A2 by its effect on the enzyme cyclooxygenase-1. Ticlopidine, clopidogrel, and prasugrel prevent the binding of adenosine diphosphate to the $P2Y_{12}$ receptor. Direct blockade is achieved through $P2Y_{12}$ blockade with ticagrelor. Combining aspirin and a $P2Y_{12}$ inhibitor results in synergistic prevention of platelet aggregation. Vorapaxar inhibits platelet activity via antagonism of the protease-activated receptor-1. Antithrombins, such as unfractionated or low molecular weight heparin, hirudin, or bivalirudin, are important in interfering with both thrombin-induced platelet activation and coagulation. The glycoprotein IIb/IIIa receptor antagonists prevent fibrinogen-mediated cross-linking of platelets, which have already become activated. ADP, adenosine diphosphate; ATP, adenosine triphosphate; COX-1, cyclooxygenase-1; GP, glycoprotein; 5-HT, 5-hydroxytryptamine; PAI, plasminogen activator inhibitor; PAR, protease-activated receptor; PDGF, platelet-derived growth factor; TXA_2, thromboxane A_2; vWF, von Willebrand factor. (Adapted from Mehta, S.R., and Yusuf, S., *J. Am. Coll. Cardiol.*, 21, 79S–88S, 2004.)

aggregation, adhesion, and platelet-induced vasoconstriction. Pharmacologic targets include inhibition of thromboxane A_2 (TXA_2), $P2Y_{12}$ receptor inhibition (directly or via adenosine diphosphate [ADP] blockade), as well as blockade of the glycoprotein (GP) IIb/IIIa receptor, the final common pathway of platelet aggregation. Dual antiplatelet therapy (DAPT)—with aspirin (a TXA_2 blocker) and a $P2Y_{12}$ receptor blocker—has become a mainstay of ACS management and early treatment following PCI.

ACETYLSALICYLIC ACID

Acetylsalicylic acid (aspirin) was the first antiplatelet therapy used clinically. Aspirin exerts its antiplatelet effect via irreversible acetylation of cyclooxygenase-1 (COX-1), which prevents arachidonic acid–induced production of TXA_2. Thereby, both TXA_2-mediated platelet aggregation and vasoconstriction are inhibited for the life of the platelet.[25] Aspirin improves cardiovascular outcomes in the setting of acute MI and stroke, and in the secondary prevention of related ischemic events.[26] Risk reduction in cardiovascular events also extends to secondary prevention among patients

with unstable angina, coronary angioplasty, transient ischemic attack (TIA), atrial fibrillation, and peripheral arterial disease.[26]

In addition to the desired therapeutic effects, inhibition of COX-1 can reduce protective gastric prostaglandin and cause direct gastric irritation, resulting in gastrointestinal bleeding. Bleeding events requiring hospitalization are infrequent[27] but are more common with aspirin doses exceeding 325 mg daily or in combination with other antiplatelet agents.[28] Therefore, use of the lowest effective aspirin dose is important. Maximal antiplatelet effects of aspirin can be achieved with as little as 30 mg oral dose once daily.[29] In secondary prevention of TIA, a daily aspirin dose as low as 30 mg is as effective as higher doses (282 mg daily), with fewer adverse effects.[30] The disadvantage of a low aspirin dose is that it may take up to 2 days to achieve maximal inhibition. Therefore, when immediate antiplatelet effect is desired, aspirin-naive patients should be administered 300 to 325 mg of non-enteric-coated aspirin.[31] For chronic therapy, 81 to 100 mg daily aspirin is recommended.

P2Y$_{12}$ INHIBITORS

A P2Y$_{12}$ inhibitor (Table 7.6) is given along with aspirin for both acute and chronic management of ACS. Thienopyridines—clopidogrel, prasugrel, and ticlopidine—irreversibly inhibit the binding of ADP to the P2Y$_{12}$ receptor on platelets, thereby preventing the transformation of a platelet to its activated form. Given its unfavorable side-effect profile compared with other thienopyridines, ticlopidine is seldom used.[32,33] Monotherapy with clopidogrel is indicated for patients with intolerance or contraindication to aspirin and for the secondary prevention of ischemic stroke. In contrast to the other P2Y$_{12}$ receptor inhibitors, ticagrelor has a binding site different from ADP, making it an allosteric antagonist, and the blockage is reversible. In aspirin-treated ACS patients, both prasugrel and ticagrelor are associated with fewer major cardiac events but increased bleeding risk than clopidogrel.[34,35]

Most commonly, a thienopyridine is used in conjunction with aspirin following coronary artery stenting or ACS. Short-term use of DAPT following placement of bare-metal stents was established in the late 1990s when studies demonstrated that concomitant administration of aspirin and a thienopyridine decreased the incidence of life-threatening subacute stent thrombosis and major adverse cardiovascular events following PCI in comparison to aspirin therapy alone.[36,37] Superior efficacy and safety of DAPT was also seen among patients undergoing PCI who were randomized to either anticoagulation (heparin bridged to phenprocoumon plus aspirin 100 mg twice daily) or antiplatelet therapy (ticlopidine 250 mg twice daily plus aspirin 100 mg twice daily) in the Intracoronary Stenting and Antithrombotic Regimen (ISAR) trial.[38] Subsequently, a clinical trial comparing aspirin alone, aspirin plus anticoagulation, and aspirin plus ticlopidine yielded similar results, with improved efficacy and less bleeding with DAPT compared to anticoagulation.[39] These trials established a minimum duration of DAPT of 30 days following bare metal stent placement.

Evidence to support DAPT beyond stent endothelization comes from several landmark clinical trials. The Clopidogrel in Unstable Angina to Prevent Recurrent Events (CURE) trial examined the effects of clopidogrel (300 mg, followed by 75 mg daily) versus placebo in addition to aspirin in 12,562 patients with ACS without ST segment elevations. The composite end point of cardiovascular death, MI, or stroke occurred less frequently with clopidogrel therapy compared with placebo (9.3% and 11.4%, respectively).[36] Also, in the Clopidogrel for the Reduction of Events During Observation (CREDO) trial, subjects who underwent planned PCI and received clopidogrel for 1 year had a lower risk of cardiovascular death, myocardial infarction (MI), and stroke compared with those treated with placebo.[37] These studies and evaluations following drug-eluting stent (DES) placement,[40–42] led to recommended use of DAPT for at least 1 year following ACS or PCI with stent placement.[43]

While clopidogrel was the early treatment of choice for DAPT, interpatient variability in its antiplatelet effects

Table 7.6 Characteristics of P2Y$_{12}$ inhibitors

	Clopidogrel	Prasugrel	Ticagrelor
Dose	LD: 300–600 mg MD: 75 mg once daily	LD: 60 mg MD: 10 mg once daily	LD: 180 mg MD: 90 mg twice daily
% ADP inhibition	50–70%	90%	90%
Onset of antiplatelet action following loading	1–8 h	30 min	30–60 min
Metabolism	Prodrug with dependent metabolism CYP3A4, CYP1A2, and CYP2C19	Prodrug rapidly metabolized/activated by esterases. Metabolized by via CYP3A4 and CYP2B6	CYP3A4 and CYP3A5
Reversibility	No	No	Yes
Duration of effect	3–10 days	5–10 days	3–4 days
Withdrawal before major elective surgery	5 days	7 days	5 days
Contraindications/ Precautions	-600 mg loading dose (not FDA approved) provides faster, greater, and more reliable platelet inhibition -CYP2C19 *2 or *3 alleles are poor metabolizers and have reduced antiplatelet effects	-Contraindicated in patients with hx CVA/TIA -Generally not recommended in patients age >75 years -Increased bleeding risk if body weight <60 kg	-Concomitant ASA dose should be <100 mg -Contraindicated if severe hepatic impairment -Avoid use with strong CYP3A inhibitors or CYP3A inducers

Note: ADP, adenosine diphosphate; ASA, aspirin; CVA, cerebrovascular accident; LD, loading dose; MD, maintenance dose; TIA, transient ischemic attack.

aroused concerns.[44] One explanation for the unpredictable response to clopidogrel is related to alterations in metabolism of this prodrug to its clinically active metabolite, which occurs via metabolism by the liver cytochromes, primarily CYP3A4, CYP1A2, and CYP2C19 isoenzymes.[45] Several potentially significant drug interactions with clopidogrel have been proposed, all involving this metabolic conversion in the liver. Atorvastatin was thought to compete with clopidogrel for CYP3A4[46]; however, this interaction was shown to be clinically irrelevant.[47–49] Likewise, decreased antiplatelet effects were observed with co-administration of proton-pump inhibitors (PPIs) and clopidogrel, likely due to the inhibition of CYP2C19.[50] Platelet assay studies and observational data from large clinical trials resulted in the FDA issuing a warning of decreased antiplatelet effects when using a combination of PPIs and clopidogrel. In contrast, the results of a large randomized placebo-controlled clinical trial showed no worsening in outcome among clopidogrel-treated patients who were also prescribed omeprazole.[51] Smoking, a known inducer of CYP1A2, may enhance the antiplatelet effects of clopidogrel by enzyme induction, though clinical relevance is not established.[52] It appears that fewer drug interactions and less interpatient variability are seen with the use of prasugrel and ticagrelor than with clopidogrel, resulting in faster, greater, and more consistent inhibition of ADP-induced platelet aggregation.[53]

These features likely contribute to the favorable clinical trial findings with prasugrel and ticagrelor compared to clopidogrel. The Therapeutic Outcomes By Optimizing Platelet Inhibition With Prasugrel Thrombolysis In Myocardial Infarction 38 (TRITON-TIMI 38) study randomized 13,608 patients with ACS and planned PCI to either prasugrel (60 mg, followed by 10 mg/day) or clopidogrel (300 mg, followed by 75 mg/day). Patients receiving prasugrel had a significant reduction in the primary composite endpoint of death from cardiovascular causes, nonfatal MI, or nonfatal stroke throughout the follow-up period of over 14 months. Increased efficacy of prasugrel over clopidogrel must be balanced with increased bleeding, including fatal bleeding, as seen in this trial.[34] Post hoc analysis revealed three groups in whom prasugrel should not be used due to excessive risk of serious bleeding: those with history of transient ischemic attack (TIA)/stroke, the elderly (>75 years), and those with a low body weight (<60 kg).

Ticagrelor, 90 or 180 mg twice daily, was compared to standard dose clopidogrel in the Platelet Inhibition And Patient Outcomes (PLATO) study[35] of 18,624 ACS patients. At 30-day and 12-month follow-up, the composite endpoint of cardiovascular death, MI, and stroke was significantly lower with ticagrelor. There was no increase in overall major bleeding; however, there was an increase in noncoronary artery bypass grafting (CABG) related bleeding. Finally, dissimilar from studies of other P2Y$_{12}$ inhibitors or GP IIb/IIIa inhibitors, there was a statistically significant reduction in all-cause mortality. A potential mechanism to explain improved outcomes over other antiplatelet agents is that ticagrelor offers other (i.e., non-ADP mediated) antiplatelet effects by inhibiting cellular uptake of adenosine, a known inhibitor of platelet aggregation.[54,55] Unfortunately, this effect is also thought to contribute to the adverse consequence of shortness of breath, seen more commonly among patients treated with ticagrelor than other P2Y$_{12}$ inhibitors.

With both prasugrel and ticagrelor showing superiority over clopidogrel with respect to thrombotic complications, questions remain on which of these agents is most effective. The Intracoronary Stenting and Antithrombotic Regimen: Rapid Early Action for Coronary Treatment (ISAR REACT) 5 study is designed to evaluate clinical outcomes comparing these two agents in patients with ACS with planned PCI.[56]

In addition to drug potency, optimal loading dose and timing of administration are important considerations. A substudy of the Clopidogrel in Unstable Angina to Prevent Recurrent Events (CURE) trial analyzed 2,658 subjects who underwent PCI.[57] Clopidogrel or placebo was started for a median of 6 days prior to PCI, with all patients receiving aspirin and thienopyridine for 4 weeks after PCI. Overall, pretreatment with clopidogrel was associated with a reduction in the composite endpoint of cardiovascular death, MI, or urgent target vessel revascularization (TVR). Similarly, a substudy of the Clopidogrel for the Reduction of Events During Observation (CREDO) trial demonstrated that patients who received a 300 mg loading dose of clopidogrel greater than 15 hours prior to PCI had a decrease in the 28-day composite endpoint of death, MI, or urgent TVR compared to those who received it at the time of PCI.[58]

Further evidence supporting clopidogrel pretreatment (particularly with a high loading dose) as an alternative to GP IIb/IIIa in low-risk patients comes from the ISAR-REACT 1[59] and ISAR-REACT 2 trials.[60] The former evaluated the use of abciximab versus placebo in 2,159 patients undergoing elective PCI, all of whom had received 600 mg of clopidogrel in advance. No difference was seen in the composite endpoint of death, MI, or urgent TVR within 30 days after randomization to abciximab or placebo (RR 1.05, 95% CI 0.69–1.59, $P = 0.82$). ISAR-REACT 2 had a similar trial design applied to 2,022 patients with non–ST elevation ACS undergoing PCI. In this higher-risk patient population, abciximab reduced the composite endpoint of death, MI, or urgent TVR at 30 days when compared with placebo (RR 0.75, 95% CI 0.58–0.97, $P = 0.03$). These studies demonstrate that clopidogrel pretreatment is sufficient for low-risk PCI; however, in patients in whom clopidogrel pretreatment is not possible or among high-risk patients (i.e., troponin positive), alternate or more potent antiplatelet strategies are needed.

Given the superior pharmacokinetic profile of newer P2Y$_{12}$ inhibitors, with both faster and more complete platelet inhibition, these agents should be preferred to support PCI. In the case of prasugrel, the TRITON design took advantage of these differences, waiting for angiography to be performed before oral administration of P2Y$_{12}$ inhibitor and potentially lending to favorable early outcomes (within the first 3 days). However, there also exists another option: the recently FDA-approved IV agent cangrelor. Cangrelor, which is similar in structure and mechanism to ticagrelor, offers several advantages. In addition to IV administration and rapid onset, it has marked and complete offset within minutes of discontinuation. While phase III clinical trials, comparing cangrelor with clopidogrel, administered before PCI (Cangrelor versus Standard Therapy to Achieve Optimal Management of Platelet Inhibition [CHAMPION] PCI) or after PCI (CHAMPION PLATFORM), failed to show clinical benefit,[61,62] the more recent CHAMPION PHOENIX demonstrated benefit in patients undergoing urgent or elective PCI compared to clopidogrel, with no significant increase in bleeding. Of note, the difference in findings is thought to be due in part to differences in definitions of peri-procedural MIs, an endpoint that drove the composite endpoint reduction in PHOENIX.[63] Cangrelor can be useful for patients undergoing urgent PCI who are not able to take oral medications.

GP IIB/IIIA RECEPTOR ANTAGONISTS

GP IIb/IIIa receptor antagonists block the final common pathway of platelet aggregation by preventing fibrinogen from binding and cross-linking platelets at the $\alpha_{IIb}\beta_3$-receptor. Interference with this process results in inhibition of approximately 80% of platelet aggregation function.[64] Three such GP IIb/IIIa inhibitor medications are FDA approved for use in conjunction with aspirin and antithrombotic therapy: abciximab, eptifibatide, and tirofiban. All are administered intravenously, providing potent antiplatelet therapy for the most critical interval following ACS diagnosis and/or stent placement. As previously mentioned, the use of clopidogrel pretreatment (which was not widespread in early GP IIb/IIIa evaluations) and newer antithrombotic regimens have lessened the role of GP IIb/IIIa inhibitors; however, they remain important for some high-risk ACS and PCI patients.[65]

The major benefits of GP IIb/IIIa inhibitors are seen among ACS patients who undergo early PCI, those with dynamic ST segment changes, and individuals with elevated troponin levels.[66] Benefit has also been established among patients with high-risk features such as diabetes.[67] Additionally, use of these agents prior to planned PCI has been established.[67-69] However, much of the trial data came from studies prior to the routine inclusion of thienopyridines. In lower-risk patient populations, no consistent benefit of GP IIb/IIIa inhibition has been observed. Mixed outcomes have resulted in the practice of preferentially treating only the highest-risk patients with upstream GP IIb/IIIa antagonists. Although no study has validated this approach recently, a meta-analysis of older studies supports this approach.[65] Individual differences in the GP IIb/IIIa antagonists and clinical trial data can guide therapy depending on the specific patient and clinical scenario.

Several important pharmacologic factors define the use of abciximab. In contrast to other GP IIb/IIIa inhibitors, abciximab is a monoclonal antibody. Following IV bolus, antiplatelet effects occur within minutes and return to normal within 48 hours in most cases.[70] Because of its general

irreversibility and slower offset compared with small-molecule GP IIb/IIIa inhibitors, abciximab is not recommended when there is a high likelihood of bleeding complications or surgical intervention. Since abciximab is an antibody, immune-mediated thrombocytopenia may occur, especially with repeated use.[71]

Eptifibatide and tirofiban are both small-molecule GP IIb/IIIa inhibitors. Tirofiban is a highly specific peptidomimetic, and eptifibatide is a synthetic cyclic heptapeptide. Both are less likely to cause hypersensitivity reactions than abciximab.[71] Additionally, these agents are preferred in patients with an increased risk of bleeding because of reversible antiplatelet activity, shorter duration of action, and lower incidence of severe thrombocytopenia as compared to abciximab.[72] These agents have been studied with favorable results in PCI-patient populations.[73-75] In addition, they have a role in ACS patients managed without PCI.

Evaluations of upstream GP IIb/IIIa inhibitor use (i.e., administered prior to angiography) in patients experiencing ST-segment elevation MI (STEMI) and undergoing primary PCI have yielded mixed results. Both the Abciximab before Direct Angioplasty and Stenting in Myocardial Infarction Regarding Acute and Long-Term Follow-up (ADMIRAL) and Randomized Early Versus Late Abciximab in Acute Myocardial Infarction Treated With Primary Coronary Intervention (RELAx-AMI) trials demonstrated that early abciximab administration resulted in improved coronary angiographic findings at the time of PCI.[76,77] However, clinical outcomes were not improved by the early administration of abciximab in the Facilitated Intervention with Enhanced Reperfusion Speed to Stop Events (FINESSE) trial.[78] In the placebo-controlled second Ongoing Tirofiban in Myocardial Evaluation (ON-TIME 2) trial, prehospital administration of tirofiban significantly improved ST-segment resolution before and after primary PCI in patients with acute STEMI.[79]

Overall, meta-analysis of trials enrolling 31,402 patients with ACS without planned PCI, showed a modest cardiovascular benefit of GP IIb/IIIa inhibitors compared with controls.[80] Boersma et al. reported a <10% relative risk reduction in death or MI at 30 days (10.8% vs. 11.8%; $P = 0.015$). With mixed trial results, growing emphasis has been placed on reducing the time from symptom onset to reperfusion, rapid-acting thienopyridine strategies, and alternative anticoagulation regimens, such as bivalirudin, while enthusiasm for upstream use of GP IIb/IIIa inhibitors has waned.

Contraindications to GP IIb/IIIa therapy are similar among abciximab, eptifibatide, and tirofiban. Given their ability to cause profound thrombocytopenia (abciximab > eptifibatide > tirofiban), a history of such reactions is a contraindication for readministration of the same GP IIb/IIIa inhibitor. Also, the patient with a platelet count of <100,000 should not receive GP IIb/IIIa therapy. Recent history of ischemic stroke (within 3 months) and any

Table 7.7 Characteristics of the glycoprotein IIb/IIIa inhibitors

	Abciximab	Eptifibatide	Tirofiban
Brand name	ReoPro	Integrilin	Aggrastat
Structure	Antibody Fab fragment	Cyclic heptapeptide	Nonpeptide
Molecular weight (kD)	48	0.8	0.5
Plasma half-life	0.3h	*2.5 h	*2 h
Excretion	Non-renal	*50% renal	*50% renal
Approved indications	PCI	ACS and PCI	ACS and PCI
Recommended dose	For PCI: 0.25 mg/kg bolus, 0.125 mcg/kg/min infusion	For ACS: 180 mcg/kg bolus, 2.0 mcg/kg/min infusion For PCI: 180 µg/kg bolus × 2, 2.0 mcg/kg/min infusion[a]	For ACS: 0.4 mcg/kg/min × 30 min, then 0.1 mcg/kg/min infusion For PCI: 25 mcg/kg bolus, 0.15 mcg/kg/min infusion

Source: Modified from Lincoff AM, et al. J Am Coll Cardiol 2000; 35(5): 1103–1115.
Note: ACS, acute coronary syndrome; MI, myocardial infarction; PCI, percutaneous coronary intervention.
[a] Eptifibatide infusion should be decreased to 1 mcg/kg/min if creatinine clearance <50 ml/min.
* Approximately, based upon preserved renal function.

history of hemorrhagic stroke warrant careful evaluation of risk versus benefits of GP IIb/IIIa inhibitor use. Administration to patients with trauma, recent surgery, and bleeding disorders should be avoided. Finally, careful attention should be paid to the dosing of these medications, particularly given the weight-based dosing and renal adjustments recommended with several of the medications. Table 7.7 shows the characteristics of the GP IIb/IIIa inhibitors.[81]

PROTEASE-ACTIVATED RECEPTOR I INHIBITOR

A third antiplatelet therapy with a novel mechanism has also been recently approved. Vorapaxar is an oral platelet protease-activated receptor 1 (PAR-1) antagonist. Unlike other available antiplatelet therapies, this medication prevents thrombin-induced platelet-activation and is approved for use in combination with DAPT (aspirin plus $P2Y_{12}$ inhibitor). Approval was based on findings of the Thrombin Receptor Antagonist in Secondary Prevention of Atherothrombotic Ischemic Events (TRA 2P)-TIMI 50 trial, which enrolled patients with history of ACS, most of whom were receiving DAPT. The addition of vorapaxar resulted in the reduction of the primary composite endpoint of cardiovascular death, MI, or stroke at the expense of increased bleeding, including intracranial hemorrhage.[82]

Currently available antiplatelet therapy reduces the risks of thrombogenicity; however, concomitant use of anticoagulation remains important for preventing clot progression, acute stent thrombosis, and subsequent ischemic events. Unfractionated heparin (UFH), low molecular weight heparin (LMWH), and bivalirudin are the most commonly used anticoagulants in PCI. Agent selection is based on clinical data, diagnosis, and patient characteristics. Benefits must be balanced with increased bleeding.

Table 7.8 enumerates currently available antithrombotic agents for PCI.

HEPARIN

Heparin is a heterogeneous mucopolysaccharide with complex effects on the coagulation pathway.[83] Heparin is a naturally occurring anticoagulant cofactor produced by human basophils and mast cells[83]; most of the pharmaceutically available heparin in the United States is derived from porcine mucosal tissue. The primary pharmacological effect is driven by the binding of heparin to antithrombin, with simultaneous binding to thrombin. The formation of a ternary complex between antithrombin, thrombin, and heparin results in the inactivation of thrombin. Heparin also exerts indirect antiplatelet effects by binding to and inhibiting von Willebrand factor. Additionally, heparin binds to plasma proteins, endothelial cells, and macrophages, which in turn inactivates heparin. These wide-ranging activities result in variable anticoagulant effects, and, as such, therapy with UFH requires close monitoring and dosing adjustments.

Heparin has been the most commonly used anticoagulant in the catheterization laboratory; however, no large-scale, prospective trials have clearly defined the optimal level of anticoagulation. Monitoring and titration of UFH during PCI can be facilitated through point-of-care testing of the activated clotting time (ACT).[84] Historically, the standard heparin regimen has been 70–100 units/kg bolus, with additional weight-based boluses to achieve and maintain an ACT of 250–350 seconds.[85] Although lacking prospective validation, retrospective data show that this approach is reasonable. Importantly, sheath removal can be accomplished with minimal bleeding risk once the ACT falls below 150–180 seconds. When UFH is administered with a GP IIb/IIIa inhibitor, ACT values of ≤200 seconds

Table 7.8 Antithrombotic therapy for PCI

Parameter	UFH	Enoxaparin	Fondaparinux	Bivalirudin	Argatroban
Route	IV	IV, subcutaneous	IV, subcutaneous	IV	IV
Clotting factors inhibited	IIa, IX, Xa	IIa, Xa	Xa	DTI	DTI
Metabolism	Unknown	Hepatic (desulfation)	NA	Hepatic and blood	Hepatic
Elimination		Renal (10% unchanged)	Renal (77% unchanged)	Renal (20% unchanged)	Renal (16% unchanged)
Half-life	1 h	2–4 h	17–21 h	25 min	30–51 min
Dose	60–100 units/kg IV prn	0.3–1.0 mg/kg IV[a]	0.5–1.0 mg/kg IV[a]	0.75 mg/kg IV then 1.75 mg/kg/h	350 mcg/kg IV then 25 mcg/kg/min
Coagulation monitoring and target for PCI	ACT (200 sec with IIb/IIIa and 300–350 sec alone)	None required, plasma antifactor Xa (if needed)	None required, plasma antifactor Xa (if needed)	ACT (>225 sec)	ACT (300–450 sec)
Reversibility	Protamine	66% by protamine, FFP	FFP	FFP	FFP

Note: ACT, activated clotting times; DTI, direct thrombin (IIa) inhibitors; FFP, fresh-frozen plasma; IV, intravenous; NA, not applicable; PCI, percutaneous coronary intervention; UFH, unfractionated heparin.

[a] Dependent on the timing of the last subcutaneous dose and concomitant IIb/IIIa use.

result in similar reductions of ischemic events as higher ACT levels with less risk for bleeding.[85,86] A different approach is used when UFH is started upstream for the medical management of ACS or administered for prevention of reocclusion following fibrinolysis. In these scenarios, UFH is traditionally administered as a 70 units/kg (maximum 5000 units) bolus followed by 1000 units/hr for up to 48 hours.[87] Rather than ACT, the activated partial thromboplastin time (aPTT) is utilized for monitoring, with a goal of 50–70 seconds or 1.5–2 times baseline.[88] Whether UFH is started before the procedure or only utilized during PCI, immediate discontinuation following successful PCI is recommended. Continued infusion after PCI has shown no benefit and results in higher rates of access site bleeding.[89,90]

LOW MOLECULAR WEIGHT HEPARINS

LMWHs are about one-third the molecular weight of UFH. Mechanistically, these shorter-chain polysaccharides bind to antithrombin and thrombin, but the binding to thrombin is to a lesser extent than with UFH. Rather, the majority of the anticoagulant effect of LMWH comes from binding to factor Xa, the catalyst for conversion of prothrombin to thrombin. As a result, LMWH has only a minimal effect on aPTT and ACT, and monitoring, if needed, requires measurement of anti-Xa activity. Since bedside monitoring of anti-Xa levels is not routinely performed, LMWH dosing recommendations are based on evidence from clinical trials.[91] LMWH has several important pharmacologic differences compared with UFH, including increased bioavailability, a prolonged route of elimination, and a more consistent anticoagulant effect. Therefore, following IV or subcutaneous (SQ) administration, LMWH offers a reasonably predictable level of anticoagulation and longer lasting antithrombotic effect than that achieved with UFH. Several LMWHs are available, though the majority of evaluations in PCI have involved enoxaparin. Like UFH, enoxaparin may be used to treat ACS with or without planned PCI and to prevent recurrent vessel occlusion following thrombolytic reperfusion.

LMWH has been compared with UFH in the setting of PCI. The Superior Yield of the New Strategy of Enoxaparin, Revascularization and GP IIb/IIIa Inhibitors (SYNERGY) trial randomized 9,978 higher-risk ACS patients with planned early invasive treatment to either UFH or enoxaparin. The results showed noninferiority, with no difference in the primary endpoint (death or MI), subacute stent thrombosis, or unsuccessful procedures.[92] These finding are in agreement with results of the subgroup analysis of patients who received PCI in the Aggrastat to Zocor (A to Z trial).[93] However, the SYNERGY trial did yield another interesting and important finding. Bleeding was increased in patients who received enoxaparin before PCI and were switched (i.e., crossed-over) to receive UFH during PCI. Therefore, "crossover" should be avoided, and, in patients who present for a catheterization procedure already receiving enoxaparin, it should be continued with subsequent doses based on the timing of the previous dose. If the last dose of enoxaparin was <8 hours prior to PCI, no additional anticoagulant is needed; if enoxaparin was administered 8 to 12 hours prior to PCI, 1.3 mg/kg IV enoxaparin should be given; and finally, if the most recent dose of enoxaparin was administered >12 hours prior to PCI, a full dose is needed or conventional therapy is indicated.[94]

The safety of enoxaparin in elective PCI was evaluated in the Safety and Efficacy of Enoxaparin in PCI Patients, an International Randomized Evaluation (STEEPLE) trial.[95] Patients undergoing PCI were randomized to 0.5 mg/kg IV, 0.75 mg/kg IV, or UFH adjusted for ACT. The primary endpoint—incidence of major or minor bleeding not related to CABG—was decreased in the 0.5 mg/kg arm. There was no difference in bleeding between the patients receiving UFH and the higher dose of enoxaparin. This trial supports the use of a single intravenous bolus of 0.5 mg/kg enoxaparin to subjects undergoing elective PCI; however, it was not sufficiently sized to assess efficacy of these regimens. Use of 0.5 mg/kg IV enoxaparin is further supported by the more recent Acute Myocardial Infarction Treated With Primary Angioplasty and Intravenous Enoxaparin or Unfractionated Heparin to Lower Ischemic and Bleeding Events at Short- and Long-Term Follow-Up (ATOLL) trial, which enrolled STEMI patients undergoing primary PCI. Investigators found a favorable reduction in 30-day composite incidence of death, complication of MI, procedure failure, or major bleeding with IV enoxaparin compared to UFH.[96]

Based on currently available data, enoxaparin seems to be slightly more effective than UFH at the expense of a modest increase in minor bleeding. Of note, although other LMWHs are approved for non-ST segment elevation (NSTE) ACS, the majority of efficacy data support enoxaparin in this setting.

DIRECT THROMBIN INHIBITORS

Direct thrombin inhibitors (DTIs) currently available in the United States include bivalirudin, argatroban, and lepirudin. DTIs inhibit soluble and clot-bound thrombin without binding to antithrombin. Another potential advantage over heparin is that DTIs do not promote platelet activity, rather the degree of thrombin inhibition decreases platelet activation. The earliest experience with DTI was in patients with known or suspected heparin-induced thrombocytopenia (HIT) who were given argatroban rather than heparin for PCI.[97] Extensive experience with bivalirudin in PCI now supports its use in high-risk patients with HIT requiring PCI.[98,99] Favorable experiences seen in these patients and inherent limitations of heparin therapy resulted in multiple evaluations of bivalirudin among patients with ACS undergoing PCI or both.

The Randomized Evaluation in PCI Linking Angiomax to Reduced Clinical Events (REPLACE-2) trial randomized 6,010 patients undergoing urgent or elective PCI to intravenous bivalirudin (0.75 mg/kg bolus plus 1.75 mg/kg/hr for the duration of PCI) or UFH with GP IIb/IIa inhibition.[100] The authors concluded that bivalirudin was noninferior to heparin and GP IIb/IIIa inhibition with regard to suppression of the primary efficacy endpoints (death, MI, or TVR) and was associated with less bleeding (2.4% vs. 4.1%; $P < 0.001$).[100] Provisional GP IIb/IIIa inhibitor therapy was administered to 7.2% of patients in the bivalirudin arm. This trial extended bivalirudin use to patients undergoing elective PCI. Bivalirudin would later demonstrate efficacy when initiated upstream from PCI in the management of NSTEMI, unstable angina, and STEMI.[101-103]

In the Acute Catheterization and Urgent Intervention Triage Strategy (ACUITY) trial, bivalirudin (with and without GP IIb/IIIa inhibition) was compared with UFH plus a GP IIb/IIIa inhibitor[101] in 13,819 patients with moderate to high-risk ACS and planned early intervention. Bivalirudin alone reduced rates of major bleeding (3% vs. 5.7%, $P < 0.001$) with similar efficacy to UFH plus GP IIb/IIIa inhibition. Similar findings were obtained from the ISAR-REACT 4 and Harmonizing Outcomes With Revascularization and Stents in Acute Myocardial Infarction (HORIZONS-AMI) trials addressing the use of bivalirudin in patients with invasively managed NSTEMI or STEMI, respectively.[102,104] The endpoints studied were major bleeding and the combination of death, reinfarction, TVR, and stroke. Anticoagulation with bivalirudin alone was compared with heparin plus a GP IIb/IIIa inhibitor and resulted in a significant decrease in bleeding and similar efficacy with regard to ischemic endpoints.

Considering the findings of ACUITY, ISAR REACT 4, and HORIZONS-AMI, bivalirudin is an attractive approach for patients undergoing elective or urgent PCI, particularly when adequate antiplatelet therapy with a DAPT is present. In these settings, with over 10,000 patient experiences in clinical trials, bivalirudin therapy continues to be noninferior to heparin plus GP IIb/IIIa inhibitor therapy with substantial reductions in bleeding. However, it is imperative to note that trials have pointed to a warning of small increases in acute stent thrombosis with bivalirudin. Combined with advancement in concomitant antiplatelet therapies limiting the use of GP IIb/IIIa inhibitors and evolution of catheterization procedures (i.e., radial access), room for reevaluation of the role of bivalirudin is warranted.

The European Ambulance Acute Coronary Syndrome Angiography (EUROMAX) trial enrolled STEMI patients to compare bivalirudin (with bailout use of GP IIb/IIIa inhibitors) to UFH or LMWH (with discretionary use of GP IIb/IIIa inhibitors).[105] Overall use of GP IIb/IIIa inhibitors was 11.5% in the bivalirudin treated patients and 69% in the heparin/LMWH arm. The composite of death or non-CABG related major bleeding was lower in the bivalirudin-treated patients; however, overall major adverse cardiovascular events were similar. An increased risk of acute stent thrombosis was observed in bivalirudin-treated patients. Later, in the Bavarian Reperfusion Alternatives Evaluation (BRAVE) 4 trial, which again enrolled STEMI patients, subjects were treated with prasugrel plus bivalirudin versus clopidogrel plus heparin; all GP IIb/IIIa inhibitor use was reserved for bailout (3% vs. 6.1% in bivalirudin and UFH groups, respectively).[106] The primary composite endpoint was similar, with neither approach demonstrating a safety or efficacy advantage. Importantly, BRAVE-4 was stopped prematurely due to slow enrollment. Also evaluating patients undergoing STEMI, the Unfractionated Heparin Versus Bivalirudin in Primary Percutaneous Coronary Intervention (HEAT-PPCI) trial randomized patients to bivalirudin or heparin and again restricted use of GP IIb/IIIa inhibitor use to bailout (13% and 15% bailout, respectively).[107] Unlike previous evaluations discussed, the type of $P2Y_{12}$ inhibitor used was at the discretion of the treating cardiologist, and was similar in both arms with ticagrelor being used most commonly (61% of study participants). The composite primary endpoint (all-cause mortality, stroke, re-infarction, or unplanned TVR) was higher with bivalirudin compared to heparin, and bleeding was similar in both groups. Similar to early trials, events in bivalirudin patients were driven by increases in stent thrombosis; bleeding was believed to be similar between treatment groups due to an increased use of radial access. With this more recent clinical trial information, the beneficial role of bivalirudin has become less certain.

FONDAPARINUX

Fondaparinux is a synthetic pentasaccharide that is an antithrombin-dependent indirect inhibitor of factor Xa. Its use as an alternative to UFH, in both the medical management of ACS and antithrombotic protection postfibrinolysis, has been evaluated. In the Fifth Organization to Assess Strategies in Ischemic Syndromes (OASIS-5) trial, 20,078 ACS patients were randomized to enoxaparin or fondaparinux. The primary short-term efficacy endpoint of death, MI, or stroke occurred at a similar frequency in both groups, with fondaparinux recipients experiencing 50% fewer bleeding events and 17% fewer deaths at 30 days. Among the 6,238 patients who underwent PCI[108] in OASIS-5, short-term rates of ischemic events were similar, and major bleeding was reduced by half. However, patients in the fondaparinux group experienced higher rates of catheter thrombosis (0.9% compared with 0.4%). Because of the risk of this potentially devastating complication, fondaparinux should not be used as the sole anticoagulant to support PCI.[85] Furthermore, fondaparinux should be avoided in patients when an early invasive strategy is planned.

ORAL ANTICOAGULANTS

There are several oral anticoagulants (e.g., rivaroxaban, apixaban, dabigatran) approved for treatment of venous thromboembolism (VTE) and for the prevention of stroke among patients with atrial fibrillation. There have been several evaluations of these agents among patients with ACS as additive therapies to DAPT. Rivaroxaban, an oral direct factor Xa inhibitor, was studied in the Anti-Xa Therapy to Lower Cardiovascular Events in Addition to Standard Therapy in Subjects with Acute Coronary Syndrome–Thrombolysis in Myocardial Infarction 46 (ATLAS ACS 2-TIMI 46) trial.[109] This trial enrolled 15,526 patients with recent (within 7 days) ACS to receive twice-daily doses of either 2.5 mg or 5 mg of rivaroxaban versus placebo. After approximately 1 year, the incidence of the composite endpoint of cardiovascular death, MI, or stroke was statistically

significantly reduced (absolute risk reduction ~1.8%) by rivaroxaban. However, major bleeding was increased by ~1.4%. Combined with concerns over missing data, the clinical utility remains questionable. Full-dose apixaban (5 mg bid) was studied in a similar patient population in the Apixaban for Prevention of Acute Ischemic Events 2 (APPRAISE-2) study.[110] This study was stopped early due to an observed increase in bleeding. Finally, the RE-DEEM trial studied dabigatran at various doses among patients with recent ACS.[111] Not surprisingly, there was a dose-related increase in bleeding; unfortunately, no significant reduction in ischemic events was observed. Further large-scale trials are underway with these agents.

CONCLUSION

Hemodynamic management of patients with cardiovascular compromise is often undertaken with intravenous vasoactive and cardioactive medications, with the goal of initial patient stabilization; longer-term strategies are implemented to allow potentially life-saving procedures to be performed. The overall pharmacologic management of patients during PCI can be remarkably complex yet vitally important to prevent both ischemic and hemorrhagic complications. Development of the ideal antithrombotic and antiplatelet regimen continues to be a goal for the cardiology community. New therapies continue to be in development and may help increase efficacy and limit adverse effects in this at-risk patient population.

REFERENCES

1. Shoemaker WC, et al. Prospective trial of supranormal values of survivors as therapeutic goals in high-risk surgical patients. *Chest* 1988; 94(6): 1176–1186.
2. Tuchschmidt J, et al. Elevation of cardiac output and oxygen delivery improves outcome in septic shock. *Chest* 1992; 102(1): 216–220.
3. The CONSENSUS Trial Study Group. Effects of enalapril on mortality in severe congestive heart failure. Results of the Cooperative North Scandinavian Enalapril Survival Study (CONSENSUS). *N Engl J Med* 1987; 316(23): 1429–1435.
4. Mullens W, et al. Sodium nitroprusside for advanced low-output heart failure. *J Am Coll Cardiol* 2008; 52(3): 200–207.
5. Opie L, Gersch B, eds. *Drugs for the Heart*. 6th ed. Philadelphia, PA: Elsevier, 2005, pp. 161–162.
6. Silver MA, et al. Effect of nesiritide versus dobutamine on short-term outcomes in the treatment of patients with acutely decompensated heart failure. *J Am Coll Cardiol* 2002; 39(5): 798–803.
7. Cuffe MS, et al. Short-term intravenous milrinone for acute exacerbation of chronic heart failure: A randomized controlled trial. *JAMA* 2002; 287(12): 1541–1547.
8. Unverferth DV, et al. Long-term benefit of dobutamine in patients with congestive cardiomyopathy. *Am Heart J* 1980; 100(5): 622–630.
9. Marino P, ed. *The ICU Book*. vol. 176, 3rd ed. Philadelphia, PA: Lippincott Williams & Wilkins, 2007, pp. 264–267.

10. Gruppo Italiano per lo Studio della Sopravvivenza nell'infarto Miocardico. GISSI-3: Effects of lisinopril and transdermal glyceryl trinitrate singly and together on 6-week mortality and ventricular function after acute myocardial infarction. *Lancet* 1994; 343(8906): 1115–1122.

11. Flather M, et al. Randomized controlled trial of oral captopril, of oral isosorbide mononitrate and of intravenous magnesium sulphate started early in acute myocardial infarction: Safety and haemodynamic effects. ISIS-4 (Fourth International Study of Infarct Survival) Pilot Study Investigators. *Eur Heart J* 1994; 15(5): 608–619.

12. Dell'Italia LJ, et al. Comparative effects of volume loading, dobutamine, and nitroprusside in patients with predominant right ventricular infarction. *Circulation* 1985; 72(6):1327–1335.

13. Berne RM. The role of adenosine in the regulation of coronary blood flow. *Circ Res* 1980; 47(6): 807–813.

14. Christensen CW, et al. Coronary vasodilator reserve. Comparison of the effects of papaverine and adenosine on coronary flow, ventricular function, and myocardial metabolism. *Circulation* 1991; 83(1): 294–303.

15. Leier CV, et al. Comparative systemic and regional hemodynamic effects of dopamine and dobutamine in patients with cardiomyopathic heart failure. *Circulation* 1978; 58(3 Pt 1): 466–475.

16. Viskin S. Long QT syndromes and torsade de pointes. *Lancet* 1999; 354(9190): 1625–1633.

17. Aranda JM, et al. Comparison of dobutamine versus milrinone therapy in hospitalized patients awaiting cardiac transplantation: a prospective, randomized trial. *Am Heart J* 2003; 145(2): 324–329.

18. Bellomo R, et al. Low-dose dopamine in patients with early renal dysfunction: A placebo-controlled randomised trial. Australian and New Zealand Intensive Care Society (ANZICS) Clinical Trials Group. *Lancet* 2000; 356(9248): 2139–2143.

19. Marik PE, Iglesias J. Low-dose dopamine does not prevent acute renal failure in patients with septic shock and oliguria. NORASEPT II Study Investigators. *Am J Med* 1999; 107(4): 387–390.

20. Kellum JA, M Decker J. Use of dopamine in acute renal failure: A meta-analysis. *Crit Care Med* 2001; 29(8): 1526–1531.

21. Bassi G, et al. Catecholamines and vasopressin during critical illness. *Endocrinol Metab Clin North Am* 2006; 35(4): 839–857.

22. Lindner KH, et al. Randomised comparison of epinephrine and vasopressin in patients with out-of-hospital ventricular fibrillation. *Lancet* 1997; 349(9051): 535–537.

23. Barrett LK, et al. Vasopressin: Mechanisms of action on the vasculature in health and in septic shock. *Crit Care Med* 2007; 35(1): 33–40.

24. Mehta SR, Yusuf S. Short- and long-term oral antiplatelet therapy in acute coronary syndromes and percutaneous coronary intervention. *J Am Coll Cardiol* 2003; 21: 79S–88S.

25. Patrono C, et al. Clinical pharmacology of platelet cyclooxygenase inhibition. *Circulation* 1985; 72(6): 1177–1184.

26. Antithrombotic Trialists' Collaboration. Collaborative meta-analysis of randomised trials of antiplatelet therapy for prevention of death, myocardial infarction, and stroke in high-risk patients. *BMJ* 2002; 324(7329): 71–86.

27. Farrell B, et al. The United Kingdom transient ischaemic attack (UK-TIA) aspirin trial: Final results. *J Neurol Neurosurg Psychiatry* 1991; 54(12): 1044–1054.

28. Roderick PJ, et al. The gastrointestinal toxicity of aspirin An overview of randomised controlled trials. *Br J Clin Pharmacol* 1993; 35(3): 219–226.

29. Patrignani P, et al. Selective cumulative inhibition of platelet thromboxane production by low-dose aspirin in healthy subjects. *J Clin Invest* 1982; 69(6): 1366–1372.

30. The Dutch TIA Trial Study Group. A comparison of two doses of aspirin (30 mg vs. 283 mg a day) in patients after a transient ischemic attack or minor ischemic stroke. *N Engl J Med* 1991; 325(18): 1261–1266.

31. Smith SC Jr, et al. ACC/AHA/ SCAI 2005 guideline update for percutaneous coronary intervention-summary article: A report of the American College of Cardiology/American Heart Association Task Force on practice guidelines (ACC/AHA/SCAI writing committee to update the 2001 guidelines for percutaneous coronary intervention). *J Am Coll Cardiol* 2006; 47(1): 216–235.

32. Bhatt DL, et al. Meta-analysis of randomized and registry comparisons of ticlopidine with clopidogrel after stenting. *J Am Coll Cardiol* 2002; 39(1): 9–14.

33. Bertrand ME, et al. Double-blind study of the safety of clopidogrel with and without a loading dose in combination with aspirin compared with ticlopidine in combination with aspirin after coronary stenting: The Clopidogrel Aspirin Stent International Cooperative Study (CLASSICS). *Circulation* 2000; 102(6): 624–629.

34. Wiviott SD, et al. Prasugrel versus clopidogrel in patients with acute coronary syndromes. *N Engl J Med* 2007; 357(20): 2001–2015.

35. Wallentin L, et al. Ticagrelor versus clopidogrel in patients with acute coronary syndromes. *N Engl J Med* 2009; 361(11): 1045–1057.

36. Yusuf S, et al. Effects of clopidogrel in addition to aspirin in patients with acute coronary syndromes without ST-segment elevation. *N Engl J Med* 2001; 345(7): 494–502.

37. Steinhubl SR, et al. Early and sustained dual oral antiplatelet therapy following percutaneous coronary intervention: A randomized controlled trial. *JAMA* 2002; 288(19): 2411–2420.

38. Schomig A, et al. A randomized comparison of antiplatelet and anticoagulant therapy after the placement of coronary-artery stents. *N Engl J Med* 1996; 334(17): 1084–1089.

39. Leon MB, et al. A clinical trial comparing three antithrombotic-drug regimens after coronary-artery stenting. Stent Anticoagulation Restenosis Study Investigators. *N Engl J Med* 1998; 339(23): 1665–1671.

40. Lagerqvist B, et al. Long-term outcomes with drug-eluting stents versus bare-metal stents in Sweden. *N Engl J Med* 2007; 356(10): 1009–1019.

41. Stone GW, et al. Safety and efficacy of sirolimus- and paclitaxel-eluting coronary stents. *N Engl J Med* 2007; 356(10): 998–1008.

42. Win HK, et al. Clinical outcomes and stent thrombosis following off-label use of drug-eluting stents. *JAMA* 2007; 297(18): 2001–2009.

43. Levine GN, et al. 2016 ACC/AHA guideline focused update on duration of dual antiplatelet therapy in patients with coronary artery disease: A report of the American College

of Cardiology/American Heart Association Task Force on Clinical Practice Guidelines. *J Am Coll Cardiol* 2016; 134(10): e123–e155.

44. Gurbel PA, et al. Clopidogrel for coronary stenting: Response variability, drug resistance, and the effect of pretreatment platelet reactivity. *Circulation* 2003; 107(23): 2908–2913.

45. Savi P, et al. The antiaggregating activity of clopidogrel is due to a metabolic activation by the hepatic cytochrome P450-1A. *Thromb Haemost* 1994; 72(2): 313–317.

46. Lau WC, et al. Atorvastatin reduces the ability of clopidogrel to inhibit platelet aggregation: A new drug-drug interaction. *Circulation* 2003; 107(1): 32–37.

47. Lotfi A, et al. High-dose atorvastatin does not negatively influence clinical outcomes among clopidogrel treated acute coronary syndrome patients—a Pravastatin or Atorvastatin Evaluation and Infection Therapy-Thrombolysis in Myocardial Infarction 22 (PROVE IT-TIMI 22) analysis. *Am Heart J* 2008; 155(5): 954–958.

48. Saw J, et al. Lack of evidence of a clopidogrel-statin interaction in the CHARISMA trial. *J Am Coll Cardiol* 2007; 50(4): 291–295.

49. Saw J, et al. Lack of adverse clopidogrel-atorvastatin clinical interaction from secondary analysis of a randomized, placebo-controlled clopidogrel trial. *Circulation* 2003; 108(8): 921–924.

50. Gilard M, et al. Influence of omeprazole on the antiplatelet action of clopidogrel associated with aspirin: The randomized, double-blind OCLA (omeprazole clopidogrel aspirin) study. *J Am Coll Cardiol* 2008; 51(3): 256–260.

51. Bhatt DL, et al. Clopidogrel with or without omeprazole in coronary artery disease. *N Engl J Med* 2010; 363(20): 1909–1917.

52. Bliden KP, et al. The association of cigarette smoking with enhanced platelet inhibition by clopidogrel. *J Am Coll Cardiol* 2008; 52(7): 531–533.

53. Wiviott SD, et al. Prasugrel compared with high loading- and maintenance-dose clopidogrel in patients with planned percutaneous coronary intervention: The prasugrel in comparison to clopidogrel for inhibition of platelet activation and aggregation-thrombolysis in myocardial infarction 44 trial. *Circulation* 2007; 116(25): 2923–2932.

54. Cannon CP, et al. Safety, tolerability, and initial efficacy of AZD6140, the first reversible oral adenosine diphosphate receptor antagonist, compared with clopidogrel, in patients with non-ST-segment elevation acute coronary syndrome: Primary results of the DISPERSE-2 trial. *J Am Coll Cardiol* 2007; 50(19): 1844–1851.

55. Armstrong D, et al. Characterization of the adenosine pharmacology of ticagrelor reveals therapeutically relevant inhibition of equilibrative nucleoside transporter 1. *J Cardiovasc Pharmacol Ther* 2014; 19(2): 209–219.

56. Schulz S, et al. Randomized comparison of ticagrelor versus prasugrel in patients with acute coronary syndrome and planned invasive strategy—Design and rationale of the iNtracoronary Stenting and Antithrombotic Regimen: Rapid Early Action for Coronary Treatment (ISAR-REACT) 5 trial. *J Cardiovasc Transl Res* 2014; 7(1): 91–100.

57. Mehta SR, et al. Effects of pretreatment with clopidogrel and aspirin followed by long-term therapy in patients undergoing percutaneous coronary intervention: The PCI-CURE study. *Lancet* 2001; 358(9281): 527–533.

58. Steinhubl SR, et al. Optimal timing for the initiation of pre-treatment with 300 mg clopidogrel before percutaneous coronary intervention. *J Am Coll Cardiol* 2006; 47(5): 939–943.

59. Kastrati A, et al. A clinical trial of abciximab in elective percutaneous coronary intervention after pretreatment with clopidogrel. *N Engl J Med* 2004; 350(3): 232–238.

60. Kastrati A, et al. Abciximab in patients with acute coronary syndromes undergoing percutaneous coronary intervention after clopidogrel pretreatment: The ISAR-REACT 2 randomized trial. *JAMA* 2006; 295(13): 1531–1538.

61. Harrington RA, et al. Platelet inhibition with cangrelor in patients undergoing PCI. *N Engl J Med* 2009; 361(24): 2318–2329.

62. Bhatt DL, et al. Intravenous platelet blockade with cangrelor during PCI. *N Engl J Med* 2009; 361(24): 2330–2341.

63. Bhatt DL, et al. Effect of platelet inhibition with cangrelor during PCI on ischemic events. *N Engl J Med* 2013; 368(14): 1303–1313.

64. Tcheng JE, et al. Pharmacodynamics of chimeric glycoprotein IIb/IIIa integrin antiplatelet antibody Fab 7E3 in high-risk coronary angioplasty. *Circulation* 1994; 90(4): 1757–1764.

65. De Luca G, et al. Risk profile and benefits from Gp IIb-IIIa inhibitors among patients with ST-segment elevation myocardial infarction treated with primary angioplasty: A meta-regression analysis of randomized trials. *Eur Heart J* 2009; 30(22): 2705–2713.

66. Heeschen C, et al. Troponin concentrations for stratification of patients with acute coronary syndromes in relation to therapeutic efficacy of tirofiban. PRISM Study Investigators. Platelet Receptor Inhibition in Ischemic Syndrome Management. *Lancet* 1999; 354(9192): 1757–1762.

67. Platelet Receptor Inhibition in Ischemic Syndrome Management (PRISM) Study Investigators. A comparison of aspirin plus tirofiban with aspirin plus heparin for unstable angina. *N Engl J Med* 1998; 338(21): 1498–1505.

68. The CAPTURE investigators. Randomised placebo-controlled trial of abciximab before and during coronary intervention in refractory unstable angina: The CAPTURE study. *Lancet* 1997; 349(9063): 1429–1435.

69. The PURSUIT Trial Investigators. Inhibition of platelet glycoprotein IIb/IIIa with eptifibatide in patients with acute coronary syndromes. Platelet glycoprotein IIb/IIIa in unstable angina: Receptor suppression using integrilin therapy. *N Engl J Med* 1998; 339(7): 436–443.

70. Mascelli MA, et al. Pharmacodynamic profile of short-term abciximab treatment demonstrates prolonged platelet inhibition with gradual recovery from GP IIb/IIIa receptor blockade. *Circulation* 1998; 97(17): 1680–1688.

71. Topol EJ, et al. Comparison of two platelet glycoprotein IIb/IIIa inhibitors, tirofiban and abciximab, for the prevention of ischemic events with percutaneous coronary revascularization. *N Engl J Med* 2001; 344(25): 1888–1894.

72. Barrett JS, et al. Pharmacokinetics and pharmacodynamics of MK-383, a selective non-peptide platelet glycoprotein-IIb/IIIa receptor antagonist, in healthy men. *Clin Pharmacol Ther* 1994; 56(4): 377–388.

73. PRICE Investigators. Comparative 30-day economic and clinical outcomes of platelet glycoprotein IIb/IIIa inhibitor use during elective percutaneous coronary intervention: Prairie ReoPro versus Integrilin Cost Evaluation (PRICE) trial. *Am Heart J* 2001; 141(3): 402–409.

74. Valgimigli M, et al. Comparison of angioplasty with infusion of tirofiban or abciximab and with implantation of sirolimus-eluting or uncoated stents for acute myocardial infarction: The MULTISTRATEGY randomized trial. *JAMA* 2008; 299(15): 1788–1799.

75. Moliterno DJ, et al. Outcomes at 6 months for the direct comparison of tirofiban and abciximab during percutaneous coronary revascularisation with stent placement: The TARGET follow-up study. *Lancet* 2002; 360(9330): 355–360.

76. Montalescot G, et al. Platelet glycoprotein IIb/IIIa inhibition with coronary stenting for acute myocardial infarction. *N Engl J Med* 2001; 344(25): 1895–1903.

77. Maioli M, et al. Randomized early versus late abciximab in acute myocardial infarction treated with primary coronary intervention (RELAx-AMI Trial). *J Am Coll Cardiol* 2007; 49(14): 1517–1524.

78. Ellis SG, et al. Facilitated PCI in patients with ST-elevation myocardial infarction. *N Engl J Med* 2008; 358(21): 2205–2217.

79. Van't Hof AW, et al. Prehospital initiation of tirofiban in patients with ST-elevation myocardial infarction undergoing primary angioplasty (On-TIME 2): A multicentre, double-blind, randomised controlled trial. *Lancet* 2008; 372(9638): 537–546.

80. Boersma E, et al. Platelet glycoprotein IIb/IIIa inhibitors in acute coronary syndromes: A meta-analysis of all major randomised clinical trials. *Lancet* 2002; 359(9302): 189–198.

81. Lincoff AM, et al. Platelet glycoprotein IIb/IIIa receptor blockade in coronary artery disease. *J Am Coll Cardiol* 2000; 35(5): 1103–1115.

82. Scirica BM, et al. Vorapaxar for secondary prevention of thrombotic events for patients with previous myocardial infarction: A prespecified subgroup analysis of the TRA 2 P-TIMI 50 trial. *Lancet* 2012; 380(9850): 1317–1324.

83. Hirsh J, et al. Heparin and low-molecular-weight heparin: Mechanisms of action, pharmacokinetics, dosing, monitoring, efficacy, and safety. *Chest* 2001; 119(1 Suppl): 64S–94S.

84. Ogilby JD, et al. Adequate heparinization during PTCA: Assessment using activated clotting times. *Cathet Cardiovasc Diagn* 1989; 18(4): 206–209.

85. Levine GN, et al. 2011 ACCF/AHA/SCAI Guideline for Percutaneous Coronary Intervention: A report of the American College of Cardiology Foundation/American Heart Association Task Force on Practice Guidelines and the Society for Cardiovascular Angiography and Interventions. *Circulation* 2011; 124(23): e574–e651.

86. Brener SJ, et al. Relationship between activated clotting time and ischemic or hemorrhagic complications: Analysis of 4 recent randomized clinical trials of percutaneous coronary intervention. *Circulation* 2004; 110(8): 994–998.

87. The Global Use of Strategies to Open Occluded Coronary Arteries (GUSTO III) Investigators. A comparison of reteplase with alteplase for acute myocardial infarction. *N Engl J Med* 1997; 337(16): 1118–1123.

88. Granger CB, et al. Activated partial thromboplastin time and outcome after thrombolytic therapy for acute myocardial infarction: Results from the GUSTO-I trial. *Circulation* 1996; 93(5): 870–878.

89. Ellis SG, et al. Effect of 18- to 24-hour heparin administration for prevention of restenosis after uncomplicated coronary angioplasty. *Am Heart J* 1989; 117(4): 777–782.

90. Friedman HZ, et al. Randomized prospective evaluation of prolonged versus abbreviated intravenous heparin therapy after coronary angioplasty. *J Am Coll Cardiol* 1994; 24(5): 1214–1219.

91. Rabah MM, et al. Usefulness of intravenous enoxaparin for percutaneous coronary intervention in stable angina pectoris. *Am J Cardiol* 1999; 84(12): 1391–1395.

92. Ferguson JJ, et al. Enoxaparin vs unfractionated heparin in high-risk patients with non-ST- segment elevation acute coronary syndromes managed with an intended early invasive strategy: Primary results of the SYNERGY randomized trial. *JAMA* 2004; 292(1): 45–54.

93. Blazing MA, et al. Safety and efficacy of enoxaparin vs unfractionated heparin in patients with non-ST-segment elevation acute coronary syndromes who receive tirofiban and aspirin: A randomized controlled trial. *JAMA* 2004; 292(1): 55–64.

94. Martin JL, et al. Reliable anticoagulation with enoxaparin in patients undergoing percutaneous coronary intervention: The pharmacokinetics of enoxaparin in PCI (PEPCI) study. *Catheter Cardiovasc Interv* 2004; 61(2): 163–170.

95. Montalescot G, et al. Enoxaparin versus unfractionated heparin in elective percutaneous coronary intervention. *N Engl J Med* 2006; 355(10): 1006–1017.

96. Montalescot G, et al. Intravenous enoxaparin or unfractionated heparin in primary percutaneous coronary intervention for ST-elevation myocardial infarction: The international randomised open-label ATOLL trial. *Lancet* 2011; 378(9792): 693–703.

97. Matthai WH Jr. Use of argatroban during percutaneous coronary interventions in patients with heparin-induced thrombocytopenia. *Semin Thromb Hemost* 1999; 25(Suppl 1): 57–60.

98. Campbell KR, et al. Bivalirudin in patients with heparin-induced thrombocytopenia undergoing percutaneous coronary intervention. *J Invasive Cardiol* 2000; 12(Suppl F): 14F–19F.

99. Mahaffey KW, et al. The anticoagulant therapy with bivalirudin to assist in the performance of percutaneous coronary intervention in patients with heparin-induced thrombocytopenia (ATBAT) study: Main results. *J Invasive Cardiol* 2003; 15(11): 611–616.

100. Lincoff AM, et al. Bivalirudin and provisional glycoprotein IIb/IIIa blockade compared with heparin and planned glycoprotein IIb/IIIa blockade during percutaneous coronary intervention: REPLACE-2 randomized trial. *JAMA* 2003; 289(7): 853–863.

101. Stone GW, et al. Bivalirudin for patients with acute coronary syndromes. *N Engl J Med* 2006; 355(21): 2203–2216.

102. Stone GW, et al. Bivalirudin during primary PCI in acute myocardial infarction. *N Engl J Med* 2008; 358(21): 2218–2230.

103. Kastrati A, et al. Bivalirudin versus unfractionated heparin during percutaneous coronary intervention. *N Engl J Med* 2008; 359(7): 688–696.

104. Kastrati A, et al. Abciximab and heparin versus bivalirudin for non–ST-elevation myocardial infarction. *N Engl J Med* 2011; 365(21); 1980–1989.

105. Steg PG, et al. Bivalirudin started during emergency transport for primary PCI. *N Engl J Med* 2013; 369(23): 2207–2217.

106. Schulz S, et al. Prasugrel plus bivalirudin vs clopidogrel plus heparin in patients with ST-segment elevation myocardial infarction. *Eur Heart J* 2014; 35(34): 2285–2294.

107. Shahzad A, et al. Unfractionated heparin versus bivalirudin in primary percutaneous coronary intervention (HEAT-PPCI): An open-label, single centre, randomised controlled trial. *Lancet* 2014; 384(9957): 1849–1858.

108. Mehta SR, et al. Efficacy and safety of fondaparinux versus enoxaparin in patients with acute coronary syndromes undergoing percutaneous coronary intervention: Results from the OASIS-5 trial. *J Am Coll Cardiol* 2007; 50(18): 1742–1751.

109. Mega JL, et al. Rivaroxaban in patients with a recent acute coronary syndrome. *N Engl J Med* 2012; 366(1): 9–19.

110. Alexander JH, et al. Apixaban with antiplatelet therapy after acute coronary syndrome. *N Engl J Med* 2011; 365(8): 699–708.

111. Oldgren J, et al. Dabigatran vs placebo in patients with acute coronary syndromes on dual antiplatelet therapy: A randomized, double-blind, phase II trial. *Eur Heart J* 2011; 32(22): 2781–2789.

8

Vascular access for percutaneous interventions and angiography

NAY HTYTE AND CHRISTOPHER J. WHITE

INTRODUCTION

A successful percutaneous vascular procedure begins before entering the catheterization laboratory with planning the details about procedural goals, including choosing an optimal vascular access site. Since access site–related complications are important causes of procedure-related morbidity,[1] securing safe and effective vessel entry is a major determinate for a complication-free case.

This chapter discusses (1) technical methods for obtaining vascular access for various arterial and venous sites; (2) access issues related to scenarios such as, obese patients, those with repeated procedures who have developed dense scar tissue, and accessing femoral bypass grafts; and (3) options for vascular site hemostasis by describing commonly used closure techniques.

BACKGROUND

Equipment and technology used in percutaneous vascular procedures continue to rapidly evolve. Dr. Sven-Ivar Seldinger's method for performing vessel puncture, first described in 1953,[2] remains the basis for current methods of vascular access. There have been two major modifications that constitute today's widely-used modified Seldinger technique. The first is the puncture of the anterior wall of the vessel instead of a through-and-through approach with subsequent withdrawal of the access needle. A second change to Seldinger's original technique is the use of an introducer sheath that maintains vascular access[3] while different catheters are exchanged.

His technique was originally described using a stylet, which is no longer used today. Instead, a hollow access needle is now used for anterior wall puncture. Once blood flow through the needle is established, a wire is advanced through it into the vessel. The needle is then withdrawn while the wire remains in the vessel. An introducer sheath is inserted into the vessel over the wire, at which point the dilator and wire can be removed.

CHOOSING THE OPTIMAL ACCESS SITE

Choosing the optimal access site affects the likelihood of procedural success. When planning access for a left- or right-sided heart catheterization, the common femoral artery (CFA) and vein are a frequent choice.[4] With percutaneous coronary intervention (PCI), the radial artery is increasingly the preferred access site by many cardiologists. For lower extremity percutaneous transluminal angioplasty (PTA), the contralateral CFA is the most common access site.[5] The brachial artery (via percutaneous approach or cutdown) is often selected for PCI or PTA. Less frequently used vascular access sites include axillary, popliteal, tibial, and carotid arteries. Access is most commonly obtained from the patient's right side due to the ergonomics of a right-handed operator and the fixed position of the monitors in the room.

Novel procedures, such as transcatheter aortic valve replacement (TAVR), endovascular abdominal aortic aneurysm repair (EVAR), and percutaneous left ventricular assist devices (pLVADs) require the placement of large-diameter catheters. The femoral artery is typically used to accommodate equipment for these procedures. However, in patients with severe aorto-iliac disease or a small femoral artery that precludes femoral access, specialized vascular access techniques may be considered, such as a transapical approach or direct aortic access via a cutdown. Another unique method is the trans-caval or cavo-aortic approach, whereby the common femoral vein (CFV) is used to access the inferior vena cava (IVC) with subsequent direct puncture of the infrarenal abdominal aorta.

One of the foremost determinates in planning and selecting vascular access is the target organ to be studied and/or treated. Catheter length and distance to the target are important considerations. For lower extremity procedures, the limitation in catheter length can be a limiting factor, especially in taller individuals. Also important is the direction of approach to the vascular branches that the equipment will traverse. Attention should be paid to the ostium of the vascular structure of interest and the angle it makes relative to the parent vessel. Examples include the visceral arterial branches—such as the celiac, superior and inferior mesenteric arteries—which often have caudally directed ostia that are more easily approached from proximal thoracic aorta or upper extremity sites.

The type of procedure to be performed and equipment to be used will dictate selection of the appropriately sized vessels. The average sizes of normal arteries and veins at various access locations are listed in Table 8.1. When planning for TAVR, EVAR, or pLVAD, noninvasive imaging modalities,

Table 8.1 Average sizes (diameters) of arteries used for percutaneous vascular access

Artery	Typical size (mm)
Radial artery	2–4
Brachial artery	5–7
Femoral artery	7–9
Popliteal artery	4–6
Dorsalis pedis artery	2–4

such as computerized tomographic angiography (CTA), may be useful for vessel sizing. Although sheath sizes can be upgraded using the over-the-wire technique, planning the correct size from the beginning can reduce procedural time. Most manufacturers include the minimal sheath size required for their equipment in their instructions for use (IFU) documentation or on their packaging. Table 8.2 lists some commonly performed PCI and PTA procedures and their required sheath sizes.

PERCUTANEOUS ARTERIAL ACCESS

Common femoral artery

ANATOMIC CONSIDERATIONS

The CFA is the continuation of the external iliac artery, which is a bifurcating branch off the common iliac artery (CIA) (Figure 8.1). The left and right CIAs originate at the distal end of the aorta, and each give rise to the internal and external iliac arteries (IIA and EIA, respectively). The medially directed internal branch supplies the organs of the pelvic and gluteal region and can be identified by its numerous tributaries. The EIA courses more laterally and transitions into the CFA as it passes the inguinal ligament into the inguinal region. The CFA extends into the lower extremity until it bifurcates into the superficial and deep (profunda) femoral arteries (SFA and PFA, respectively).

EXTERNAL LANDMARKS

The optimal entry for femoral artery access is an anterior wall puncture into the CFA. This should be proximal to the femoral bifurcation and distal to a horizontal line drawn from the inferior-most point of the inferior epigastric artery (most distal branch of the EIA) (Figure 8.2). This region frequently lies anterior to the bony surface of the infero-lateral pelvic girdle and femoral head right at the hip joint, making it ideal for compressive hemostasis when needed. When available, reviewing prior femoral angiograms will allow proper identification of the CFA as well as valuable anatomic information, such as high bifurcations.

Several techniques have been described for identification of an ideal location for CFA access. These variations include using the skin or inguinal crease, identifying palpable bony landmarks, finding the point of maximal pulse, and/or

Table 8.2 Common percutaneous coronary and peripheral procedures and required sheath sizes

Procedure type	Required sheath sizes (Fr)
Diagnostic Angiography	4
Cardiac Procedures	
PCI for most Type A lesions	6
Complex PCI/bifurcation stenting	8
Balloon valvuloplasty	11–14
Intra-aortic balloon pump	7.5–8
Impella® pLVAD device	13 (2.5) or 14 (CP®)
TandemHeart® pVAD	21
AngioJet™ (coronary)	6–7
Laser atherectomy ELCA™	4–7
Rotablator™	6–10
TAVR	22–26
Swan Ganz catheterization	7
Transvenous pacemaker	5
Right heart biopsy	9
ASD/PFO closure	6–12
Watchman™ LAA closure device	14
Mitral clip	24
Peripheral Procedures	
Most lower extremity angioplasty	6
Peripheral Rotablator	4–8
Orbital atherectomy with Diamondback 360®	6
Directional atherectomy TurboHawk™	6–8
pEVAR (TriVascular® Ovation™ device)	14
Angiojet™ (peripheral)	4–8
Laser atherectomy Turbo-Power™	7
AngioVac™	22
Carotid artery stenting with Mo.Ma® proximal protection	9
Carotid artery stenting with distal protection	4–6

Note: ASD, atrial septal defect; ELCA, excimer laser coronary angioplasty; Fr, French; LAA, left atrial appendage; PCI, percutaneous coronary intervention; pEVAR, percutaneous endovascular aneurysm repair; PFO, patent foramen ovale; pLVAD, percutaneous left ventricular assist device; pVAD, percutaneous ventricular assist device; TAVR, transcatheter aortic valve replacement.

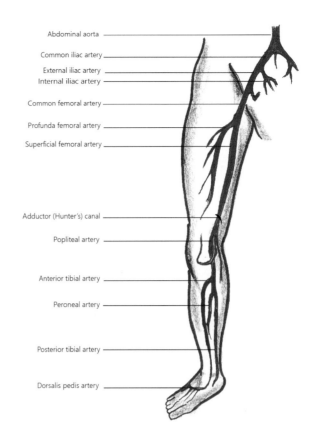

Figure 8.1 Major arteries of the lower extremity.

using image-guidance such as fluoroscopy or ultrasound. While these techniques can be combined, when used as a single method, other than ultrasound, these are not reliable methods.

The inguinal ligament anatomically demarcates the transition of EIA and CFA. However, it often does not correspond with the inguinal crease. In a study of 100 patients, Lechner et al. showed the distance between the inguinal ligament and the inguinal crease varied between 0 and 11 cm, and in three quarters of the patients, the CFA bifurcated above the inguinal crease.[6] Consequently, using the inguinal crease as a landmark for femoral access is not advisable. Nevertheless, a survey[7] of interventionalists revealed that 40% of the time the inguinal crease was used to obtain femoral access and bony landmarks were used only 13% of the time.

Palpation of the anterior superior iliac spine (ASIS) and symphysis pubis identifies the two anatomic locations that are connected by the inguinal ligament. An imaginary line connecting these two points identifies the superior border of the CFA. The artery usually takes its course through the inguinal canal at the medial one-third along this line.

The point of maximum palpation of the femoral pulse is less reliable for identifying the CFA. Because the impulse can be affected by the amount of overlying soft tissue, areas with a lesser amount of subcutaneous fat will result in a more forceful impulse, however, may not correspond to the ideal site. Therefore, this method is not suitable as a sole technique to guide needle puncture.

The femoral head is an important bony landmark to identify. In a study of patients undergoing femoral artery puncture, the bifurcation of the femoral artery was below the inferior border of the femoral head (Figure 8.3) in 55% and at the inferior border in 22%. However, the center of

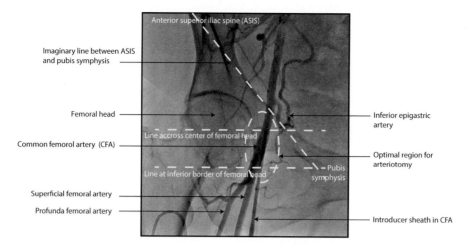

Figure 8.2 Fluoroscopic landmarks for common femoral artery puncture.

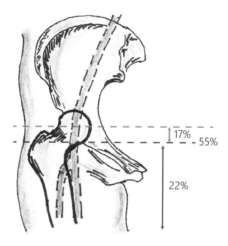

Figure 8.3 The common femoral artery bifurcation lies below the level of the center of the femoral head in 94% of patients found in a survey conducted by Schnyder et al.[8]

the femoral head was above the CFA bifurcation in 94% of patients.[8] This was confirmed in another study that showed optimal CFA puncture in 99% of patients when the needle entered at the level of the middle of the femoral head.[9]

The intended arteriotomy site is below the inferior epigastric artery; however, this vascular landmark cannot guide access but can only be used to confirm ideal entry after puncture and a femoral angiogram is performed. Nevertheless, it serves as an important landmark since this vessel does not cross the inguinal ligament[10] and functions as a surrogate marker for the origin of the CFA.

Many variations in the origin of the CFA have been described, including its origin from the gluteal or IIA, duplication of the femoral artery below the bifurcation with reuniting in the distal thigh, and location behind the thigh.[11] One important variation of the CFA is its length, ranging from 2.5 to 5 cm from the inguinal ligament, which translates to occurrence of high bifurcation.[10]

ULTRASOUND GUIDANCE

Ultrasound-guided arterial access allows direct visualization of needle entry, thus decreasing the number of needle passes through the artery and inadvertent venous puncture. The femoral artery is viewed in cross section using this technique (Figure 8.4a). Preparation for using ultrasound guidance adds to the total procedural time; however, actual time to access is shorter relative to the fluoroscopic method. In a study comparing fluoroscopic to ultrasound-guided access to the CFA, utilization of ultrasonography reduced the number of attempted punctures, time to arterial access, risk of venous puncture, and vascular complications.[12]

The ultrasound probe is held at the femoral location of intended puncture (Figure 8.4b). Directing it caudally enables visualization of the femoral bifurcation while directing it cranially allows identification of the CFA. Various characteristics differentiate the CFA from the CFV. The CFA is not compressible with the probe while the vein is easily compressed. Blood flow direction can also distinguish the artery from the vein. In addition, a triphasic pulse is observed in the artery with Doppler, while a monophasic signal is seen with venous flow.[13] With the probe held in place with one hand, needle puncture can be observed in real-time, allowing accurate entry on first pass. Using this technique, femoral arterial access is reportedly successful in >95% of patients undergoing percutaneous peripheral intervention.[14]

TECHNIQUE FOR RETROGRADE PUNCTURE

Although various techniques are available, as previously described, image guidance is recommended as it allows better identification of proper landmarks. Using fluoroscopy to identify the femoral head, a radiopaque marker—such as a hemostat tip—should be placed on the skin surface no higher than the midpoint of the femoral head and no lower than its inferior third. After palpating the femoral pulse at this location, the hemostat marker is replaced by the index, middle, and ring fingers of the left hand. At this point, removal or movement of these fingers is avoided as

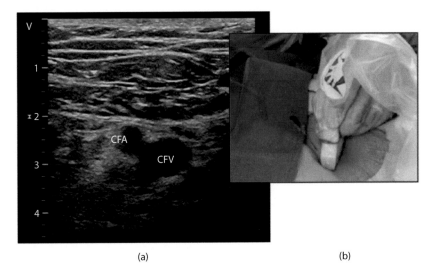

Figure 8.4 **(a)** Cross-sectional view of common femoral artery (CFA) and vein (CFV) seen by ultrasound imaging. **(b)** Ultrasound-guided needle puncture.

they mark the optimal arteriotomy site. Using three fingers enables palpation of the course of the artery lateral to medial as it courses cranially.

Subcutaneous infiltration of 1% lidocaine should adequately anesthetize the skin at the access site. Entry of the lidocaine needle should be in the same trajectory angle as the puncture needle to be used for access. After adequate infiltration of lidocaine subcutaneously, the access needle should be advanced into the anterior vessel wall along the same tract.

Many catheterization laboratories use the 18G Cook needle for arterial puncture because its entry into the artery is apparent as pulsating blood flow through the needle lumen. Alternatively, a 21G micropuncture needle can be used to gain vascular access.[15] This 7-cm-long access needle accommodates a 0.014-in nitinol wire that is packaged in a Micro-Introducer kit (Vascular Solutions, Minneapolis, MN) along with a 4- or 5-Fr sheath and dilator (Figure 8.5). This sheath can subsequently be exchanged for a larger diameter one over a 0.035-in wire. The use of a micropuncture sheath affords the opportunity for repeat arterial puncture with minimal bleeding risk should the arteriotomy be suboptimal. All equipment and needles should be flushed and prepped before use.

With the left-hand fingers positioned over the course of the artery, the access needle should puncture the skin at a 30° to 45° angle with its tip directed cranially. This allows optimal entry for the sheath to be secured in the arterial lumen without kinking or bending acutely at the arteriotomy site. Steep entry of the needle into the artery may result in an unwanted bend in the sheath, while a shallow angle of entry may result in a "high stick" with the needle entering the EIA.

Bright red blood return through the needle lumen is observed with anterior wall puncture; if a micropuncture needle is used, blood flow will be much slower. The wire is advanced through the needle lumen, and the needle is then removed over the wire while the left hand maintains hemostasis. Insertion of the micropuncture sheath facilitates

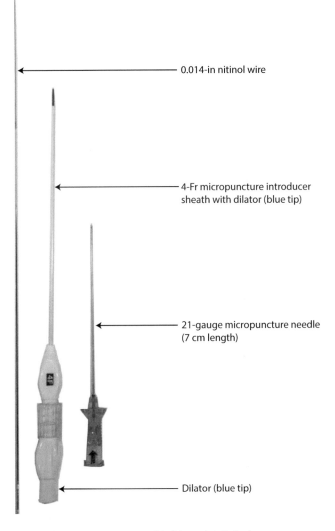

0.014-in nitinol wire

4-Fr micropuncture introducer sheath with dilator (blue tip)

21-gauge micropuncture needle (7 cm length)

Dilator (blue tip)

Figure 8.5 Micropuncture kit (Vascular Solutions, Minneapolis, MN).

femoral angiography using a 50/50 contrast/saline solution to identify improper puncture site, local bleeding, or vessel dissection. If any of these occur, the micropuncture sheath can be removed and manual compression applied in order to facilitate a repeat attempt at vascular access. When optimal access without complication is confirmed, the micropuncture sheath can be exchanged over a 0.035-in wire for the desired introducer sheath. Finally, the wire and dilator are removed and the sheath sidearm is aspirated and flushed, confirming good blood return.

COMPLICATIONS

CFA vascular access site complication is a significant cause of morbidity in percutaneous cases. Improvement in equipment and technical experience has contributed to a reduction in the incidence of complications. Although closure devices have resulted in faster patient recovery time after a procedure using the CFA, there is no evidence of a decrease in vascular complications.[16] Vascular site bleeding varies from 0.5%[17–20] to <3.5%.[21,22]

In addition to vessel dissection during guidewire or sheath insertion, complications at the femoral site can occur if arterial puncture is proximal or distal to the CFA. Puncture above the inguinal ligament results in entry of the EIA, which increases the risk for retroperitoneal hemorrhage due to lack of a bony surface for adequate compression of the artery for hemostasis. This life-threatening complication has been observed to occur in 0.5% to 0.75% of procedures performed via the femoral approach.[23,24] Female sex, older age, and low body weight are also risk factors for retroperitoneal hemorrhage.[24] When the puncture site is below the CFA in the PFA or SFA, there is an increased risk for pseudoaneurysm formation, which occurs in <2% of femoral access procedures.[19] Inadequate manual pressure postprocedure can also lead to a pseudoaneurysm. When the time for holding manual pressure is extended by 5 minutes over the standard time, the incidence rate for pseudoaneurysm can be reduced to 1%.[25] Other complications that may occur with femoral access include arteriovenous fistula (AVF) formation—at an incidence of <1%[26]—dissections, thrombosis, and embolism (Table 8.3).

With careful access, the CFA can be used for almost all percutaneous coronary or peripheral procedures. Since the access is centrally located, commonly used catheter equipment can be used to reach target organs. The CFA's larger lumen relative to other access sites can accommodate sheath sizes up to 24-Fr without occluding the vessel; therefore, it is preferred for procedures that require larger equipment such as TAVR, EVAR, or pLVAD. Equipment used for coronary and peripheral interventions and their associated sheath size requirements are listed in Table 8.2.

ANTEGRADE ACCESS

Antegrade CFA access is useful for ipsilateral lower extremity endovascular interventions, particularly those performed in infrapopliteal arteries.[27] Similar to retrograde access, complications related to location of arterial entry

Table 8.3 Rates of various femoral access site complications from a report of the NCDR CathPCI Registry

Type of complication	Incidence (%)
Access site bleed	0.82
Retroperitoneal bleed	0.29
Femoral artery occlusion	0.04
Embolization	0.04
Femoral artery dissection	0.24
Pseudoaneurysm	0.41
Arteriovenous fistula	0.06
All bleeding	1.08
All vascular complications	0.76

Source: Tavris, et al., *J. Invasive Cardiol.,* 24(7), pp. 328–334, 2012. With permission.

Note: NCDR, National Cardiovascular Data Registry; PCI, percutaneous coronary intervention.

occur such that retroperitoneal bleeding is associated with high EIA insertions, while pseudoaneurysms or AVFs occur more frequently if puncture occurs in the SFA.

A major difference between antegrade and retrograde access is the location of the skin incision. With the antegrade approach, after the midline of the femoral head is located fluoroscopically and marked using a hemostat tip, anesthetization with lidocaine and a skin incision is made superior or cephalad to the marker. Subsequently, the needle is directed caudally at a 45° angle, and extra precaution is taken for wire advancement into the SFA. Fluoroscopic guidance allows passage of the guidewire into the SFA prior to sheath insertion. The SFA and PFA can be differentiated fluoroscopically with a 30° to 45° oblique view.

Complications related to antegrade access are usually from a high arterial puncture, which places the patient at an increased risk for retroperitoneal hemorrhage.[27] Obese patients are at increased risk for these complications, and extra caution should be taken to locate the femoral head fluoroscopically as the inguinal crease is an unreliable marker for locating the CFA.[6]

ADVANTAGES OF FEMORAL OVER RADIAL ACCESS

There are advantages to femoral artery access over the radial approach. The femoral artery is central to most target organs and more catheter equipment is available for use from this access site. The average size of the CFA allows insertion of larger sheath sizes (i.e., up to 24-Fr). The CFA is less susceptible to spasm than the radial artery, allowing the operator to complete the procedure without concern for vessel collapse and occlusion around catheters, which may interfere with their positioning.

DISADVANTAGES OF FEMORAL COMPARED TO RADIAL ACCESS

Disadvantages of femoral access compared to a radial approach include longer postprocedural immobilization and recovery time. With the advent and increased use of closure devices, this issue is less concerning; however, post-procedure recovery is still quicker with radial artery access. Additionally, there is an increased risk for access site bleeding complications with femoral access.

Radial artery access

ANATOMY

The brachial artery bifurcates into the radial and ulnar arteries proximal to the elbow (Figure 8.6). These vessels continue parallel to one another, with the ulnar traveling along the medial aspect of the forearm and the radial artery laterally.[28] Access and sheath entry for procedures performed at the radial site are obtained in the distal forearm proximal to the wrist (Figure 8.7).

Most radial arterial anatomic variations occur at the level of bifurcation with high branching of the radial artery being a common anomaly. In an occasional patient, the ulnar artery may be absent,[11] making the radial artery the only major blood supply to the hand and inadvisable for procedural use. An incomplete palmar arch is another anatomic variant that places the hand at risk for ischemia when the radial artery is used for access. Its occurrence has been reported to range from 3%[29] to 21%.[30] However, in the most

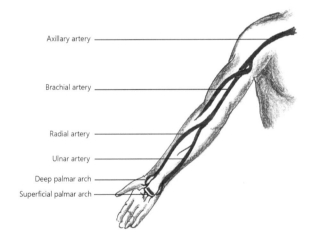

Figure 8.6 Arteries of the upper extremity.

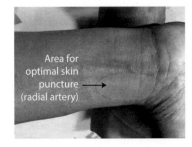

Figure 8.7 Optimal area for radial artery puncture. Slight hyperextension of the wrist can maximize palpation of the radial artery.

common subtype of this noncollateralized palmar artery of the hand, the ulnar branch supplies most of the superficial arch.

Radial artery access has increasingly been used in many catheterization labs and is the most commonly used site for PCI in many other countries.[31] Its capacity to safely secure a 6-Fr × 11 cm sheath enables many diagnostic and interventional procedures to be performed. However, complex interventions requiring large lumen sheaths and catheters for hemodynamic support, or procedures needing multiple wires and simultaneous stent placement—as in bifurcation lesion angioplasty—may not be amenable to radial access. The radial artery is susceptible to spasm, and there is an inherent risk for thrombosis, which is not a factor for diagnostic cases performed femorally.[32]

ALLEN TEST

The Allen test is a simple physical examination used to evaluate competent collateral blood flow to the hand. Circulation to the hand is temporarily occluded with pressure applied to the ulnar and radial arteries simultaneously. Clenching of the fist will cause blanching of the hand. Each artery is then released sequentially in turn to determine patency of the other. If sufficient collateral flow is present through a competent ulnar artery, there will be restoration of perfusion within 10 seconds while manual pressure is maintained on the radial artery.[2,33]

In a modified version of the Allen test, a pulse oximeter is used to observe the waveform as patency of collateral blood flow is tested and the Barbeau classification is applied; the time of the normal waveform to return is used to grade differing Barbeau responses to occlusion of the radial artery. Patients with Barbeau A or B (Figure 8.8) responses should tolerate radial access with little risk of compromised collateral flow, while Barbeau C and D patients have increased risk of inadequate collateral blood flow.[34]

INDICATIONS

There are situations in which the radial or brachial arteries offer procedural advantages over the femoral approach. These include patients with severely diseased aorto-iliac arteries in whom lower extremity intervention is needed, visceral arterial interventions with caudally-oriented main branches, morbid obesity, or compromised femoral sites (i.e., due to infection or excessive scar tissue). Primary PCI is commonly performed using radial artery access and has been shown to have similar outcomes as femoral access in patients presenting with chronic stable ischemic heart disease or acute coronary syndromes, including ST-segment elevation myocardial infarction (STEMI).[35,36]

TECHNICAL METHODS FOR RADIAL ARTERY ACCESS

Proper positioning of the patient and preparation of the forearm, with the wrist supernated, is important to maximize radial artery exposure. In preparing the patient for radial artery puncture, the arm should be positioned

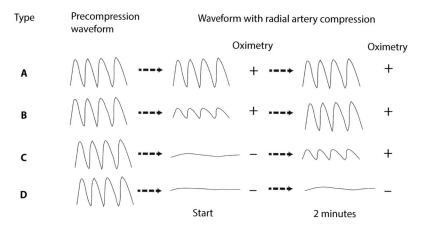

Figure 8.8 Barbeau classification for testing patency of collateral blood flow to the hand. Pulse oximetry is assessed while occlusive pressure is applied to the radial artery.

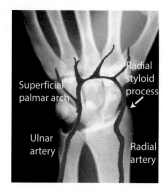

Figure 8.9 Distal radial artery near styloid process of the wrist joint.

parallel to the body. A towel rolled up into a cylinder can be placed under the wrist (Figure 8.7). This will allow slight hyperextension of the wrist and straightening of the radial artery, thereby allowing optimal palpation for the pulse. Arterial puncture can occur between 4 cm proximally from the wrist to 1 cm distal to the styloid process. However, the most distal part of the vessel before the bony prominence of the radial styloid may present a challenge (Figure 8.9), because the vessel often takes a course that is slightly angulated, becoming coaxial with the trajectory of the needle entry. This carries the potential for the puncture needle to contact the vessel at a very shallow angle making insertion suboptimal and shearing the vessel wall, thus increasing the risk for dissection.

Palpation for the pulse can be done using two or three fingers to delineate the course of the artery. After anesthetizing the skin puncture site with 1% lidocaine, the area is ready for needle entry. The access needle should enter the skin at a 30° angle with the goal being an anterior wall puncture. Once blood flow is observed through the needle lumen, a 0.014-in nitinol guidewire can be advanced through it. The wire should advance smoothly with vigilant attention for any resistance. Once the wire is adequately advanced, the needle can be exchanged for

a radial 5- or 6-Fr hydrophilic sheath over the wire. After the sheath is safely secured, the sidearm should be flushed with a spasmolytic solution (verapamil 2.5 mg and/or nitroglycerine 0.1–0.4 mg, in saline) and a heparin bolus to prevent vessel thrombosis.[37]

Ultrasound-guided radial artery puncture is not routinely used, and there are no randomized prospective studies comparing palpation of radial pulse versus sonography-assisted access. One single-center study using this image-guided technique reported a median access time of 35 seconds and a success rate of 80% with the first puncture attempt and 92% on a subsequent attempt.[38] First-time success rates with palpation have been reported to be as low as 34% with a median time to access of 314 seconds[39] in other small observational studies comparing the two methods. A more recent prospective small study among experienced cardiac anesthesiologists showed no difference in time for successful access, number of attempts, or bleeding complications with palpation versus image-guided radial access.[40] Larger comparative studies will be required to demonstrate the benefits of ultrasound-guided radial access.

COMPLICATIONS

Radial access has been reported to be safer than femoral arterial access, primarily driven by fewer access site–related bleeding complications. Safety benefits of radial arterial access have been observed with primary PCI of patients with STEMI with lower mortality, decreased combined death/myocardial infarction (MI)/stroke, and less major bleeding compared to femoral access.[41] Local bleeding is easier to manage for radial arterial access because of its superficial location and proximity to bony structures that allow relatively easy compressive hemostasis. However, there is a learning curve for passage of the catheter through the vasculature of the upper arm and neck that presents a challenge of added risk for injury and vascular perforation away from the access site that is not present with procedures performed from the femoral artery.[42] Other complications, such as bleeding after sheath removal, radial artery spasm, thrombosis, sterile abscess formation, pseudoaneurysm, and AVFs have been described, occurring at rates <5%.[43] Hand ischemia, forearm vessel perforation, and sterile abscess formation are discussed further in this chapter.

Brachial and axillary artery access

Anatomically, the axillary artery transitions into the brachial artery distal to the inferior border of the teres major muscle. It lies medial to the humerus and biceps tendon and its point of maximal pulsation can be palpated proximal to the antecubital fossa before reaching the neck of the radius where the radial and ulnar artery bifurcation occurs (Figure 8.6). Some variations in vascular anatomy include high location of this bifurcation or anomalous branching of these arteries from the axillary or high brachial artery.[44]

Relative to the radial site, brachial and axillary arteries provide vascular access that is closer in proximity to visceral and lower extremity vasculature and can be used for patients whose femoral site is inaccessible. Additionally, brachial and axillary arteries can accommodate slightly larger sheath sizes (i.e., up to 7-Fr) than the radial artery with minimal risk for limb ischemia.[45]

TECHNICAL METHOD

For adequate exposure of the brachial artery, the arm should be positioned slightly abducted and extended with some elevation relative to the patient. The hand can be placed behind the patient's head or outstretched on a table. Ultrasound guidance can augment proper identification of the vessel and decrease complication risks;[46] however, the point of maximal pulsation above the antecubital fossa is adequate in most cases. The modified Seldinger technique has now replaced the traditional practice of an arterial cutdown. A 4-cm long 21G micropuncture needle is recommended for arterial puncture, which will allow passage of a 0.014 in nitinol wire through the needle lumen. After the needle has been exchanged for a micropuncture (4- or 5-Fr) sheath over the nitinol wire, a 0.035-in wire can then be substituted for the nitinol wire to allow insertion of a larger sheath. As in the radial artery, the brachial artery is also susceptible to spasm and thrombosis and, therefore, using vasodilators (nitroglycerin, verapamil) and anticoagulation is recommended.

COMPLICATIONS

Bleeding and hematoma formation is a major complication that can occur with brachial artery access; however, local access site complication rates are comparable to femoral arterial access at <2%.[47] Pseudoaneurysm formation, local thrombosis, AVFs, and median nerve injury have all been reported as possible complications at the brachial access site with incidence rates of <2%.[45] Vessel occlusion

and thrombosis leading to arm ischemia have been reported at up to 6%.[48] In one series—with the use of an introducer sheath and adequate anticoagulation—vessel occlusion occurred in <1% and was more frequent in females than males (1.24% vs. 0.28%, respectively).[49] Other complications seen with brachial artery access include hematoma formation with median nerve compression and arterial dissection.[47]

Popliteal artery access

INDICATION

There are special cases when puncture of the popliteal artery will facilitate procedural success, including percutaneous recanalization of ostial SFA lesions on the ipsilateral leg, CFA stenosis, accessing aorto-femoral bypass graft lesions, difficult contralateral access, and with multiple lesions in SFA and iliac arteries on both sides. For proximal lesions, the popliteal artery should be accessed in the retrograde direction. Antegrade popliteal access directed distally is indicated in percutaneous interventions for critical limb ischemia (CLI) and limb salvage procedures.[50]

ANATOMY

The popliteal artery lies within the popliteal fossa in the posterior knee. It originates as the SFA, exits Hunter's canal, and continues distally to form the tibial-peroneal trunk as it branches into the arteries of the lower part of the leg. Within the fossa, the popliteal artery lies medial to the popliteal vein (Figure 8.10a).

TECHNICAL METHODS

Patency of the popliteal artery should be established before planning its access. Contrast injection should be performed initially through ipsilateral or contralateral CFA access to allow angiographic visualization of the popliteal artery. Therefore, obtaining CFA access with a 4-Fr sheath should precede positioning of the patient for posterior access. Once the sheath has been sutured in place, the patient should then be turned to the prone position followed by prepping and draping of the popliteal fossa. A fluoroscopic road map of the popliteal artery using the angiogram performed from the CFA sheath will allow visual guidance for popliteal access (Figure 8.11). Alternatively, ultrasonographic imaging can be used.

The popliteal artery and vein lie within the popliteal fossa in an anterior to posterior relationship. When using ultrasound imaging, the artery will be seen deeper to the vein and more medial (Figure 8.10b). Pressing down on the vessels with the probe will cause the vein to compress, thereby allowing its proper identification (Figure 8.10c). After adequately anesthetizing an area caudal to the probe, the micropuncture access needle should be advanced with direct visualization of the arterial puncture. The popliteal artery can facilitate sheath sizes up to 6-Fr with minimal risk for limb ischemia.

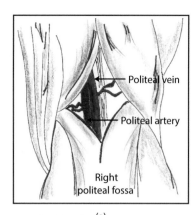

(a)

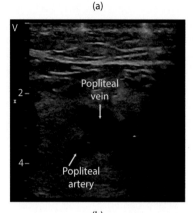

(b)

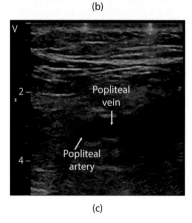

(c)

Figure 8.10 **(a)** Popliteal fossa showing location of popliteal artery and vein. Note popliteal vein is more posterior and lateral within the fossa. **(b)** Ultrasound of popliteal artery and vein. **(c)** Ultrasound showing easily compressible popliteal vein.

Tibial artery access

INDICATION

The tibial artery is the access site of choice in special cases of CLI with below the knee (infrapopliteal) occlusions involving the tibial artery. Other situations where this access site can be helpful include SFA recanalization where femoral or popliteal access is unobtainable. The success rate for recanalization of patients with CLI or Rutherford II-III claudication symptoms using tibial access has been reported around 64% with very little complication and 100% patency rate of the access artery

at 1-month follow-up.[51] This could serve as a feasible alternative for access, especially when performed for limb salvage purposes.

ANATOMY

The anterior tibial artery transitions into the dorsalis pedis at the ankle and is one of two major arteries supplying the plantar arch and arteries of the foot. Using ultrasound guidance enables visualization and entry into the vessel. The dorsalis pedis or anterior tibial arteries lie superficially and can be easily accessed for this reason.

TECHNICAL METHODS

Ultrasound guidance should be used for identification of the tibial artery (Figure 8.12). After locating the artery, a 4-cm long 21G micropuncture needle is used to puncture the artery and facilitate insertion of a 4-Fr sheath. An antispasmodic solution (2.5 mg verapamil with 100 mcg of nitroglycerin) should then be injected to prevent vessel spasm. A 6-Fr Glidesheath Slender introducer sheath (Terumo Medical Corp, Somerset, NJ) can be placed in the tibial artery with little risk for vascular occlusion[51] since it has an outer diameter of a standard 5-Fr sheath.

Carotid artery access

Specific indications for direct transcervical carotid artery access include carotid artery stenting (CAS) in situations where excessive vascular tortuosity or stenosis prohibit canalization of the carotid artery from the femoral approach, or when there is higher risk for embolic events with manipulation of catheters around an aortic arch that has severe atheromatous disease. Femoral artery occlusive disease, severe aorto-iliac stenosis, prior aortic or femoral vascular surgery, and severe obesity present challenges to carotid arterial access and, therefore, may benefit from direct carotid artery access. Technical success for CAS via direct access to cervical vasculature, with or without embolic protection devices (EPDs), has been reported as high as 96.3%.[52] When combined with an EPD, such as the MICHI Neuroprotection System (Silk Road Medical, Inc., Sunnyvale, CA) (Figure 8.13), this access technique may be superior to femoral arterial access in decreasing the risk for stroke with CAS because catheter negotiation of the aortic arch can be avoided.[53] However, this requires a mini-incision and surgical cutdown for carotid artery access. For the purpose of this chapter, focus will be made on percutaneous direct trans-cervical puncture.

ANATOMIC CONSIDERATIONS

The internal carotid artery (ICA) originates at the bifurcation of the common carotid artery (CCA) on either side of the neck (Figure 8.14). It can be identified angiographically by having no branches, while the external carotid artery has several vascular distributions to regions of the head and neck. The carotid bulb lies at the bifurcation of the CCA as a nerve bundle abutting the wall of the ICA. One anatomic

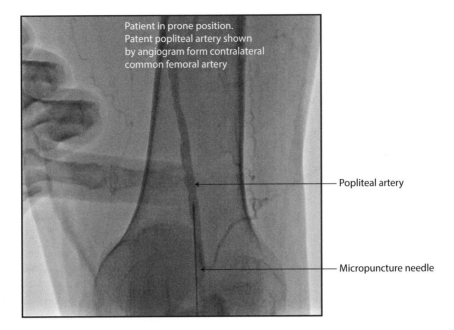

Patient in prone position.
Patent popliteal artery shown
by angiogram form contralateral
common femoral artery

— Popliteal artery

— Micropuncture needle

Figure 8.11 Fluoroscopy-guided popliteal arterial puncture.

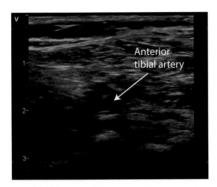

Anterior
tibial artery

Figure 8.12 Ultrasound image of anterior tibial artery.

difference between the left and right CCA is the origin of the left occurs from the aortic arch in the chest while the right branches from the brachiocephalic artery at the neck. Rare anomalies can be found such as the left CCA originating from a common trunk with the brachiocephalic artery.[54]

TECHNICAL METHODS

Ultrasound imaging can guide entry of a micropuncture needle into the CCA. The patient should be positioned in Trendelenburg with the base of the neck adequately exposed. Once needle entry into the CCA is achieved, an angiogram can be performed through the lumen of the needle or the 4- or 5-Fr micropuncture sheath. A 6-Fr sheath can be inserted into the CCA and secured in place, which will accommodate filter-type EPDs.

Trans-caval aortic access

With the increased use of new percutaneous therapeutic options such as TAVR, there is potential need for access with large-diameter sheaths and catheters. In such situations where access to the proximal aorta and femoral artery access is prohibitive, a trans-aortic approach using the IVC can be pursued. In this technique, the femoral vein, which is a more compliant vessel than the artery, accommodates large sheath entry, which can then be advanced into the aorta in the lumbar region. This technique has been used in transcatheter implantation and replacement of the aortic valve in patients with inaccessible femoral arteries and frailty scores that preclude safe surgical valve replacement.

ANATOMIC CONSIDERATIONS

The IVC lies in close proximity to the adjoining abdominal aorta. Because of its low pressure, the risk of bleeding into the surrounding confined space during arterial perforation is low and will avert hemorrhagic occurrence by venous decompression. Additionally, acquired aorto-caval fistulas are not emergently life-threatening.[55,56]

TECHNICAL METHODS

Contrast-enhanced computed tomography (CT) of the abdominal aorta is a critical part of planning for caval-aortic access. This allows identification of landmarks in relation to the lumbar spine during the procedure and selection of the crossing trajectory into the least calcified region in the aorta.

Access through the IVC into the aorta begins with a simultaneous aortogram and venogram (Figure 8.15); therefore, femoral venous and arterial access is secured at the beginning of the procedure. It is important to use heparin for adequate anticoagulation throughout the procedure. A gooseneck snare is placed in the aorta at the region of the needle entry from the IVC and functions as a target for the guidewire as it is advanced into the abdominal aorta from

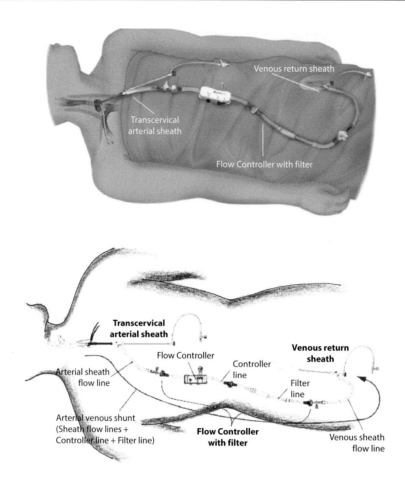

Figure 8.13 MICHI Neuroprotective system (Silk Road Medical Inc., Sunnyvale, CA).

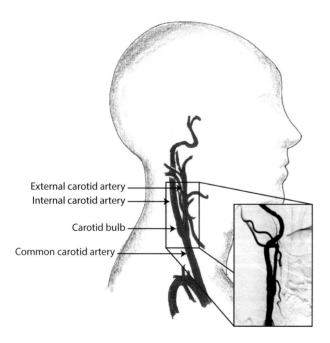

Figure 8.14 Anatomy of the common carotid artery bifurcation and the internal and external carotid arteries. The external carotid artery has several branches within the neck while the internal carotid does not branch until it becomes intracranial.

the IVC. The snare will then be used to grab the guidewire as it crosses into the aorta. A coaxial crossing system is used for transcaval puncture, which consists of a stiff 0.014-in guidewire (Asahi ConfianzaPro12, Abbott Vascular, Santa Clara, CA) inside a 0.035-in wire converter (Piggyback, Vascular Solutions, Minneapolis, MN) inside a support catheter (Navicross, Terumo, Somerset, NJ), which is then advanced through a guiding catheter. This crossing system is inserted into the IVC and directed toward the snare (Figure 8.16a). A Bovie or electrocautery electrode tip is connected to the proximal end of the stiff guidewire with forceps and then put on cutting mode. While energized, the distal end of the wire is advanced toward the snare target. Once the wire has crossed into the aorta and insertion into the snare is confirmed, securing the distal end of the wire by cinching the snare will enable the crossing system to be advanced into the aorta (Figure 8.16b through 8.16f). A more rigid 0.035-in guidewire, such as the Lunderquist (Cook, Bloomington, IN), can then be placed through the system, which will allow enough support for delivery of large sheaths through the cavo-aortic tract.[56] This access tract is closed with a nitinol occluder device that is used for closing ductus arteriosus (Amplatzer Duct Occluder, St. Jude Medical, St. Paul, MN). Similar successful closure can be achieved with a ventricular septal defect (VSD) closure device (Figure 8.17) (Amplatzer muscular VSD occluder, St. Jude Medical, St. Paul, MN).

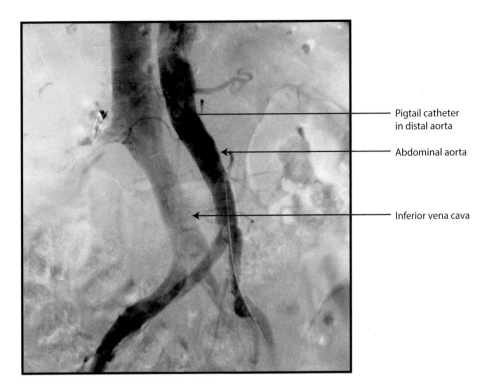

Pigtail catheter
in distal aorta

Abdominal aorta

Inferior vena cava

Figure 8.15 Simultaneous aortogram and venogram for trans-caval access.

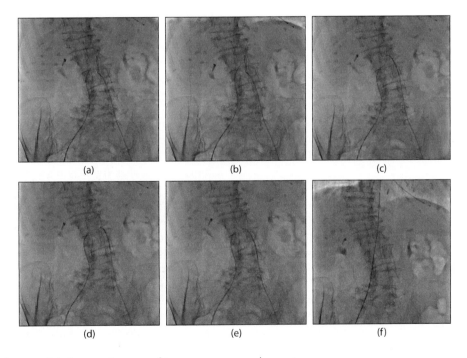

Figure 8.16 **(a–f)** Sequential cine-angiogram of trans-venous caval puncture.

This is a relatively novel technique and allows percutaneous procedures with large-diameter sheaths to be performed in patients who otherwise cannot accommodate their passage through the femoral artery. Greenbaum et al.[56] reported a series of 19 TAVR patients in whom sheath sizes up to 24-Fr were successfully placed via the caval-aortic technique, including closure device implantation.

PERCUTANEOUS VENOUS ACCESS

The veins of the lower extremity run parallel to the arterial tree and the anatomic nomenclature is analogous to the arterial counterpart. The relationship in anatomic location between the artery and vein within specific regions is important to know when attempting access in order to avoid accidental entry into the artery.

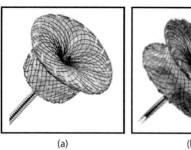
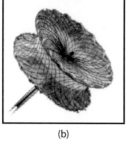

(a)   (b)

Figure 8.17 Amplatzer occluder devices (St. Jude Medical, St. Paul, MN).

General technical considerations

The modified Seldinger technique is recommended for percutaneous venous access. Although the underlying concept of exchanging a sheath over a wire after vascular puncture with a needle is the same as with percutaneous arterial access, the low pressure and blood flow direction of the venous system requires the use of a syringe attached to the needle with continuous aspiration for confirmation of vessel entry and adequate flow. The syringe should contain saline or heparinized saline to prevent inadvertent entry of air into the vessel as the needle is advanced. For all percutaneous access sites, needle entry into the skin should be made 2–3 cm distal to the expected vessel wall puncture.

Technical methods are similar in most access sites, including the CFV, superficial femoral vein (SFV), popliteal, internal jugular (IJ), and subclavian vein (SCV). However, the antecubital site does not require use of ultrasound guidance and can be accessed by insertion of an 18G IV into the median cubital vein with subsequent entry into the basilic vein.

Common femoral vein access

Indications for CFV access include right heart catheterization, placement of an IVC filter, diagnostic and intervention procedures of the superior vena cava (SVC), transseptal puncture to access the left atrium (i.e., for balloon mitral valvuloplasty, percutaneous mitral valve repair, or left atrial appendage closure device implantation), intracardiac procedures such as closure of a patent foramen ovale (PFO) or atrial septal defect (ASD), temporary transvenous pacemaker (TVP) placement, trans-caval access or central venous access for administration of medications.

ANATOMY

In the distal lower extremity, the deep and superficial veins drain into the popliteal vein, which then traverses the popliteal fossa into Hunter's canal where it becomes the SFV. The superficial and deep femoral veins (DFVs) join to become the CFV within the femoral triangle (Figure 8.18). The inguinal ligament forms the superior border of the

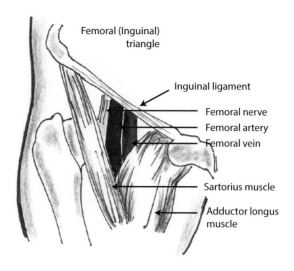

Figure 8.18 Femoral triangle. The femoral vein, artery, and nerve are found medial to lateral bordered by the inguinal ligament superiorly, adductor longus muscle medially, and sartorius muscle laterally.

triangle while the sartorius muscle and adductor longus muscle make up the lateral and medial borders, respectively. The neurovascular bundle within this femoral triangle consists of the femoral vein, artery, and nerve from medial to lateral.[28]

The external landmarks used to identify the inguinal ligament described earlier in the section for CFA access can be used. Additionally, palpation of the point of maximum impulse in this area identifies the femoral artery. Once this location has been identified, an area 1 cm medial and 1–2 cm distal should be chosen for skin puncture. However, care should be taken that, as the vessels travel more distally, the location of the vein is posterior to the femoral artery, thereby increasing the risk for inadvertent arterial puncture.

After adequately anesthetizing the skin with infiltration of 1% lidocaine, a micropuncture needle attached to a syringe with 1–2 mL of saline should be advanced at a 45° angle with continuous aspiration. Once adequate blood return is confirmed, a 0.014-in nitinol wire is passed through the needle lumen, paying close attention for resistance. Fluoroscopically, the path of the wire right of the patient's spine (left on viewing monitor) confirms appropriate venous access. A 4- or 5-Fr micropuncture sheath is advanced over the wire, which is then exchanged for a 0.035-in J-tipped wire that facilitates placement of a larger sheath. The larger vessel diameter of the CFV compared to the CFA allows accommodation of sheath sizes.

Although ultrasound guidance can assist with direct visualization of the femoral vein (Figure 8.19a through 8.19c) and reduce the number of puncture attempts or inadvertent arterial puncture, its use for CFV access is infrequent. When both the CFV and artery are to be accessed, it is recommended that venous access be attempted first.[57]

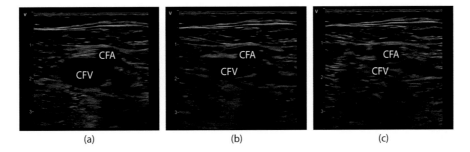

Figure 8.19 (a–c) Ultrasound of common femoral vein. Note that the vein is easily compressible compared to the artery. Left common femoral vein (CFV) and artery (CFA) shown.

Popliteal vein access

ANATOMY

The popliteal vein forms with the joining of tibial and saphenous veins below the patella and traverses the popliteal fossa into Hunter's canal (also known as adductor canal) at which point it transitions into the SFV. Within the popliteal fossa, the popliteal vein lies lateral to the popliteal artery (Figure 8.10a) and courses posterior to the artery as it crosses from medial to lateral within the fossa.

The SFV joins with the DFV then subsequently receives drainage from the great saphenous vein (a second major venous drainage of the lower leg) to form the CFV.

INDICATION

Superficial femoral and popliteal veins can be accessed using similar techniques as arterial access. Ultrasound guidance is recommended. Access at these vascular locations is desirable for percutaneous thrombolysis or thrombectomy procedures involving the proximal deep veins of the lower extremity, such as the common or external iliac veins.

TECHNICAL METHODS

Popliteal vein access is obtained with ultrasound guidance using a similar technique as with CFV access. The patient is positioned in the prone position with the popliteal fossa prepped and draped. Under ultrasound imaging, the vein will lie posteriorly within the fossa relative to the artery and will compress easily with the ultrasound probe (Figure 8.10b and 8.10c). With the patient in the prone position, the vein lies on top of the artery on ultrasound imaging and closer to the probe. Once the vessel is verified, the skin entry site for the needle, approximately 1 cm inferior to the ultrasound probe, should be anesthetized with 1% lidocaine. After adequate infiltration is achieved with local anesthesia, the access needle attached to a syringe with 1–2 mL of saline should be advanced while aspirating. Once adequate blood return is obtained, the syringe can be removed and a 0.035-in J-tipped wire can be advanced through the needle lumen. Fluoroscopic visualization will aid insertion of the wire and further advancement. The needle is then removed, and an introducer sheath can then be entered over the wire and subsequently secured in place.

The SFV can be accessed using a similar technique described above. However, the patient should be in the supine position. Ultrasound imaging will provide adequate visualization and guidance for accurate identification of the vascular structures. Needle entry, infiltration of local anesthesia, and introducer sheath insertion techniques do not vary from the described method for popliteal vein access.

COMPLICATIONS

Local hemorrhage and bleeding are complications that can occur with SFV and popliteal vein access. Compartment syndrome with compression of neurovascular structures is a major complication that requires surgical intervention. Severe pain and neuromotor impairment after access should alert potential for this complication, and the patient should be evaluated promptly. An intracompartmental pressure greater than 30 mmHg is high risk for developing this potentially limb-threatening complication.

Internal jugular vein access

INDICATION

The IJ vein is accessed for indications that range from central venous access for medication administration and multiple sampling of venous blood for monitoring of electrolytes and hematologic trends, to right heart catheterization procedures, including pulmonary artery catheter placement for continuous hemodynamic monitoring, TVP placement, and IV interventions of the upper thoracic veins. There is no absolute contraindication for IJ vein access. However, relative contraindications include IJ thrombosis and presence of overlying skin infection.

ANATOMY

The IJ veins receive blood from the sigmoid dural and inferior petrosal sinuses of the head and begin at the jugular foramen at the base of the skull on both sides and unite with the SCVs to form the innominate veins. The left and right innominate veins combine to form the SVC. The IJ drains blood from the head and neck as it travels vertically down the side of the neck.

Although external landmarks can be used to access the IJ vein, ultrasound-guided vessel entry is now recommended for routine use.[58,13] It has been shown to reduce the number of unsuccessful attempts, vein thrombosis, and infection rates for indwelling access lines.[13]

TECHNICAL METHOD

The IJ vein is usually found between the two clavicular heads of the sternocleidomastoid muscle. Skin entry is recommended at the apex of the triangle formed by the clavicular heads and the clavicle. However, the use of ultrasound imaging allows needle entry along the lower length of the vein. The patient should be positioned in Trendelenburg with the head slightly turned in the contralateral direction. With imaging, the vessel is viewed in cross section and can be seen lateral to the carotid artery (Figure 8.20). The vein will compress easily by applying moderate pressure of the probe to the skin.

Once the area of entry has been selected, the skin should be anesthetized by infiltrating with 1% lidocaine. Vessel puncture can be performed using the micropuncture kit or a regular 18G access needle attached to a syringe with 1 mL or 2 mL saline. Holding the ultrasound probe in place, the needle should be advanced with continuous aspiration in an acute angle to the ultrasound probe for visualization as it enters. Directing it slightly lateral will avoid accidental arterial puncture. Once vascular access is obtained, an introducer sheath can be placed using the modified Seldinger technique and secured in place.

Sonographic imaging to identify the IJ vein and guide needle entry is commonly used for central venous access at this site. This minimizes risk for inadvertent entry into the carotid artery, or in rare cases, accidental lung puncture leading to pneumothorax.

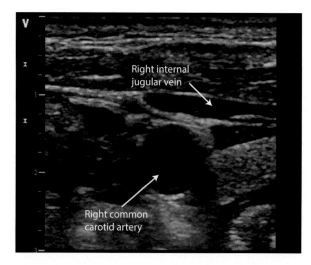

Figure 8.20 Ultrasound image of right internal jugular vein and common carotid artery. The internal jugular vein is easily compressible.

COMPLICATIONS

Complications while attempting IJ vein access include accidental puncture of the carotid artery, local bleeding and hematoma formation, air embolism, hemothorax, pneumothorax, ventricular arrhythmias, damage of nearby structures such as the trachea, vagus, or recurrent laryngeal nerves and, in rare cases, cardiac perforation or tamponade.

Subclavian vein access

INDICATION

Similar to the IJ vein, the SCV can be used for indwelling central venous access in a critically ill patient. This is desirable for administration of medications directly into the circulation, intracardiac access, hemodialysis, and plasmapheresis, or tunneled catheter placement for long-term IV medical infusion therapy such as chemotherapeutic agents. Diagnostic and interventional procedures involving the deep veins of the thorax can also indicate access at this site.

ANATOMY

The SCV courses superior to the first rib and inferior to the clavicle. These bony landmarks can be identified by palpation. The location for needle puncture can be identified along the medial one-third of the clavicle where it makes a slight bend.

TECHNICAL METHODS

The patient should be placed in Trendelenburg position. This maximizes venous filling as well as decreases the risk for stroke caused by air embolism. The clavicle is palpated for the point when it transitions from the medial one-third to the lateral two-thirds. At this location, the clavicle has a slight angle, which can be identified visually as well as by palpation. Once found, the skin puncture site should be 1 cm lateral and caudal to it, and the needle should be directed at an angle posterior to the clavicle, parallel to the "floor" or inferior surface of the clavicle. Using a syringe with 1–2 mL saline attached to the access needle, it should be advanced while aspirating until the vein is entered.

An alternative approach for canalizing the SCV involves a supraclavicular approach. For this method, the junction of the lateral border of the sternocleidomastoid muscle and the clavicle should be identified. The needle should puncture the skin 1 cm superior and 1 cm lateral to this junction and be directed in a slight posterior angle along a line that bisects the junction in half.

COMPLICATIONS

Infection, bleeding, hematoma formation, pneumothorax, and hemothorax are some of the complications that can occur. Other rare complications include thrombosis, air embolization, arrhythmias, nerve injury, cardiac perforation, and tamponade. Inadvertent subclavian artery puncture can also occur.

CONTRAINDICATIONS

Caution should be taken in patients with bleeding disorders, as hemostasis can be difficult due to the SCV position posterior to bony structures. It is also advisable to avoid access if there is known thrombosis at the target site. Patients on assisted ventilation with high end-expiratory pressures can be at higher risk for pneumothorax with attempted SCV puncture.

Antecubital access

The antecubital fossa contains several neuromuscular and vascular structures. The median cubital vein, cephalic vein, and basilic vein course superficial in the cubital fossa. These vessels make up the major draining tributaries of the forearm and upper arm. Although direct central venous access is not obtained through the antecubital fossa, catheters can be advanced for various indications, including Swan Ganz catheter placement and hemodynamic catheterization. The median cubital vein is desired for more direct access into the basilic vein, which is the deeper and larger vein of the upper arm.

TECHNICAL METHODS

An 18G access needle for routine IV access or 21G micropuncture needle can be used to gain initial access in the antecubital fossa. The superficial median cubital vein is frequently palpable and can be found coursing in the lateral to medial direction as it drains cranially. Once vessel puncture is made and blood flow is confirmed, a 0.014-in nitinol wire can be used to insert a micropuncture sheath that allows a 0.035-in wire for exchanging to a larger sheath size (i.e., up to 8-Fr).

SPECIFIC ACCESS ISSUES

Access in the anticoagulated patient

Vascular access bleeding is one of the most common issues that can lead to significant morbidity. Some vascular access sites—such as the radial artery—have a decreased incidence of local bleeding because of their superficial location in an area with easy compressibility. However, this does not circumvent the issue of bleeding in vessels or organs distant to the access site.

Review of the patient's anticoagulation status is as important as planning the procedure and choosing an optimal access site. Newer antithrombotic agents, like direct thrombin inhibitors, present a challenge to the interventionalist as they currently have no diagnostic testing to assess level of anticoagulation. However, current recommendations suggest withholding these agents at least 3 days prior to any elective major invasive procedure.

Difficult femoral artery access

FEMORAL BYPASS GRAFT

Vascular access in patients who have significant peripheral arterial disease (PAD) can be challenging. Those with prior femoral bypass grafts present a unique situation when it is necessary to gain percutaneous entry into the graft. One notable concern is risk of hemorrhage that cannot be controlled, as there is an increased risk of local bleeding and hematoma formation at the access site. In such individuals, the operator should attempt vessel puncture as proximal and close to the inguinal ligament as possible. Fluoroscopic visualization as the needle is advanced can aid in achieving this. Avoid bending of the catheter by inserting the access needle at a shallow angle (30° to 45°) relative to the graft.[59] It is also possible for wires to pass easily into the graft lumen; however, when attempting to enter the introducer sheath or dilator, it causes the wire to kink. When this occurs, advancing the wire farther into the vessel and using the stiffer part of the wire can allow a dilator to advance into the graft. However, if there is too much kinking of the wire, it should be exchanged for a stiffer one.[59]

Other complications that can occur include disruption of the anastomotic suture, pseudoaneurysm formation, infection at the access site, and scar tissue formation that can disrupt the graft patency. In most graft access cases, using vascular closure devices (VCDs) is not recommended and hemostasis should be achieved with manual compression.

DENSE SCAR TISSUE

Dense scar tissue can form when multiple prior access attempts have been performed. Patients after heart transplant who have had numerous surveillance procedures as follow-up are examples of such situations. Scar tissue can also form with previous surgery, chronic groin infection, hip flexion deformity, and an aneurysmal CFA.

In these situations, using skin incision followed by dilatation of the needle tract with a hemostat prior to needle entry can facilitate advancement of the sheath. Using a stiff guidewire, such as an Amplatz Stiff with a J-tip (Boston Scientific, Marlborough, MA) or Supra Core (Abbott Vascular, Abbott Park, IL), is recommended to facilitate sheath insertion through the dense scar tissue. Using sequential dilation with progressively larger dilators can help to prepare the tract for the desired sheath. Generally, a dilator that is one Fr size larger than the selected sheath size can adequately provide an accommodating tract.

STENTED COMMON FEMORAL ARTERY

Although surgical intervention used to be the recommended treatment for functionally limiting CFA lesions, endovascular angioplasty and provisional stenting has been shown to be an effective alternative.[60,61] Therefore, these patients can present with other endovascular procedures where femoral access is needed. When a patient has had a prior CFA stent, it is preferable to use the contralateral CFA site for additional procedures, unless otherwise unavoidable. In such circumstances, knowledge of the type and timing of stent placement will determine if re-entry into the stent should be attempted. If a prior femoral angiogram is available, this should be reviewed prior to access. In situations where prior imaging is not available, obtaining noninvasive imaging can be helpful to identify the location of the stent in the CFA. Access should be obtained under fluoroscopic guidance.

OBESE PATIENTS

Femoral arterial access in the obese patient can be challenging as the inguinal crease is often notably lower than the inguinal ligament and an unreliable landmark for arterial access.[6] Additional preparation by retraction and taping abdominal tissue and pannus up toward the chest may allow better exposure of the femoral region and prevent kinking or bending of the sheath by the thick subcutaneous tissue. In these challenging situations, using visual guidance by ultrasound imaging can decrease inadvertent punctures too superior or below the CFA bifurcation and the number of access attempts. Achieving hemostasis can also be challenging, so multiple access punctures should be avoided. When clinically possible, choosing radial access in this population may allow safe vascular access and decrease local bleeding risk.[62]

AORTO-ILIAC STENOSIS

Patients with aorto-iliac stenosis present a situation when CFA access for vascular beds proximal to the aortic bifurcation cannot be used. Careful planning is needed to determine feasibility of CFA access for provisional aorto-iliac angioplasty with stent placement prior to continuation with the primary procedure, especially when upper extremity access is not procedurally feasible.

Large-bore cannulae

As percutaneous procedures become increasingly complex and advancement of transcatheter techniques continue, the need for larger-diameter access has increased. Sheath sizes as large as 24-Fr may be needed for extracorporeal bypass equipment for endovascular thrombus removal, such as the AngioVac System (Angiodynamics, Latham, NY); pLVADs such as the Impella CP (Abiomed, Danvers, MA); intra-aortic balloon pump (IABP); percutaneous aortic valve replace (PAVR); or endovascular aortic aneurysm repair.

When these accesses are required, preprocedure planning is critical. Noninvasive imaging, such as CT angiography of the distal aorta and aorto-iliac bifurcation, is necessary to make precise measurements in determining procedure feasibility.

Serial incremental dilator insertions using a stiff wire allow progressive entry of larger-bore cannulae up to the desired sheath size without vessel rupture. The vascular closure technique using the Perclose ProGlide Suture-Mediated Closure device (Abbott Vascular, Abbott Park, IL) is recommended for procedures with large-bore cannulae, especially if the femoral artery is used. For sheath sizes larger than 8-Fr, it is recommended that two Perclose devices be deployed.

Severe aorto-iliac disease, small-caliber iliac and femoral arteries and highly calcified PAD at the access site are relative contraindications and may preclude vascular access.

Left radial artery access: Optimal techniques

The left radial artery allows vascular entry that is optimal for left internal mammary artery cannulation. It has been shown to be successful in accommodating coronary graft angiograms safely with no additional time delay compared to the transfemoral approach.[63] It can also be used for other vascular procedures in patients with a hemodialysis fistula in their right arm, which would be a relative contraindication for right radial artery access. Other situations where access from the left arm is desirable include left axillary balloon pump placement, in which case a road map can serve as initial fluoroscopic guidance. The proximity of the left subclavian artery to the descending aorta, and thus to the lower extremities, is another advantage of left radial access.

Positioning the patient properly can affect ergonomic convenience for the operator. There are two commonly used positions. In the first, the patient's left arm is placed outstretched on an arm board abducted away from the body, and the operator stands between the arm and the body (Figure 8.21a). Alternatively, the patient's arm is placed along the side of the body, and the operator works from the right side of the patient (Figure 8.21b). A variation of this method exists where the left arm is placed over the patient's body slightly crossing over toward the right leg (Figure 8.21c).

Left radial artery access is similar to the transfemoral approach for catheter selection and manipulation in performing native coronary artery angiograms/angioplasty.

TREATMENT OF COMMON VASCULAR ACCESS COMPLICATIONS

Complications regarding each access site have been mentioned briefly in prior sections. Because common femoral and radial arteries are the most frequently used access locations for percutaneous procedures, special attention will be focused on common complications that occur at these sites, and ways to treat and resolve them will be discussed.

CFA puncture can lead to retroperitoneal hemorrhage, pseudoaneurysm formation, and AVFs. While local access bleeding is better controlled with radial artery access than with femoral access, this technique has increased risk for hand ischemia, forearm vessel perforation, and formation of a sterile abscess.

Common femoral artery complications

RETROPERITONEAL HEMORRHAGE

Retroperitoneal hemorrhage can occur with femoral artery access, with higher risk when antegrade access is attempted. One known procedural cause for this bleeding to occur is a high-puncture site, such as entry of the EIA, where there is inadequate bony surface for achieving hemostasis with manual pressure. Accordingly, it is important to secure

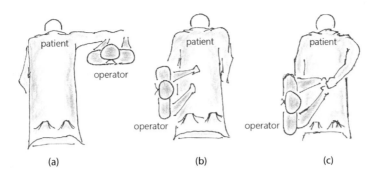

(a)   (b)   (c)

Figure 8.21 Various patient positions for left radial artery access. **(a)** Left arm extended outward with the operator standing adjacent to the arm. This initial setup is used for securing access. **(b)** The arm is then placed along on the side. **(c)** A variation where the left arm is crossed over the body in order to allow more ergonomic comfort within reach of the operator.

proper CFA vessel entry by identifying helpful landmarks and using visual guidance through fluoroscopy or ultrasound imaging. Ultrasound guidance has been shown to decrease the number of needle puncture attempts and inadvertent high sticks.

Should a retroperitoneal bleed occur, it is important to recognize it quickly to prevent potentially fatal progression. Clinical signs associated with a retroperitoneal bleed are hypotension, tachycardia, pallor, lower abdominal pain, back pain, and neurologic changes in the leg where the arterial puncture was made.

PSEUDOANEURYSM

Pseudoaneurysm, or false aneurysm formation, at the femoral artery site has been reported at an incidence of less than 2%–4%.[19] Inadequate manual pressure postprocedure has been described as a risk factor, and increasing the length of time for manual compression decreases the incidence.

A pseudoaneurysm can be managed in several ways. If <2 cm in size by ultrasound, it can usually be managed without surgical intervention.[64] Thrombin injection into the pseudoaneurysm,[65] or manual compression,[66] both using ultrasound imaging, have been successful in reducing them. Percutaneous placement of a covered stent to exclude the pseudoaneurysm can also successfully treat this complication.[64]

ARTERIOVENOUS FISTULA

Communication between the femoral artery and vein can occur when the needle passes through one vessel and into the other. Inadvertent vessel puncture leading to fistula formation is more likely to occur with femoral access if the initial entry point is selected more caudally because of the anterior to posterior relationship of the artery and vein. In contrast, these vessels lie next to each other in a side-by-side relationship as the CFA and vein. Using image guidance—such as ultrasound visualization—can reduce inadvertent, inappropriate vessel puncture and thus AVF formation.

This complication has been reported to occur at a rate of <1%.[19] A continuous thrill or bruit at the access location on physical exam is a finding that is consistent with AVF formation. Confirmation is achieved with Doppler ultrasound or contrast CT imaging. Rarely is an intervention needed as most resolve spontaneously. However, surgical correction or closure of the fistula can be performed for patients with high-output heart failure or symptoms due to the fistula. Endovascular exclusion of the fistula using a covered stent has also been described.[64]

Radial artery complications

HAND ISCHEMIA

Although CLI from transradial access is not typically observed if access is properly obtained,[67] it is a possible complication if the palmar arch circulation is obstructed from occlusion of the radial artery when collateral supply is inadequate. The radial artery is susceptible to spasm as well as thrombotic occlusion. Thromboembolic complication after radial access can manifest with gangrenous digits and pain at ischemic regions. Routine administration of heparin after sheath insertion and successful guidewire advancement to the target vascular bed decreases the risk of acute thrombosis of the vessel.[37] Partial occlusive pressure for hemostasis at the end of the procedure reduces the occurrence of acute and chronic radial artery occlusion as well.[43]

FOREARM VESSEL PERFORATION

Vessel perforation of the proximal radial artery away from the arteriotomy site can lead to bleeding and hematoma into the neuromuscular compartments of the forearm or upper arm. Caution should be taken when hydrophilic guidewires are used as these wires have a higher risk for causing vessel perforation. Bleeding into the forearm can raise intracompartmental pressure, leading to ischemic compression of nerves and vessels contained within the compartment. Permanent neurologic damage can occur with compartment syndrome without decompressive open fasciotomy. Loss of motor and/or sensory function associated with increased pain and swelling in the upper arm or forearm should raise suspicion for hemorrhage and should be promptly evaluated.

STERILE ABSCESS

Abscess formation at the site of sheath insertion is a rare complication that can occur as a result of an inflammatory response to the silicon material on the coating of the introducer sheath.[68] It has been speculated that the silicon material can get trapped in the dermis leading to inflammation and granuloma formation. Although sterile, it is difficult to differentiate sterile abscesses from those formed by bacterial infection. Therefore, a short course of antibiotics can be added to the otherwise supportive and conservative management. The acute phase can last 2 weeks, and the resulting chronic granuloma will usually resolve fully after a year. These can cause chronic pain and tenderness at the site. Wiping the sheath with gauze soaked in saline can reduce such reactions from occurring.[68]

HEMOSTASIS

Achieving hemostasis safely and efficiently is as important as securing vascular access. Local bleeding can lead to patient discomfort and significant morbidity. The advent of VCDs has led to faster recovery time and quicker hemostasis following the procedure, thus facilitating early ambulation. However, VCDs have not been shown to decrease the incidence of vascular complications.

The two major methods for obtaining hemostasis are by manual compression or by using various available VCDs. These include mechanical compression equipment, such as Femstop (St. Jude Medical, St. Paul, MN); external collagen plugs, such as the Angio-Seal (St. Jude Medical, St. Paul, MN); external "glue," such as Mynx (Cardinal Health, Dublin, OH); and suturing devices like the Perclose ProGlide SMC System (Abbott Vascular, Abbott Park, IL). VCDs have also been designed for CFA closure when accessed in retrograde.

Manual pressure

Adequate hemostasis using manual compression can be achieved at most arterial and venous access sites with the exception of the subclavian artery and vein. Traditionally, manual pressure has been used to obtain hemostasis for arteriotomy closure and requires prolonged immobilization of the patient and close monitoring for spontaneous bleeding. One important consideration is the status of anticoagulation in patients in whom percutaneous intervention has just been completed. Safe periprocedural instrumentation requires an activated clotting time (ACT) >250 seconds in heparinized patients, which increases the bleeding risk at vascular access sites. Therefore, prior to sheath removal it

is important to check the ACT. Reversal of anticoagulation with heparin is typically achieved through administration of protamine sulfate (heparin [1-1.5 mg per 100 USP units of heparin; not to exceed 50 mg]), which is recommended to be given if ACT is >200 seconds. A small test dose should be given in order to avoid protamine reactions, which are more common in diabetics who have previously received neutral protamine Hagedorn (NPH) insulin. Symptoms include shaking, flushing, chills, back, or chest pain, and in rare cases, vasomotor instability. Protamine reactions are usually self-limited and last less than 1 hour. Supportive care through symptom management by administration of morphine, meperidine, diphenhydramine, and saline administration can be adequate.

Once ACT is at an acceptable level of <180–200 seconds, the sheath can be removed and manual compression applied. If this method is chosen for hemostasis, pressure should be placed on the arteriotomy site and not the skin puncture. This is commonly more cranial or proximal to skin entry. Firm manual pressure on the artery should be kept for 15–20 minutes with patent occlusive pressure to allow some residual pulse distally. Compressive pressure should be decreased every 5 minutes with constant examination of distal pulses and the puncture site.

Vascular closure devices

VCDs have been increasingly used and can provide faster time for recovery after a percutaneous access from the femoral sites. Most of these devices have been designed for use at the femoral access site and usage in any puncture sites other than the CFA is considered "off-label" use of the device.

RADIAL BANDS

Radial access hemostasis is commonly achieved by using bands that are placed around the wrist and fastened in place to maintain compressive pressure. The R-Band (Vascular Solutions, Minneapolis, MN) and TR-Band (Terumo, Somerset, NJ) use inflation pressure at the arteriotomy site, while the D-Stat (Vascular Solutions, Minneapolis, MN) functions by a snap-belt system—similar to a plastic tie cable—with attached dry hemostatic bandages that cover the arteriotomy and skin puncture site. All devices require slow release of pressure over 2 hours before removal.

FEMOSTOP

The Femostop (St. Jude Medical, St. Paul, MN) VCD is designed specifically for the femoral artery or vein. It is used to apply constant compressive pressure at the arteriotomy or venous entry site by a fastening mechanism that is wrapped around the patient's body. An inflatable pressure balloon is inflated over the access site, which is then slowly deflated at regular time intervals according to a protocol, thereby decreasing the amount of force applied on the vessel. This is effective when prolonged manual pressure is necessary after removal of larger sheaths.

EXTERNAL COLLAGEN PLUG (ANGIO-SEAL)

Angio-Seal (St. Jude Medical, St. Paul, MN) is a collagen-based sealing system that uses an intra-arterial anchor to create a plug at the arteriotomy site. It comes in a 6- or 8-Fr sheath size, and can be used for hemostasis in procedures using up to 8-Fr sheaths. Detailed step-by-step methods for deployment can be found on the Angio-Seal product site online, along with an instructional video. Some complications that can occur include bleeding or hematoma, AVF, pseudoaneurysm formation, infection, allergic reaction, foreign body reaction, inflammation, or edema.

EXTERNAL "GLUE" (MYNX [CARDINAL HEALTH, DUBLIN, OH])

This type of closure device is similar in concept to the collagen plug used in the Angio-Seal system. However, it differs with respect to the use of a GRIP sealant or external "glue" that is bioabsorbable and a balloon that is inflated within the vessel at the puncture site, which forms a mechanical seal as it is retracted upward against the vascular wall. This device can be used for arterial or venous closures for 5- or 7-Fr access sizes.

Suture-mediated

Suture-mediated closure systems allow vascular closure by delivery of a suture. One example of such a device is the Perclose ProGlide SMC System (Abbott, Santa Clara, CA), which inserts a single monofilament polypropylene suture. This system uses a sheath that houses a footplate for apposition of suture to the vessel wall and a needle system with precise controls for placement of needles around a puncture site. The sheath is advanced over 0.038-in wire for proper insertion into the vessel. The mechanism of delivering the suture places a knot that is subsequently fastened against the vascular wall using accessories that comes with each device. It is recommended for use in procedures that have used sheaths larger than 8-Fr and up to 21-Fr in size.

Although there is no known absolute contraindication to using this device, some special patient populations where safety and effectiveness of this device have not been established include <5-Fr or >21-Fr access sizes; patients with femoral arteries <5 mm in diameter; "high" femoral vascular access (i.e., above the inferior epigastric artery); calcified vessel at the suture site; and patients with hematoma, pseudoaneurysm, or AVF prior to sheath removal.

Some known potential adverse events from SMC device use include allergic reaction or hypersensitivity to device components, AVF, bleeding, hematoma, device entrapment, diminished pulses distal to the closure, embolism, infection, inflammation, nerve injury, perforation, pseudoaneurysm, thrombus formation, and wound dehiscence.

Preclose technique

The preclose technique allows initial implantation of Perclose sutures at the arteriotomy site at the beginning of a percutaneous procedure during initial access puncture. The sutures are then closed with securing down of the knots at the completion of the procedure. This technique is useful when large access sizes are used. Two Perclose SMC devices are recommended for closure of an access site that has accommodated a sheath >8-Fr in size. Jaffian et al 2013[69] showed vascular hemostasis success rates of 94% using the preclose technique in percutaneous endovascular aortic repair (pEVAR) procedures with vascular sheath sizes up to 20-Fr. TAVR procedures using 24-Fr femoral sheaths have also included use of the preclose technique. This allows safe delivery of sutures prior to establishing a larger arteriotomy or venotomy. For details on this technique and proper use of the Perclose ProGlide SMC device, refer to the product information guide.

Contraindications to vascular closure devices

There are no absolute contraindications to using VCDs. However, there is increased risk for ischemia when a VCD is used in situations of low arterial puncture at the bifurcation of the CFA, including SFA or PFA puncture; in patients with moderate to severe PAD at the site; and in small-diameter (<4 mm) vessels.[70] Patients prone to infections—such as those with uncontrolled diabetes or post-transplant patients on chronic immune suppressant therapy—deserve thoughtful consideration for infection risk prior to placing a VCD. Allergies to beef products or polyglycolic polymers (Angio-Seal) should also warrant avoidance of using such devices. It is important to remember that most of the VCDs described in this chapter are intended for use at the femoral artery access site. Therefore, using these tools in other vascular locations is considered off-label use and should be carried out with extra caution.

CONCLUSION

Choosing an optimal site when planning percutaneous vascular procedures is as important as mastering the techniques for securing access. The CFA is still most frequently used, accommodates most interventional and diagnostic tools, and is centrally located for most vascular beds. However, the radial artery has increasingly become more popular, especially for coronary procedures where it has been shown to be safe and effective.[41] While understanding vascular anatomy and knowledge of common variations is fundamental in selection of vessel access and decreasing the number of puncture attempts, routine supplementation with fluoroscopic and/or sonographic guidance can augment likelihood for a successful procedure and reduce access site–related complications.

REFERENCES

1. Sherev DA, et al. Angiographic predictors of femoral access site complications: Implication for planned percutaneous coronary intervention. *Catheter Cardiovasc Interv* 2005;65(2):196–202.

2. Seldinger SI. Catheter replacement of the needle in percutaneous arteriography: A new technique. *Acta Radiol* 1953;39(5):368–376.

3. Barry WH, et al. Left heart catheterization and angiography via the percutaneous femoral approach using an arterial sheath. *Cathet Cardiovasc Diagn* 1979;5(4):401–409.

4. Irani F, et al. Common femoral artery access techniques: A review. *J Cardiovasc Med (Hagerstown)* 2009;10(7):517–522.

5. Narins CR. Access strategies for peripheral arterial intervention. *Cardiol J* 2009;16(1):88–97.

6. Lechner G, et al. The relationship between the common femoral artery, the inguinal crease, and the inguinal ligament: A guide to accurate angiographic puncture. *Cardiovasc Intervent Radiol* 1988;11(3):165–169.

7. Grier D, Hartnell G. Percutaneous femoral artery puncture: Practice and anatomy. *Br J Radiol* 1990;63(752):602–604.

8. Schnyder G, et al. Common femoral artery anatomy is influenced by demographics and comorbidity: Implications for cardiac and peripheral invasive studies. *Catheter Cardiovasc Interv* 2001;53(3):289–295.

9. Garrett PD, et al. Fluoroscopic localization of the femoral head as a landmark for common femoral artery cannulation. *Catheter Cardiovasc Interv* 2005;65(2):205–207.

10. Standring S, Gray H. *Gray's Anatomy: The Anatomical Basis of Clinical Practice*. 39th ed. Edinburgh: Elsevier Churchill Livingstone, 2005, p. 1627.

11. Bergman RA. *Compendium of human anatomic variation: Text, atlas, and world literature*. Baltimore, MD: Urban & Schwarzenberg, 1988(XIV), p. 593.

12. Seto AH, et al. Real-time ultrasound guidance facilitates femoral arterial access and reduces vascular complications: FAUST (Femoral Arterial Access With Ultrasound Trial). *JACC Cardiovasc Interv* 2010;3(7):751–758.

13. Augoustides JG, Cheung AT. Pro: Ultrasound should be the standard of care for central catheter insertion. *J Cardiothorac Vasc Anesth* 2009;23(5):720–724.

14. Yeow KM, et al. Sonographically guided antegrade common femoral artery access. *J Ultrasound Med* 2002;21(12):1413–1416.

15. Ben-Dor I, et al. A novel, minimally invasive access technique versus standard 18-gauge needle set for femoral access. *Catheter Cardiovasc Interv* 2012;79(7):1180–1185.

16. Turi ZG. An evidence-based approach to femoral arterial access and closure. *Rev Cardiovasc Med* 2008;9(1):7–18.

17. Wyman RM, et al. Current complications of diagnostic and therapeutic cardiac catheterization. *J Am Coll Cardiol* 1988;12(6):1400–1406.

18. Oweida SW, et al. Postcatheterization vascular complications associated with percutaneous transluminal coronary angioplasty. *J Vasc Surg* 1990;12(3):310–315.

19. Tavakol M, et al. Risks and complications of coronary angiography: A comprehensive review. *Glob J Health Sci* 2012;4(1):65–93.

20. Tavris DR, et al. Bleeding and vascular complications at the femoral access site following percutaneous coronary intervention (PCI): An evaluation of hemostasis strategies. *J Invasive Cardiol* 2012;24(7):328–334.

21. Doyle BJ, et al. Major femoral bleeding complications after percutaneous coronary intervention: Incidence, predictors, and impact on long-term survival among 17,901 patients treated at the Mayo Clinic from 1994 to 2005. *JACC Cardiovasc Interv* 2008;1(2):202–209.

22. Rao SV, et al. Trends in the prevalence and outcomes of radial and femoral approaches to percutaneous coronary intervention: A report from the National Cardiovascular Data Registry. *JACC Cardiovasc Interv* 2008;1(4):379–386.

23. Ellis SG, et al. Correlates and outcomes of retroperitoneal hemorrhage complicating percutaneous coronary intervention. *Catheter Cardiovasc Interv* 2006;67(4):541–545.

24. Farouque HM, et al. Risk factors for the development of retroperitoneal hematoma after percutaneous coronary intervention in the era of glycoprotein IIb/IIIa inhibitors and vascular closure devices. *J Am Coll Cardiol* 2005;45(3):363–368.

25. Katzenschlager R, et al. Incidence of pseudoaneurysm after diagnostic and therapeutic angiography. *Radiology* 1995;195(2):463–466.

26. Kelm M, et al. Incidence and clinical outcome of iatrogenic femoral arteriovenous fistulas: Implications for risk stratification and treatment. *J Am Coll Cardiol* 2002;40(2):291–297.

27. Biondi-Zoccai GG, et al. Mastering the antegrade femoral artery access in patients with symptomatic lower limb ischemia: Learning curve, complications, and technical tips and tricks. *Catheter Cardiovasc Interv* 2006;68(6):835–842.

28. Hansen JT, Netter FH. *Netter's clinical anatomy*. 2nd ed. Philadelphia, PA: Saunders/Elsevier, 2010(XVIII), p. 470

29. Coleman SS, Anson BJ. Arterial patterns in the hand based upon a study of 650 specimens. *Surg Gynecol Obstet* 1961;113:409–424.

30. Al-Turk M, Metcalf WK. A study of the superficial palmar arteries using the Doppler Ultrasonic Flowmeter. *J Anat* 1984;138(1):27–32.

31. Nathan S, Rao SV. Radial versus femoral access for percutaneous coronary intervention: Implications for vascular complications and bleeding. *Curr Cardiol Rep* 2012;14(4):502–509.

32. Agostoni P, et al. Radial versus femoral approach for percutaneous coronary diagnostic and interventional procedures; Systematic overview and meta-analysis of randomized trials. *J Am Coll Cardiol* 2004;44(2):349–356.

33. Kern M. *The Cardiac Catheterization Handbook*. 5th ed. Philadelphia, PA: Elsevier, 2015, pp. 40–42

34. Barbeau GR, et al. Evaluation of the ulnopalmar arterial arches with pulse oximetry and plethysmography: Comparison with the Allen's test in 1010 patients. *Am Heart J* 2004;147(3):489–493.

35. Jolly SS, et al. Radial versus femoral access for coronary angiography and intervention in patients with acute coronary syndromes (RIVAL): A randomised, parallel group, multicentre trial. *Lancet* 2011;377(9775):1409–1420.

36. Romagnoli E, et al. Radial versus femoral randomized investigation in ST-segment elevation acute coronary syndrome: The RIFLE-STEACS (Radial Versus Femoral Randomized Investigation in ST-Elevation Acute Coronary Syndrome) study. *J Am Coll Cardiol* 2012;60(24):2481–2489.

37. Plante S, et al. Comparison of bivalirudin versus heparin on radial artery occlusion after transradial catheterization. *Catheter Cardiovasc Interv* 2010;76(5):654–658.

38. Roberts J, Manur R. Ultrasound-guided radial artery access by a non-ultrasound trained interventional cardiologist improved first-attempt success rates and shortened time for successful radial artery cannulation. *J Invasive Cardiol* 2013;25(12):676–679.

39. Shiver S, et al. A prospective comparison of ultrasound-guided and blindly placed radial arterial catheters. *Acad Emerg Med* 2006;13(12):1275–1279.

40. Peters C, et al. Ultrasound guidance versus direct palpation for radial artery catheterization by expert operators: A randomized trial among Canadian cardiac anesthesiologists. *Can J Anaesth* 2015;62(11):1161–1168.

41. Mehta SR, et al. Effects of radial versus femoral artery access in patients with acute coronary syndromes with or without ST-segment elevation. *J Am Coll Cardiol* 2012;60(24):2490–2499.

42. Rao SV, et al. Best practices for transradial angiography and intervention: A consensus statement from the society for cardiovascular angiography and intervention's transradial working group. *Catheter Cardiovasc Interv* 2013;83(2):228–236.

43. Pancholy S, et al. Prevention of radial artery occlusion-patent hemostasis evaluation trial (PROPHET study): A randomized comparison of traditional versus patency documented hemostasis after transradial catheterization. *Catheter Cardiovasc Interv* 2008;72(3):335–340.

44. Casserly IP, et al. *Practical Peripheral Vascular Intervention*. Philadelphia, PA: Lippincott Williams & Wilkins, 2011, pp. 60–74.

45. Campeau L. Entry sites for coronary angiography and therapeutic interventions: From the proximal to the distal radial artery. *Can J Cardiol* 2001;17(3):319–325.

46. Sos TA. Brachial and axillary arterial access. *Endovascular Today* 2010;5:55–58.

47. Kiemeneij F, et al. A randomized comparison of percutaneous transluminal coronary angioplasty by the radial, brachial and femoral approaches: The access study. *J Am Coll Cardiol* 1997;29(6):1269–1275.

48. Basche S, et al. Transbrachial angiography: An effective and safe approach. *Vasa* 2004;33(4):231–234.

49. Armstrong PJ, et al. Complication rates of percutaneous brachial artery access in peripheral vascular angiography. *Ann Vasc Surg* 2003;17(1):107–110.

50. Feiring AJ, Wesolowski AA. Antegrade popliteal artery approach for the treatment of critical limb ischemia in patients with occluded superficial femoral arteries. *Catheter Cardiovasc Interv* 2007;69(5):665–670.

51. Kwan TW, et al. Feasibility and safety of routine transpedal arterial access for treatment of peripheral artery disease. *J Invasive Cardiol* 2015;27(7):327–330.

52. Sfyroeras GS, et al. Results of carotid artery stenting with transcervical access. *J Vasc Surg* 2013;58(5):1402–1407.

53. Pinter L, et al. Safety and feasibility of a novel transcervical access neuroprotection system for carotid artery stenting in the PROOF Study. *J Vasc Surg* 2011;54(5):1317–1323.

54. Muller M, et al. Variations of the aortic arch—A study on the most common branching patterns. *Acta Radiol* 2011;52(7):738–742.

55. Martinez-Clark PO, et al. Transcaval retrograde transcatheter aortic valve replacement for patients with no other access: First-in-man experience with CoreValve. *JACC Cardiovasc Interv* 2014;7(9):1075–1077.

56. Greenbaum AB, et al. Caval-aortic access to allow transcatheter aortic valve replacement in otherwise ineligible patients: Initial human experience. *J Am Coll Cardiol* 2014;63(25 Pt A)2795–2804.

57. Kern MJ. *Cardiac Catheterization Handbook*. 6th ed. Atlanta: Elsevier, 2015, p. 64.

58. Lamperti M, et al. International evidence-based recommendations on ultrasound-guided vascular access. *Intensive Care Med* 2012;38(7):1105–1117.

59. Chisholm RJ. Femoral artery catheterization in patients with previous bifemoral grafting. *Cathet Cardiovasc Diagn* 1993;30(4):313.

60. Silva JA, et al. Percutaneous revascularization of the common femoral artery for limb ischemia. *Catheter Cardiovasc Interv* 2004;62(2):230–233.

61. Davies RS, et al. Endovascular treatment of the common femoral artery for limb ischemia. *Vasc Endovascular Surg* 2013;47(8):639–644.

62. Achenbach S, et al. Transradial versus transfemoral approach for coronary angiography and intervention in patients above 75 years of age. *Catheter Cardiovasc Interv* 2008;72(5):629–635.

63. Sanmartin M, et al. Transradial cardiac catheterization in patients with coronary bypass grafts: Feasibility analysis and comparison with transfemoral approach. *Catheter Cardiovasc Interv* 2006;67(4):580–584.

64. Samal AK, White CJ. Percutaneous management of access site complications. *Catheter Cardiovasc Interv* 2002;57(1):12–23.

65. Kuma S, et al. Ultrasound-guided percutaneous thrombin injection for post-catheterization pseudoaneurysm. *Circ J* 2015;79(6):1277–1281.

66. Coley BD, et al. Postangiographic femoral artery pseudoaneurysms: Further experience with US-guided compression repair. *Radiology* 1995;194(2):307–311.

67. Uhlemann M, et al. The Leipzig prospective vascular ultrasound registry in radial artery catheterization: Impact of sheath size on vascular complications. *JACC Cardiovasc Interv* 2012;5(1):36–43.

68. Kozak M, et al. Sterile inflammation associated with transradial catheterization and hydrophilic sheaths. *Catheter Cardiovasc Interv* 2003;59(2):207–213.

69. Jaffan AA, et al. The preclose technique in percutaneous endovascular aortic repair: A systematic literature review and meta-analysis. *Cardiovasc Intervent Radiol* 2013;36(3):567–577.

70. Bangalore S, Bhatt DL. Femoral arterial access and closure. *Circulation* 2011;124(5):e147–e156.

PART 2

Hemodynamic Assessment and Endomyocardial Biopsy

9

Right heart catheterization: Cardiac output, vascular resistance, shunt detection, and quantification

FRANZ R. EBERLI

INTRODUCTION

In addition to Doppler echocardiography and cardiac magnetic resonance imaging (MRI), right heart catheterization is a complementary, but indispensable procedure for hemodynamic assessment and diagnosis of many cardiac diseases. Right heart catheterization provides data on the pressures and oxygen saturations in the right heart chambers and the pulmonary artery (PA), including PA occlusion pressure, or "wedge" pressure. Combined with data obtained during simultaneous left heart catheterization, cardiac output, pulmonary and systemic vascular resistances, and ejection fractions are calculated, and shunt detection and quantification in structural heart disease can be performed. From these measurements, information about preload, afterload, and contractility are derived.

Hemodynamic responses to changes in loading conditions and/or to pharmacologic interventions are often noted for accurate evaluation of the physiology of a specific condition. This information is particularly valuable in the assessment of adult congenital heart disease and pulmonary hypertension prior to any therapeutic intervention or operation.[1,2]

In contrast to right heart catheterization's undisputed value as a diagnostic tool in the cardiac catheterization laboratory, the bedside use of a pulmonary artery catheter (PAC) in critically ill patients is controversial. Reports that its use leads to increased mortality and morbidity[3] have resulted in careful evaluations of the use of bedside right heart catheterization in patients with cardiac disease.[4] Following these reports, two randomized trials (PAC-MAN and ESCAPE) have found no increased mortality with the use of PACs in critically ill patients and have concluded they are safe for use in appropriate patient populations.[5,6]

ANATOMIC CONSIDERATIONS AND FUNDAMENTALS

Access to the right heart can be gained via the inferior or superior vena cava (SVC). The SVC is accessed from the internal jugular vein, the subclavian vein, or an antecubital vein. If left heart catheterization is performed simultaneously, however, right heart catheterization is generally performed via femoral access. With the widespread switch from transfemoral to transradial access for left heart catheterization, right heart catheterization, including endomyocardial biopsy, is increasingly performed via an antecubital vein.[7,8] Apart from operator experience and preference, certain conditions make a SVC approach preferable. Such conditions are as follows: suspected femoral vein/iliac vein thrombosis, renal vein thrombus, inferior vena cava (IVC) filter, and anomalous IVC. Other conditions, such as massive dilation of the right-sided chambers, severe tricuspid or pulmonary regurgitation, and pulmonary hypertension, are technically easier to assess by a SVC approach.

The PAC (Figure 9.1) is advanced through the right atrium (RA), the right ventricle (RV), and the PA until a PA occlusion pressure is reached (Figure 9.2). The static column of blood between the tip of the PAC and the pulmonary vein will transmit the pressure from the left atrium (LA). During diastole, when the mitral valve is open, the measured pressure corresponds to the left ventricular diastolic pressure (Figure 9.2). A prerequisite of a correct measurement is that the pulmonary venous pressure exceeds the pulmonary alveolar pressure. This is more likely the case when the catheter tip is directed into the lower lobe.[9] The lung tissue between the tip of the catheter and the left heart results in damping (2–4 mmHg) and delay (100–150 msec) of the pressure wave in the pulmonary capillary wedge tracing compared with the left ventricular (LV) or LA pressure (Figure 9.3).

Cardiac output measurements are usually performed by thermodilution or by the Fick method. Thermodilution is more accurate in normal and high output states, whereas the Fick method is more accurate in low output states, valvular regurgitation, or intracardiac shunts. Shunt detection and quantification is complementary to echocardiography results. Echocardiographic findings should be reviewed before performing right heart catheterization so that the invasive procedure can be tailored toward unresolved and specific questions. This will allow the investigator to shorten the oximetry run and plan a potentially valuable pharmacologic intervention or volume load.

INDICATIONS

Right heart catheterization is no longer part of every diagnostic heart catheterization. Echocardiography, other imaging modalities, and noninvasive hemodynamic measurements have reduced the need for right heart catheterization. Nevertheless, direct measurements of pressure, flow, and oxygen saturations are often necessary to correctly diagnose or quantify cardiac diseases.[10] For example, despite indisputable achievements, Doppler echocardiography has its limitations for correct assessment of pressures.[11] Interestingly, Doppler estimation of PA hypertension more often overestimates pulmonary pressures, particularly when right heart pathology or lung disease is present.[11] Therefore, right heart catheterization remains the gold standard for diagnosing pulmonary hypertension.[2] The indications for right heart catheterization can be divided into two main categories:

1. Diagnostic catheterization for establishing a diagnosis and for planning and guiding a therapeutic intervention.
2. Monitoring and guiding intensive medical care or perioperative hemodynamics (Table 9.1).[12]

CONTRAINDICATIONS

Absolute contraindications to right heart catheterization are mechanical tricuspid or pulmonic valve prostheses or terminal illness. Relative contraindications are endocarditis, a tumor or thrombus in the right heart chambers, and newly implanted pacemaker or defibrillator leads. A profound coagulopathy with an international normalized ratio (INR) > 3 or low platelet count (<20,000/mm³) increases bleeding risk, particularly when a jugular vein or subclavian vein approach is chosen. Periprocedural administration of fresh frozen plasma or platelets might be considered under such circumstances.

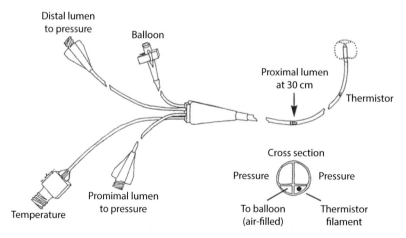

Figure 9.1 Diagram depicting the pulmonary artery catheter (PAC). A PAC with two pressure monitor lumens is depicted. The distal lumen goes to the tip of the catheter to measure pulmonary artery pressure and, if the balloon is inflated and the pulmonary artery occluded, the pulmonary capillary wedge pressure (PCWP) is measured. A thermistor near the catheter tip measures pulmonary artery blood temperature and is used for thermodilution cardiac output measurements. The proximal lumen is located 30 cm from the tip of the catheter and usually lies within the right atrium. This lumen is also used for injection of cold saline for thermodilution cardiac output measurements. In the cross section, the distribution of the four lumens within the catheter are depicted.

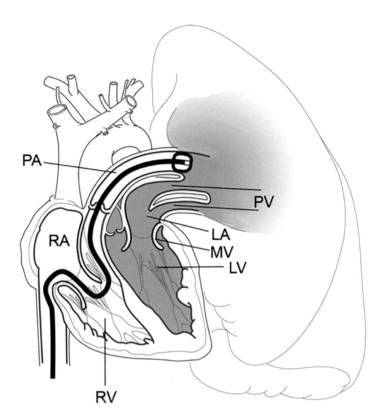

Figure 9.2 Principles of right heart catheterization. The balloon-tipped right heart catheter is inserted from an inferior vena cava approach into the right atrium (RA), through the tricuspid valve into the right ventricle (RV) and up into the pulmonary artery (PA) and "wedged" into the distal pulmonary artery. Distal to the inflated balloon, a blood column is present between the pulmonary vein (PV) and the catheter. The PV is connected to the left atrium (LA) and, importantly, if the mitral valve (MV) is open, it is connected to the left ventricle (LV). According to the law of pressures in communicating vessels, the left ventricular end-diastolic pressure corresponds to LA pressure, which in turn corresponds to PV pressure and pulmonary capillary wedge pressure (PCWP).

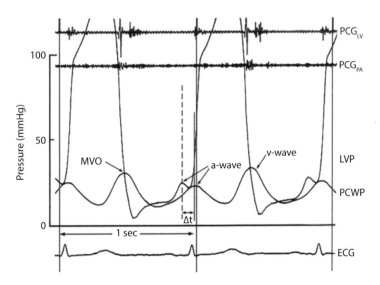

Figure 9.3 Simultaneous left ventricular (LV) and pulmonary capillary wedge pressures (PCWP). This figure depicts the simultaneous pressure measurement with a tip manometer catheter (Millar catheter) in the left ventricle (LV) and in pulmonary capillary wedge position. The left atrial contraction results in an a-wave that is transmitted into the LV and retrogradely into the PCWP (the time delay [Δt] is usually 80 to 140 msec). Similarly, the v-wave is delayed and dampened (2 to 4 mmHg). After mitral valve opening (MVO), the v-wave should decrease simultaneously with the LV pressure. The recorded delayed pressure decay is the result of the dampening of the pressure transmission through the lung tissue. ECG, electrocardiogram; LVP, left ventricular pressure; PCG$_{LV}$, phonocardiogram left ventricle; PCG$_{PA}$, phonocardiogram pulmonary artery; PCWP, pulmonary capillary wedge pressure.

Table 9.1 Indications for right heart catheterization

A. Diagnosis and Planning of Therapeutic Interventions

1. Valvular heart disease

   Assessment of severity of valve disease and concomitant pulmonary hypertension. Planning of surgical or interventional valve interventions

2. Intracardiac shunts

   Shunt detection and quantification. Assessment of concomitant pulmonary hypertension. Exploratory balloon occlusion of the defect. Vasoreactivity test in case of pulmonary hypertension

3. Left heart failure

   To differentiate between cardiogenic or non-cardiogenic edema. Guide therapy in acute and chronic heart failure. Differentiate between diastolic and systolic dysfunction. Test for reversible pulmonary hypertension in transplant candidates

4. Shock states

   Differentiate shock states. Cardiogenic versus non-cardiogenic, hypovolemic, or septic shock

5. Acute myocardial infarction

   Complicated by hypotension, unclear volume status (acute myocardial infarction and bleeding, acute myocardial infarction and renal insufficiency). Right ventricular infarction. Mechanical complications (ventricular septal defect, papillary muscle rupture)

6. Pulmonary hypertension

   Diagnostic gold standard. Assessment of etiology of pulmonary hypertension. Determination of severity. Testing for vasoreactivity

7. Pericardial diseases

   Differentiation between constrictive and restrictive physiology. Cardiac tamponade (only when echocardiography is unavailable or non-diagnostic)

B. Monitoring of Intensive Medical Therapy

1. Heart failure

   Guidance of vasodilator, positive inotrope, and diuretic therapy. Perioperative management of patients with decompensated heart failure

2. Myocardial infarction

   Guidance of pharmacological and mechanical support. Management of pulmonary edema that does not respond to usual medical treatment

3. Perioperative use in cardiac surgery

   To determine etiology of low cardiac output, differentiate between left and right heart failure, management of pulmonary hypertension

4. Severe acute respiratory distress syndrome

   Assess cardiac output during positive end-expiratory pressure trials

TECHNIQUE

Equipment

The most widely used and safest catheter for right heart catheterization is a multilumen, balloon-tipped flotation catheter, the so-called Swan-Ganz catheter (Figure 9.1). When used from a SVC approach, the catheter floats easily through the right heart chambers and the balloon wedges into the distal PA (Figure 9.2). The distal and proximal lumen of the catheter allow measurement of pressures in the PA and in the RA; the built-in thermistors allow measurements of cardiac output by thermodilution technique. The standard PAC is 110 cm long and has a distal and proximal lumen (ending 30 cm from the catheter tip) that, in most patients, will lie within the RA. It also has a thermistor filament near the tip. For diagnostic purposes in the catheterization laboratory, double-lumen catheters are often employed. In the intensive care unit, more sophisticated catheters with a built-in oxygen probe and continuous cardiac output measurements are used. In these 8-Fr catheters, a thermal filament in the RV heats the surrounding blood (7.5 W energy transformed to heat the blood to 39°C–43°C). The heat change at the thermistor near the tip of the catheter is cross-correlated with the RV thermal input to produce a thermodilution washout curve from which cardiac output is calculated.

The soft PAC has a low risk of injury. However, when floated from the femoral vein, it is not easily guided by torquing. Maneuverability is improved with guidewires (usually 0.021–0.032 inches). Unfortunately, the soft catheter with a small diameter has a poor frequency response that might impede pressure measurements.[13] Instead of a PAC, multipurpose catheters or stiffer (woven Dacron) Goodale-Lubin or Cournand catheters might be used in the cardiac catheterization laboratory. If a PA or pulmonary vein angiography is to be performed, a regular pigtail catheter or an angled (Grolman) pigtail catheter is the preferred catheter. A Berman catheter can also be used. This is a balloon-tipped catheter specifically designed for right-sided angiography. It has no end-holes but several side-holes proximal to the balloon. The inflated balloon stabilizes the catheter and the large lumen allows flows similar to that of pigtail catheters. The flow and injection rate on the right side should be somewhat lower than on the left side, and the maximal pressure of injection should be reduced to 600 psi.

Venous access

The femoral vein is the preferred point of access when right heart catheterization is part of a diagnostic or interventional procedure in the catheterization laboratory. For a description of gaining access and inserting the sheath, see Chapter 8. The advantages of femoral access are the ease of cannulation and the absence of the risk of a pneumothorax. Disadvantages are increased technical difficulties guiding and advancing the catheter, the risk of femoral artery puncture, the long time to ambulation, and bleeding complications.[8] For long-term monitoring, there are additional disadvantages to femoral vein access, particularly patient immobility, a higher risk of thrombosis, and infection.

If internal jugular vein access is used, the right side is the preferred side, since it provides direct access to the RA. Furthermore, the left internal jugular vein sometimes has a venous valve at the entrance into the subclavian vein. The advantages of a jugular vein approach are the easy compressibility of the access site and the low risk of a pneumothorax. The disadvantage is the risk of carotid artery puncture. The internal jugular vein is the preferred access point for hemodynamic monitoring in the intensive care unit and perioperatively. In the cardiac catheterization laboratory, it is often preferred when myocardial biopsy (e.g., in post-transplant patients) is simultaneously performed, or when IVC access is impossible.

The great advantage of subclavian access is patient comfort and reduced infection rate compared with other access sites. The disadvantages are the danger of subclavian artery puncture and the risk of a pneumothorax. Subclavian access is seldom used in the catheterization laboratory; it is mainly reserved for long-term hemodynamic monitoring in the intensive care unit.

The antecubital vein, usually the brachial vein, can be accessed in conjunction with transradial left heart catheterization. Compared with femoral access, antecubital vein access reduces time to ambulation, fluoroscopic time, and heparin dose.[8] However, it may sometimes be difficult to access the SVC from a brachial approach.

Pulmonary artery catheter insertion

FEMORAL VEIN

After flushing, the PAC is introduced into the sheath and advanced into the common iliac vein where the balloon is inflated under fluoroscopy. Inflation of the balloon in a side branch should be avoided. When the balloon is inflated without fluoroscopic control, the catheter should be attached to the pressure manifold so that the balloon may be deflated immediately if pressure damping is detected. During advancement, deviation from the straight path along the spine usually suggests entry into a renal or hepatic vein. The catheter is then withdrawn, rotated, and advanced further. When right heart catheterization is performed to detect or quantify a left-to-right shunt, the catheter should first be advanced into the SVC. In order to do this, the balloon is best deflated and the catheter rotated to the lateral wall. It is then advanced in a counterclockwise rotation movement. Alternatively, a guidewire within the PAC can be used to access the SVC. Once the catheter is advanced into the SVC, blood samples are drawn from the high SVC and at the entrance into the RA (for detection or exclusion of anomalous pulmonary venous return).

Advancement of the PAC from the RA into the RV and PA is usually done by passing directly, or medially, across the tricuspid valve into the RV. This directs the tip of the catheter toward the apex of the RV. Then, the catheter has to be pulled back slightly and rotated further clockwise. In order to transmit the torque, it is important to maintain pressure on the catheter and use slight forward and backward movements. When the balloon tip is pointing upward toward the RV outflow tract, the catheter is quickly advanced into the PA. Deep inspiration might help to advance the catheter up into the PA and to advance the tip of the catheter into a wedge position in the distal PA.

When the RA is enlarged, advancement of the PAC into the PA can be difficult. It is sometimes necessary to loop the catheter. In order to do that, one can bend it against the lateral wall of the RA or engage the ostium of the hepatic vein. The catheter is then advanced and rotated clockwise. This will help advance the catheter into the tricuspid valve. If the tip of the catheter reaches the RV outflow tract, it can usually be advanced easily into the PA and wedge position. Occasionally, the balloon is so soft that it will not advance across the tricuspid valve and into the RV, despite a nice loop in the RA. Introducing a guidewire into the loop, but not to the tip of the catheter, can assist advancement into the PA.

If both PAs need to be engaged for a procedure, a guidewire can be introduced into the PAC with an appropriate bend such that the catheter can be advanced into each artery. It is often necessary to use the stiff end of the guidewire to assure an appropriate bend. In such a case, the guidewire is never to be advanced to the tip of the PAC. The stiff end of a guidewire has a very high risk of perforation and should never be exposed in the right heart or in the PA. Even the soft end of the guidewire carries a certain risk of perforation in the PA and should not be routinely used.

After recording the pulmonary wedge pressure, the balloon is deflated under slight tension, such that no abrupt forward movement of the catheter tip occurs. Then, the PA pressure is measured and blood oxygen saturation samples are taken simultaneously from the PA and from a systemic artery (femoral or radial) to measure cardiac output according to the Fick formula. Pressure measurements (and if needed, oxygen saturations) are recorded during withdrawal of the catheter from the PA to the RV and RA by counterclockwise rotation and pulling.

Advancing a multipurpose catheter from the femoral vein to the PA is done using the same technique. In the RA, the guidewire is withdrawn and the tip of the multipurpose catheter is directed medially toward the tricuspid valve and advanced into the RV. Under clockwise rotation, it is then advanced up to the PA and gently brought forward into a wedge position.

When advancing the catheters, anatomical variants and anomalies, such as patent foramen ovale (PFO), a persistent left SVC, and anomalous returning pulmonary veins might direct the catheter into an unwanted cavity. Fluoroscopy, contrast injection, and oximetry help to correctly locate the position of the catheter. Erroneous catheter placement into the LA and pulmonary vein is recognized by a path through the heart and deviation into a posterior position on a lateral view and can be confirmed by oxygen saturation measurements. Catheter position in the coronary sinus is detected using fluoroscopy and confirmed by oxygen saturation measurements that range from 20% to 30%.

JUGULAR OR SUBCLAVIAN VEIN

Cannulation of the internal jugular vein is often done with ultrasound guidance because it provides faster and safer access than landmark-based access. Ultrasound-guided cannulation of the subclavian vein is not established. Insertion of the PAC from a SVC is usually done with an inflated balloon connected to a pressure transducer. The distance marker on the catheter (every 10 cm) is helpful for orientation. After 15 to 20 cm, right atrial tracing is seen, and with the inflated balloon, the catheter is advanced across the tricuspid valve. The catheter is then advanced into the PA and into wedge position. This position should be reached after about 50 to 55 cm. If no wedge position is reached at this distance, the catheter might be coiled in the RV. The operator should deflate the balloon, withdraw the catheter into the RA, and start the process again.

ANTECUBITAL VEIN

The most commonly used technique to gain access to an antecubital vein is to insert a 20-gauge cannula in either the cephalic or basilica vein and then to exchange the cannula for a 6-Fr sheath. The basilica vein is preferred because the cephalic vein sometimes narrows in the *musculus deltoideus*, making advancement of the catheter impossible. The PAC is advanced into the SVC without inflating the balloon. In case of difficulties accessing the SVC, a guidewire can provide support.[14]

COMPLICATIONS

The complications of PAC insertion can be divided into issues related to vascular access, to catheter insertion, and to catheter residence (Table 9.2).[15] Additional complications are related to vasoreactivity testing, volume loading, and pulmonary or RV angiography (see Chapters 10 and 22).[16] The risk of catheter-related complications seems to have declined over time. In earlier reports, serious complications were found in approximately 5% of cases.[17-19] In recent studies, serious complications were encountered in less than 1%, even in patients with pulmonary hypertension.[6,16]

Hemodynamic monitoring in critically ill patients carries additional risks related to medium- to long-term indwelling lines. Thromboembolism and infection are the most frequent complications encountered in these patients.[20] In the ESCAPE trial, 4.2% of patients suffered PAC-related complications, of which two-thirds were attributed to long-term dwell time. The complications were infection and pulmonary infarction/haemorrhage.[5]

The most serious complication is PA rupture. In a prospective study, the rate of PA rupture was 0.2%; in retrospective studies, it varied between 0.001 to 0.47%.[17,21] Elderly patients and patients on chronic steroid therapy are at increased risk, whereas pulmonary hypertension does not constitute a higher risk for this complication.[22,23] The rupture may cause an asymptomatic pseudoaneurysm, hemoptysis that stops spontaneously, or hemoptysis

Table 9.2 Complications of pulmonary artery catheterization

Vascular Access Complications
- Vasovagal reaction
- Arterial puncture
- Arteriovenous fistula
- Bleeding from insertion site
- Nerve injury
- Air embolism
- Pneumothorax, hemothorax (subclavian, internal jugular vein approach)

Related to Catheter Insertion
- Arrhythmias (supraventricular tachycardia, ventricular premature beats, VT, VF)
- Right bundle branch block or complete heart block
- Injury to chordae in right ventricle
- Tricuspid regurgitation
- Dislodgement of pacemaker leads
- Pulmonary artery rupture/right ventricular perforation

Related to Catheter Residence
- Pulmonary artery rupture
- Pulmonary infarction
- Thrombosis
- Infection/endocarditis/thrombophlebitis
- Balloon rupture/embolization

Note: VF, ventricular fibrillation; VT, ventricular tachycardia.

and hemothorax.[21] In case of hemoptysis and hemothorax, the mortality rate is reportedly between 45% and 70%. Diagnosis should be suspected with the onset of chest pain related to catheter advancement or balloon inflation, frank hemoptysis, and dyspnea. If frank hemoptysis is present, immediate selective intubation of the uninjured lung should be performed. If no hemothorax is present, techniques such as balloon tamponade of the ruptured artery, tamponade of the bleeding lung by bronchoscopy, and embolization of the ruptured artery, have all been used to control the bleeding.[24] In case of hemothorax, the treatment is mostly surgical, with lobectomy or pneumectomy sometimes the only option to stop the bleeding.[25] To avoid this most serious complication, the balloon should only be inflated in the large proximal PA; the time of the balloon in "wedge" position should be minimized; and traction on the catheter when deflating the balloon should be maintained to prevent a rapid forward movement of the catheter tip.[21]

Insertion of a PAC in patients with preexisting left bundle branch block is complicated in approximately 3% to 5% by the occurrence of additional right bundle branch block that can result in complete heart block.[18,19] Therefore, when inserting a PAC in a patient with a left bundle branch block, a temporary pacemaker should be available for emergency pacing.

PRESSURE MEASUREMENTS AND PRESSURE WAVEFORMS

A prerequisite for accurate pressure measurements is a pressure recorder with a satisfactory frequency response and few artefacts. The most common problem in right-sided pressure recording is related to the quality of the soft catheters. The long, soft tubing results in over-damping of the pressure waveforms similar to air bubbles or to kinking in the catheter. Stiffer catheters and hyperdynamic states result in underdamping. Whipping the catheter against the septum results in pressure artefacts. Therefore, it is important to carefully examine the position of the pressure

transducer, the quality of the waveform, and the simultaneously recorded electrocardiogram. A crisp, dicrotic notch on the PA pressure waveform usually indicates a properly responsive pressure system.

The intracardiac and transmural pressures are greatly influenced by intrathoracic pressures. Intrathoracic pressure is transmitted to intracardiac pressures and thus pressures will vary with respiration. In normal physiology, inspiration will decrease intrathoracic pressure and increase venous return. The RA and ventricle being rather elastic will accommodate this increased volume without greatly increasing intracardiac pressure. Thus, in normal hearts, the net effect of inspiration is a decrease in right-sided pressures and an increase during expiration.[26] At end-expiration, the intrathoracic pressure is almost zero and closest to atmospheric pressure. Therefore, all pressures should be recorded at end-expiration. For an optimal, steady recording, ask the patient to stop breathing at the end of a nonlabored expiration. Intrathoracic pressures are reversed in a mechanically ventilated patient. On a mechanical ventilator, intrathoracic pressures are increased and venous return impaired during inspiration, and conversely, intrathoracic pressures are decreased and venous return increased during expiration. However, as is the case in normal respiration, the intrathoracic pressures are closest to atmospheric pressure at the end of expiration and should be measured at this point, also.[26]

The normal pressure waveforms are depicted in Figures 9.3 through 9.6. If there is an impairment to filling (e.g., restrictive physiology) or a great increase in right-heart filling (e.g., decompensated heart failure), the pressures will not vary with respiration. RA pressures may remain flat (and elevated) throughout the respiratory cycle or even increase during inspiration (Kussmaul's sign) (Figure 9.7).

The pulmonary capillary wedge pressure (PCWP) is particularly sensitive to pathologic intrathoracic pressures. Since PCWP is an indirect measurement of LA pressure, transmitted by a blood column from the LA to the tip of the catheter, any changes in intrathoracic pressure that

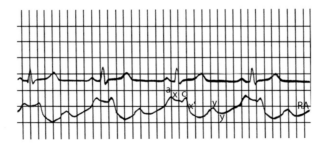

Figure 9.4 Right atrial (RA) pressure. The right atrial systole follows the P-wave on the electrocardiogram (ECG). The a-wave indicates atrial contraction and is followed by the x descent that corresponds to atrial relaxation. The closure of the tricuspid valve produces a slight upward deflection of the x descent and is called the c-wave. The x descent represents the descent of the atrioventricular ring during ventricular systole and atrial relaxation. The c-wave is not always present and the waveform is than reduced to the a-wave and the x descent. Following the T-wave on the ECG, a v-wave is present. The v-wave represents the atrial filling during diastole. The v-wave is followed by the y descent that marks the opening of the tricuspid valve and the emptying of the atrium during the rapid diastolic ventricular filling.

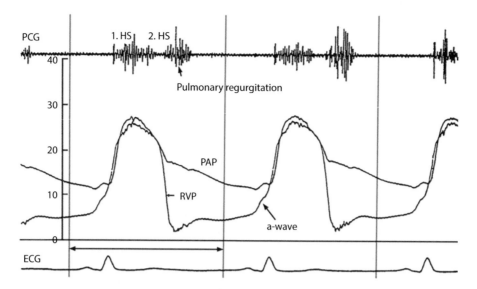

Figure 9.5 Right ventricular and pulmonary artery pressures. The right ventricular (RVP) and pulmonary artery pressures (PAP) are simultaneously recorded by a tip manometer (Millar catheter). Also recorded are the phonocardiogram (PCG) and the electrocardiogram (ECG). The patient has minimal pulmonic stenosis and mild pulmonary regurgitation. The atrial contraction results in an a-wave that occurs after the P-wave of the ECG. The end of the a-wave marks closure of the tricuspid valve as evidence by the first heart sound and represents right ventricular end-diastolic pressure. This is followed by ventricular systole. Ventricular relaxation results in closure of the pulmonary valve that induces the second heart sound (2. HS) and the dicrotic notch in the pressure tracing of the pulmonary artery. The isovolumic relaxation of the right ventricle (RV) continues until the tricuspid valve opens and rapid diastolic filling of the RV occurs. Usually RV end-diastolic pressure and peak RV systolic pressure are measured. Systolic and diastolic PAPs are measured and mean pressure is calculated.

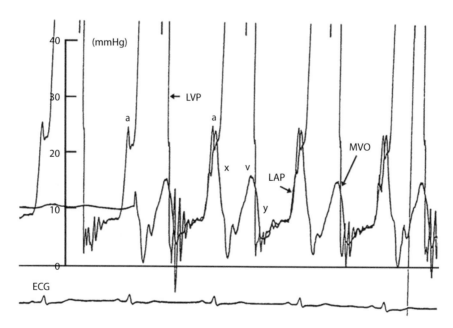

Figure 9.6 Simultaneous left ventricle (LVP) and left atrial (LAP) pressures. Depicted are the pressure waveforms recorded by fluid-filled catheters in the LV and the LA. The LA pressure is initially recorded as mean pressure and then in a phasic condition. The a-wave of the LA contraction is followed by the x descent that marks the descent of the atrioventricular ring during ventricular systole and atrial relaxation. The filling of the left atrium produces the v-wave and the rapid emptying of the LA after mitral valve opening (MVO) results in the y descent. Atrial and left ventricular pressures are overlapping during diastasis of diastole. The a-wave of atrial contraction is transmitted into the LV and results in the a-wave of the LV pressure tracing. The trough after the a-wave marks left ventricular end-diastolic pressure. Uncharacteristically, in this example, the a-wave is larger than the v-wave. Normally in LA pressures the v-wave is larger than the a-wave.

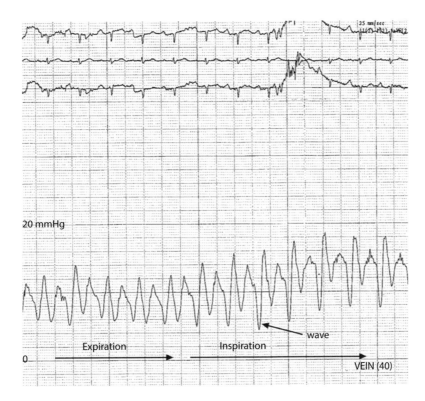

20 mmHg

Expiration

Inspiration

wave

0

VEIN (40)

Figure 9.7 Kussmaul's Sign. The right atrial pressure tracing of a patient with restrictive cardiomyopathy is depicted. Right atrial pressure is elevated. The prominent x and y descents give the waveform the characteristic *M*- over *W*-shaped appearance. During inspiration, right atrial pressure increases and the y descent is further augmented. This paradoxical increase in right atrial pressure during inspiration is called Kussmaul's sign.

influence this fluid column will change PCWP. An increase in intra-alveolar pressure (e.g., chronic obstructive lung disease, positive end-expiratory pressure) will lead to an overestimation of LA filling pressure.

CARDIAC OUTPUT MEASUREMENT

The volume of blood pumped to the body per minute is termed *cardiac output*. Cardiac output is dependent on metabolic state, body size, age, and a number of other factors, such as posture, anxiety, and body temperature.[27] Baseline cardiac output is mainly determined by metabolic rate, and baseline metabolic rate is closely correlated with body surface area (BSA). It has therefore become common practice to normalize cardiac output to BSA as the cardiac index (liters/minute/m^2). In the cardiac catheterization laboratory, cardiac output is most often determined by the Fick oxygen consumption method, or the thermodilution technique. In addition, angiographic cardiac output measurements (stroke volume × heart rate) might be used.

Fick technique

The Fick principle states that the total uptake or release of a substance by any organ is the product of the arteriovenous concentration difference of the substance and the blood flow

to that organ.[27] In the lungs, the released substance is oxygen, and the pulmonary blood flow can be calculated from the measured differences in arterial and venous oxygen saturations and the oxygen uptake by the lungs per minute. In the absence of intracardiac shunts, pulmonary flow equals systemic flow.

The arteriovenous oxygen gradient is calculated from the difference in oxygen saturation between arterial and mixed venous blood. Mixed venous blood is best obtained from the PA, or alternatively from an RV blood sample. For correct measurement of blood oxygenation in the lungs, a pulmonary venous sample should be measured. For practical reasons, a sample from the LV or the femoral artery is taken. The small decrease in saturation due to bronchial and thebesian vein drainage is negligible. In the arterial and venous samples, oxygen saturation is measured. The calculation of the oxygen content assumes that red cells with 100% oxygen saturation carry 1.36 mL of oxygen per gram of hemoglobin. Oxygen content (mL O_2/L blood) = % oxygen saturation × 1.36 (mL of O_2/g hemoglobin) × hemoglobin (g/dL) × 10 (converts from dL to L).

Oxygen consumption can be measured by a metabolic rate meter (polarographic cell method) where the patient breathes ambient room air in a steady state for several minutes and the metabolic rate meter gives a readout of oxygen consumption in liters per minute. Alternatively, basal oxygen consumption can be assumed from BSA, age, and sex.

In young patients, a basal oxygen consumption of 3 mL/kg body weight or 125 mL/m^2 BSA is often used. For elderly patients, an oxygen consumption of 110 mL/m^2 is normal. It is important, however, to understand the limitations of this assumption. Baseline oxygen consumption can vary by as much as 25% between patients.[28] A poor correlation has been found between cardiac output determination by the Fick method measuring oxygen consumption or estimating oxygen consumption.[29] This imprecision may lead to misclassification of disease states.[30] If the patient is not in a steady state because of anxiety, dyspnea, tachycardia, or is oversedated and breathes shallowly, oxygen consumption is either increased or decreased to an unpredicted level. The error is greatest in tachycardic patients. Caution is therefore warranted when cardiac output is calculated using an assumed oxygen consumption, and consequently, also when this value is used to calculate valve areas or vascular resistances.

Another important source of error in calculating cardiac output by the Fick method is the administration of supplemental oxygen to the patient. This makes it almost impossible to calculate oxygen content (dissolved oxygen in plasma!) and hence cardiac output. Therefore, if possible, supplemental oxygen should be discontinued at least 15 minutes before determination of cardiac output by the Fick oxygen consumption technique.

Thermodilution technique

The thermodilution technique to measure cardiac output is an indicator-dilution method with cold fluid as the indicator. It is based on the Stewart-Hamilton principle: A known quantity of an indicator is injected as a bolus into the circulating system and after thorough mixing, a concentration-time curve is sampled downstream.[31] Cold saline is injected via the proximal lumen of the PAC (Figure 9.1) and the transient drop in blood temperature is sensed by the thermistor at the distal end of the catheter. The cardiac output computer generates a thermodilution curve by plotting the decline in temperature (°C) versus time in seconds. The area under the curve is inversely related to cardiac output and is measured to calculate cardiac output. Because the body acts as a large heat sink, there is no recirculation. Hence, successive measurements can be made without waiting. Usually, five measurements are performed. The lowest and the highest measurements are discarded and the mean of the three remaining measurements is recorded as cardiac output.

Apart from proper calibration of the different catheters, correct onset of recording and checking the correct position of the catheters, two additional main limitations of the thermodilution technique have to be considered. Commercially available systems are designed to prevent warming of the injectate by the hands of the operator. However, warming of the cold solution caused by prolonged stay of the injectate in the RA, secondary to severe tricuspid regurgitation or low cardiac output, makes the thermodilution method unreliable.[32] Similarly, heavy respiration might induce PA temperature changes and result in inaccurate thermodilution cardiac output measurements.[26]

VASCULAR RESISTANCE

Ohm's law defines hydraulic resistance as the ratio of mean pressure drop (ΔP) across the hydraulic system to laminar flow through it. In such a system, the resistance to flow depends solely on the diameter of the tubing and the viscosity of the fluid. The concept of vascular resistance was established in analogy to Ohm's law. However, the cardiovascular system differs in a number of ways from a hydraulic system. For example, it is a pulsatile system; the blood is an inhomogeneous fluid (i.e., the vessels are elastic); and pressure waves are reflected. Therefore, the concept of vascular resistance is questionable. Vascular impedance, defined as the ratio of pulsatile pressure to pulsatile flow, would be a more accurate concept to describe the resistance and elasticity of the cardiovascular system.[27] Nevertheless, the concept of systemic and pulmonary vascular resistance has gained wide acceptance. Its usefulness to assess pathophysiological conditions has been established by empirical data. Calculation of vascular resistance is now widely used for clinical decision-making.

Systemic or pulmonary vascular resistance might also be termed *systemic or pulmonary arteriolar resistance*. However, only about 60% of the pressure drop across the system occurs at the arteriolar level; the other 40% occurs at other sites in the vascular bed.[27] Therefore, *systemic and pulmonary vascular resistance* is the preferred term.

Systemic vascular resistance is calculated as the ratio of the pressure drop from aorta to RA (mean aortic pressure–mean right atrial pressure), to systemic flow (Q_s). The result of this ratio is expressed either in an arbitrary resistance unit (mmHg/L/min), also called hybrid resistance unit, or Wood unit (according to its first introduction by Dr. Paul Wood). This hybrid resistance unit is used in pediatric cardiology. In adult cardiology, it is usually converted into metric resistance units, expressed in dynes $\times$ sec $\times$ cm^5 by use of the conversion factor 80 (Table 9.3). In pediatric cardiology, the resistance is also usually normalized for BSA, thus resulting in a vascular resistance index. The resistance index is obtained by dividing the mean pressure drop by the cardiac index (not obtained by dividing the resistance by BSA).

Pulmonary vascular resistance is calculated as the ratio of the pressure drop from the PA to the LA, to pulmonary flow (Q_p). LA pressure is, in most cases, substituted by PCWP. The mean pressure drop from the PA to the LA or the pulmonary capillaries is termed *transpulmonary pressure gradient* (TPG) (Figure 9.8). In a normal pulmonary vascular bed, the TPG is no larger than 12 mmHg.[33,34] However, it has been recognized that TPG is a composite variable that is highly sensitive to changes in both flow and filling pressures.[33,34] Diastolic pressure gradient (DPG), that is the diastolic pressure of the PA pressure minus the mean wedge pressure, is another parameter that describes the gradient across the pulmonary vasculature (Figure 9.8). DPG lies between 1

Table 9.3 Formulas for calculation of cardiac output and vascular resistances

Oxygen content = O_2 saturation $\times 1.36 \times Hgb \times 10$ = ml/L

Cardiac output (CO) by the Fick oxygen consumption method: $CO = \dfrac{O_2 \text{ consumption (ml / min)}}{AVO_2 \text{ difference (ml } O_2 \text{ / 100 ml blood)} \times 10}$

$CO = \dfrac{Wt \times 3 \text{ ml } O_2 / kg \text{ BW}}{(AO_2\% - VO_2\%) \times 1.36 \times Hgb \times 10}$ = L/min (Wt, weight in kilograms; $AO_2\%$, arterial oxygen saturation; $VO_2\%$, venous oxygen saturation; Hgb, hemoglobin concentration in g/dl)

Cardiac index (CI) $= \dfrac{CO}{BSA}$ = L / min/ m^2 (BSA, body surface area in m^2)

Stroke volume $(SV) = \dfrac{CO \text{ (ml / min)}}{\text{Heart rate (beats / min)}}$ = ml / beat

Stroke index $(SI) = \dfrac{SV \text{ (ml / beat)}}{BSA \text{ } (m^2)}$ = ml / beat / m^2 (BSA, body surface area; SV, stroke volume)

Transpulmonary pressure gradient = mean PAP − mean PCWP = mmHg

Diastolic pressure gradient = diastolic PAP − mean PCWP = mmHg (PAP, pulmonary artery pressure; PCWP, pulmonary capillary wedge pressure)

Pulmonary vascular resistance $(PVR) = \dfrac{\text{mean PAP} - \text{mean PCWP}}{CO} \times 80$ = dynes $\times$ sec $\times cm^5$ 80 = factor to convert into metric units (dynes $\times$ sec $\times cm^5$)

Systemic vascular resistance (SVR) $= \dfrac{\text{mean aortic pressure} - \text{mean RAP}}{CO} \times 80$ = dynes $\times$ sec $\times cm^5$ (RAP, right atrial pressure)

Systemic vascular resistance index (SVRI) $= \dfrac{\text{mean aortic pressure} - \text{mean RAP}}{CI} \times 80$ = dynes $\times$ sec $\times cm^5$ / m^2 (CI, cardiac index)

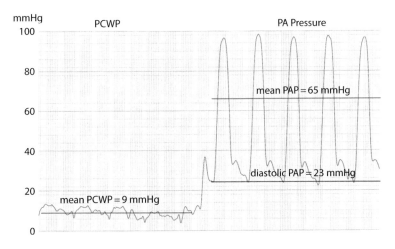

Figure 9.8 Transpulmonary pressure gradient (TPG) and diastolic pressure gradient (DPG). The measurement of pulmonary capillary wedge pressure (PCWP) and pulmonary artery (PA) pressure in a patient with pulmonary hypertension is depicted. TPG is defined as mean pulmonary artery pressure (mPAP) minus mean PCWP. Diastolic pressure gradient (DPG) is defined as diastolic PAP minus mean PCWP. TPG is influenced by flow, resistance, and left heart filling pressures. DPG is minimally influenced by flow or filling pressures. Therefore, DPG has replaced TPG to assess concomitant pulmonary vascular disease in cases of pulmonary hypertension secondary to left heart failure.

and 3 mmHg and almost never exceeds 5 mmHg in normal subjects.[33] DPG is only minimally influenced by flow or filling pressures.[33] In case of increased PA pressures, TPG and DPG have been used to assess vascular remodeling and pulmonary vascular disease (Figure 9.8).[35] Since DPG is much better suited then TPG to assess these pulmonary vascular changes independent of hemodynamic changes, DPG is now the recommended parameter to define and classify pulmonary hypertension, particularly in pulmonary hypertension secondary to left heart failure.[2,33,34,36] An increase of

DPG of 7 mmHg or more indicates pathologic pulmonary vascular changes and a precapillary component to pulmonary hypertension (Figure 9.8). For hemodynamic evaluation and testing of pulmonary vascular reactivity in case of pulmonary hypertension, see Chapter 10.

SHUNT DETECTION

Patients with clinically suspected intracardiac shunts usually undergo echocardiography that reveals the location and quantification of the shunt. Even hemodynamically insignificant shunts through a small atrial defect or a PFO are visualized by contrast echocardiography or color Doppler echocardiography. Accordingly, the main purposes of right heart catheterization in patients with known intracardiac shunts are their quantification, the assessment of relative shunt volumes in bidirectional shunts, or the evaluation of concomitant pulmonary hypertension. Nevertheless, unsuspected intracardiac shunts are occasionally found during routine right heart catheterization. A left-to-right shunt should be suspected when PA oxygen saturation is ≥80%, and a right-to-left shunt when arterial oxygen saturation is below 90% or approaches 80% without apparent underlying heart failure, pulmonic disorder, or alveolar hypoventilation. In case of suspected right-to-left shunt, alveolar hypoventilation should be excluded by making the patient cough and take deep breaths. If arterial desaturation persists, oxygen should be given by face mask to achieve full arterial oxygenation. If full arterial oxygenation cannot be achieved by providing oxygen, right-to-left shunt is presumed to be present.

Oximetry run

If a left-to-right shunt or a right-to-left shunt is suspected, it should be localized and quantified. In the case of a left-to-right shunt, the receiving heart chamber gets an admixture of arterial blood that will increase its oxygen saturation compared with the upstream chamber (Table 9.4). The simplest way to screen for a left-to-right shunt is to search for an oxygen saturation step-up over the entire right-sided heart by sampling the SVC and the PA. If an oxygenation step-up of more than 8% is detected, a left-to-right shunt may be present. For exact localization (atrial, ventricular, great vessels) of the shunt, an oximetry run is performed. An oxygen saturation step-up of ≥7% at the atrial level and ≥5% at the ventricular or great vessel level indicates a left-to-right shunt.[37]

The oximetry run should be performed with a large-bore end-hole or side-hole catheter, usually the PAC or a multipurpose catheter. The saturation run should be started in the PA, and samples should be obtained in the various locations after verification of the position of the catheter by fluoroscopy. The possible sample sites are listed in Table 9.5. It is advisable to obtain two samples from the most important sites and to sample the receiving chambers several times and average the values. The oximetry run is performed during steady-state conditions within a few minutes. In equivocal cases, increasing systemic flow with exercise will increase the likelihood of detection of a small left-to-right shunt.[37] Importantly, supplemental oxygen should be withheld, if possible. If a significant step-up and thus a left-to-right shunt is detected, the blood oxygen saturation is used to calculate the shunt magnitude.

However, it is important to understand that the step-up indicates a net left-to-right shunt. A concomitant right-to-left shunt may be present. For example, in large atrial septal defects (ASDs), a right-to-left shunt of varying magnitude is always present. In analogy to the step-up of the oxygen saturation of the left-to-right shunt, a right-to-left shunt is detected by a step-down of oxygen saturation in the chambers of the left heart. To detect and to calculate the magnitude of a right-to-left shunt, an oxygen saturation sample of the pulmonary vein, LA, LV, and aorta (below the insertion of the ductus arteriosus) is obtained.

Calculation of shunt size

If an intracardiac shunt is present, pulmonary flow (Qp) no longer equals systemic flow (Qs). In the presence of a

Table 9.4 Detection of left-to-right shunt by oxygen saturation step-up

Level of Shunt (chambers)	O$_2$ % Saturation Step-Up	Possible Causes of Step-Up
Atrial (SVC/IVC to RA)	≥7	ASD, sinus venosus defects, partial anomalous pulmonary venous drainage, coronary or other arteriovenous fistula to the RA, ruptured sinus valsalva, VSD with TR
Ventricular (RA to RV)	≥5	VSD, primum ASD, fistula to RV, PDA with PR
Great vessel (RV to PA)	≥5	Patent ductus arteriosus, aorto-pulmonic window, aberrant coronary artery origin

Source: Adapted from Grossman, W., Shunt detection and quantification, In: Baim, D.S., ed., *Grossman's Cardiac Catheterization, Angiography, and Intervention*, 7 edn, Lippincott, Williams & Wilkins, Philadelphia, PA, 2006, pp. 163–172.

Note: ASD, atrial septal defect; IVC, inferior vena cava; PA, pulmonary artery; PDA, patent ductus arteriosus; PR, pulmonary regurgitation; RA, right atrium; RV, right ventricle; SVC, superior vena cava; TR, tricuspid regurgitation; VSD, ventricular septal defect.

Table 9.5 Sample sites for oxygen saturation during diagnostic oximetry run

1. Left and/or right pulmonary artery
2. Main pulmonary artery
3. Right ventricular outflow tract
4. Right ventricular, mid
5. Right ventricular, apex
6. Right atrium, low or near tricuspid valve
7. Right atrium, mid
8. Right atrium, high (near junction with superior vena cava)
9. Superior vena cava, low (near junction with right atrium)
10. Superior vena cava, high
11. Inferior vena cava, high (just beneath heart, above hepatic vein)
12. Inferior vena cava, low (above renal vein, below hepatic vein)
13. Pulmonary vein
14. Left atrium
15. Left ventricle
16. Aorta (distal to insertion of ductus)

left-to-right shunt, pulmonary flow is increased by the shunt volume, and conversely, in the presence of a right-to-left shunt, pulmonary flow relative to systemic flow is decreased by the shunt volume. The shunt fraction is then the ratio of the pulmonary flow to the systemic flow (Qp/Qs).

CALCULATION OF PULMONIC FLOW

The pulmonary flow is calculated according to the Fick formula:

$$\text{Pulmonary flow}(Qp) = \frac{\text{oxygen consumption}}{\left(\text{pulmonary vein-pulmonary artery oxygen saturation}\right) \times 1.36 \times \text{Hgb} \times 10}$$

in l/min

If no pulmonary vein sample has been obtained, arterial oxygen saturation may be used. A prerequisite for the use of an arterial oxygen saturation as substitute for pulmonary vein saturation is the exclusion of a right-to-left shunt and an arterial oxygen saturation of ≥95%. If a right-to-left shunt is present, an assumed oxygen saturation of 98% should be used for the calculation of pulmonary blood flow.[38]

CALCULATION OF SYSTEMIC FLOW

Systemic flow is calculated according to the following formula:

$$\text{Systemic flow}(Qs) = \frac{\text{oxygen consumption}}{\left(\text{systemic arterial-mixed venous oxygen saturation}\right) \times 1.36 \times \text{Hgb} \times 10}$$

in l/min

Mixed venous oxygen saturation refers to the oxygen saturation of the heart chamber upstream to the chamber receiving the shunt. For shunts on the atrial level, the mixed venous oxygen saturation is therefore the oxygen saturation of the SVC and IVC. For shunts at the ventricular and great vessel level, the mixed venous saturation used for flow calculation is the oxygen saturation of the RA and RV, respectively.

In adults, the mixed venous oxygen saturation is calculated as the sum of three times the SVC oxygen saturation, plus one times the oxygen saturation of the IVC divided by four.[39] (In pediatric cardiology, the saturation difference between the SVC and IVC is ignored, and the saturation of the SVC is usually used as venous oxygen saturation.) The increased weighing of the more desaturated blood of the SVC is due to the fact that the admixture of the heavily desaturated blood from the coronary sinus is not measured. The empiric formula has proven to best approximate the mixed venous saturation in adults at rest.[39] During exercise, however, oxygen saturation of the IVC weighs more prominently on mixed venous oxygen saturation. During exercise, mixed venous oxygen saturation therefore is computed as the sum of the oxygen saturation of the SVC, plus two times the oxygen saturation of the IVC divided by three.[39]

Quantification of left-to-right and right-to-left shunts

In the absence of a right-to-left shunt, the left-to-right shunt is calculated as pulmonic flow (Qp) minus systemic flow (Qs). The magnitude of the left-to-right shunt can be expressed as the ratio of pulmonic to systemic flow (Qp/Qs). The ratio Qp/Qs can be calculated by knowing the oxygen saturations alone (Table 9.6). The Qp/Qs ratio derived from the oximetry data is routinely compared to the Qp/Qs ratio obtained from echocardiographic shunt quantification. Shunt ratios between 1 and 1.5 indicate a

Table 9.6 Formulas for shunt calculation

Mixed venous oxygen saturation (%) $= \dfrac{3\,SVC_{sat} + 1\,IVC_{sat}}{4}$

Pulmonary flow $\left(\mathbf{Q_p}\right) = \dfrac{O_2 \text{ consumption}}{\left(PV_{sat} - PA_{sat}\right) \times 1.36 \times Hgb \times 10} = L/min$

Systemic flow $\left(\mathbf{Q_s}\right) = \dfrac{O_2 \text{ consumption}}{\left(Art_{sat} - \text{Mixed venous}_{sat}\right) \times 1.36 \times Hgb \times 10} = L/min$

$\mathbf{Q_p / Q_s} = \dfrac{Art_{sat} - \text{mixed venous}_{sat}}{Pv_{sat} - PA_{sat}}$

$\mathbf{Q_p \text{effective}}\ \left(\mathbf{Q_s \text{effective}}\right) = \dfrac{O_2 \text{ consumption}}{\left(PV_{sat} - \text{Mixed venous}_{sat}\right) \times 1.36 \times Hgb \times 10} = l/min$

Left–right shunt $(\mathbf{Q_{left-right}}) = Q_p - Q_p \text{ effective} = L/min$

Right–left shunt $(\mathbf{Q_{right-left}}) = Q_s - Q_s \text{ effective} = L/min$

% left − to − right shunt $= \dfrac{PA_{sat} - \text{mixed venous}_{sat}}{PV_{sat} - \text{mixed venous}_{sat}} \times 100 = \%$

% right − to − left shunt $= \dfrac{PV_{sat} - Art_{sat}}{PV_{sat} - \text{mixed venous}_{sat}} \times 100 = \%$

Note: Art, arterial; Hgb, hemoglobin; IVC, inferior vena cava; PA, pulmonary artery; PV, pulmonary vein; SAT, saturation; SVC, superior vena cava.

Table 9.7 Anticipated normal values

Right atrium	a-Wave	2–10 mmHg
	v-Wave	2–10 mmHg
	Mean	0–8 mmHg
Right ventricle	Systolic	15–30 mmHg
	End-diastolic	0–8 mmHg
Pulmonary artery	Systolic	15–30 mmHg
	End-diastolic	3–12 mmHg
	Mean	10–21 mmHg
Left atrium or pulmonary capillary wedge pressure	a-Wave	4–15 mmHg
	v-Wave	4–15 mmHg
	Mean	4–12 mmHg
Transpulmonary pressure gradient		4–12 mmHg
Diastolic pressure gradient	Mean	1–5 mmHg
Cardiac output		5–10 L/min
Cardiac index		3–5 L/min/m²
Stroke volume		80–160 ml
Stroke volume index		40–160 ml/m²
Mixed venous oxygen saturation		65–75%
Systemic vascular resistance		770–1500 dynes × sec × cm⁵
Pulmonary vascular resistance		20–120 dynes × sec × cm⁵

Note: Normal values are expected values in average-sized adults at rest.[31,40]

small left-to-right shunt, between 1.5 and 2 an intermediate shunt, and greater than 2 indicates a large shunt. Surgical or percutaneous defect closure is recommended in large and most intermediate shunts. Of note, shunt size is not equal to defect size. In the case of increased right heart pressures, left-to-right shunts might be small despite a large ASD.

In the presence of a right-to-left shunt or a bidirectional shunt (simultaneous left-to-right and right-to-left shunt), the magnitude of each shunt can be calculated by the additional quantification of the hypothetic effective pulmonic and systemic blood flow. The effective blood flow is the blood flow that would exist in a pulmonic or systemic vascular system in the absence of any left-to-right or right-to-left shunt. The effective blood flow is as follows:

$$\left(Q_{\text{eff}}\right) = \frac{\text{oxygen consumption}}{\left(\text{pulmonic vein saturation-mixed venous saturation}\right) \times 1.36 \times \text{Hgb} \times 10}$$

The left-to-right shunt then equals $Q_p - Q_{\text{eff}}$, and conversely, the right-to-left shunt equals $Q_s - Q_{\text{eff}}$.

Knowing the effective blood flow allows for the calculation of the percentage of shunt volumes. The percentage left-to-right shunt is computed as $1 - Q$ effective/ Q_p and the percentage right-to-left shunt is computed as $1 - Q$ effective/Q_s. A simplified formula to calculate percentage of shunts is obtained by factoring out variables, such as oxygen consumption, from these formulas. The percentage of the respective shunt volumes can then be calculated by using the blood oxygen saturations alone (Table 9.7).

REFERENCES

1. Deanfield J, et al. Management of grown up congenital heart disease. *Eur Heart J* 2003;24(11):1035–1084.
2. Galie N, et al. 2015 ESC/ERS Guidelines for the diagnosis and treatment of pulmonary hypertension: The Joint Task Force for the Diagnosis and Treatment of Pulmonary Hypertension of the European Society of Cardiology (ESC) and the European Respiratory Society (ERS): Endorsed by: Association for European Paediatric and Congenital Cardiology (AEPC), International Society for Heart and Lung Transplantation (ISHLT). *Eur Heart J* 2016;37:67–119.
3. Connors AF Jr, et al. The effectiveness of right heart catheterization in the initial care of critically ill patients. SUPPORT Investigators. *JAMA* 1996;276(11):889–897.
4. Mueller HS, et al. ACC expert consensus document. Present use of bedside right heart catheterization in patients with cardiac disease. American College of Cardiology. *J Am Coll Cardiol* 1998;32(3):840–864.
5. Binanay C, et al. Evaluation study of congestive heart failure and pulmonary artery catheterization effectiveness: The ESCAPE trial. *JAMA* 2005;294(13):1625–1633.
6. Harvey S, et al. Assessment of the clinical effectiveness of pulmonary artery catheters in management of patients in intensive care (PAC-Man): A randomised controlled trial. *Lancet* 2005;366(9484):472–477.
7. Harwani N, et al. Comparison of brachial vein versus internal jugular vein approach for access to the right side of the heart with or without myocardial biopsy. *Am J Cardiol* 2015;116(5):740–743.
8. Speiser B, et al. Compared to femoral venous access, upper extremity right heart catheterization reduces time to ambulation: A single center experience. *Catheter Cardiovasc Interv* 2017;89(4):658–664.
9. O'Quin R, Marini JJ. Pulmonary artery occlusion pressure: Clinical physiology, measurement, and interpretation. *Am Rev Respir Dis* 1983;128(2):319–326.
10. Callan P, Clark AL. Right heart catheterisation: Indications and interpretation. *Heart* 2016;102(2):147–157.
11. Finkelhor RS, et al. Limitations and strengths of Doppler/echo pulmonary artery systolic pressure-right heart catheterization correlations: A systematic literature review. *Echocardiography* 2015;32(1):10–18.
12. Cotter G, et al. Hemodynamic monitoring in acute heart failure. *Crit Care Med* 2008;36(1 Suppl):S40–S43.
13. Grossmann W. Pressure Measurement. In: Baim DS, ed. *Grossman's Cardiac Catheterization, Angiography, and Intervention.* 7 edn. Philadelphia: Lippincott Williams & Wilkins; 2006:133–147.
14. Lee SH, et al. Right cardiac catheterization using the antecubital fossa vein in Korean patients. *Korean Circ J* 2016;46(2):207–212.
15. Kellan EA, Cho L. Right Heart Catheterization. In: Griffin PB, Topol EJ, Nair D, Ashley K, eds. *Manual of Cardiovascular Medicine.* 3 edn. Philadelphia: Lippincott Williams & Wilkins; 2009:744–758.
16. Hoeper MM, et al. Complications of right heart catheterization procedures in patients with pulmonary hypertension in experienced centers. *J Am Coll Cardiol* 2006;48(12):2546–2552.
17. Boyd KD, et al. A prospective study of complications of pulmonary artery catheterizations in 500 consecutive patients. *Chest* 1983;84(3):245–249.
18. Gupta PK, Haft JI. Complete heart block complicating cardiac catheterization. *Chest* 1972;61(2):185–187.
19. Sprung CL, et al. Risk of right bundle-branch block and complete heart block during pulmonary artery catheterization. *Crit Care Med* 1989;17(1):1–3.
20. Burns KE, McLaren A. A critical review of thromboembolic complications associated with central venous catheters. *Can J Anaesth* 2008;55(8):532–541.
21. Poplausky MR, et al. Swan-Ganz catheter-induced pulmonary artery pseudoaneurysm formation: Three case reports and a review of the literature. *Chest* 2001;120(6):2105–2111.
22. Hardy JF, et al. Pathophysiology of rupture of the pulmonary artery by pulmonary artery balloon-tipped catheters. *Anesth Analg* 1983;62(10):925–930.
23. Lois JF, et al. Vessel rupture by balloon catheters complicating chronic steroid therapy. *AJR Am J Roentgenol* 1985;144(5):1073–1074.
24. Kaiser CA, et al. Selective embolization of a pulmonary artery rupture caused by a Cournand catheter. *Catheter Cardiovasc Interv* 2004;61(3):317–319.

25. Mullerworth MH, et al. Recognition and management of catheter-induced pulmonary artery rupture. *Ann Thorac Surg* 1998;66(4):1242–1245.

26. Tuman KJ, et al. Pitfalls in interpretation of pulmonary artery catheter data. *J Cardiothorac Anesth* 1989;3(5):625–641.

27. Grossmann W. Blood Flow Measurement: Cardiac Output and Vascular Resistance. In: Baim DS, ed. *Grossman's Cardiac Catheterization, Angiography, and Intervention*. Philadelphia, PA: Lippincott, Williams & Wilkins; 2006:148–162.

28. Kendrick AH, et al. Direct Fick cardiac output: Are assumed values of oxygen consumption acceptable? *Eur Heart J* 1988;9(3):337–342.

29. Fanari Z, et al. Cardiac output determination using a widely available direct continuous oxygen consumption measuring device: A practical way to get back to the gold standard. *Cardiovasc Revasc Med* 2016;17(4):256–261.

30. Boland JE, et al. Impact of cardiac output imprecision on the clinical interpretation of haemodynamic variables in the cardiac catheterisation laboratory. *Int J Cardiol* 2016;210:63–65.

31. Spiller P, Webb-Peploe MM. Blood flow. *Eur Heart J* 1985;6 Suppl C:11–18.

32. Cigarroa RG, et al. Underestimation of cardiac output by thermodilution in patients with tricuspid regurgitation. *Am J Med* 1989;86(4):417–420.

33. Naeije R, et al. The transpulmonary pressure gradient for the diagnosis of pulmonary vascular disease. *Eur Respir J* 2013;41(1):217–223.

34. Vachiery JL, et al. Pulmonary hypertension due to left heart diseases. *J Am Coll Cardiol* 2013;62(25 Suppl):D100–D108.

35. Delgado JF, et al. Pulmonary vascular remodeling in pulmonary hypertension due to chronic heart failure. *Eur J Heart Fail* 2005;7(6):1011–1016.

36. Rosenkranz S, Preston IR. Right heart catheterisation: Best practice and pitfalls in pulmonary hypertension. *Eur Respir Rev* 2015;24(138):642–652.

37. Antman EM, et al. Blood oxygen measurements in the assessment of intracardiac left to right shunts: A critical appraisal of methodology. *Am J Cardiol* 1980;46(2):265–271.

38. Grossman W. Shunt Detection and Quantification. In: Baim DS, ed. *Grossman's Cardiac Catheterization, Angiography, and Intervention*. 7 edn. Philadelphia: Lippincott, Williams & Wilkins; 2006:163–172.

39. Flamm MD, et al. Measurement of systemic cardiac output at rest and exercise in patients with atrial septal defect. *Am J Cardiol* 1969;23(2):258–265.

40. Kovacs G, et al. Pulmonary arterial pressure during rest and exercise in healthy subjects: A systematic review. *Eur Respir J* 2009;34(4):888–894.

10

Pulmonary hypertension: Hemodynamic assessment and response to vasodilators

MYUNG H. PARK AND VALLERIE V. MCLAUGHLIN

INTRODUCTION

The first observation of patients with pulmonary hypertension (PH) was described by German physician Dr. Ernst von Romberg as "sclerosis of the pulmonary arteries" from autopsy findings.[1] The term *primary pulmonary hypertension* (PPH) was used by Dresdale et al. in 1951, describing a hypertensive vasculopathy of pulmonary vessels of unknown cause.[2] Paul Wood contributed to understanding the possible etiology of this disease by observing that a reduction in pulmonary artery pressure (PAP) was seen in response to intravenous (IV) administration of acetylcholine in patients with PH secondary to mitral stenosis, eliciting a proposal that a "vaso-constrictive factor" may be the cause.[3]

However, it was an outbreak of aminorex-induced PH in the 1960s in Europe that prompted the World Health Organization (WHO) to assemble a group of experts to determine the current state of knowledge of PPH.[4] The National Heart, Lung, and Blood Institute (NHLBI) created a National Registry of Patients with PPH from 1981 to 1987, enrolling 187 patients from 32 clinical centers. This registry had a monumental impact in elucidating clinical, epidemiological, and pathophysiological information and promoted subsequent research. The registry revealed that PPH occurred more frequently in women than men (1.7:1), with a mean age at diagnosis of 36 years; when left untreated, it was a progressive disease with a median survival of 2.8 years.[5,6] In addition, a significant delay was noted in making the diagnosis from onset of symptoms (2.5 years), a factor that has prompted efforts to increase awareness of PH.

The second WHO meeting was held in Evian, France in 1998, commemorating the 25th anniversary of the first meeting in Geneva. The experts developed a classification system categorizing PH into five groups based on different etiologies. However, the most comprehensive changes were made during the third world symposium in Venice, Italy, held in 2003. This meeting was heralded by tremendous advances in the field of molecular and genetic sciences, as well as the development of effective therapies that changed the understanding and practice of PH. The 2003 Venice Classification of Pulmonary Hypertension replaced the term PPH with idiopathic pulmonary arterial hypertension (IPAH), along with modifications of the five categories previously established.[7] In 2008, the fourth World Symposium on Pulmonary Hypertension took place in

Dana Point, California, where current research and clinical trials were evaluated, resulting in an updated classification system and treatment guidelines (see "Clinical Aspects").[8,9]

FUNDAMENTALS

Pathobiology of pulmonary arterial hypertension

The pulmonary vasculature is a low-pressure system with a normal systolic PAP range of 15–30 mmHg and mean PAP of 9–18 mmHg, essentially functioning at less than one-tenth the resistance to flow observed in the systemic vascular bed, in part because of the large cross-sectional area of the pulmonary circulation.[10]

The current definition of pulmonary arterial hypertension (PAH) from the fourth world symposium is mean PAP >25 mmHg and pulmonary capillary wedge pressure (PCWP) ≤15 mmHg.[11] PAH is characterized by structural changes in the pulmonary vascular bed resulting in pulmonary arterial obstruction due to vascular proliferation and remodeling. This leads to a progressive increase in PAP and pulmonary vascular resistance (PVR), resulting in right ventricular (RV) failure and death. The predominant cause of increased PVR is the loss of vascular luminal cross-sectional area due to pulmonary vascular remodeling. This process involves all layers of the vessel wall and is characterized by intimal hyperplasia, medial hypertrophy, adventitial proliferation, and *in situ* thrombosis.

The process by which pulmonary vasculopathy is initiated results from the interaction of a predisposing state and one or more inciting stimuli, a concept known as the "multiple-hit hypothesis."[12,13] Two or more "hits" is thought to consist of a genetic abnormality or substrate that renders an individual susceptible. The second hit may be either a systemic disorder (i.e., connective tissue disease [CTD], human immunodeficiency virus [HIV]), an environmental trigger (i.e., hypoxic state, ingestion of an anorexigen), or additional genetic conditions (i.e., mutation, polymorphism). Once a combination of factors affects a susceptible individual, various mechanisms are activated which result in vasoconstriction, cellular proliferation, and a prothrombotic state leading to PAH.

Molecular and cellular mechanisms

PROSTACYCLIN AND THROMBOXANE A2

The two prostanoids, prostacyclin (PGI2) and thromboxane A2, are the main metabolites of arachidonic acid. PGI2, produced by the action of PGI2 synthase, is a potent vasodilator and a strong inhibitor of platelet aggregation and smooth muscle cell proliferation. Thromboxane A2 is a potent vasoconstrictor and promotes platelet activation. In PAH, PGI2 synthase activity and PGI2 levels are reduced, whereas thromboxane levels are increased, thereby resulting in vasoconstriction, cellular proliferation, and thrombosis (Figure 10.1).[14–16]

ENDOTHELIN-1

Endothelin (ET)-1 is a 21-amino peptide that is produced by endothelium-converting enzymes from big endothelium. ET-1 is a potent vasoconstrictor and smooth muscle mitogen, and it exerts its effects through two receptors, ET_A (located on smooth muscle cells) and ET_B receptors (located on vascular endothelial cells and smooth muscle cells).[17,18] Activation of the ET_A and ET_B receptors on smooth muscle cells induces vasoconstriction and cellular proliferation and hypertrophy, whereas stimulation of ET_B receptors on endothelial cells results in production of vasodilators (nitric oxide [NO] and PGI2). ET_B receptors are also involved in the clearance of ET-1 from the circulatory system.[18] In PAH patients, plasma levels of ET-1 are increased and its level has been shown to be inversely proportional to the magnitude of the pulmonary blood flow and cardiac output (CO) (Figure 10.1).[19,20]

NITRIC OXIDE PATHWAY

NO, produced from arginine by NO synthase in endothelial cells, is a potent and selective pulmonary vasodilator. It exerts its effects through its second messenger, cyclic guanosine monophosphate (cGMP), which is degraded by phosphodiesterase-5 (PDE-5). Patients with PAH have decreased NO synthase activity, thus promoting vasoconstriction and cellular proliferation.[21] PDE-5 inhibitors (PDE5-Inhs) act by selectively blocking this enzyme, thus promoting the accumulation of intracellular cGMP and enhancing NO-mediated effects (Figure 10.1).

SEROTONIN

Serotonin (5-hydroxytryptamine) is a vasoconstrictor that promotes smooth muscle cell hypertrophy and hyperplasia.[22] Elevated plasma serotonin and reduced content of serotonin in platelets have been reported in IAPH and PAH associated with ingestion of dexfenfluramine, which increases the release of serotonin from platelets and inhibits its reuptake.[23,24] Furthermore, mutations in the serotonin transporter (5-HTT) and its receptor 5-HT2B have been described in PAH patients.[25] However, it is not certain whether elevated serotonin levels are implicated in PAH since selective serotonin reuptake inhibitors (SSRIs) are not associated with an increased incidence of PH and may even be protective against hypoxic PH.[26]

ADDITIONAL MECHANISMS

Inhibition of voltage-dependent potassium channels (Kv) has been linked to factors that promote PAH, such as hypoxia and fenfluramine derivatives.[27,28] Abnormalities of the coagulant cascade, including increased levels of von Willebrand factor, plasminogen activator inhibitor-1, and plasma fibrino-peptide, have been reported in PAH patients.[29] Furthermore, inflammatory factors such as proinflammatory cytokines and autoantibodies have been implicated in PAH.[30]

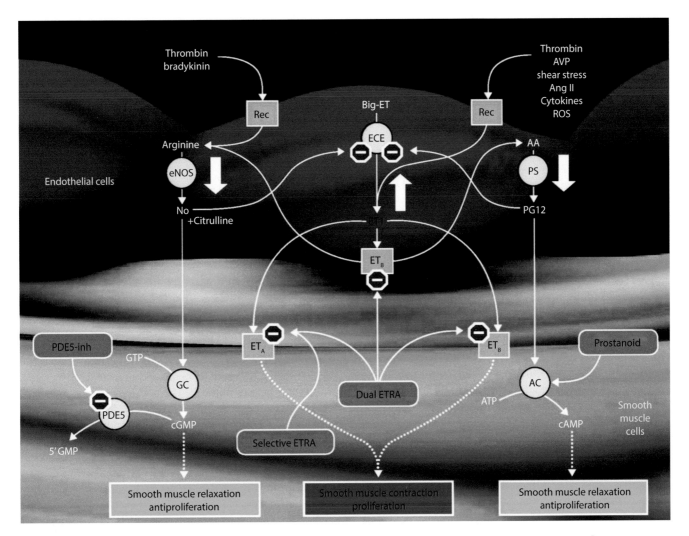

Figure 10.1 Three major mechanistic pathways are known to be perturbed in patients with PAH. (1) The NO pathway: NO is created in endothelial cells by type III NO synthase (eNOS), which in turn induces guanylate cyclase (GC) to convert guanosine triphosphate (GTP) to cyclic guanosine monophosphate, a second messenger that constitutively maintains PASMC relaxation and inhibition of PASMC proliferation. (2) The ET pathway: Big-ET (or pro-ET) is converted in endothelial cells to ET-1 (21 amino acids) by endothelin-converting enzyme (ECE). ET-1 binds to PASMC ET_A and ET_B receptors, which ultimately leads to PASMC contraction, proliferation, and hypertrophy. ET-1 also binds to endothelial cell ET_B receptors. (3) The prostacyclin pathway: The production of PGI2 is catalyzed by prostacyclin synthase (PS) in endothelial cells. In PASMCs, PGI_2 stimulates adenylate cyclase (AC), thus increasing production from ATP of cAMP, another second messenger that maintains PASMC relaxation and inhibition of PASMC proliferation. Importantly, the pathways interact as illustrated, modulating the effect of any single pathway. They also are impacted by transmitters and stimuli that act at cell membrane receptors (Rec). Examples of these include but are not limited to thrombin, bradykinin, arginine vasopressin (AVP), vessel wall shear stress, angiotensin II (Ang II), cytokines, and reactive oxygen species (ROS). In addition, the effect of a transmitter depends on its specific site of action (such as PASMC ET_A or ET_B receptors vs. endothelial cell ET_B receptor). The large white arrows depict aberrations observed in these pathways among patients with PAH. The PDE5-inh, dual and selective ETRA, and prostanoids are agents that have reported clinically beneficial effects in patients with PAH. PDE5-Inh indicates phosphodiesterase-5 inhibitor, for example, sildenafil; ETRA, endothelin receptor antagonist, for example, bosentan (dual), ambrosentan, and sitaxsentan (Receptor A selective). Prostanoids, for example, epoprostenol, treprostinil, and iloprost, supplement exogenously deficient levels of PGI_2. The dashed lines in the octagonal figure signify an inhibitory effect of depicted agents. Dotted arrows depict pathways with known and unknown intervening steps that are not shown. AA, arachidonic acid; ATP, adenosine triphosphate; cAMP, cyclic adenosine monophosphate; cGMP, cyclic guanosine monophosphate; ET, endothelin; NO nitric oxide; PAH, pulmonary arterial hypertension; PASMC, pulmonary artery smooth muscle cell; PGI_2, prostacyclin. (From McLaughlin, V.V., and McGoon, M.D., *Circulation*, 114(13), 1417–1531, 2006. With permission.)

GENETIC SUBSTRATES

Molecular genetic studies have identified mutations in a receptor in the transforming growth factor b (TGFb) receptor pathway—named bone morphogenetic protein receptor 2 (BMPR2)—in certain patients identified with heritable pulmonary arterial hypertension (HPAH).[31,32] The mutation in the BMPR2 receptor protein results in aberrations of signal transduction in the pulmonary smooth muscle cell which leads to cellular proliferation. Less common mutations associated with PAH occur in activin receptor-like kinase (Alk1), another TGFb receptor implicated in patients with hereditary hemorrhagic telangiectasia and PAH.[33]

The right ventricle in pulmonary hypertension

Although it is the pulmonary arterial vasculature where the pathological processes take place in PAH, the ability of the RV to function under increased pressure and resistance determines symptoms and survival. The RV is a thin-walled, compliant, crescent-shaped structure formed by the RV free wall (connected to the left ventricle [LV] by the anterior and posterior septum) and the interventricular septum. Because of the low resistance of the pulmonary vasculature, the compliant RV is able to pump the same stroke volume as the LV with much less work.[34,35]

The RV must be able to adapt to increased afterload for survival in PAH. The initial adaptive response is usually RV hypertrophy, which has been seen within 96 hours of inducing PH in animal models.[36] RV hypertrophy can be followed by contractile dysfunction and/or RV dilatation for further compensatory adaptation to maintain CO by increasing preload to offset the decrease in fractional shortening. Continued remodeling of the RV soon causes alterations in RV shape from crescent to concentric and flattens the septum. Because of interventricular dependence, these changes cause LV diastolic dysfunction and decrease LV end-diastolic volume, resulting in further decline in stroke volume and deterioration of end organ function.[37]

However, the development of RV failure due to PAH is quite variable and the reasons why some RVs maintain adequate CO for prolonged periods of time while others decompensate remain unclear. Several mechanisms have been proposed, including retention of the "fetal" genotype believed to be a contributory factor for favorable survival of PAH associated with congenital heart disease (CHD), polymorphisms in genes related to the rennin-angiotensin aldosterone system, and differences in the degree of ischemia and apoptosis.[35,38,39] Resurgence of interest in determining mechanisms of RV failure and more effective methods of imaging the RV are currently underway. As for now, one fact remains clear, which is that RV function is the single most important determinant of survival in patients with PAH.

INDICATIONS FOR RIGHT HEART CATHETERIZATION IN PULMONARY ARTERIAL HYPERTENSION

Right heart catheterization (RHC) is necessary to establish diagnosis, perform acute vasodilator testing, assess prognosis, and guide therapy in PAH. While echocardiography is the single most important screening tool in PH, it lacks diagnostic accuracy in PAH.

Establishing diagnosis in pulmonary arterial hypertension

MEASURING PULMONARY ARTERY PRESSURE: LIMITATIONS OF ECHOCARDIOGRAPHY

The most widely used screening test for PH is the peak systolic velocity of the tricuspid regurgitation (TR) jet with continuous-wave spectral Doppler. An estimation of RV systolic pressure (RVSP) is generated by adding an assessment of right atrial pressure (RAP) to the gradient using the modified Bernoulli equation: $RVSP = 4v^2 + RAP$, in which v is the velocity of the tricuspid jet in meters per second.[10,11,40]

Several factors influence the accuracy of this measurement. First, the pressure estimation is RVSP rather than systolic PAP, which is a valid assumption in the absence of obstruction to RV outflow (pulmonic valve stenosis or outflow tract obstruction). Second, the accuracy of RAP estimation can greatly influence the RVSP value. Some centers use an arbitrarily fixed value for RAP, while others employ a clinically estimated value derived from the jugular venous pulse.[40,41] Another commonly used method is to make an estimation on the basis of the degree of inferior vena cava collapse during spontaneous respiration. One study suggested that ≥50% or <50% collapse reflects RAP values of <10 mmHg or ≥10 mmHg, respectively.[42]

Inability to obtain TR jets is a limitation; studies have demonstrated that the Doppler profile was insufficient to measure RV to right atrium (RA) pressure gradients in 10%–70% of patients referred for PH evaluation, mainly because of poor acoustic windows.[43–45] Patients with advanced lung disease are particularly challenging in this regard. Furthermore, age and weight also affect systolic PAP in normal individuals. In a large-scale study of 3,790 subjects from 1 to 89 years of age, a systolic PAP >40 mmHg was found in 6% of those >50 years old and 5% of those with a body mass index (BMI) >30 kg/m²·[46] The level of physical training has also been shown to affect systolic PAP. Comparing a group of highly-trained athletes versus normal males, systolic PAP was higher among the trained individuals both at rest and with exercise, largely because of increases in stroke volume affecting PAP.[47] While some studies comparing Doppler-derived systolic PAP with catheterization have reported good correlation, others have demonstrated substantial discrepancy between the techniques.[44,48–54] In patients with severe PH, Doppler-derived systolic PAP has been shown to commonly underestimate pressures.[50] With advanced lung disease and PH, systolic PAP measurements frequently overestimated true PAP, leading to overdiagnosis.[51–53] A similar lack of adequate correlation was reported in patients with PH associated with systemic sclerosis.[54]

Essential components of a complete hemodynamic assessment in pulmonary arterial hypertension

Although the basic principles of RHC were discussed in Chapter 9, some comments specific to PAH are appropriate. The most common RAP abnormality in PAH is due to TR, which can produce an attenuated *x* descent, a prominent *c-v* wave, and a deep and rapid *y* descent (Figure 10.2).[55,56] In severe TR, ventricularization of RAP may occur where RAP is nearly indistinguishable from the RV pressure contour (Figure 10.2). In PAH with RV hypertrophy and volume overload, a prominent *a* wave may appear on the ventricular waveform at end-diastole indicative of RA contracting against a noncompliant RV. A careful assessment of RAP is imperative since RAP carries significant prognostic importance in PAH. In advanced PAH, the PAP can be elevated to various degrees and can reach systemic levels (Figure 10.3). The pulmonary artery (PA) diastolic pressure does not

correlate well with the mean PCWP in the presence of pulmonary vascular disease.

Accurate measurement of left heart filling pressure is critical for correct diagnosis of PAH. Definition of PAH requires both elevation of mean PAP (>25 mmHg) and normal PCWP (or LVEDP ≤15 mmHg). The difference between these two measurements calculates the transpulmonary gradient (TPG = mean PAP-PCWP). Elevated PCWP is characteristic of PH in the setting of chronically elevated left-sided cardiac filling pressure, termed pulmonary venous hypertension (PVH), and is classified as WHO Group 2 PH.[8] PVH usually results from systolic and/or diastolic cardiac dysfunction or valvular disease. Thus, therapeutic decisions can be significantly different on the basis of the left-sided filling pressure measurement. PAH is characterized by elevated PAP, normal PCWP, and elevated TPG, whereas in PVH, PAP is elevated but TPG is normal because of elevated PCWP.

Careful attention to waveforms and timing of measurement are essential for accuracy. The most common mistake is "underwedging," which occurs with incomplete advancement of the PA catheter, resulting in a hybrid tracing of PAP and PCWP. This usually results in a falsely elevated PCWP, leading to misdiagnosing a patient as PVH. If an operator is suspicious that the PCWP being measured is greater than

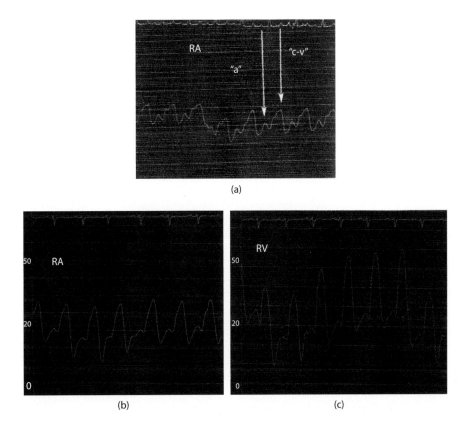

Figure 10.2 **(a)** Right atrial waveform from a patient with secondary tricuspid regurgitation from associated severe left-sided heart failure and right-sided heart failure. Attenuation of the *x* descent is present, leading to prominent *c-v* wave. **(b)** These tracings are from a patient with severe tricuspid regurgitation. The right atrial waveform shows ventricularization. **(c)** Compare with the right ventricle (RV) waveform from the same patient. RA, right atrium. (From Ragosta, M., Right sided heart disorders, in Ragosta, M., (Ed.), *Textbook of Clinical Hemodynamics*, WB Saunders, Philadelphia, PA, 2008, pp. 109–122. With permission.)

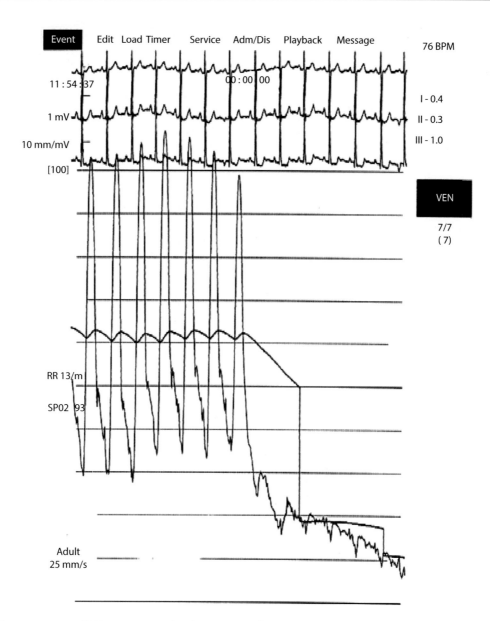

Figure 10.3 Pulmonary artery (PA) pressure and pulmonary capillary wedge pressure (PCWP) from a patient with severe PA hypertension. PA pressure 102/34-millimeters of mercury with mean of 63 mmHg and PCWP 70 mmHg. Each line represents 10 mmHg. (Image Courtesy of Myung H. Park.) BPM, beats per minute.

expected on the basis of clinical assessment, an oxygen saturation measurement can be done from the distal port with the catheter in the wedge position. Its measurement should be equal or close to the systemic arterial oxygen saturation (usually >90%) done by pulse oximetry. If it is markedly lower, the catheter is most likely underwedged. In patients with significant PAP elevation and/or PA dilation, placing the catheter in the correct anatomic position for optimal PCWP measurement can be challenging. One helpful maneuver is to deflate the balloon, allowing the catheter to migrate distally, and carefully reinflating the balloon following the pressure tracings closely. Usually with this approach, optimal placement is obtained with the balloon partially inflated. An intraluminal guidewire can also aid in advancing the catheter to a more distal position. All these

maneuvers should be performed very cautiously and under direct fluoroscopic visualization since patients with PAH are at increased risk of PA rupture, a potentially fatal event.

Factors that can aid in obtaining an accurate PCWP measurement include the following:[55–57] (1) distinct *a* and *v* waves should be present, except in atrial fibrillation where the *a* wave will be absent; (2) waiting for steady state in the PCWP tracing to occur (not immediately after the balloon is inflated) and recording at end expiration; (3) a distinct, immediate rise in pressure should occur when the balloon is deflated out of the wedge position; (4) the catheter tip should be stable in the PA when viewed under fluoroscopy with the balloon inflated (not moving back and forth); (5) an oxygen saturation measured in PCWP should be >90%; and (6) multiple measurements of PCWP should produce similar results. If these maneuvers fail to obtain a reliable PCWP, a left heart catheterization should be performed to measure left ventricular end-diastolic pressure (LVEDP).

Although less common, the catheter can also be "overwedged" with excessive inflation of the balloon relative to the size of the vessel. This should be avoided not only because of inaccurate pressure measurement but also because of increased risk of arterial rupture. In bedside catheter measurements, the potential for PA catheter migration also needs to be kept in mind. The balloon should be slowly inflated at every measurement with close monitoring of the pressure tracings, with inflation stopped when a PCWP tracing is obtained.

The presence of a "large" v wave can also lead to an inaccurate reading of PCWP. The v wave is a normal finding on the wedge tracing and normally higher than the a wave, so what measurement constitutes a large v wave is subjective. Common causes of a large v wave include mitral regurgitation (MR), though the height of the v wave is neither a sensitive nor a specific indicator of the degree of MR.[58,59] Other causes include situations that increase volume or flow into a noncompliant left atrium (LA), such as ventricular septal defect, mitral stenosis, cardiomyopathy of any etiology, or postoperative surgical conditions.

Accurate CO measurement is critical in calculating PVR and assessing prognosis in PAH. The total pulmonary resistance (TPR) calculates the relationship between the mean PAP and CO: TPR = mean PAP × 80/CO; the normal TPR is 100 to 300 dynes-s/cm[5]. The PVR measures the resistance to flow imposed by pulmonary vasculature without the influence of the left-sided filling pressure: PVR = (mean PAP - PCWP) × 80/ CO or PVR = TPG × 80/CO; the normal PVR is 20 to 130 dynes-s/cm[5]. Elevated PAP and low CO is a marker of poor prognosis (see Assessment of Prognosis).[6]

Chronic left-to-right intracardiac shunting can result in PAH. Echocardiography with agitated saline contrast can detect right-to-left shunts, but can fail to detect left-to-right shunts. Multiple measurements of oxygen saturations from superior and inferior vena cavae, RA, and PA can detect and quantify shunts (see Chapter 9). If the shunt has reversed, the typical "step-up" may not be present. A detailed oxygen saturation study is a crucial part of RHC in a patient with clinical or echocardiographic suspicion of intracardiac shunting.

Assessment of prognosis

Since PAH is a disease manifested by an increase in afterload leading to progressive RV dysfunction and failure, hemodynamic markers are considered to be the gold standard for indicating prognosis. This was first demonstrated in a National Institutes of Health (NIH) registry where the investigators concluded that "mortality in primary pulmonary hypertension appears to correlate best with indices of right ventricular hemodynamic functions of three independent variables: pulmonary artery pressure, right atrial pressure, and cardiac index."[6] Specifically, RAP ≥20 mmHg, mean PAP ≥85 mmHg, and cardiac index (CI) <2 L/min/m^2 were associated with an increased risk of death. The data obtained were the basis of formulating the regression equation to calculate survival on the basis of hemodynamics, which was validated in a prospective study.[60] Subsequent studies have corroborated the importance of elevated RAP and low CO as determinants of poor outcome.[61] The relevance of mean PAP on prognosis has been variable. In a retrospective study among patients treated with epoprostenol, patients with lower mean PAP correlated with poor outcome, which may indicate that mean PAP per se is not a reliable surrogate for RV function, but needs to be assessed as part of PVR (mean PAP/CO).[62]

Acute vasodilator testing

The purpose of evaluating PAH patients with a short-acting vasodilator is to determine the degree in which pulmonary vasoconstriction is contributing to the elevated PAP. Vasodilator responsiveness identifies patients with a better prognosis and those who are more likely to have a sustained beneficial response to oral calcium channel blockers (CCBs).

IV epoprostenol and IV adenosine have both been studied as acute vasodilators. Both are short-acting, potent vasodilators, and investigators have reported different degrees of responsiveness depending on the criteria used.[63–65] However, because both agents have the potential to cause systemic hypotension and side effects, using inhaled NO emerged as the vasodilator of choice because of its pulmonary selectivity, short half-life, and lack of systemic side effects (Table 10.1).[66] However, it is expensive and requires trained respiratory personnel to administer.

Table 10.1 Agents used in acute vasodilator testing in patients with pulmonary arterial hypertension

	Nitric oxide	Epoprostenol	Adenosine
Route of administration	Inhaled	IV	IV
Dose range	10–80 ppm	2–10 ng/kg/min	50–250 µg/kg/min
Dosing increments	None to variable titration (10–80 ppm for 5–10 min)	1–2 ng/kg/min every 10–15 min	50 µg/kg/min every 2 min
Side effects	Increased left-sided filling pressure in susceptible patients	Hypotension, headache, flushing, nausea, lightheadedness	Chest tightness, dyspnea, atrioventricular block, hypotension

Source: From McLaughlin, V.V., et al., *J. Am. Coll. Cardiol.*, 53(17), 1573–1619, 2009. With permission. IV, intravenous.

The definition of what constitutes an acute vasodilator "responder" has undergone changes over the years. The current consensus definition is a fall in mean PAP of at least 10 mmHg to ≤40 mmHg, with an increased or unchanged CO.[67,68] If a patient meets this acute criteria, they should be treated with oral CCBs; however, the patient needs to be followed closely for a clinical response. Those who improve to functional class (FC) I or II without the need for additional therapy are likely to do well; however, this response is rare, accounting for only approximately 6.8% of IPAH patients in a large French series.[67] Patients who do not meet the definition of an acute response should not be treated with CCBs.

Acute vasodilator response is rare in patients with associated forms of PAH. Patients with advanced disease such as FC IV symptoms, overt right heart failure, or hemodynamic markers of advanced disease (high RAP and/or reduced CO, systemic hypotension) should not undergo acute vasodilator testing since these patients need prompt treatment with PAH-approved therapies and are not appropriate candidates for CCBs. The development of acute pulmonary edema during vasodilator testing should raise the suspicion of veno-occlusive disease or pulmonary capillary hemangiomatosis, in which therapy with pulmonary vasodilators is contraindicated.[69]

Risks associated with right heart catheterization in pulmonary arterial hypertension patients

Although RHC is necessary for the correct diagnosis of PAH, concerns regarding risks in this population have been raised. A recent multicenter study, which included 15 PAH centers over a 5-year period with >7,000 procedures, evaluated the safety and risks of this procedure.[70] The overall incidence of serious adverse events was 1.1%. The most frequent complications were related to venous access; others included arrhythmia and hypotension due to vagal reactions or pulmonary vasoreactivity testing. Thus, the authors concluded that when performed in experienced centers, RHC in PAH patients are safe and associated with low morbidity rates.

The following maneuvers can enhance safety of the procedure. When accessing from an internal jugular approach, use of an ultrasound device to visualize the size and depth of the vein greatly assists in gaining access safely. Since PAH patients often have dilated right-sided chambers, which can make maneuvering the catheter difficult, especially under high-pressure systems and under significant tricuspid valvular regurgitation, performing the procedure under fluoroscopy reduces the risks of catheter "coiling" and inducing arrhythmia. Direct visualization also assists in placing the catheter in the safe and optimal "wedge" position to avoid PA rupture, "overwedging," and migration of the catheter. Fluoroscopy is also necessary in patients with intracardiac devices. Furthermore, having peripheral IV access in patients prior to starting the procedure is recommended to promptly deliver treatment in the event of vagal episodes, which can lead to significant clinical deterioration in PAH patients.

Evaluating pulmonary hypertension with left-sided heart disease

DIASTOLIC DYSFUNCTION AND PULMONARY HYPERTENSION

Diastolic heart failure (DHF) refers to a clinical syndrome in which patients present with heart failure symptoms with preserved LV systolic function. Epidemiological studies have shown high prevalence of DHF (40%–70%) among symptomatic patients and the risk factors have been well elucidated (age >65 years, hypertension, elevated pulse pressure, obesity, coronary artery disease, diabetes mellitus, atrial fibrillation).[71,72] The predominant underlying structural abnormalities in DHF are concentric remodeling and hypertrophy of the LV caused by chronic pressure overload, usually due to systemic hypertension. These alterations produce abnormalities in both relaxation and filling, which can be a precursor to LV systolic dysfunction or be the main structural abnormality producing symptoms and signs of heart failure.[73,74]

Diastolic dysfunction with PH is a common clinical dilemma and can be very challenging to distinguish from PAH. Up to 70% of patients with LV diastolic dysfunction may develop PH, the presence of which is associated with a poor prognosis.[75] The presentations are similar to PAH and include dyspnea and/or signs and symptoms of heart failure. Echocardiographic findings suggestive of LV diastolic dysfunction include left atrial enlargement, LV hypertrophy, and elevated LV filling pressure (Grade II-IV diastolic dysfunction) (Table 10.2).[68,76]

Table 10.2 Risk factors favoring diagnosis of diastolic heart failure

Clinical features
- Age >65 years
- Elevated systolic blood pressure
- Elevated pulse pressure
- Obesity
- Hypertension
- Coronary artery disease
- Diabetes mellitus
- Atrial fibrillation

Echocardiography
- Left atrial enlargement
- Concentric remodeling (relative wall thickness >0.45)
- Left ventricular hypertrophy
- Elevated left ventricular filling pressures (Grade II–IV diastolic dysfunction)

Interim evaluation (after echocardiography)
- Symptomatic response to diuretic drugs
- Exaggerated increase in systolic blood pressure with exercise
- Re-review of chest radiograph consistent with heart failure

Source: From Hoeper, M.M., et al., *J. Am. Coll. Cardiol.,* 54(1 Suppl), S85–S96, 2009. With permission.

At this juncture, it is critical to perform RHC to measure the left-sided filling pressure and calculate the TPG and PVR. It needs to be emphasized that attention must be paid to the quality of the PCWP tracing for a correct diagnosis to be made. Misinterpretation of either "underwedged" or hybrid tracing as true PCWP (thereby misdiagnosing as diastolic dysfunction because of falsely elevated PCWP) or recorded measurements from improper placement of the catheter can lead to the wrong diagnosis. The possible results obtained fall into one of three categories:

1. PCWP is normal (<15 mmHg) and TPG and PVR are elevated (≥3 Wood units). The patient has PAH and treatment needs to be considered after full evaluation. If the patient has clinical risk factors and/or echo findings suggestive of diastolic dysfunction, PCWP or LVEDP can be normal after treatment with diuretics. Some investigators have advocated for fluid challenge or exercise to assess response as a measure of LV compliance. Although there are no definite standards, the recently published American College of Cardiology Foundation (ACCF)/American Heart Association (AHA) Expert Consensus Document on Pulmonary Hypertension and reports from the fourth World Symposium on Pulmonary Hypertension outline consensus-based recommendations for the evaluation of patients presenting with both syndromes (Figure 10.4).[68,76]

2. PCWP is elevated (>15 mmHg) and PVR is <3 Wood units, and TPG is normal. The patient has diastolic dysfunction, and therapy should be aimed at optimizing volume status, heart rate, and systemic blood pressure.

3. If the PCWP and the PVR are both elevated (the TPG can be normal or elevated), careful evaluation and intervention need to be made to determine if the elevated PVR is passive (because of elevated filling pressure and thus responsive to diuretics and/or systemic vasodilator) or fixed (remains elevated, despite normalizing PCWP and systemic blood pressure). If the PCWP and PVR both decrease (TPG normal) with optimal heart failure therapy, then patients need to be treated aggressively with that regimen. If the PCWP normalizes but PVR remains elevated (elevated TPG), this may be indicative of pulmonary arteriopathy being the dominant disorder with structural changes in pulmonary vasculature along with diastolic dysfunction.

No PAH-specific therapies have been systematically studied for PH associated with diastolic dysfunction. In patients with chronic heart failure, treatments with epoprostenol and

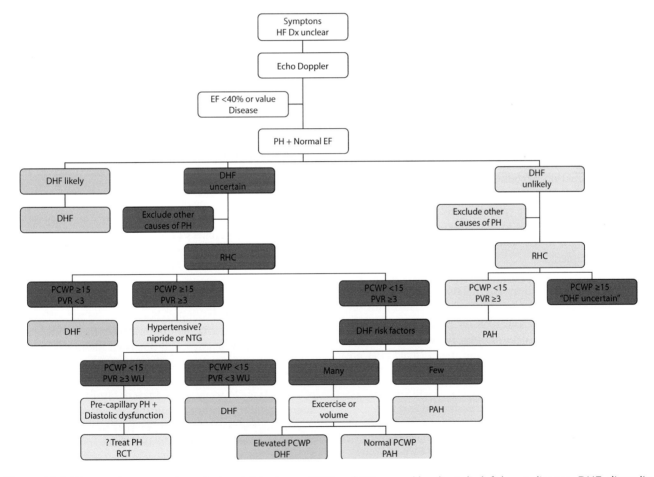

Figure 10.4 Diagnostic approach to distinguish between PAH and PH caused by diastolic left heart disease. DHF, diastolic heart failure; Dx, diagnosis; EF, ejection fraction; HF, heart failure; NTG, nitroglycerin; OMT, optimal medical therapy; PAH, pulmonary arterial hypertension; PCWP, pulmonary capillary wedge pressure; PH, pulmonary hypertension; PVR, pulmonary vascular resistance; RCT, randomized controlled trial; RHC, right heart catheterization; WU, Wood units. (From Hoeper, M.M., et al., J. Am. Coll. Cardiol., 54(1 Suppl), S85–S96, 2009. With permission.)

endothelin receptor antagonists (ERAs) have failed to show beneficial effects, although these trials did not specifically target patients with heart failure and PH.[77–79] The PDE5-Inh sildenafil showed improvement in LV systolic and diastolic function, as well as systemic vasoreactivity in animal models of heart failure.[80,81] Recent small, short-term studies evaluating patients with chronic systolic heart failure and PH using sildenafil have demonstrated improvement in exercise capacity and quality of life.[82,83] However, data from a well-designed trial studying long-term benefits are necessary before any recommendations can be made in regard to use of sildenafil in patients with heart failure and PH.

SYSTOLIC HEART FAILURE AND PULMONARY HYPERTENSION: EVALUATION FOR CARDIAC TRANSPLANTATION

PH secondary to LV systolic dysfunction is a common complication in patients presenting with advanced heart failure and RV dysfunction.[75,84] This process is mainly due to a chronic increase in left-sided filling pressure, resulting in perturbations in vascular mediators, leading to an increase in vascular tone and structural remodeling. Typically, the duration and severity of heart failure is an important determinant that governs the degree of these changes, with abnormalities in vascular tone being the early phase that is manageable with vasodilator agents (reversible PH), and structural changes appearing at more advanced stage, usually not amenable to pharmacological maneuvers (fixed PH).[85,86]

Preoperative assessment of PH is a critical part of heart transplant (HTx) evaluation since preoperative PVR is an independent risk factor for early mortality after HTx.[87] The degree of pulmonary vascular changes in the recipient is a major factor that determines RV function post-transplant and RV dysfunction accounts for both early deaths and postoperative complications.[88] It is imperative to determine if the elevation in PVR is reversible and manageable with pharmacological therapies to avoid donor heart RV failure from subjecting it to the acute rise in pulmonary vascular tone of the recipient.

There is no absolute or reliable hemodynamic threshold below which RV failure is avoidable or beyond which it is certain to occur. The risk of death correlates with the increase in systolic PAP and PVR for early and late transplant outcomes.[88] In determining hemodynamics, the values reported to define "reversible" from "fixed" PH are variable and center dependent:

1. Systolic PAP >50 mmHg despite optimal vasodilation has been reported to be a relative contraindication to HTx.[89]
2. Different PVR values have been reported to be associated with adverse outcomes. PVR >4 Wood units is an independent predictor of early post-transplant mortality.[90] PVR <5 Wood units at rest or <3 Wood units with maximal vasodilatation is considered favorable.
3. TPG is viewed by some centers to be a more reliable marker for pulmonary vascular tone since it does not rely on CO. TPG >15 mmHg increases the risk of postoperative RV failure.[84]

Agents used to test vasoreactivity differ widely, ranging from systemic vasodilators to more selective pulmonary vasodilators. One needs to consider various factors, including systemic blood pressure, severity of PH, CO, and clinical stability to determine the optimal agent.[91,92] Some investigators have also advocated combining more than one agent to target multiple hemodynamic abnormalities to determine degree of reversibility. For patients with severe PH, despite maximal medical therapy, mechanical unloading with a left ventricular assist device (LVAD) is the next step. Mechanical unloading of the LV has been shown to decrease PVR by inducing reverse remodeling of pulmonary vascular through alleviating chronic elevation of left-sided filling pressures and by improving oxygenation and CO. These effects are not immediate, with optimal changes reported to occur after 2–6 months of support. Successful orthotopic HTx after LVAD placement in patients with fixed PH has been reported.[93–95] Both pulsatile and continuous flow ventricular assist device (VAD) systems have been used.

CLINICAL ASPECTS

Classification of pulmonary hypertension

The clinical classification of PH from the fourth World Symposium on Pulmonary Hypertension has several modifications from the prior classification (Table 10.3).[8] Key changes included subclassification of heritable PH and the addition of chronic hemolytic anemia and schistosomiasis to the associated PAH category under WHO Group 1.

PULMONARY ARTERIAL HYPERTENSION

IPAH is PAH of unknown cause, a diagnosis of exclusion determined after a thorough evaluation. IPAH is more common among young females as reported from the NIH registry (F:M 1.7:1, mean age 37 years), though the age of affected individuals appears to be increasing, likely reflecting increased awareness of the disease and improved survival with therapy.[5,8,9] Heritable PAH has been reported in 6%–10% of patients with PAH.[5] It is characterized by autosomal dominant transmission, incomplete penetrance, and genetic anticipation, in which family members of the successive generation develop PAH at an earlier age with a more aggressive disease course. The mutation in BMPR2 loci is the most widely studied and has been identified not only in patients with familial PAH (50%–90%) but also among 25% of IPAH patients, raising the possibility of spontaneous mutations in some individuals or familial transmission among members without clinically evidenced disease.[13,96,97]

Although the incidence of IPAH is rare, PAH has been identified to occur with increased frequency in the presence of CTD, HIV, portal hypertension, and CHD. Patients with CTD, especially the scleroderma spectrum, comprise the largest subgroup of population affected. Patients with PAH associated with CTD have poorer survival than IPAH patients. Median survival of 12 months has been reported compared with 2.6 years in IPAH patients.[5,98]

Table 10.3 Updated classification of pulmonary hypertension

1. Pulmonary arterial hypertension
    1.1 Idiopathic PAH
    1.2 Heritable PAH
    1.2.1 BMPR2
    1.2.2 ALK-1, ENG, **SMAD9, CAVÍ, KCNK3**
    1.2.3 Unknown
    1.3 Drug and toxin induced
    1.4 Associated with:
    1.4.1 Connective tissue disease
    1.4.2 HIV infection
    1.4.3 Portal hypertension
    1.4.4 Congenital heart diseases
    1.4.5 Schistosomiasis
1'. Pulmonary veno-occlusive disease and/or pulmonary capillary hemangiomatosis
1". **Persistent pulmonary hypertension of the newborn (PPHN)**
2. Pulmonary hypertension due to left heart disease
    2.1 Left ventricular systolic dysfunction
    2.2 Left ventricular diastolic dysfunction
    2.3 Valvular disease
    2.4 **Congenital/acquired left heart inflow/outflow tract obstruction and congenital cardiomyopathies**
3. Pulmonary hypertension due to lung diseases and/or hypoxia
    3.1 Chronic obstructive pulmonary disease
    3.2 Interstitial lung disease
    3.3 Other pulmonary diseases with mixed restrictive and obstructive pattern
    3.4 Sleep-disordered breathing
    3.5 Alveolar hypoventilation disorders
    3.6 Chronic exposure to high altitude
    3.7 Developmental lung diseases
4. Chronic thromboembolic pulmonary hypertension **(CTEPH)**
5. Pulmonary hypertension with unclear multifactorial mechanisms
    5.1 Hematologic disorders: **chronic hemolytic anemia,** myeloproliferative disorders, splenectomy
    5.2 Systemic disorders: sarcoidosis, pulmonary histiocytosis, lymphangioleiomyomatosis
    5.3 Metabolic disorders: glycogen storage disease, Gaucher disease, thyroid disorders
    5.4 Others: tumoral obstruction, fibrosing mediastinitis, chronic renal failure, **segmental PH**

Source: From Simonneau, G., et al., *J. Am. Coll. Cardiol.,* 62(25 Suppl), D34–D41, 2013. With permission.
5th World Symposium on Pulmonary Hypertension, Nice, France, 2013. Main modifications to the previous Dana Point classification are in **bold**. ALK-1, activin receptor-like kinase 1; BMPR2, bone morphogenic protein receptor type II; CAVI, caveolin-1; ENG, endoglin; HIV, human immunodeficiency virus; KCNK3, potassium channel subfamily K member 3; PAH, pulmonary arterial hypertension; PH, pulmonary hypertension; SMAD9, Mothers against decapentaplegic homolog 9.

Furthermore, current therapies are less effective in CTD patients compared with IPAH patients.[99]

PAH associated with CHD occurs as a result of high pulmonary blood flow from systemic-to-pulmonary shunts and from smaller lesions such as atrial septal defect. Portopulmonary hypertension is PAH that occurs in association with liver disease and portal hypertension and is reported in 4%–15% of patients being evaluated for liver transplantation.[100,101] Portal hypertension results in a high CO state, so in general, the COs of portopulmonary hypertension patients tend to be higher than other types of PAH. A normal CO in a portopulmonary hypertension patient suggests RV dysfunction. Mean PAP >35 mmHg has significant impact on peritransplant morbidity and survival.[102] Regarding toxic agents, a definite association between ingestion of amphetamine-derived drugs and PAH has been established, the most notable ones being appetite suppressants aminorex, fenfluramine, and dexfenfluramine.[24] All of these agents have been removed from the market after studies demonstrated linkage between these drugs and PAH. An association between methamphetamine use and PAH has been reported recently as well.[8,103] HIV infection is a risk for PAH with approximately 1 of 200 patients being affected.[104] Among patients with PAH, survival is the worst for patients with CTD and HIV.[61]

Evaluation of pulmonary arterial hypertension

Evaluating patients with suspected PH encompasses recognizing at-risk populations, screening for PH, identifying the underlying cause or associated disease, and confirming diagnosis and assessing prognosis. A diagnostic approach, including pivotal and contingent tests and rationale, is shown in Figure 10.5. RHC is required to make the diagnosis of PAH.

Prognostic indicators in pulmonary arterial hypertension

Prognosis in PAH is related to RV function and indicators used to assess this include WHO FC, exercise capacity, and hemodynamics.[16] The importance of RAP, mean PAP, and CO as critical determinants of outcome, as initially shown in the NIH registry, has been discussed in a prior section (Assessment of Prognosis). The NIH registry also demonstrated that survival correlated directly with FC; for patients who were in FC I or II at presentation, the median survival was almost 6 years, versus 2.5 years for patients in FC III, and 6 months for patients presenting in FC IV.[6] Even on therapy, FC was shown to be an important determinant in two large retrospective studies among IPAH patients receiving epoprostenol, in that prognosis was worse for patients who were initiated on therapy with more advanced symptoms.[62,105] Furthermore, patients who improved to FC I or II after the initial period (3–17 months) had a significantly better long-term prognosis than those who remained in FC III or IV on IV epoprostenol.

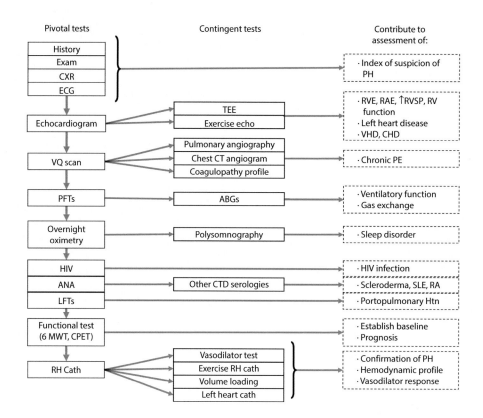

Figure 10.5 Diagnostic approach to pulmonary arterial hypertension (PAH). General guidelines for the evaluation of PH. Since the suspicion of PH may arise in various ways, the sequence of tests may vary. However, the diagnosis of PAH requires that certain data support a specific diagnosis. In addition, the diagnosis of idiopathic pulmonary arterial hypertension is one of excluding all other reasonable possibilities. Pivotal tests are those that are essential to establishing a diagnosis of any type of PAH either by identification of criteria of associated disease or exclusion of diagnosis other than IPAH. All pivotal tests are required for a definitive diagnosis and baseline characterization. An abnormality of one assessment (such as obstructive pulmonary disease on PFTs), does not preclude that another abnormality (chronic thromboembolic disease on VQ scan and pulmonary angiogram) is contributing or predominant. Contingent tests are recommended to elucidate or confirm results of the pivotal tests, and need only be performed in the appropriate clinical context. The combination of pivotal and appropriate contingent tests contributes to assessment of the differential diagnosis in the right-hand column. It should be recognized that the definitive diagnosis may require additional specific evaluation not necessarily included in this general guideline. 6MWT, 6-minute walk test; ABGs, arterial blood gases; ANA, antinuclear antibody serology; CHD, congenital heart disease; CPET, cardiopulmonary exercise test; CT, computed tomography; CTD, connective tissue disease; CXR, chest X-ray; ECG, electrocardiogram; HIV, human immunodeficiency virus screening; Htn, hypertension; LFT, liver function test; PE, pulmonary embolism; PFT, pulmonary function test; PH, pulmonary hypertension; RA, rheumatoid arthritis; RAE, right atrial enlargement; RH Cath, right heart catheterization; RVE, right ventricular enlargement; RVSP, right ventricular systolic pressure; SLE, systemic lupus erythematosus; TEE, transesophageal echocardiography; VHD, valvular heart disease; VQ scan, ventilation-perfusion scintigram. (From McLaughlin, V.V., et al., *J. Am. Coll. Cardiol.*, 53(17), 1573–1619, 2009. With permission.)

The 6-minute walk distance (6MWD) is the most commonly used test to evaluate exercise capacity in PAH. In the first PAH trial evaluating treatment with epoprostenol, baseline 6MWD was a powerful predictor of survival.[106] Sitbon et al. report among patients treated with epoprostenol, the 6MWD performed after 3 months of therapy correlated with long-term survival; specifically, patients who walked ≥380 m demonstrated a significantly better outcome than the cohorts who did not.[62] Used less commonly, mainly because of patient limitations, cardiopulmonary exercise testing has also been studied, and one study demonstrated that maximum oxygen consumption of >10.4 mL/kg/min and peak systolic BP of >120 mmHg to be favorable indicators.[107]

Echocardiographic findings correlating with prognosis include measurements reflecting right-sided cardiac function (RA and RV size, Doppler parameters and indices of RV function, eccentricity index) and presence of pericardial effusion.[108,109] Biomarkers, specifically brain natriuretic peptide (BNP) and N-terminal pro-BNP (NT-pro-BNP), have been shown to correlate with outcome, though the specifics of how to utilize this marker is still under investigation.[110–112] It is recommended that a composite of subjective and objective data be used to determine risk of the patient, which can be used to choose appropriate therapy and as a guide to determine response to treatment (Table 10.4).[16,68]

Table 10.4 Risk assessment for pulmonary arterial hypertension

Determinates of risk	Lower risk (good prognosis)	Higher risk (poor prognosis)
Clinical evidence of RV failure	No	Yes
Progression of symptoms	Gradual	Rapid (and/or presence of syncope)
WHO class[a]	II, III	IV
6MW distance[b]	Longer (>400 m)	Shorter (<300 m)
CPET	Peak VO$_2$ >10.4 mL/kg/min	Peak VO$_2$ <10.4 mL/kg/min
Echocardiography	Minimal RV dysfunction	Pericardial effusion, significant RV enlargement/dysfunction, right atrial enlargement, TAPSE <1.5 cm
Hemodynamics	RAP <10 mmHg, CI >2.5 L/min/m^2	RAP >15 mmHg, CI <2.0 L/min/m^2
BNP[c]	Minimally elevated	Significantly elevated

Source: From McLaughlin, V.V., et al., *J. Am. Coll. Cardiol.*, 53(17), 1573–1619, 2009. With permission. 6MW, 6-minute walk; BNP, brain natriuretic peptide; CI, cardiac index; CPET, cardiopulmonary exercise testing; IPAH, idiopathic pulmonary arterial hypertension; IV, intravenous; PAH, pulmonary arterial hypertension peak; RAP, right atrial pressure; RV, right ventricle; TAPSE, tricuspid annular plane systolic excursion; VO$_2$, ventilatory oxygen uptake; WHO, World Health Organization.

Note: Most data available pertain to IPAH. Little data are available for other forms of PAH. One should not rely on any single factor to make risk predictions.

[a] WHO class is the functional classification for PAH and is a modification of the New York Heart Association functional class.

[b] 6MW distance is also influenced by age, gender, and height.

[c] As there is currently limited data regarding the influence of BNP on prognosis, and many factors including renal function, weight, age, and gender may influence BNP, absolute numbers are not given for this variable.

Treatment of pulmonary arterial hypertension

PROSTANOIDS

Epoprostenol. IV epoprostenol improves FC, exercise capacity, hemodynamics, and survival in IPAH, which was demonstrated in an open-label, randomized trial of 81 FC III and IV IPAH patients comparing IV epoprostenol with conventional treatment.[106] All eight deaths during the 12-week trial period occurred among patients who were randomized to conventional therapy, which resulted in a survival benefit ($P = 0.003$). IV epoprostenol has also been studied in PAH associated with CTD, demonstrating marked improvements in 6MWD and hemodynamics but no effect on mortality in a 12-week, open-label randomized trial.[113] Observational studies have also reported beneficial effects of IV epoprostenol in patients with PAH related to HIV, CHD, and portopulmonary hypertension.[114–116] Two longer-term observational studies have confirmed the chronic benefits of IV epoprostenol in IPAH patients, specifically improvements in survival compared with historical controls, FC, 6MWD, and hemodynamics.[62,105]

IV epoprostenol is a challenging therapy to implement because of its short half-life (<6 minutes) and the need for continuous IV infusion via a tunneled catheter. Each patient must learn the techniques of sterile preparation of the medication, operation of the ambulatory infusion pump, and care of the central venous catheter. Incidence of sepsis and catheter-related infections are not negligible (0.1–0.6 cases per patient year) and can cause significant morbidity.[105] Any interruption of the drug infusion can be potentially life-threatening because of the short half-life of epoprostenol and the potential for rebound PH. IV epoprostenol is commonly started in the hospital at a dose of 2-ng/kg/min and titrated on the basis of PAH symptoms and side effects. Most experts consider the optimal dose of chronic therapy to be between 25 and 40 ng/kg/min. Chronic overdose can lead to high CO failure and recurrent symptoms.[117] Common side effects include headache, jaw pain, diarrhea, nausea, flushing, rash, and musculoskeletal pain. Because of the complexity of administering this therapy, epoprostenol, use should be limited to experienced centers (Table 10.5).[118]

Treprostinil. Treprostinil is a PGI2 analogue with a half-life of 4 hours. It was studied as a continuous subcutaneous infusion in a 12-week, placebo-controlled, randomized trial of 470 patients with FC II, III, or IV PAH.[119] There was a modest but statistically significant median increase of 16 m in 6MWD; the improvement was dose related, and patients in the highest dose quartile reported close to 40 m improvement. However, the major hindrance of using subcutaneous treprostinil is pain and erythema at the infusion site, which was reported by 85% of the patients and limited the dose increases. It is now recognized that site pain is not dose related, and that some patients feel better after proper dose escalation, which helps them to improve their PAH symptoms.

Because of limitations of the subcutaneous delivery system, IV treprostnil was studied in a 12-week open-label trial of 16 patients.[120] It demonstrated improvements in 6MWD (82 m) and hemodynamics. In another open-label trial, 31 FC II and III PAH patients on IV epoprostenol were transitioned to IV treprostinil.[121] Twenty-seven patients completed the transition, and four were transitioned back to epoprostenol. 6MWD measurements were maintained among patients who completed the transition; however, there was a modest increase in mean PAP and decrease in CI. Noteworthy is that the dose of IV treprostinil at the end of the study period was more than twice the dose

Table 10.5 U.S. Food and Drug Administration approved therapies for the treatment of pulmonary arterial hypertension

Drug trial name (N)	Trial outcomes	Clinical pearls
Endothelin receptor antagonists		
Bosentan BREATHE-1 (213)	Improved 6 MW distance Improved dyspnea Delayed clinical worsening	Hepatic toxicity Teratogenic Fluid retention, peripheral edema, anemia, nasal congestion, sinusitis, flushing Monthly transaminase monitoring required
Ambrisentan ARIES-1 (202) ARIES-2 (192)	Improved 6 MW walk distance Delayed clinical worsening Improved hemodynamics No effect on transaminases	Teratogenic Fluid retention, peripheral edema, anemia, nasal congestion, sinusitis, flushing
Macitentan SERAPHIN (742)	Reduced incidence of composite endpoint of death, atrial septostomy, lung transplantation, intravenous or SQ prostanoid therapy or worsening PAH	Teratogenic Headache, nasopharyngitis, anemia
Phosphodiesterase-5 inhibitors		
Sildenafil SUPER-1 (278)	Improved 6 MW walk distance Improved dyspnea Improved hemodynamics	No delay in clinical worsening end point Headache, flushing, dyspepsia, epistaxis, visual disturbance Interactions with protease inhibitors
Tadalafil PHIRST (405)	Improved 6 MW distance Improved time to clinical worsening Improved hemodynamics Improved quality of life	Headache, myalgias, flushing, dyspepsia, epistaxis, visual disturbance
Soluble quanylate cyclase aqonists		
Riociguat PATENT-1 and 2 (443)	Improved 6 MW distance Improved hemodynamics Improved time to clinical worsening Improved quality of life Reduced brain natriuretic peptide Improved WHO class Improved dyspnea	Teratogenic Headache, dyspepsia, edema, dyspepsia, nausea, dizziness Severe hypotension with PDE-5 inhibitors
Prostanoids		
Epoprostenol, intravenous (81)	Improved 6 MW distance Improved dyspnea Improved hemodynamics Improved survival	Indwelling central line Pump malfunction Flushing, jaw pain, thrombocytopenia, headache, dizziness, nausea/vomiting/ diarrhea, abdominal pain, hypotension, rash
Treprostinil, intravenous or subcutaneous (70)	Improved 6 MW distance Improved dyspnea Improved hemodynamics	Indwelling central line or subcutaneous catheter Pain, erythema at infusion site (subcutaneous) Flushing, jaw pain, thrombocytopenia headache, dizziness, nausea/vomiting/ diarrhea, abdominal pain, hypotension, rash
Treprostinil, inhaled Triumph (470)	Improved 6 MW distance Improved quality of life Administration four times daily	No delay in clinical worsening or dyspnea No change in functional class Cough, headache, nausea, dizziness, flushing, throat irritation or pain

(Continued)

Table 10.5 (Continued) U.S. Food and Drug Administration approved therapies for the treatment of pulmonary arterial hypertension

Drug trial name (N)	Trial outcomes	Clinical pearls
Treprostinil, oral FREEDOM-M (349)	Improved 6 MW distance	No additional benefits when added to PDE-5 or ERA. Headache, nausea, diarrhea, jaw pain
Iloprost, inhaled (203)	Improved composite endpoint of 6 MW distance and dyspnea	Administration 6–9 times daily Cough, headache, nausea, dizziness, flushing, throat irritation or pain
IP Prostacyclin receptor agonist		
Selexipag GRIPHON (1156)	Reduced incidence of composite endpoint of any complication of PAH or death	Headache, diarrhea, nausea, jaw pain.

Source: From Barnett, C.F., et al., Cardiol. Clin., 34(3), 375–389, 2016. With permission.
Note: ERA, endothelin-receptor antagonist; MW, minute walk; PAH, pulmonary arterial hypertension; PDE-5, phosphodiesterase type 5; SQ, continous subcutaneous; WHO, World Health Organization.

of epoprostenol at the start of the study. Inhaled treprostinil was recently approved by the U.S. Food and Drug Administration (FDA), and oral treprostinil is currently undergoing active clinical investigation (Table 10.5).

Inhaled Iloprost. Iloprost is a stable PGI2 analogue that is delivered via an aerosolized device six to nine times per day. Iloprost was studied in a 12-week, multicenter, placebo-controlled, randomized trial of 207 FC III and IV patients with either IPAH, PAH associated with CTD or appetite suppressants, or PH related to inoperable chronic thromboembolic disease.[122] Treatment with iloprost resulted in meeting a novel composite end point of improvement in FC by at least one level and increase in 6MWD by at least 10% in the absence of clinical deterioration (16.8% vs. 4.9%, treated vs. placebo, $P = 0.007$). It was generally well-tolerated with coughing, headache, and flushing as the most common side effects (Table 10.5).

Selexipag is an oral prostacyclin IP receptor agonist, which as a diphenylpyrazine moiety, is chemically distinct from prostacyclin and prostanoid analogues. Selexipag becomes hydrolyzed via enzymatic actions to a long-acting active metabolite that has a half-life of about 8 hours. Distinct from other prostanoid analogues, it has been shown to be highly selective for the human prostacyclin IP receptor. In the Prostacyclin (PGI2) Receptor Agonist in Pulmonary Arterial Hypertension (GRIPHON) trial, the primary endpoint of morbidity and mortality occurred in 27% of selexipag-treated patients and 41.6% of patients receiving placebo (hazard ratio 0.6; $P < 0.001$), mostly driven by a decrease in morbidity. There was no significant effect on 6MWD. Adverse effects were consistent with that of prostacyclins, namely headache, jaw pain, diarrhea, and nausea.

Endothelin receptor antagonists

BOSENTAN

Bosentan, a nonselective endothelin receptor blocker, was the first orally available therapy approved for PAH. It was studied in two placebo-controlled, randomized trials of FC III or IV patients.[123,124] In the pivotal Bosentan: Randomized Trial of Endothelin Receptor Antagonist Therapy for Pulmonary Hypertension 1 (BREATHE-1) trial, bosentan improved the primary endpoint of 6MWD by 36 m, whereas placebo patients deteriorated by 8 m ($P = 0.0002$). Bosentan also improved the composite endpoint of time to clinical worsening, which was defined as death, initiation of IV epoprostenol, hospitalization for worsening PAH, lung transplantation, or atrial septostomy. Long-term observational results have shown improved survival compared with expected outcome based on the NIH registry equation.[125] Bosentan was shown to be effective in mildly symptomatic patients in the Treatment of Patients with Mildly Symptomatic Pulmonary Arterial Hypertension with Bosentan (EARLY) study, a 6-month, multicenter, placebo-controlled trial, which enrolled 168 FC II PAH patients.[126] The results demonstrated a significant decrease in PVR, which was the primary endpoint to evaluate treatment effects on vascular remodeling, and a significant delay in clinical worsening.

Bosentan is mainly metabolized through the hepatic P450 enzymes and an increase in hepatic transaminases more than three times the upper limit of normal has been reported in 10%–12% of patients.[124] Bosentan is teratogenic and may decrease the efficacy of hormonal contraception; women of child-bearing age must be counseled to use dual contraception for birth control. Other side effects include headache, flushing, lower-extremity edema, and anemia. Treatment with bosentan requires monitoring of liver function with tests on a monthly basis, pregnancy tests on women of child-bearing potential on a monthly basis, and hemoglobin/hematocrit tests on a quarterly basis. Patients should be counseled regarding potential for lower-extremity edema, especially in the initial weeks of therapy, and possible need for diuretic adjustments. Glyburide and cyclosporine A are contraindicated with bosentan because of significant drug-drug interactions (Table 10.5).

AMBRISENTAN

Ambrisentan is a selective ET_A receptor antagonist studied in two placebo-controlled, randomized, 12-week studies of WHO Group I patients (ARIES-1 and ARIES-2). The studies were conducted in the United States and Europe/South America, respectively.[127] Treatment resulted in a significant improvement in 6MWD and delay in time to clinical worsening in all treatment groups. Ambrisentan is available in 5 mg and 10 mg oral tablets taken once a day.

The incidence of hepatic transaminase elevation more than three times the upper limit of normal was 0.8% for patients receiving ambrisentan.[127] This was further investigated in a recently published study of 36 patients who did not tolerate bosentan or sitaxsentan because of hepatic transaminase increases and were placed on ambrisentan therapy.[128] Ambrisentan therapy was tolerated well in this group. Peripheral edema is another side effect of the ERA class and was reported in mild to moderate severity in the clinical trials.[127] An increased incidence of peripheral edema during postmarketing use prompted the FDA to issue a labeled warning for elderly patients.[129] The mechanisms behind this observed edema is currently undergoing evaluation. No drug interaction was found with sildenafil.[129] Ambrisentan is teratogenic. Monthly blood tests for liver function and pregnancy tests for women of child-bearing age are required (Table 10.5).

MACITENTAN

Macitentan is a dual ET_A and ET_B endothelin receptor blocker designed to have enhanced tissue penetration, mainly due to an increased proportion of the nonionized form of the molecule improving its ability to cross the lipophilic cell membranes. Macitentan was well-tolerated in a Phase II study among healthy volunteers demonstrating dose-dependent pharmacokinetics. The pivotal Phase III Study with an Endothelin Receptor Antagonist in Pulmonary Arterial Hypertension to Improve Clinical Outcome (SERAPHIN) is the first clinical trial in PAH that defined morbidity and mortality as the primary endpoint. This double-blind placebo-controlled study enrolled 742 patients within 180 participating centers in over 40 countries. Patients were randomized to receive placebo or macitanten (10 mg once a day or 3 mg once a day). Most of the patients were classified as New York Heart Association (NYHA) FC II or III (97%) with idiopathic PAH or PAH due to CTD (87%). Baseline hemodynamics were consistent with severe PH with mean PAP 55 mmHg, CI 2.3 L/min/m², and PVR 12.5 Wood units. The majority of patients were on background therapy, most of which was sildenafil (64%). The mean study duration of treatment was 85 weeks.

Compared with placebo, the hazard ratio for reaching the composite primary endpoint of death and disease progression for the 3 mg of macitentan was 0.70 (95% CI, 0.52 to 0.96; $P = 0.01$) and the hazard ratio for the 10 mg dose compared with placebo was 0.55 (97.5% CI 0.39 to 0.76;

$P < 0.001$), irrespective of background therapy. In the subset of patients who underwent hemodynamic study at baseline and at 6 months, significant decrease in PVR and improvement in CI were observed compared with placebo. Only the 10 mg dose was approved for WHO Group 1 patients to delay disease progression. The main side effects reported were anemia, nasopharyngitis, and headache. The incidence of liver transaminase elevation in the SERAPHIN study was greater than three times the upper limits of normal range in 3.4% of patients treated with macitanten versus 4.5% for placebo. Liver function testing needs to be performed prior to initiation of treatment and repeated during therapy as indicated; however, monthly liver function testing is not mandated. For patients with anemia, macitanten use should be done with close monitoring for its known side effects of decreasing hemoglobin.

Phosphodiesterase-5 inhibitor

SILDENAFIL

Sildenafil was studied in a 12-week randomized placebo-controlled study of 278 symptomatic PAH patients.[130] The primary endpoint of 6MWD improved by 45, 46, and 50 m in the 20, 40, and 80 mg groups, respectively ($P < 0.001$). There was no change in the time to clinical worsening at week 12. The result of 222 patients who completed 1 year of treatment demonstrated that the 6MWD improvement was maintained; however, nearly all patients were titrated up to a dose of 80 mg three times a day. Side effects include headache, flushing, dyspepsia, and epistaxis (Table 10.5).

TADALAFIL

Tadalafil, a PDE5-inhibitor with a longer half-life than sildenafil, was recently studied in a 16-week, double-blind, placebo-controlled trial among 405 PAH patients using 2.5, 10, 20, and 40 mg tablets once a day.[131] The highest dose of tadalafil demonstrated a 41 m increase in 6MWD compared with a 9 m increase for placebo ($P < 0.001$). There was also a delay in the time to clinical worsening (defined as death, hospitalization, initiation of new PAH therapy, worsening WHO FC). Side effects include headache, diarrhea, nausea, back pain, dizziness, dyspepsia, and flushing (Table 10.5).

Soluble guanylate cyclase stimulators

RIOCIGUAT

Riociguat is the first agent within the soluble guanylate cyclase stimulator pathway approved for Group 1 PAH. It is also the first and only therapy approved for treatment of chronic thromboembolic pulmonary hypertension (CTEPH: Group 4 PAH). Riociguat works with dual mechanisms to increase the soluble guanylate cyclase stimulator. It directly stimulates the soluble guanylate cyclase stimulator, independent of nitric oxide, and enhances the sensitivity of soluble guanylate cyclase stimulator to nitric oxide. The pivotal Phase III clinical trial Pulmonary Arterial

Hypertension Soluble Guanylate Cyclase-Stimulator Trial 1 (PATENT-1) enrolled 443 patients with PAH in an 12-week trial. Most of the patients had idiopathic PAH (61%) and an NYHA FC of II or III (95%). The majority of the patients were on background therapy (44% previously treated with ERA and 6% with inhaled prostanoids). Riociguat was given in doses of 0.5–2.5 mg three times daily, and the primary outcome was the placebo-corrected change from baseline in 6MWD. The results showed a significant increase in 6MWD from a baseline of 35.8 m with riociguat versus placebo (95% CI 20.1–51.5 m, $P < 0.0001$) and the results were similar between treatment-naïve patients versus patients on background therapy. Significant improvements were also seen in PVR ($P < 0.0001$) and clinical deterioration ($P = 0.0046$). The most common reported side effects included headache, gastritis/reflux, dizziness, and hypotension. Cases of hemoptysis were also reported. Concomitant use of riociguat and PDE-5 inhibitors is contraindicated due to hypotension.

The Pulmonary Arterial Hypertension Soluble Guanylate Cyclase-Stimulator Trial 2 (PATENT-2) evaluated the long-term safety and efficacy of riociguat in an open-label extension study that enrolled 396 patients from the PATENT-1 study. Patients received individually adjusted doses, with up to a maximum dose of 2.5 mg three times daily.[10] The study showed that the improvements in the 6MWD and WHO FC observed in PATENT-1 were maintained for up to 1 year in PATENT-2. The 6MWD increased by 51±74 m and WHO FC improved in 33%, stabilized in 61%, and worsened in 6% of the patients compared with the PATENT-1 baseline. Riociguat was well-tolerated with a long-term safety profile similar to that observed in PATENT-1 with cases of hemoptysis and pulmonary hemorrhage reported.

The Chronic Thromboembolic Pulmonary Hypertension Soluble Guanylate Cyclase-Stimulator Trial 1 (CHEST-1) study enrolled 261 patients with inoperable CTEPH or persistent or recurrent PH after pulmonary thromboendarterectomy (PTE) to receive either riociguat (0.5 to 2.5 mg, three times daily) or placebo. The CHEST-1 trial met its primary endpoint of showing significant improvement in 6MWD in CTEPH patients treated with riociguat, the first therapy ever to demonstrate such improvement in this population. It also demonstrated improvement in relevant secondary endpoints, including improvement in PVR and WHO FC. The most common reported side effects include headache, gastritis/reflux, dizziness, and hypotension. Cases of hemoptysis have also been reported. Riociguat received dual indications in PH, namely for patients with WHO Group 1 PH to improve exercise capacity, FC, and help delay clinical worsening; and for WHO Group 4 patients with inoperable CTEPH or recurrent or persistent PH post-thromboendarterectomy. It must also be noted that all patients with surgically accessible lesions should undergo surgical evaluation and that riociguat cannot replace surgical treatment that can restore normal cardiopulmonary status.

Conventional treatment

CCBs are recommended for patients who demonstrate responsiveness during acute vasodilator testing (see Acute Vasodilator Test). Patients with IPAH who meet the criteria may be considered for treatment with CCBs. Long-acting nifedipine, diltiazem, or amlodipine are suggested. Verapamil should be avoided because of its potentially negative inotropic effects. Patients need to be followed closely for efficacy and safety. If a patient does not improve to FC I or II with CCBs, the patient should not be considered a chronic responder and PAH-directed treatment should be initiated.

Anticoagulation has been studied in two small, uncontrolled trials in IPAH patients. On the basis of these studies, most experts recommend warfarin anticoagulation.[68,132] The recommended international normalized ratio (INR) varies from 2 to 2.5 and 2 to 3 to 1.5 to 2 in some centers. In patients with associated pulmonary arterial hypertension (APAH), anticoagulation is controversial with few data to support its use. In CTD and portopulmonary patients, the risk of gastrointestinal bleeding may be increased. Most experts recommend warfarin anticoagulation in APAH patients being treated with IV prostanoids in the absence of contraindicating factors.

Hypoxemia is a potent pulmonary vasoconstrictor and thus can contribute to progression of PAH. It is recommended that patients with PAH maintain oxygen saturation >90% at all times, though the use of supplemental oxygen in patients with Eisenmenger physiology is controversial. Diuretics are used to treat volume overload because of right heart failure. For diuretic naive patients, slow initiation and monitoring of renal function are recommended with the goal of attaining near-normal intravascular volume. In acute decompensated right heart failure and/or in the presence of diuretic resistance, IV diuretics are needed. Although digoxin has not been well studied in patients with PAH, it is used with careful monitoring in low doses in the setting of refractory right heart failure and/or atrial arrhythmia.

Combination therapy in pulmonary arterial hypertension

With the approval of therapies targeting different pathways, utilizing a combination approach has attracted marked interest. The potential to increase efficacy by utilizing combination therapy must be measured against possible toxicity and drug-drug interactions. Several small, open-label observational studies reported potential benefits.[133,134] An initial study evaluating combining bosentan or placebo to FC III or IV patients receiving IV epoprostenol failed to show benefit, though this study was underpowered.[135] Two studies evaluated adding inhaled iloprost to bosentan therapy in a randomized, double-blind, placebo-controlled design. The STEP study enrolled 67 patients in a 12-week study, which demonstrated safety, as well as improvement in 6MWD (26 m, $P = 0.051$); the COMBI study, which evaluated 40 patients, failed to demonstrate benefit and the study was terminated.[136,137] The largest completed combination trial in PAH to date is the Pulmonary Arterial Hypertension Combination Study of Epoprostenol and Sildenafil (PACES) study, with sildenafil as add-on therapy to IV epoprostenol.[138] This 16-week, multinational, double-blind, placebo-controlled study enrolled 267 patients who were on stable epoprostenol therapy. Patients were randomized to receive 20 mg three times a day titrated to 40 and 80 mg three times daily at 4-week intervals, or the corresponding placebo. At the end of 16 weeks, more than 80% of patients had reached the 80 mg, three times daily dosing level. The primary endpoint was change in 6MWD, and there was an increase of 26 m in the subjects who received sildenafil. There were seven deaths in the placebo group and none among patients receiving sildenafil. Clinical worsening events defined as death, transplant, hospitalization, or an increase in epoprostenol dose were significantly different in favor of the treated group. Several large studies

are currently underway evaluating the effect of combining different classes of oral regimen, including the Effects of Combination of Bosentan and Sildenafil versus Sildenafil Monotherapy on Morbidity and Mortality in Symptomatic Patients with PAH (COMPASS-2) trial, which is the first morbidity/mortality-driven trial focusing on combination therapy in PAH.

Treatment algorithm and assessing response to therapy

The most recent treatment guideline from the Dana Point meeting is shown in Figure 10.6.[9] Incorporating a risk-based approach by combining known factors that determine prognosis in PAH in selecting therapy has been recommended and is widely utilized by clinicians (Figure 10.7).[16] The ACCF/AHA 2009 Expert Consensus Document published a guideline outlining recommendations in assessing response and following patients on therapy (Table 10.6).[68]

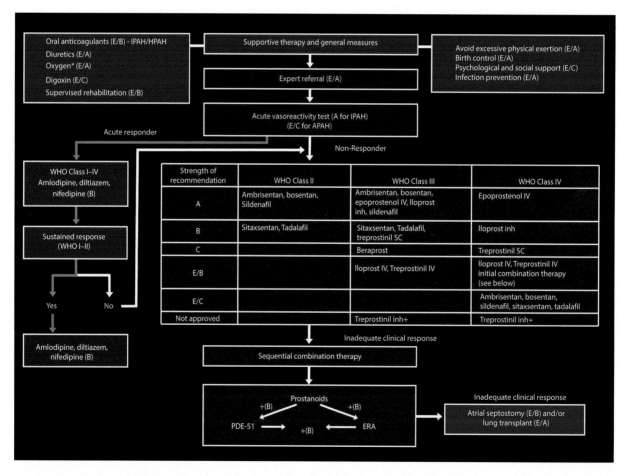

Figure 10.6 PAH evidence-based treatment algorithm. Drugs within the same grade of evidence are listed in alphabetical order and not order of preference. Not all agents listed are approved or available for use in all countries. *To maintain oxygen at 92%. +Investigational, under regulatory review. APAH, associated pulmonary arterial hypertension; ERA, endothelin receptor antagonist; HPAH, heritable pulmonary arterial hypertension; inh, inhibitor; IPAH, idiopathic pulmonary arterial hypertension; IV, intravenous; PAH, pulmonary arterial hypertension; PDE-5, phosphodiesterase type 5; SC, subcutaneous; WHO, World Health Organization. (From Barst, R.J., et al., *J. Am. Coll. Cardiol.*, 54(1 Suppl), S78–S84, 2009. With permission.)

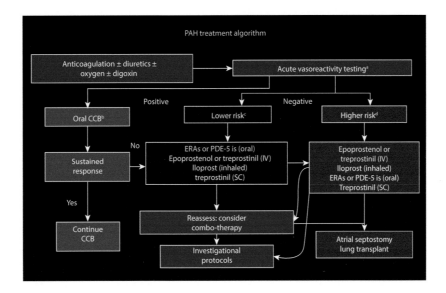

Figure 10.7 PAH treatment algorithm based on risk assessment. Background therapies include warfarin anticoagulation, which is recommended in all patients with IPAH without contraindication. Diuretics are used for management of right heart failure. Oxygen is recommended to maintain oxygen saturation greater than 90%.

a   Acute vasodilator testing should be performed in all IPAH patients who may be potential candidates for long-term therapy with CCBs. Patients with PAH due to conditions other than IPAH have a very low rate of long-term responsiveness to oral CCBs, and the value of acute vasodilator testing in such patients needs to be individualized. IPAH patients in whom CCB therapy would not be considered, such as those with right heart failure or hemodynamic instability, should not undergo acute vasodilator testing.

b   CCBs are indicated only for patients who have a positive acute vasodilator response, and such patients need to be followed closely for both safety and efficacy.

c   For patients who did not have positive acute vasodilator testing and are considered lower risk on the basis of clinical assessment (Table 10.4), oral therapy with endothelin receptor antagonist (ERA) or phosphodiesterase-5 inhibitor (PDE-5 I) would be the first line of therapy recommended. If an oral regimen is not appropriate, other treatments would need to be considered on the basis of patient's profile and the side effects and risk of each therapy.

d   For patients who are considered high risk on the basis of clinical assessment (Table 10.4), continuous treatment with intravenous (IV) prostacyclin (epoprostenol or treprostinil) would be the first line of therapy recommended. Combination therapy should be considered when patients are not responding adequately to initial monotherapy. Timing for lung transplantation and/or atrial septostomy is challenging and is reserved for patients who progress despite optimal medical treatment.

CCBs, calcium channel blockers; IPAH, idiopathic pulmonary arterial hypertension; PAH, pulmonary arterial hypertension; SC, subcutaneous. (From McLaughlin, V.V., et al., *J. Am. Coll. Cardiol.*, 53(17), 1573-1619, 2009. With permission.)

Table 10.6 Longitudinal evaluation of pulmonary arterial hypertension patients on therapy

Clinical course	Stable	Unstable
	• No increase in symptoms and/or decompensation	• Increase in symptoms and/or decompensation
	• No evidence of right heart failure	• Signs of right heart failure
	• FC I/II	• FC IV[a]
	• 6MWD >400 m	• 6MWD <300 m[a]
	• RV size/function normal	• RV enlargement/dysfunction
	• RAP normal; CI normal	• RAP high; CI low
	• BNP normal/stable or decreasing	• BNP elevated/increasing
	• Oral therapy	• IV prostacyclin and/or combination treatment
Frequency of evaluation	Q 3–6 mo[b]	Q 1–3 mo
FC assessment	Every clinic visit	Every clinic visit
6MWD	Every clinic visit	Every clinic visit

(Continued)

Table 10.6 (Continued) Longitudinal evaluation of pulmonary arterial hypertension patients on therapy

Clinical course	Stable	Unstable
Echocardiogram[c]	Q 12 mo or center dependent	Q 6–12 mo or center dependent
BNP[d]	Center dependent	Center dependent
Right heart catheterization	Clinical deterioration and center dependent	Q 6–12 mo or clinical deterioration

Source: From McLaughlin, V.V., et al., *J. Am. Coll. Cardiol.*, 53(17), 1573–1619, 2009. With permission. 6MWD, 6-min walk distance; BNP, brain natriuretic peptide; CI, cardiac index; FC, functional class; IV, intravenous; mo, months; PASP, systolic pulmonary artery pressure; PH, pulmonary hypertension; Q, every; RAP, right atrial pressure; RV, right ventricle.

Note: For patients in the high-risk category, consider a referral to a PH specialty center for consideration for advanced therapies, clinical trials, and/or lung transplantation.

[a] The frequency of follow-up evaluation for patients in FC III and/or 6MWD between 300 and 400 m depends on composite of detailed assessments on other clinical and objective characteristics listed.

[b] For patient who remains stable on established therapy, follow-up assessments can be performed by referring physician(s) or PH specialty centers.

[c] Echocardiographic measurement of PASP is estimation only and it is strongly advised not to rely on its evaluation as the sole parameter to make therapeutics decisions.

[d] The utility of serial BNP levels to guide management in individual patients has not established.

CONCLUSION

PAH has become a major treatment focus with 10 approved drugs. Accurate diagnosis requires RHC. Continued efforts are being pursued to study other pathways in PAH and develop novel therapies, to update current epidemiology and treatment patterns, and to evaluate the efficacy and safety of combination therapies in this complex disease. Patients with underlying hypoxic lung disease, left-sided heart disease, and chronic thromboembolic disease need further study.

REFERENCES

1. Romberg E. Ueber sklerose der lungen arterie. *Dsch Arch Klin Med* 1891;48:197–206.
2. Dresdale DT, et al. Primary pulmonary hypertension: I. Clinical and hemodynamic study. *Am J Med* 1951;11(6):686–705.
3. Wood P, et al. The effect of acetylcholine on pulmonary vascular resistance and left atrial pressure in mitral stenosis. *Br Heart J* 1957;19(2):276–286.
4. Hatano S, Strasser R, eds. *Primary Pulmonary Hypertension.* Geneva: World Health Organization, 1975.
5. Rich S, et al. Primary pulmonary hypertension: A national prospective study. *Ann Intern Med* 1987;107(2):216–223.
6. D'Alonzo GE, et al. Survival in patients with primary pulmonary hypertension: Results from a national prospective registry. *Ann Intern Med* 1991;115(5):343–349.
7. Simonneau G, et al. Clinical classification of pulmonary hypertension. *J Am Coll Cardiol* 2004;43 (12 Suppl, S):S5–12S.
8. Simonneau G, et al. Updated clinical classification of pulmonary hypertension. *J Am Coll Cardiol* 2009;54(1 Suppl):S43–S54.
9. Barst RJ, et al. Updated evidence-based treatment algorithm in pulmonary arterial hypertension. *J Am Coll Cardiol* 2009;54(1 Suppl):S78–S84.
10. Grossman W, Barry WH. Cardiac catheterization. In: Braunwald E, ed. *Heart Disease: A Textbook of Cardiovascular Medicine.* Philadelphia: WB Saunders, 1988:247–252.
11. Badesch DB, et al. Diagnosis and assessment of pulmonary arterial hypertension. *J Am Coll Cardiol* 2009; 54(1 Suppl):S55–S66.
12. Yuan JXJ, Rubin LJ. Pathogenesis of pulmonary arterial hypertension: The need for multiple hits. *Circulation* 2005;111(5):534–538.
13. Machado RD, et al. Investigation of a second genetic hits at the BMPR2 locus as a modulator of disease progression in familial pulmonary arterial hypertension. *Circulation* 2005;111(5):607–613.
14. Christman BW, et al. An imbalance between the excretion of thromboxane and prostacyclin metabolites in pulmonary hypertension. *N Engl J Med* 1992;327(2):70–75.
15. Tuder RM, et al. Prostacyclin synthase expression is decreased in lungs from patients with severe pulmonary hypertension. *Am J Respir Crit Care Med* 1999;159(6):1925–1932.
16. McLaughlin VV, McGoon MD. Pulmonary arterial hypertension. *Circulation* 2006;114(13):1417–1531.
17. Yanagisawa M, et al. A novel potent vasoconstrictor peptide produced by vascular endothelial cells. *Nature* 1988;332(6163):411–415.
18. Ogawa Y, et al. Molecular cloning of a non-isopeptide-selective human endothelin receptor. *Biochem Biophys Res Commun* 1991;178(1):248–255.
19. Giad A, et al. Expression of endothelin-1 in the lungs of patients with pulmonary hypertension. *N Engl J Med* 1993;328(24):1732–1739.
20. Rubens C, et al. Big endothelin-1 and endothelin-1 plasma levels are correlated with the severity of primary pulmonary hypertension. *Chest* 2001;120(5):1562–1569.
21. Giaid A, Saleh D. Reduced expression of endothelial nitric oxide synthase in the lungs of paients with pulmonary hypertension. *N Engl J Med* 1995;333(4):214–221.
22. Lee SL, et al. Serotonin produces both hyperplasia and hypertrophy of bovine pulmonary artery smooth muscle cell in culture. *Am J Physiol* 1994;66(1 Pt 1):L46–L52.

23. Herve P, et al. Increased plasma serotonin in primary pulmonary hypertension. *Am J Med* 1995;99(3):249–254.

24. Abenhaim L, et al. Appetite-suppressant drugs and the risk of primary pulmonary hypertension. *N Engl J Med* 1996;335(9):609–616.

25. Eddahibi S, et al. Serotonin transporter over expression is responsible for pulmonary artery smooth muscle hyperplasia in primary pulmonary hypertension. *J Clin Invest* 2001;108(8):1141–1150.

26. Marcos E, et al. Serotonin transporter inhibitors protect against hypoxic pulmonary hypertension. *Am J Respir Crit Care Med* 2003;168(4):487–493.

27. Yuan JJ, et al. Dysfunctional voltage-gated Kþ channels in pulmonary artery smooth muscle cells of patients with primary pulmonary hypertension. *Circulation* 1998;98(14):1400–1406.

28. Weir EK, et al. Anorexic agents aminorex, fenfluramine, and dexfenfluramine inhibit potassium current in rat pulmonary vascular smooth muscle and cause pulmonary vasoconstriction. *Circulation* 1996;94(9):2216–2230.

29. Welsh CH, et al. Coagulation and fibrinolytic profiles in patients with severe pulmonary hypertension. *Chest* 1996;110(3):710–717.

30. Tuder RM, et al. Exuberant endothelial cell growth and elements of inflammation are present in plexiform lesions in pulmonary hypertension. *Am J Pathol* 1994;144(2):275–285.

31. Lane KB, et al. Heterozygous germline mutations in BMPR2, encoding a TGF-b receptor, cause familial primary pulmonary hypertension: The International PPH Consortium. *Nat Genet* 2000;26(1):81–84.

32. Deng Z, et al. Familial primary pulmonary hypertension (gene PPH1) is caused by mutations in the bone morphogenetic protein receptor-II gene. *Am J Hum Genet* 2000;67(3):737–744.

33. Trembath R, et al. Clinical and molecular genetic features of pulmonary hypertension in patients with hereditary hemorrhagic telangiectasia. *N Engl J Med* 2001;345(5):325–334.

34. Kukulski T, et al. Normal regional right ventricular function and its changes with age: A Doppler myocardial imaging study. *J Am Soc Echocardiogr* 2000;13(3):194–204.

35. Voekel NF, et al. Right ventricular function and failure: Report of a National Heart, Lung, and Blood Institute working group on cellular and molecular mechanisms of right heart failure. *Circulation* 2006;114(17):1883–1891.

36. Dias CA, et al. Reversible pulmonary trunk banding, II: An experimental model for rapid pulmonary ventricular hypertrophy. *J Thorac Cardiovasc Surg* 2002;124(5):999–1006.

37. Louie EK, et al. Pressure and volume loading of the right ventricle have opposite effects on left ventricular ejection fraction. *Circulation* 1995;92(4):819–824.

38. Hopkins WE, Waggoner AD. Severe pulmonary hypertension without right ventricular failure: The unique hearts of patients with Eisenmenger syndrome. *Am J Cardiol* 2002;89(1):34–38.

39. Busjahn A, et al. Angiotensin-converting enzyme DD genotype in patients with primary pulmonary hypertension: Increased frequency and association with preserved hemodynamics. *J Renin Angiotensin Aldosterone Syst* 2003;4(1):27–30.

40. Masuyama T, et al. Continuous-wave Doppler echocardiographic detection of pulmonary regurgitation and its application to noninvasive estimation of pulmonary artery pressure. *Circulation* 1986;74(3):484–492.

41. Weir EK, et al. Pulmonary hypertension. In: Willerson JT, Cohn JN, eds. *Cardiovascular Medicine.* 2nd edn. Philadelphia, PA: Churchill Livingstone, 2000:1856–1884.

42. Kircher BJ, et al. Noninvasive estimation of right atrial pressure from the inspiratory collapse of the inferior vena cava. *Am J Cardiol* 1990;15(4):493–496.

43. Hinderliter AL, et al. Frequency and severity of tricuspid regurgitation determined by Doppler echocardiography in primary pulmonary hypertension. *Am J Cardiolol* 2003;91(8):1033–1037.

44. Currie PJ, et al. Continuous wave Doppler determination of right ventricular pressure: A simultaneous Doppler-catheterization study in 127 patients. *J Am Coll Cardiol* 1985;6(4):750–756.

45. Hinderliter AL, et al. Effects of long-term infusion of prostacyclin (epoprostenol) on echocardiographic measures of right ventricular structure and function in primary pulmonary hypertension: Primary Pulmonary Hypertension Study Group. *Circulation* 1997;95(6):1479–1486.

46. McQuillan BM, et al. Clinical correlates and reference intervals for pulmonary artery systolic pressure among echocardiographically normal subjects. *Circulation* 2001;104(23):2797–2802.

47. Bossone E, et al. Range of tricuspid regurgitation velocity at rest and during exercise in normal adult men: Implications for the diagnosis of pulmonary hypertension. *J Am Coll Cardiol* 1999;33(6):1662–1666.

48. Chan KL, et al. Comparison of three Doppler ultrasound methods in the prediction of pulmonary artery pressure. *J Am Coll Cardiol* 1987;9(3):549–554.

49. Yock PG, Popp RL. Noninvasive estimation of right ventricular systolic pressure by Doppler ultrasound in patients with tricuspid regurgitation. *Circulation* 1984;70(4):657–662.

50. Brecher SJ, et al. Comparison of Doppler derived hemodynamic variables and stimultaneous high fidelity pressure measurements in severe pulmonary hypertension. *Br Heart J* 1994;72(4):384–389.

51. Arcasoy SM, et al. Echocardiographic assessment of pulmonary hypertension in patients with advanced lung disease. *Am J Respir Crit Care Med* 2003;167(5):735–740.

52. Homma A, et al. Pulmonary artery systolic pressures estimated by echocardiogram vs cardiac catheterization in patients awaiting lung transplantation. *J Heart Lung Transplant* 2001;20(8):833–839.

53. Tramarin R, et al. Doppler echocardiographic evaluation of pulmonary artery pressure in chronic obstructive pulmonary disease. A European multicenter study. *Eur Heart J* 1991;12(2):103–111.

54. Denton CP, et al. Comparison of Doppler echocardiography and right heart catheterization to assess pulmonary hypertension in systemic sclerosis. *Br J Rheumatol* 1997;36(2):239–243.

55. Pepine CJ, et al. Pressure measurement and determination of vascular resistance. In: Pepine CJ, Hill JA, Lambert CR, eds. *Diagnostic and Therapeutic Cardiac Catheterization.* 2nd edn. Philadelphia: Williams & Wilkins, 1994:355–371.

56. Ragosta M. Right sided heart disorders. In: Ragosta M, ed. *Textbook of Clinical Hemodyanmics*. Philadelphia, PA: Saunders, 2008:109–122.

57. Ragosta M. Normal waveforms, artifacts, and pitfalls. In: Ragosta M, ed. *Textbook of Clinical Hemodynamics*. Philadelphia: Saunders, Inc., 2008:16–37.

58. Pichard AD, et al. Large V waves in the pulmonary wedge pressure tracing in the absence of mitral regurgitation. *Am J Cardiol* 1982;50(5):1044–1050.

59. Fuchs RM, et al. Limitation of pulmonary wedge V waves in diagnosing mitral regurgitation. *Am J Cardiol* 1982;49(4):849–854.

60. Sandoval J, et al. Survival in primary pulmonary hypertension: Validation of a prognostic equation. *Circulation* 1999;89(4):1733–1744.

61. McLaughlin VV, et al. Prognosis of Pulmonary arterial hypertension: ACCP evidence-based clinical practice guidelines. *Chest* 2004;126(1 Suppl):78S–92S.

62. Sitbon O, et al. Long-term intravenous epoprostenol infusion in primary pulmonary hypertension: Prognostic factors and survival. *J Am Coll Cardiol* 2002;40(4):780–788.

63. Groves BM, et al. Correlation of acute prostacyclin response in primary (unexplained) pulmonary hypertension with efficacy of treatemt with calcium channel blockers and survival. In: Weir K, ed. *Ion Flux in Pulmonary Vascular Control*. New York: Plenum Press, 1993:317–330.

64. Sitbon O, et al. Inhaled nitric oxide as a screening vasodilator agent in primary pulmonary hypertension: A dose-response study and comparison with prostacyclin. *Am J Respir Crit Care Med* 1995;151(2 Pt 1):384–389.

65. Schrader BJ, et al. Comparison of the effects of adenosine and nifedipine in pulmonary hypertension. *J Am Coll Cardiol* 1992;19(5):1060–1064.

66. Sitbon O, et al. Inhaled nitric oxide as a screening agent for safely identifying responders to oral calcium-channel blockers in primary pulmonary hypertension. *Eur Respir J* 1998;12(2):265–270.

67. Sitbon O, et al. Long-term response to calcium channel blockers in idiopathic pulmonary arterial hypertension. *Circulation* 2005;111(23):3105–3111.

68. McLaughlin VV, et al. ACCF/AHA 2009 expert consensus document on pulmonary hypertension: A report of the American College of Cardiology Foundation Task Force on Expert Consensus Documents. *J Am Coll Cardiol* 2009;53(17):1573–1619.

69. Palmer SM, et al. Massive pulmonary edema and death after prostacyclin infusion in a patient with pulmonary veno-occlusive disease. *Chest* 1998;113(1):237–240.

70. Hoeper MM, et al. Complications of right heart catheterization procedures in patients with pulmonary hypertension in experienced centers. *J Am Coll Cardiol* 2006;48(12):2546–2552.

71. Senni M, et al. Congestive heart failure in the community: A study of all incident cases in Olmsted County, Minnesota, in 1991. *Circulation* 1998;98(21):2282–2289.

72. Higg K, et al. Heart failure with preserved left ventricular systolic function. *J Am Coll Cardiol* 2004;43(3):317–327.

73. Kitzman DW, et al. Pathophysiological characterization of isolated diastolic heart failure in comparison to systolic heart failure. *JAMA* 2002;288(17):2144–2150.

74. Zile MR, Brutsaert DL. New concepts in diastolic dysfunction and diastolic heart failure. Part II: Causal mechanisms and treatment. *Circulation* 2002;105(12):1503–1508.

75. Ghio S, et al. Independent and additive prognostic value of right ventricular systolic function and pulmonary artery pressure in patients with chronic heart failure. *J Am Coll Cardiol* 2001;37(1):183–188.

76. Hoeper MM, et al. Diagnosis, assessment, and treatment of non-pulmonary arterial hypertension pulmonary hypertension. *J Am Coll Cardiol* 2009;54(1 Suppl):S85–S96.

77. Califf RM, et al. A randomized controlled trial of epoprostenol therapy for severe congestive heart failure: The Flolan International Randomized Survival Trial (FIRST). *Am Heart J* 1997;134(1):44–54.

78. Mylona P, Cleland JG. Update of REACH-1 and MERIT-HF clinical trials in heart failure. *Eur J Heart Fail* 1999;1(2):197–200.

79. Teerlink JR. Recent heart failure trials of neurohormonal modulation (OVERTURE and ENABLE): Approaching the asymptote of efficacy? *J Card Fail* 2002;8(3):124–127.

80. Lewis GD, Semigran MJ. The emerging role for type 5 phosphodiesterase inhibition in heart failure. *Curr Hear Fail Rep* 2006;3(3):123–128.

81. Salloum FN, et al. Sildenafil (Viagra) attenuates ischemic cardiomyopathy and improves left ventricular function in mice. *Am J Physiol Heart Circ Phyiol* 2008;294(3):H1398–H1406.

82. Lewis GD, et al. Sildenafil improves exercise hemodynamics and oxygen uptake in patients with systolic heart failure. *Circulation* 2007;115(1):59–66.

83. Lewis GD, et al. Sildenafil improves exercise capacity and quality of life in patients with systolic heart failure and secondary pulmonary hypertension. *Circulation* 2007;116(14):1555–1562.

84. Butler J, et al. Pulmonary hypertension and exercise intolerance in patients with heart failure. *J Am Coll Cardiol* 1999;34(6):1802–1806.

85. Kingsbury MP, et al. Structural remodeling of lungs in chronic heart failure. *Basic Res Cardiol* 2003;98(5):295–303.

86. Todorovich-Hunter L, et al. Increased pulmonary artery elastolytic activity in adult rats with monocrotaline induced progressive hypertensive pulmonary vascular disease compared with infant rats with nonprogressive disease. *Am Rev Respir Dis* 1992;146(1):213–223.

87. Chen JM, et al. Reevaluating the significance of pulmonary hypertension before cardiac transplantation: Determination of optimal thresholds and quantification of the effect of reversibility on perioperative mortality. *J Thorac Cardiovasc Surg* 1997; 114(4):627–634.

88. Taylor DO, et al. Registry of the International Society for Heart and Lung Transplantation: Twenty-fifth official adult heart transplantation report—2008. *J Heart Lung Transplant* 2008;27(9):943–956.

89. Kormos RL, et al. Utility of preoperative right heart catheterization data as a predictor of survival after heart transplantation. *J Heart Lung Transplant* 1986;5:391.

90. Tsai FC, et al. Recent trends in early outcomes of adult patients after transplantation: A single-institution review of 251 transplants using standard donor organs. *Am J Transplant* 2002;2(6):539–545.

91. Radovancevic B, et al. Nitric oxide versus prostaglandin E1 for reduction of pulmonary hypertension in heart transplant candidates. *J Heart Lung Transplant* 2005;24(6):690–695.

92. Natale ME, Pina IL. Evaluation of pulmonary hypertension in heart transplant candidates. *Curr Opin Cardiol* 2003;18(2):136–140.

93. Zimpler D, et al. Left ventricular assist devices decrease fixed pulmonary hypertension in cardiac transplant candidates. *J Thorac Cardiovasc Surg* 2007;133(3):689–695.

94. Klotz S, et al. Left ventricular pressure and volume unloading during pulsatile versus nonpulsatile left ventricular assist device support. *Ann Thorac Surg* 2004;77(1):143–149.

95. Garatti A, et al. Is fixed severe pulmonary hypertension still a contraindication to heart transplant in the modern era of mechanical circulatory support? A review. *J Cardiovasc Med* 2008;9(10):1059–1062.

96. Cogan JD, et al. Gross BMPR2 gene rearrangements constitute a new cause for primary pulmonary hypertension. *Genet Med* 2005;7(3):169–174.

97. Thomson JR, et al. Sporadic primary pulmonary hypertension is associated with germline mutations of the gene encoding BMPR-II, a receptor member of the TGF-B family. *J Med Genet* 2000;37(10):741–745.

98. Koh ET, et al. Pulmonary hypertension in systemic sclerosis: An analysis of 17 patients. *Br J Rheumatol* 1996;35(10):989–993.

99. Kuhn KP, et al. Outcome in 91 consecutive patients with pulmonary arterial hypertension receiving epoprostenol. *Am J Respir Crit Care Med* 2003;167(4):580–586.

100. Kuo PC, et al. Distinctive clinical features of portopulmonary hypertension. *Chest* 1997;112(4):980–986.

101. Colle IO, et al. Diagnosis of portopulmonary hypertension in candidates for liver transplantation: A prospective study. *Hepatology* 2003;37(2):401–409.

102. Krowka M, et al. Pulmonary hemodynamics and perioperative cardiopulmonary mortality in patients with portopulmonary hypertension undergoing liver transplantation. *Liver Transpl* 2000;6(4):443–450.

103. Walker AM, et al. Temporal trends and drug exposures in pulmonary hypertension: An American experience. *Am Heart J* 2006;152(3):521–526.

104. Opravil M, et al. HIV-associated primary pulmonary hypertension: A case control study: Swiss HIV Cohort Study. *Am J Respir Crit Care Med* 1997;155(3):990–995.

105. McLaughlin VV, et al. Survival in primary pulmonary hypertension: The impact of epoprostenol therapy. *Circulation* 2002;106(12):1477–1482.

106. Barst RJ, et al. A comparison of continuous intravenous epoprostenol (prostacyclin) with conventional therapy for primary pulmonary hypertension. The Primary Pulmonary Hypertension Study Group. *N Engl J Med* 1996;334(5):296–302.

107. Wensel R, et al. Assessment of survival in patients with primary pulmonary hypertension: Importance of cardiopulmonary exercise testing. *Circulation* 2002;106(3):319–324.

108. Raymond RL, et al. Echocardiographic predictors of adverse outcomes in primary pulmonary hypertension. *J Am Coll Cardiol* 2002;39(7):1214–1219.

109. Hinderliter A, et al. Frequency and prognostic significance of pericardial effusion in primary pulmonary hypertension. PPH Study Group. *Am J Cardiol* 1999;84(4):481–484, A10.

110. Nagaya N, et al. Plasma brain natriuretic peptide as a prognostic indicator in patients with primary pulmonary hypertension. *Circulation* 2000;102(8):865–870.

111. Park MH, et al. Usefulness of B-type natriuretic peptide as a predictor of treatment outcome in pulmonary arterial hypertension. *Congest Heart Fail* 2004;10(5):221–225.

112. Andreassen A, et al. N-terminal pro-B-type natriuretic peptide as an indicator of disease severity in a heterogeneous group of patients with chronic precapillary pulmonary hypertension. *Am J Cardiol* 2006;98(4):525–529.

113. Badesch DB, et al. Continuous intravenous epoprostenol for pulmonary hypertension due to the scleroderma spectrum of disease: A randomized, controlled trial. *Ann Intern Med* 2000;132(6):425–434.

114. Aguilar RV, Farber HW. Epoprostenol (prostacyclin) therapy in HIV-associated pulmonary hypertension. *Am J Respir Crit Care Med* 2000;162(5):1846–1850.

115. Rosenzweig EB, et al. Long-term prostacyclin for pulmonary hypertension with associated congenital heart defects. *Circulation* 1999;99(14):1858–1865.

116. Kuo PC, et al. Continuous intravenous infusion of epoprostenol for the treatment of portopulmonary hypertension. *Transplantation* 1997;63(4):604–616.

117. Rich S, McLauglin VV. The effects of chronic prostacyclin therapy on cardiac output and symptoms in primary pulmonary hypertension. *J Am Coll Cardiol* 1999;34(4):1184–1187.

118. Park MH. Pharmacotherapeutic options for pulmonary arterial hypertension. *Current Medical Literature: Pulmonary Hypertension* 2009;1:1–21.

119. Simonneau G, et al. Continuous subcutaneous infusion of treprostinil, a prostacyclin analogue, in patients with pulmonary arterial hypertension. *Am J Respir Crit Care Med* 2002;165(6):800–804.

120. Tapson VF, et al. Safety and efficacy of IV treprostinil for pulmonary arterial hypertension: A prospective, multicenter, open-label, 12-week trial. *Chest* 2006;129(3):683–688.

121. Gomberg-Maitland M, et al. Transition from intravenous epoprotenol to intravenous treprostinil in pulmonary hypertension. *Am J Respir Crit Care Med* 2005;172(12):1586–1589.

122. Olschewski H, et al. Inhaled iloprost for severe pulmonary hypertension. *N Engl J Med* 2002;347(5):322–329.

123. Channick RN, et al. Effects of the dual endothelin-receptor antagonist bosentan in patients with pulmonary hypertension: A randomized placebo-controlled study. *Lancet* 2001;358(9288):1119–1123.

124. Rubin LJ, et al. Bosentan therapy for pulmonary arterial hypertension. *N Engl J Med* 2002;346(12):896–903.

125. McLaughlin VV, et al. Survival with first-line bosentan in patients with primary pulmonary hypertension. *Eur Respir J* 2005;25(2):244–249.

126. Galie N, et al. Treatment of patients with mildly symptomatic pulmonary arterial hypertension with bosentan (EARLY study): A double-blind, randomized controlled trial. *Lancet* 2008;317(9630):2093–2100.

127. Galie N, et al. Ambrisentan for the treatment of pulmonary arterial hypertension. Results of the ambrisentan in pulmonary arterial hypertension, randomized, double-blind, placebo-controlled, multicenter, efficacy (ARIES) study 1 and 2. *Circulation* 2008;117(23):3010–3019.

128. McGoon M, et al. Ambrisentan therapy in patients with pulmonary arterial hypertension who discontinued bosentan or sitaxsentan due to liver function test abnormalities. *Chest* 2009;135(1):122–129.

129. *Highlights of prescribing information Letairis.* Available at: http://www.gilead.com/pdf/letairis_pi.pdf (accessed 10 January, 2007).

130. Galie N, et al. Sildenafil citrate therapy for pulmonary arterial hypertension. *N Engl J Med* 2005;353(20):2148–2157.

131. Galie N, et al. Tadalafil therapy for pulmonary arterial hypertension. *Circulation* 2009;119(22):2894–2903.

132. Fuster V, et al. Primary pulmonary hypertension: Natural history and the importance of thrombosis. *Circulation* 1984;70(4):580–587.

133. Hoeper MM, et al. Combination therapy with bosentan and sildenafil in idiopathic pulmonary arterial hypertension. *Eur Respir J* 2004; 24(6):1007–1010.

134. Ghofrani HA, et al. Oral sildenafil as long-term adjunct therapy in severe pulmonary arterial hypertension. *J Am Coll Cardiol* 2003;42(1):158–164.

135. Humbert M, et al. Combination of bosentan with epoprostenolol in pulmonary arterial hypertension: BREATHE-2. *Eur Respir J* 2004;24(3);353–359.

136. McLaughlin VV, et al. Randomized study adding inhaled iloprost to existing bosentan in pulmonary arterial hypertension. *Am J Respir Crit Care Med* 2006;174(11):1257–1263

137. Hoper MM, et al. Combining inhaled iloprost with bosentan in patients with idiopathic pulmonary hypertension. *Eur Repir J* 2006;28(4):691–694.

138. Simonneau G, et al. Addition of sildenafil to long-term intravenous epoprostenol therapy in patients with pulmonary arterial hypertension. *Ann Intern Med* 2008;149(8)SS521–530.

11

Valvular heart disease: Measurement of valve orifice area and quantification of regurgitation

BLASE A. CARABELLO

INTRODUCTION

In 1929, Werner Forssmann published a radiograph of a successful right heart catheterization he performed on himself.[1] Subsequently, Dickinson Richards and André Cournand used the heart catheter to make a series of seminal hemodynamic measurements in man, resulting in the three men winning the Nobel Prize in Medicine in 1956 for their accomplishments. In 1951, the Gorlin formula[2] for calculating cardiac valve area was published, and for the next three decades, invasive hemodynamics held sway as the gold standard for assessing cardiac physiology and pathophysiology.

In the 1980s, the use of Doppler interrogation of the heart made assessment of cardiac physiology easily applied noninvasively. While at first there was serious debate about whether noninvasive measurements could reliably be substituted for invasive hemodynamics, the echocardiogram was eventually accepted; it then largely supplanted invasive hemodynamics. In fact, the 2006 American Heart Association (AHA)/American College of Cardiology (ACC) Guidelines for the Management of Patients with Valvular Heart Disease[3] gives invasive assessment of valve disease a class III recommendation (not indicated and possibly harmful) when there is no doubt about the diagnosis following

clinical and noninvasive evaluation. While this recommendation was dropped in the 2014 guidelines,[4] the point is worth making that current practice generally relies upon noninvasive assessment of stenosis severity. On the other hand, it is a Class I recommendation (indicated and beneficial) to obtain invasive hemodynamic data when the diagnosis is unclear. Thus, we currently rely on a progressively less practiced modality to help us solve our most important diagnostic dilemmas. The problem is compounded by a relative lack of teaching of hemodynamic principles in our cardiovascular medicine fellowships and by computers that allow calculations to be made without the operator understanding the pitfalls of such calculations. Thus, the gold standard of cardiac diagnosis is threatened with a good deal of tarnish. In light of this, the following is a summary of the modern use of invasive hemodynamics in the assessment of valvular heart disease (VHD).

ASSESSMENT OF STENOTIC VALVES

Normal cardiac valves permit unidirectional circulatory flow at low resistance with equal pressure on both sides of an open valve. Even when these valves are narrowed to 50% of their normal aperture, only a small pressure gradient exists during flow. However, further narrowing results in progressively greater obstruction to flow and persistently higher and higher transvalvular pressure gradients. Because pressure gradient varies with flow, a gradient by itself may be an unreliable indicator of stenosis severity. Knowledge of this concept led to the use of valve area to help quantify stenosis severity.

Both invasive and noninvasive assessments of stenosis severity use the same hemodynamic principle to calculate valve area: Flow (*F*) = valve area (*A*) × flow velocity (*V*). Thus, $A = F/V$. In the echo laboratory, *V* is measured directly by Doppler ultrasonography. When using invasive hemodynamics, the pressure gradient across the valve is measured and converted to velocity, where

$$V = \sqrt{2g}\, P_1 - P_2$$

Here, $P1 - P2$ is the mean pressure gradient and *g* is the acceleration due to gravity. This last term is incorporated because pressure is expressed in mmHg, which depends on the specific weight of mercury—mass × acceleration. Thus, in the catheterization laboratory, accurate calculation of valve area relies on an accurately determined pressure gradient, an accurate determination of flow [cardiac output (CO)], and an accurate formula that relates the two together.

AORTIC STENOSIS

Accurate pressure gradient assessment

To record an accurate transaortic valvular pressure gradient, two properly placed catheters must be connected to two properly calibrated transducers, reporting to an accurate recording device. Alternatively, a pressure gradient may be recorded in patients in sinus rhythm during pullback of the catheter from the left ventricle (LV) to the aorta, recognizing that a pullback determination is a "one-time" opportunity. If premature beats or any technical problems arise during the pullback, the data are lost, necessitating re-crossing the valve or abandoning the measurement.

PROPER CATHETER PLACEMENT

Figure 11.1 depicts potential positions that might be used in recording a transvalvular pressure gradient; most of them create erroneous data.[5] Of the two potential positions for the LV catheter, the proper one is with the lumen placed in the body of the LV. As shown in Figure 11.2, in most patients with aortic stenosis (AS), a subvalvular gradient usually exists between the body of the LV and the LV outflow tract.[6] This gradient does not represent subvalvular AS, but rather occurs as blood normally accelerates into the outflow tract, which is narrower than the body of the LV. If the LV catheter is placed in the outflow tract, or if the natural ejection of blood pushes the catheter there, the true LV-aortic (Ao) gradient can be underestimated by as much as 20–40 mmHg. The distal catheter should be placed in the proximal ascending Ao just distal to the valve. For convenience, some operators have used the side port on the femoral sheath to record

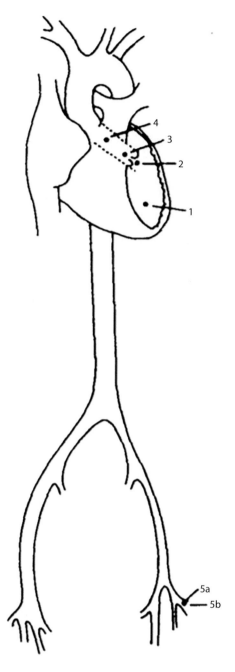

Figure 11.1 Various catheter positions that could be used to obtain the transvalvular gradient in aortic stenosis. 1, left ventricular body; 2, left ventricular outflow tract; 3, ascending aorta, coronary level; 4, ascending aorta, distal to coronaries; and 5, femoral artery sheath. The most accurate data are obtained when the left ventricle catheter is placed in Position 1 and the aortic catheter is placed in Position 4. (From Assey, M.E., et al., *Cathet. Cardiovasc. Diagn.*, 30(4), 287–292, 1993. With permission.)

the distal pressure. This practice is fraught with difficulty and should be avoided.[7] By the time the pulse reaches the femoral artery (FA), the turbulent flow present above the valve has become relaminarized, causing pressure recovery and a reduced pressure gradient. Because it takes a finite period of time for the pulse to reach the FA, it is impossible

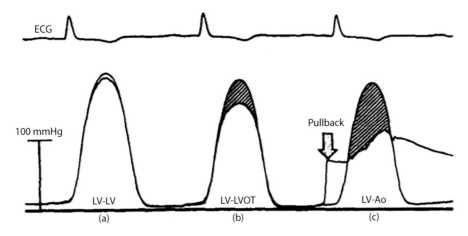

Figure 11.2 Pressure tracings taken from high-fidelity micromanometer-tipped catheters. Both transducers are placed in the body of the LV and no gradient exists **(a)**. Both transducers are inside the LV, and both record an LV pressure; however, one transducer is in the body of the LV, while the other is in the LV outflow tract, recording the pressure gradient between the two positions **(b)**. The true gradient between LV body and Ao is recorded **(c)**. Ao, aortic; ECG, electrocardiogram; LV, left ventricle; LVOT, left ventricular outflow tract. (From Pasipoularides, A., *J. Am. Coll. Cardiol.*, 15(4), 859–882, 1990. With permission.)

for LV and FA pressures to be simultaneous. This requisite misalignment overestimates the true pressure gradient. Unfortunately, manual realignment causes substantial underestimation of the gradient. Because invasive hemodynamics are only recorded when the diagnosis is in doubt, it is crucial to obtain the best data possible. This is done by obtaining pressures from two properly placed lumens (or transducers, if micromanometer catheters are used). To place the lumens properly, either two separate catheters can be employed or a double lumen catheter is used. In either case, scrupulous attention to proper damping and catheter flushing is necessary to obtain an accurate gradient.

ACCURATE TRANSDUCER CALIBRATION

The most effective way to ensure accurate transducer calibration is to connect the transducer to a mercury manometer because pressure is defined as mmHg. The pressure displayed from the transducer must be identical to the reading from the mercury manometer, or if not, adjusted to be so. Frankly, this procedure is ignored in many laboratories, which rely instead on the pressure recorder's internal calibration device. If internal calibration is used, two absolute tenets must be observed. First, after the catheters (or double lumen catheter) are placed in the circulation, the closely approximated lumens must record identical pressures because in that position there can be no gradient. If the pressures are not identical, (1) ensure that the lines connecting the catheters to the transducers are properly flushed and free of kinks, (2) be sure the zero references of the two transducers are accurate and identical, and (3) recalibrate both transducers. If these steps do not mitigate the errors in the pressure being recorded, mercury calibration is then necessary. Second, the above process only proves that the catheters are recording identical pressures, but not necessarily that the pressures are accurate. To be certain that the pressures recorded invasively are at least in the "ballpark"

of accuracy, their pressure should be similar to cuff pressure measured by a sphygmomanometer.

It should be recognized that some recording devices falsely "assume" that the operator is going to use the FA as the distal recording site despite its inaccuracies. The recorder then offsets the distal pressure to compensate for the expected delay in registering it. The result will be that the upstroke of the Ao pressure will actually precede that of the LV pressure, an obviously physiologic impossibility leading to inaccurate pressure recording.

Accurate cardiac output determination

The second datum crucial to the accurate assessment of stenosis severity is the CO. The gold standard for this determination is use of the Fick principle, which states that the oxygen consumed by the body is the product of O_2 delivery (CO) and O_2 extraction by the tissues. Thus, O_2 consumption = CO × (arterial O_2 – venous O_2 content, i.e., AO_2 – $VO_2\Delta$). Rearranging the terms, CO = O_2 consumption/AO_2 – $VO_2\Delta$. Expanding the latter term, AO_2 – $VO_2\Delta$ = (arterial O_2 saturation – venous O_2 saturation) × hemoglobin (Hb) concentration (g/dL) × 1.36 cc O_2/g Hb × 10 dL/L. The principles for the use of the Fick principle are (1) an accurate measurement of O_2 consumption, (2) accurate measurements of O_2 saturations in arterial and venous blood (the latter best taken from the pulmonary artery where mixing is ideal), and (3) an accurate measurement of hemoglobin concentration. Unfortunately, O_2 consumption is rarely measured today but rather is assumed from standard tables usually estimated as function of body size and habitus in normal subjects. However, the patient with severe valve disease is hardly normal and significant error in CO determination and hence valve area determination arise when O_2 consumption is estimated rather than measured by actual analysis of expired air.[8] This error can be as much as 50%.

By far, the most commonly used method to determine CO is thermodilution:

$$CO_{TD} = \frac{V_I(T_B - T_I)(S_I \cdot C_I / S_B \cdot C_B)60(sec/min)}{\int_0^\infty \Delta T_B(t)dt}$$

where T_B is the temperature of blood before injection; T_I is the temperature of the injected saline; S_I and S_B are the specific gravities of the injectate and blood, respectively; C_I and C_B are the specific heats of the injectate and blood, respectively; and

$$\int_0^\infty \Delta T_B(t)dt$$

is the area under the time–temperature curve recorded by the thermister at the end of the thermodilution catheter. When cold saline is injected into the pulmonary artery, the saline mixes with the blood and cools it. The larger the blood pool and the faster the blood flow is, the smaller the change in downstream blood temperature, thus the area under the time–temperature curve will be smaller causing the calculated CO to be larger than when the blood volume and rate of flow are less. In general, thermodilution is accurate, but pitfalls exist. The tacit assumption is that all of the coldness of the injectate is transferred to the bloodstream. However, when CO is low (an obvious consequence of severe AS), the right atrium (RA) and ventricle absorb some of the cold, warming up the blood so that the time-temperature curve area will be factiously small. Other causes of inaccuracy include faulty thermisters, tricuspid regurgitation, and intracardiac shunts.

The Gorlin Formula

In 1951, the Gorlins published their formula for calculating valve area (A):

$$A = \frac{F}{C_v\sqrt{2gh \cdot C_c}} = \frac{F}{C_vC_c\sqrt{2 \cdot 980 \cdot h}} = \frac{F}{(C)(44.3)\sqrt{h}}$$

where F is flow; Cv is the constant of velocity dissipation; Cc is the constant of orifice contraction; g is acceleration due to gravity; and h is the transvalvular pressure gradient.[3] Cv accounts for the loss of energy as blood flows through the valve since not all of the driving gradient is converted to flow. Cc accounts for the fact that as blood flows through an orifice it tends to stream through the middle so that the physiologic aperture is less than the anatomic one. Because flow only occurs when the valve is open during each beat, flow = CO/heart rate × flow duration. Aortic valve area (AVA) is as follows:

$$AVA = \frac{CO/(SEP)(HR)}{44.3C\sqrt{\Delta P}}$$

where SEP is systolic ejection period.

When the Gorlins devised their formula it was considered malpractice to cross the Ao valve retrogradely as is done today; other methods for entering the LV had not yet been perfected. Their formula was vetted against data from patients with *mitral* stenosis (MS) where they assumed a LV end diastolic pressure of 10 mmHg and substituted wedge pressure for left atrial pressure (LAP) to obtain the transmitral gradient. The actual mitral valve area (MVA) was measured from autopsy or surgical specimens and the data compared with their calculations. They then substituted an empirical constant (C) for Cv and Cc. The empirical constant simply reduced the calculated valve area to a value closer to the actual measured valve area. However, the Gorlins had no data for developing a similar empiric constant for the Ao valve, so they simply assumed a constant of 1, warning that when data became available, the constant should be calculated, but it never has been calculated.

Flow dependence of calculated aortic valve area

It has been well demonstrated that calculated Ao valve area may be quite flow-dependent at COs <5.0 L/min, with AVA varying directly with flow.[9] Increased AVA with increasing flow may be real or factitious. It could be that low CO produced by a weakened LV is unable to fully open a moderately but not severely stenotic Ao valve. As output is increased by exercise or infusion of positive inotropic drugs, the valve is opened more widely and output increases more than gradient, causing an increase in calculated AVA that truly reflects increased orifice area. Conversely, it may be that problems with the Gorlin formula cause calculated AVA to be flow dependent, either because it assumes constant flow or because the discharge coefficients were never calculated. Existing data support both viewpoints. One recommended method for circumventing this problem is to calculate AVA at increasing outputs, constructing a relationship to project what the AVA would be at an output of 5 L/min, where AVA becomes less flow dependent.[9] Flow dependence of calculated AVA is rarely a problem when mean gradient exceeds 40 mmHg since in such cases AVA almost always falls in the severe range of AS irrespective of CO.

Discrepancies in the definition of "severe" aortic stenosis

The 2014 ACC/AHA guidelines for the management of VHD define severe AS as a valve area of <1 cm², a peak jet velocity of >4 m/sec, or a mean transvalvular gradient of >40 mmHg. It should be noted that while each parameter has literary support for the benchmark, the benchmarks often do not agree with each other.[10] In Figure 11.3, only 39% of patients with normal LV function in the lower right-hand corner of the graph have concordant pressure gradients and valve areas consistent with the current definitions of "severe" AS. In fact, a mean pressure gradient of 40 mmHg fits better with an AVA of 0.8 cm² than it does with a valve area of 1 cm². Thus, it is important to keep in mind that our man-made definitions of "severe" are not always obeyed by the actual physiology of our patients.

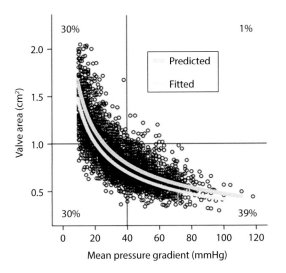

Figure 11.3 The relationship between valve area and mean pressure gradient for over 2,000 patients with aortic stenosis and normal left ventricular function is demonstrated. Valve area predicted by the Gorlin formula using a fixed cardiac output plotted against increasing gradients (blue line) fit closely with actual data fitted to the curve (yellow line). Importantly, only 39% of patients (right lower quadrant) had concordantly small valve areas and high-pressure gradients consistent with the definitions of severe aortic stenosis. (From Minners, J., et al., *Eur. Heart J.*, 29(8), 1043–1048, 2008. With permission.)

Assessment of inotropic reserve

The outcome of aortic valve replacement (AVR) for patients with AS is usually excellent, resulting in substantial prolongation of life, a dramatic improvement in symptoms, and an improvement in LV function.[11] Even when preoperative ejection is markedly reduced, LV ejection fraction (EF) may return to normal following removal of a large transvalvular gradient and the afterload that accompanies such a gradient.[12] However, this is not the case in patients with a low gradient (<30 mmHg mean gradient) and low EF (<0.30).[13,14] Such patients have severe myocardial dysfunction and a poor prognosis. However, some such patients may improve substantially following AVR. Many are patients that have inotropic reserve (Figure 11.4).[15] If stroke volume increases by 20% or more during the infusion of dobutamine and gradient increases concomitantly, prognosis following AVR is acceptable. For patients lacking inotropic reserve, operative risk is as high as 30% although even then some patients still improve if they survive AVR. Predicting who falls into this group is still problematic. A fourth group of patients exists where stroke volume increases but gradient does not, resulting in a large increase in calculated AVA.[16] It is thought that such patients have moderate but not severe AS and primary myocardial disease. When increased output is pushed through such a valve, it opens more widely (see above). In such cases (termed pseudo-AS),[17] it is believed, but not certain, that AVR would not be of benefit since myocardial disease, rather than valve disease, lies at the crux of the problem. Guideline-directed therapy for heart failure seems to benefit this group (Figure 11.5).[18] While inotropic reserve is often tested for in the echocardiography laboratory, the catheterization laboratory is also ideal for making

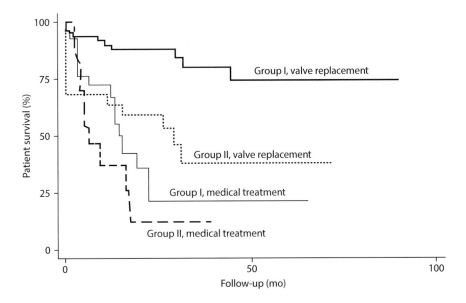

Figure 11.4 The outcome of aortic stenosis patients with low gradient and low ejection fraction according to inotropic reserve and therapy. Group I patients had inotropic reserve and a satisfactory outcome with AVR—far better than with medical therapy. Group II failed to have inotropic reserve and had a very high operative risk, although they still did better with AVR than with medical therapy. AVR, aortic valve replacement. (From Monin, J.L., et al., *Circulation*, 108(3), 319–324, 2003. With permission.)

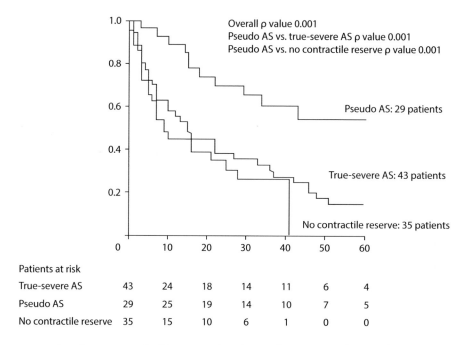

Figure 11.5 The outcome of patients treated without aortic valve replacement with pseudo-aortic stenosis (AS); those with true AS and patients without inotropic reserve is demonstrated. Survival for true AS without mechanical intervention is almost universally fatal. The prognosis for pseudo-AS while not good, is similar to that of heart failure in general. (From Fougères, E., et al., *Eur. Heart J.*, 33(19), 2426–2433, 2012. With permission.)

such determinations since careful hemodynamic measurements can be made before and during the inotropic challenge. Further, one cause of failed inotropic reserve can be the presence of obstructive coronary artery disease where increasing inotropy can induce ischemia, leading to misinterpretation of test results. In the catheterization laboratory, coronary arteriography can be performed to establish the presence or absence of coronary disease, allowing for better understanding of the results of the inotropic challenge.

MITRAL STENOSIS

The hemodynamic determination of MVA in MS employs the same principles as the hemodynamic determination of AS severity. It requires an accurate transmitral valvular gradient, an accurate CO, and an accurate formula relating the two.

Accurate pressure gradient

In common practice, the transmitral gradient is obtained using direct measurement of LV pressure, while pulmonary capillary wedge pressure (PCWP) is used as a surrogate for LAP. While PCWP may overestimate LAP and therefore overestimate the gradient and the severity of MS, overestimation is minimized to a few millimeters of mercury when careful technique is followed.[19] In most labs, PCWP is obtained using a pulmonary artery balloon-tipped catheter. Once the balloon is inflated, the catheter is advanced to the wedge position at which time the pressure waveform changes from that of a pulmonary artery tracing to that of the PCWP. However, the change in waveform does not by itself guarantee that the catheter is fully wedged and that an accurate LAP is being measured. To ensure that the catheter is truly wedged, it is necessary to confirm the wedge position by withdrawing highly oxygen-saturated left atrial blood from the catheter while it is wedged. When comparison of PCWP with direct measurement of LAP is made using this technique, the difference is usually less than 3 mmHg, while comparisons made in the absence of oxymetric confirmation show larger overestimation of LAP by PCWP.[20]

Exact calibration and zeroing of the transducers is crucial to establishing the transmitral gradient. Whereas an error of 3–4 mmHg would only rarely affect clinical decisions in AS, this magnitude of gradient could be one-third of the total in MS and lead to serious misdiagnosis.

The Gorlin formula in mitral stenosis

The Gorlin formula applied to the mitral valve is

$$MVA = \frac{CO/(DFP)(HR)}{44.3 \times 0.85 \times \sqrt{\Delta P}}$$

where DFP is the diastolic filling period and 0.85 is the empiric constant derived by the Gorlins. MVA calculated by the Gorlin formula is generally less flow dependent than calculated AVA, and calculated MVA usually compares well to actual planimetered measurements of MVA.[20] Why there is better agreement with invasive data used to calculate MVA and noninvasive techniques than for AVA is uncertain. Perhaps it is due to employment of the empiric constant, or perhaps the MVA changes less than AVA with flow, or perhaps it is a combination of both phenomena.

Shortcut for calculating aortic valve area and mitral valve area: The Hakki formula

Because the heart rate, filling time, and square root of the acceleration due to gravity typically equal a similar constant in most patients, a rough approximation of valve area can be made simply by dividing the CO (in liters) by the square root of the gradient.[21] This shortcut is useful in making a quick ballpark estimate of valve stenosis severity in the catheterization laboratory before offline calculations can be employed.

TRICUSPID STENOSIS

Tricuspid stenosis (TS) is rare today in developed nations because its major cause, rheumatic heart disease, is also rare. TS may also result from carcinoid syndrome. The diagnosis is usually made by echocardiography, and its clinical significance is usually well defined at the bedside by examination of the neck veins from which central venous pressure can be estimated. If the diagnosis is uncertain, invasive hemodynamics may be helpful. A double lumen catheter (or separate right atrial and right ventricular catheters) is advanced across the tricuspid valve so that one lumen is positioned on either side of the valve and the gradient is recorded. Since there is no agreed upon valve area that constitutes severe TS, severity is estimated from the gradient alone. A mean gradient of >5 mmHg is clinically important as it will yield a systemic venous pressure of >10 mmHg at rest, usually enough venous hypertension to cause symptoms.

PULMONIC STENOSIS

The severity of pulmonic stenosis is inferred from the magnitude of the transvalvular gradient. Mean gradients of less than 25 mmHg are considered hemodynamically insignificant, while gradients in excess of 50 mmHg indicate severe disease, requiring intervention. Mean gradients between 25 and 50 mmHg are intermediate with a decision to intervene based on symptomatology.[22]

VALVULAR REGURGITATION

Both the invasive and noninvasive assessment of lesion severity for regurgitant lesions tend to be less accurate than the assessment of valvular stenosis. While relatively precise methods for regurgitation severity are available, they are more difficult to apply than the quantitative approaches to stenosis severity. Noninvasive assessment of mitral regurgitation (MR) uses an integrated approach, summing up several parameters to estimate whether MR is mild, moderate, or severe.[4] Nonetheless, there may still be uncertainty regarding lesion severity, even after a careful integrative, noninvasive approach—in turn, necessitating invasive evaluation. In the catheterization laboratory, evaluation of pressures and waveforms at rest and with exercise, quantification of regurgitant flow and regurgitant fraction (RF), and visualization of the regurgitant flow, contribute to the assessment of regurgitant severity.

Waveforms

AORTIC REGURGITATION

Figure 11.6 shows some of the classic features of the hemodynamics of aortic regurgitation (AR).[23] FA systolic pressure is about 50 mmHg greater than LV systolic pressure (Hill's sign). The mechanism of this phenomenon is not entirely clear. It is postulated that standing waves along the Ao periphery sum with the systolic pressure wave produced by the increased total stroke volume (SVt) of AR to augment Ao systolic pressure as it moves down the aorta to the FA.

Ao diastolic pressure and LV diastolic pressure equalize (diastasis) because the physical barrier between the aorta

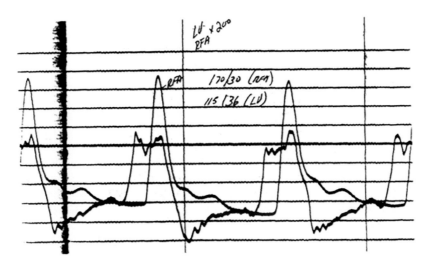

Figure 11.6 Simultaneous recording of left ventricular and right femoral artery pressures in a patient with severe aortic regurgitation. LV, left ventricle; RFA, right femoral artery. (From Carabello, B.A., et al., *Aortic Regurgitation in Cardiology Pearls*, Hanley & Belfus, Philadelphia, PA, 46.)

and LV is largely removed. In turn, there is a rapid rise in LV diastolic pressure because the LV is filling from both the LA and from the aorta. In chronic AR, there is usually a very wide pulse pressure indicative of the large SVt ejected into the aorta.

MITRAL REGURGITATION

Much has been written about the implications of a large V wave in the LA (or PCWP) pressure tracing with regard to the severity of MR.[24] In fact, the presence of a large V wave is neither sensitive nor specific for the presence of severe MR. The V wave height is related to LA systolic volume and compliance. A large regurgitant volume (RV) and normal or low LA compliance will yield a large V wave. However, when severe MR coexists with a large compliant LA, the V wave may be of normal amplitude. On the other hand, large V waves may occur in acute heart failure without MR and also with ventricular septal defects.

Angiography

AORTIC REGURGITATION

Aortography has the potential to add significant data in the evaluation of the patient with AR. Whereas Doppler interrogation of the valve images only the velocity of the regurgitant jet, injection of contrast medium into the aorta during aortography visualizes actual flow of opacified blood from the aorta across the leaking valve into the LV. The severity of AR is classified on the basis of the density of this opacification. Mild AR (1+) is diagnosed when the regurgitant contrast medium fails to opacify the whole LV. Moderate AR (2+) is thought present when contrast faintly opacifies the entire LV cavity. Moderately severe AR (3+) is present when opacification of the LV is equal to that of the aorta, and severe AR (4+) is present when opacification of the LV exceeds that of the aorta. In performing aortography, it is important to inject enough contrast to fully opacify the aorta and the enlarged LV, usually 60 cc of contrast injected over 3 seconds.

MITRAL REGURGITATION

Ventriculography has a similar advantage in visualizing MR as aortography does in AR; it images actual flow instead of flow velocity. Severity is judged by the level of left atrium (LA) opacification during injection of contrast into the LV. The scale used for MR is similar to that for AR, grading the density of contrast in the LA instead of in the LV. However, the tendency of ventriculography to cause ventricular ectopy (which by itself causes MR) has made the use of ventriculography uncommon in assessing MR severity. However, a diagnostic ventriculogram may be obtained by placing the injection catheter just underneath the mitral valve and using a test injection to evaluate the potential for ectopy. If the test is unsatisfactory, the catheter is repositioned and the injection repeated. As with AR, enough contrast must be injected to opacify the two enlarged chambers of interest.

Volumetric quantification

More precise assessment of the amount of AR or MR can be made by measuring the RV, which is the difference between total and forward stroke volume (SVf). SVt is all that is ejected from the LV and can be calculated as end diastolic minus end systolic volume, where the volumes are determined angiographically (see Chapter 21). SVf is determined as the CO from the Fick or thermodilution principles, divided by the heart rate. The volume regurgitated back into the receiving chamber (the LV in AR and the LA in MR), RV, is the difference between SVt and SVf (SVt-SVf). RF = RV/SVt. RF >0.50 or regurgitant flow >60 cc is considered to be severe AR or MR.[4]

Exercise testing

In most cases, symptoms develop during exercise, yet hemodynamics are measured at rest. Therefore, exercise testing during hemodynamic recording can be very illuminating. Either supine bicycle exercise or isometric handgrip exercise can be employed. Handgrip exercise is well suited for evaluation of valvular regurgitation because it increases afterload by raising mean arterial blood pressure by 10–20 mmHg.[25] Normal subjects and patients with well-compensated AR or MR maintain normal LV filling pressure and increase CO with handgrip. Conversely, in poorly compensated patients, filling pressure may increase dramatically, giving insight into the mechanism of the patient's symptoms and supporting the need for intervention.

Indications for surgery

Surgery is recommended either when symptoms are due to severe valve disease or when there is evidence of LV dysfunction[4] in the case of the AR and MR. Symptomatology is based on obtaining a good history. However, if the source of the dyspnea, the most common symptom of VHD, is unclear, invasive hemodynamics can be helpful in establishing cause. If the filling pressures are normal both at rest and during exercise, it is likely that the dyspnea is coming from a noncardiac source. If the patient has both lung and heart disease, examining PCWP and pulmonary artery pressure (PAP) at rest and exercise can be diagnostic. A normal PCWP and high PAP suggests severe lung disease with increased pulmonary vascular resistance, a condition unlikely to be improved by valve surgery. On the other hand, a high PCWP indicates LV failure as the culprit.

LV dysfunction is inferred from the LVEF at ventriculography. An EF of <0.50 for AR and <0.60 for MR is considered evidence of LV dysfunction and an indication for valve replacement or repair.[4]

SUMMARY

The diagnosis of VHD is usually made at the bedside and is confirmed by echocardiography. However, in some cases, the severity of disease is still in doubt following noninvasive testing. In such cases, careful hemodynamic evaluation at rest and/or with exercise can be diagnostic. Further, invasively based angiography can contribute diagnostic information especially for the regurgitant lesions.

Our modern understanding of cardiac function is based on hemodynamic information obtained invasively from pressure and flow measurement. These principles still have an important diagnostic role to play even in the 21st century, but for them to be useful, the careful techniques of 60 years ago must still be employed.

REFERENCES

1. Forssmann W. Uber Kontrastdarstellung der Hohlen des lebenden rechten Herzens und der Lungenschlagader. *Munchen Med Wochenschr* 1931;1974:489–492.

2. Gorlin R, Gorlin SG. Hydraulic formula for calculation of the area of the stenotic mitral valve, other cardiac valves, and central circulatory shunts. I. *Am Heart J* 1951;41(1):1–29.

3. Bonow RO, et al. ACC/AHA 2006 guidelines for the management of patients with valvular heart disease: A report of the American College of Cardiology/American Heart Association Task Force on Practice Guidelines (writing committee to revise the 1998 Guidelines for the Management of Patients With Valvular Heart Disease): Developed in collaboration with the Society of Cardiovascular Anesthesiologists: Endorsed by the Society for Cardiovascular Angiography and Interventions and the Society of Thoracic Surgeons. *Circulation* 2006;114(5):e84–e231.

4. Nishimura RA, et al. 2014 AHA/ACC guideline for the management of patients with valvular heart disease: Executive summary: A report of the American College of Cardiology/American Heart Association Task Force on Practice Guidelines. *J Am Coll Cardiol* 2014;63(22):2438–2488.

5. Assey ME, et al. Effect of catheter positioning on the variability of measured gradient in aortic stenosis. *Cathet Cardiovasc Diagn* 1993;30(4):287–292.

6. Pasipoularides A. Clinical assessment of ventricular ejection dynamics with and without outflow obstruction. *J Am Coll Cardiol* 1990;15(4):859–882.

7. Folland ED, et al. Is peripheral arterial pressure a satisfactory substitute for ascending aortic pressure when measuring aortic valve gradients? *J Am Coll Cardiol* 1984;4(6):1207–1212.

8. Hillis LD, et al. Analysis of factors affecting the variability of Fick versus indicator dilution measurements of cardiac output. *Am J Cardiol* 1985;56(12):764–768.

9. Blais C, et al. Projected valve area at normal flow rate improves the assessment of stenosis severity in patients with low-flow, low-gradient aortic stenosis: The multicenter TOPAS (Truly or Pseudo-Severe Aortic Stenosis) study. *Circulation* 2006;113(5):711–721.

10. Minners J, et al. Inconsistencies of echocardiographic criteria for the grading of aortic valve stenosis. *Eur Heart J* 2008;29(8):1043–1048.

11. Schwarz F, et al. The effect of aortic valve replacement on survival. *Circulation* 1982;66(5):1105–1110.

12. Smith N, et al. Severe aortic stenosis with impaired left ventricular function and clinical heart failure: Results of valve replacement. *Circulation* 1978;58(2):255–264.

13. Carabello BA, et al. Hemodynamic determinants of prognosis of aortic valve replacement in critical aortic stenosis and advanced congestive heart failure. *Circulation* 1980;62(1):42–48.

14. Connolly HM, et al. Severe aortic stenosis with low transvalvular gradient and severe left ventricular dysfunction: Result of aortic valve replacement in 52 patients. *Circulation* 2000;101(16):1940–1946.

15. Monin JL, et al. Low-gradient aortic stenosis: Operative risk stratification and predictors for long-term outcome: A multicenter study using dobutamine stress hemodynamics. *Circulation* 2003;108(3):319–324.

16. Nishimura RA, et al. Low-output, low-gradient aortic stenosis in patients with depressed left ventricular systolic function: The clinical utility of the dobutamine challenge in the catheterization laboratory. *Circulation* 2002;106(7):809–813.

17. Carabello BA, et al. *Cardiology Pearls*. Philadelphia: Hanley & Belfus, 1994.

18. Fougères E, et al. Outcomes of pseudo-severe aortic stenosis under conservative treatment. *Eur Heart J* 2012;33(19):2426–2433.

19. Lange RA, et al. Use of pulmonary capillary wedge pressure to assess severity of mitral stenosis: Is true left atrial pressure needed in this condition? *J Am Coll Cardiol* 1989;13(4):825–831.

20. Wang A, et al. Assessing the severity of mitral stenosis: Variability between noninvasive and invasive measurements in patients with symptomatic mitral valve stenosis. *Am Heart J* 1999;138(4 Pt 1):777–784.

21. Hakki AH, et al. A simplified valve formula for the calculation of stenotic cardiac valve areas. *Circulation* 1981;63(5):1050–1055.

22. Johnson LW, et al. Pulmonic stenosis in the adult. Long-term follow-up results. *N Engl J Med* 1972;287(23):1159–1163.

23. Carabello BA, et al. *Aortic Regurgitation in Cardiology Pearls*. 1st edn. Philadelphia, PA: Hanley & Belfus, 1994:46.

24. Fuchs RM, et al. Limitations of pulmonary wedge V waves in diagnosing mitral regurgitation. *Am J Cardiol* 1982;49(4):849–854.

25. Grossman W. Stress testing during cardiac catheterization: Exercise and pacing tachycardia. In: Baim DS, ed. *Grossman's Cardiac Catheterization, Angiography, and Intervention*. 7th edn. Philadelphia, PA: Lippincott, Williams & Wilkins, 2006:283–303.

12

Hemodynamic assessment for restriction, constriction, hypertrophic cardiomyopathy, and cardiac tamponade

BRINDER KANDA, MARIO GÖSSL, AND PAUL SORAJJA

INTRODUCTION

Whereas the cardiac hemodynamics of myocardial and pericardial disease can be examined in many patients with noninvasive testing, cardiac catheterization remains the gold standard for these assessments. Cardiac catheterization provides data through direct determination of flow and intracardiac pressures, whose measurement with Doppler echocardiography or other noninvasive evaluations remains limited. The principal indication for invasive hemodynamic catheterization is to resolve discrepant clinical and noninvasive findings when the data will incrementally impact the management of the patient. In patients with multiple or complex lesions, cardiac catheterization may be the only reliable and accurate method for hemodynamic assessment.

APPROACH TO HEMODYNAMIC ASSESSMENT

General considerations

For patients with myocardial or pericardial disease, the approach to the invasive hemodynamic assessment should be individualized. Proper planning of the procedure requires full knowledge of what data are known, what clinically relevant information is required, and a comprehensive differential diagnosis of the patient's problems. The vascular access sites and approach to gathering data should be delineated fully before proceeding (Tables 12.1 and 12.2).

While all patients should be fasting before the cardiac catheterization, intravenous (IV) fluids should be administered to patients who have a long waiting period between their last oral intake and the procedure. This prevents the hemodynamic measurements from being taken during a low-output, low-volume state. Patients can be lightly sedated, but should be awake to simulate the hemodynamic milieu of their outpatient state with close approximation to the heart rate and blood pressure that occurs in their usual daily activities. No parenteral oxygen should be administered prior to the procedure to allow measurements of oxygen saturations.

Right and left heart catheterization is recommended for assessment of pericardial disease, restrictive cardiomyopathy, and hypertrophic cardiomyopathy (HCM). Examination for disorders of diastolic dysfunction and cardiac tamponade does not require left heart catheterization, though these abnormalities are readily assessable with left ventricular and left atrial pressures. For arterial and venous access, the femoral sites can be utilized in most situations; however, the internal jugular approach will facilitate the performance of right heart catheterization in cases involving severe tricuspid regurgitation with enlarged right-sided chambers. The internal jugular approach should also be favored when an endomyocardial biopsy is required (e.g., suspicion of infiltrative cardiomyopathy), and if hemodynamic information during supine bicycle exercise is desired. For patients with HCM,

Table 12.1 Indications for hemodynamic assessment

Hypertrophic cardiomyopathy

Assess LVOT obstruction; assess severity of mitral regurgitation; evaluate diastolic function and perform alcohol septal ablation

Restrictive cardiomyopathy

Confirm diagnosis and rule out other potential causes of heart failure (e.g., constrictive pericarditis, cor pulmonale); measure pulmonary arteriolar resistance for potential transplant candidates; perform endomyocardial biopsy

Constrictive pericarditis

Establish the diagnosis and examine for other potential causes of heart failure

Cardiac tamponade

Invasive assessment is not necessary for the diagnosis of tamponade, but the typical hemodynamic findings of tamponade during cardiac catheterization need to be understood.

Note: LVOT, left ventricular outflow tract.

transseptal catheterization should be considered in the evaluation of left ventricular outflow tract (LVOT) obstruction. The advantages of transseptal catheterization over a retroaortic approach are discussed separately in the section on HCM.

Equipment

Accurate measurement of intracardiac pressures with fluid-filled catheters requires the use of rigid, large-bore catheters with minimization of the tubing length between the catheter and pressure transducer. Awareness of potential errors of measurement due to catheter whip, entrapment, damping, and other artifacts is always necessary during an invasive hemodynamic study. The use of coronary catheters with single-end holes and the potential for entrapment (e.g., right Judkins catheter) should be avoided. In patients with intracavitary gradients (e.g., HCM and known or suspected left ventricular outflow tract ([LVOT]) obstruction), multiple shaft side holes on a left ventriculography catheter (i.e., pigtail) also will lead to errors in the measurement of the subaortic pressure and thus should not be used in these patients.

Fluid-filled catheters can reliably measure mean and absolute intracardiac pressures. For analysis of pressure waveforms, however, instantaneous recordings with high-fidelity micromanometer tip catheters should be utilized (Millar Instruments, Houston, TX). These catheters should be calibrated to fluid-filled pressures at baseline, and calibration needs to be repeated following any catheter repositioning. For right heart pressure measurements, a 6- or 7-Fr single-lumen balloon wedge catheter (Arrow International, Teleflex Medical, Research Triangle Park, NC) is relatively

Table 12.2 Fundamentals of hemodynamic assessment

- A comprehensive differential diagnosis of the patient's clinical problems aids in planning the invasive hemodynamic evaluation.
- LVOT obstruction in HCM is dynamic and highly dependent on ventricular load and contractile state. Physical or pharmacological provocation should be performed to determine the presence of latent obstruction in symptomatic patients with no evidence of significant LVOT gradient at rest.
- In patients with obstructive HCM, the typical response on the post-PVC beat is a decrease in the pulse pressure and an increase in the LVOT gradient (Brockenbrough sign). In patients with fixed aortic stenosis, the pulse pressure increases on the post-PVC beat.
- Transseptal catheterization provides the most complete and accurate hemodynamic information in patients with HCM. A retroaortic approach can also be used with the understanding of the potential pitfalls.
- Invasive assessment of restrictive cardiomyopathy and constrictive pericarditis should entail the use of high-fidelity, micromanometer tip catheters to avoid artifacts due to overdamping.
- Early rapid ventricular filling (i.e., dip and plateau pattern) can be seen in patients with restrictive cardiomyopathy, constrictive pericarditis, or any volume overload state that results in a decrease in effective myocardial or pericardial compliance.
- Both traditional and respiratory criteria should be utilized to distinguish restrictive cardiomyopathy from constrictive pericarditis. Respiratory criteria are: (i) *dissociation* of intrathoracic and intracavitary pressures and (ii) *discordance* of the right and left ventricular systolic pressures.
- The hemodynamic hallmarks of cardiac tamponade are pulsus paradoxus and loss of the descent in the atrial waveform.
- Endomyocardial biopsy has low clinical yield and does not significantly impact therapy in most cardiac disease states. However, endomyocardial biopsy should be considered in patients with possible acute fulminant giant cell myocarditis, where immunosuppressive therapy may be beneficial.
- Accurate determination of PAR and its reversibility is an essential component of the comprehensive invasive hemodynamic evaluation.
- With few exceptions, pericardiocentesis is best performed under echocardiographic guidance.

Note: HCM, hypertrophic cardiomyopathy; LVOT, left ventricular outflow tract; PAR, pulmonary arteriolar resistance; PVC, premature ventricular contraction.

rigid with a large bore that will accommodate a 2-Fr high-fidelity micromanometer tip catheter.

For patients with irregular heart rates (e.g., atrial fibrillation), temporary pacing should be considered to maintain consistent R–R intervals to improve the diagnostic interpretation of the hemodynamic findings. If possible, continuous recording of all hemodynamic pressures should be made to allow retrospective review of these pressures throughout the entire study.

Cardiac catheterization

The following sequence of catheter placement and advancement allows prospective examination of the relation of pressures between the left- and right-sided chambers:

1. Following vascular access, the right heart catheter is used to acquire oxygen saturations from the inferior and superior vena cavae to calculate mixed venous oxygen content and to screen for intracardiac shunts.
2. The right atrial pressure is measured with the catheter in the mid-portion of the right atrium (RA) and turned to the lateral wall to avoid prolapse across the tricuspid valve.
3. Ascending aortic pressure is then measured by placement of a left heart catheter, followed by advancement of the catheter into the left ventricle (LV) to measure simultaneous left ventricular and right atrial pressures.
4. The right heart catheter is then advanced into the right ventricle (RV) to measure simultaneous right ventricular and left ventricular pressures.
5. The right heart catheter is then placed into the pulmonary artery (PA). Simultaneous saturations from the PA and LV are obtained for calculation of cardiac output by the Fick method.
6. Finally, the PA wedge pressure is obtained with position confirmation by oxygen saturation. Pulmonary arteriolar resistance (PAR) is then calculated from these measurements.

HYPERTROPHIC CARDIOMYOPATHY

HCM is a common, inheritable cardiac disorder with a prevalence of 1 in 500 in the general population. Hundreds of causative mutations in over 14 different genes have been identified.[1]

Pathophysiology

Diastolic abnormalities are the major pathophysiological mechanisms contributing to signs and symptoms for patients with HCM. These abnormalities arise from impaired myocardial relaxation and poor compliance in the presence of altered loading conditions, ventricular non-uniformity, myocardial ischemia, and severe hypertrophy. The cumulative result of diastolic dysfunction is an increase in left ventricular filling pressures, which leads to typical symptoms of dyspnea and angina. In patients with HCM, there may be a significant discrepancy between the left atrial pressure and left ventricular end-diastolic pressure.

Therefore, measurements of both of these pressures should be made if possible.

Dynamic LVOT obstruction is present in three-quarters of patients with HCM.[2] Because the presence of LVOT obstruction serves as the basis for therapy, it is important to document the presence and severity of the LVOT gradient. Two mechanisms lead to the development of dynamic LVOT obstruction: (1) septal hypertrophy and narrowing of the LVOT promote the generation of Venturi forces that accelerate during ventricular emptying and pull the mitral apparatus anteriorly;[2] and (2) anterior papillary muscle displacement subjects the mitral leaflets to systolic intraventricular currents that drag the apparatus anteriorly. Decreased mitral leaflet coaptation occurs because of systolic anterior motion of the mitral valve, leading to mitral regurgitation in patients with LVOT obstruction.[3] It is important to note the dynamic nature of LVOT obstruction and secondary mitral regurgitation, and the marked sensitivity of these abnormalities to changes in preload, afterload, and the contractile state of the LV. Mitral regurgitation may be related to intrinsic valve abnormalities in a subset of patients, and such abnormalities have implications for septal reduction therapy. Intrinsic abnormalities of the mitral valve with elongated leaflets and abnormal papillary muscle insertion have been increasingly recognized in recent studies of HCM patients.[4]

During catheterization, HCM should be suspected when there is a small, hypertrophied LV with hyperdynamic systolic function on left ventriculography. Left ventriculography may demonstrate regional hypertrophy, such as basal septal hypertrophy (Figure 12.1). In patients with the apical form of HCM, a typical spade-shaped configuration is seen on left ventriculography (Figure 12.2). A dynamic LVOT obstruction can also be suspected if there is a gradient between the left ventricular apex and base, or if a "spike and dome" pattern is present on the aortic pressure trace.

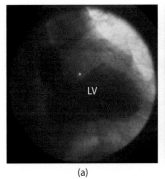 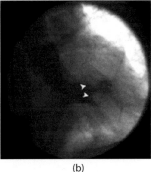

(a)   (b)

Figure 12.1 Left ventriculogram from a patient with severe basal septal hypertrophy due to hypertrophic cardiomyopathy. End-diastolic frame showing severe basal septal hypertrophy (asterisk) **(a)**. End-systolic frame showing hyperdynamic systolic function with papillary muscle hypertrophy (arrowheads) **(b)**. LV, left ventricle. (From Sorajja, P., Nishimura, R.A., *Myocardial and pericardial disease assessment and management, CathSAP-3*. American College of Cardiology Foundation. With permission.)

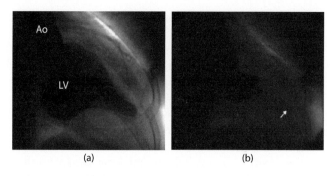

Figure 12.2 Left ventriculogram from a patient with severe apical hypertrophy due to hypertrophic cardiomyopathy. End-diastolic frame shows the typical "spade-shaped" configuration seen on ventriculography **(a)**. End-systolic frame of the same patient showing systolic obliteration of the left ventricular cavity with a small apical pouch (arrow) **(b)**. Ao, ascending aorta; LV, left ventricle. (From Sorajja P, Nishimura RA. *Myocardial and pericardial disease assessment and management, CathSAP-3.* American College of Cardiology Foundation. With permission.)

Indications for cardiac catheterization

For the majority of patients with HCM, two-dimensional (2D) and Doppler echocardiography reliably assess the presence and severity of LVOT obstruction.[5] However, in some circumstances, echocardiography may be inaccurate or significantly limited. Mitral regurgitation frequently accompanies LVOT obstruction in HCM. The presence of mitral regurgitation may contaminate the LVOT signal, resulting in erroneous or inaccurate estimates of the LVOT gradient (Figure 12.3). The velocity jet of mitral regurgitation that occurs secondary to LVOT obstruction also is eccentric, and thus, mitral regurgitation is difficult

to quantify with current noninvasive methods in patients with HCM. In some patients, a high intracavitary velocity can be mistaken on Doppler echocardiography for a significant LVOT gradient, and may require further invasive assessment.[6] For patients with combined valvular stenosis and subaortic obstruction, cardiac catheterization may be necessary to assess the relative contributions of these different levels of obstruction. For patients with cardiovascular symptoms and no evidence of significant LVOT obstruction at rest, cardiac catheterization with provocative maneuvers is utilized to delineate the presence of latent LVOT obstruction.[7]

Cardiac catheterization

Measurement of the LVOT gradient should be made with simultaneous ascending aortic and left ventricular pressures. Because of peripheral amplification, femoral tracing should not be used. In patients with significant LVOT obstruction, a typical spike and dome pattern appears in the ascending aortic pressure (Figure 12.4). The optimal method for measurement of LVOT obstruction is to measure the left ventricular pressure via a transseptal approach to avoid catheter entrapment. The catheter can be placed in the left ventricular inflow region immediately distal to the opening of the mitral valve leaflets (Figure 12.5). Using a transseptal sheath with a side arm, simultaneous left atrial pressure also can be obtained (Figure 12.4).

If transseptal catheterization cannot be performed, left ventricular pressure is obtained by a retrograde approach across the aortic valve. In these instances, a pigtail catheter with shaft side holes should not be used. Importantly, catheter entrapment may occur with left ventricular pressure measured from a retrograde approach and may falsely elevate

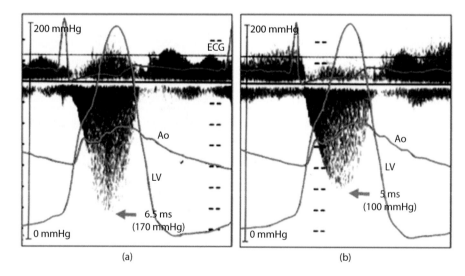

Figure 12.3 Contamination of the Doppler left ventricular outflow tract signal with mitral regurgitation in a patient with obstructive hypertrophic cardiomyopathy. Contamination from mitral regurgitation leads to an erroneous calculation of the left ventricular outflow tract gradient **(a)**. The correct Doppler left ventricular outflow tract gradient **(b)**. Cardiac catheterization is indicated when it is difficult to separate the velocities and the severity of left ventricular outflow tract obstruction is unclear. Ao, ascending aorta pressure; ECG, electrocardiogram; LV, left ventricular pressure.

the LVOT gradient. If catheter entrapment is present, there will be a lack of systolic pulsation when the catheter is disconnected and the left ventricular pressure contour will be dampened. In the retrograde approach, it is also important to confirm that the catheter position is beneath the level of

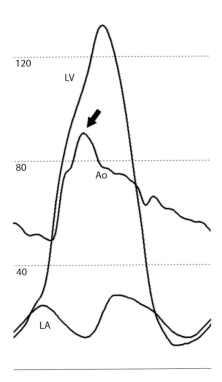

Figure 12.4 Dynamic left ventricular outflow obstruction in hypertrophic cardiomyopathy. Arrow indicates typical "spike and dome" configuration, indicating dynamic systolic obstruction. Ao, ascending aorta; LA, left atrium; LV, left ventricle.

LVOT obstruction (Figure 12.6). A hand contrast injection should be performed to ensure that the end of the catheter is floating freely within the left ventricular cavity.

The dynamic nature of LVOT obstruction due to HCM will lead to a Brockenbrough response. On the beat following a premature contraction, the LVOT gradient increases and the pulse pressure decreases (Figure 12.7). Because of its high sensitivity to loading conditions, variation of the LVOT gradient may also be seen in different phases of respiration (Figure 12.8).

If the resting LVOT gradient is <50 mmHg in a patient with HCM, provocative maneuvers should be performed in the catheterization laboratory. These maneuvers include the Valsalva maneuver, amyl nitrate inhalation, and drug provocation. The optimal drug to use for provoking LVOT obstruction is isoproterenol because of its beta-1 and beta-2 agonist activity.[8] Simultaneous echocardiography should be performed during isoproterenol infusion to determine the location of obstruction (e.g., systolic anterior motion of the mitral valve, and mid-cavitary obstruction) when a gradient is detected during these maneuvers. It is the subset of patients who have both systolic anterior motion and LVOT gradient >50 mmHg (either at rest or during provocation) who will benefit from septal reduction therapy.[5]

RESTRICTIVE CARDIOMYOPATHY

Restrictive cardiomyopathy is characterized by a nondilated, rigid ventricle that results in severe diastolic dysfunction and restrictive filling. Desmin and troponin I mutations have been described in patients with restrictive cardiomyopathy.[9-11] Infiltrative cardiomyopathies, such as amyloidosis, hemochromatosis, and sarcoidosis, can present as restrictive cardiomyopathy.

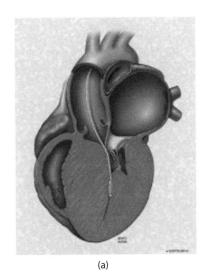 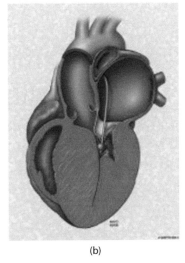

(a)   (b)

Figure 12.5 Transseptal versus retrograde approach for assessment of left ventricular outflow tract obstruction in hypertrophic cardiomyopathy. In the retrograde approach, the catheter becomes easily entrapped and leads to erroneous left ventricular pressure measurements (a). In the transseptal approach, the left ventricular catheter can be easily positioned near the mitral inflow (b). This catheter position leads to the most accurate measurements of left ventricular pressure in patients with subaortic obstruction. (From Elesber, A., et al., *Am. J. Cardiol.*, 101(4), 516–520, 2008. With permission.)

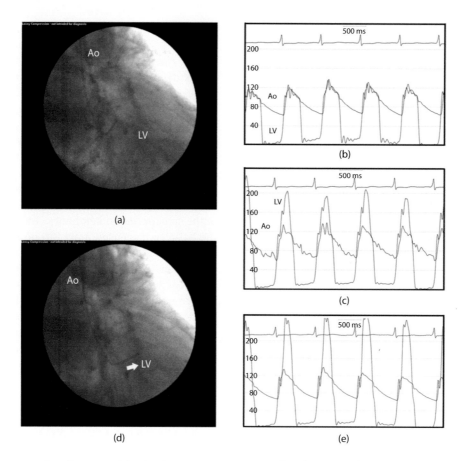

Figure 12.6 Importance of catheter position in the retroaortic approach in hypertrophic cardiomyopathy. When a retroaortic approach is utilized for assessment of LVOT obstruction in hypertrophic cardiomyopathy, it is important to confirm that the catheter position is beneath the level of LVOT obstruction. A catheter in the ascending aorta and a catheter in the left ventricle **(a)**. With the catheter in this position, the LVOT gradient is either not detected **(b)** or measured to be approximately 80 mmHg **(c)**. However, the true gradient is obtained by advancing the left ventricular catheter further into the chamber **(d)**, leading to the correct LVOT gradient of 120 mmHg **(e)**. Ao, ascending aorta; LV, left ventricle; LVOT, left ventricular outflow tract.

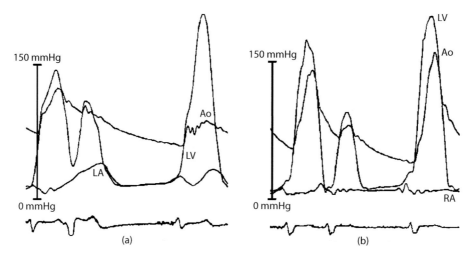

Figure 12.7 Dynamic left ventricular outflow obstruction (Brockenbrough sign) in hypertrophic cardiomyopathy **(a)** versus a patient with aortic stenosis **(b)**. On the beat after a premature ventricular contraction, the increased inotropy leads to dynamic outflow tract obstruction. The left ventricular outflow tract gradient increases and the pulse pressure decreases. Conversely, in a patient with aortic stenosis, the increase in contractility leads to an increase in stroke volume and pulse pressure. Ao, ascending aorta; LA, left atrium; LV, left ventricle; RA, right atrium. (From Sorajja P., Nishimura, R.A. The assessment and therapy of valvular heart disease in the cardiac catheterization laboratory. In: Willerson, J.P., Cohn, J.N., Wellens, H.H., et al., eds. *Cardiovascular Medicine. 3rd ed.* London: Springer, 2007:463–486. With permission.)

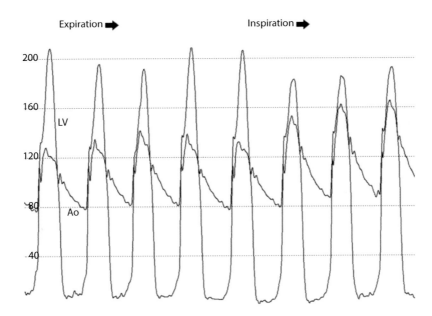

Figure 12.8 Respiratory variation of the LVOT gradient in hypertrophic cardiomyopathy. LVOT obstruction in hypertrophic cardiomyopathy is highly sensitive to ventricular load. This sensitivity is evident in this patient during quiet respiration. In expiration, the transmural pressure decreases, leading to a decrease in afterload and an increase in LVOT obstruction. During inspiration, the drop in thoracic pressure leads to an increase in transmural pressure and afterload, leading to a decrease in LVOT obstruction. Ao, ascending aorta; LV, left ventricle; LVOT, left ventricular outflow tract.

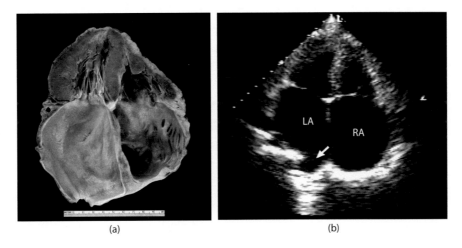

Figure 12.9 Gross specimen showing severe biatrial enlargement due to restrictive cardiomyopathy in panel **(a)**. Biatrial enlargement is easily seen on echocardiography (apical four-chamber transthoracic view) in panel **(b)**; arrow shows dilated pulmonary vein that suggests elevated diastolic filling pressures. LA, left atrium; RA, right atrium. (Courtesy of William D. Edwards, M.D., Mayo Clinic.)

Endomyocardial biopsy can be performed for patients in whom restrictive cardiomyopathy due to infiltrative disorders is suspected (see section entitled "Endomyocardial Biopsy"). Restrictive cardiomyopathy may also result from radiation therapy and eosinophilia syndromes (Figure 12.9).

The diagnosis of restrictive cardiomyopathy is made by the presence of diastolic dysfunction, dilated atria, and the absence of ventricular hypertrophy or dilatation on noninvasive imaging. In these patients, systolic function is preserved or out of proportion to the degree of diastolic dysfunction. For patients presenting with restrictive cardiomyopathy, the major differential diagnosis that must be considered is constrictive pericarditis. If constrictive pericarditis is present, complete pericardiectomy can result in relief of symptoms and improvement of longevity.[12] However, for patients with idiopathic restrictive cardiomyopathy, there is no curative treatment apart from cardiac transplantation.[13] During cardiac catheterization, it is also important to evaluate other potential causes of heart failure.

The presence of severe intrinsic pulmonary hypertension, tricuspid regurgitation, and left ventricular or right ventricular failure will lead to symptoms and signs similar to those of constrictive pericarditis and restrictive cardiomyopathy.

Cardiac catheterization

The major abnormality in restrictive cardiomyopathy is the presence of significantly elevated filling pressures in all four cardiac chambers. Early rapid ventricular filling leads to a "dip and plateau" pattern or "square root sign" in the ventricular pressure curves during early diastole, and rapid x and y descents on the atrial pressure curves (Figure 12.10).[14] Because underdamping from fluid-filled catheters can mimic early rapid ventricular filling, high-fidelity micromanometer catheters should be used if early rapid ventricular filling is suspected.[15]

Both restrictive cardiomyopathy and constrictive pericarditis present with evidence of early rapid diastolic filling and elevation of diastolic pressures that are out of proportion to systolic dysfunction. Traditional criteria for differentiation of restrictive cardiomyopathy from constrictive pericarditis have included the following:

- Left ventricular end-diastolic pressure exceeds right ventricular end-diastolic pressure by <5 mmHg.
- PA systolic pressure is >50 mmHg.
- In the RV, end-diastolic pressure is <0.3 of systolic pressure.

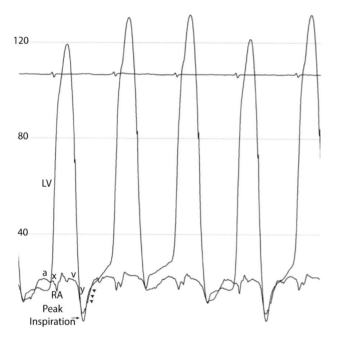

Figure 12.10 Early rapid ventricular filling. In the right atrial tracing, there are rapid x and y descents. The y descent of the right atrial pressure tracing corresponds to the early rapid filling phase of the ventricular pressure tracing, which demonstrates the typical dip and plateau pattern (arrow). These hemodynamic tracings were taken using high-fidelity micromanometer catheters from a patient with constrictive pericarditis. LV, left ventricle; RA, right atrium. (Courtesy of Paul Sorajja, M.D.)

Nonetheless, these traditional criteria have been found to have poor specificity, and they cannot be used in isolation to differentiate restrictive cardiomyopathy from constrictive pericarditis. Conversely, changes in the hemodynamic pressure relationships during respiration have been shown to be useful in distinguishing between these two disorders (see section entitled "Constrictive Pericarditis").

CONSTRICTIVE PERICARDITIS

Constrictive pericarditis results from pericardial inflammation, fibrosis, and possibly calcification with subsequent loss of elasticity.[16] Radiation therapy, cardiac surgery, trauma, and systemic diseases that affect the pericardium (e.g., connective tissue disease, tuberculosis, and malignancy) can lead to constrictive pericarditis.[17]

In patients with constrictive pericarditis, the noncompliant pericardium is rigid, impairs diastolic filling, and prevents the complete transmission of intrathoracic pressure to the intracardiac cavities. Ventricular filling rapidly occurs in early diastole and terminates abruptly because of pericardial restraint. The diastolic pressures become equalized, or nearly equalized, in all four cardiac chambers. The total intracardiac volume is fixed by the noncompliant pericardium. Because the ventricular septum is not affected in constrictive pericarditis, bulging of the septum toward the LV occurs during inspiration and returns toward the RV during expiration, leading to marked enhancement of ventricular interaction. This ventricular interaction leads to reciprocal changes in the filling and emptying of the RVs and LVs.

Cardiac catheterization

Hemodynamic evaluation of the patient with suspected constrictive pericarditis is accomplished with comprehensive, simultaneous right and left heart catheterization. High-fidelity micromanometer catheters should be utilized to avoid underdamping artifact.[14] For patients with atrial fibrillation, temporary pacing should be performed to create constant heart rate intervals during the study.

Criteria for the diagnosis of constrictive pericarditis include both traditional hemodynamic criteria and dynamic respiratory criteria. Respiration affects ventricular filling in constrictive pericarditis in a manner that is distinct from restrictive cardiomyopathy.[18,19]

- In patients with constriction, the inspiratory fall in thoracic pressure affects the pulmonary wedge pressure, but the ventricular pressure is shielded from respiratory pressure changes by pericardial constriction. By lowering pulmonary wedge pressure and presumably left atrial pressure, inspiration leads to a decrease in pressure gradient for ventricular filling. Reciprocal changes occur in right ventricular filling that are mediated by the ventricular septum (not by increased systemic venous return). These findings are described as *dissociation* of the intrathoracic and intracavitary pressures (Figure 12.11).[20]

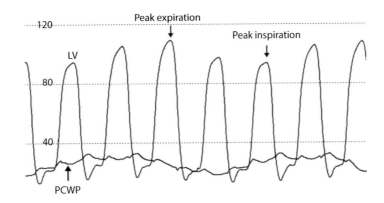

Figure 12.11 Dissociation of intracavitary and intrathoracic pressures in constrictive pericarditis. In patients with constrictive pericarditis, inspiration leads to a decrease in ventricular filling by decreasing intrathoracic pressure relative to ventricular diastolic pressure. Conversely, during expiration, positive intrathoracic pressure leads to an increase in ventricular filling. These respiratory effects can be seen by examining the changes in the pressure gradient between the PCWP and ventricular early diastolic pressure (gray). LV, left ventricle; PCWP, pulmonary capillary wedge pressure. (Courtesy of Paul Sorajja, M.D.)

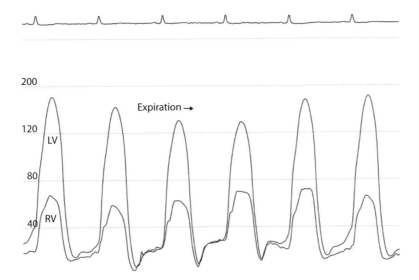

Figure 12.12 Enhancement of ventricular interdependence. In patients with constrictive pericarditis, the total ventricular volume is fixed by the noncompliant pericardium. Thus, reciprocal respiratory changes in the filling of each ventricle occur. These changes are described as discordance in pulse pressure, systolic pressure, or stroke volume between the right and left ventricles during the respiration. LV, left ventricle; RV, right ventricle. (Courtesy of Paul Sorajja, M.D.)

- In patients with constriction, the enhancement of ventricular interaction leads to *discordant* right and left ventricular pressures. This discordance typically manifests as reciprocal changes in stroke volume, pulse pressure, or peak systolic pressure during respiration (Figure 12.12).

Both dissociation of intrathoracic and intracavitary pressures and enhancement of ventricular interaction are not present in patients with restrictive cardiomyopathy. In these patients, inspiration lowers the pulmonary wedge and left ventricular diastolic pressures equally. Thus, the pressure gradient for ventricular filling is virtually unchanged during respiration. Because ventricular interaction is not enhanced, the left ventricular and right ventricular pressures are *concordant* throughout the respiratory cycle in patients with restrictive cardiomyopathy.

Equalization of pressures in all cardiac chambers is commonly said to be a major criterion for constrictive pericarditis but is nonspecific. This equalization also may be present in patients with restrictive cardiomyopathy or other disease states when acute volume overload leads to pericardial restraint. Examples of this phenomenon include right ventricular dilatation after right ventricular infarction, severe decompensated left heart failure, severe tricuspid insufficiency, and acute mitral regurgitation secondary to chordal rupture. In addition, equalization of diastolic pressures may not be present in a patient with constrictive pericarditis who has been diuresed and has low to normal right atrial pressure. In these patients, the cardiac output will be low, and fluid challenge will be necessary to unveil the hemodynamic findings of constrictive pericarditis.[20]

Tricuspid regurgitation

The differentiation between tricuspid regurgitation, restrictive cardiomyopathy, and constrictive pericarditis can be difficult due to similar hemodynamic findings. Enhancement of ventricular interaction (see above) certainly helps differentiate constriction from restriction but can also be seen in severe tricuspid regurgitation with right heart failure. Patients with severe tricuspid regurgitation and constrictive pericarditis both show early rapid filling waves and elevation and equalization of left and right ventricular end-diastolic pressures (Figure 12.13).

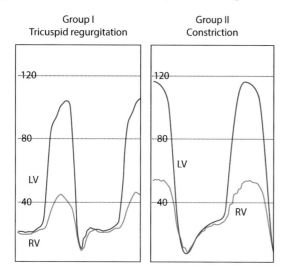

Figure 12.13 Representative hemodynamic tracings from patients with severe tricuspid regurgitation and constrictive pericarditis. Early rapid filling waves and elevation and equalization of left and right ventricular end-diastolic pressures are seen in both subsets of patients. LV, left ventricle; RV, right ventricle. (From Jaber, W.A., et al., *Heart*, 95(17), 1449–1454, 2009. With permission.)

With deep inspiration, however, diastolic pressures separate in patients with severe tricuspid regurgitation with a significantly higher right ventricular diastolic pressure. In addition, the rapid right ventricular filling wave becomes deeper and steeper (Figure 12.14). This is in contrast to patients with constrictive pericarditis where left ventricular diastolic pressure and right ventricular rapid filling do not change significantly.[21]

In a comparison of patients with severe tricuspid regurgitation or constrictive pericarditis, the most reliable difference was the change in left and right ventricular diastolic pressures (Figure 12.15). In contrast, elevated right atrial pressure, early rapid ventricular filling, expiratory equalization of ventricular diastolic pressures, and even interventricular dependence, were similar in both groups.

CARDIAC TAMPONADE

Cardiac tamponade may result from any disorder that causes a pericardial effusion. The pericardium normally contains 15–50 mL of fluid between its parietal and visceral layers, and the intrapericardial pressure approximates intrapleural pressure (–5 to +5 cm H_2O). Tamponade occurs when intrapericardial pressure exceeds intracardiac pressure.[22] The hemodynamic effect of a pericardial effusion may be acute or gradual, depending on the amount and rate of fluid accumulation. The most common etiology of tamponade is malignancy, with breast and lung cancer being the most frequent. Other important etiologies are idiopathic or viral pericarditis, aortic dissection with disruption of the aortic valve annulus, complications of invasive cardiac procedures, uremia, tuberculosis, and pericarditis or myocardial rupture from

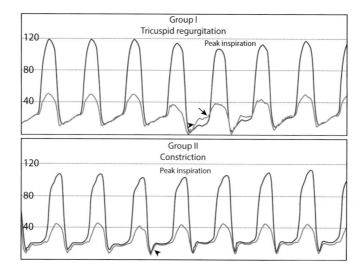

Figure 12.14 Representative hemodynamic tracings from patients with severe tricuspid regurgitation and constrictive pericarditis within a respiratory cycle. In patients with severe tricuspid regurgitation (upper panel) deep inspiration leads to separation of diastolic pressures (arrow) and the rapid right ventricular filling wave becomes deeper and steeper (arrowhead). (From Sorajja, P., *Cardiol. Clin.*, 29(2), 191–199, 2011. With permission.)

myocardial infarction (MI). Unusual manifestations of cardiac tamponade include the following:

- *Low-pressure tamponade*, which is tamponade without elevated jugular venous pressure because the intracardiac filling pressures are low. Examples of this manifestation are patients with malignancy or tuberculosis that is complicated by severe dehydration.
- *Localized tamponade*, which occurs when a loculated pericardial effusion is tactically located to cause impairment of ventricular filling. An example of this manifestation is in the postoperative setting, where a loculated effusion is present in the posterior pericardial space adjacent to the atria. A posterior effusion may not be seen with transesophageal echocardiography (TEE) and must be carefully sought in a postoperative patient with hemodynamic instability.
- *Pneumopericardium*, which may be caused by gas-forming bacterial pericarditis following penetrating chest trauma.

Cardiac tamponade should be considered when there is a compatible history, hypotension, and an elevated jugular

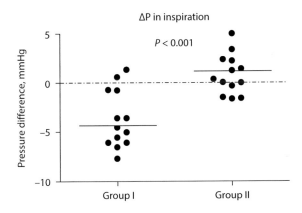

Figure 12.15 Scatterplot of the difference between left (LVEDP) and right ventricular end-diastolic pressure (RVEDP) during deep inspiration. On average LVEDP is lower than RVEDP in patients with tricuspid regurgitation. (From Jaber, W.A., et al., *Heart*, 95(17), 1449–1454, 2009. With permission.)

venous pressure or pulsus paradoxus.[23] The chest X-ray (e.g., "water bottle heart") and electrocardiography (e.g., electrical alternans, sinus tachycardia) may be helpful. However, echocardiography is the primary test for the diagnosis. Specific signs include collapse of the RA and RV, ventricular septal shifting with respiration, and enlargement of the inferior vena cava. Respiratory variation in Doppler mitral inflow velocities occurs early in the evolution of tamponade. The changes in mitral inflow are highly sensitive, and can precede changes in cardiac output, blood pressure, and other echocardiographic evidence of tamponade.

Cardiac catheterization

Although cardiac catheterization is usually not needed to make the diagnosis of cardiac tamponade, recognition of the typical hemodynamic findings has gained renewed importance in the era of increasingly complex cardiac interventions. When performed, the right atrial pressure tracing in tamponade will demonstrate a prominent *x*-descent and blunted or obliterated *y*-descent (Figure 12.16).[19] Preservation of the x-descent occurs because systolic ejection decreases the intracardiac volume and leads to a transient reduction in intrapericardial and right atrial pressures. During the remainder of the cardiac cycle, elevated intrapericardial pressure impairs ventricular filling and leads to blunting or obliteration of the *y*-descent. Intrapericardial pressure rises with fluid accumulation and pericardial restraint. Venous return becomes impaired once the intrapericardial pressure exceeds the filling pressure of the heart. This impairment leads to a reduction in cardiac output, followed by increases in pulmonary venous and jugular venous pressures. During inspiration, there is a fall in the driving pressure to fill the LV, followed by a reduction in ventricular filling, stroke volume, and consequently, the pulse pressure. These events during inspiration cause the hallmark finding of *pulsus paradoxus* in patients with tamponade.

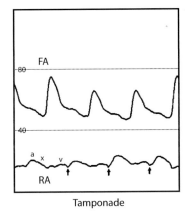

Tamponade

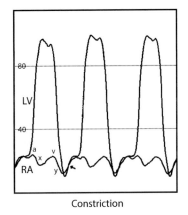

Constriction

Figure 12.16 Tamponade versus constrictive pericarditis. In cardiac tamponade, the *y* descent in the right atrial pressure tracing becomes blunted because of impairment of ventricular filling (arrows). The FA pressure tracing also demonstrates pulsus paradoxus seen on the second and third full systolic tracings. However, in patients with constrictive pericarditis, there is early rapid diastolic filling that manifests as a prominent *y* descent in the right atrial tracing and as a "dip and plateau" sign in the left ventricular pressure tracing (arrow). FA, femoral artery; LV, left ventricle; RA, right atrium.

SPECIAL ISSUES

Endomyocardial biopsy

Endomyocardial biopsy provides myocardial tissue for microscopic analysis and can be safely performed using either an internal jugular or femoral venous access.[24] Particular care must be taken to target the apical septum, and to avoid sampling from the right ventricular free wall and the tricuspid valve (Figure 12.17). Biplane fluoroscopy and/or simultaneous echocardiography are helpful in preventing this from occurring. Complications are infrequent (<1%), but include tricuspid valve injury and tamponade from cardiac perforation.

Before proceeding with endomyocardial biopsy, it is important to consider both the expected yield of the biopsy, risks of the procedure, and its therapeutic implications. Endomyocardial biopsy can diagnose myocarditis and infiltrative disorders causing cardiomyopathy. However, its sensitivity is limited in disorders with patchy myocardial involvement (e.g., sarcoidosis and lymphocytic myocarditis). Moreover, the histological findings, even if positive, may not alter therapy in other disorders. Thus, few indications for endomyocardial biopsy exist in patients with left ventricular systolic dysfunction. For infiltrative cardiomyopathies, there are usually clinical clues in the history, electrocardiography, and laboratory testing, such as iron studies, protein electrophoresis, and peripheral eosinophilia. In patients presenting with acute fulminant myocarditis, endomyocardial biopsy may identify giant cell myocarditis, which may respond favorably to immunosuppressive therapy.

Pulmonary arteriolar resistance

Patients being considered for cardiac transplantation require cardiac catheterization to ensure suitability for cardiac transplantation. In these patients, an accurate measurement of PAR is critically important in their evaluation. In other patients, measurement of PAR also can be helpful to determine appropriate medical therapy (e.g., vasodilators). Thus, determination of PAR should be a routine component of a comprehensive invasive hemodynamic evaluation. Calculation of the PAR is made with measurements of the PA pressure, left atrial pressure, and cardiac output. The pulmonary capillary wedge pressure (PCWP) approximates left atrial pressure except in rare circumstances (e.g., cor triatriatum, pulmonary veno-occlusive disease).

$$PAR(Wood\ units) = \frac{mean\ PA\ pressure - mean\ LA\ pressure\ (or\ PCWP)}{Pulmonary\ flow\ (or\ cardiac\ output)}$$

For patients with elevated PAR, cardiac transplantation has a poor outcome due to the high afterload imposed on the RV. When the PAR is elevated, vasodilators or inhaled

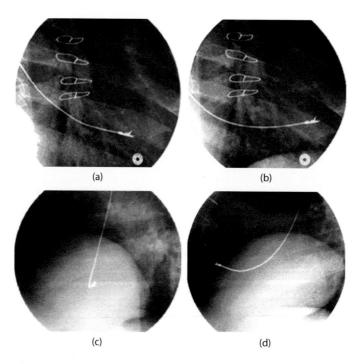

(a)   (b)

(c)   (d)

Figure 12.17 Proper technique for performing endomyocardial biopsy of the right ventricle. Images **(a)** and **(c)** are from one patient; images **(b)** and **(d)** are from a second patient. The bioptome is in a similar position on the anteroposterior view in both patients **(a)** and **(b)**. However, in the lateral views, the bioptome is safely positioned against the septum only in the patient on the left **(c)**. In the patient on the right **(d)**, the bioptome is directed anteriorly against the right ventricular free wall. This could result in perforation and cardiac tamponade. (Courtesy of Paul Sorajja, M.D.)

nitric oxide should be used to determine the degree of its reversibility. For patients with normal to mildly elevated filling pressures (left atrial pressure <20 mmHg), nitric oxide, epoprostenol, or nitroprusside may be administered. For patients with elevated filling pressures, nitroprusside primarily is used. Repeat measurements of PA pressure, left atrial pressure or PA wedge pressure, and cardiac output should be made after each increase in infusion rate. The endpoint of the infusion should be either a PAR <4 Wood units or a systolic blood pressure <75 mmHg.

Several technical considerations when measuring PAR include the following:

- The measurements of PA pressure and left atrial pressure (or PCWP) should be near simultaneous and at held end-expiration.
- If PCWP is used in place of direct left atrial pressure, its accuracy must be confirmed. Phasic respiratory changes in the pressure and confirmation by >95% oxygen saturation be oximetry should be present.
- Cardiac output is a critical measurement, and should be confirmed by at least two methods. The Fick method requires steady-state conditions and measurement of myocardial oxygen consumption. The thermodilution technique is better for acute changes in cardiac output.

PERICARDIOCENTESIS

Historically, pericardiocentesis was performed in a blinded or electrocardiographic-guided fashion, usually from a subxyphoid approach. Although these techniques are still used in some situations (e.g., cardiogenic shock), echocardiographic guidance is strongly preferred because of the high incidence of complications. Care should also be taken to avoid pericardiocentesis for tamponade that occurs with aortic dissection as the abrupt return of ventricular ejection may extend the dissection and lead to acute decompensation.

Echocardiography is used to determine the most appropriate portal of entry and needle direction into the pericardial effusion, typically the window closest to the effusion. This site frequently is apical, but other locations that have been used are axillary, left or right parasternal, and the subxyphoid window. The needle trajectory is transfixed in the operator's mind. Care should be taken to avoid the internal mammary or intercostal arteries by passing superior to the ribs. The entry site can be marked with an indelible pen.

- Local anesthesia is administered.
- Using the predetermined angulation, a Polytef-sheathed needle is inserted at the entry site and advanced with gentle aspiration into the pericardial space. Once fluid is obtained, the needle is advanced slightly further (2 mm). The Polytef sheath then is advanced over the needle, followed by withdrawal of the needle. The needle should not be re-advanced forward into the sheath once it has been removed.
- Agitated saline is injected into the Polytef sheath via a three-way stopcock under echocardiographic monitoring. If contrast does not opacify the pericardial space, then the catheter should be repositioned by withdrawal or another needle passage. As previously noted, the needle should not be advanced back into the sheath once it has been removed.

- Once the intrapericardial position of the Polytef sheath is confirmed, it is exchanged over a guidewire for a 5- to 6-Fr introducer sheath followed by placement of a pigtail catheter in the pericardial space. The introducer sheath is subsequently removed to leave only the smooth walled pigtail catheter in place. If needed, reconfirmation of the catheter location and measurement of intrapericardial pressure can be performed with saline injection.
- The pericardial effusion is removed using either manual techniques and/or vacuum bottle. Fluid removal is monitored with echocardiography. If drainage stops despite residual effusion on echocardiography, the pigtail is repositioned.
- The pigtail catheter is aspirated and flushed with heparinized saline every 4–6 hours. Reapposition of the parietal and visceral pericardial surfaces in this manner promotes adhesions that prevent fluid recurrence. The catheter is removed when the drainage is minimal (<25 cc/24 hr) and repeat echocardiography reveals no significant residual effusion.

Infrequently, the tense pericardium will discharge its fluid into the pleural space during attempts at needle passage and relieve tamponade. This effect is recognized on echocardiography, and may obviate further attempts at pericardiocentesis. While the majority of pericardial effusions can be treated percutaneously, some still require subxyphoid surgical drainage, especially if they are viscous or loculated. Bacterial infections in the pericardium also usually require large drainage. Recent hemorrhage into the pericardium may result in clot formation that can be difficult to remove percutaneously. A true posterior effusion may be difficult to approach from any thoracic window and may require surgery.

REFERENCES

1. Geisterfer-Lowrance AA, et al. A molecular basis for familial hypertrophic cardiomyopathy: A beta cardiac myosin heavy chain gene missense mutation. *Cell* 1990;62(2):999–1006.
2. Maron MS, et al. Hypertrophic cardiomyopathy is predominantly a disease of left ventricular outflow tract obstruction. *Circulation* 2006;114(21):2232–2239.
3. Levine RA, et al. Papillary muscle displacement causes systolic anterior motion of the mitral valve. Experimental validation and insights into the mechanism of subaortic obstruction. *Circulation* 1995;91(4):1189–1195.
4. Sherrid MV, et al. The mitral valve in obstructive hypertrophic cardiomyopathy: A test in context. *J Am Coll Cardiol* 2016;67(15):1846–1858.
5. Gersh BJ, et al. 2011 ACCF/AHA guideline for the diagnosis and treatment of hypertrophic cardiomyopathy: A report of the American College of Cardiology Foundation/American Heart Association Task Force on Practice Guidelines. *Circulation* 2011;124(24):e783–831.
6. Jaber WA, et al. Not all systolic velocities indicate obstruction in hypertrophic cardiomyopathy: A simultaneous Doppler catheterization study. *J Am Soc Echocardiogr* 2007;20(8):1009 e5–e7.
7. Bishu K, et al. The role of hemodynamic catheterization in the evaluation of hypertrophic obstructive cardiomyopathy: A case series. *Catheter Cardiovasc Interv* 2015;86(5):903–912.

8. Elesber A, et al. Utility of isoproterenol to provoke outflow tract gradients in patients with hypertrophic cardiomyopathy. *Am J Cardiol* 2008;101(4):516–520.

9. Arbustini E, et al. Restrictive cardiomyopathy, atrioventricular block and mild to subclinical myopathy in patients with desmin-immunoreactive material deposits. *J Am Coll Cardiol* 1998;31(3):645–653.

10. Mogensen J, et al. Idiopathic restrictive cardiomyopathy is part of the clinical expression of cardiac troponin I mutations. *J Clin Invest* 2003;111(2):209–216.

11. Zhang J, et al. Clinical and molecular studies of a large family with desmin-associated restrictive cardiomyopathy. *Clin Genet* 2001;59(4):248–256.

12. McCaughan BC, et al. Early and late results of pericardiectomy for constrictive pericarditis. *J Thorac Cardiovasc Surg* 1985;89(3):340–350.

13. Ammash NM, et al. Clinical profile and outcome of idiopathic restrictive cardiomyopathy. *Circulation* 2000;101(21):2490–2496.

14. Sorajja P, Nishimura R. Assessment and therapy of valvular heart disease in the cardiac catheterization laboratory. In: Willerson JT, ed. *Cardiovascular Medicine*. 3rd edn. London, UK: Springer; 2007:463–486.

15. Sorajja P, Nishimura R. *Myocardial and pericardial disease assessment and management*. CathSap3, American College of Cardiology Foundation; 2008.

16. Khandaker MH, et al. Pericardial disease: Diagnosis and management. *Mayo Clin Proc* 2010;85(6):572–593.

17. Talreja DR, et al. Constrictive pericarditis in the modern era: Novel criteria for diagnosis in the cardiac catheterization laboratory. *J Am Coll Cardiol* 2008;51(3):315–319.

18. Doshi S, et al. Invasive hemodynamics of constrictive pericarditis. *Indian Heart J* 2015;67(2):175–182.

19. Goldstein JA. Cardiac tamponade, constrictive pericarditis, and restrictive cardiomyopathy. *Curr Probl Cardiol* 2004;29(9):503–567.

20. Sorajja P. Invasive hemodynamics of constrictive pericarditis, restrictive cardiomyopathy, and cardiac tamponade. *Cardiol Clin* 2011;29(2):191–199.

21. Jaber WA, et al. Differentiation of tricuspid regurgitation from constrictive pericarditis: Novel criteria for diagnosis in the cardiac catheterisation laboratory. *Heart* 2009;95(17):1449–1454.

22. Sagrista-Sauleda J, et al. Low-pressure cardiac tamponade: Clinical and hemodynamic profile. *Circulation* 2006;114(9):945–952.

23. Spodick DH. Acute cardiac tamponade. *N Engl J Med* 2003;349(7):684–690.

24. Shields RC, et al. The role of right ventricular endomyocardial biopsy for idiopathic giant cell myocarditis. *J Card Fail* 2002;8(2):74–78.

13

Endomyocardial biopsy: Indications and procedures

GREGG F. ROSNER, GARRICK C. STEWART, AND KENNETH L. BAUGHMAN*

INTRODUCTION

Disorders of the heart muscle remain among the most poorly understood disease processes in all of cardiovascular medicine. Endomyocardial biopsy techniques have now been available for over 50 years to evaluate underlying primary myocardial pathology. Cardiac biopsy has been particularly useful in establishing diagnosis and prognosis in patients with recent-onset or rapidly deteriorating cardiomyopathy and in monitoring patients for rejection after cardiac transplantation. The role of endomyocardial biopsy continues to evolve as novel molecular and genetic analyses are being performed on biopsy specimens. This chapter will review the history of endomyocardial biopsy, define the anatomic considerations and basic biopsy technique, and discuss the indications, complications, and future directions of this important procedure.

History of endomyocardial biopsy

Techniques for biopsying cardiac tissue outside the operating room have been available now for nearly 60 years. In 1958, Weinberg, Fell, and Lynfield first performed heart

biopsies through a small incision in the left intercostal space. After dissection, samples of pericardium, epicardium, and myocardium were obtained, revealing inflammatory and restrictive cardiac disorders, and tubercular and traumatic causes of pericardial constriction.[1] Because of the need for open incision and surgical extraction, the technique was not widely adopted. The first closed percutaneous biopsy was performed by Sutton and Sutton in 1960 using a needle introduced through the chest wall at the point of maximal impulse to sample myocardial tissue at the left ventricular apex.[2] This method, and other early percutaneous techniques, had only modest diagnostic yield and were plagued by high complication rates, including cardiac tamponade, arrhythmia, and postpericardiectomy syndrome.[3,4]

In 1965, Bulloch introduced the concept of passing a biopsy needle through the jugular vein, which allowed sampling of the right interventricular septum using a cutting blade.[5] Though no longer in use, this technique established several principles central to endomyocardial biopsy today, including use of the right internal jugular vein, designation of the heart boundaries by right heart catheterization prior to biopsy attempt, rotation of a curved biopsy sheath to avoid trauma to

* Deceased

the tricuspid valve or coronary sinus, and appropriate angulation of the biopsy device in the right interventricular septum.

Sakakibara and Konno introduced a flexible bioptome with sharpened cups allowing biopsy by a pinching technique rather than advancement of a cutting needle.[6] The original Konno bioptome is now infrequently used because of its lack of durability and a stiff, large caliber shaft often requiring venous cutdown for access. In the early 1970s, Caves made a series of modifications to the Konno biopsy forceps to allow percutaneous biopsy through the right internal jugular vein with only local anesthesia and rapid serial tissue sampling through a preformed sheath.[7,8] Pioneered at Stanford University, the Stanford-Caves-Schulz bioptome became central to monitoring cardiac transplant patients for rejection and served as the standard device for endomyocardial biopsy from 1975 to 1995. The biopsy forceps were more flexible and had features allowing the operator to adjust the force applied to the forceps using a surgery-like clamp. The Stanford-Caves-Schulz device was also reusable. This led to the requirement for frequent retooling and resharpening, along with concerns about protecting patients from infection and pyrogen reaction. Richardson in 1974, and Kawai in 1977, added special features to the bioptome for right or left ventricular sampling by increasing sheath flexibility, electrocardiographic monitoring, and intracardiac maneuverability.[9,10]

Modern bioptomes in use since the mid-1990s are disposable, single-use devices eliminating concerns about disease transmission, pyrogen reactions, or cutting edge resharpening (Figure 13.1). Bioptomes are made in standard lengths of 50 cm for use in the neck and chest central venous system, or over 100 cm, for use in the femoral vein or artery. The 50 cm bioptomes may be preshaped to facilitate transit across the tricuspid valve or unshaped to be inserted through a preformed sheath. The preformed sheath is generally guided into the ventricular cavity over an angled pigtail or balloon flotation catheter. This sheath remains in the ventricular cavity through the biopsy procedure, increasing risk of arrhythmia or perforation and reducing operator control of the bioptome's path and biopsy site. In contrast, preshaped bioptomes are introduced through a short venous sheath, giving operators greater control of biopsy site selection. The degree of bioptome curvature may be modified to facilitate entry into either the right or left ventricles (RVs or LVs). Disposable bioptomes and sheaths are available for use from the right or left jugular, the subclavian and femoral veins, as well as the femoral arteries, and vary in length, degree of angulation, diameter, and jaw size.

ANATOMIC CONSIDERATIONS

Vascular access

RIGHT INTERNAL JUGULAR VEIN

The right internal jugular vein is the most common site for performance of right ventricular endomyocardial biopsy procedures.[11] With the patient's head turned to the left 30° to 45°, the internal jugular vein is located lateral to the carotid artery within the anterior triangle of the neck formed by the sternal and clavicular heads of the sternocleidomastoid muscle and the clavicle (Figure 13.2). This triangle may be clearly outlined by having the patient raise his or her head off the table briefly to tense the muscular boundaries. Entry into the jugular vein in the upper third of this triangle, well above the clavicle, will lessen the risk of pneumothorax and allow for easier compression of accidental carotid punctures, as well as the venous access site after the procedure. Routine use of ultrasonography is encouraged to identify the location and size of the jugular vein prior to access attempt, particularly in patients with challenging surface anatomy (Figure 13.3). The jugular vein is most commonly located lateral to the carotid artery, is easily compressible when pressure is applied to the ultrasound transducer, and lacks the pulsatility of the artery, which may be confirmed by color or pulse wave Doppler.[13] Use of sonography during venous access has been shown to improve access time and decrease complication rates.[14]

Once anatomic landmarks have been identified, the patient's neck is prepared with standard antibacterial solutions and the region is isolated with sterile towels or drapes with the patient's head resting in a comfortable position. In patients with low venous pressure or a small jugular vein, the legs may be elevated or the patient placed in Trendelenburg position to increase jugular venous filling and augment the puncture target. A 22- or 25-gauge needle is used to introduce local anesthetic (2% lidocaine) intradermally and subcutaneously along the planned route of access needle entry. After successful local anesthesia is applied, a small 1–2 mm superficial incision is made at the anticipated entry site using a surgical blade and may be expanded using a mosquito clamp. This incision prevents the venous sheath from meeting resistance when passing through the skin.

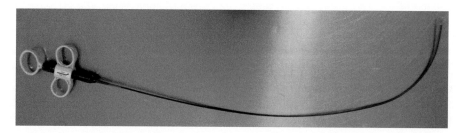

Figure 13.1 Modern bioptome.

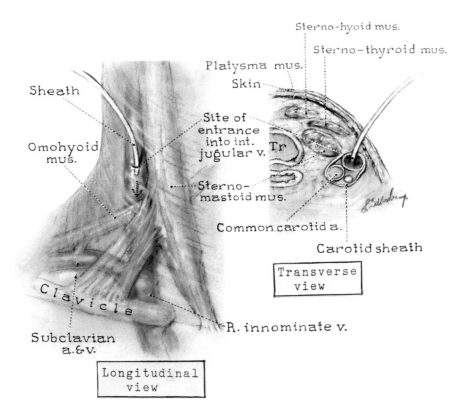

Figure 13.2 Surface anatomy of the neck and jugular vein access. (Courtesy of Leon Schlossberg, from Baumgartner, W.A., et al., *Heart and Lung Transplantation*, 2nd ed., WB Saunders, Philadelphia, PA, 2002.)

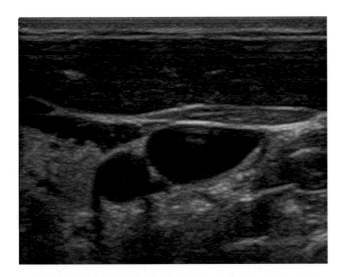

Figure 13.3 Ultrasound visualization of the internal jugular vein (lateral) (*right*) and the carotid artery (medial) (*left*).

In the classic approach, the 22-gauge needle is directed in small increments toward the venous entry site at an angle of 30°–40° from vertical and 20° right of the sagittal plane. This aims the finder needle away from the more medially located carotid artery. After each advancement, the needle should be aspirated before infusing small amounts of lidocaine. Excess anesthetic infiltration is discouraged as it may compress the jugular vein, obscure landmarks, or infiltrate into the carotid sheath or vocal cords resulting in transient

Horner's syndrome or hoarseness. Once venous blood is aspirated, the operator notes the position and an 18-gauge single wall puncture needle with a syringe attached is advanced along the prior pathway of the finder needle. Continuous aspiration should be applied as the 18-gauge needle is advanced in small increments until there is a "give" of the vein wall and blood return is evident. A J-tipped guidewire is introduced followed by the appropriate sheath.

Alternatively, we now frequently use a 22-gauge micropuncture needle as the probe and entry device for jugular venous access. This needle is very atraumatic and accepts a 0.021-in mandril guidewire over which a coaxial 5-Fr double dilator guide sheath is advanced. Once this has entered the jugular vein and superior vena cava (SVC), the inner cannula and guidewire are withdrawn and a conventional guidewire (0.038-in) is inserted through the outer cannula. This remaining cannula is then removed and a 7- or 8-Fr self-sealing sheath is introduced over the guidewire. This sheath may be preformed for right ventricular biopsy, or standard length to allow for preshaped bioptome use. Once the sheath is appropriately positioned, the guidewire may be removed and the sheath may be aspirated, flushed, and then is available for endomyocardial biopsy.

If initial attempts at venous access are unsuccessful, the probing or micropuncture needle should be retracted to just beneath the skin and redirected more laterally. If there is still no venous return, medial redirection toward the carotid may be attempted. Should arterial puncture occur at any point, the probing needle or micropuncture needle syringe will fill with well-oxygenated blood. The needle must be removed immediately and the area compressed for 5 minutes or until hemostasis is achieved. This problem may be avoided by using simultaneous ultrasonographic guidance during puncture attempt.

RIGHT SUBCLAVIAN VEIN

The right subclavian vein may be used in those rare cases where anatomic abnormalities preclude use of the internal jugular or femoral vein approaches. The entry point should be more lateral than for routine subclavian venous access and should be from an infraclavicular approach past the bend of the clavicle. This more lateral approach is required so that the subclavian to vena-caval angle will not be too acute, preventing the relatively stiff bioptome from being positioned into the right heart. Application of local anesthetic and needle entry are similar to internal jugular vein access. A standard single-wall needle or micropuncture kit may be used. If cannulation is unsuccessful, a more inferior approach with a steeper angle may be required. In both the internal jugular and subclavian techniques, fluoroscopy should be used to ensure that the guidewire is directed down the vena cava toward the right atrium (RA) rather that superiorly to the head.

FEMORAL VEIN AND ARTERY

Despite relatively easy cannulation, biopsy from the femoral vein can be challenging.[15] The femoral vein is located medial to the femoral artery and the entry site should be below the inguinal ligament. The Amplatz, Seldinger, or micropuncture techniques may be used for venous access. A guide sheath is introduced into the inferior vena cava (IVC) via the femoral vein. The femoral artery may be accessed in a similar fashion and is the site of entry for most left ventricular biopsy attempts. Left ventricular biopsies, though rare, may be indicated in patients with specific intraventricular masses or isolated left ventricular pathology, such as myocarditis or infiltrative disease.[16] After femoral arterial sheath insertion, a constant infusion of heparinized saline should be maintained through the sheath to prevent thrombus formation within these long catheters.

FUNDAMENTALS

Biopsy techniques

GUIDANCE METHODOLOGY

Endomyocardial biopsies are most easily performed under fluoroscopic guidance to define the heart borders and easily visualize the course of the sheath and/or bioptome into the heart. Some investigators advocate the use of two-dimensional (2D) echocardiography to guide biopsy to reduce radiation exposure and risk of perforation.[17] Echocardiographic guidance may be particularly useful in biopsying intracardiac masses in either the left or right heart.[18] It is often technically challenging to obtain adequate

windows and visualize the biopsy forceps with echocardiography. Compared with 2D echocardiography, fluoroscopy provides the operator with superior information about the course of the bioptome and biopsy site. Widespread use of newer technologies, such as cardiac magnetic resonance imaging (MRI), may allow the detection of a focal disease process in the RV or LV. This information can then be used to direct endomyocardial biopsy to a location most likely to demonstrate underlying pathology.[19] Advances in three-dimensional (3D) echocardiography may improve visualization of myocardium during biopsy, thereby reducing the reliance on fluoroscopic imaging.[20]

RIGHT INTERNAL JUGULAR VEIN APPROACH: PRESHAPED BIOPTOME

The preshaped 50 cm bioptome is introduced through the venous sheath with the bioptome tip directed toward the lateral wall of the RA. The bioptome is slowly advanced and in the mid-RA, it is rotated counterclockwise to facilitate passage across the tricuspid valve, avoiding the coronary sinus and tricuspid apparatus. The bioptome tip and handle have concordant motion and angulation, but positioning should always be confirmed fluoroscopically. Continued advancement and counterclockwise rotation allow passage into the mid-RV with the bioptome forceps directed toward the septum (Figure 13.4). Extreme care should be taken to avoid perforation of the relatively thin RA, vena cava, or RV with the stiff bioptome. If there is any resistance to bioptome passage, it should be withdrawn slightly and a different angle of entry attempted. Bioptome forceps must never be forced or prolapsed into the ventricle. If passage into the RV remains difficult, the path across the tricuspid valve may be defined by the passage of a balloon-tipped pulmonary artery (PA) catheter.

Once the bioptome is in the RV, the tip should lie against the interventricular septum. On anterior-posterior fluoroscopy, the bioptome should lie across the vertebral bodies and is usually directed inferiorly below and to the left of the tricuspid valve plane. Bioptome position may be confirmed by fluoroscopy in the 30° right anterior oblique (RAO) and the 60° left anterior oblique (LAO) projection. These views will confirm that the bioptome is on the ventricular side of the atrioventricular groove and pointed toward the septum. The absence of ectopy or fluoroscopy showing a position within the atrioventricular (AV) groove suggests the bioptome has entered the coronary sinus and must be withdrawn and repositioned before any biopsy is attempted. Even within the RV, the thin right ventricular free wall must be avoided by directing the bioptome toward the septum (Figure 13.5). The interventricular septum lies on a plane 45° from the chest wall, corresponding to a bioptome handle orientation posteriorly and to the left. In patients with right ventricular enlargement, the handle may be straight posterior.

Contact with the interventricular septum is confirmed by premature ventricular beats. The biopsy forceps should be withdrawn 1–2 cm, opened, and advanced slowly to engage the septum. The forceps head is then closed slowly to collect

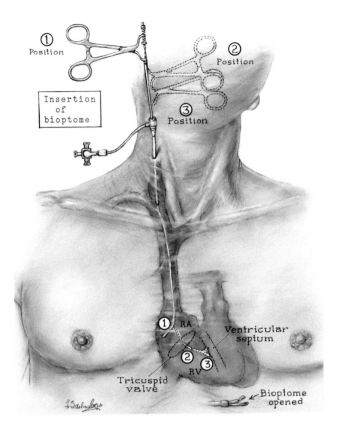

Figure 13.4 Bioptome position for right ventricular septal biopsy from the internal jugular vein approach. RA, right atrium; RV, right ventricle. (Courtesy of Leon Schlossberg, from Baumgartner, W.A., et al., *Heart and Lung Transplantation*, 2nd ed., WB Saunders, Philadelphia, PA, 2002.)

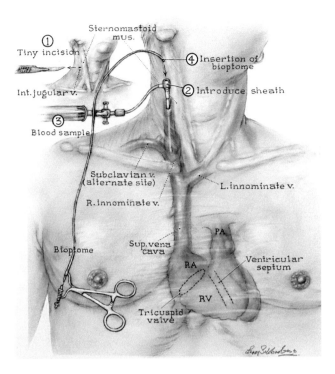

Figure 13.5 Right ventricular free wall. PA, pulmonary artery; RA, right atrium; RV, right ventricle. (Courtesy of Leon Schlossberg, from Baumgartner, W.A., et al., *Heart and Lung Transplantation*, 2nd ed., WB Saunders, Philadelphia, PA, 2002.)

the endomyocardial specimen. Given the trabeculations within the ventricle, gentle forward pressure should be applied during jaw closure to maintain contact with myocardium. Septal engagement may be marked by transmission of ventricular pulsations in post-transplant patients or in those with restrictive cardiomyopathy. Patients with idiopathic dilated cardiomyopathies may have no engagement sensation and contact with the septum can be confirmed only by the presence of premature ventricular beats.

The bioptome jaws must be closed to perform the biopsy and pressure must be maintained on the forceps closure device after the sample has been obtained and during withdrawal from the RV, atrium, vena cava, and sheath to prevent the jaws from opening (Figure 13.6). There may be a slight release of traction once the specimen is removed from the septum. Excessive resistance in bioptome withdrawal suggests entrapment on the tricuspid valve apparatus or an area of scar tissue. When this occurs, the forceps jaws should be opened, the bioptome withdrawn, and the bioptome repositioned to secure another biopsy site. During routine biopsy, it is not uncommon for patients to experience a tugging sensation during specimen acquisition. Sharp chest pain, however, implies cardiac perforation. Other evidence that perforation may have occurred includes persistence

of premature beats, excessive retraction of the ventricular septum during biopsy, and a sample that floats in fixative, implying epicardial fat content. Any of these clues should prompt close hemodynamic monitoring and fluoroscopy of the heart borders to detect tamponade.

Perforation is less likely in patients with prior cardiac surgery and advanced cardiomyopathy, and more so in nonsurgical patients with normal chamber size and systolic function. At the end of every biopsy procedure, the heart borders should be examined with fluoroscopy to exclude tamponade prior to removal of venous access.

RIGHT INTERNAL JUGULAR VEIN: PREFORMED SHEATH

In this method, the preformed sheath, rather than the bioptome itself, is advanced into the right ventricle. The sheath directs a flexible straight bioptome to the desired biopsy site. A 7-Fr 45 cm preformed sheath may be inserted in the internal jugular vein. The performed sheath is positioned into the RV with the aid of a guidewire or balloon-tipped catheter. Once in the RV, the guidewire or catheter is removed and the sheath flushed with heparinized saline and connected to an infusion port to maintain patency. The sheath should be free-floating and not abutting ventricular myocardium. The distal segment of a flexible bioptome should be angulated or curved before insertion to avoid straightening the preformed sheath. Precurved bioptomes may also be used through the preshaped sheath.

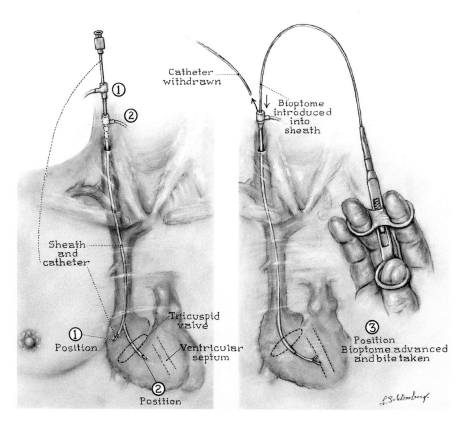

Figure 13.6 Bioptome position and tissue sample acquisition from the internal jugular approach. (Courtesy of Leon Schlossberg, from Baumgartner, W.A., et al., *Heart and Lung Transplantation*, 2nd ed., WB Saunders, Philadelphia, PA, 2002.)

The bioptome jaws should be opened immediately upon exiting the sheath to reduce risk of perforation. The bioptome is directed posteriorly, perpendicular to the interventricular septum. Gentle pressure is applied as the jaws are closed, then the sample may be removed as described above. The sheath should be flushed with saline and repeat biopsy performed as indicated.

FEMORAL VEIN APPROACH: PREFORMED SHEATH

From the femoral vein, a 7-Fr preformed guiding sheath can be introduced into the RV using a balloon-tipped catheter, pigtail catheter, or guidewire. Rarely, in children, the femoral venous approach may be used to facilitate left ventricular biopsy by transseptal puncture.[21] The standard preformed femoral sheath has a 130° angle from the RA into the RV to facilitate positioning. The preshaped sheath may increase the risk of perforation because the operator may have less control of the direction of the bioptome to the cardiac septum. The femoral sheath must be evaluated before insertion to ensure that the sheath length after the angulation does not exceed the anatomic distance from the RA to ventricle for a given patient because of risk of perforation. This may be confirmed by placing the sheath on the exterior of the patient on a sterile field and imaging under fluoroscopy. Once the sheath is inserted, it should be flushed to avoid clot formation. If there is any question about the position of the sheath tip, hand injection of contrast dye and hemodynamic monitoring may be helpful.

After sheath insertion, the unshaped bioptome should be curved, similar to the jugular approach, to avoid straightening the preformed sheath when inserted. Posterior angulation of the bioptome tip out of the plane relative to the broad proximal curvature of the sheath can help direct the bioptome toward the interventricular septum upon exiting the sheath (Figure 13.7).

Fluoroscopy can be used to track bioptome passage through the sheath and can confirm interventricular septal position. Bioptome jaws should be opened just as the bioptome exits the preformed sheath to avoid perforation. After slow advancement to the septum, the jaws are slowly closed while forward pressure is maintained. If the sheath tip is resting against the septum, the bioptome jaws can be exposed by retracting the sheath while maintaining the forceps in a stable position. After the forceps are withdrawn, the sheath can be repositioned within the ventricle for another biopsy attempt.

LEFT VENTRICULAR BIOPSY: FEMORAL ARTERY PREFORMED SHEATH

The femoral artery approach usually requires insertion of a 9-Fr self-sealing sheath through which a preformed 7-Fr biopsy sheath is inserted to allow bioptome sheath manipulation. All femoral artery sheaths must be maintained with continuous infusion of heparinized saline to avoid embolic phenomenon. The preformed sheath is gently inserted into the LV across the aortic valve using a guidewire and pigtail

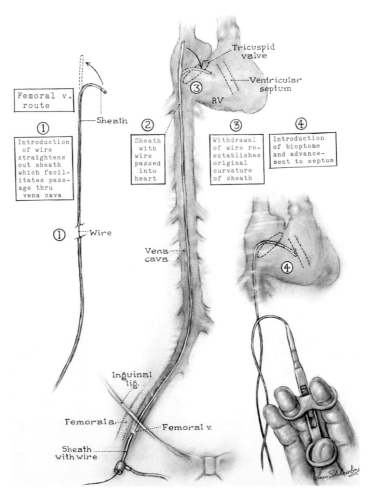

Figure 13.7 Endomyocardial biopsy from the femoral vein. RV, right ventricle. (Courtesy of Leon Schlossberg, from Baumgartner, W.A., et al., *Heart and Lung Transplantation*, 2nd ed., WB Saunders, Philadelphia, PA, 2002.)

catheter. Once in the LV, areas of prior myocardial infarction (MI) and inferior-posterior positions should be avoided to reduce the perforation risk in these relatively thin-walled sites. After the sheath is cleared of debris by aspiration and flushing, a 104 cm bioptome is inserted into the left ventricular cavity. The biopsy forceps should be directed away from the mitral valve apparatus. The jaws are opened upon exiting the sheath, directed toward the ventricular wall, the specimen is encapsulated, and the jaws are closed firmly while extracting the sample. The sheath is maintained within the LV and repositioned to ensure sampling from several different sites. Since most myocardial disease processes affect both ventricles, right ventricular biopsy is preferred because of greater ease, shorter procedure time, and reduced likelihood of morbidity. In diseases with confirmed selective left ventricular involvement or in patients in whom right ventricular biopsy has been unsuccessful, left ventricular biopsy may be attempted. In general, left ventricular biopsy is reserved for cases with selective left ventricular involvement, such as in endomyocardial fibrosis, scleroderma, left heart radiation, and cardiac fibroelastosis of infants and newborns.

POSTPROCEDURE CARE

After biopsy sheath removal, pressure must be applied to prevent local bleeding complications. After uncomplicated biopsy, patients with biopsies from the jugular vein may be discharged home after 1 hour of observation. Patients who had femoral venous entry require 2–3 hours of supine bed rest before safely attempting ambulation. Patients with femoral arterial access require several hours of bed rest with or without use of a vascular closure device before ambulation. All patients must be monitored for bleeding and hemodynamic changes. The bandage applied to the vascular access site may be removed in 24 hours and oral intake may resume once patients can sit up.

INDICATIONS

Transplant rejection

Endomyocardial biopsy has been the cornerstone of monitoring patients for rejection after heart or heart-lung transplantion.[22,23] Early rejection may be detected on endomyocardial biopsy before clinical manifestations. Regular post-transplantation biopsies monitor antirejection therapy and can confirm the adequacy of pulsed immuno-suppressive therapy for episodes of acute rejection. Despite promising research, no single methodology has had the predictive accuracy to replace endomyocardial biopsy in the assessment of cellular and humoral rejection.[24-26] Because rejection is a diffuse immune-mediated phenomenon, sampling errors are rare. The severity of rejection on biopsy has been divided into four grades as established by the International Society of Heart and Lung Transplantation.[27] Grade 0R represents no rejection, Grade 1R is mild rejection, and Grade 2R is moderate rejection. Severe rejection (Grade 3R) is marked by multifocal aggressive infiltrates and/or myocyte damage or diffuse polymorphous infiltrate with necrosis and a variable degree of edema, hemorrhage, or vasculitis. More severe rejection requires aggressive immunosuppression even in asymptomatic patients.

Biopsy in the management of cardiovascular disease

Routine use of endomyocardial biopsy to inform management of a variety of cardiovascular diseases in patients without a heart transplant remains controversial. Decisions to proceed with endomyocardial biopsy are most often made on the basis of clinical presentation, not the underlying pathologic diagnosis which is known only after biopsy. Few randomized, controlled treatment trials have evaluated the utility of heart biopsy in disease management, and recommendations are made on the basis of case-control series and expert opinion. A comprehensive scientific statement from the American Heart Association (AHA), American College of Cardiology (ACC), and European Society of Cardiology (ESC) was published in 2007 that outlines the appropriate role of endomyocardial biopsy outside the post-transplant setting (Table 13.1).[28] Biopsy does have an important role in the evaluation of unexplained heart failure.[29-31] Heart failure is considered to be unexplained when comprehensive testing, including electrocardiogram (ECG), chest radiography, echocardiography, and coronary angiography, fails to reveal a diagnosis. Standard evaluations of patients with new-onset cardiomyopathy are informative, but as many as half of this population has no diagnosis after routine testing.[32] The potential value of direct assessment of heart muscle tissue in patients with new-onset heart failure may be more valuable in this population.

Table 13.1 Recommendations for endomyocardial biopsy

Class I—Conditions for which there is evidence or general agreement that biopsy is beneficial, useful, and effective
- New onset heart failure of <2 weeks duration associated with a normal-sized or dilated left ventricle and hemodynamic compromise.
- New-onset heart failure of 2 weeks to 3 months duration associated with a dilated left ventricle and new ventricular arrhythmias, second- or third-degree heart block, or failure to respond to usual care within 1–2 weeks.

Class IIa—Conditions for which the weight of evidence/opinion is in favor of usefulness/efficacy
- Heart failure of >3 months duration associated with a dilated left ventricle and new ventricular arrhythmias, second- or third-degree heart block, or failure to respond to usual care within 1–2 weeks.
- Heart failure associated with a dilated cardiomyopathy of any duration association with suspected allergic reaction and/or eosinophilia.
- Heart failure associated with suspected anthracycline cardiomyopathy.
- Heart failure associated with unexplained restrictive cardiomyopathy.
- Suspected cardiac tumors.
- Unexplained cardiomyopathy in children.

Class IIb—Conditions for which usefulness/efficacy of biopsy is less well-established by evidence/opinion
- New-onset heart failure of 2 weeks to 3 months duration associated with a dilated left ventricle, without new ventricular arrhythmias, second- or third-degree heart block, that responds to usual care within 1–2 weeks.
- Heart failure of >3 months duration associated with a dilated left ventricle and new ventricular arrhythmias, second- or third-degree heart block, that responds to usual care within 1–2 weeks.
- Heart failure associated with unexplained hypertrophic cardiomyopathy.
- Suspected arrhythmogenic right ventricular dysplasia/cardiomyopathy.
- Unexplained ventricular arrhythmias.

Class III—Conditions for which there is evidence and/or general agreement that biopsy is not useful
- Unexplained atrial fibrillation.

Source: Adapted from Cooper, L.T., et al., *Circulation*, 116(19), 2216–2233, 2007. With permission.

Table 13.2 Cardiac disorders with specific findings on biopsy

Immune or inflammatory disease states	Infiltrative
Myocarditis	Amyloidosis
Cardiac allograft rejection	Gaucher's disease
Sarcoidosis	Hemochromatosis
Cytomegalovirus infection	Fabry's disease
Toxoplasmosis	Glycogen storage disease
Rheumatic carditis	
Chagas disease	
Kawasaki disease	
Degenerative	**Ischemic**
Idiopathic cardiomyopathy	Acute myocardial infarction
Anthracycline cardiomyopathy	Chronic ischemic cardiomyopathy
Radiation cardiomyopathy	Schonlein–Henoch purpura
	Cancer
	Primary cardiac cancer
	Metastatic cardiac cancer

Table 13.3 Restrictive cardiomyopathies

Myocardial	Endocardial
Non-infiltrative	Fibrosis
Idiopathic	Hypereosinophilic
Familial	Carcinoid
Hypertrophic	Metastatic cancer
Scleroderma	Radiation
Diabetic	Anthracyclines
Infiltrative	Drugs
Amyloid	
Sarcoid	
Gaucher's	
Hurler's	
Fatty	
Storage	
Hemochromatosis	
Fabry's	
Glycogen	

Patients most appropriate for biopsy are those with new-onset heart failure of less than 2 weeks duration accompanied by hemodynamic compromise, or those with heart failure of 2 weeks to 3 months duration who have heart failure or dysrhythmias that fail to respond to standard therapies. Patients with severe cardiac compromise and duration of less than 2 weeks often have fulminant lymphocytic myocarditis and a good prognosis.[33–35] These cases must be distinguished from similarly aggressive disorders, such as giant cell myocarditis and necrotizing eosinophilic myocarditis, which have a similarly fulminant course, often requiring permanent mechanical support or consideration of cardiac transplantation.[36,37] Giant cell myocarditis in particular may be associated with both ventricular tachycardia and AV block.[38] Confirmation of histologic diagnosis of either giant cell or necrotizing eosinophilic myocarditis would lead to immunosuppressive treatment, while fulminant lymphocytic myocarditis resolves without such agents. Studies are ongoing to define the appropriate diagnostic criteria for myocarditis and guide appropriate immune-modulating therapies.[39,40]

Patients with long-term and established dilated cardiomyopathy responding to usual heart failure treatments have less to gain from endomyocardial biopsy. In these subjects, biopsy generally displays nonspecific findings of myocyte hypertrophy, interstitial and replacement fibrosis, and endocardial thickening.[41,42] Such findings do not establish etiology, long-term prognosis, or guide-specific therapies. Nevertheless, there is a subset of patients with dilated cardiomyopathy who may have specific disease processes identified on biopsy, particularly those who fail to respond to standard heart failure therapies and have refractory symptoms (Table 13.2). Patients with suspected cardiac sarcoidosis or myocarditis should be considered for heart biopsy.

Endomyocardial biopsy is also recommended for patients with cardiomyopathy from suspected anthracycline toxicity, cardiomyopathy associated with allergic or eosinophilic reaction, patients with unexplained ventricular tachycardia or conduction disease, or children with unexplained cardiomyopathy.[28] Endomyocardial biopsy may also help establish a diagnosis in patients with underlying restrictive physiology, a common entity seen in patients with heart failure and a preserved ejection fraction. By helping distinguish between restrictive cardiomyopathy and constrictive pericarditis, biopsy can help spare patients inappropriate medical or surgical therapies.[43] Disorders causing a restrictive cardiomyopathy include primary amyloidosis, Loeffler endomyocardial fibrosis, carcinoid-related heart disease, Fabry disease, and glycogen storage diseases (Table 13.3).[44,45]

CLINICAL ASPECTS

Equipment needed for endomyocardial biopsy are listed in Table 13.4.

Biopsy complications

Complications associated with endomyocardial biopsy are considered either acute (while the patient is still in the catheterization laboratory) or delayed. The vast majority of complications fall into the acute category. Potential acute complications include ventricular perforation and pericardial tamponade, malignant ventricular or supraventricular arrhythmias, transient complete heart block, pneumothorax, central artery puncture, nerve paresis, thromboembolism, systemic platelet embolization associated with left ventricular biopsy, venous or arterial hematoma, damage of the tricuspid or mitral valve, and creation of arterial venous fistula within the heart. Delayed complications include access site bleeding and damage to the tricuspid valve from repeated trauma associated with transplant

Table 13.4 Equipment

18-gauge Amplatz needle or 22-gauge micropuncture needle
250 mL of flush solution (with heparin unless allergic)
4- or 5-Fr micropuncture sheath
7-, 8-, or 9-Fr self-sealing introducer with 0.038-in guidewire
Assorted syringes (1, 5, 10, and 20 mL)
Automatic intermittent cutaneous or invasive blood pressure monitor
Continuous electrocardiographic monitor
Continuous oxygen saturation monitor
Defibrillator
Dry ice
Emergency equipment
Ether screen or drape support (optional)
Formalin
Glutaraldehyde
Lidocaine—1% or 2%, 15 mL
Micropuncture wire, 0.021-in
Mosquito clamp or small-tipped instrument
No. 11 surgical blade and handle
One 25-gauge, one 22-gauge, and three to four 18-gauge needles
Pacemaker and pacing leads
Pericardiocentesis set
Plastic or cloth drape set
Povidone–iodine, alcohol, or both
Resuscitation drugs and equipment
Tissue preservativeVascular ultrasound machine (i.e., SonoSite M-turbo)

rejection surveillance. Factors associated with endomyocardial biopsy complication risk include operator experience, patient clinical status, indication for biopsy, access site, underlying cardiac conduction disease (presence of a left bundle branch block [LBBB]), and possibly bioptome, since allergic reactions to reusable bioptomes have been reported. Fowles and Mason reported a complication rate of <1% in over 4,000 transplant and cardiomyopathy patients biopsied at Stanford University.[46] They reported no deaths in their series. Cardiac tamponade occurred in four patients (<0.14%), none of whom needed thoracotomy. Other complications included atrial fibrillation (AF) in three patients, and sustained ventricular arrhythmia in one patient. Complications related to the internal jugular vein approach included pneumothorax in three patients, uncomplicated air embolism in six patients, transient right recurrent laryngeal nerve paresis in two patients, and Horner's syndrome in one patient. Similarly, Sekiguchi and Take reported, by questionnaire, an overall complication rate of 1.17% in 6,739 worldwide patients, including perforation in 28 patients (0.42%) and death in 2 patients (0.03%).[47]

Deckers et al. prospectively recorded complications of right heart biopsy from 546 procedures in 464 consecutive patients with new-onset idiopathic cardiomyopathy.[48] The internal jugular vein was the primary site of access in 96% of cases. An overall complication rate of 6% occurred in this series. Of these complications, 15 (2.7%) occurred during catheter insertion including 12 arterial punctures (2%), 2 vasovagal reactions (0.4%), and 1 episode of prolonged bleeding (0.2%), all without sequelae. There were 18 (3.3%) complications during the actual biopsy, including six arrhythmias (1.1%), 5 conduction abnormalities (1%), 4 possible perforations (0.7%), and 3 definite perforations (0.5%) (pericardial fluid). Two (0.4%) of the three patients with definite perforation died.

Biopsy complications occur at a similar rate when echocardiography rather than fluoroscopy is used to guide the procedure. Han et al. prospectively recorded complications of right heart biopsy in 90 consecutive nontransplant patients who underwent 2D echocardiography-guided transfemoral biopsy.[49] The overall complication rate was 5.6%, and no deaths occurred in this cohort. Myocardial perforation occurred in three patients but did not progress to cardiac tamponade requiring pericardiocentesis in any patient. Unstable ventricular tachycardia occurred in one patient, and a new and persistent right bundle branch block (RBBB) occurred in one patient.

Baraldi-Junkins et al. reviewed 2,454 endomyocardial biopsies performed in 133 cardiac transplant patients.[50] An overall complication rate of 3% occurred; however, no perforations or deaths were observed in this cohort. Of these, 56 (2.3%) complications were associated with catheter insertion, including carotid puncture (1.8%), vasovagal reaction (0.1%), and prolonged bleeding (0.4%). Complications during biopsy included arrhythmias (0.25%) and conduction abnormalities (0.2%). Additional complications included five episodes (three patients) of allergic reaction to a reusable bioptome and one case of pacemaker dislodgement.

Recently, Holzmann et al. reported results of a retrospective and prospective study examining the incidence of major and minor complications of right ventricular endomyocardial biopsies via the right femoral vein approach at a single center in Germany.[51] In their study, 1,919 patients underwent 2,505 endomyocardial biopsy procedures, retrospectively evaluated between January 1995 and December 2003, and 496 patients underwent 543 endomyocardial biopsy procedures, prospectively assessed between January 2004 and December 2005. Major complications (pericardial tamponade requiring pericardiocentesis, pneumothorax or hemothorax, permanent pacemaker support, cases requiring emergency cardiac surgery, or death) were extremely rare in both the retrospective study (0.12%) and the prospective study (0%). No deaths were reported during either study (total of 3,048 endomyocardial biopsies). Major complications reported during the retrospective study included cardiac perforation in two cases (0.08%) and permanent pacemaker in one patient (0.04%). No major complications occurred during the prospective study. A difference was reported in the incidence of minor complications (hemodynamically insignificant pericardial effusion, conduction abnormalities not requiring permanent pacemaker, or arrhythmias not requiring advanced cardiac life support

[ACLS]) between the retrospective and prospective studies. Minor complications occurred in 0.2% of the endomyocardial procedures in the retrospective study and 5.5% in the prospective study. Five patients (0.2%) developed complete heart block requiring temporary pacing during the retrospective study. Minor complications seen during the prospective study included 4 cases (0.74%) of hemodynamically insignificant pericardial effusion, conduction abnormality not requiring temporary pacing in 12 patients (1.84%), temporary pacing requirement in 8 cases (1.47%), and AF in 6 patients (1.1%). The authors believed the most likely reason for the increased minor complication rate observed during the prospective study compared with the retrospective study was a more detailed documentation sheet initiated during the prospective study.

The risk of endomyocardial biopsy in children was studied by Pophal et al. in a retrospective review of 1,000 consecutive heart biopsies in 194 children.[52] The mean age at the time of biopsy was 8.6 years (8 days–18 years), mean weight was 30 kg (2.8–127 kg), mean height was 121 cm (48–187 cm), and mean body surface area was 0.98 m² (0.18–2.05 m²). Indications for heart biopsy included heart transplant rejection surveillance (84.6%) and the evaluation of cardiomyopathy or arrhythmia for possible myocarditis (15.4%). The overall incidence of a serious complication from endomyocardial biopsy was 1.9%. There were nine perforations (0.9%) and one death (0.1%) secondary to perforation. In the evaluation of cardiomyopathy/myocarditis, the incidence of complication was 9.1%, perforation was 5.2%, and mortality was 0.6%. In patients undergoing biopsy for transplant rejection surveillance, the incidence of complication was 0.6%, perforation was 0.1%, and no deaths occurred.

No reported series has estimated complication rates from left ventricular biopsies. In addition to the risk of arterial versus venous access, these patients require antiplatelet therapy and heparinized sheaths, which may increase the risk of bleeding. Platelet emboli into the systemic arterial bed place patients at increased risk for central nervous system complications. The risk of perforation from left ventricular biopsy is probably not decreased compared with the right ventricular approach.

On the basis of these studies, the estimated risk of complication related to endomyocardial biopsy for the evaluation of cardiomyopathy or for possible myocarditis is 1%–6%. The risk of fatal complication is 0 to 0.4%. Of note, there appears to be a lower risk of morbidity and mortality related to endomyocardial biopsy for the purpose of heart transplant rejection surveillance.

PERFORATION

The greatest risk to patients undergoing endomyocardial biopsy is ventricular perforation. If hemodynamically significant and left uncorrected, such perforation can lead to pericardial tamponade and death.[53] Factors associated with an increased likelihood of perforation include bleeding diathesis, recent receipt of heparin, pulmonary hypertension, and increased right ventricular systolic pressures or right ventricular enlargement. Patients with a prothrombin time of >18 seconds or who have received heparin without reversal within the prior 2 hours should probably not undergo endomyocardial biopsy. Perforation is usually a complication of injury to the right ventricular free wall, which is only 1–2 mm thick. Interestingly, performance of left ventricular biopsy shares similar perforation complication rates despite significantly thicker ventricular walls.

It is critical that clinicians who perform endomyocardial biopsy have a high index of suspicion for cardiac perforation. To this end, any patient complaining of pain during the performance of the endomyocardial biopsy should be considered to have experienced cardiac perforation. Typically, patients with perforation immediately complain of a visceral pain and within 1–2 minutes may develop vagal symptoms, including bradycardia and hypotension. Despite the excess parasympathetic tone thought to underlie these symptoms, limited benefit is achieved by atropine administration. Further biopsy attempts are contraindicated until a thorough investigation into the patient's complaints has been completed. If cardiac perforation is suspected, continuous evaluation of right atrial pressure and the pulsatility of the right and left heart borders by fluoroscopy should be performed. Increased right atrial pressure and loss of pulsation of heart borders are strong indicators for pericardial tamponade. Emergent transthoracic echocardiography (TTE) should be obtained to determine the presence and severity of pericardial blood accumulation.

Cardiovascular collapse or electrical mechanical disassociation (pulseless electrical activity (PEA) arrest) in the setting of a biopsy should be considered to be presumptive evidence of pericardial tamponade, and mandates immediate pericardiocentesis, even in the absence of echocardiographic confirmation of tamponade. Occasionally, acute bleeding into the pericardial space will clot and prevent adequate draining by pericardiocentesis. Should this situation arise in a hemodynamically unstable patient, it may be necessary that the pericardial space be surgically evacuated occasionally in the catheterization laboratory. Because of the risk of tamponade, a pericardiocentesis tray should always be available in the procedure room where endomyocardial biopsies are performed.

MALIGNANT VENTRICULAR ARRHYTHMIAS

Ventricular ectopy is an expected consequence of cannulation and mechanical stimulation of the cardiac chambers by the sheath or bioptome. In fact, premature ventricular contractions are utilized as an indication of appropriate placement of the bioptome or biopsy sheath within the ventricular cavity. Rarely, sustained malignant ventricular arrhythmias may develop during the biopsy procedure. Risk factors for this complication include cardiomyopathy and preexistent ventricular arrhythmias. Treatment begins with immediate withdrawal of the bioptome or biopsy sheath from the ventricular cavity. Should this fail to stop the arrhythmia, medical therapy with antiarrhythmic agents or cardioversion may be necessary.

SUPRAVENTRICULAR ARRHYTHMIAS

During instrumentation of the RA, the atrial wall may be stimulated leading to supraventricular arrhythmias. Risk factors for this complication include prior history of supraventricular arrhythmia or elevated right-sided filling pressures. Operators should try to avoid right atrial wall contact, particularly in patients identified at risk. In the event that a supraventricular tachycardia develops, mechanical interruption of the circus rhythm may be attempted by touching the right atrial wall with the bioptome. However, this may lead to an increased risk of cardiac perforation.

Heart block

Occasionally, patients with preexistent LBBB may develop complete heart block during manipulation of instruments within the right heart. Pressure against the septum near the tricuspid apparatus may "stun" the right bundle, resulting in a new RBBB. In patients with a preexistent LBBB, the addition of a new RBBB results in progression to complete heart block. Removal of the offending bioptome or catheter often resolves the complete heart block; however, should complete heart block persist, a temporary pacing catheter can be inserted into the right ventricular cavity. For this reason, a temporary pacemaker and pacing wire should be immediately available in the catheterization laboratory for emergent use if needed, particularly in patients with a preexistent LBBB.

Pneumothorax and hemothorax

Puncture of the lung pleura during performance of internal jugular or subclavian venous access may result in a pneumothorax or hemothorax. On the basis of a large meta-analysis of 17 prospective comparative trials, including data on 2,085 jugular and 2,428 subclavian catheters, the risk of one of these complications has been estimated at 1.5% for subclavian venous access and 1.3% for internal jugular venous access.[54] Several strategies can be utilized to minimize this risk. A growing body of literature supports the use of real-time 2D ultrasound guidance for internal jugular venous access.[55,56] Secondly, strict attention to detail should be maintained during insertion. This includes performing a "higher" internal jugular stick with avoidance of the immediate supraclavicular region, continuous aspiration of the needle plunger during every attempt at venous entry, and also during subclavian venous access the operator should never let the needle drop below the horizontal plane. Immediate investigation with fluoroscopy of the lung margins should be performed in any patient undergoing endomyocardial biopsy who complains of spontaneous shortness of breath. Urgent pneumothorax or hemothorax evacuation should be performed as needed.

Puncture of the carotid, subclavian, or femoral artery

Central veins lie adjacent to their corresponding arteries. The risk of carotid, subclavian, and femoral artery puncture

has been estimated to be approximately 3%, 0.5% to 5%, and 9%, respectively.[54,57] Under most circumstances, the operator can easily distinguish an arterial puncture from a venous puncture by the red color and pulsatile flow of arterial blood. In patients with significant hypoxemia and/or reduced cardiac output (i.e., cardiomyopathy), this distinction can sometimes be difficult. To help distinguish between arterial and venous blood, the operator may send a sample of blood for blood gas analysis. Alternatively, the operator can insert a small 18-gauge catheter over the guidewire and then determine the pressure waveform of the cannulated vessel. Puncture of an artery utilizing the finder or micropuncture needle should be addressed by withdrawal of the needle and compression of the vessel until hemostasis is obtained. This does not preclude performance of a safe venous approach. Cannulation of an artery with a large (7- to 9-Fr) sheath is a more serious complication that requires urgent vascular surgery consultation. In this situation, the sheath should not be removed before surgical consultation because of the risk of hemorrhage.

THROMBOEMBOLIC PHENOMENON

Patients with preformed sheaths that are not continuously flushed may develop a clot within the sheath during the performance of the endomyocardial biopsy.[58] As the bioptome is advanced through the clot-containing sheath, this can lead to expulsion of the clot into the patient's circulation. When this occurs during right ventricular biopsy it can lead to pulmonary embolization. Should this occur during a left ventricular biopsy or during a right ventricular biopsy in a patient with a right-to-left shunt, systemic embolization can occur. A risk unique to left ventricular biopsy is systemic platelet embolization. The incidence of platelet emboli during left heart biopsy has not been reported. Some operators suggest use of antiplatelet therapy such as aspirin prior to performing a biopsy in the left heart.

NERVE PARESIS

Infiltration of local anesthesia into the jugular venous or carotid sheath may result in Horner's syndrome, vocal cord paresis, or rarely, diaphragmatic weakness.[59,60] These complications typically last a few hours (on the basis of the half-life of the local anesthetic used) unless direct nerve trauma has occurred from the needle itself.

TRICUSPID VALVE DAMAGE

Tricuspid regurgitation is a well-recognized complication of endomyocardial biopsy.[61] In fact, tricuspid regurgitation is the most common valvular lesion after orthotopic heart transplantation. The most common etiology of significant tricuspid regurgitation in the post-transplant patient is endomyocardial biopsy performed to detect allograft rejection. Endomyocardial biopsy can lead to direct anatomic disruption of the valve apparatus, such as ruptured chordae tendinae or torn leaflet.[62] In their study of 98 post-transplant patients, Mielniczuk et al. found histologic evidence of chordal tissue in 9% of endomyocardial biopsy specimens, which accounted for 47% of patients with significant tricuspid regurgitation in their cohort.[63] Nguyen et al. examined whether there was a correlation between the number of endomyocardial biopsies and the risk of severe tricuspid valvular regurgitation.[64] In their study of 101 post-transplant patients, they found 60% of patients with more than 31 endomyocardial biopsies had developed severe tricuspid regurgitation, whereas none of the patients with fewer than 18 endomyocardial biopsies had severe tricuspid regurgitation.

HEMATOMA

A venous or arterial hematoma may form as a result of excessive movement of the sheath during the biopsy procedure, inadequate compression of the vascular access site after removal of the sheath, or late bleeding due to a transient or sustained increase in right atrial or mean arterial pressure. Patients with coagulopathy or who are on anticoagulant therapy as well as aspirin are at increased risk for hematoma formation and should be monitored more closely.

ARTERIAL-VENTRICULAR FISTULA

Occasionally arterial-ventricular fistulas develop between small branches of a coronary artery and the RV in postcardiac transplant patients.[65] These are caused by inadvertent biopsy of septal branches of a coronary artery and subsequent arterial communication into the RV. Several studies have shown that these fistulae are of no clinical consequence and can be followed conservatively.

LIMITATIONS

Sampling error

One limitation of endomyocardial biopsy as a diagnostic tool for myocarditis or transplant rejection is that it is prone to sampling error. Since myocarditis, and to a lesser extent transplant rejection, tend to be focal processes, accurate diagnosis depends on adequate sampling of the myocardium. Standard bioptomes sample approximately $1-2$ mm^3 (30 mg) of endomyocardium with each biopsy. Researchers have demonstrated on *ex vivo* hearts with histologically proven myocarditis (either postmortem or explanted) that sampling error contributes appreciably to false-negative results.[66] Chow et al. demonstrated that from a single endomyocardial biopsy, histologic myocarditis could be demonstrated in only 25% of samples.[67] With more than five random samples, Dallas criteria myocarditis could be diagnosed in approximately two-thirds of subjects. Most recently, Mahrholdt et al. demonstrated by cardiovascular MRI that the earliest myocardial inflammatory abnormalities in myocarditis are located in the lateral wall of the LV, a site that is not available to biopsy with the standard approach.[19] For transplant rejection surveillance, the sensitivity of detecting transplant rejection approaches 98% when five adequate biopsy samples are obtained.[68]

Limitations of the Dallas criteria

Originally proposed in 1986, the Dallas criteria established a histopathologic categorization by which the diagnosis of myocarditis could be made.[69] According to the Dallas criteria, active myocarditis requires an inflammatory infiltrate and associated myocyte necrosis or damage uncharacteristic of an ischemic event. Borderline myocarditis requires a less intense inflammatory infiltrate and no light microscopic evidence of myocyte destruction. Data from the Myocarditis Treatment Trial reveal that approximately 10% of patients (214 out of 2,233) with clinically suspected myocarditis (new-onset unexplained heart failure during the 2 years preceding enrollment) who underwent endomyocardial biopsy were diagnosed by the current histopathologic Dallas criteria.[40]

To compound this further, the Dallas criteria require that biopsy specimens be examined by qualified cardiac pathologists. Additionally, even when specimens are examined by expert cardiac pathologists, there are variations in the interpretation of histologic samples. In the Myocarditis Treatment Trial, only 64% of the 111 patients diagnosed with myocarditis by endomyocardial biopsy had their diagnosis confirmed by the expert pathology panel during review of the same biopsy samples at a later date. In a separate analysis of interobserver variability, Shane et al. submitted endomyocardial biopsy specimens from 16 patients with dilated cardiomyopathy to seven expert cardiac pathologists. Their assessments varied remarkably with respect to significant fibrosis (25%–69%), hypertrophy (19%–88%), nuclear changes (31%–94%), lymphocyte count per high-power field (0–38%), and the diagnosis of myocarditis. Definite or probable myocarditis was diagnosed in 11 of 16 patients by at least one pathologist. However, of the 11 patients, three of seven pathologists agreed on the diagnosis in 3 patients, and two of seven pathologists, agreed on the diagnosis in 5 patients.

Several researchers have demonstrated the presence of cardiotropic virus in myocardium in the absence of Dallas criteria myocarditis. Martin et al. utilized polymerase chain reaction (PCR) to analyze myocardial tissue samples from 34 patients with suspected acute viral myocarditis. They demonstrated that 26 heart biopsy samples were positive for viral pathogens, and 13 of the 26 positive samples had no evidence of Dallas criteria myocarditis.[70] Pauschinger et al. found either adenoviral or enteroviral PCR positivity in 24 myocardial tissue samples (none of which showed histopathologic evidence of myocarditis) from 94 patients with "idiopathic" dilated cardiomyopathy.[71] In a separate study of 45 patients with left ventricular dysfunction and suspected myocarditis, Paushchinger et al. demonstrated enterovirus ribonucleic acid (RNA) in 18 (40%) of the 45 patients. Of the 18 patients with enterovirus RNA detected, 10 were found to have active viral replication as well.[72] In this study, 13% of the biopsy samples were diagnosed as having Dallas criteria borderline myocarditis; however, histopathology did not help to distinguish between patients with and those without enteroviral positivity. Why et al. showed in their cohort of 120 patients with idiopathic dilated cardiomyopathy that the 34% who were enteroviral positive had a significantly worse outcome over 2 years compared with those who were enteroviral negative.[73] Taken together, the virus can exist in the myocardium (even in a replicative form) in the absence of histopathologic findings adequate to meet Dallas criteria and may adversely affect outcome.

Another limitation in the usefulness of the Dallas criteria is the dissociation between histopathology findings and response to immune modulation therapy. For instance, in the Myocarditis Treatment Trial, there was no difference in 1- or 5-year survival or improvement of left ventricular ejection fraction (LVEF) at 28 weeks in patients with Dallas criteria myocarditis treated with immunosuppressive therapy or placebo. Other authors have used alternative criteria to diagnose immune-related heart disease such as human leucocyte antigen (HLA) upregulation on endomyocardial biopsy. Wojnicz et al. found HLA upregulation in cardiac biopsy samples from 84 of 202 patients (41.6%) with new-onset cardiomyopathy, while only 27% were positive by Dallas criteria for myocarditis.[74] HLA-identified patients were randomized to receive treatment with either immunosuppressive therapy or placebo. After 2 years of follow-up, there was no significant difference in the primary endpoint (a composite of death, heart transplantation, and hospital readmission) between the study groups (22.8% for the immunosuppression group and 20.5% for the placebo group); however, the ejection fraction in the immunosuppressive group increased from 24% to 36%, whereas it remained unchanged in the placebo group (25%–27%).

Despite the presence of Dallas criteria myocarditis, response to treatment may be influenced by the presence of virus or immunologic response to infection. This was most clearly demonstrated by Frustaci et al. in their study of immunosuppressive therapy in patients with Dallas criteria myocarditis who failed to respond to conventional therapy.[75] Out of 652 patients who underwent endomyocardial biopsy, 112 were identified with Dallas criteria myocarditis. Of these 112 patients, 41 had progressive congestive heart failure (CHF) despite standard medical therapy and were treated with prednisone and azathioprine for 6 months. Twenty-one patients responded to treatment with improvement of LVEF from 25.7% to 47.1%, and showed evidence of healed myocarditis on follow-up biopsy. Twenty patients failed to respond to treatment and showed a histologic evolution toward dilated cardiomyopathy. Viral genomes were present in endomyocardial biopsy specimens in 85% of nonresponders versus 15% of responders. Circulating cardiac antibodies were present in 90% of responders versus 0% of nonresponders.

Given that the Dallas criteria are prone to sampling error, interobserver variability, variance with other markers of viral infection and immune activation in the heart, and variance with treatment outcomes, we suggest that the Dallas criteria should no longer be used to diagnose myocarditis in isolation. Instead, myocarditis should be diagnosed on the basis of a combination of clinical presentation, histopathology, immunohistochemistry, viral polymerase chain reaction (PCR), cardiac antibody assessment, and imaging results.

SPECIAL ISSUES

Tissue processing

The clinician performing the endomyocardial biopsy is responsible for obtaining adequate tissue for analysis and ensuring the tissue is placed in the appropriate preservative. The number of specimens obtained depends on the clinical situation and studies to be performed. Adequate diagnostic yield from repeated biopsy must be balanced against the risk of the biopsy procedure. It is generally recommended that at least five separate specimens, each 1–2 mm^3 in size, be obtained from more than one region to minimize sampling error. For transplant rejection surveillance, the International Society of Heart and Lung Transplantation requires a minimum of four biopsy specimens, each with less than 50% of the sample being fibrous tissue, thrombus, or other uninterpretable tissues, such as those with crush artifact. The sensitivity of detecting transplant rejection approaches 98% when the pathologist reviews five adequate biopsy samples.[76]

To avoid contamination of the biopsy specimen, once the bioptome forceps have been removed from the venous sheath and the jaws are opened, the sample should be gently extracted with a sterile needle and placed immediately into preservative solution (10% neutral buffered formalin).[77,78] Fixative should be at room temperature to prevent contraction band artifacts.[79] Excessive traction or crushing of the sample, as well as cutting a single larger sample into many, should be avoided because it may disrupt histologic architecture. Additional samples may be submitted for transmission electron microscopy to evaluate infiltrative diseases or anthracycline toxicity.[80] For transmission electron microscopy, pieces are fixed in 4% glutaraldehyde at room temperature. One or more samples may be frozen for molecular analysis, immunofluorescence, immunohistochemistry, or viral genome analysis. To prepare frozen specimens in the catheterization laboratory, samples should be placed in embedding solution then snap frozen in optical cutting temperature (OCT)-embedding medium or alternatively placed in RNA later solution and stored at −80°F. These study samples may be required for suspected myocarditis, amyloid classification, tumor typing, or viral genome analysis. Additional sample preparation may be individualized for evaluation of specific disease states (e.g., amyloid, iron staining). It is the operator's responsibility to ensure timely delivery of biopsy samples to the appropriate pathologic laboratory.

Cardiac pathologist

Experienced cardiac pathologists are central to any biopsy program. The safest and most pristine biopsy specimen is useless without an experienced cardiac pathologist who is fully trained in the evaluation of biopsy-obtained tissue and conversant with the latest classification schemes. Crush artifacts or contraction bands are frequently present in biopsy specimens and may be incorrectly interpreted by an inexperienced or noncardiac pathologist. The operator may assist the pathologist through careful handling of the biopsy specimen in the catheterization laboratory, by ensuring that the heart biopsy specimens obtained are delivered to the appropriate laboratory for analysis, and by reviewing the slide material obtained with the pathologist to provide clinical details and to ensure that special studies are obtained as needed.

Light microscopic examination and stains

Endomyocardial biopsy tissue that is going to be examined by routine light microscopy is embedded in paraffin and serially sectioned into 4 mm thick layers mounted on sequentially numbered glass slides. In cases of suspected myocarditis, most laboratories stain every third slide with hematoxylin and eosin for histomorphologic characterization. Two slides are typically stained with Movat or elastic trichrome stain to visualize collagen and elastic tissue. In addition, many laboratories will stain one slide for iron on specimens from men and all postmenopausal women. Congo red staining is performed on a 10 to 15 mm section in all patients over the age of 50 to identify cardiac amyloidosis. Table 13.5 summarizes the stains that are occasionally used in the evaluation of heart biopsy samples depending on the clinical situation.

Table 13.5 Special stains for endomyocardial biopsy

Stain	Frequent Indication
Methyl green pyronin	Lymphocytes (myocarditis/allograft rejection)
Movat pentachrome	
Masson elastic trichrome	Connective tissue/vasculature
Prussian blue	
Sulfated Alcian blue	Connective tissue/vasculature
Congo red	Iron
Ziehl–Neelsen	Iron and amyloid
Periodic acid Schiff	Amyloid
Gram	Granulomas (acid-fast bacilli)
Gomori methenamine silver	Intramyocardial glycogen/vasculture/fungi
Hematoxylin phloxine saffron	Bacteria (endocarditis) Fungi
Methyl violet	Connective tissue Amyloid

Source: Reproduced from Veinot, J., et al., Light microscopy and ultra-structure of the blood vessel and heart, In: Silver, M., et al., *Cardiovascular Pathology*, 3rd edn, Churchill Livingstone, New York, 2001, pp. 30–53. With permission.

Molecular studies

Increasingly, molecular techniques are available that improve the clinical utility of endomyocardial biopsy above and beyond the simple histopathologic and biochemical analysis that has been available to this point. Advances in PCR techniques allow pathologists or investigators to determine whether or not the patient's cardiomyopathy or myocarditis is associated with a preexistent or ongoing viral infection.[72] Current PCR techniques can detect fewer than 10 gene copies of viral pathogens in an endomyocardial biopsy sample. For PCR analysis to be considered reliable, the biopsy sample must be rapidly and properly transported to the laboratory for analysis. Proper handling of the sample includes the use of pathogen-free biopsy devices and storage vials and the transportation of biopsy samples in RNA later solution on dry ice at room temperature.

Over the past 20 years, the use of PCR has increased our understanding of possible cardiotropic viruses in patients with unexplained cardiomyopathy. Numerous studies of patients with myocarditis or dilated cardiomyopathy have reported a wide range of viruses, including enteroviruses (most commonly Coxsackie B virus), adenoviruses, Parvovirus B19, cytomegalovirus, influenza and respiratory syncytial virus, Ebstein–Barr virus, HIV, Hepatitis C virus, and human herpes virus 6.[81–87] There are several limitations to the widespread use of PCR in screening endomyocardial biopsy samples for cardiotropic viruses. Currently available PCR-based viral isolation techniques remain labor intensive and costly, and lack standardization. Existing PCR screening methods are also restricted to a limited number of predetermined candidate viruses. Because the number of biopsy samples needed to attain a clinically acceptable sensitivity for cardiotropic viruses is not known, a positive PCR is diagnostic of viral infection; however, a negative PCR does not exclude viral infection. Most importantly, the presence of viral genomic material in biopsy specimens does not prove causality of cardiomyopathy and currently does not change management strategy.

Molecular studies can also be utilized to look for immune markers, such as HLA upregulation and immune deposition, to identify those patients who have an autoimmune process that may be perpetuating ventricular dysfunction.[74] Molecular studies are not limited to diagnostic evaluation, but have also been shown to have prognostic implications in patients with new-onset idiopathic cardiomyopathy. Heidecker et al. demonstrated that microarray technology could be utilized to generate a transcriptomic signature (45 genes) from a single endomyocardial biopsy, which could predict prognosis in patients with new-onset heart failure of unclear etiology with very high specificity (90%).[88]

Future directions

The clinical utility of endomyocardial biopsy will no doubt be strengthened by the application of highly specific molecular probes and microarray deoxyribonucleic acid (DNA) technology used to look for viral genomic material and autoimmunity in heart biopsy specimens. Our current understanding of idiopathic cardiomyopathies is that they are the consequence of a complex interplay between inflammatory, infectious, autoimmune, and genetic factors ultimately resulting in myocardial injury and remodeling. With the improvement and increased availability of techniques to define immune upregulation and viral persistence, it is likely that endomyocardial biopsies will redefine myocarditis and its appropriate treatment. Only through a detailed understanding of the pathobiology of idiopathic cardiomyopathies will we be able to develop novel therapies targeted at these important disorders.

CONCLUSIONS

Endomyocardial biopsy remains an integral mode of investigation for diagnosing many primary and secondary myocardial conditions. The modern approach to endomyocardial biopsy was introduced by Sakakibara and Konno in the early 1960s and then modified and popularized by the Stanford group in the early 1970s as a means to monitor graft rejection following cardiac transplantation. Since then, the right ventricular heart biopsy procedure has gained acceptance as a useful investigative tool for nontransplant cardiac pathology. The indications for endomyocardial biopsy have been outlined in a consensus statement published in 2007 by the AHA, ACC, and the ESC.[28] Indications for endomyocardial biopsy include post-transplant rejection surveillance, investigation of infiltrative disorders of the myocardium, primary cardiomyopathies, myocarditis, endocardial fibrosis (as a way to help distinguish between constrictive and restrictive pathology), drug toxicity, ventricular arrhythmias, unexplained heart failure in children, and suspected cardiac neoplasia. Cardiac biopsy is extremely safe when performed by an experienced operator. Complication rates are reduced by appropriate patient selection, careful biopsy technique guided by fluoroscopy and ultrasound, as well as close patient monitoring. The role of endomyocardial biopsy continues to evolve as novel molecular and genetic analyses shed new light on heart muscle disorders.

REFERENCES

1. Weinberg M, et al. Diagnostic biopsy of the pericardium and myocardium. *AMA Arch Surg* 1958;76(5):825–829.
2. Sutton DC, Sutton GC. Needle biopsy of the human ventricular myocardium: Review of 54 consecutive cases. *Am Heart J* 1960;60:364–370.
3. Shirey EK, et al. Percutaneous myocardial biopsy of the left ventricle. Experience in 198 patients. *Circulation* 1972;46(1):112–122.
4. Timmis GC, et al. Percutaneous myocardial biopsy. *Am Heart J* 1965;70(4):499–504.
5. Bulloch RT, et al. Intracardiac needle biopsy of the ventricular septum. *Am J Cardiol* 1965;16:227–233.
6. Sakakibara S, Konno S. Endomyocardial biopsy. *Jpn Heart J* 1962;3:537–543.
7. Caves PK, et al. New instrument for transvenous cardiac biopsy. *Am J Cardiol* 1974;33(2):264–267.
8. Caves PK, et al. Percutaneous transvenous endomyocardial biopsy. *JAMA* 1973;225(3):288–291.
9. Kawai C, Kitaura Y. New endomyocardial biopsy catheter for the left ventricle. *Am J Cardiol* 1977;40(1):63–65.
10. Richardson PJ. King's endomyocardial bioptome. *Lancet* 1974;1(7859): 660–661.
11. Baughman K, Baim D. Endomyocardial biopsy. In: Baim D, ed. *Grossman's Cardiac Catheterization, Angiography, and Intervention.* 7th edn. Philadelphia: Lippincott Williams and Wilkins, 2006:395–412.
12. Baumgartner WA, et al. *Heart and Lung Transplantation.* 2nd edn. Philadelphia, PA: W. B. Saunders Company, 2002.
13. Denys BG, et al. An ultrasound method for safe and rapid central venous access. *N Engl J Med* 1991;324(8):566.
14. Denys BG, et al. Ultrasound-assisted cannulation of the internal jugular vein. A prospective comparison to the external landmark-guided technique. *Circulation* 1993;87(5):1557–1562.
15. Anderson JL, Marshall HW. The femoral venous approach to endomyocardial biopsy: Comparison with internal jugular and transarterial approaches. *Am J Cardiol* 1984;53(6):833–837.
16. Brooksby IA, et al. Left-ventricular endomyocardial biopsy. *Lancet* 1974; 2:1222–1225.
17. Pierard L, et al. Two-dimensional echocardiographic guiding of endomyocardial biopsy. *Chest* 1984;85:759–762.
18. Miller LW, et al. Echocardiography-guided endomyocardial biopsy. A 5-year experience. *Circulation* 1988;78(5 Pt 2):III99–III102.
19. Mahrholdt H, et al. Cardiovascular magnetic resonance assessment of human myocarditis: A comparison to histology and molecular pathology. *Circulation* 2004;109(10):1250–1258.
20. Amitai ME, et al. Comparison of three-dimensional echocardiography to two-dimensional echocardiography and fluoroscopy for monitoring of endomyocardial biopsy. *Am J Cardiol* 2007;99(6):864–866.
21. Rios B, et al. Left ventricular endomyocardial biopsy in children with the transseptal long sheath technique. *Cathet Cardiovasc Diagn* 1984;10(4):417–423.
22. Hunt SA, Haddad F. The changing face of heart transplantation. *J Am Coll Cardiol* 2008;52(8):587–598.
23. Miller LW, et al. 24th Bethesda conference: Cardiac transplantation. Task force 5: Complications. *J Am Coll Cardiol* 1993;22:41–54.
24. Ballester M, et al. Evaluation of biopsy classification for rejection: Relation to detection of myocardial damage by monoclonal antimyosin antibody imaging. *J Am Coll Cardiol* 1998;31(6):1357–1361.
25. Deng MC, et al. Noninvasive discrimination of rejection in cardiac allograft recipients using gene expression profiling. *Am J Transplant* 2006;6(1):150–160.
26. Pham MX, et al. Molecular testing for long-term rejection surveillance in heart transplant recipients: Design of the Invasive Monitoring Attenuation Through Gene Expression (IMAGE) trial. *J Heart Lung Transplant* 2007;26(8):808–814.

27. Stewart S, et al. Revision of the 1990 working formulation for the standardization of nomenclature in the diagnosis of heart rejection. *J Heart Lung Transplant* 2005;24(11):1710–1720.

28. Cooper LT, et al. The role of endomyocardial biopsy in the management of cardiovascular disease: A scientific statement from the American Heart Association, the American College of Cardiology, and the European Society of Cardiology. *Circulation* 2007;116(19):2216–2233.

29. Heart Failure Society of America. HFSA 2006 Comprehensive Heart Failure Practice Guideline. *J Card Fail* 2006;12:e1–e2.

30. Hunt SA. ACC/AHA 2005 guideline update for the diagnosis and management of chronic heart failure in the adult: A report of the American College of Cardiology/American Heart Association Task Force on Practice Guidelines (Writing Committee to Update the 2001 Guidelines for the Evaluation and Management of Heart Failure). *J Am Coll Cardiol* 2005; 46(6):e1–e82.

31. Swedberg K, et al. Guidelines for the diagnosis and treatment of chronic heart failure: Executive summary (update 2005): The Task Force for the Diagnosis and Treatment of Chronic Heart Failure of the European Society of Cardiology. *Eur Heart J* 2005;26(11):1115–1140.

32. Felker GM, et al. Underlying causes and long-term survival in patients with initially unexplained cardiomyopathy. *N Engl J Med* 2000;342(15):1077–1084.

33. Amabile N, et al. Outcome of acute fulminant myocarditis in children. *Heart* 2006;92(9):1269–1273.

34. Dec GW Jr., et al. Active myocarditis in the spectrum of acute dilated cardiomyopathies. Clinical features, histologic correlates, and clinical outcome. *N Engl J Med* 1985;312(14):885–890.

35. McCarthy RE III, et al. Long-term outcome of fulminant myocarditis as compared with acute (non-fulminant) myocarditis. *N Engl J Med* 2000;342(10):690–695.

36. Cooper LT Jr., et al. Idiopathic giant-cell myocarditis—natural history and treatment. Multicenter Giant Cell Myocardi tis Study Group Investigators. *N Engl J Med* 1997;336:1860–1866.

37. Cooper LT, Zehr KJ. Biventricular assist device placement and immunosuppression as therapy for necrotizing eosinophilic myocarditis. *Nat Clin Pract Cardiovasc Med* 2005;2(10):544–548.

38. Okura Y, et al. A clinical and histopathologic comparison of cardiac sarcoidosis and idiopathic giant cell myocarditis. *J Am Coll Cardiol* 2003;41(2):322–329.

39. Baughman KL. Diagnosis of myocarditis: Death of Dallas criteria. *Circulation* 2006;113(4):593–595.

40. Mason JW, et al. A clinical trial of immunosuppressive therapy for myocarditis. The Myocarditis Treatment Trial Investigators. *N Engl J Med* 1995;333(5):269–275.

41. Dec GW, Fuster V. Idiopathic dilated cardiomyopathy. *N Engl J Med* 1994;331(23):1564–1575.

42. Felker GM, et al. The spectrum of dilated cardiomyopathy. The Johns Hopkins experience with 1,278 patients. *Medicine (Baltimore)* 1999;78(4):270–283.

43. Schoenfeld MH, et al. Restrictive cardiomyopathy versus constrictive pericarditis: Role of endomyocardial biopsy in avoiding unnecessary thoracotomy. *Circulation* 1987;75(5):1012–1017.

44. Arad M, et al. Glycogen storage diseases presenting as hypertrophic cardiomyopathy. *N Engl J Med* 2005;352(4):362–372.

45. Falk RH. Diagnosis and management of the cardiac amyloidoses. *Circulation* 2005;112(13):2047–2060.

46. Fowles RE, Mason JW. Endomyocardial biopsy. *Ann Intern Med* 1982;97(6):885–894.

47. Sekiguchi M, Take M. World survey of catheter biopsy of the heart. In: Sekiguchi M, Olsen E, eds. *Cardiomyopathy: Clinical, Pathological and Theoretical Aspects.* Baltimore, MA: University Park Press, 1980:217–225.

48. Deckers JW, et al. Complications of transvenous right ventricular endomyocardial biopsy in adult patients with cardiomyopathy: A seven-year survey of 546 consecutive diagnostic procedures in a tertiary referral center. *J Am Coll Cardiol* 1992;19(1):43–47.

49. Han J, et al. Complications of 2-D echocardiography guided transfemoral right ventricular endomyocardial biopsy. *J Korean Med Sci* 2006;21(6):989–994.

50. Baraldi-Junkins C, et al. Complications of endomyocardial biopsy in heart transplant patients. *J Heart Lung Transplant* 1993;12(1 Pt 1):63–67.

51. Holzmann M, et al. Complication rate of right ventricular endomyocardial biopsy via the femoral approach: A retrospective and prospective study analyzing 3048 diagnostic procedures over an 11-year period. *Circulation* 2008;118(17):1722–1728.

52. Pophal SG, et al. Complications of endomyocardial biopsy in children. *J Am Coll Cardiol* 1999;34(7):2105–2110.

53. Friedrich SP, et al. Myocardial perforation in the cardiac catheterization laboratory: Incidence, presentation, diagnosis, and management. *Cathet Cardiovasc Diagn* 1994;32(2):99–107.

54. Ruesch S, et al. Complications of central venous catheters: Internal jugular versus subclavian access—a systematic review. *Crit Care Med* 2002;30(2):454–460.

55. Hind D, et al. Ultrasonic locating devices for central venous cannulation: Meta-analysis. *BMJ* 2003;327(7411):361.

56. Karakitsos D, et al. Real-time ultrasound-guided catheterisation of the internal jugular vein: A prospective comparison with the landmark technique in critical care patients. *Crit Care* 2006;10(6):R162.

57. Merrer J, et al. Complications of femoral and subclavian venous catheterization in critically ill patients: A randomized controlled trial. *JAMA* 2001;286(6):700–707.

58. Kreher SK, et al. Frequent occurrence of occult pulmonary embolism from venous sheaths during endomyocardial biopsy. *J Am Coll Cardiol* 1992;19(3):581–585.

59. Bell RL, et al. Traumatic and iatrogenic Horner syndrome: Case reports and review of the literature. *J Trauma* 2001;51(2):400–404.

60. Martin-Hirsch DP, Newbegin CJ. Right vocal fold paralysis as a result of central venous catheterization. *J Laryngol Otol* 1995;109(11):1107–1108.

61. Wong RC, et al. Tricuspid regurgitation after cardiac transplantation: An old problem revisited. *J Heart Lung Transplant* 2008;27(3):247–252.

62. Braverman AC, et al. Ruptured chordae tendineae of the tricuspid valve as a complication of endomyocardial biopsy in heart transplant patients. *Am J Cardiol* 1990;66(1):111–113.

63. Mielniczuk L, et al. Tricuspid valve chordal tissue in endomyocardial biopsy specimens of patients with significant tricuspid regurgitation. *J Heart Lung Transplant* 2005;24(10):1586–1590.

64. Nguyen V, et al. Tricuspid regurgitation after cardiac transplantation: How many biopsies are too many? *J Heart Lung Transplant* 2005;24(7 Suppl):S227–S231.

65. Sandhu JS, et al. Coronary artery fistula in the heart transplant patient. A potential complication of endomyocardial biopsy. *Circulation* 1989;79(2):350–356.

66. Hauck AJ, et al. Evaluation of postmortem endomyocardial biopsy specimens from 38 patients with lymphocytic myocarditis: Implications for role of sampling error. *Mayo Clin Proc* 1989;64(10):1235–1245.

67. Chow LH, et al. Insensitivity of right ventricular endomyocardial biopsy in the diagnosis of myocarditis. *J Am Coll Cardiol* 1989;14(4):915–920.

68. Winters G, Schoen F. Pathology of cardiac transplantation. In: Silver M, Gotlieb A, Schoen F, eds. *Cardiovascular Pathology*. Philadelphia, PA: Churchill Livingstone, 2001:725–759.

69. Aretz HT, et al. Myocarditis. A histopathologic definition and classification. *Am J Cardiovasc Pathol* 1987;1(1):3–14.

70. Martin AB, et al. Acute myocarditis. Rapid diagnosis by PCR in children. *Circulation* 1994;90(1):330–339.

71. Pauschinger M, et al. Detection of adenoviral genome in the myocardium of adult patients with idiopathic left ventricular dysfunction. *Circulation* 1999;99(10):1348–1354.

72. Pauschinger M, et al. Enteroviral RNA replication in the myocardium of patients with left ventricular dysfunction and clinically suspected myocarditis. *Circulation* 1999;99(7):889–895.

73. Why HJ, et al. Clinical and prognostic significance of detection of enteroviral RNA in the myocardium of patients with myocarditis or dilated cardiomyopathy. *Circulation* 1994;89(6):2582–2589.

74. Wojnicz R, et al. Randomized, placebo-controlled study for immunosuppressive treatment of inflammatory dilated cardiomyopathy: Two-year follow-up results. *Circulation* 2001;104(1):39–45.

75. Frustaci A, et al. Immunosuppressive therapy for active lymphocytic myocarditis: Virological and immunologic profile of responders versus nonresponders. *Circulation* 2003;107(6):857–863.

76. Billingham M. Pathology of heart transplantation. In: Solez K, Racusen L, Billingham M, eds. *Solid Organ Transplant Rejection: Mechanisms, Pathology and Diagnosis*. New York: Marcel Dekker, Inc., 1996:137–159.

77. Virmani R, et al. *Cardiovascular Pathology*. 2nd edn. Philadelphia, PA: Saunders, 2001.

78. Veinot J, et al. Light microscopy and ultra- structure of the blood vessel and heart. In: Silver M, Gotlieb A, Schoen F, eds. *Cardiovascular Pathology*. 3rd edn. New York: Churchill Livingstone, 2001:30–53.

79. Cunningham KS, et al. An approach to endomyocardial biopsy interpretation. *J Clin Pathol* 2006;59(2):121–129.

80. Billingham ME, et al. Anthracycline cardiomyopathy monitored by morphologic changes. *Cancer Treat Rep* 1978;62(6):865–872.

81. Bowles NE, et al. Detection of viruses in myocardial tissues by polymerase chain reaction. Evidence of adenovirus as a common cause of myocarditis in children and adults. *J Am Coll Cardiol* 2003; 42(3):466–472.

82. Grasso M, et al. Search for Coxsackievirus B3 RNA in idiopathic dilated cardiomyopathy using gene amplification by polymerase chain reaction. *Am J Cardiol* 1992;69(6):658–664.

83. Jin O, et al. Detection of enterovirus RNA in myocardial biopsies from patients with myocarditis and cardiomyopathy using gene amplification by polymerase chain reaction. *Circulation* 1990;82(1):8–16.

84. Kuhl U, et al. High prevalence of viral genomes and multiple viral infections in the myocardium of adults with "idiopathic" left ventricular dysfunction. *Circulation* 2005;111(7):887–893.

85. Matsumori A. Hepatitis C virus infection and cardiomyopathies. *Circ Res* 2005;96(2):144–147.

86. Muir P, et al. Rapid diagnosis of enterovirus infection by magnetic bead extraction and polymerase chain reaction detection of enterovirus RNA in clinical specimens. *J Clin Microbiol* 1993;31(1):31–38.

87. Tschope C, et al. High prevalence of cardiac parvovirus B19 infection in patients with isolated left ventricular diastolic dysfunction. *Circulation* 2005;111(7):879–886.

88. Heidecker B, et al. Transcriptomic biomarkers for individual risk assessment in new-onset heart failure. *Circulation* 2008;118(3):238–246.

14

Pericardiocentesis

CARL L. TOMMASO

INTRODUCTION

Pericardiocentesis is the transcutaneous drainage of fluid from the pericardial space. The first reported pericardiocentesis was by Johannes Riolanus in 1648 who performed the procedure via a hole drilled in the sternum. Franz Schuh is credited with the first indirect pericardiocentesis in 1840.[1]

Pericardiocentesis is performed for both diagnostic and therapeutic indications. Elective pericardiocentesis may be necessary if bacterial infection is suspected or the source of the pericardial effusion is unknown. Therapeutic pericardiocentesis for pericardial tamponade may be emergent and life-saving. More recently, other indications for entry into the pericardial space, namely, epicardial ventricular tachycardia ablation and left atrial appendage ligation, have emerged. These procedures are usually performed in patients without pericardial effusion.

ANATOMIC CONSIDERATIONS

The pericardium consists of two layers, the visceral pericardium that is adherent to the epicardium and the parietal pericardium that normally is about 1–2 mm thick. The parietal pericardium has attachments to the diaphragm, the sternum, and the anterior mediastinum, and holds the heart in a relatively fixed position during respiration and changes in body position. The two layers are continuous and form a "sac" that surrounds most of the heart except for the left atrium that is mostly extrapericardial. The pericardial reflection includes the origins of the vena cavae and the great arteries. The phrenic nerves are the only nonvascular structures included within the pericardium.

The inferior vena cava and right ventricle are the most anterior cardiac structures and attempted pericardiocentesis

risks entering either of these structures. The left anterior descending coronary artery is the most anterior of the coronary arteries and can rarely be punctured during pericardiocentesis. The internal mammary (thoracic) arteries are located on the posterior surface of the chest wall in the midclavicular line. Although not usually in the path of a pericardiocentesis needle, they can be punctured during lateral attempts at a loculated effusion (Figure 14.1).

Within the normal pericardial sac is less than 50 mL of serous fluid. The normal pericardium is relatively inelastic and small amounts of additional fluid (<100 mL) may compromise filling of cardiac chambers (cardiac tamponade). However, with chronic fluid accumulation, the pericardium may progressively stretch, become elastic, and accommodate large amounts of fluid without hemodynamic alteration.

When pericardial effusions occur, the fluid may be distributed throughout the pericardial space, or may be loculated, depending on the etiology of the effusion (Table 14.1) and prior pericardial disease or surgery.

CLINICAL ASPECTS

Chest pain, dyspnea at rest or with exertion, pleuritic pain, or palpitations may be associated with pericardial effusion, but there are no specific symptoms.

Cardiac tamponade also has nonspecific physical findings, including paradoxical pulse, and inspiratory decrease in systemic venous pressure. Distant heart sounds when noted with the other physical findings are a further clue; however, this constellation of findings may be present in other disease states including severe obstructive lung disease. Hemodynamic compromise includes hypotension (or a relative decrease from baseline pressure) and tachycardia

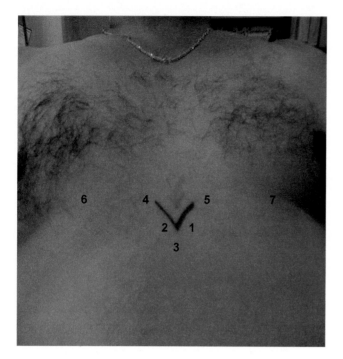

Figure 14.1 Locations for needle insertion for peri-cardiocentesis. Location 1 is just left (*patient's left*) of the xiphoid and is the most common location used. Alternatives include Location 2, to the right of the xiphoid, and Location 3, below the xiphoid. Locations 4 and 5 are in the fifth intercostal space on either side of the sternum, and 6 and 7 are in the mid-clavicular line as the insertion site for lateral loculated effusions.

Table 14.1 Causes of pericardial effusions

1. Collagen vascular disease
2. Iatrogenic
   a. Cardiac surgery
   b. CVP catheter insertion
   c. Endomyocardial biopsy
   d. Pacemaker lead (temporary or permanent)
   e. Percutaneous coronary intervention
      i. Cutting balloon
      ii. Glycoprotein IIb/IIIa inhibitors
      iii. Guidewire perforation
      iv. Saphenous vein graft rupture
   f. Radiofrequency ablation
   g. Trans-septal puncture
   h. Valvuloplasty
   i. Ventriculogram
3. Infection
4. Malignancy
5. Trauma
6. Uremia

(which may be masked by the presence of beta-blockers). As right-sided cardiac chamber filling decreases, so does stroke volume. The heart rate increases in an effort to maintain cardiac output. The most common noninvasive method of determining the presence of tamponade is echocardiography. The presence of diastolic right heart chamber collapse on echocardiography is sensitive for tamponade.[2,3]

"Asymptomatic" pericardial effusions can be suspected by an abnormal chest X-ray with a typical water-bottle configuration of the cardiac silhouette. The chest X-ray findings can be confirmed by echocardiography, chest computed tomography (CT), or magnetic resonance imaging, or initially can be detected with these imaging modalities.

The most accurate test for the presence of cardiac tamponade is the hemodynamic assessment of intracardiac pressures simultaneous with the measurement of intrapericardial pressure. In the presence of tamponade, there will be diastolic equilibration of the pressures equal to the intrapericardial pressure (Chapter 12).

The treatment for cardiac tamponade is pericardiocentesis or surgical drainage. The advantage of pericardiocentesis over surgical drainage is that it can be performed at the bedside if necessary. Given the mechanical nature of tamponade, there is no other treatment option. Diuretics may worsen the situation by reducing the intracardiac pressures and worsening filling of the heart. Balloon pericardiotomy is occasionally performed, particularly for recurrent effusions due to cancer.[4]

In cardiac tamponade there is a reduced stroke volume, so a compensatory increase in heart rate can initially maintain cardiac output and blood pressure. In the event that there is a delay in performing pericardiocentesis, administration of fluid volume and increasing the heart rate with isoproterenol or dopamine may be necessary for the short-term support of blood pressure.

Once the pericardial catheter has been placed, the amount of pericardial fluid drainage is monitored within the collection system. In addition, serial echocardiography may be performed. If fluid continues to drain, but no reduction in the size of the effusion is noted, surgical intervention may be necessary.

INDICATIONS

The most common indication for pericardiocentesis is to discern the etiology of a chronic effusion. Pericardial effusion can be inflammatory, uremic, infectious, or oncologic, or due to congestive heart failure or trauma (closed chest or iatrogenic).[5] Pericardial effusions may be due to fluid (transudate), pus, blood (or thrombus), or air.

Therapeutic pericardiocentesis is performed for the relief of cardiac tamponade. Tamponade may be due to any of the above etiologies, but is increasingly more commonly due to perforation of a cardiac structure during a therapeutic intervention[6] (particularly in patients receiving anticoagulation or antiplatelet agents) or from closed chest trauma, such as cardiopulmonary resuscitation. At one time, motor vehicle accidents were a common cause of pericardial effusion, but this has become less common since the universal adaptation of air bags. In one recent large study of pericarditis, trauma was the leading etiology.[7]

A scoring system for the urgency of pericardiocentesis has been developed and is based on the etiology, clinical presentation, and results of imaging.[8,9] The scoring system calculates whether the procedure should be done urgently or can be deferred for 12–24 hours.

Urgent surgical drainage and repair of the underlying cause are indicated for cardiac tamponade when it is due to Type A aortic dissection, ventricular free wall rupture due to myocardial infarction, severe chest trauma, or any cause where the etiology cannot be controlled with pericardiocentesis.

EQUIPMENT

In elective pericardiocentesis, an echocardiogram at the bedside is necessary for quantitating and localizing the effusion, and determining needle placement.

The preferred position for most pericardiocentesis procedures is to have the patient supine at a 30°–45° angle. This is best accomplished by a wedge placed behind the patient, or if done in bed, by elevating the backrest (Figure 14.2). To monitor needle position, an electrocardiogram (EKG) or cardiac monitor with a unipolar lead is necessary. The other equipment is usually provided in a commercially available prepackaged pericardiocentesis kit, the contents of which are outlined in Table 14.2.

APPROACH

There are several approaches to the performance of pericardiocentesis, including subxiphoid, parsternal, and apical. Similarly, there are several imaging techniques to guide pericardiocentesis: electrocardiography, echocardiography, fluoroscopy, and CT.

The initial technique of pericardiocentesis used the EKG as a guide. An alligator clip was connected from the needle to a unipolar EKG lead and monitoring of the EKG was done as the needle was inserted. If the needle touched

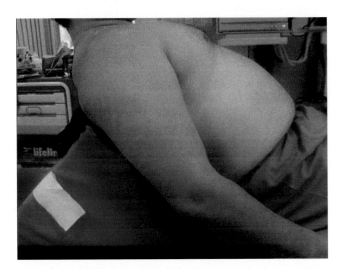

Figure 14.2 Patient positioned in semi-upright (30°–45°) position in preparation for pericardiocentesis.

the myocardium, an injury current (ST elevation) would develop on the EKG indicating the needle had been inserted too far.

The presence of bedside hand-held echo machines, nearly ubiquitous in the emergency department, have facilitated the diagnosis of pericardial effusion.[10] The current most common approach is the echocardiographically guided subxiphoid approach.[8] Prior to the procedure, an echocardiogram is obtained to ascertain the size and location of the effusion. A small or noncompressive effusion may not be necessary to drain under most circumstances. The echo-guided approach has the advantage of identifying the effusion to the closest portion of the chest wall so that an alternate approach may be used. It also can identify whether the needle is in the pericardial space or cardiac structure by noting "bubbles" when agitated saline is administered.

An alternate imaging approach is fluoroscopy. Once the operator has entered the pericardial space using a needle attached to a syringe of contrast, injection can be performed and fluoroscopy used to ascertain contrast presence in the pericardial space. Some institutions have substituted CT imaging for the echocardiogram, which may be as effective, but the portability and ease of the echocardiogram make it the imaging modality of choice.

Most effusions are free-flowing within the pericardial space and may be accessed from an anterior approach, but the few loculated effusions that occur will need to be accessed with a different technique (described below).[11] A unique imaging approach to a posterior loculated effusion is transesophageal ultrasound.[12]

In an elective procedure, right heart catheterization with simultaneous measurement of pulmonary capillary wedge, right atrial, and intrapericardial pressures is an elegant method of diagnosing pericardial tamponade, but may not be necessary. In an emergency, such as a vascular or chamber perforation during a cardiac intervention with free-flowing blood into the pericardium and resultant hemodynamic

Table 14.2 Equipment (much of this is packaged together in a disposable pericardial tray)

- 0.038-in guidewire
- 18-gauge 1.5-in needle
- 21-gauge skin needle
- 30°–45° wedge
- 4- to 5-in long 18-gauge needle
- 6-Fr dilator
- 6-Fr pigtail or specialized pericardial drain
- Alligator clip
- Echocardiogram machine
- EKG machine or monitor
- Lidocaine
- Skin cleansing agent
- Sterile drapes
- Stopcock, tubing, and drainage bag
- Tubes for chemistry and culture

deterioration, no imaging is necessary and pericardiocentesis should be performed as quickly as possible.

In order to bring the effusion inferior and closer to the chest wall, especially in free-flowing effusions, the elective procedure is best done in a sitting-up position of at least 30°–45°. In loculated effusions, the patient should be positioned to bring the effusion closest to the chest wall and may require the patient being placed in an extreme lateral decubitus position.[13]

Local anesthesia is administered as a skin wheal with a 21-gauge needle and then deeper anesthesia is infused with a 1.5-in 18-gauge needle. On occasion, this needle will enter the pericardial space as signaled by straw-colored fluid return. This needle can be used as a guide and the pericardiocentesis needle inserted alongside of it.

The typical location for skin entry is at the left xiphoid notch aiming toward the left mid-clavicle (Figures 14.1 and 14.3 through 14.5). The needle is initially advanced vertically and, once under the rib cage, angled horizontally toward the clavicle. The entry position may be altered depending on the presence of fluid loculation and an alternative positioning and puncture site may be needed. The needle that has been utilized in the past is a 7–10-in 18-gauge needle, which is commonly provided in most prepackaged pericardiocentesis trays. More recently, a 7-in micropuncture needle has become the needle of choice. The needle is often bent to a 45°–60° angle to facilitate passage under the rib cage into the pericardial space. A syringe is placed on the needle and gentle suction is applied as the needle is advanced.

Other sites of entry include the fifth or sixth intercostal space at the left or right of the sternum. Using this approach, the patient should be in the 30°–45° upright position and the needle angled to the mid-clavicle. The potential advantage of this approach is that the puncture site is already above the diaphragm, thus abdominal contents/organs are avoided.

The apical approach is also occasionally used. Since the point of maximal impact will not be present in the setting of a pericardial effusion, the apex is identified by echocardiography, and the needle inserted toward the largest accumulation of fluid identified by the echocardiogram. The approach to lateral loculated pericardial effusions is also through puncture at the mid-clavicular line. The key to puncturing a loculated lateral effusion, whether right or left sided, is to position the patient to bring the effusion as close as possible to the chest wall as determined by the echocardiogram.[14]

Since the pericardium is thick, resistance may be felt and a "pop" noted upon entering the pericardial space. Depending on the etiology of the pericardial fluid, it may be serous or bloody. An old adage that can no longer be trusted to distinguish pericardial blood from intracardiac blood is that "blood in the pericardium will not clot" since patients may be on potent antiplatelet and anticoagulant medications. Pressure measurement can be helpful, but the pressures in the right atrium and vena cava may be identical to pericardial pressure, although a right ventricular pressure tracing will be obvious.[15]

If needle location is in doubt, injection of nonionic contrast with fluoroscopy visualization, or saline administration with echocardiographic visualization, will be helpful in ensuring the presence in the pericardial space (Figure 14.6). Once the needle position has been ascertained, measurement

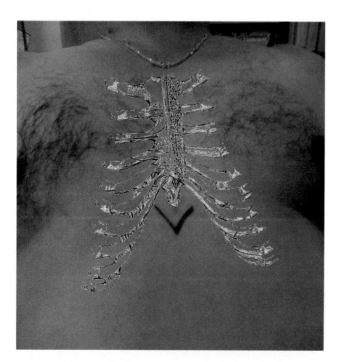

Figure 14.3 Bony landmarks superimposed on the trunk.

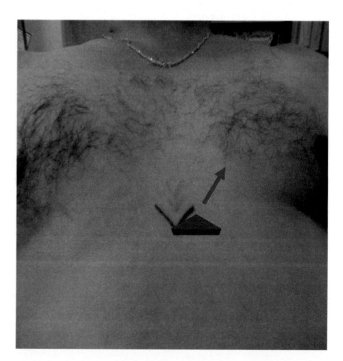

Figure 14.4 Direction of the needle. The broad arrow is the initial insertion, "walking above the diaphragm," and the narrow arrow indicates aiming toward the left mid-clavicle.

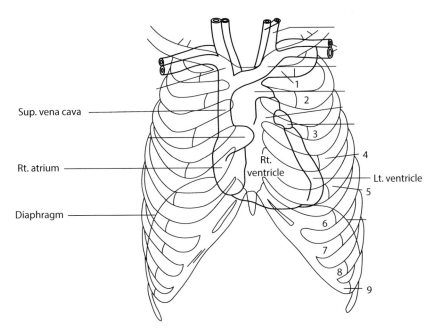

Sup. vena cava

Rt. atrium

Diaphragm

Rt. ventricle

Lt. ventricle

Figure 14.5 Bony structures of the thorax with the location of the cardiac structure behind to demonstrate the cardiac structures that can be punctured or lacerated during pericardiocentesis.

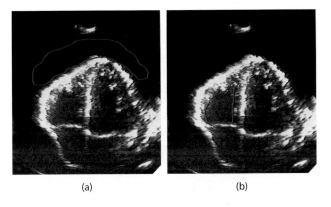

(a)   (b)

Figure 14.6 Depiction by echocardiogram **(a)** when needle is placed properly in pericardium and saline is injected and **(b)** when needle is placed in the right ventricle and saline Is Injected. The marked area in frame **(a)** represents pericardial space and in frame **(b)** represents right ventricular cavity.

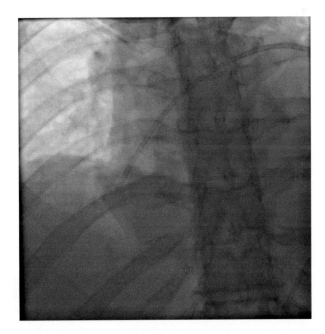

Figure 14.7 Chest X-ray of appropriate position of pericardial drainage catheter.

of the intrapericardial pressure to compare with the right atrial pressure can be made to confirm the presence of tamponade. Withdrawal of as little as 50–100 mL of fluid may be adequate to relieve the pressure within the pericardium and restore normal hemodynamics in the presence of cardiac tamponade.

If diagnostic pericardiocentesis is being performed for a large effusion, adequate specimens may be withdrawn through the needle; however, it is probably best to first exchange the needle for a soft tip catheter or introducer sheath before fluid aspiration.

When a drainage catheter is to be placed, a 0.035-in guidewire is inserted through the needle and confirmed in the pericardial space by fluoroscopy. A 6- or 7-Fr tapered dilator is first advanced to facilitate insertion of the catheter. The dilator can be used to withdraw fluid when only a diagnostic pericardiocentesis is being performed. A pigtail-shaped or straight catheter with multiple side holes is then inserted. The optimum location for this catheter is inferior or posterior to the heart (Figure 14.7). To ascertain position, nonionic contrast may be injected.

If a micropuncture needle is used, the micropuncture compatible wire can be inserted and upsized to a 0.035-in wire to facilitate catheter placement.

The drainage catheter is then connected to a drainage bag via a plastic tube.[16] Hand withdrawal of fluid may be necessary to withdraw enough fluid to decompress the tamponade. Once the drainage catheter position is confirmed and hemodynamic stability has been restored, the catheter is sutured in place, and gravity or low negative pressure drainage begun.

The pericardial fluid is usually sent for cell count, cell differential, chemistries (total protein, pH, LDH, glucose, etc.), serologies, culture, and cytology. Recent data suggest that the differentiation between exudative and transudative effusions is not relevant to determine etiology.[17]

Depending on the situation, the pericardial catheter is left in place for 12 hours or longer, and once the pericardial effusion has stopped draining, as confirmed by echocardiography, it can be removed.

CONTRAINDICATIONS

The contraindications to pericardiocentesis include the following:

1. Lack of or inadequate amount of pericardial fluid. Particularly in situations of acute/chronic pericarditis, there may be rapid resolution of the effusion, so echocardiography immediately prior to pericardiocentesis is necessary.
2. Coagulopathy. When performing an elective diagnostic pericardiocentesis, there should be correction of any coagulopathy to reduce the risk of iatrogenic bleeding. However, in the presence of tamponade, pericardiocentesis, even in the presence of coagulopathy, may be life-saving.
3. Loculated lateral or posterior effusions. These may be difficult or impossible to reach with a needle, and surgical drainage should be considered.

COMPLICATIONS

Complications of pericardiocentesis include laceration of cardiac or noncardiac structures. Because the right ventricle and inferior vena cava lie anterior, they are the most common cardiac structures that can be inadvertently punctured, but coronary arteries, coronary veins, and the internal thoracic artery can also be lacerated. Serous-colored fluid that quickly turns bloody may be an indication of laceration of a cardiac structure. While rare, noncardiac structures, including the liver, spleen, and stomach, can be lacerated.

The easiest way to avoid inadvertent puncture of these structures is to carefully select the path of the pericardiocentesis needle and inject iodinated contrast or saline with X-ray or echocardiographic imaging to demonstrate the location of the puncture.[18]

Occasionally, congestive heart failure or pulmonary edema due to transient left ventricular dysfunction may result after drainage of a large pericardial effusion (post-decompression syndrome). Echocardiography may be necessary to differentiate these symptoms from reaccumulation of pericardial fluid. A rare phenomenon after relief of pericardial effusion is biventricular decompensation. The etiology of this is uncertain, it is usually transient, and it

may require vasopressors or mechanical support for a short period of time.

Dysrhythmias can occur during pericardiocentesis, and may be due to the irritation from the needle or catheter on the epicardium.

REFERENCES

1. Owens WC, et al. Pericardiocentesis: Insertion of a pericardial catheter. *Cathet Cardiovasc Diagn* 1975;1:317–321.
2. Kronzon I, et al. Diastolic atrial compression: A sensitive echocardiographic sign of cardiac tamponade. *J Am Coll Cardiol* 1983;2:770–775.
3. Armstrong WF, et al. Diastolic collapse of the right ventricle with cardiac tamponade: An echocardiographic study. *Circulation* 1982;65:1491–1496.
4. Bhardwaj R, et al. Evaluation of safety and feasibility of percutaneous balloon pericardiotomy in hemodynamically significant pericardial effusion (review of 10-years experience in single center). *J Interv Cardiol* 2015;28;409–414.
5. Vaitkus PT, et al. Treatment of malignant pericardial effusion. *JAMA* 1994;272:59–64.
6. Tsang T, et al. Rescue echocardiographically guided pericardiocentesis for cardiac perforation complicating catheter-based procedures: The Mayo Clinic experience. *J Am Coll Cardiol* 1998;32:1345–1350.
7. Gouriet F, et al. Etiology of pericarditis in a prospective cohort of 1162 cases. *Am J Med* 2015;128;784.e1–e8.
8. Halpern DG, et al. A novel pericardial effusion scoring index to guide decision for drainage. *Crit Pathw Cardiol* 2012;2:85–88.
9. Ristić AD, et al. Triage strategy for urgent management of cardiac tamponade: A position statement of the European Society of Cardiology Working Group on Myocardial and Pericardial Diseases. *Eur Heart J* 2014;35:2279–2284.
10. Ceriani E, Cogliati C. Update on bedside ultrasound diagnosis of pericardial effusion. *Intern Emerg Med* 2016;1(3):477–480.
11. Callahan JA, et al. Cardiac tamponade: Pericardiocentesis directed by two-dimensional echocardiography. *Mayo Clin Proc* 1985;60:344–347.
12. Hashimoto Y, Inoue K. Endoscopic ultrasound-guided transesophageal pericardiocentesis: An alternative approach to a pericardial effusion. *Endoscopy* 2016;48 Suppl 1:E71–72.
13. Tsang T, et al. Echocardiographically guided pericardiocentesis: Evolution and state-of-the-art technique. *Mayo Clin Proc* 1998;73:647–652.
14. Tsang TS, et al. Consecutive 1127 therapeutic echocardiographically guided pericardiocenteses: Clinical profile, practice patterns, and outcomes spanning 21 years. *Mayo Clin Proc* 2002;77:429–436.
15. Kilpatrick ZM, Chapman CB. On pericardiocentesis. *Am J Cardiol* 1965;16:722–728.
16. Kopecky SL, et al. Percutaneous pericardial catheter drainage: Report of 42 consecutive cases. *Am J Cardiol* 1986;58:633–635.
17. Akyuz S, et al. Differentiation between transudate and exudate in pericardial effusion has almost no diagnostic value in contemporary medicine. *Clin Lab* 2015;61:957–963.
18. Duvernoy O, et al. Complications of percutaneous pericardiocentesis under fluoroscopic guidance. *Acta Radiol* 1992;33:309–313.

15

Catheterization of the cardiac venous system

AMARTYA KUNDU, CHIRAG BAVISHI, PARTHA SARDAR, AND SAURAV CHATTERJEE

INTRODUCTION

With advancing medical knowledge and the advent of newer technologies, the coronary sinus (CS)—a structure that was once thought to be nothing more than an obscure source of passive venous drainage—is now recognized as an important gateway for an array of clinical interventions. Although vascular cardiology has historically focused on coronary artery circulation, there has recently been an increased emphasis on catheterization of the cardiac venous system for a number of interventional procedures, such as cardiac resynchronization therapy (CRT), gene therapy, and structural interventions, including valvular procedures. Interventional cardiologists would benefit from expanding their repertoire to be familiar with CS anatomy, and also learning the necessary procedural skills to catheterize the CS and its branches.

This paradigm shift began after CRT emerged as a ground-breaking therapy that revolutionized the management of patients with systolic heart failure. The main purpose of CRT is to restore left ventricular (LV) synchrony in patients with dilated cardiomyopathy and a widened QRS, predominantly a result of left bundle branch block (LBBB), in order to improve mechanical LV function. CRT has been shown to improve functional status, as demonstrated by the 6-minute walk test, peak oxygen uptake, and the New York Heart Association (NYHA) classification system, as well as health-related quality of life.[1] Recent trials have also shown a significant reduction in the combined endpoint of all-cause mortality and hospitalization.[2] However, the success of CRT is operator-dependent and requires the delivery of an LV pacing lead to the CS in a position that is stable and free from phrenic nerve stimulation. This requires a comprehensive understanding of the anatomy of the cardiac venous system. While CRT has provided most of the incentive to develop tools and techniques to catheterize the CS and the cardiac veins, other reasons for venous catheterization have become popular in recent times and will be discussed.

ANATOMIC CONSIDERATIONS

Venous drainage of the myocardium comprises two interconnecting systems, the thebesian system and the epicardial system, which is further divided into the CS and the branch epicardial veins. The branch veins may additionally be classified into those that are always present and those that are variably present.

Thebesian venous system

In the first half of the eighteenth century, Raymond Vieussens and Adam Thebesius discovered the vasa cordis minima, which is known today as thebesian veins. The thebesian veins form the smaller (or "lesser") of the two cardiac venous systems. They consist of small, valveless venous branches that drain the subendocardium into the nearest cardiac chamber. They are primarily composed of endothelial cells that are continuous with the lining of the chambers of the heart.[3] These veins are found throughout all four chambers of the heart but are more prominent on the right.[4]

They produce a small, physiologic right-to-left shunt capable of carrying approximately 0.3% of aortic flow.[5,6] In addition, this venous system provides drainage to the right atrial appendage (RAA) and a significant segment of the muscular ventricular septum.[4]

If the epicardial venous system is compromised for some reason, the thebesian system provides an alternate collateral network for venous drainage of the myocardium. This is probably why balloon-occlusion venography does not impair venous outflow, and why retrograde contrast injections are well-tolerated, even in patients with advanced heart failure.[7] When major epicardial veins get obstructed by traumatic injury or pacing leads, the thebesian network can facilitate vein-to-vein collateralization. This protective collateralization may account for the relative immunity of the atrial and right ventricular free wall to ischemic injury. The thebesian network is also clinically important for retrograde myocardial perfusion, drug delivery, and gene therapy.

The thebesian venous system can be visualized during alcohol septal ablation for hypertrophic cardiomyopathy when echo contrast injected into a septal perforator artery flows into the ventricles. It can also be seen during coronary angiography as plumes of contrast entering the ventricles. It is important to recognize this as normal anatomy and not a vascular malformation.

The coronary sinus

The CS is an extremely important structure to recognize for safe and efficient catheterization of the cardiac venous system, and should be considered as the fifth chamber of the heart.

It is a small, contractile chamber that lies in the atrioventricular (AV) groove behind the left atrium (LA), just above the location of the circumflex artery. The CS begins proximally at the RA orifice and ends distally at the Vieussens valve.[4] It has its own myocardium, valves, and electric conduction system. It receives blood from the ventricular veins during ventricular systole and drains into the RA during atrial systole. The length of the CS ranges from 3 to 5.5 cm and depends on the site of drainage of the posterolateral vein.[8] Its diameter is variable and depends on preload, extent of atrial myocardium with the coronary vein, prior cardiac surgery, and presence of existing cardiac pathology.

Embryologically, the CS develops through differentiation of the sinus venosus. Initially, the sinus venosus opens into the posterior wall of the RA and differentiates into right and left horns, which gives rise to the venous network entering the RA. The right horn is absorbed and persists as the smooth portion of the superior vena cava (SVC) and the adjacent area extending into the CS ostium. The left horn undergoes degenerative changes and gives rise to the CS.[4]

Like other chambers of the heart, the CS internally consists of three layers—epicardium, myocardium, and endocardium. The myocardium consists of striated cardiac muscle with intercalated disks enabling the CS to contract in synchrony with the atria.[9] These contractions can be observed during the venous phase of coronary arteriography and transthoracic or intracardiac ultrasound (Figure 15.1).[10] Normal contractility can often be mistaken for strictures and lead to unnecessary balloon dilatation. Contractions of the CS are surprisingly forceful and can even eject balloon occlusion catheters during venography.

Electrically conductive muscle bands connect the CS to both atrial chambers and provide inputs for activation of the CS myocardium.[11] It is therefore not surprising that rhythmic contractions of the CS are absent in patients with atrial fibrillation (AF). The electrically active bridges, however, predispose the CS to participate in re-entrant atrial arrhythmias by forming accessory pathways that are difficult to ablate. The CS also receives additional inputs from the vein of Marshall, which is a known trigger for AF. The vein of Marshall may give rise to AF either by virtue of myocardial extensions into the structure or as a result of node-like remnants within the vein, or by virtue of the rich autonomic innervation that typically encapsulates the structure.[4] Last, myocytes within the CS may also be capable of intrinsic automaticity.[12]

Similar to the rest of the cardiac venous system, the CS contains various valves, the most common of which is the thebesian valve at the ostium of the CS.[13] The thebesian valve is a crescent-shaped structure guarding the mouth of the CS where it opens to the RA. It is a highly variable structure that may sometimes present as an obstruction during cannulation of the CS.[14] It is always attached posteriorly and open anteriorly, directing flow from the CS to the tricuspid valve. The CS also contains Vieussens valve at the distal end of the vein. It is an important structure to recognize, as it can often be mistaken for an occlusion or stenosis. The Vieussens valve also marks the division between the contractile CS and the noncontractile great cardiac vein (GCV), which is a clinically important structure during balloon-occlusion venography. Each of the major veins emptying into the CS can contain valves near their opening, which may obstruct the passage of leads and catheters during interventional procedures. The CS ostium is 5–15 mm in diameter and is located on the posterior interatrial septum anterior to the Eustachian ridge and posterior to the tricuspid annulus.[15] The thebesian valve usually covers the superior and posterior surfaces of the ostium, but may be covered completely

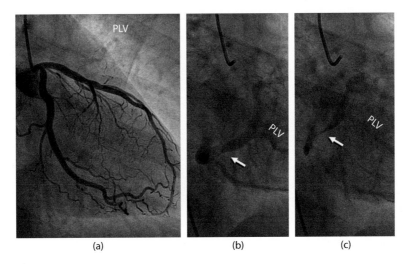

Figure 15.1 Normal contractility of the CS observed during coronary arteriography. **(a)** Arterial phase. **(b)** Venous phase in atrial diastole. The junction of the CS and GCV is indicated by a subtle annular narrowing (arrow). **(c)** Venous phase during atrial systole. The distinction between contractile CS and noncontractile GCV is apparent (arrow). A large posterolateral vein draining to the GCV provides a position reference. CS, coronary sinus; GCV, great cardiac vein; PLV, posterior left ventricle.

with formation of fenestrations. In rare instances, the valve may cover the inferior hemi-circumference.

Atrial venous drainage

The atrial myocardium drains into the CS via a number of atrial veins and the vein of Marshall. The largest of these venous branches, an embryological remnant of the left SVC, courses opposite the posterolateral vein between the anterior surface of the pulmonary veins and the posterior surface of the left atrial appendage (LAA). When completely patent, it is known as a persistent left superior vena cava (SVC). When it is patent only in its atrial course, it is known as the vein of Marshall. When it is occluded either completely or partially, it is known as the oblique vein of Marshall.[16] The left atrial veins can be used for atrial pacing, especially when thresholds are poor in the RA or specific left atrial-left ventricular synchrony is desired.

Epicardial venous system

The epicardial veins carry most of the venous return from the LV to the CS, which empties into the RA. They provide a transvenous path to the LV that can be utilized for cardiac resynchronization, myocardial perfusion, drug delivery, and gene therapy. Unlike the CS, the epicardial veins vary significantly in size, number, and location.

ANTERIOR INTERVENTRICULAR VEIN

The anterior interventricular vein (AIV) is the largest and most consistent of the cardiac veins. It courses in the interventricular groove next to the left anterior descending (LAD) artery. The AIV is the most anterior vein seen

in the right anterior oblique (RAO) projection. As it flows to the base of the heart, the AIV receives branches from the anterolateral LV free wall and the interventricular septum. At the base of the heart near the origin of the LAD, the AIV courses laterally, following the circumflex artery toward the AV groove to form the GCV. The GCV usually receives tributaries from the lateral LV free wall before emptying into the CS.

LATERAL CARDIAC VEINS

Three distinct veins drain the lateral wall of the LV. The largest and most consistent of these is the posterolateral vein, which flows directly opposite the vein of Marshall.[8,15,17] The other veins in the lateral wall are highly variable in character and location. They include the straight lateral vein and the anterior lateral vein.

MIDDLE CARDIAC VEIN

The middle cardiac vein (MCV), also known as the posterior interventricular vein (PIV), is the largest proximal tributary of the CS (Figure 15.2). It receives tributaries from the anterior veins in addition to branches from the inferior ventricular walls and septum. The MCV courses with the posterior descending artery in the posterior interventricular groove and can be considered to be its venous equivalent. It eventually drains into the CS close to the RA orifice. The MCV also has a varied number of branches, the most important of which are the left marginal and inferior veins.[18] The MCV can be specifically used for placing an LV lead.

The AIV and MCV connect at the apex, forming a semicircle that establishes the plane of the interventricular septum. The GCV and the CS form another semicircle that establishes the plane of the mitral annulus.

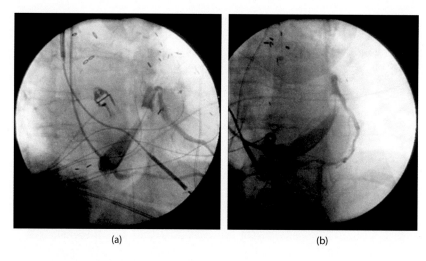

Figure 15.2 Posterolateral and middle cardiac vein. Right anterior oblique **(a)** and left anterior oblique **(b)** projections showing a typical anastomotic vein between the posterior and anterior circulation that traverses the lateral wall. (From Constans, M.M., and Asirvatham, S.J., *Indian Pacing Electrophysiol. J.*, 8(Suppl. 1), S105–S121, 2008. With permission.)

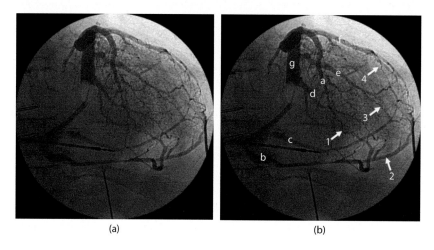

Figure 15.3 **(a)** Typical branches and **(b)** collateral loops. Epicardial veins of the left ventricle include anterior interventricular **[a]**, posterior interventricular or middle cardiac **[b]**, posterior **[c]**, lateral **[d and e]**, anterolateral **[f]**, and great cardiac **[g]**. Collateral loops include anterior interventricular vein to PIV at the apex [1], apical-lateral branch of PIV [2], posterior to lateral [3], and anterolateral to lateral [4]. PIV, posterior interventricular vein.

The intersection of these two semicircles establishes the outline of the LV and provides a frame of reference for orienting all other veins.

POSTERIOR VENTRICULAR VEIN

The posterior ventricular vein courses with the posterolateral branches of the right coronary artery along the later ventricular wall, and drains the diaphragmatic and lateral walls of the LV. It is sometimes mistaken for a branch of the MCV. In approximately 25% of patients, the posterior ventricular vein and the MCV share a common ostium.[15,17,19]

SURFACE COLLATERALS

The surface veins of the LV are connected by a network of collateral channels, most of which are too small to be visualized by venography. Four of these channels make collateral loops that are large enough and consistent enough to

be clinically useful. The collateral loops can be utilized for guidewire and lead placements. Loop 1 connects the AIV and MCV at the apex. Loop 2 connects the apical-lateral branch of the MCV to posterior and lateral veins. Loop 3 connects posterior to lateral veins. Loop 4 connects lateral to anterolateral veins (Figure 15.3).

FUNDAMENTALS

Catheterization techniques: A brief overview

Catheterizing the CS is an operator-dependent process that requires a thorough understanding of the venous anatomy, more so than manual skill and dexterity. With experience, operators learn to make purposeful advances toward a specific target utilizing known anatomical landmarks.

CS interventions are usually performed with internal jugular or subclavian access. The manipulations are the same for left-sided and right-sided approaches. The direction of rotation is from the operator's perspective. Successful catheterization of the CS is a two-step process.

FINDING THE CS OSTIUM

Having a clear understanding of the orientation of the CS and great veins with the RA is of paramount importance. That being said, the anatomical relationships are very consistent in nature. The SVC is oriented anteriorly toward the tricuspid valve and enters the posterior aspect of the RA. The inferior vena cava (IVC) is directed toward the fossa ovalis of the atrial septum. The CS enters the RA between the IVC and the tricuspid valve, with its opening directed anteriorly toward the tricuspid valve. Between the IVC and the tricuspid annulus lies a recess of RA free wall known as the Eustachian fossa. The Eustachian fossa, the tricuspid annulus, and the Eustachian ridge are easily identifiable landmarks that aid in localizing the CS. Of note, it should be remembered that the SVC does not enter the RA vertically as seen in two-dimensional (2D) fluoroscopy. Manipulations to engage catheters via the SVC do not always align with the CS ostium and reorientation is usually required. The catheter is first advanced near the tricuspid valve until it reaches the tricuspid annulus. It is then rotated counterclockwise so that the tip of the catheter contacts the heart. It is imperative that rotation proceeds in a counterclockwise manner as clockwise rotations cause the catheter tip to engage the Eustachian ridge and valve, deflecting away from the CS. Following this step, the catheter is withdrawn while maintaining counterclockwise torque so that the tip of the catheter rides over the tricuspid annulus into the recess between the annulus and the Eustachian ridge. Injecting contrast media at this point confirms the position of the CS and forward advancement engages the CS ostium.

If the CS is not engaged immediately, it is likely that the catheter tip is in one of two possible locations, which can be confirmed by injecting contrast media. The catheter tip may be in the Eustachian fossa, in which case it is too inferior and the operator needs to repeat the counterclockwise maneuver from a more superior starting point. Alternatively, the catheter tip may be in body of the RA, in which case, it is too superior, and the operator is required to advance the catheter and repeat the counterclockwise maneuver from a more inferior starting point.

Entering the Great Cardiac Vein

It is important to know how to catheterize the GCV as most therapeutic procedures depend on a guide-catheter or delivery system that has been inserted deeply enough to be stable.

After locating the CS ostium, several changes in direction must be navigated to enter the body of the CS and the GCV. It is difficult to advance catheters using a 2D fluoroscopic image to negotiate into a three-dimensional (3D) structure, which is why a crystal clear understanding of

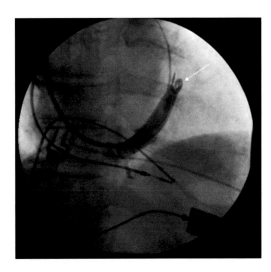

Figure 15.4 Left anterior oblique coronary sinus angiogram demonstrating a near occlusive valve about 3 cm from the coronary sinus. This is a frequent site to find the valve of Vieussens. (From Constans, M.M., and Asirvatham, S.J., *Indian Pacing Electrophysiol. J.*, 8(Suppl. 1), S105–S121, 2008. With permission.)

the venous anatomy is essential. Forceful advancement of catheters should be avoided as they can cause complications such as dissection or perforation.

The CS forms a flat, C-shaped loop around the mitral annulus on venography in the left anterior oblique (LAO) projection. From the RAO view, to enter the CS, a catheter is directed down, left, and posterior using counterclockwise rotation from a superior approach. After passing the contractile portion of the CS, the catheter must be redirected upward and anterior using clockwise rotation. The catheter will eventually turn rightward with the GCV, reaching the base of the heart at the anterior interventricular groove. Resistance at the level of Vieussens valve is common and easily overcome (Figure 15.4). This is fairly easy to recognize and occurs when the tip of the catheter enters a valve cusp and retrograde force closes the valve. This resistance to catheter advancement may be misinterpreted as a fixed stenosis or an occlusion. The valve will not yield to force, but it can always be crossed by gently probing with a steerable, hydrophilic guidewire. The guidewire will hold the pliable valve aside, allowing easy passage of catheters and delivery systems. The initial insertion should be beyond the area of interest, making subsequent manipulations more precise as pull-back removes slack and improves stability while avoiding injury at the same time.

INDICATIONS

Electrophysiology

The cardiac venous system has been used by electrophysiologists for a number of procedures, such as accessing the ventricles for pacing, defibrillation, arrhythmia mapping, and radiofrequency ablation.[4] CRT, which involves the process of placing a pacing lead in an LV vein, has been shown to improve quality of life in patients with severe symptomatic (NYHA III) chronic heart failure (CHF) who are already receiving optimal medical therapy.[1] The combination of biventricular pacing and an implantable cardiac defibrillator in patients with CHF has been shown to reduce all-cause mortality.[2]

Coronary sinus reducer stent

In patients with refractory angina who are not candidates for revascularization, increased pressure in the CS can facilitate redistribution of blood from normal to ischemic areas via the thebesian veins. This can be achieved with the help of a CS reducer stent. The Coronary Sinus Reducer stent (Neovasc Medical, Inc., Or Yehuda, Israel) is a stainless steel balloon expandable stent designed to establish narrowing of the CS. It is implanted via a percutaneous transverse approach and introduced into the CS through the right internal jugular vein. An open-label, multicenter, nonrandomized, prospective study showed significant reductions in angina and improvements in objective measures of myocardial perfusion without adverse events.[20] While these results are promising, further studies are necessary to establish the CS Reducer stent as a definitive therapy for refractory angina.

Drug delivery

Studies have investigated the efficacy of retrograde perfusion of pharmacologic agents into the coronary veins. Intact nonischemic myocardium drug concentrations after retro-infusion are comparable to that obtained via intravenous (IV) administration. However, in the setting of myocardial ischemia, retroinfusion achieves higher levels of drug concentration in tissue than IV delivery with the advantage of lower peak systemic concentrations and reduced or absent systemic effects.[21,22] This is probably due to the improved access to low-pressure capillary beds, and less washout of drugs in the presence of reduced anterograde blood flow. Fibrinolytic agents given directly into the coronary veins act more rapidly, reduce final infarct size more effectively, and improve recovery.

Gene therapy

Gene delivery to the heart has been attempted by using both viral and nonviral vectors. Adenovirus is the most effective viral vector used, although its usage may be limited by the host immune responses. The delivery of genes to the myocardium by retrograde venous perfusion was demonstrated to be superior to surgical and percutaneous myocardial gene transfer.[23]

In addition, angiogenic growth factors, such as basic fibroblast growth factor (FGF-2) and vascular endothelial growth factor (VEGF), have been shown to induce the growth of coronary collaterals.[24] These growth factors can be introduced into the myocardium by techniques such as direct injection into the myocardium, infusion into the coronary artery, and repeated intracoronary bolus administration.[24,25]

Mitral annuloplasty

The purpose of mitral annuloplasty is to treat functional mitral regurgitation secondary to dilated cardiomyopathy via a percutaneous approach, thereby avoiding the risks of open surgery. This is possible because of the proximity of the CS to the mitral valve annulus. The procedure mimics surgical annuloplasty by shortening the anterior-posterior dimensions of the mitral annulus.

A number of devices have been used for percutaneous mitral annuloplasty. The VIKING and MONARC devices (Edwards Life Sciences, Irvine, CA) consist of two nitinol anchor stents connected by a spring-like bridge. One anchor is deployed in the GCV and the other near the CS ostium.[26] The bridge spring contracts as biodegradable spacers slowly dissolve, pulling the stents together and shortening the annulus. The CARILLON device (Cardiac Dimensions, Kirkland, WI) is similar, with two self-expanding anchors connected by a tensioning ribbon.[27] The design of this device allows tension to be adjusted at the time of implantation.

Although initial human trials with these devices have demonstrated significant short-term reductions in the degree of mitral regurgitation, the long-term safety and efficacy of annuloplasty remain to be established. Design enhancements for both devices have improved mechanical stability and durability. Two issues remain with CS annuloplasty. First, the CS frequently lies along the LA free wall, well above the mitral annulus, and it is not yet known if this geometric variability affects outcomes. Second, the GCV frequently crosses the circumflex artery or a major marginal branch, and extrinsic compression by the device can lead to ischemia.

Percutaneous *in situ* coronary venous arterialization

The cardiac venous system has been used as a passage to perfuse ischemic regions because of the extensive arteriovenous communications within the myocardium.

Percutaneous *in situ* coronary venous arterialization (PICVA) is a percutaneous approach to coronary artery bypass that redirects arterial blood flow from an artery into an adjacent coronary vein, arterializing the vein and providing retroperfusion to ischemic myocardium.[28,29] It takes advantage of the fact that the venous system is generally free of atherosclerosis and that individual veins are dispensable due to a redundant drainage system. The technique was inspired by early studies of coronary retroperfusion from the 1940s and 1970s, which left anecdotal evidence of partial or complete relief of angina in patients. The procedure employs specially designed catheters and implantable devices to create a fistula between the artery and vein, and force retroperfusion through the vein.

Cardiac endoscopy

Placement of electrophysiology catheters and pacing leads in the CS is challenging in some patients, particularly those with dilated cardiomyopathy. Direct visualization of the CS ostium and branches is possible through infrared endoscopy.[30] This is a novel but invasive method for better visualization of the cardiac venous system, which can help facilitate other interventional procedures.

EQUIPMENT

Catheters used to cannulate the CS have mostly been tailored to facilitate CRT. Widespread availability of modern equipment has made CRT safer and more reliable, but despite an extensive array of catheters, the success of the procedure is operator-based and depends to a large degree on a good working knowledge of venous anatomy.

Guide catheters are used to help place LV pacing leads by providing a framework to securely wedge the leads firmly into the branch veins. Complete delivery packages are now commonly available and include deflectable guide catheters, catheters for selective cannulation of branch veins, catheters of various shapes to cannulate the CS, guidewires, and other tools (Figure 15.5). Depending on operator preference, deflectable electrophysiology catheters or fixed-curve angiographic catheters are commonly used. Angiographic catheters have the advantages of being available in a variety of shapes, are less expensive, and also enable injections of contrast, making them ideal for negotiating complex structures.

In patients with advanced heart failure and dilated chambers, use of special catheters can help overcome technical challenges. Telescoping catheter systems are frequently used and include an outer guide catheter and an inner angiographic catheter such that each catheter can be maneuvered independently, thereby providing a nearly complete range of tip trajectories. In most cases, the outer guide catheter provides the anterior and superior starting position for the angiographic catheter. The outer guide catheter can be directed toward the anterior RA using clockwise rotation while the inner angiographic catheter is directed toward the CS using counterclockwise rotation. The addition of a guidewire creates a triple telescoping system that is useful in cases of extreme RA enlargement.

However, even patients with chamber dilatation have fixed anatomical relationships where the CS always opens into the same location in the RA, and can therefore be cannulated with the use of conventional catheters. Moreover, the CS, which is approximately 10 mm in diameter at the ostium, is even larger in patients with CHF, allowing fairly easy access for the operator. Regardless of which catheters are used, the objective is the same—to place a delivery system into a stable, deep, coaxial position inside the body of the CS.

CLINICAL ASPECTS

Catheterization of the CS is performed under fluoroscopic guidance. Venography should be performed in as many projections as necessary to fully define the anatomy. The anteroposterior (AP) projection has several advantages including lower X-ray dose rate, more comfortable posture for the operator, and better preservation of the sterile field. The LAO projection provides left-right perspective, while the RAO projection provides anterior-posterior perspective.

Reconciliation of images from different projections requires proper identification of two planes: the plane of the mitral valve outlined by the CS and GCV, and the plane of the interventricular septum outlined by the anterior and PIV. A 3D perspective can be obtained by visualizing the LV as a spherical fishbowl, with veins curving across the outer surface and the neck representing the mitral valve plane (Figure 15.6).

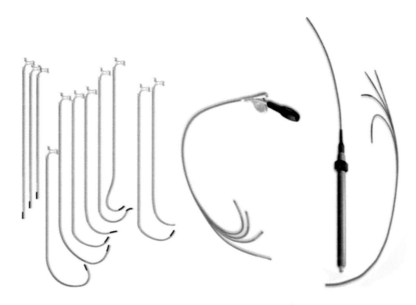

Figure 15.5 Catheters for coronary sinus cannulation. (Courtesy of Medtronic, Inc.)

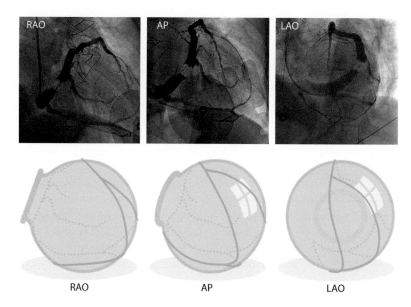

Figure 15.6 Visualizing epicardial veins. The surface veins are distributed over the free hemisphere of left ventricle. AP, anteroposterior; LAO, left anterior oblique; RAO, right anterior oblique.

The CS can also be localized with the venous phase of coronary arteriography. The femoral approach to CS catheterization is used for angiography procedures that do not require the backup support needed to deliver pacing leads into branch veins, and for diagnostic electrophysiology and blood sampling.

The best way to visualize the cardiac veins at the time of LV lead placement is with the help of balloon-occlusion venography, which helps to identify branch veins that are most suitable for placement of an LV pacing lead. It is the only method capable of effectively visualizing all potential target veins and is the cornerstone for proper CRT.

LIMITATIONS

Complications of coronary sinus catheterization

The CS is relatively thin-walled compared to other chambers of the heart and hence easily susceptible to traumatic injury.[31,32] CS injuries are usually preventable and can be avoided by having a detailed understanding of cardiac venous anatomy, by choosing curved catheters or steerable guidewires to negotiate changes in direction so as to remain coaxial with the vessel lumen, and by injecting small volumes of contrast for orientation. Despite these measures, the following complications are frequently seen.

Perforations

Perforations occur when force is directed perpendicular to the vessel wall after a catheter inadvertently enters a branch vein. In contrast to arterial perforations, low pressures in the cardiac venous system help these perforations seal spontaneously when the catheter is removed. Tamponade is extremely rare and should raise suspicion for other explanations, such as perforation of the right ventricular apex by a pacing lead.

Dissection

Dissections occur when a lead or catheter is advanced forcefully in a different direction or to overcome resistance at sites such as branch veins or valves. Dissections can also result from balloon inflation in an undersized branch vein. Common locations for dissection include the origin of the MCV, the origin of the vein of Marshall, Vieussens valve, and the origin of lateral branch veins. The most dangerous consequence of dissection is that it can prevent cannulation of branch veins needed for CRT.

Contrast extravasation

Contrast extravasation is seen during balloon-occluded venography due to injection through an end-hole catheter when the tip lies against a vessel wall.

Most catheter-related CS injuries may appear dangerous at first but are usually benign and often clinically silent. The most common way of recognizing injury is looking for extravasated contrast during venography. These are usually contained by the epicardial fat around the CS and do not communicate with the pericardial space. Extravasation makes visualization of branch vessel anatomy extremely difficult, and operators should stop injecting contrast at the first sign of extravasation. Retrograde dissections close spontaneously when the offending catheter is removed.[33]

Whatever the type of injury to the CS, it is not necessarily a reason to terminate a procedure. After recognizing an injury, the operator can safely continue as long as the true lumen can be visualized. This may require a brief waiting period (5–10 minutes), a different choice of catheters and guidewires, and alternate imaging projections. In some instances, the procedure may have to be stopped altogether and redone on a different day. Most CS injuries heal with time, without any intervention.

Abnormalities of the coronary sinus

Although the CS is a fairly consistent structure, some anomalies are encountered that can make catheterization of the CS difficult.

PLSVC is the most common anomaly of the thoracic vein.[34–38] The hallmark finding is a markedly dilated CS due to increased flow. PLSVC is usually an incidental finding by echocardiography or chest computed tomography (CT), but it may be discovered while passing catheters or pacing leads from the left subclavian or jugular approach. PLSVC can also be discovered during right heart catheterization from the femoral approach. The markedly enlarged CS is easily entered, and catheters may appear to enter the pulmonary artery (PA). The unusual trajectory can make manipulation of pacing leads difficult. Blood flow with PLSVC is physiologic, so there are no clinical consequences.

Unroofed CS is a rare form of atrial septal defect (ASD) where the normal separation between the LA and the CS is absent.[39–47] The CS forms a connection between the left and right atria, allowing the left-to-right shunt that is typical of an ASD. The condition is commonly associated with a PLSVC. The clinical features of unroofed CS include right heart failure from chronic volume overload, cyanosis, and paradoxical embolism. The diagnosis can be made by echocardiography and/or angiography, but imaging modalities such as magnetic resonance imaging (MRI) and CT can also be used. Treatment involves percutaneous catheter-based interventions aimed at covering the defect or occluding the left vena cava.[48–50]

A CS diverticulum is usually discovered by contrast venography at the time of electrophysiology procedures for posterior-septal accessory pathways.[51] It can be associated with arrhythmias and sudden cardiac death.[52,53] On rare occasions, a CS diverticulum is seen merely as an incidental finding and carries no clinical significance.[54]

CONTRAINDICATIONS

Cardiac catheterization techniques have greatly evolved in recent years and the procedure is generally well-tolerated, even in patients with myocardial infarction (MI), cardiogenic shock, and ventricular tachycardia. Few of the relative contraindications to catheterization of the cardiac venous system include the following: acute pulmonary edema, severe uncontrolled hypertension, severe anemia, decompensated systolic heart failure, acute kidney injury with or without dialysis, allergy to contrast, and bleeding disorders and/or anticoagulation therapy.

CONCLUSIONS

The CS and the cardiac venous system have become a vital gateway for a number of interventions. Successful catheterization requires good understanding of anatomy, indications/contraindications, and procedural techniques.

REFERENCES

1. Strickberger SA, et al. Patient selection for cardiac resynchronization therapy: From the Council on Clinical Cardiology Subcommittee on Electrocardiography and Arrhythmias and the Quality of Care and Outcomes Research Interdisciplinary Working Group, in collaboration with the Heart Rhythm Society. *Circulation* 2005;111(16):2146–2150.
2. Bristow MR, et al. Cardiac-resynchronization therapy with or without an implantable defibrillator in advanced chronic heart failure. *N Engl J Med* 2004;350(21):2140–2150.
3. von Ludinghausen M, et al. Atrial veins of the human heart. *Clin Anat* 1995;8(3):169–189.
4. Habib A, et al. The anatomy of the coronary sinus venous system for the cardiac electrophysiologist. *Europace* 2009;11 Suppl 5:v15–21.
5. Ansari A. Anatomy and clinical significance of ventricular Thebesian veins. *Clin Anat* 2001;14(2):102–110.
6. Ravin MB, et al. Contribution of thebesian veins to the physiologic shunt in anesthetized man. *J Appl Physiol* 1965;20(6):1148–1152.
7. Faxon DP, et al. Coronary sinus occlusion pressure and its relation to intracardiac pressure. *Am J Cardiol* 1985;56(7):457–460.
8. Von Ludinghausen M. Clinical anatomy of cardiac veins, Vv. cardiacae. *Surg Radiol Anat* 1987;9(2):159–168.
9. Chauvin M, et al. The anatomic basis of connections between the coronary sinus musculature and the left atrium in humans. *Circulation* 2000;101(6):647–652.
10. D'Cruz IA, et al. Dynamic cyclic changes in coronary sinus caliber in patients with and without congestive heart failure. *Am J Cardiol* 1999;83(2):275–277.
11. Antz M, et al. Electrical conduction between the right atrium and the left atrium via the musculature of the coronary sinus. *Circulation* 1998;98(17):1790–1795.
12. Eckardt L. Automaticity in the coronary sinus. *J Cardiovasc Electrophysiol* 2002;13(3):288–289.
13. Dobosz PM, et al. Anatomy of the valve of the coronary (Thebesian valve). *Clin Anat* 1995;8(6):438–439.
14. Gami AS, et al. Electrophysiological anatomy of typical atrial flutter: The posterior boundary and causes for difficulty with ablation. *J Cardiovasc Electrophysiol* 2010;21(2):144–149.
15. Ortale JR, et al. The anatomy of the coronary sinus and its tributaries. *Surg Radiol Anat* 2001;23(1):15–21.
16. Hwang C, et al. Vein of Marshall cannulation for the analysis of electrical activity in patients with focal atrial fibrillation. *Circulation* 2000;101(3):1503–1505.
17. Duda B, Grzybiak M. Main tributaries of the CS in the adult human heart. *Folia Morphol (Warsz)* 1998;57:363–369.
18. Jongbloed MR, et al. Noninvasive visualization of the cardiac venous system using multislice computed tomography. *J Am Coll Cardiol* 2005;45(5):749–753.

19. Ludinghausen M, et al. Myocardial coverage of the CS and related veins. *Clin Anat* 1992;5:1–15.

20. Banai S, et al. Coronary sinus reducer stent for the treatment of chronic refractory angina pectoris: A prospective, open-label, multicenter, safety feasibility first-in-man study. *J Am Coll Cardiol* 2007;49(17):1783–1789.

21. Haga Y, et al. Ischemic and nonischemic tissue concentrations of felodipine after coronary venous retroinfusion during myocardial ischemia and reperfusion: An experimental study in pigs. *J Cardiovasc Pharm* 1994;24(2):298–302.

22. Ryden L, et al. Pharmacokinetic analysis of coronary venous retroinfusion: A comparison with anterograde coronary artery drug administration using metoprolol as a tracer. *J Am Coll Cardiol* 1991;18(2):603–612.

23. Raake P, et al. Myocardial gene transfer by selective pressure-regulated retroinfusion of coronary veins: Comparison with surgical and percutaneous intramyocardial gene delivery. *J Am Coll Cardiol* 2004;44(5):1124–1129.

24. Schumacher B, et al. Induction of neoangiogenesis in ischemic myocardium by human growth factors: First clinical results of a new treatment of coronary heart disease. *Circulation* 1998;97(7):645–650.

25. Sato K, et al. Efficacy of intracoronary or intravenous VEGF165 in a pig model of chronic myocardial ischemia. *J Am Coll Cardiol* 2001;37(2):616–623.

26. Webb JG, et al. Percutaneous transvenous mitral annuloplasty: Initial human experience with device implantation in the coronary sinus. *Circulation* 2006;113(6):851–855.

27. Schofer J, et al. Percutaneous mitral annuloplasty for functional mitral regurgitation: Results of the CARILLON Mitral Annuloplasty Device European Union Study. *Circulation* 2009;120(4):326–333.

28. Reifart N. Percutaneous in situ coronary venous arterialization: A catheter-based procedure for coronary artery bypass. *J Interv Cardiol* 2005;18(6):491–495.

29. Oesterle SN, et al. Percutaneous in situ coronary venous arterialization: Report of the first human catheter-based coronary artery bypass. *Circulation* 2001;103(21):2539–2543.

30. Nazarian S, et al. Direct visualization of coronary sinus ostium and branches with a flexible steerable fiberoptic infrared endoscope. *Heart Rhythm* 2005;2(8):844–848.

31. Johnson WB, et al. Incidence of coronary sinus dissection and perforation complications from coronary sinus venograms in a large multicenter trial. *Pacing Clin Electrophysiol* 2003;26:S56.

32. Walker S, et al. Dissection of the coronary sinus secondary to pacemaker lead manipulation. *Pacing Clin Electrophysiol* 2000;23(4 Pt 1):541–543

33. de Cock CC, et al. Major dissection of the coronary sinus and its tributaries during lead implantation for biventricular stimulation: Angiographic follow-up. *Europace* 2004;6(1):43–47.

34. Alam M, et al. Persistent left superior vena cava: An incidental finding. *J Am Coll Cardiol* 2009;53(13):1159.

35. Ho KL, Tan JL. Persistent left sided superior vena cava. *Heart* 2006;92(8):1046.

36. Schulz HU, et al. Persistent left superior vena cava. *Lancet* 2003;361(9357):560.

37. Gerber TC, Kuzo RS. Images in cardiovascular medicine. Persistent left superior vena cava demonstrated with multislice spiral computed tomography. *Circulation* 2002;105(14):e79.

38. Tahir T, et al. Persistent left superior vena cava: Incidence, significance and clinical correlates. *Int J Cardiol* 2002;82(1):91–93.

39. Nakatani S, et al. Images in cardiology. Unroofed coronary sinus. *Heart* 2002;87(3):278.

40. Piacentini G, et al. Persistent left superior vena cava into unroofed coronary sinus. *Lancet* 2006;368(9551):1963–1964.

41. Sueyoshi E, et al. Persistent left superior vena cava into left atrium. *Lancet* 2006;368(9543):1270.

42. Kwok OH, Chan JK. Unroofed coronary sinus defect. *Hong Kong Med J* 2008;14(4):331–332.

43. Huang XS. Images in cardiovascular medicine. Partially unroofed coronary sinus. *Circulation* 2007;116(15):e373.

44. Acar P, et al. Unroofed coronary sinus with persistent left superior vena cava assessed by 3D echocardiography. *Echocardiography* 2008;25(6):666–667.

45. Thangaroopan M, et al. Images in cardiovascular medicine. Rare case of an unroofed coronary sinus: Diagnosis by multidetector computed tomography. *Circulation* 2009;119(16):e518–e520.

46. Oyama N, et al. Volume-rendering and endocardial views of partially unroofed coronary sinus with 64-slice multidetector CT. *J Cardiovasc Comput Tomogr* 2009;3(5):346–347.

47. Low SC, et al. Magnetic resonance imaging of unroofed coronary sinus. *Heart* 2009;95(9):720.

48. Heng JT, De Giovanni JV. Occlusion of persistent left superior vena cava to unroofed coronary sinus using vena cava filter and coils. *Heart* 1997;77(6):579–580.

49. Geggel RL, et al. Left superior vena cava connection to unroofed coronary sinus associated with positional cyanosis: Successful transcatheter treatment using Gianturco-Grifka vascular occlusion device. *Catheter Cardiovasc Interv* 1999;48(4):369–373.

50. Torres A, et al. Closure of unroofed coronary sinus with a covered stent in a symptomatic infant. *Catheter Cardiovasc Interv* 2007;70(5):745–748.

51. Sun Y, et al. Coronary sinus-ventricular accessory connections producing posteroseptal and left posterior accessory pathways: Incidence and electrophysiological identification. *Circulation* 2002;106(11):1362–1367.

52. Guiraudon GM, et al. The coronary sinus diverticulum: A pathologic entity associated with the Wolff-Parkinson-White syndrome. *Am J Cardiol* 1988;62(10 Pt 1):733–735.

53. Blank R, et al. Images in cardiovascular medicine. Wolff-Parkinson-White syndrome and atrial fibrillation in a patient with a coronary sinus diverticulum. *Circulation* 2007;115(20):e469–e471.

54. Thal S, et al. Coronary sinus diverticulum complicating CRT device implantation. *Pacing Clin Electrophysiol* 2008;31(9):1184–1185.

PART 3

Coronary Angiographic Assessment

16

Coronary arterial anatomy: Normal, variants, and well-described collaterals

JOHN P. ERWIN, EVAN L. HARDEGREE, AND GREGORY J. DEHMER

INTRODUCTION

The practice of medicine requires an understanding of normal physiologic function, plus the pathophysiology of disease. To fully understand coronary artery disease, a solid knowledge base of normal coronary anatomy is required. During coronary angiography, the anatomy of the epicardial coronary arteries, including collateral vessels, is the main focus. However, with the development of percutaneous techniques to treat epicardial coronary artery stenoses, an understanding of the normal anatomic structure of a coronary artery is also important. Although this chapter focuses mainly on the normal and variant anatomy of the epicardial coronary system, a brief review of the structure of a normal coronary artery is appropriate.

CORONARY ARTERY ANATOMY

A normal coronary artery consists of three histologically distinct layers (Figure 16.1). The innermost layer is the *tunica intima* or simply the *intima*. It is composed of a single layer of endothelial cells bounded by the lumen on one side and the internal elastic lamina on the other side. The endothelial layer is vital for maintaining vascular health and has three distinctive roles. First, it is a metabolically active tissue that secretes both vasodilator substances (such as prostacyclin, nitric oxide, and endothelial-derived hyperpolarizing factors) and vasoconstrictor substances (endothelin and vasoconstrictor prostanoids).[1,2] Endothelial cells also secrete certain components of the extracellular matrix, such as elastin, glycosaminoglycans, and fibronectin, and, along with smooth muscle cells, secrete matrix metalloproteinases, which are critical in arterial remodeling.[3,4] Certain growth factors that control smooth muscle proliferation are also secreted by endothelial cells. Second, normal quiescent endothelial cells have an antithrombotic surface that inhibits platelet adhesion and coagulation.[5] However, when stimulated by cytokines or other inflammatory mediators, the endothelium can produce various prothrombotic factors. Endothelial cells produce von Willebrand factor, Factor VIII antigen, prostacyclin, nitric oxide, tissue factor, Antithrombin III, heparin-like molecules, and tissue plasminogen activator, which all have roles in coagulation and fibrinolysis. Although the endothelium normally exists in a functional state of balance between thrombotic and antithrombotic factors, injury or inflammation enhances the prothrombotic state of the endothelium. Third, the normal endothelium provides a barrier to the indiscriminate

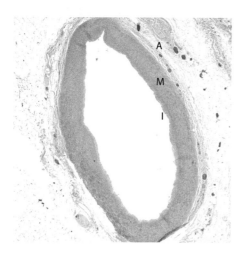

Figure 16.1 Normal human coronary artery (hematoxylin and eosin stain at 40 power magnification) showing the intima (I), media (M), and adventitia (A). (Courtesy of Dr. V.O. Speights, Department of Pathology, Scott & White Medical Center.)

passage of blood constituents into the arterial wall. Fluid and macromolecular transport functions of the endothelium are dependent on vessel size. There are two major mechanisms that regulate the endothelial barrier function: One involves cell-to-cell contacts, allowing transport in the junctions between cells, and the other involves vesicular transport directly through the cell.

The next layer is the *tunica media* or simply *media*. It surrounds the internal elastic lamina, and its composition depends on the type of artery. Large arteries have additional circumferential layers of elastic tissue within the media and are referred to as elastic arteries. The epicardial coronary arteries are elastic arteries, as are the carotids, cerebral arteries, and the aorta. However, at the point the epicardial arteries turn into the myocardium, usually at a right angle from the parent vessel, they become more muscular arteries with few, if any, elastic fibers.[6] In normal arteries, the vessel lumen diameter can be altered by contraction or relaxation of the medial vascular smooth muscle in response to a variety of systemic signals and locally released factors. The final layer is the *tunica adventitia* or simply *adventitia*, which is a layer of loose connective tissue surrounding the media.[6] In elastic arteries, this is demarcated by a layer of elastic fibers termed the *external elastic lamina*. The adventitia contains a network of small blood vessels (vaso vasorum), which are responsible for nutrition of the outer two-thirds of the artery. The inner third of the artery derives nutrition by diffusion through the endothelium. The adventitia also contains nerves that control the constriction and relaxation of the artery. In various locations within the adventitia, and associated with the outermost elastic layer, are pressure receptors. These pressure or baroreceptors have a phasic discharge rate in harmony with the arterial stretching associated with the pulse wave. Impulses from the baroreceptors are integrated centrally and when increased or decreased cause appropriate alterations in many vascular beds.

BASIC ANATOMY OF THE CORONARY CIRCULATION

The anatomy of the coronary arteries was described by Raymond Vieussens about 300 years ago. Careful postmortem studies have provided greater detail of the normal coronary anatomy. The Latin term "corona," or crown, aptly describes coronary arteries as the coronary branches that traverse the atrioventricular and interventricular sulci in the shape of a crown.[6] In humans and other mammals, the major epicardial vessels are the left main and right main coronary arteries (RCA). The left and right coronary arteries originate at the base (root) of the aorta from openings called the coronary ostia, which are located in the left and right sinus of Valsalva, respectively. The ostia usually originate at the center of each sinus just below or no more than 1 cm above the superior edge of the aortic cusp. The left coronary orifice normally arises from the left sinus of Valsalva, midway between the posterior portion of the pulmonary artery and the left atrial appendage, just above the level of the free margin of the aortic valve leaflet and generally below the sinotubular junction.

The left coronary ostium is usually single, giving rise to a short, common left coronary artery (LCA) trunk (the left main artery) that courses in the epicardial fat for distances varying from a few millimeters to several centimeters before bifurcating into the left anterior descending (LAD) and left circumflex (LCx) coronary arteries. The length of the left main artery derived from pathologic examinations is 1 ± 0.3 cm.[7] Some studies have suggested that patients with bicuspid aortic valves have shorter left main segments, but this is not universally accepted.[8,9] No correlation of left main coronary artery length with age, gender, heart weight, extent of coronary artery disease, or left ventricular (LV) wall thickness was found in one autopsy series.[9] Histologically, the left main ostium lacks an adventitia and has a greater portion of elastic tissue than other segments of the coronary tree. This may account for some of the differences in response to coronary interventions involving this segment of the left main. Moreover, since the left main ostium technically lies within the wall of the aorta, it is subject to diseases affecting the aortic wall, such as syphilitic aortitis, radiation-induced aortitis, and Takayasu arteritis.[10] In some individuals, there is a trifurcation of the left main with a third branch arising in the crotch between the LAD and LCx. This third artery, called a *ramus intermedius* or simply a *ramus* branch, acts functionally as a circumflex branch, supplying a portion of the obtuse margin of the heart between the LAD and LCx. In one series, a ramus intermedius occurred in 37% of the general population, and was considered a normal variant.[11] In another series of 150 hearts, the left main bifurcated in 55%, trifurcated in 39%, and had a quadrification (ramus and separate diagonal) in 7%.[12] A trifurcation pattern was found in 60% of nonwhite females. The length of the ramus varies from 20 to 50 mm and its relative length varied from 21% to 50% of the length of the LV.

The normal location of the RCA ostium is more variable. It usually arises from the middle of the right coronary sinus just below the sinotubular junction of the right sinus of Valsalva, but it can arise lower, near the valve, to higher, near the sinotubular ridge. The right and left coronary arteries are usually the only vessels arising immediately above the free margin of aortic valve, but in one-third of angiograms, the artery to the pulmonary outflow tract (conus artery) may originate as a separate ostium rather than its usual position as a branch of the proximal RCA. Common variations of the location of the coronary ostia exist, which can have clinical implications as will be discussed later in this chapter.

Coronary dominance

The coronary artery from which the posterior descending artery (PDA) arises is considered the dominant coronary artery (Figure 16.2). The PDA traverses the posterior interventricular sulcus and supplies the posterior part of the ventricular septum and often a portion of the posterolateral wall of the LV. Most humans are right dominant, but the frequency of right dominance varies in the literature from a low of 70% to a high of 90%.[13] In a right-dominant circulation, the RCA crosses the interventricular groove and continues in the atrioventricular groove beyond the origin of the PDA to supply one or more posterolateral LV branches. The artery to the atrioventricular node usually arises from the RCA at an area called the crux, which represents the intersection of the interventricular and atrioventricular grooves on the inferior surface of the heart. This is noted on the posterior surface of the heart by a small indentation or dimple.

If the PDA arises from the terminal portion of the LCx, the term *left dominance* is applied to the circulation. The frequency of a left-dominant circulation in the literature varies from 8% to 15%.[13] In some individuals, the posterior septum is supplied by branches arising from both the RCA and LCx. In this situation the circulation is said to be "balanced" or codominant with dual PDAs (one from the RCA and the other from the LCx) or no clear PDA with multiple smaller branches arising from both arteries. It is important to note that anatomic dominance does not imply the vessel is of greater physiologic importance and thus is somewhat a misnomer. Although the RCA is most frequently the dominant artery, the LCA almost always supplies a greater myocardial mass.[14]

Left anterior descending artery

The LAD is a direct continuation of the left main artery with its course along the anterior interventricular groove. When the heart is viewed frontally, the LAD is seen as it curves around and emerges from behind the pulmonary artery (Figure 16.3). The LAD, in combination with the left main, forms a curve that resembles a reverse "S" shape. The tight upper curve brings the LAD around the pulmonary artery to the uppermost portions of the interventricular septum, and the lower portion curves in the opposite direction as it follows the interventricular septum toward the apex. Several normal variations in the length and distribution of the LAD have been recognized. The LAD may fail to reach the apex and have relatively few branches over the anterolateral wall of the ventricle.[14] Alternatively, the LAD may course well around the apex ("wraparound" LAD) and supply a substantial portion of the posterior septum and even replace the PDA.[15] Some individuals may have dual or bifid LAD

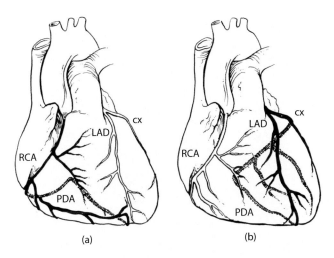

(a)   (b)

Figure 16.2 **(a)** Right and **(b)** left dominant coronary anatomy. The dominant coronary artery is the one from which the posterior descending coronary artery arises. (Reproduced from Giuliani, E.R., et al., (Eds.), *Mayo Clinic Practice of Cardiology*, 3rd ed., Mosby, 1996, p. 341. Used with permission of Mayo Foundation for Medical Education and Research.)

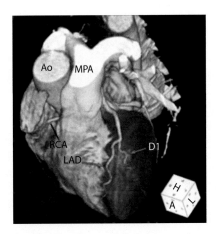

Figure 16.3 Three-dimensional reconstruction of a 64-slice CT angiogram illustrating the coronary tree in a left anterior oblique view with cranial angulation. Ao, aorta; D1, first diagonal artery; LAD, left anterior descending artery; MPA, main pulmonary artery; RCA, right coronary artery. (Courtesy of Dr. John Rumberger, Princeton Longevity Center, Princeton, NJ.)

systems with one vessel almost exclusively supplying the septum and the other vessel running almost parallel, giving rise to all of the diagonal arteries.[16] Along its course toward the cardiac apex, the LAD gives rise to anterior septal perforating branches and diagonal branches. As these branches arise from the LAD, the lumen diameter of the LAD is progressively reduced toward the cardiac apex. Small branches may arise from the LAD to supply a small portion of the anterior wall of the right ventricle with isolated reports of larger vessels termed a *right ventricular descending branch*.[17]

DIAGONAL ARTERIES

Diagonal artery branches arise from the LAD and course at downward angles to supply the anterolateral free wall of the LV (Figure 16.3). Most individuals have one to three diagonal arteries, but up to six small diagonals may be present. The larger diagonal arteries arise from the upper portion of the LAD and the caliber of the branches becomes progressively smaller as the LAD approaches the apex. The diagonals roughly run parallel to each other and also parallel to a ramus branch if one is present.

SEPTAL PERFORATING BRANCHES

In over 99% of individuals, the blood supply to the anterior interventricular septum is from the LAD.[18] Septal perforating branches arise at nearly right angles from the LAD and penetrate deep into the interventricular septum. In 38% of individuals, a large dominant septal perforator is present and is usually the first septal, whereas in the remainder, there is no dominant septal artery.[18] Septal perforator arteries may bifurcate and trifurcate, but the branching pattern is somewhat unordered and may take the appearance of a pitchfork with multiple branches off one central point of the trunk. Septal arteries are occasionally seen arising from other arteries, such as the first diagonal, proximal RCA or LCx, and as a separate ostium from the right sinus of Valsalva.[19]

Left circumflex artery

The LCx artery arises from the left main artery at its bifurcation and courses posteriorly under the left atrial appendage to reach the left atrioventricular groove (Figure 16.4). The LCx origin is often at nearly a right angle from the left main, but in some patients may have a greater or lesser degree of angulation at its origin. The LCx remains in the atrioventricular groove circumscribing the mitral valve annulus, giving rise to as many as four obtuse marginal arteries. The extent and distribution of the LCx and marginal arteries is usually reciprocal with that of the RCA. If the LCx has an extensive distribution over the posterior and inferior walls, the RCA will typically be small with fewer branches in this region and vice versa. Atrial branches may arise from the LCx coronary artery and supply the sinus node in 37% of patients.[20] Although the circumflex sinus node artery usually arises near the origin of the LCx, in approximately 20% of individuals who have a circumflex origin of this artery, the artery is an S-shaped vessel that originates from the posterolateral branch of the circumflex.

OBTUSE MARGINAL ARTERIES

Marginal arteries arise from the LCx and supply the lateral wall of the LV. The nomenclature of the marginal arteries is based on their origin from the LCx—that is, first marginal, second marginal, and so forth. There is considerable anatomic variation in the number and size of the marginal arteries, but there is at least one marginal branch present in most individuals (Figure 16.5). When a single large

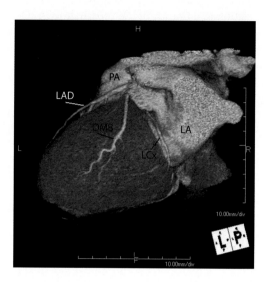

Figure 16.4 Three-dimensional reconstruction of 64-slice CT angiogram illustrating the coronary tree in a left posterior oblique projection. Note the circumflex running posteriorly under the left atrial appendage to reach the left atrioventricular groove. LA, left atrium; LAD, left anterior descending; LCx, left circumflex; OMB, obtuse marginal branch; PA, pulmonary artery. (Courtesy of Dr. John Rumberger, Princeton Longevity Center, Princeton, NJ.)

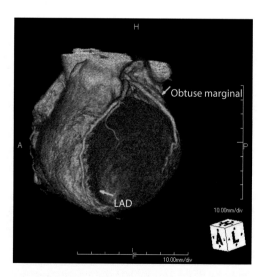

Figure 16.5 Three-dimensional reconstruction of 64-slice CT angiogram illustrating the left anterior descending artery and an obtuse marginal branch in a left anterior oblique view with cranial angulation. LAD, left anterior descending. (Courtesy of Dr. John Rumberger, Princeton Longevity Center, Princeton, NJ.)

marginal branch is present, there is usually extensive secondary and tertiary branching of the vessel. The most common pattern is to have two or three marginal branches of similar size with less extensive secondary branching. There is also a reciprocal relationship between the diagonal arteries and circumflex marginal arteries such that when there are only a few small and short diagonals, there should be large marginal branches of the LCx, which course quite anterior to supply a portion of the anterolateral wall. Failure to see this pattern may be a hint that there is a flush occlusion of a vessel and an area of nonperfused myocardium. If a large ramus branch is present, then the proximal diagonal branches are smaller and few in number and only supply the territory close to the LAD. The ramus supplies the next more lateral segment of the LV wall and then the LCx marginal branches supply the territory of the posterolateral LV free wall.

Right coronary artery

The RCA courses in the right atrioventricular groove and circumscribes the tricuspid valve annulus (Figure 16.6). The first branch arising from the RCA is frequently the conus or infundibular branch; it courses anteriorly to supply the muscular right ventricular outflow tract or infundibulum. Alternatively, in 30%–50% of angiograms, the conus artery may arise from a separate ostium close to the RCA ostium or from a common aortic ostium shared with the RCA.[14] Another important proximal branch of the RCA is the sinus node artery. The sinus node artery arises from the proximal RCA in 50%–70% of individuals with a dual blood supply from both the RCA and LCx in 3%.[21] In its mid-portion, the RCA provides one or more branches that supply the right

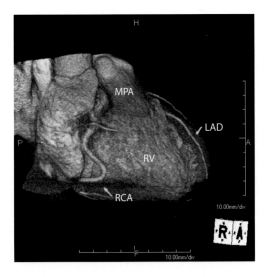

Figure 16.6 Three-dimensional reconstruction of 64-slice CT angiogram illustrating the right coronary artery in a right anterior oblique view. LAD = left anterior descending artery; MPA = main pulmonary artery; RCA = right coronary artery; RV = right ventricle. (Courtesy of Dr. John Rumberger, Princeton Longevity Center, Princeton, NJ.)

ventricular free wall (right ventricular marginal branches). The RCA also supplies blood to the atria with a highly variable pattern of small branches. The anatomy of the distal RCA is quite variable. In those with a right dominant pattern, the PDA arises at or near the crux in 50%–60% of individuals. In the remaining individuals with right dominance, the PDA originates more proximally, either at the acute margin (13%) or between the acute margin and the crux (19%).[22] An anomalous origin of the PDA from the first septal perforator without ischemic complications has also been reported.[23]

The blood supply to the papillary muscles is clinically important. The anterolateral papillary muscle more frequently has a dual blood supply from the diagonal branches of the LAD and marginal branches of the LCx. Accordingly, it is more protected from ischemic dysfunction. In contrast, the posteromedial papillary muscle is usually supplied only by the PDA, making it more vulnerable. Thus, myocardial infarction involving the PDA is more likely to cause mitral regurgitation.[24]

Coronary microcirculation

Because they lie on the surface of the heart, the left and right coronary arteries and their major branches are referred to as the epicardial coronary arteries. However, the entire coronary arterial system is composed of three distinct components that have different physiologic functions. A detailed description of coronary microvascular anatomy and function is beyond the scope of this chapter, but an overview is important to understanding the coronary circulation. Although there are three components of the coronary circulation, these are not demarcated by distinct anatomic borders. The most proximal component comprises the large epicardial coronary arteries. These function primarily as conduits offering little resistance to coronary blood flow under normal conditions, but are subject to flow-mediated dilation. Therefore, the pressure drop along these conduit or conductive arteries is negligible in the absence of a coronary stenosis. In general, epicardial coronary arteries vary in diameter from 1 to 5 mm, but arteries as small as 500 μm can still be found on the epicardial surface. Pathologic degrees of spasm may also occur in the epicardial coronary arteries.

The next component in series is the prearteriole, which range in size from 100 to 500 μm. Because of their location and wall thickness, these vessels are not directly affected by products of myocardial metabolism. Their role is to maintain pressure at the origin of the arterioles within a narrow range in response to changes in epicardial coronary perfusion pressure and flow, a function that is often referred to as the autoregulation of coronary blood flow.

The final component is the network of intramural arterioles, which have diameters less than 100 μm. The arteriole wall consists of an endothelial layer facing the blood surrounded by a layer of circumferentially oriented smooth muscle cells. These are encased by connective tissue containing a rich plexus of sympathetic and parasympathetic fibers. The smooth muscle cells are able to constrict the lumen of an arteriole and frequently do under physiologic and pathologic stimuli. Their role is to regulate myocardial blood supply to match myocardial oxygen consumption. This function is especially marked at their junction with the capillaries, thus blood passage into the capillaries is carefully controlled. The arterioles have a high resting tone and dilate in response to metabolites released by the myocardium at times of increased oxygen demand.[25] Blood flow can increase by 200% or more over resting values in many capillary beds by the relaxation of the arteriolar constrictors. Therefore, by regulating the resistances in the prearterioles and arterioles, blood flow is matched with oxygen requirements in the coronary circulation.[26]

The arterioles branch into numerous capillaries that lie adjacent to the cardiac myocytes. The capillaries measure 10–15 μm in diameter and are the site of metabolic exchange. A high capillary-to-cardiomyocyte ratio and short diffusion distance ensure adequate oxygen delivery to the myocytes and removal of metabolic waste products from the cells. Capillaries are composed of a single layer of endothelium with surrounding basement membrane and an incomplete layer of pericytes. Pericytes, also known as Rouget cells or mural cells, are mesenchymal-like cells associated with the walls of small blood vessels. As a relatively undifferentiated cell, they support the small vessel but can differentiate into a fibroblast, smooth muscle cell, or macrophage. They are important in angiogenesis and have been implicated in blood flow regulation at the capillary level. Capillaries are also surrounded by a loosely formed adventitia of collagen, elastic fibers, and matrix.

Just as the epicardial coronary arteries are affected by atherosclerosis, the coronary microcirculation is affected in a variety of systemic and cardiac disorders. These consist of functional alterations, involving changes in the responsiveness of the coronary microvasculature, and structural changes involving alterations in the number and diameter of the coronary microvessels. A proposed classification of the pathogenic mechanisms of coronary microvascular dysfunction is shown in Table 16.1.[27]

Coronary venous anatomy

The capillaries terminate in small venules that have a diameter of approximately 15 μm. Other than size, the morphologic change from capillary to venule is not very distinctive. Small venules have an endothelial lining, a surrounding basement membrane, and collagen connections from the basement membrane to the surrounding matrix. In contrast to capillaries, vasoactive compounds like histamine, various kinins, and serotonin can affect the separation of the endothelial cell tight junctions in venules, resulting in leakage of large molecular weight substances. Veins of about 0.5 mm in diameter begin to acquire a muscular coat and eventually form small epicardial veins that run in parallel with the visible epicardial arterial branches.

There is considerable variability in cardiac venous anatomy, but there are some consistent venous structures (Figure 16.7).[28] The most notable of these is the great

Table 16.1 Pathogenic mechanisms of coronary microvascular dysfunction

Alterations	Causes
Structural	
Luminal obstruction	Microembolization in acute coronary syndromes or after recanalization
Vascular-wall infiltration	Infiltrative heart disease (e.g., Anderson–Fabry cardiomyopathy)
Vascular remodeling	Hypertrophic cardiomyopathy, arterial hypertension
Vascular rarefaction	Aortic stenosis, arterial hypertension
Perivascular fibrosis	Aortic stenosis, arterial hypertension
Functional	
Endothelial dysfunction	Smoking, hyperlipidemia, diabetes
Dysfunction of smooth muscle cell	Hypertrophic cardiomyopathy, arterial hypertension
Autonomic dysfunction	Coronary recanalization
Extravascular	
Extramural compression	Aortic stenosis, hypertrophic cardiomyopathy, arterial hypertension
Reduction in diastolic perfusion time	Aortic stenosis

Source: Adapted from Camici, P.G., Crea, F., *N. Engl. J. Med.*, 356(8), 830–840, 2007.

(or anterior) cardiac vein, which begins at the apex of the heart and ascends along the anterior interventricular groove to the base of the ventricles parallel to the LAD. It connects with diagonal veins draining the lateral and anterolateral portion of the LV and turns posterior at the left atrioventricular groove, wrapping around the left side of the heart parallel to the LCx coronary artery.[29] In addition to several smaller tributaries from the left atrium and ventricles, the great cardiac vein receives two main branches, the large left marginal vein along the lateral border of the heart and the posterior LV branch (also known as the posterolateral branch). The great cardiac vein terminates in the coronary sinus, a junction defined by the presence of the left atrial oblique vein. This transition point is usually marked by the presence of intravenous valves, which can obstruct catheter and pacemaker lead placement. Another fairly consistent branch is the middle cardiac vein, which runs in the posterior interventricular groove, parallel to the posterior descending coronary artery. Of all of the branches of the coronary venous system, the great cardiac and middle cardiac veins are the two most consistently present branches seen in more than 90% of individuals.[30] However, unlike the middle cardiac vein, the great

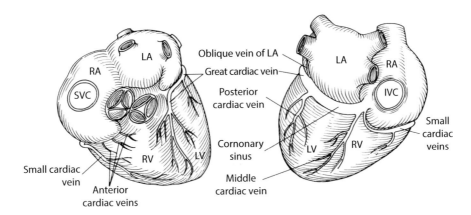

Figure 16.7 Cardiac venous anatomy shown in an anterior (left) and posterior (right) views. (Reproduced from Murphy, J.G., Applied anatomy of the Heart and Great Vessels, in Murphy, J.G. (Ed.), *Mayo Clinic Cardiology Review*, 2nd ed., Lippincott Williams & Wilkins, Philadelphia, PA, 2005, p. 948. Used with permission of the Mayo Foundation for Medical Education and Research.)

cardiac vein varies considerably in its course.[31] Lateral and posterior venous branches together are seen in less than 50% of human hearts.

The coronary sinus is the most constant feature of the cardiac venous system, although several congenital anomalies have been described.[32,33] The coronary sinus lies in the atrioventricular groove on the posterior surface of the heart and receives veins from the lateral wall, which are referred to as marginal veins. Although the coronary sinus invariably lies in the atrioventricular groove, its branches and their locations are far more variable than those of the coronary arterial system.[33] The coronary sinus opens into the right atrium, posteromedially, just superior to the septal leaflet of the tricuspid valve. At the ostium of the coronary sinus is the thebesian valve, a semicircular fold of the lining membrane of the atrium. The valve may vary in size or be completely absent and acts to prevent regurgitation of blood into the coronary sinus during contraction of the atrium. The valve can also hinder cannulation of the coronary sinus.[34] The coronary sinus and its tributaries drain approximately two-thirds of the LV myocardium, but they do not drain the superior part of the interventricular septum, the right atrium and ventricle, or the myocardium of the roof of the left atrium. These are drained by the right cardiac (or anterior cardiac) venous system. These veins originate on the anterolateral surface of the right ventricle and drain directly into the right atrium. In addition, there are also thebesian veins that drain directly into the cardiac chambers. They are more common on the interventricular and interauricular septum, particularly on the right side of the heart, but prominent thebesian veins are occasionally seen entering the LV. Other variable features of the coronary venous anatomy include the presence of ostial valves of the cardiac veins (Vieussens valves).

Knowledge of cardiac venous structures is becoming increasingly important in the field of cardiac electrophysiology to properly place mapping catheters and LV pacing leads. Coronary sinus pacing leads are usually positioned in the lateral and posterior branches, which are quite variable

Table 16.2 Myocardial regions associated with epicardial coronary arteries

Region	Coronary artery most likely associated
Inferior	Right coronary artery or distal circumflex
Anteroseptal	Left anterior descending
Anteroapical	Distal left anterior descending
Anterolateral	Diagonal branches of left anterior descending or obtuse marginal arteries

in their number, tortuosity, dimensions, and angulation with respect to the main trunk of the atrioventricular venous ring.[35]

VARIATIONS IN CORONARY ANATOMY

Although there is considerable heterogeneity in coronary anatomy among individuals, there is greater consistency in the regions of the heart generally supplied by the different coronary arteries (Table 16.2). This anatomic distribution is important because these cardiac regions are assessed by 12-lead electrocardiograms to help localize ischemic or infarcted segments of the myocardium. This, in turn, can be loosely associated with specific coronary vessels, but because of vessel heterogeneity, the specific vessel involvement requires verification by coronary angiography or other imaging techniques.

Embryology of the coronary arteries

Although a detailed description of the formation of the coronary vasculature is beyond the scope of this chapter, some fundamental principles are important for understanding variations in coronary anatomy and coronary anomalies. During the earliest stages of cardiogenesis, the heart is formed as an endothelial tube within a muscular tube. The lateral plate mesoderm is the source of both the endothelium and the muscle layers, and these are the only two cardiac cell types generated. Anteriorly, in the region that will eventually become the ventricles, myogenic cells proliferate and form extensive trabeculae. However, in posterior regions, extensive trabeculations are not formed by proliferating myocytes, and this region eventually becomes the atria. By the end of the first 24 days in humans, the heart has an endocardium and a myocardium but lacks an epicardium, and there are no rudimentary blood vessels.[36]

All the cells that form the coronary vascular system come from outside the heart and then differentiate into blood vessels only when they are within the heart. All of this occurs without interaction with the blood coursing through the primitive heart lumen.[37] Three major anatomic components are important in the development of the coronary arteries.[14,37] First, the myocardial sinusoids are an elongation of the trabeculae into the primitive, loosely packed myocardium and thus communicate with the heart cavities. These sinusoids are the earliest sites of metabolic exchange nourishing the developing myocardium. As the myocardium becomes more compact, the sinusoids disappear, but persistence of these sinusoids may lead to coronary artery-cameral fistulaes. Second, a separate *in situ* vascular network begins to develop. This primitive network of arteries, veins, and capillaries may have connections with other mediastinal vessels, which can be a source for coronary artery fistulae. Third, as the coronary artery system evolves, endothelial buds arise from the base of the truncus arteriosus as septation is occurring. It is still unclear if there are initially only two buds or six buds, one from each potential cusp of the aortic and pulmonary sinuses with later involution of all but two buds. These buds grow and, after septation is complete, fuse with the developing *in situ* coronary vessels to form the coronary artery system (Figure 16.8).

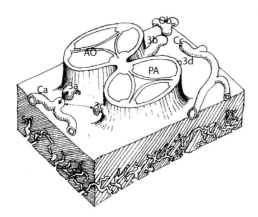

Figure 16.8 Basic components involved in the embryogenesis of coronary arteries. Aorta (AO) and pulmonary (PA) trunks are shown at completion of septation; coronary buds (3a, 3b, 3c, 3d) emerge from semilunar sinuses. Rudiments of right (Ca), circumflex (Cb), and left anterior descending (Cc), coronary arteries are shown as isolated *in situ* vascular networks. At this stage sinusoids (Sn) are site of metabolic exchanges between intracavitary blood and cardiac jelly. (From Angelini, P., *Am. Heart J.*, 117(2), 418–434, 1989. With permission.)

Variations in coronary anatomy of minimal clinical significance

RIGHT CORONARY ARTERY

Normally, there are two main coronary ostia but several common variations may occur. In 30% to 50% of angiograms, the conus branch of the RCA arises separately from the right sinus rather than its usual position as a branch of the proximal RCA.[14,22] Two right conus branches have also been reported. A separate conus branch usually has an ostial diameter varying from 0.5 to 1.9 mm and may give rise to preventricular and ventricular branches, which nourish more than just the infundibular myocardium of the outflow tract. In patients with occlusion of the LAD or RCA, the conus artery often serves as a principal source of collateral circulation. In such patients, it is important to visualize the conus artery well to adequately visualize the collateralized vessels.[38]

The location of the RCA ostium is more variable than the left ostium. This variability makes it difficult to define the exact normal location, but an origin below the aortic ring is definitely "low," and more than 1 cm above the sinotubular ridge is definitely a "high" takeoff. A high origin of the RCA is generally thought to be of no clinical consequence, but sudden death was reported in an amateur athlete with a high origin of the RCA plus small, hypoplastic right and LCx arteries.[39] Furthermore, instead of the usual location in the middle of the sinus, the RCA ostium can be located closer to the aortic valve commissures. This causes a slight alteration in the usual course of the vessel but has no other clinical significance. The RCA may arise from the posterior (noncoronary) sinus, but this is a rare anomaly, which has never been associated with symptoms or complications.[40] Finally, a RCA arising from the mid-segment of the LAD has been described and presumed not to cause ischemic complications.[41]

LEFT CORONARY ARTERY

The left coronary orifice usually arises from the center of the left sinus of Valsalva just above the free margin of the aortic valve leaflet. Malposition of the left coronary ostium either high or low in the sinus or near the aortic valve commissures occurs less often compared with the RCA but should be suspected when standard angiographic catheters or manipulations fail to cannulate the artery. Similar to a high origin of the RCA, a high takeoff of the left main is not generally felt to have any clinical significance, but there is one older report showing morphologic evidence of chronic ischemia and LV scarring in a patient with a high takeoff of the left main.[42] A very high origin of the left main should be noted if cardiac surgery is planned so as to avoid accidentally cross-clamping or transecting the vessel during surgery. Similar to the RCA, the origin of the left coronary has been rarely observed from the noncoronary cusp but has never been associated with symptoms or complications in this location.[40]

The left coronary ostium is usually single and is the origin of the left main coronary artery. The most frequent minor variation observed is absence of the left coronary, which results in the LAD and LCx arising directly from the aortic root as separate vessels. The vessels are otherwise normal in their respective distributions. The incidence of truly separate ostia varies from 0.5% to 8% in otherwise normal hearts.[43] Variation in the occurrence of this finding in the literature is, in part, related to the absence of a consistent definition for this entity. If defined as two separate ostia from the aorta, the incidence is probably less than 1%. However, if it is defined simply as the absence of a proper left main trunk, the incidence is higher. Rather than two distinctly separate vessels, the more common observation is a single ostium, shared by the origins of the LAD and LCx.

Variation in coronary size

Various techniques have been used to determine the size of normal coronary arteries. Size measurements from autopsy specimens do not correlate well with measurements made *in vivo*.[44] Some of this discrepancy is due to the techniques used for fixation of the autopsy specimens.[45] Moreover, since atherosclerosis is a diffuse process, it can sometimes be difficult for angiography to distinguish a diffusely diseased segment from one that is just normally small in diameter. Coronary artery diameters at multiple locations were determined in carefully selected normal coronary arteries using computer-based quantitative measurements (Table 16.3).[46] Using these and other measurements,[47] the size of specific normal coronary segments can be estimated, but the wide standard deviation makes application of these to an individual patient difficult. Nevertheless, some associations are noted. For example, the RCA or LCx is significantly larger when it is the dominant vessel, but the PDA is similar in size whether it arises from the RCA or LCx. Furthermore, coronary arterial diameter in women is about 9% ± 8% smaller than in men, even after normalization for body surface area. The smaller

arterial size of the left main and proximal LAD in women was confirmed in a more recent study using intravascular ultrasound.[48] Other studies have shown a good correlation between the lumen area of a coronary artery along its length and the corresponding summed distal branch lengths and regional myocardial mass in patients with and without coronary disease; thus, the greater amount of distal territory supplied, the larger is the caliber of the artery lumen.[49]

ABSENT CIRCUMFLEX OR RCA

At the extreme of variations in coronary size are the rare anomalies of an absent LCx or RCA. With an absent LCx, the RCA is a very large vessel (superdominant), which crosses the crux and ascends in the atrioventricular groove on the left to supply the posterior and lateral myocardium. With an absent RCA, the LCx continues in the atrioventricular groove in the course typical of the normal RCA.[50] The LAD is usually normal in its size and distribution. Neither of these anomalies appears to be of clinical significance in the absence of coronary artery disease.

Variations in the course of coronary arteries

MYOCARDIAL BRIDGING

One of the most common variations in the course of a coronary artery occurs when a segment of the epicardial artery dips into the myocardium, resulting in the overlying myocardium compressing the artery during systole.[51] The muscle overlying the intramyocardial segment is called a myocardial bridge and the artery coursing through the myocardium is called a tunneled artery. The most frequent site of bridging is the mid-segment of the LAD. A typical muscular bridge in this segment is 10–20 mm long and 2–4 mm thick, but segments up to 50 mm in length have been observed. Muscular bridges may exist over diagonal

Table 16.3 Diameter measurements of the major epicardial coronary arteries in normal men

Location	Right dominant (mm)	Left dominant (mm)
Left main Midway between ostium and bifurcation	4.5 ± 0.5	4.6 ± 0.4
LAD (first segment) Midway between its origin and first septal	3.6 ± 0.5	3.7 ± 0.2
LAD (third segment) Midway between the third septal and apex	1.7 ± 0.5	2.0 ± 0.3
LCx (first segment) Midway between its origin and the first marginal	3.4 ± 0.5	4.2 ± 0.6
LCx (third segment) Midway between the first marginal and most distal marginal	1.6 ± 0.6	3.2 ± 0.5
RCA (first segment) Midway between its origin and the first acute marginal	3.9 ± 0.6	2.8 ± 0.5
RCA (third segment) Midway between the third acute marginal (if present) and posterior descending	3.1 ± 0.5	1.1 ± 0.4

Source: Adapted from Dodge, J.T., Jr, et al., *Circulation*, 86(1), 232–246, 1992.
Note: LAD, left anterior descending; LCx, left circumflex artery; RCA, right coronary artery.

arteries, the left main, LCx, marginal branches, and the RCA. Angiographic studies show a prevalence of bridging varying from 0.5% to 7.5% of studies, whereas autopsy studies show a prevalence as high as 60% in the LAD and 6% to 50% in other vessels.[52,53] Factors such as the length of the tunneled segment, the degree of systolic compression, and the heart rate have all been postulated to explain the difference between angiographic and autopsy studies. In addition, for systolic narrowing to occur, the external muscular compressive force must exceed the arterial pressure and the intrinsic arterial wall stiffness. During angiography, the increased intraluminal pressure related to the contrast injection may diminish the appearance of systolic compression and thus the appreciation of a myocardial bridge. Anatomic variation in bridges also exists. Arteries located in the atrioventricular groove (proximal RCA and LCx) may be surrounded by scattered muscular fibers continuous with the atrial myocardium and may have systolic compression, but these are referred to as myocardial loops rather than classic myocardial bridges. Also, arteries such as an obtuse marginal branch or ramus located over the free wall of the LV may dive into the myocardium and not resurface.

Myocardial bridges and tunneled arteries have long been recognized clinically and are usually felt to be a benign incidental finding as the majority of coronary flow in the left coronary occurs during diastole when there is no compression.[51,54] However, there are case reports describing typical angina with anterior wall ischemia during tachycardia, myocardial perfusion defects, acute myocardial infarction, abnormal ventricular repolarization, and sudden cardiac death attributed to myocardial bridges.[55–58] More elegant studies using intravascular ultrasound and Doppler flow velocity have documented altered intracoronary hemodynamics in both symptomatic and asymptomatic patients with myocardial bridging in the mid-portion of the LAD.[59,60] In symptomatic patients, treatment by either stent placement or surgical transsection of the muscle bridge has relieved both symptoms and objective findings of myocardial ischemia.[60,61] Several anatomic studies have reported a "protective" effect of myocardial bridging on the development of atherosclerosis. The mechanism of this effect is unknown but is postulated to be from a reduction in systolic wall stress in the tunneled segment. In humans, myocardial bridges may slightly increase the occurrence of proximal atherosclerosis while protecting the bridged segment and the distal artery. Careful autopsy studies have shown that when myocardial bridging is present, intimal thickening and macroscopic raised atherosclerotic plaques are increased just proximal to the bridge.[62]

CROSSING EPICARDIAL CORONARY ARTERIES

Rarely, two coronary artery branches may cross over each other on the epicardial surface. The true incidence of this minor variation in coronary anatomy is unknown, and it is not believed to have any functional significance.[63] Crossing of two right ventricular branches, an acute marginal branch of the RCA with the RCA in the atrioventricular groove, a

diagonal and circumflex marginal branch, two obtuse marginal branches of the circumflex, and the LAD and a diagonal have all been reported.

INTERCORONARY CONTINUITY

Intercoronary artery continuity or "coronary arcade" is a rare variant of the coronary circulation. The true incidence is unknown, but in one report it was seen in 0.02% of nearly 10,000 coronary angiograms.[64] Arterial continuities exist in other areas, such as the superficial volar arch in the hand, intestinal branches of the superior mesenteric artery, and the circle of Willis. Communications between the distal LCx and the distal RCA in the posterior atrioventricular groove and between the LAD and PDA in the distal interventricular groove have both been observed (Figure 16.9). These connections occur in the absence of obstructive coronary disease and are pathologically distinct from coronary collaterals.[65] Compared with collaterals, these connections have a well-defined muscular layer, are larger in diameter (>1 mm), and are extramural.

SMALL CORONARY ARTERY FISTULAS

A coronary artery fistula is an abnormal communication between an epicardial coronary artery and a cardiac chamber, major vessel, or other vascular structure. Small coronary artery fistulas occur in 0.1%–0.2% of patients undergoing coronary angiography and usually drain into a single cardiac structure.[66] One of the most commonly observed small fistulas in adults is a communication between the LAD and the main pulmonary artery. Small fistulas are usually not associated with continuous murmurs or detectable intracardiac shunts and have a benign course. A few

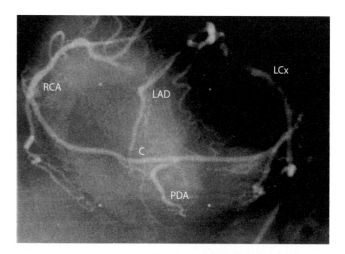

Figure 16.9 Coronary angiogram of the right coronary artery in a left anterior oblique view with cranial angulation. The catheter is in the right coronary artery and a forceful injection used to visualize the entire coronary circulation with reflux of contrast into the aorta. LAD, left anterior descending artery LCx, left circumflex artery; PDA, posterior descending artery; RCA, right coronary artery. (From Carangal, V.P., and Dehmer, G.J., *Clin. Cardiol.*, 23(2), 125–126, 2003. With permission.)

patients have undergone serial angiographic studies demonstrating no increase in fistula size over time and patients have been followed for up to 11 years without complications attributable to their fistula.[67] The detection of small fistulas in the elderly confirms their benign nature. The majority of coronary fistulas are congenital and arise from two defects in coronary artery embryogenesis. Fistulas can arise from failure of the embryonal intramyocardial sinusoids to obliterate, resulting in a gradual enlargement of one of these channels or from enlargement of a thebesian vein.[66] Alternatively, as in the case of a fistula involving the pulmonary artery, it may evolve from persistence of a vascular bud that remains attached to the pulmonary artery as it separates from the aorta early in embryogenesis. Patients with small asymptomatic fistulas require no special treatment and can simply be followed clinically. Small fistulas can also be acquired and have been reported secondary to deceleration injuries, coronary angioplasty, repeated myocardial biopsies in heart transplant patients, pacemaker leads, and after cardiac surgery.

CORONARY ARTERY ANOMALIES

The true incidence of coronary anomalies is unknown. The reported incidence varies depending on the methods used to detect the anomalies, the population assessed, and what is included as a coronary anomaly as opposed to a variant of normal. Some sources classify several of the anatomic variations described above as anomalies while other sources simply consider these to be variants of normal. In general, congenital coronary artery anomalies in the absence of other cardiac congenital anomalies have been described in approximately 1% of patients who undergo coronary angiography and approximately 0.3% of patients at autopsy (Table 16.4).[68–72]

There are several congenital syndromes associated with coronary anomalies. Patients with Williams syndrome (elfin facies, infantile hypercalcemia, hypoplastic teeth) may have coronary ostial narrowing as a component of supravalvar aortic stenosis, which is characteristic of this disease. Patients with congenital aortic valve disease commonly have variants in coronary ostial origin. Coronary anomalies may be commonly associated with other congenital cardiac malformations, most notably, transposition of the great arteries, tetralogy of Fallot, and different forms of pulmonary atresia.[73,74]

Table 16.4 Incidence of coronary anomalies detected by angiography

Authors	Patients (n)	Incidence (%)
Yamanaka and Hobbs[72]	126,595	1.3
Wilkins et al.[71]	10,661	0.78
Baltaxe and Wixson[68]	1000	0.9
Chaitman et al.[69]	3750	0.83
Engle et al.[70]	4250	1.2

Coronary anomalies not associated with ischemic complications

ORIGIN OF THE LEFT CIRCUMFLEX FROM THE RIGHT CORONARY SINUS

This anomaly is said to be the most common anomaly of coronary arterial origin in adults with an incidence of about 0.3% when assessed by coronary angiography and autopsy.[71,72] The aberrant LCx can arise from either the proximal segment of the RCA or a separate ostium near the origin of the RCA (Figure 16.10). The LAD and RCA are normal in their distribution, and the anomalous LCx invariably courses posterior to the aorta and then to its normal distribution over the lateral wall of the heart (Figure 16.11). Most patients have no other associated anomalies. This anomaly should be suspected when angiography of the left coronary shows an unusually long, nonbranching proximal segment and no obvious LCx vessel.[75] This anomaly can be missed during angiography of the RCA if the tip of the catheter is beyond the origin of the anomalous vessel and the force of the injection is inadequate to fill the aberrant LCx by the reflux of contrast. It can also be suspected if a "dot sign" is seen in a right anterior oblique left ventriculogram or supravalvular aortagram (Figure 16.12). This anomaly has traditionally been considered of little clinical significance unless the operator incorrectly assumes the LCx is occluded or an important stenosis in the aberrant artery is not visualized. However, there are a few case reports where ischemic complications have been associated with this anomaly.[76,77] Furthermore, it has been reported that the stenosis severity in this anomaly is greater than in control subjects matched for age, gender, symptoms, and degree of atherosclerosis in nonanomalous coronary arteries.[78] Compression of the anomalous LCx has been reported from the fixation rings of a prosthetic valve.[79]

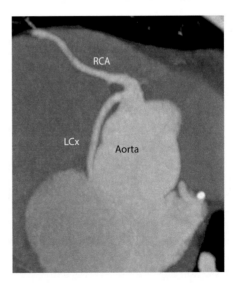

Figure 16.10 A 64-slice CT coronary angiogram of left circumflex (LCx) arising from the right coronary artery (RCA) and traversing posterior to aorta (Ao). (Courtesy of Dr. John Rumberger, Princeton Longevity Center, Princeton, NJ.)

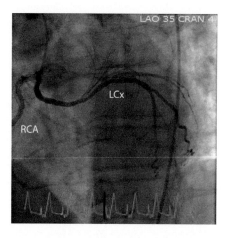

Figure 16.11 Anomalous left circumflex coronary artery. Injection of the right coronary artery (RCA) in the left anterior oblique projection slight cranial angulation shows the anomalous left circumflex (LCx) with a typical course posterior to the aorta. (Courtesy of Dr. Gregory J. Dehmer, Cardiac Catheterization Laboratory, Scott & White Medical Center, Temple, Texas.)

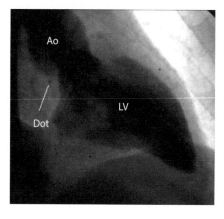

Figure 16.12 The "dot" sign is seen on a right anterior oblique left ventriculogram or supravalvular aortagram and represents the anomalous circumflex in its course posterior to the aorta. Ao, aorta; LV, left ventricle.

ORIGIN OF A CORONARY ARTERY FROM THE POSTERIOR SINUS OF VALSALVA

Either the RCA or the left main coronary artery can arise from the posterior sinus of Valsalva (the noncoronary sinus). Both of these variants are extremely rare, although the RCA from this location is said to be more frequent.[40] Origin of the left main from the posterior cusp has not been reported in the absence of other anomalies of the heart and great vessels, and the simultaneous origin of both arteries from this location has never been reported.[40,71,72]

VARIATIONS OF A SINGLE CORONARY ARTERY

There are many variations of a single coronary artery and several anatomic classifications have been proposed.[80,81]

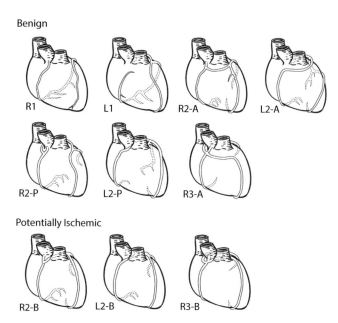

Figure 16.13 Classification of single coronary artery anomalies. In this classification, the letters "R" and "L" indicate whether the single artery arises from the right or left aortic sinus and the letters "A," "B," and "P" signify whether the "transverse" branch courses anterior, between, or posterior to the great vessels, respectively. The associated number in this classification indicates the number of major branches somewhat mimicking the right and left circumflex and left anterior descending arteries. In the diagram, the great vessels from front to back are the pulmonary artery, aorta, and superior vena cava. Those anomalies not typically associated with complications (benign) are shown on the top and those potentially associated with ischemia are on the bottom. (Adapted from Wilkins, C.E., et al., *Texas Heart Inst. J.*, 15, 166–173, 1988. With permission. Copyright 1988 by the Texas Heart Institute, Houston.)

In the classification proposed by Lipton, the letters "R" and "L" indicate whether the single artery arises from the right or left aortic sinus and the letters "A," "B," and "P" signify whether the "transverse" branch courses anterior, between, or posterior to the great vessels, respectively (Figure 16.13).[80] The associated number in this classification indicates the number of major branches somewhat mimicking the RCA, LCx, and LAD. When found in a younger age group (<20 years), a single coronary artery is frequently associated with other anomalies of the heart and great vessels, but when identified later in life, associated anomalies are infrequent.[40] From the cases reported, there is a slight male predominance (male-to-female ratio 1.4:1) with a similar frequency of arteries arising from the right or left sinuses of Valsalva. Single coronary arteries where no vessel courses between the great vessels are not usually associated with clinical complications (Figure 16.13, top). However, should coronary atherosclerosis develop in the main trunk of a single artery, the complications of atherosclerosis can be devastating.

Coronary anomalies associated with clinical complications

ORIGIN OF ONE OR MORE ARTERIES FROM THE PULMONARY TRUNK

One of the most serious congenital coronary artery anomalies is a coronary artery arising from the pulmonary artery. This frequently results in death during infancy and only a few individuals survive to adulthood.[82,83] Either the left or right coronary artery, both major coronary arteries, or rarely, the LAD or LCx may originate from the pulmonary artery. Occasionally, the conus artery may arise from the pulmonary artery. The most frequent variety of this anomaly, known as Bland-White-Garland syndrome, is origin of the left coronary from the pulmonary artery with a normal positioned RCA (Figure 16.14).[84] Children with this anomaly usually present between 8 and 16 weeks after birth, but adult presentation is occasionally seen.[85] During fetal life, systemic pressure and oxygenation in the pulmonary artery provide adequate perfusion to the LV. However, within days after birth, the pressure and oxygen content of the pulmonary artery decline so that the LV is underperfused. It is not clear why the clinical presentation is delayed for several weeks, but persistence of collaterals and a delayed fall in pulmonary artery pressure are possible explanations. If a substantial collateral circulation between the RCA and the anomalous LCA persists, survival into adulthood is possible with a left-to-right shunt from the RCA to the pulmonary artery.

In the most common infantile presentation of this anomaly, collaterals are inadequate to support the LV and the child presents with tachypnea, cough, wheezing, pallor, and cyanosis. Signs of myocardial ischemia and anterior infarction with the associated complications of aneurysm formation, mitral regurgitation, and congestive heart failure are present.[82] Angiography is frequently necessary to confirm the diagnosis. Prompt surgical therapy is indicated as survival without surgery is <20% in symptomatic infants.[86] Some reports suggest that up to 20% of patients with this anomaly may survive into adulthood and remain asymptomatic or have a late presentation with mitral regurgitation, angina, or congestive heart failure (CHF).[87] Sudden death is a complication in both infants and adults. The clinical course of the patient tends to be more favorable if extensive collateral circulation exists.

Anomalous origin to the RCA from the pulmonary artery is much less common and has fewer clinical consequences; the same is true for a conus branch arising from the pulmonary trunk. If the LAD alone arises from the pulmonary artery, the presentation in both children and adults is often similar to that of the left main in this position. Depending on the extent of collaterals, symptoms and signs of myocardial ischemia may occur in infancy or be delayed until adulthood and surgical repair is often necessary.[40] In some cases of this anomaly, only ligation of the anomalous LAD is performed, while in other cases, ligation and some form of bypass are used. Anomalous origin of the circumflex alone has been reported in children with other cardiac abnormalities, but no adults have been reported with this anomaly.[40]

ORIGIN OF BOTH RIGHT AND LEFT CORONARY ARTERIES FROM THE SAME SINUS OF VALSALVA

When either the RCA arises from the left sinus of Valsalva (Figure 16.15) or the left coronary arises from the right sinus of Valsalva (Figure 16.16), the anomalous vessel traverses the base of the heart in one of four possible paths. The anomalous vessel can pass *A*nterior to the pulmonary trunk (Type A) (Figure 16.16), *B*etween the aorta and pulmonary trunk (Type B), through the *C*rista supraventricularis (within the ventricular septum, beneath the right ventricular infundibulum) (Type C), or posterior or *D*orsal to the aorta (Type D) (Figure 16.17).[40,80] The angiographic appearance of these various courses has been well described (Figure 16.18).[88] There is now agreement that the course of an anomalous coronary

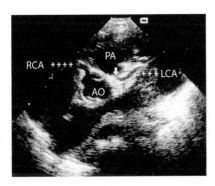

Figure 16.14 Two-dimensional echocardiographic image in a short axis view of an infant who has an anomalous origin of the left coronary artery from the pulmonary artery. The anomalous left coronary artery (LCA) can be seen arising from the pulmonary artery (PA), whereas the mildly dilated right coronary artery (RCA) arises from its normal position off the aorta (AO). (From Frommelt, P.C., and Frommelt, M.A., *Pediatr. Clin. North Am.*, 51(5), 1273–1288, 2004. With permission.)

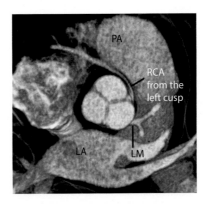

Figure 16.15 A 64-slice CT coronary angiogram of the right coronary artery (RCA) arising from the left coronary cusp and coursing posterior to the pulmonary artery (PA). LA = left atrium; LM = left main coronary artery. (Courtesy of Dr. John Rumberger, Princeton Longevity Center, Princeton, NJ.)

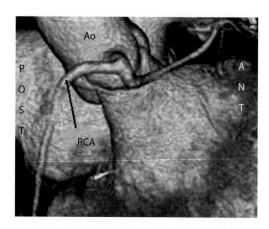

Figure 16.16 Three-dimensional 64-slice computerized tomography (CT) coronary angiogram illustrating the left main (LM) arising from the right coronary artery (RCA) and traversing anterior to the aorta (Ao) and posterior to the pulmonary artery. In this reconstructed image, the pulmonary artery has been cut away and is not shown to allow visualization of the left main. (Courtesy of Dr. John Rumberger, Princeton Longevity Center, Princeton, NJ.)

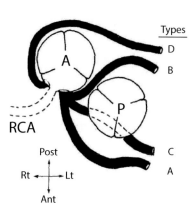

Figure 16.17 Anomalous left main coronary artery from the right sinus of Valsalva. The anomalous vessel traverses the base of the heart in one of four possible paths: *Anterior* to the pulmonary trunk (Type A), *Between* the aorta and pulmonary trunk, through the *Crista* supraventricularis (within the ventricular septum beneath the right ventricular infundibulum) (Type C), and posterior or *Dorsal* to the aorta (Type D). (Adapted from Ishikawa, T., and Brandt, P.W., *Am. J.Cardio.*, 55(6), 770–776, 1985. With permission.)

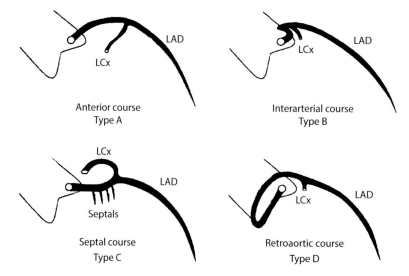

Figure 16.18 Diagrams of the angiographic appearance of an anomalous left main coronary artery arising from the right sinus of Valsalva shown in a 30° right anterior oblique projection. These illustrate the general appearance and relationship of the anomalous left main to the aorta, the left anterior descending (LAD), and the left circumflex (LCx). In the anterior course (Type A) the LCx is inferior to the left main and proximal LAD when there is no cranial angulation used. With the interarterial course (Type B), the left main may appear "on-end" as a dot as it courses around the aorta anteriorly and the LCx arises with a caudal orientation. With the course via the crista supraventricularis or septum (Type C), the LCx forms a cranial loop with respect to the left main and the proximal left main gives rise to one or more septal vessels. Finally, the retroaortic, or dorsal (Type D) course is easily identified in the projection by the caudal and posterior initial course of the anomalous left main. (Adapted from Ishikawa, T., and Brandt, P.W., *Am. J. Cardiol.*, 55(6), 770–776, 1985. With permission.)

artery, rather than the location of the coronary ostium, is a major discriminating factor for the anomaly being benign or associated with clinical complications such as angina, ventricular arrhythmias, syncope, or sudden death.[40,72] Adverse outcomes occur more frequently when the anomalous coronary artery has a course that passes between the aorta and the pulmonary artery, or less commonly via a septal pathway.

The mechanism of ischemia, infarction, or sudden death in this situation appears related to the shape of the anomalous coronary ostium rather than compression of the anomalous vessel by the aorta and pulmonary artery during systole. Normally, the coronary ostia are round to oval shaped, but in these anomalies the transverse course of the vessel to the opposite side of the heart results in an acute-angle takeoff that

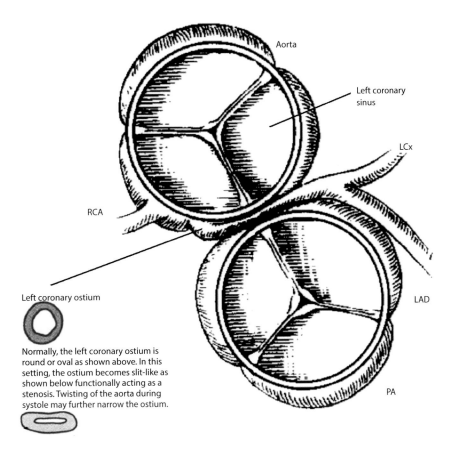

Normally, the left coronary ostium is round or oval as shown above. In this setting, the ostium becomes slit-like as shown below functionally acting as a stenosis. Twisting of the aorta during systole may further narrow the ostium.

Figure 16.19 Diagram showing the course of an anomalous left main arising from the right sinus of Valsalva. When either the right or, as in this illustration, left coronary artery arises from the opposite sinus of Valsalva and courses between the aorta and pulmonary artery (PA), the anomalous artery has an acute angle takeoff and the normal round to oval coronary ostium is converted into a slit-like shape. LAD = left anterior descending artery; LCx = left circumflex artery; RCA = right coronary artery. (Adapted from Kragel, A.H., and Roberts, W.C., *Am. J. Cardiol.*, 62(10 Pt 1), 771–777, 1988.)

converts the ostium into a slit-like shape (Figure 16.19).[89,90] Clinical events, in particular sudden death, are usually seen during exertion in young individuals in the absence of coronary atherosclerosis or other cardiac abnormalities. The increased cardiac output during exercise dilates and stretches the aortic wall, resulting in further distortion and compromise of the slit-like opening, thereby causing a transient limitation of coronary blood flow.

A left main artery arising from the right sinus of Valsalva and coursing between the aorta and pulmonary artery is the most threatening variety in this group of anomalies.[40,91] Complications have not been associated with a course of the LCA that is either behind the aorta or anterior to the pulmonary artery, but there are reports of ischemic complications when the course is through the upper septum.[40,72,92] Although there are other anatomic possibilities, a right coronary artery arising from the left sinus of Valsalva or the proximal left main almost invariably (>99%) will pass between the aorta and pulmonary artery.[72] The clinical course in these patients is variable with some having no symptoms or evidence of cardiac dysfunction and others having complications including angina, myocardial infarction, syncope, and sudden death.[93] There is some suggestion

that a familial clustering of anomalous origin of a coronary artery from the wrong aortic sinus with an intra-arterial course may exist. An additional variation of this anomaly occurs when the LAD alone arises from the right sinus of Valsalva or the proximal RCA. This is a rare anomaly and several varieties have been recognized. The anomalous LAD can course anterior to the pulmonary artery, and this is often seen in association with tetralogy of Fallot. It is important to identify this course in children undergoing repair of the tetralogy of Fallot so as to avoid damage to this branch during surgery. Although this course is usually not associated with clinical complications in adults, isolated case reports of ischemic complications exist.[94,95] Ischemic complications have also been reported to occur when the LAD courses between the aorta and pulmonary artery[96] or has a course within the interventricular septum.[97] Certain variations of a single coronary artery are quite similar to a wrong-sided coronary artery and are also associated with ischemic complications (Figure 16.13).[98]

Unfortunately, many patients with these anomalies present with sudden cardiac death, usually occurring during or immediately after intense athletic activity. In one large series of cases presenting with sudden cardiac death, and proven at autopsy to have either the left or right coronary artery arising from the wrong side and passing between the aorta and pulmonary artery, only 45% had premonitory symptoms of chest pain or syncope.[99] In those who had some type of cardiovascular test before death, all tests were within normal limits, including 12-lead electrocardiograms, stress ECG with maximal exercise, and LV wall motion and cardiac dimensions by two-dimensional echocardiography. If there is a suspicion of this anomaly, visualization of the coronary arteries by some imaging method is usually necessary.[100,101]

Coronary atresia

Atresia or hypoplasia of the left main or RCA is a rare cause of ischemia and myocardial infarction in infancy and early childhood.[102] Survival to adulthood depends on the development of adequate collateral flow from the other main coronary artery. Atresia of a coronary artery can occur as an isolated lesion or in association with other congenital diseases such as supravalvular aortic stenosis, homocystinuria, Friedreich's ataxia, Hurler's syndrome, progeria, and pulmonary atresia.[103] Successful surgical repair is possible.[104]

Large coronary artery fistulas

As described earlier, a coronary artery fistula is an abnormal micro- or macrovascular connection between a coronary artery and a cardiac chamber, vein, or another artery. Fistulas between a coronary artery and a cardiac chamber are also called *coronary-cameral fistulas*, and those between a coronary artery and vein are termed *coronary arteriovenous fistulas*. Small fistulas rarely are associated with

clinical findings or complications and are usually detected as an incidental finding on angiography.[66] Prominent thebesian veins are an example of small fistulas between a coronary artery and cardiac chamber (Figure 16.20, including Video 16.1a). About half of the patients with a coronary artery fistula are asymptomatic, but the clinical presentation in those with large fistulas depends on the type of fistula, shunt volume, site of the shunt, and presence of other cardiac conditions. Detection of a continuous murmur, dyspnea with exertion, fatigue, congestive heart failure, arrhythmias, pulmonary hypertension, infective endocarditis, or myocardial ischemia are common presentations in symptomatic patients.[66,105] Large fistulas are associated with the development of very tortuous ectatic coronary arteries proximal to the origin of the fistula. Fistulae can arise from any of the coronary arteries, but about 50% arise from the RCA, 42% from the left coronary and 5% from both arteries.[106] The most common sites for drainage of the fistulas are the coronary sinus, right atrium, or pulmonary artery, but many other locations have been reported (Figure 16.20, including Video 16.1b). Echocardiography with Doppler studies can suggest the presence of a fistula, but confirmation requires computed tomographic or invasive angiographic imaging, the latter often coupled with quantification of the shunt volume. If therapy is felt necessary, the treatment should obliterate the fistula yet maintain antegrade coronary flow.[107] Traditional coronary artery bypass or coronary reimplantation with closure of the fistula have been used, but percutaneous methods, such as catheter embolization, are now being considered as an alternative.[108,109] Multiple coronary-cameral fistulas causing myocardial ischemia have been reported in some patients.[110] In these patients, coronary angiography shows diffuse endocardial opacification and filling of the ventricular cavity.

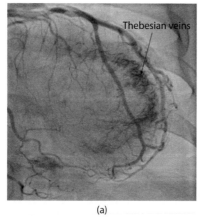

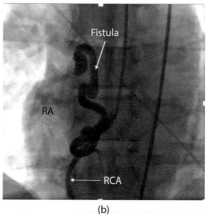

(a)

(b)

Figure 16.20 Coronary-cameral fistula. **(a)** Right anterior oblique (RAO) view showing the blush from multiple thebesian veins emptying into the left ventricle. The accompanying video shows a left anterior oblique (LAO) view of thebesian veins emptying into the left ventricle. **(b)** LAO view of a large coronary cameral fistula arising from the proximal right coronary artery (RCA) and emptying into the right atrium (RA) near the junction with the superior vena cava. The accompanying video shows the angiogram of the fistula in an LAO view and more clearly shows emptying into the RA. (Images provided by Jeffrey Schussler, M.D., Baylor Heart and Vascular Hospital, Dallas, TX, and the Cardiac Catheterization Image Archive, Mayo Clinic, Rochester, MN.)

CORONARY COLLATERAL BLOOD VESSSELS

Normal embryologic development of the coronary circulation includes the formation of collateral vessels, which connect different components of the coronary arterial circulation. In the normal adult heart, the collateral channels are small, thin-walled channels, usually less than 50 μm in diameter, that contribute little to total coronary blood flow. However, in response to coronary arterial narrowing and myocardial ischemia, these collateral channels can increase in diameter to 200–600 μm or greater, develop muscular media, and transport a substantial proportion of blood flow.[111] The enlargement of native channels is termed *vasculogenesis*, but collaterals can also develop from the growth of new vessels (angiogenesis). Limited data exist regarding the conditions required to induce collateral growth in humans. Several clinical factors, including coronary occlusion and ischemia, hypoxia, and anemia, have been identified as stimulating collateral development and evidence suggests this is mediated by the release of certain growth factors, cytokines, and proteases from activated monocytes.[112] Collateral

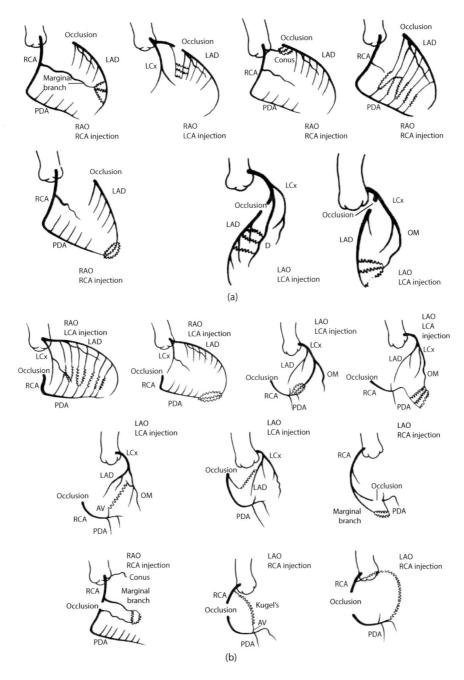

Figure 16.21 Common routes of collateral supply to the three major coronary arteries. **(a)** Collateral channels that develop with occlusion of the left anterior descending (LAD). **(b)** Collateral channels that develop with occlusion of the right coronary artery (RCA).

(Continued)

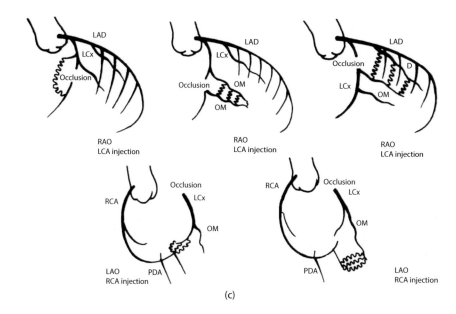

(c)

Figure 16.21 (Continued) Common routes of collateral supply to the three major coronary arteries. **(c)** Collateral channels that develop with occlusion of the left circumflex (LCx). AV, atrioventricular branch; D, diagonal branch; LAO, left anterior oblique; LCA, left coronary artery; OM, obtuse marginal; PDA, posterior descending artery; RAO, right anterior oblique. (Adapted from Levin, D.C., *Circulation*, 50(4), 831–837, 1974.)

development can occur quickly. At the time of acute coronary occlusion resulting in myocardial infarction, only 16% of patients had angiographically evident collateral vessels. Serial angiography showed that effective collaterals were present in 50% of the patients by 2 weeks and 66% of patients by 7 weeks following the infarction.[113] Functioning collaterals can maintain a coronary artery wedge pressure that averages nearly 40% of the mean aortic pressure, thereby maintaining myocardial viability.[114] The angiographic demonstration of collateral flow into the distribution of an occluded coronary artery is one of the strongest indicators on myocardial viability in the affected area.

Functional collaterals can develop between the terminal extensions of two coronary arteries, between the side branches of the two coronary arteries, between branches of the same artery, or within the same branch via the vasa vasorum. Common routes for collateral blood flow to the three main coronary arteries were elegantly defined by Levin in the early days of coronary angiography and are still relevant today (Figure 16.21).[115] Certain collaterals have been specifically identified such as Kugel's artery.[116] Although originally described as arising from the proximal LCx, most now consider a Kugel's artery as a collateral arising from either the proximal RCA, the sinus node artery, or LCx that traverses the intra-atrial septum to anastomose with the atrioventricular node artery, thus supplying the distal RCA or LCx branches. It is identified in 3%–6% of angiograms in patients with significant coronary atherosclerosis.[117] Another specifically identified collateral is a Vieussens' ring.[118] This is a collateral connection between the conus artery of the RCA and a proximal right ventricular branch of the LAD. This collateral circle provides flow to reconstitute a proximally occluded LAD or, less frequently, a proximally occluded RCA.

VIDEOS

- **Video 16.1a (https://youtu.be/1wZ5bTpO4oY)**; Thesbian veins emptying onto the left ventricle.
- **Video 16.1b (https://youtu.be/l536w00RXUg)**; Coronary-cameral fistula from the right coronary artery (RCA) emptying into the right atrium (RA).

REFERENCES

1. Furchgott RF, Zawadzki JV. The obligatory role of endothelial cells in the relaxation of arterial smooth muscle by acetylcholine. *Nature* 1980;288(5789):373–376.
2. Moncada S, Vane JR. Arachidonic acid metabolites and the interactions between platelets and blood-vessel walls. *N Engl J Med* 1979;300(20):1142–1147.
3. Galis ZS, et al. Cytokine-stimulated human vascular smooth muscle cells synthesize a complement of enzymes required for extracellular matrix digestion. *Circ Res* 1994;75(1):181–189.
4. Sato T, et al. Role of glycosaminoglycan and fibronectin in endothelial cell growth. *Exp Mol Pathol* 1987;47(2):202–210.
5. Rosenberg RD, Rosenberg JS. Natural anticoagulant mechanisms. *J Clin Invest* 1984; 74(1):1–6.
6. James TN. *Anatomy of the Coronary Arteries*. New York: P.B. Hoeber, 1961.
7. Kronzon I, et al. Length of the left main coronary artery: Its relation to the pattern of coronary arterial distribution. *Am J Cardiol* 1974;34(7):787–789.
8. Green GE, et al. The length of the left main coronary artery. *Surgery* 1967;62(6):1021–1024.
9. Virmani R, et al. Length of left main coronary artery. Lack of correlation to coronary artery dominance and bicuspid aortic valve: An autopsy study of 54 cases. *Arch Pathol Lab Med* 1984;108(8):638–641.

10. Bergelson BA, Tommaso CL. Left main coronary artery disease: Assessment, diagnosis, and therapy. *Am Heart J* 1995;129(2):350–359.

11. Levin DC, et al. Anatomic variations of the coronary arteries supplying the anterolateral aspect of the left ventricle: Possible explanation for the "unexplained" anterior aneurysm. *Invest Radiol* 1982;17(5):458–462.

12. Baptista CA, et al. Types of division of the left coronary artery and the ramus diagonalis of the human heart. *Jpn Heart J* 1991;32(3):323–335.

13. Allwork SP. The applied anatomy of the arterial blood supply to the heart in man. *J Anat* 1987;153:1–16.

14. Angelini P. Normal and anomalous coronary arteries: Definitions and classification. *Am Heart J* 1989;117(2):418–434.

15. Musselman DR, Tate DA. Left coronary dominance due to direct continuation of the left anterior descending to form the posterior descending coronary artery. *Chest* 1992;102(1):319–320.

16. Spindola-Franco H, et al. Dual left anterior descending coronary artery: Angiographic description of important variants and surgical implications. *Am Heart J* 1983;105(3):445–455.

17. Yoshikai M, et al. A very rare anatomic variation of the right ventricular branch: Right ventricular descending branch from the anterior interventricular branch. *Surg Radiol Anat* 2004;26(6):512–514.

18. Ilia R, et al. Variations in blood supply to the anterior interventricular septum: Incidence and possible clinical importance. *Cathet Cardiovasc Diagn* 1991;24(4):277–282.

19. Rath S, et al. Frequency and clinical significance of anomalous origin of septal perforator coronary artery. *Am J Cardiol* 1986;58(7):657–658.

20. Nerantzis C, Avgoustakis D. An S-shaped atrial artery supplying the sinus node area. An anatomical study. *Chest* 1980;78(2):274–278.

21. Kyriakidis MK, et al. Sinus node coronary arteries studied with angiography. *Am J Cardiol* 1983;51(5):749–750.

22. Adams J, Treasure T. Variable anatomy of the right coronary artery supply to the left ventricle. *Thorax* 1985;40(8):618–620.

23. Errichetti A, et al. Anomalous origin of the posterior descending artery from the first septal perforator. *Cathet Cardiovasc Diagn* 1986;12(6):402–404.

24. Voci P, et al. Papillary muscle perfusion pattern. A hypothesis for ischemic papillary muscle dysfunction. *Circulation* 1995;91(6):1714–1718.

25. Kuo L, et al. Coronary arteriolar myogenic response is independent of endothelium. *Circ Res* 1990;66(3):860–866.

26. Chilian WM. Coronary microcirculation in health and disease. Summary of an NHLBI workshop. *Circulation* 1997;95(2):522–528.

27. Camici PG, Crea F. Coronary microvascular dysfunction. *N Engl J Med* 2007;356(8):830–840.

28. von Lüdinghausen M. The venous drainage of the human myocardium. *Adv Anat Embryol Cell Biol* 2003;168:1–104.

29. Hood WB Jr. Regional venous drainage of the human heart. *Br Heart J* 1968;30(1):105–109.

30. Gilard M, et al. Angiographic anatomy of the coronary sinus and its tributaries. *Pacing Clin Electrophysiol* 1998;21(11 Pt 2):2280–2284.

31. Bales GS. Great cardiac vein variations. *Clin Anat* 2004;17(5):436–443.

32. Mantini E, et al. Congenital anomalies involving the coronary sinus. *Circulation* 1966;33(2):317–327.

33. Ortale JR, et al. The anatomy of the coronary sinus and its tributaries. *Surg Radiol Anat* 2001;23(1):15–21.

34. Shinbane JS, et al. Thebesian valve imaging with electron beam CT angiography: Implications for resynchronization therapy. *Pacing Clin Electrophysiol* 2004;27(11):1566–1567.

35. Singh JP, et al. The coronary venous anatomy: A segmental approach to aid cardiac resynchronization therapy. *J Am Coll Cardiol* 2005;46(1):68–74.

36. Manasek FJ. Embryonic development of the heart. I. A light and electron microscopic study of myocardial development in the early chick embryo. *J Morphol* 1968;125(3):329–365.

37. Reese DE, et al. Development of the coronary vessel system. *Circ Res* 2002;91(9):761–768.

38. Levin DC, et al. Frequency and clinical significance of failure to visualize the conus artery during coronary arteriography. *Circulation* 1981;63(4):833–837.

39. Menke DM, et al. Hypoplastic coronary arteries and high takeoff position of the right coronary ostium. A fatal combination of congenital coronary artery anomalies in an amateur athlete. *Chest* 1985;88(2):299–301.

40. Roberts WC. Major anomalies of coronary arterial origin seen in adulthood. *Am Heart J* 1986;111(5):941–963.

41. Rath S, Battler A. Anomalous origin of the right coronary artery from the left anterior descending coronary artery. *Cathet Cardiovasc Diagn* 1998;44(3):328–329.

42. Alexander RW, Griffith GC. Anomalies of the coronary arteries and their clinical significance. *Circulation* 1956;14(5):800–805.

43. Dicicco BS, et al. Separate aortic ostium of the left anterior descending and left circumflex coronary arteries from the left aortic sinus of Valsalva (absent left main coronary artery). *Am Heart J* 1982;104(1):153–154.

44. Arnett EN, et al. Coronary artery narrowing in coronary heart disease: Comparison of cineangiographic and necropsy findings. *Ann Intern Med* 1979; 91(3):350–356.

45. Siegel RJ, et al. Limitations of postmortem assessment of human coronary artery size and luminal narrowing: Differential effects of tissue fixation and processing on vessels with different degrees of atherosclerosis. *J Am Coll Cardiol* 1985;5(2 Pt 1):342–346.

46. Dodge JT Jr, et al. Lumen diameter of normal human coronary arteries. Influence of age, sex, anatomic variation, and left ventricular hypertrophy or dilation. *Circulation* 1992;86(1):232–246.

47. Vieweg WV, et al. Caliber and distribution of normal coronary arterial anatomy. *Cathet Cardiovasc Diagn* 1976;2(3):269–280.

48. Sheifer SE, et al. Sex differences in coronary artery size assessed by intravascular ultrasound. *Am Heart J* 2000;139(4):649–653.

49. Seiler C, et al. Basic structure-function relations of the epicardial coronary vascular tree. Basis of quantitative coronary arteriography for diffuse coronary artery disease. *Circulation* 1992;85(6):1987–2003.

50. Ayala F, et al. Right coronary ostium agenesis with anomalous origin of the right coronary artery from an ectatic circumflex artery. A case report. *Angiology* 1995;46(7):637–639.

51. Kramer JR, et al. Clinical significance of isolated coronary bridges: Benign and frequent condition involving the left anterior descending artery. *Am Heart J* 1982;103(2):283–288.

52. Angelini P, et al. Myocardial bridges: A review. *Prog Cardiovasc Dis* 1983;26(1):75–88.

53. Irvin RG. The angiographic prevalence of myocardial bridging in man. *Chest* 1982; 81(2):198–202.

54. Roberts WC, et al. Origin of the left main from the right coronary artery or from the right aortic sinus with intramyocardial tunneling to the left side of the heart via the ventricular septum. The case against clinical significance of myocardial bridge or coronary tunnel. *Am Heart J* 1982;104(2 Pt 1): 303–305.

55. Berry JF, et al. Systolic compression of the left anterior descending coronary artery: A case series, review of the literature, and therapeutic options including stenting. *Catheter Cardiovasc Interv* 2002;56(1):58–63.

56. Chee TP, et al. Myocardial bridging of the left anterior descending coronary artery resulting in subendocardial infarction. *Arch Intern Med* 1981;141(12):1703–1704.

57. Cutler D, Wallace JM. Myocardial bridging in a young patient with sudden death. *Clin Cardiol* 1997;20(6):581–583.

58. Faruqui AM, et al. Symptomatic myocardial bridging of coronary artery. *Am J Cardiol* 1978;41(7):1305–1310.

59. Ge J, et al. Comparison of intravascular ultrasound and angiography in the assessment of myocardial bridging. *Circulation* 1994;89(4):1725–1732.

60. Klues HG, et al. Disturbed intracoronary hemodynamics in myocardial bridging: Early normalization by intracoronary stent placement. *Circulation* 1997;96(9):2905–2913.

61. Vogt PR, et al. Images in cardiovascular medicine. Muscle bridging of the left anterior descending coronary artery. *Circulation* 1996;93(3):614.

62. Ishii T, et al. The significance of myocardial bridge upon atherosclerosis in the left anterior descending coronary artery. *J Pathol* 1986;148(4):279–291.

63. Muyldermans LL, et al. Epicardial crossing of coronary arteries: A variation of coronary arterial anatomy. *Int J Cardiol* 1985;7(4):416–419.

64. Carangal VP, Dehmer GJ. Intercoronary communication between the circumflex and right coronary arteries. *Clin Cardiol* 2000;23(2):125–126.

65. Donaldson RF, Isner JM. Intercoronary continuity: An anatomic basis for bidirectional coronary blood flow distinct from coronary collaterals. *Am J Cardiol* 1984;53(2):351–352.

66. Sapin P, et al. Coronary artery fistula: An abnormality affecting all age groups. *Medicine (Baltimore)* 1990;69(2):101–113.

67. Hobbs RE, et al. Coronary artery fistulae: A 10-year review. *Cleve Clin Q* 1982;49(4):191–197.

68. Baltaxe HA, Wixson D. The incidence of congenital anomalies of the coronary arteries in the adult population. *Radiology* 1977;122(1):47–52.

69. Chaitman BR, et al. Clinical, angiographic, and hemodynamic findings in patients with anomalous origin of the coronary arteries. *Circulation* 1976;53(1):122–131.

70. Engel HJ, et al. Major variations in anatomical origin of the coronary arteries: Angiographic observations in 4,250 patients without associated congenital heart disease. *Cathet Cardiovasc Diagn* 1975;1(2):157–169.

71. Wilkins CE, et al. Coronary artery anomalies: A review of more than 10,000 patients from the Clayton Cardiovascular Laboratories. *Tex Heart Inst J* 1988;15(3):166–173.

72. Yamanaka O, Hobbs RE. Coronary artery anomalies in 126,595 patients undergoing coronary arteriography. *Cathet Cardiovasc Diagn* 1990;21(1):28–40.

73. Hanley FL, et al. Outcomes in neonatal pulmonary atresia with intact ventricular septum. A multiinstitutional study. *J Thorac Cardiovasc Surg* 1993;105(3):406–427.

74. Sim EK, et al. Coronary artery anatomy in complete transposition of the great arteries. *Ann Thorac Surg* 1994;57(4):890–894.

75. Page HL Jr, et al. Anomalous origin of the left circumflex coronary artery. Recognition, angiographic demonstration and clinical significance. *Circulation* 1974;50:768–773.

76. Piovesana P, et al. Morbidity associated with anomalous origin of the left circumflex coronary artery from the right aortic sinus. *Am J Cardiol* 1989;63(11):762–763.

77. Rozenman Y, et al. Anomalous origin of the circumflex coronary artery from the right sinus of Valsalva as a cause of ischemia at old age. *Clin Cardiol* 1993;16(12):900–901.

78. Click RL, et al. Anomalous coronary arteries: Location, degree of atherosclerosis and effect on survival—a report from the Coronary Artery Surgery Study. *J Am Coll Cardiol* 1989;13(3):531–537.

79. Roberts WC, Morrow AG. Compression of anomalous left circumflex coronary arteries by prosthetic valve fixation rings. *J Thorac Cardiovasc Surg* 1969;57(6):834–838.

80. Lipton MJ, et al. Isolated single coronary artery: Diagnosis, angiographic classification, and clinical significance. *Radiology* 1979;130(1):39–47.

81. Ogden JA, Goodyer AV. Patterns of distribution of the single coronary artery. *Yale J Biol Med* 1970;43(1):11–21.

82. Wesselhoeft H, et al. Anomalous origin of the left coronary artery from the pulmonary trunk. Its clinical spectrum, pathology, and pathophysiology, based on a review of 140 cases with seven further cases. *Circulation* 1968;38(2):403–425.

83. Frommelt PC, Frommelt MA. Congenital coronary artery anomalies. *Pediatr Clin North Am* 2004;51(5):1273–1288.

84. Bland E, et al. Congenital anomalies of the coronary arteries: Report of an unusual case associated with cardiac hypertrophy. *Am Heart J* 1933;8(6):787–801.

85. Thomas CS Jr, et al. Complete repair of anomalous origin of the left coronary artery in the adult. *J Thorac Cardiovasc Surg* 1973;66(3):439–446.

86. Michielon G, et al. Anomalous coronary artery origin from the pulmonary artery: Correlation between surgical timing and left ventricular function recovery. *Ann Thorac Surg* 2003;76(2):581–588.

87. Kandzari DE, et al. An anomalous left coronary artery originating from the pulmonary artery in a 72-year-old woman: Diagnosis by color flow myocardial blush and coronary arteriography. *J Invasive Cardiol* 2002;14(2):96–99.

88. Ishikawa T, Brandt PW. Anomalous origin of the left main coronary artery from the right anterior aortic sinus: Angiographic definition of anomalous course. *Am J Cardiol* 1985;55(6):770–776.

89. Kragel AH, Roberts WC. Anomalous origin of either the right or left main coronary artery from the aorta with subsequent coursing between aorta and pulmonary trunk: Analysis of 32 necropsy cases. *Am J Cardiol* 1988;62(10 Pt 1):771–777.

90. Taylor AJ, et al. Sudden cardiac death associated with isolated congenital coronary artery anomalies. *J Am Coll Cardiol* 1992;20(3):640–647.

91. Barth CW III, Roberts WC. Left main coronary artery originating from the right sinus of Valsalva and coursing between the aorta and pulmonary trunk. *J Am Coll Cardiol* 1986;7(2):366–373.

92. Roberts WC, Kragel AH. Anomalous origin of either the right or left main coronary artery from the aorta without coursing of the anomalistically arising artery between aorta and pulmonary trunk. *Am J Cardiol* 1988;62(17):1263–1267.

93. Roberts WC, et al. Origin of the right coronary artery from the left sinus of Valsalva and its functional consequences: Analysis of 10 necropsy patients. *Am J Cardiol* 1982;49(4):863–868.

94. Coyle L, Thomas WJ. Anomalous left anterior descending coronary artery: Malignant hospital course of a not so benign anomaly. *Catheter Cardiovasc Interv* 2000;51(4):468–470.

95. Tuncer C, et al. Origin and distribution anomalies of the left anterior descending artery in 70,850 adult patients: Multicenter data collection. *Catheter Cardiovasc Interv* 2006;68(4):574–585.

96. Roynard JL, et al. Anomalous course of the left anterior descending coronary artery between the aorta and pulmonary trunk: A rare cause of myocardial ischaemia at rest. *Br Heart J* 1994;72(4):397–399.

97. Takenaka T, et al. Anomalous origin of the left anterior descending coronary artery from the right sinus of Valsalva associated with effort angina pectoris. *Eur Heart J* 1993;14(1):29–31.

98. Brothers JA, et al. The Congenital Heart Surgeons' Society Registry of Anomalous Aortic Origin of a Coronary Artery: An update. *Cardiol Young* 2015;25(8):1567–71.

99. Basso C, et al. Clinical profile of congenital coronary artery anomalies with origin from the wrong aortic sinus leading to sudden death in young competitive athletes. *J Am Coll Cardiol* 2000;35(6):1493–1501.

100. Angelini P, Flamm SD. Newer concepts for imaging anomalous aortic origin of the coronary arteries in adults. *Catheter Cardiovasc Interv* 2007;69(7):942–954.

101. Deibler AR, et al. Imaging of congenital coronary anomalies with multislice computed tomography. *Mayo Clin Proc* 2004;79(8):1017–1023.

102. Byrum CJ, et al. Congenital atresia of the left coronary ostium and hypoplasia of the left main coronary artery. *Am Heart J* 1980;99(3):354–358.

103. Ueda K, et al. Absence of proximal coronary arteries associated with pulmonary atresia. *Am Heart J* 1983;106(3):596–598.

104. Musiani A, et al. Left main coronary artery atresia: Literature review and therapeutical considerations. *Eur J Cardiothorac Surg* 1997;11(3):505–514.

105. Luo L, et al. Coronary artery fistulae. *Am J Med Sci* 2006;332(2):79–84.

106. Levin DC, et al. Hemodynamically significant primary anomalies of the coronary arteries. Angiographic aspects. *Circulation* 1978;58(1):25–34.

107. Rittenhouse EA, et al. Congenital coronary artery-cardiac chamber fistula. Review of operative management. *Ann Thorac Surg* 1975;20(4):468–485.

108. Perry SB, et al. Transcatheter closure of coronary artery fistulas. *J Am Coll Cardiol* 1992;20(1):205–209.

109. Urrutia SC, et al. Surgical management of 56 patients with congenital coronary artery fistulas. *Ann Thorac Surg* 1983;35(3):300–307.

110. Wolf A, Rockson SG. Myocardial ischemia and infarction due to multiple coronary-cameral fistulae: Two case reports and review of the literature. *Cathet Cardiovasc Diagn* 1998;43(2):179–183.

111. Gregg DE, Patterson RE. Functional importance of the coronary collaterals. *N Engl J Med* 1980;303(24):1404–1406.

112. Lazarous DF, et al. Effects of chronic systemic administration of basic fibroblast growth factor on collateral development in the canine heart. *Circulation* 1995;91(1):145–153.

113. Schwartz H, et al. Temporal evolution of the human coronary collateral circulation after myocardial infarction. *J Am Coll Cardiol* 1984;4(6):1088–1093.

114. Seiler C, et al. Coronary collateral quantitation in patients with coronary artery disease using intravascular flow velocity or pressure measurements. *J Am Coll Cardiol* 1998;32(5):1272–1279.

115. Levin DC. Pathways and functional significance of the coronary collateral circulation. *Circulation* 1974;50(4):831–837.

116. Kugel M. Anatomical studies on the coronary arteries and their branches. I. Arteria anastomotica auricularis magna. *Am Heart J* 1927;3(3):260–270.

117. Grollman JH Jr, Heger L. Angiographic anatomy of the left Kugel's artery. *Cathet Cardiovasc Diagn* 1978;4(2):127–133.

118. O'Leary EL, et al. Images in cardiovascular medicine. Vieussens' ring. *Circulation* 1998;98(5):487–488.

17

Diagnostic angiographic catheters: Coronary and vascular

MICHAEL J. LIM

INTRODUCTION

The fundamental aspect of performing an angiogram requires the use of a catheter—a hollow tube that comes in various shapes that can be manipulated to an appropriate place; a center lumen allows fluid to be injected (i.e., contrast) or pressures to be measured. Over the past 50 years, very little change has occurred in the design of diagnostic catheters, leaving most operators to focus on the shapes and sizes rather than the design and specifications of a particular catheter. This chapter attempts to provide a practical guide to many of the most important "workhorse" catheters that are in use today. It is not intended to provide an exhaustive list of all available catheters but discusses the principal catheters utilized in the fields of coronary angiography, ventriculography, and peripheral angiography.

HISTORY OF SELECTIVE ANGIOGRAPHIC CATHETERS

Mason Sones conducted the first diagnostic coronary angiogram in 1958. He later developed a standard technique from a brachial cutdown approach with the design of his own catheters. Sones helped to develop a single catheter with a stiff body that would allow for torquability. A tapered tip allowed the catheter to be manipulated against the aortic cusps to take a primary curve in order to engage the coronary ostia. This tapered tip also prevented the tip of the catheter from completely obstructing the coronary ostia. This is known as the Sones catheter and the technique for engaging the coronary ostia through a brachial cutdown is known as the Sones technique.

The next major milestone in coronary catheter design came from Melvin Judkins, who developed pre-shaped, selective coronary catheters based on chest radiographs. These catheters are now known as the Judkins left and right catheters, and his technique of inserting these catheters from a percutaneous femoral approach is known as the Judkins technique. With the influence of pioneers like Sones and Judkins, the percutaneous approach and standardized preformed catheters are now the standard for both femoral and arm (radial and brachial) access for coronary and peripheral angiography.

GENERAL DIAGNOSTIC CATHETER DESIGN

Modern vascular diagnostic catheters are typically polymer-blended catheters made of nylon, polyurethane, or other proprietary polymers. These polymer catheters are reinforced with braided steel that promotes torque transmission from the distal end to the catheter tip. The tip of the catheter is usually tapered with a nonbraided polymer, which allows for increased flexibility and less trauma when being manipulated into a vessel ostium (Figure 17.1). Some catheters may incorporate a radiopaque tip for maximal visualization. The standard selective diagnostic coronary catheters are 100 cm in length and range in diameters from 4- to 6-Fr. While larger catheter sizes can deliver larger volumes and increased flow rates of contrast, allowing for better visualization of the selected vessel, smaller catheters are less traumatic to the selected vessel and allow for smaller percutaneous entry sheaths. Standard selective peripheral arterial catheters are similar in construction but they come in smaller lengths as well. Most diagnostic catheters are rated to accept a maximum of 1,200 pounds per square inch (psi) of contrast injection.

CATHETERS TYPICALLY USED FOR CARDIAC CATHETERIZATION FROM THE FEMORAL APPROACH

Left coronary catheters

More than two-thirds of the mortality risk associated with diagnostic coronary catheterization is related to trauma of the left main coronary artery.[1] Therefore, proper diagnostic catheter selection and proper engagement of the left main coronary artery are of critical importance. The most common coronary diagnostic catheter used to engage the ostium of the left main is the Judkins left coronary catheter. It is an endhole catheter with a 90° primary curve that allows the tip to enter the coronary ostium and a 180° secondary curve that allows backup support from the opposing wall of the aorta. Depending on the manufacturer, it might go by different brand names or abbreviations, but it is usually abbreviated as "JL" for Judkins left. The length of the segment between the primary and secondary curve is denoted by the number, so the "4" in JL4 means that there is 4 cm in length between the primary and secondary curves. The Judkins left catheter comes typically in sizes ranging from 3.5 to 6 cm (Figure 17.2). Bigger sizes are needed for bigger patients with dilatation of the aortic arch.

JL catheters are the most commonly used because very little manipulation is needed to engage most left main arteries. Generally, the catheter is advanced under fluoroscopy to the ascending aorta over a wire. After the wire is removed, the catheter will tend to move cranially and leftward to engage the left main artery. The left main can be engaged usually with only a slight advancement of the catheter forward at the introducer sheath, seen as a "pop" of the catheter into the left main while watching on fluoroscopy. Rarely, the left main can be out of plane either anteriorly or

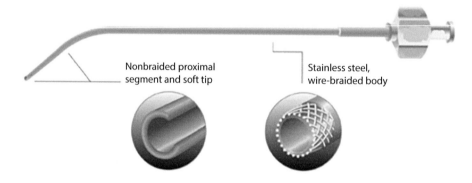

Figure 17.1 Catheters are created out of polymer and reinforced with braided steel that allows torque transmission. The tip of the catheter is usually tapered with a nonbraided polymer, which allows for increased flexibility and less trauma.

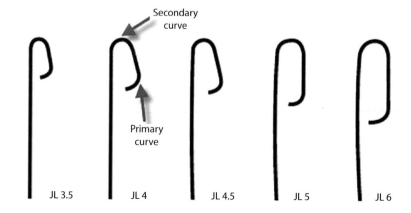

Figure 17.2 Judkins left coronary catheters in common sizes.

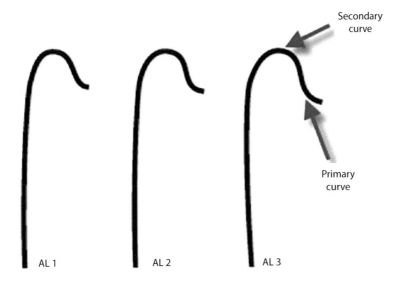

Figure 17.3 Amplatz left catheters in typical sizes reflective of the diameter of their secondary curve.

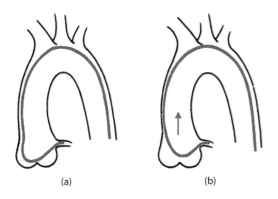

Figure 17.4 Technique for cannulating the coronary arteries utilizing the Amplatz left catheter. **(a)** The catheter is advanced until the secondary curve rests in the noncoronary or posterior aortic cusp and its tip is pointing toward the left coronary artery. **(b)** The catheter is then gently advanced and retracted until the ostium of the coronary is engaged. (Modified from Schoonmaker, F.W., King, S.B., *Circulation.*, 50(4), 735–740, 1974.)

posteriorly, and then either a slight clockwise or counterclockwise torque, respectively, may be used to engage the artery. Another common problem is choosing the wrong initial size of the Judkins left catheter.

When the left main cannot be cannulated with a Judkins curve, other catheter shapes must be considered to allow for a successful and safe procedure. This situation can occur when the left main orifice is too high, too out of plane anteriorly or posteriorly, or there is a very short left main where selective injection of the left anterior descending (LAD) and left circumflex are needed (Figure 17.3). In these cases, a more torquable catheter, such as the Amplatz left catheter, invented by Kurt Amplatz, can be used. The most common sizes of the Amplatz left diagnostic catheters are the AL1, AL2, and AL3. They are sized based on the diameter of their secondary curve (Figure 17.4). The larger-sized Amplatz catheters have more "reach" to engage more superior takeoffs of coronary ostia.

Typically the AL2 is used as the standard size to engage the left main coronary ostia, but higher or more superior directed left main ostia require longer catheters.

The Amplatz left catheters require slightly more manipulation, with subsequent increased risk for coronary dissection for engagement and disengagement than the standard Judkins left catheters, making them secondary choices for engaging the left main. They are inserted into the ascending aorta in standard fashion over a wire. When the wire is removed, often the catheter will be pointed with its tip down to the aortic valve. If the tip is tilted toward the right cusp, then the catheter must be rotated so that the tip looks toward the left cusp. The catheter must then be advanced so that the secondary curve is sitting on the aortic valve with the tip climbing up the aortic wall and now pointing slightly upward. At this point, the catheter can now be torqued either clockwise or counterclockwise (tip anterior or posterior) to engage the ostium of the left main (Figure 17.5).

There are various methods to disengage an Amplatz left diagnostic catheter. Commonly, it is said that once the Amplatz left catheter is engaged in the left main, pushing the catheter will advance the front of the secondary curve against the aortic wall, thereby backing out the tip of the catheter. In contrast, it is commonly described that pulling the catheter will force the tip of the catheter deeper into the left main, which will increase the risk of catheter dissection. Depending on how the secondary curve of the catheter is sitting on the aortic root or how deeply the tip is engaged, then this "withdrawal paradox" may not always occur.

Right coronary catheters

The most commonly used diagnostic right coronary catheter is the Judkins right catheter. Its primary curve is a 90° bend to allow the catheter to enter the right coronary ostium. The secondary bend is a gradual 30° bend. Depending on the manufacturer, it might go by different brand names

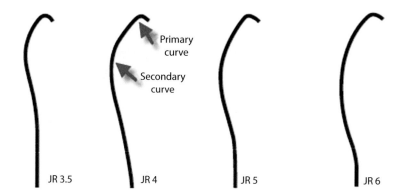

Figure 17.5 Judkins right catheters in typically available sizes.

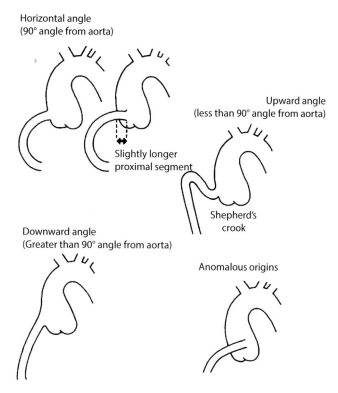

Figure 17.6 Typical variations that may be found in the origination and proximal course of the right coronary artery. (Modified from Myler, R.K., et al., *Catheter. Cardiovasc. Diag.*, 19(1), 58–67, 1990. With permission.)

or abbreviations, but it is usually abbreviated as "JR" for Judkins right, followed by the length of the distance between the primary and secondary curves. For example, for most typical adults, a JR4 catheter is used to engage the right coronary artery. The Judkins right catheter comes typically in sizes ranging from 3.5 to 6 cm (Figure 17.6). Bigger sizes (i.e., JR5 or JR6A) are needed for patients with larger or dilated ascending aortas. Unlike the Judkins left catheter, the Judkins right catheter requires more manipulation in order for it to engage the coronary ostium. The standard approach involves inserting the catheter so that it rests on the cusps of the aortic valve. The tip of the catheter starts facing toward the right of the viewing monitor (toward the

patient's left). The catheter is then pulled up to the level where it is assumed the right coronary comes off (usually a centimeter or two above the right coronary cusp), while torque in a clockwise direction is simultaneously applied to spin the tip so it slowly looks toward the left of the screen and engages the ostium of the right coronary artery. Sometimes, it will not be possible to engage from the level of the ostium, as the ostium lies right below the sinotubular junction. In some patients, the sinotubular junction of the aorta is more pronounced and acts as a ridge that deflects the catheter tip away from the ostium. An alternative approach can be taken by starting with the catheter slightly above the level of the right coronary ostium, and the catheter is clockwise torqued while simultaneously advanced downward toward the aortic valve.

In some patients, the JR4 catheter might not torque adequately with clockwise rotation. In these cases, the catheter is first torqued counterclockwise to see if that resolves the problem. It is important to avoid vigorous torquing of the catheter, as this can lead to kinking of the catheter. This will be recognized by a sudden dampening of the arterial pressure waveform, despite little movement of the catheter itself. If the JR4 catheter cannot engage the right coronary artery, then the operator must consider looking for the origin of the vessel in an anterior, posterior, or superior position, and/or consider changing to an alternative catheter. A typical second-choice catheter for use in right coronary artery cannulation is the "no-torque" right catheter, also known as a Williams right or a 3DRC catheter. This was a catheter that was designed to engage the right coronary ostium without any significant manipulation, unlike the JR4. It has a third curve out of plane of the primary and secondary curves of the usual JR4 that gives it a three-dimensional (3D) shape and allows it to engage the right coronary ostium without significant torque.

In some patients, the right coronary ostium has an alternative anatomic takeoff compared to the usual orthogonal takeoff at the level of the free margin of the aortic cusp.[2] Common variants include a superior takeoff that mimics the shape of the head of a shepherd's crook, or orthogonal takeoffs from a more anterior position of the aortic wall (Figure 17.7). In the case of a shepherd's crook origin, a catheter that has a tip that

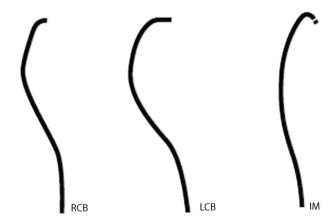

Figure 17.7 Catheters frequently used for cannulation of bypass grafts. IM, internal mammary; LCB, left coronary bypass; RCB, right coronary bypass.

looks superior is necessary. One example of this is an internal mammary artery (IMA) catheter. The internal mammary (IM) catheter is a modified JR4 with an 80° primary curve and a longer distal tip. This 10° difference in angle between the JR4 allows for a slight superior engagement. For a more superior angled takeoff, a hockey stick catheter or the El Gamal catheter (longer tip than the hockey stick) can be tried. Its primary curve can vary but typically is 75°, allowing engagement of a more superior takeoff.

For a more anterior takeoff of the right coronary ostium, initial catheter choice can be a Williams right catheter as described above. If the takeoff has a more significant anterior and superior takeoff, then an Amplatz right modified catheter can be tried. It resembles the duckbill shape of the Amplatz left catheter, but it has a much smaller secondary curve diameter. If more you need more reach for an even higher and more anterior takeoff of the right coronary artery, then an Amplatz left catheter will be needed.

BYPASS GRAFT CATHETERS

Common grafts that need to be engaged include the left internal mammary artery (LIMA), the right internal mammary artery (RIMA), free radial or saphenous vein grafts (SVGs) off of the anterior aorta that can course to any of the major epicardial vessels, or rarely, a gastroepiploic artery. Typically, the JR4 catheter is utilized as the "work-horse" in angiography of grafts. While the JR4 can commonly engage most of the free grafts off of the anterior aorta going to the left-sided epicardial vessels, it may not provide engagement of the usually inferior directed takeoff of a graft to the right coronary artery. Also, the angle of the tip is sometimes not acute enough to selectively engage the ostium of the left and right internal thoracic arteries. In the cases where selective engagement of the grafts cannot be accomplished with a JR4, then specialty diagnostic catheters must be used.

Free grafts to the distal right coronary artery, or patent ductus arteriosus (PDA), tend to have an inferior takeoff coming from the right and anterior wall of the ascending

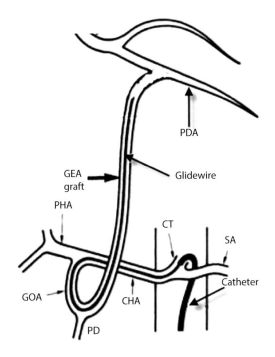

Figure 17.8 Selective engagement of the GEA. First, a diagnostic catheter is used to engage the CT. An exchange length angled Glidewire is then used to advance to the distal GEA graft. From here (not pictured), the original diagnostic catheter can be walked out and exchanged for a long glide catheter. The other branches of the CT depicted are the SA, CHA, GDA, PHA, and the PD. CHA, common hepatic artery; CT, celiac trunk; GDA, gastroduodenal artery; GEA, gastroepiploic artery; PD, pancreatoduodenal artery; PDA, posterior descending artery; PHA, proper hepatic artery; SA, splenic artery. (Adapted from Isshiki T, Yamaguchi T, Tamura T, et al. *J Am Coll Cardiol*, 1993; 22:727–732. With permission.)

aorta. Most frequently, a multipurpose catheter is the first choice for engaging this graft. It is brought over a wire with the image intensifier in the left anterior oblique (LAO) 30° position. The catheter begins with its tip high in the ascending aorta and is then turned so its tip faces the aortic wall to the left of the viewing screen (right of the patient). The tip of the catheter then slowly is advanced downward while applying torque until it is seen or felt to fall into the right-sided graft. The multipurpose catheter tends to work best in grafts that come off with a significant downward takeoff. For more subtle inferior takeoffs, an Amplatz right modified catheter or a right coronary bypass (RCB) catheter can be helpful (Figure 17.8). The RCB resembles a JR4 with a tip curved greater than 90° so that when it comes up and around the aorta, the tip of the catheter points slightly inferiorly.

For grafts to the LAD or left circumflex arteries or their branches, a JR4 catheter is the first choice catheter and will typically engage selectively. These grafts come off above the left main ostium, with the LAD grafts typically in the lowest position followed by the diagonal grafts and then left circumflex grafts most superior. In the cases where the grafts are coming off with a more upward takeoff, then the second choice is a left coronary bypass (LCB) catheter. The primary curve is 90° like a JR4, but the secondary curve is 70° (as compared to the gentle 30° secondary curve of the JR4), which gives the catheter more reach to the left side of the aorta, as well as a slightly superior oriented tip of the catheter (Figure 17.8). For grafts that cannot be engaged with a JR4 or LCB catheter, then manipulation of a Amplatz left 2 or 3, or multipurpose catheter frequently achieves the ability to selectively engage and image the vessel.

For engaging the IMAs, again a JR4 can be tried for initial engagement, as these will often selectively engage both the RIMA and LIMA and can save a step of catheter exchange. To manipulate the JR4 to the right subclavian, the catheter is pulled back to the top of the ascending aorta in the LAO 30° view, which lays out the aorta without foreshortening or the branch vessels. In this view, the tip of the JR4 is usually pointed caudally; it is then rotated 180° to point in a cranial direction while the catheter is then pulled back slightly to engage the takeoff of the right subclavian artery. It is important to adjust the torque of the catheter as it is being pulled back to always keep the tip of the catheter pointed directly cranial. The catheter tip will otherwise have a natural tendency to torque out of plane, resulting in the catheter being pulled back into the descending aorta without engagement of the arch vessels. Once the catheter is seen to jump into the brachiocephalic trunk, a test injection is given to confirm the location and to get an idea of the takeoff of the RIMA. The catheter tip can be manipulated to point more toward the right subclavian as compared to the right carotid. A J-wire is then placed deep into the right subclavian and the JR4 can be advanced to the midportion of the right subclavian, at least 1–2 cm distal to where the suspected takeoff of the RIMA is located. With frequent test injections, the JR4 is slowly pulled back and torqued as needed to engage the RIMA. If the angle of takeoff is steeper than can be engaged by the JR4, then an exchange length guidewire is needed to exchange the JR4 for the internal mammary diagnostic catheter. The 80° primary curve on the tip of the internal mammary catheter as compared to the 90° tip of the JR4 should allow successful selective engagement (Figure 17.8).

In a manner similar to engagement of the brachiocephalic trunk, the JR4 catheter can be used to engage the left subclavian artery. Some operators prefer to engage the brachiocephalic trunk as described above, and then while keeping a cranial angulation of the catheter tip, the catheter is pulled back until it is seen to jump into the left carotid artery, and then pulled back again until a second jump is seen into the left subclavian. Alternatively, some operators prefer to avoid engagement of the carotid artery in any capacity, so the JR4 is brought with the tip oriented caudally around to the proximal portion of the aortic arch. From there, the tip is pointed cranially in order to directly engage the left subclavian. With either technique, a test injection is done to confirm the catheter is in the left subclavian and to assess the general position of the takeoff of the LIMA. A J-wire is then advanced into the left subclavian artery and the JR4 can be placed in the midportion of the left subclavian, at least 1–2 cm distal to where the suspected takeoff

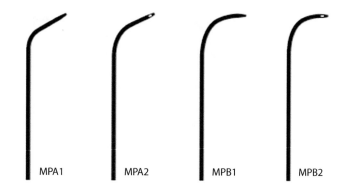

Figure 17.9 Commonly available multipurpose catheters. MP, multipurpose.

of the LIMA is. At this point, the image intensifier can be moved to the pulmonary artery (PA) position if preferred. With frequent test injections, the JR4 is slowly pulled back and torqued as needed to engage the LIMA. If the angle of takeoff is steeper than can be engaged by the JR4, then an exchange length guidewire is needed to exchange for the internal mammary artery diagnostic catheter.

Uncommonly, the right gastroepiploic artery might be used as a bypass graft to the posterior descending artery.[3] The right gastroepiploic artery originates as a branch of the gastroduodenal artery, which is a branch of the common hepatic artery from the celiac trunk. Selective engagement of the celiac trunk will provide "nonselective" angiography of the right gastroduodenal artery. The celiac trunk originates from the anterior aorta just below the diaphragm at the level of the T12 vertebral body. Lateral angiography provides the best views of the takeoff of the celiac trunk to allow for selective engagement with a JR4 or internal mammary artery catheter. When those catheters will not selectively engage the celiac trunk, then visceral catheters such as the Cobra or SOS catheters (see section entitled Peripheral Diagnostic Catheters) can be used. If poor visualization of the distal graft anatomy and runoff is seen with nonselective angiography, then super-selective angiography must be performed. This requires using an exchange length angled Terumo Glidewire to advance selectively into the right gastroepiploic (Figure 17.9). The supporting diagnostic catheter can then be exchanged for a 4-Fr soft Glide Catheter (Terumo) that is small and soft enough to be positioned deep into the right gastroepiploic without causing any trauma. Its 4-Fr size will allow for adequate angiography when it is selectively engaged.

MULTIPURPOSE CATHETER

As previously mentioned, the multipurpose catheter is similar in shape to the original Sones catheter, with a straight tip and only one curve, and was developed by Spencer King and Fred Schoonmaker.[4] There are four types of common multipurpose catheters: the MPA1, MPA2, MPB1, and MPB2 (Figure 17.10). The "A" curved catheters have approximately a 120° curve, while the B catheters have a 90° gradual curve.

The "1" designation refers to endhole only catheters, and the "2" designation refers to the addition to two sideholes to the endhole. The benefit of the sideholes allows for ventriculography on top of selective coronary angiography. Similar to the original Sones technique, an operator can complete an entire diagnostic cardiac catheterization with just the multipurpose catheter. The soft tip allows it to be easily manipulated into a "J" shape when pressed against the aortic valve, thereby allowing it to more easily selectively cannulate the left and right coronary ostium. Because the tip is long, it can tend to more deeply engage the coronaries, and care must be taken to avoid this predilection. With sideholes, a multipurpose catheter can be manipulated into the left ventricle and left ventricular angiography can also be performed. Since the invention of more selective catheters as described above, this technique has fallen out of favor. In today's practice, it is most commonly used as described above as a first or second choice for an RCB graft angiography or when multiple catheters have tried and failed to engage a native coronary or bypass graft; then the multipurpose can usually be manipulated into selective engagement with trial and error.

Catheters for a radial (or brachial) approach

In recent years, operators have begun to more commonly choose the radial approach for catheterization after it was pioneered in Europe and found to be safer (decreased bleeding complications) and have better patient tolerance (no requirement for lying flat postprocedure). The right radial approach is usually preferred, as it allows the operator to stand in the usual position on the right side of the normally positioned patient. Also, approaches from the right arm allow direct access into the ascending aorta, whereas left arm approaches end in the takeoff of the left subclavian artery, which will frequently direct wires and catheters down the descending aorta preferentially. Depending on which arm is used for access, different types and sizes of catheters can be used. In general, since the left arm approach takes the same approach across the aortic arch and down the descending aorta as a femoral approach, then the typical coronary catheters as described above can be used. Typically, a JL4 and JR4 can successfully be used for coronary angiography from a left arm access.

From a right arm access, because of the straight trajectory into the ascending aorta, choosing a Judkins left catheter that is a half size smaller should be used than would normally be used if approaching from the femoral (JL 3.5 to start). For engaging the right coronary artery, a size larger, the JR5, tends to engage the right coronary artery better than the JR4.

The multipurpose A catheter can be used in either arm approach for inferiorly directed takeoffs, while the multipurpose B catheter can be more useful for horizontal and superior directed takeoffs. A modified version of the multipurpose A catheter is the Barbeau catheter. This catheter adds a 135° primary curved tip to the end of the typical multipurpose catheter, which allows for better engagement of the right coronary artery and bypass grafts from the right arm approach.

Typically, current practice has relied upon catheters that have been developed to engage both the right and left coronary ostium from arm access without switching catheters. The Kimny curve diagnostic catheter (Schneider), invented by Ferdinand Kiemeneij, has three curves: the primary curve is 145°, a secondary curve of 90°, and a tertiary curve of 133° (Figure 17.11). These curves allow backup support from the opposing aortic wall while allowing coaxial engagement of the left main, right coronary ostium, or vein grafts. To engage

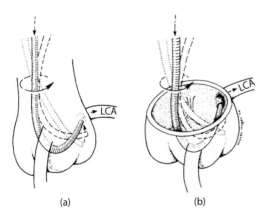

(a)   (b)

Figure 17.10 (a) Technique of multipurpose catheter manipulation for cannulation of the left coronary artery in the 30° RAO projection. The tip of the catheter is slowly advanced off of the left coronary cusp with simultaneous counterclockwise rotation until in engages the left coronary ostium. (b) Catheter manipulation for engagement of the right coronary artery ostium from the 60° LAO projection. LCA, left coronary artery; LAO, left anterior oblique; RAO, right anterior oblique. (Adapted from Schoonmaker, F.W., King, S.B., Circulation., 50(4), 735–740, 1974. With permission.)

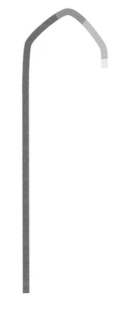

Figure 17.11 Angulation and design of the Kimny curved catheter.

a Kimny curve catheter into the left main or right coronary artery, two general techniques can be used (Figures 17.12 and 17.13).[5] The first technique involves bringing the catheter tip down to the level of the ipsilateral coronary cusp to the ostium that is to be engaged. From there, the catheter can be withdrawn and turned counterclockwise or clockwise to engage the left coronary or right coronary, respectively. The second technique involves the same torque but instead of withdrawing the catheter, it is advanced forward against the respective cusps to point the tip up and into the coronary ostium similar to the Amplatz catheter. Similarly shaped catheters from other companies (Jacky, Tiger II, and Sarah catheters from Terumo, and the Radial Brachial catheter from Cordis) also exist to engage both coronary ostium.[6]

To engage aortocoronary SVGs from a transradial approach is more difficult than a typical transfemoral approach as described previously.[7] From the left radial approach, as this is generally taking the same curve around the aortic arch as the femoral approach, typical catheters for bypass grafts can be tried first (multipurpose for right bypass, JR4 or LCB for left bypasses). If the JR4 or LCB is not working for the left-sided grafts, then an Amplatz Left, Judkins left, or multipurpose can be tried as a second option. For the right radial approach, for grafts originating on the right side of the aorta (usually that have distal anastomoses in the right coronary artery), again, a typical approach with a multipurpose or internal mammary artery catheter can be used. For left-sided aortic anastomoses of SVGs a JR4 or LCB will not have enough reach coming from the right radial approach. In this case, an Amplatz left catheter can be very helpful.

To engage a LIMA from the right arm approach is difficult. The Yumiko catheter (Goodman, Nagoya, Japan) was invented specially for this purpose (Figure 17.14).[8] It must be advanced

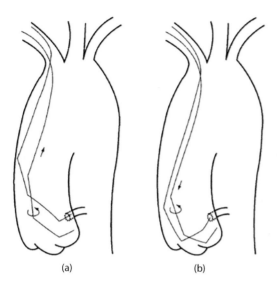

Figure 17.12 Technique for catheterizing the left coronary artery in the posteroanterior (PA) view using the Kimny catheter. The catheter is advanced so that the tip enters the left sinus of Valsalva. (a) The catheter tip is rotated counterclockwise and withdrawn until it enters the left coronary ostium. (b) The body of the catheter is rotated counterclockwise and advanced gradually until the tip rises to enter the left coronary ostium. (From Shibata Y, et al. *Cathet Cardiovasc Diagn*, 1998;4 (3):344–351. With permission.))

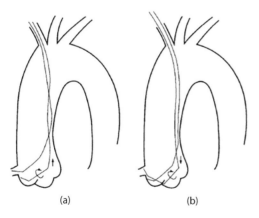

Figure 17.13 Technique for catheterizing the right coronary artery in the left anterior oblique (LAO) view using the Kimny catheter. The catheter is advanced so that the tip enters the right sinus of Valsalva. (a) The catheter tip is rotated clockwise and withdrawn slightly until the tip enters the right coronary ostium. (b) The body of the catheter is rotated clockwise and advanced gradually until the tip rises to enter the right coronary ostium. (From Shibata Y, et al. *Cathet Cardiovasc Diagn*, 1998;43(3):344–351. With permission.)

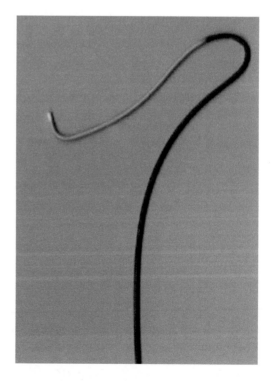

Figure 17.14 Yumiko diagnostic catheter design allows for selective cannulation of the left internal mammary artery via the right radial approach. (Adapted from Miyake, Y., et al., *Am. J. Cardiol.*, 89(8), 984–986, 2002. With permission.)

against the aortic valve so its tip points upward. It is then torqued into the left subclavian artery, at which point the catheter is pulled back, which takes out slack in the aortic looped portion of the catheter allowing it to dive forward and engage the LIMA (Figure 17.15). This catheter is not readily available in the United States, but the special LIMA1 catheter (Cordis) has a similar shape and is available in the United States (Figure 17.16). Alternatively, in the absence of a specially designed catheter, an angled Glidewire (Terumo) can be manipulated from an internal mammary catheter from right arm access to aim up the left subclavian.[9] The wire is extended out into the left subclavian and the internal mammary catheter is used to track over it, past the takeoff of the LIMA. After that, the wire is removed and the catheter is flushed and hooked to the manifold. Test injections are given as the internal mammary catheter is pulled back. If the internal mammary catheter cannot initially aim the J wire into the left subclavian, a Judkins left catheter can be used to send an exchange length guidewire into the left subclavian, at which point the Judkins left catheter can be exchanged for an internal mammary catheter for selective angiography. A similar method can be used to engage the RIMA from left arm access.

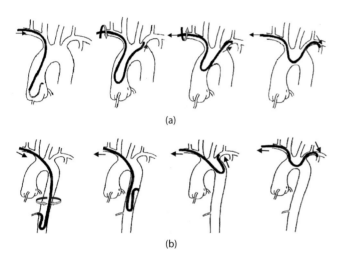

(a)

(b)

Figure 17.15 **(a)** The technique of advancing the YUMIKO-LITA catheter into the LITA via the ascending aorta. The catheter is advanced to the ascending aorta using a guidewire (*first image*). After the guidewire is removed, the catheter is rotated to direct the tip toward the left subclavian artery. The tip easily selects the left subclavian artery by a slight clockwise rotation (*second image*). Pulling the catheter with a slight counterclockwise rotation, the tip is advanced to the distal subclavian artery (*third image*). Further pulling of the catheter enables the tip to be engaged into the LITA (*fourth image*). **(b)** The technique for advancing the YUMIKO-LITA catheter into the LITA via the descending aorta. The catheter is advanced to the descending aorta using a guidewire. After guidewire removal, the catheter is turned, hanging the tip on the side branch of the descending aorta at the celiac trunk or renal artery (*first image*). By pulling the catheter tip to be directed to the left (*second image*), the tip is advanced toward the left subclavian artery (*third image*). Further pulling enables the tip to be engaged into the LITA (*fourth image*). LITA, left internal throacic artery. (From Miyake, Y., et al., *Am. J. Cardiol.*, 89(8), 984–986, 2002. With permission.)

VENTRICULAR ANGIOGRAPHIC CATHETERS

Although performed far less frequently in the current era, left ventriculography remains a component of diagnostic catheterization and is typically performed with a pigtail catheter. A pigtail catheter has an endhole, plus multiple sideholes, that will inject contrast in multiple planes, allowing for better filling of the ventricle with contrast. The catheter has a straight shaft with a circular tip that is usually 1 cm in diameter. The circular tip is a safety feature to minimize the chance of ventricular trauma and myocardial staining with contrast, as compared to a straight endhole catheter like the multipurpose. Since the contrast is focused over multiple ejection points, the catheter will usually sit relatively quietly in the left ventricle, as compared to an endhole catheter, which will shoot backward with a power injection. Common variations on the typical pigtail design include 145° and 155° angled shafts to allow the catheter to favor a mid-ventricle position rather than favoring the inferior wall, which can be common with a straight shafted pigtail (Figure 17.17). A mid-ventricle position of the catheter is important to allow for even angiography and to avoid ventricular ectopy. There are also catheters available with radiopaque markers along its shaft to assist in quantitative angiography. As mentioned above, the "b" type multipurpose catheter can be used for ventriculography as well. However, since the catheter has fewer sideholes and a straight tip, there is more chance of myocardial staining, ventricular ectopy, and catheter movement as compared to a pigtail. In general, less flow rate is recommended through a multipurpose catheter to minimize these complications, but this can lead to poor ventricular visualization.

Right ventriculography is less commonly done in adult catheterization but still is a technique that is useful when there are adult patients with congenital heart disease, such as pulmonic stenosis, or if PA angiography is warranted.

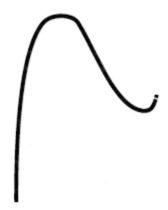

Figure 17.16 The LIMA1 catheter is used to engage the LIMA from right radial access, similar to a Yumiko catheter. LIMA, left internal mammary artery.

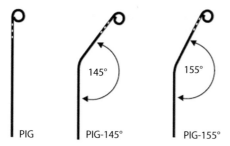

Figure 17.17 Straight and angled pigtail catheters. PIG, pigtail.

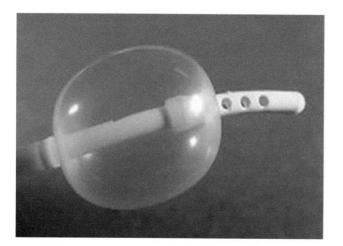

Figure 17.18 Berman angiographic balloon floatation catheter.

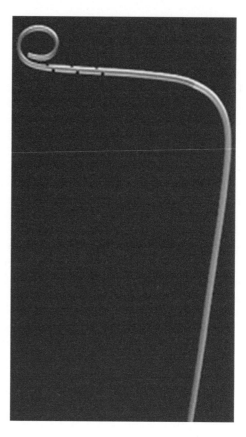

Figure 17.19 Grollman pigtail catheter.

The modern catheter of choice for right ventriculography is a Berman angiographic catheter developed by Michael Berman. This is a sidehole-only catheter with a balloon flotation tip (Figure 17.18). The balloon flotation mechanism allows safe and easy passage into the right ventricle without the risk of trauma to the right atrium or ventricle with catheter manipulation. There is no endhole so catheter recoil with injection is not an issue. The catheter is inserted through the femoral vein and up the inferior vena cava (IVC) with the use of the balloon flotation in as exact manner as a PA flotation catheter can be inserted. If the right ventricular chamber is to be visualized, the balloon is kept inflated to stabilize the catheter and a power injection is given. The Berman catheter can accept flow rates and PSI similar to the typical left ventricular pigtail catheter. It can also be floated easily into the main PA for selective PA angiography.

A second choice for right ventricle and pulmonary angiography is the Grollman catheter, developed by Julius Grollman. It is a modified pigtail catheter with a reversed 90° secondary curve 3 cm from the catheter tip (Figure 17.19). This reversed curve allows it to engage the right ventricle and be advanced to the PA if needed. Because this catheter requires more manipulation in order to advance into the right ventricle or PA, it is the second choice behind the Berman angiographic catheter.

PERIPHERAL DIAGNOSTIC CATHETERS

Peripheral diagnostic catheters have a similar design to coronary catheters, and in some cases, coronary diagnostic catheters are used for a wide variety of peripheral angiography as described below. There are also specialty-designed catheters for accessing challenging anatomy, such as the carotid arteries and the visceral abdominal vessels. Frequently, a nonselective angiogram is used to visualize anatomic takeoffs of branch vessels, and then more specialized catheters are used to engage for selective diagnostic catheterization. We will present common peripheral angiographic catheters based on the anatomic location where they are used.

Carotid

Typically, an angiogram of the aortic arch using a straight-bodied pigtail catheter is used for initial information about the location of the takeoffs of the carotid arteries, and to see if there is any ostial stenosis that might make selective engagement of diagnostic catheters dangerous. In most aortic arches, a JR4 can be used to selectively engage and perform angiography of the common carotids. As described in the above section for graft anatomy, the Judkins right 4 catheter can be advanced to the top of the ascending aorta in the LAO 30° view, which lays out the aorta and ensures its branch vessels are not foreshortened. The JR4 can then be advanced safely over the stiff Glidewire to the proximal carotid for selective angiography. Any catheter with one simple primary curve can be replaced for the JR4 for carotid angiography, with the choice currently being very operator dependent. Examples include an angled Glide catheter (Terumo), a internal mammary artery catheter, a vertebral catheter, or a headhunter catheter. A headhunter catheter has a slight secondary curve as well, but it still functions as a "simple curve" catheter to be used for normal type 1 and 2 arches and its manipulation remains the same as the JR4 catheter. In cases of tortuous anatomy or a type 3 aortic arch, then preformed complex curved catheters such as the Simmons or Vitek catheter will be necessary for selective engagement.[10]

The Simmons sidewinder (SS) catheter was named after Charles Simmons, and typically comes in three sizes based on the length of the catheter from the "knee" portion (secondary curve) to the tip.[11] The Simmons 2 catheter is the most common size used for carotid angiography and has a 4.5 cm distance from knee to tip. The head of a Simmons catheter looks like a shepherd's crook. To be used, it first must be reformed and positioned in the ascending aorta. The preferred technique[12] for reformation involves pushing the catheter (with the guidewire removed) over the aortic arch so that its tip is in the ascending aorta looking caudally, and the secondary curve of the catheter lies over the highest point of the aortic arch. At this point, the catheter is rotated clockwise rapidly, which causes the catheter to buckle and loop over on itself at the secondary curve, resembling the shape of a scissor. With continuing rotation, the catheter tip will loop back over from the ascending to the descending aorta. At this point, the catheter's secondary curve is pushed over the arch and is allowed to rest on the aortic valve. With counterclockwise rotation, the catheter is unwound and resumes its preformed packaged shape. Alternatively, it can be reformed in the ascending aorta against the aortic valve to its preformed shape like an Amplatz catheter (usually by following a stiff wire that has prolapsed over the aortic valve). Once the Simmons is reformed in the aortic root, the catheter should be rotated if needed so that the tip is pointing to the right of the patient and anterior in the aortic root. The catheter is then pulled back until the tip engages the brachiocephalic trunk. This might require some clockwise or counterclockwise manipulation to successfully engage. Once the Simmons catheter tip has engaged, it is pulled back further which will extend the tip cranially into the great vessel. This should always be done over a guidewire. A stiff-angled Glidewire is ideal. The angled tip allows for directional advancement, and the stiff body allows straightening and advancement of the complex curved catheter. A softer guidewire would let the complex curve keep its shape and prolapse into the aorta with further advancement. For engagement of the left common carotid, the Simmons catheter is advanced without a guidewire to prolapse its body back into the ascending aorta. From here, the tip is rotated 180° to look caudally so the catheter can be pulled back past the takeoff of the brachiocephalic trunk. Then the tip is rotated back 180° to look cranial, and the catheter is pulled backward until the tip pops into the left carotid artery. The Simmons catheter tends to loop on itself or get knotted, and particular attention must be paid to avoid this complication.

The Vitek (Cook) catheter is a modified Simmons catheter with a 90° reverse curve of the shepherd's crook tip (Figure 17.20). This allows for the catheter to more easily reform in the descending aorta or distal aortic arch, unlike the Simmons catheter. It is placed over a guidewire into the top of the descending thoracic aorta. As the guidewire is removed, it reforms to its preformed shape. It is pushed proximally across the arch until it engages one of the great vessels where the tip of the catheter will jump cranially into the vessel. At this point, the catheter is pulled back, which straightens out the tip of the catheter, sending it further cranially. In the case of left carotid angiography, no further manipulation needs to be done. If right carotid angiography is needed, then at this point the Vitek catheter has selectively engaged the brachiocephalic trunk. From this point, a stiff-angled Glidewire can be advanced into the appropriate vessel, and the Vitek catheter will track over this for selective angiography. The big difference between a Simmons and Vitek catheter is location of reformation of the preformed shape. Based on location, the Vitek becomes a "push" catheter to engage the arch vessels while the Simmons catheter becomes a "pull" catheter in order to engage the vessels. Also, once the Vitek has engaged the brachiocephalic trunk, the tip of the catheter is pointed cranially and slightly rightward, which allows easier wire manipulation into the right carotid, whereas the Simmons tip will point slightly leftward, requiring slightly more manipulation to engage the right common carotid. For these reasons, the Vitek catheter usually requires less manipulation than a Simmons catheter and is generally preferred as the first choice for difficult arch anatomy.

For a bovine arch with the left carotid coming off low in the brachiocephalic trunk, the Vitek catheter is best used to selectively engage the left carotid. As described above, upon engagement of the brachiocephalic trunk, the Vitek tip naturally points cranially and to the right. Once the Vitek is engaged in the brachiocephalic trunk as described above, if the tip is already above the left carotid takeoff, then the catheter is advanced forward until the tip moves down the brachiocephalic trunk.

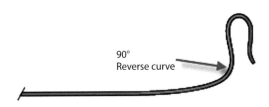

90°
Reverse curve

Figure 17.20 The Vitek catheter has a similar hooked tip as the Simmons catheter, but it has a 90° reversed curve, which makes it a "push" catheter for engagement.

Then a stiff-angled Glidewire can be used to selectively engage the left carotid. The catheter can then be pulled backward, which will advance the tip selectively over the wire into the "bovine" left carotid. A Simmons catheter requires significantly more manipulation into a bovine left carotid as the initial tip looks rightward and should not be used.

Vertebral

Angiography of the vertebral arteries is considered part of a complete cerebral circulation study (along with carotid angiography with anterior cerebral runoff) in order to fully evaluate posterior cerebral circulation. Again, the first choice for selective vertebral angiography remains a simple curve catheter with the JR4 being the first choice. Other choices include the internal mammary artery catheter, the Angled Glide catheter, or a vertebral catheter based on operator training and preference. The vertebral catheter has the gentlest primary curve of 150° (i.e., the tip is only angled 30° from a completely straight position) (Figure 17.21).

Subclavian and upper extremity

Similar to carotid angiography, an aortic angiogram in the LAO 30°–45° view will give a nonselective view of the takeoff of the right and left subclavian arteries. As described in the section on carotid angiography, a JR4 or other simple curved catheter can usually be manipulated for selective left and right subclavian angiography. In the cases of tortuous or Type III arches, then a Vitek or Simmons catheter is the catheter of choice to engage the left or right subclavian. Once selective subclavian angiography is performed,

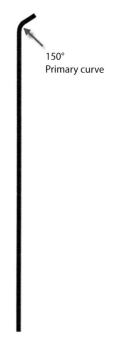

150°
Primary curve

Figure 17.21 Vertebral catheter.

runoff to the upper extremity can be visualized with panning of the angiographic table. For more selective angiography of the upper extremities, a simple curved catheter like a JR4 or internal mammary artery catheter can be used and advanced over a wire more distally in the arm. If a complex curve catheter is used for initial angiography, then an exchange length Wholey or Glidewire can be placed distally in the arm. Following this, the original diagnostic catheter is walked out, and can be exchanged for a straight or angled Glide catheter or a multipurpose catheter.

Renal

Renal angiography begins with a nonselective descending aortic angiogram (utilizing a straight pigtail catheter) at the level of the takeoff of the renal arteries. The renal arteries typically branch off of the descending aorta at the interspace between the L1 and L2 vertebrae. The sideholes of the pigtail catheter thus will be at the level of the renal ostia. The right renal artery usually comes off at a slightly higher level than the left renal artery. The pulmonary angiogram will give useful information regarding the orientation of the renal ostia or anatomic variants such as an accessory renal artery. Since many patients whose renal arteries are being assessed have renal insufficiency, the pigtail angiogram can be done with minimal contrast (only 10 cc needed at high flows). At this point, the operator can proceed with selective angiography. Typically, the renal arteries have a fairly orthogonal takeoff of the lateral aspect of the aorta. The right renal artery has a slightly anterior takeoff as well. The JR4 catheter, again, is very useful as the first choice catheter to engage the laterally directed renal ostia. Alternatively, a Cobra catheter (invented by Melvin Judkins) can be used to selectively engage the renal arteries. The shape of this catheter looks like a cobra head or question mark and is similar in shape to the LCB catheter described above; it has three curves. The primary curve has a 90° tip angled from the shaft of the secondary portion of the catheter. Along with about a 70° secondary curve in the same direction, the tip points slightly downward to be able to hook into visceral ostia (Figure 17.22). Finally, there is a very broad tertiary curve that is angled in the opposite direction of the primary and secondary curves. This reversed tertiary curve allows contralateral support from the opposite aortic wall. If a renal artery has an inferiorly directed takeoff and the Cobra catheter cannot engage, then an IM catheter, which has a more acutely angled tip, might be able to engage. If the takeoff is extremely inferior, then a shepherd's crook-shaped catheter ("hooked" end similar to a Simmons catheter as described above but with a smaller overall curve radius), such as the SOS OMNI (Angiodynamics), can be useful (Figure 17.23). It is named after its inventor, Tom Sos, who practices interventional radiology at Cornell University, New York. Similar to a Simmons catheter, this hooked catheter requires a "pull" technique to engage the renal ostia. The catheter is brought above the level of the renal ostium over a wire. As the

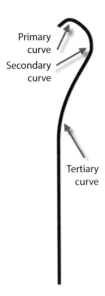

Figure 17.22 Cobra catheter.

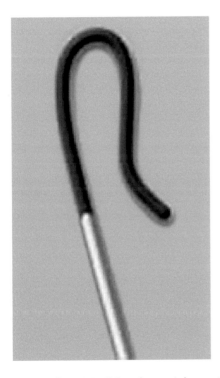

Figure 17.23 Tip of SOS OMNI catheter. It has a similar hooked shape as a Simmons catheter, but it has a much tighter radius of curvature, allowing for easier reformation of its primary shape.

wire is removed, the catheter will reform to its prepackaged shape in the abdominal aorta since it has such a tight curve. The catheter is then manipulated either clockwise or counterclockwise in order to look to the lateral wall of the aorta. The catheter is then brought down and when it is thought to hook a renal ostium, a test injection is given.

Another method called the "flick" technique allows engagement of a renal artery without multiple injections of contrast. This method involves reforming the SOS

OMNI catheter in the abdominal aorta below the level of the renal arteries. A soft-tipped straight guidewire like the Bentson guidewire is left in the preformed catheter with 1 cm extending from the catheter tip. Because the tip of the Bentson guidewire is very floppy, the catheter remains in its preformed shape, despite having the guidewire extending from its tip. This floppy tip also allows for minimal aortic trauma. The catheter then will engage the renal ostium with a push technique. The tip of the guidewire remains parallel to the aortic wall until the catheter is pushed high enough so that the wire will "flick" laterally into the selective renal artery. At this point, the catheter can be advanced to the vessel ostium, and the wire can be pulled out.

Visceral

Angiography of the major abdominal aortic branches (celiac trunk, superior mesenteric artery, and inferior mesenteric artery) begins with a nonselective abdominal aortic angiogram with a nonselective flush catheter, like a pigtail. Angiography is done in the lateral orientation to identify the origin of the appropriate vessel, as they have takeoffs from the anterior aorta. The tip of the pigtail should be placed above the level of T11 so that the celiac trunk can be visualized at the level of T12. Runoff should visualize the takeoff of the superior mesenteric artery at the level of L1 and the internal mammary artery at the level of T3. After nonselective angiography is performed, then selective angiography is usually performed with a simple curved catheter like a JR4 or internal mammary artery catheter. If the JR4 or internal mammary artery catheter is unable to hook the vessel, then a more complex curved catheter like a Sos or Cobra catheter can be helpful. In order to hook the appropriate vessel, the catheter is positioned at a level above the artery that is intended to be studied with a guidewire. The guidewire is removed allowing the complex curved catheter to reform in the descending aorta. The catheter is pulled back and rotated with its tip toward the anterior aorta (tip looking laterally in the lateral fluoroscopic angulation) until it is seen and felt to hook into a visceral ostium.

Lower extremity

Lower extremity angiography usually begins with a nonselective angiogram with a pigtail catheter in the distal descending aorta above the level of the iliac bifurcation. Nonselective angiography is performed, and the table is panned to view runoff from the iliac artery all the way to the below the knee runoff. If a stenosis is visualized, then more selective angiography can be performed with catheters selectively placed in any of the vessels (contralateral to the access sheath) or through the sheath in the femoral artery (to image the ipsilateral vessels). The common iliac arteries are usually spaced about 90° apart, so a catheter with around a 90° tip, like a JR4 or internal mammary artery, is the primary choice to selectively cannulate contralateral vessels. If the angle between the iliac arteries is

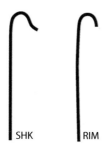

Figure 17.24 The SHK and RIM catheter can be used to access a contralateral iliac artery in the "up and over" approach. SHK, shepherd's hook.

less than 90°, then a hook-shaped catheter head can be more useful to hook the ostium of the ipsilateral iliac. Examples of this include the SOS, Shepherd's hook, or Rim catheters (Figure 17.24). Once a wire is advanced from the diagnostic catheter up and over, then the diagnostic catheter is walked out, and a long flexible sheath is placed up and over to the contralateral iliac artery. At this point, more selective angiography can be performed through the sheath itself or through a straight Glide catheter inserted distally from the guidewire to the area of interest artery.

REFERENCES

1. Devlin G, et al. Mortality related to diagnostic cardiac catheterization. The importance of left main coronary disease and catheter induced trauma. *Int J Card Imaging* 1997;13(5):379–384.
2. Myler RK, et al. Guiding catheter selection for right coronary artery angioplasty. *Cathet Cardiovasc Diagn* 1990;19(1):58–67.
3. Tamnimoto Y, et al. Angiography of right gastroepiploic artery for coronary artery bypass graft. *Cathet Cardiovasc Diagn* 1989;16(1):35–38.
4. Schoonmaker FW, King SB. Coronary angiography by the single catheter percutaneous femoral technique: Experience in 6,800 cases. *Circulation* 1974;50(4):735–740.
5. Shibata Y, et al. New guiding catheter for transradial PTCA. *Cathet Cardiovasc Diagn* 1998;43(3):344–351.
6. Kim SM, et al. Novel diagnostic catheter specifically designed for both coronary arteries via the right transradial approach. A prospective, randomized trial of Tiger II vs. Judkins catheters. *Int J Cardiovasc Imaging* 2006;22(3–4):295–303.
7. Burzotta F, et al. Transradial approach for coronary angiography and interventions in patients with coronary bypass grafts: Tips and tricks. *Catheter Cardiovasc Interv* 2008;72(2):263–272.
8. Kim MH, et al. Bilateral selective internal mammary artery angiography via right radial approach: Clinical experience with newly designed Yumiko catheter. *Cathet Cardiovasc Interv* 2001;54(1):19–24.
9. Zheng H, et al. Bilateral internal mammary angiography through a right radial approach: A case report. *Cathet Cardiovasc Diagn* 1998;45(2):188–190.
10. Simmons CR, et al. Angiographic approach to the difficult aortic arch: A new technique for transfemoral cerebral angiography in the aged. *Am J Roentgenol Radium Ther Nucl Med* 1973;119(3):605–612.
11. Grable GS, Smith DC. The use of the Simmons "Sidewinder" catheter in percutaneous transluminal angioplasty of the renal arteries. *Radiology* 1980;137(2):541–543.
12. Smith DC, Simmons CR. The quick aortic turn: A rapid method for reformation of the Simmons sidewinder catheter. *Radiology* 1985;155(1):247–248.

18

Coronary imaging: Angiography, computed tomography angiography, and magnetic resonance coronary angiography

JOEL A. GARCIA FERNANDEZ AND JOHN D. CARROLL

INTRODUCTION

The central diagnostic goal of contemporary imaging is to completely visualize the coronary artery tree to understand the anatomy and to recognize and characterize pathologic findings. Beyond its diagnostic role, imaging is used to plan and execute treatment using recognition and quantification of a variety of vessel and lesion features prior to interventions. The therapeutic planning goals are to develop an equipment strategy for each lesion to be treated. Likewise, an imaging strategy is developed before interventions that allows for a working view to provide real-time visualization during the procedure.

Finally, at the completion of the intervention, coronary imaging is used to confirm and quantify therapeutic changes to the coronary tree and detect any complications.

While the imaging technologies of computed tomography angiography (CTA) and magnetic resonance coronary angiography (MRCA) are available and used clinically, catheter-based standard coronary angiography (SCA) remains the gold standard. SCA is not only widely available but also provides the highest spatial and temporal resolution for coronary imaging in current practice. SCA provides reliable angiographic information with vast experience over multiple decades of use. It is routinely used to determine the appropriateness of percutaneous coronary interventions (PCIs), coronary artery bypass grafting (CABG), or medical therapy. Coronary angiography, first performed by Mason Sones in 1959, has been a cornerstone in the development of the concept of transluminal angioplasty and revascularization therapies. This includes the work of Charles Dotter who performed the first transluminal angioplasty in 1964, Rene Favaloro who performed the first CABG in 1967, and Andreas Gruentzig who performed the first percutaneous coronary angioplasty in 1977.[1-3] The use of diagnostic coronary angiography has significantly increased in the last three decades due to the high prevalence of coronary artery disease (CAD) in the industrialized world as well as its increasing prevalence in the remainder of the world. This chapter focuses on traditional catheter-based coronary angiography and two revolutionizing noninvasive technologies that also define the coronary anatomy: CTA and MRCA.

Standard coronary angiography

Coronary angiography clearly delineates the course and size of the coronary arteries, identifies anomalies, and provides information on the location, characteristics and degree of obstructions. It provides information on coronary origin, vessel size, artery pathway, branches, lesion presence, collateral circulation, and myocardial bridging. Aneurysmal segments, thrombotic lesions, thrombus burden, and vessel spasm can be evaluated.[1,2] Access to the aorta is commonly obtained by cannulation of the femoral or radial artery, though brachial and axillary approaches are infrequently used. Vascular access is described in detail in Chapter 8. Shape-specific catheters are then advanced via the aorta to the ostium of the coronary arteries over a guidewire. Once the wire is removed and the catheter is engaged, the injection of contrast with the subsequent radiographic acquisition results in an angiographic image. Hemodynamic parameters are constantly recorded (before, during, and after injections). Diagnostic catheters are the focus of Chapter 17.

The two-dimensional (2D) nature of SCA requires that multiple single-view angiographic acquisitions are performed in various projections. These views are obtained by rotating the imaging system around the patient who lies supine in a radiolucent table.[1,2] The imaging system can be rotated from left anterior oblique (LAO) to right anterior oblique (RAO) with an angulation toward the head (cranial) or an angulation toward the legs (caudal). While a wide array of potential combinations of rotation and angulation is possible, several standard approaches result in a comprehensive and mostly complete visualization of the coronary anatomy.

The methods of performing coronary angiography have evolved substantially. Smaller catheters are currently used, resulting in minimization of vascular risk, early ambulation, and discharge.[2] Images were traditionally stored on 35 mm cinefilm but now are almost exclusively digital recordings stored on local hard drives, servers, and occasionally compact disc (CD) or digital video disc (DVD) media.

Coronary anatomic considerations

The individual variability of the coronary anatomy requires that the acquisition techniques allow the ability to perform various combinations of angulation and rotation that result in a gantry position that acquires a clinically useful image. Multiple gantry positions are used in an effort to minimize the imaging inaccuracies resulting from viewing a three-dimensional (3D) structure in 2D. These imaging inaccuracies and misrepresentations are mostly related to vessel overlap, ostial lesion characterization, and foreshortening (Figure 18.1). Overlap results from the superimposed image of a vessel on another one. The same concept applies for "opening" an ostial lesion that may be obscured by the main vessel. Foreshortening results from the relationship of a vessel segment's longitudinal path in relation to the path of the X-ray beam. This can result in a projection image that may minimize the true length of a vessel segment as well as a coronary artery lesion.

Standard coronary angiography limitations

Although SCA has significantly improved over the past 30 years in terms of the quality of the image, postprocessing enhancement, display on high-quality monitors, and tools for replay and lesion quantification, it is still hampered by limitations inherent to 2D projection images of the opacified inner diameter (lumen) and the obvious risk of exposure to contrast media and radiation (Table 18.1).[4,5] These limitations and the so-called "luminology" evaluation of the vessel have resulted in the need to have alternative technologies

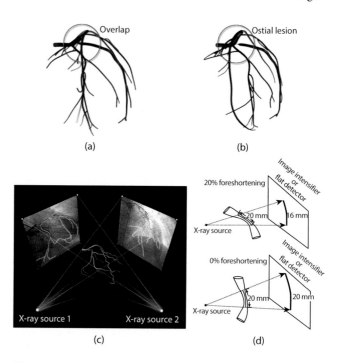

Figure 18.1 Standard coronary angiography imaging inaccuracies and 3D modeling. **(a)** Representation of overlap as a common imaging limitation; **(b)** ostial lesion representation; **(c)** 3D modeling concept; and **(d)** vessel foreshortening representation.

Table 18.1 Standard coronary angiography imaging and safety limitations

Imaging limitations	Safety limitations
Vessel foreshortening	Invasive procedure
Vessel overlap	Contrast administration
Ostial and bifurcation lesion evaluation	Radiation exposure
Lesion eccentricity evaluation	

that allow for a more precise characterization of vessel anatomy, lesions, and stents. Intravascular ultrasound (IVUS) is one widely available technology that complements SCA by providing a more precise coronary evaluation. Another group of technologies enhances the projection images to highlight certain structures like coronary stents, and other technologies transform the 2D images into 3D models and reconstructions. These will be discussed subsequently.

IMAGE INTENSIFIERS AND FLAT PANEL DETECTORS

Imaging related coronary fundamentals and limitations

The development of techniques for imaging the vasculature over the last 100 years has revolutionized the understanding and treatment of patients with cardiovascular, cerebrovascular, and peripheral vascular disease (PVD). The history of vascular imaging began shortly after the development of radiography when, in 1896, Hascheck and Lindenthal injected and imaged the vasculature of an amputated hand with a mixture of salts. Soon thereafter, femoral and cerebral arteriography using sodium bromide and strontium bromide injections were described in 1924 and 1927. With the development of less toxic contrast agents and better imaging equipment, these initial experiences resulted in surgical interventions to treat peripheral and cerebrovascular disease and formed the historical foundation for the field of interventional radiology.[3]

Contemporary medicine has evolved along with current imaging techniques and X-ray equipment. Image intensifiers (IIs) have evolved into flat-panel detectors that allow for the most advanced vessel evaluations. Images are digitally enhanced and the equipment software constantly adjusts settings to provide a superior evaluation. The traditional 2D planar imaging evaluation is now complemented by advanced imaging systems like biplane angiography, rotational angiography, single- and dual-axis RA, CTA, and MRCA. Most of these techniques and technologies allow for the representation of vessels in 3D utilizing workstations with advanced graphics capabilities.

3D acquisition and 3D visualization

The display and quantification of 3D vessel properties has been a recent development in coronary imaging. Modeling and/or reconstructive techniques based on SCA have made

a significant leap forward in visualizing vessels in 3D and some approaches have become commercially available (Figure 18.1c).[6-8] The ability to produce 3D coronary models and reconstructions has led to quantification of clinically relevant 3D vessel properties, such as tortuosity, bifurcation angles, takeoff angles, vessel ostium orientation, and accurate segment length determination.

The coronary tree rests on the epicardial surface of the heart, moves with the underlying myocardium, and as a result, changes in 3D shape. Attempts to quantify the specific dynamic behavior of a coronary vessel throughout the cardiac cycle (i.e., 4D shape changes), using traditional SCA have previously been unsuccessful. The clinical relevance of 4D shape changes has come to light with problems such as stent-induced conformational changes in coronary artery shape (i.e., straightening) and the risk of stent fracture from repetitive deformation. A multimodality 3D vessel quantification algorithm will likely be part of all future endovascular therapies.

CORONARY CONTRAST DELIVERY METHODS

Optimizing coronary angiography requires reliable, adequate, and steady injections of contrast media during image acquisition. Furthermore, the use of RA for volumetric reconstruction requires a longer coronary contrast injection. The traditional manifold allows for the injection of contrast media but suffers from the inherent limitations of being unable to provide a standard amount of flow (mL/s). This is also coupled to the fact that the manifold total contrast volume (mL) is fixed and dependent on the setup. Newer power injectors or control injectors allow for the combination of a variety of flows and volumes that can be predetermined by the operator.[9,10] The safety of these longer injections (<7.1 seconds) to provide longer acquisitions that allow vessel reconstruction has been evaluated.[9]

STANDARD CORONARY ANGIOGRAPHY

Indications

The American College of Cardiology (ACC) and American Heart Association (AHA) Task Force has delineated the indications for coronary angiography in patients with known or suspected CAD (Table 18.2).[2,10,11] Please refer to Chapter 5 for a full review of cardiac catheterization patient selection, including patients with stable angina.

Table 18.2 CTA/MRCA appropriateness criteria

	CAD PTP	HRF NIT	ECG	Exercise	ECG changes	Cardiac markers	Prior CTA	Risk	CTA	MRCA	SCA
Chest pain syndrome	Interm	–	Interp	Able	–	–	–	–	U(5)	I(2)	–
	Interm	–	Interp	Unable	–	–	–	–	A(7)	I(2)	Class I (if refractory to MT)
	High	–	–	–	–	–	–	–	I(2)	I(1)	Class I
	–	–	–	–	–	–	–	–	A(7–9)	A(8)	–
Coronary anomaly suspected/CHD/ new onset CHF (CTA only)	Low	Y	–	–	N	–	–	–	U(5)	–	Class I (if no HRF IIb)
Acute chest pain/USA	Interm	–	–	–	N	Neg	–	–	A(7)	U(6)	Class I
	High	–	–	–	N	Neg	–	–	U(6)	–	Class I
	High	–	–	–	Y	Pos	–	–	I(1)	I(1)	Class I
	Interm	–	–	–	Y	Pos	–	–	U(4)	–	–
Triple rule out/NSTEMI	–	–	–	–	–	–	–	–	U(4)	–	–
Asymptomatic	–	–	–	–	–	–	–	Low	I(1)	–	Class III
	–	–	–	–	–	–	–	Mod	I(2)	–	Class III
	–	–	–	–	–	–	–	High	U(4)	–	Class III
Uninterpretable test (ETT, perfusion, stress echo)	–	–	–	–	–	–	–	–	A(8)	–	–
Moderate–severe ischemia	–	–	–	–	–	–	–	–	I(2)	–	Class III
Risk assessment (asymptomatic)	–	–	–	–	–	–	<2 years (NOD)	High	I(2)	–	Class III
	–	–	–	–	–	–	Ca score >400	High	I(3)	–	Class III (as screening test)
Pre-operative evaluation (NCS)											
• Low-risk surgery	–	–	–	–	–	–	–	Interm	I(1)	–	
• High-risk surgery	–	–	–	–	–	–	–	Interm	U(4)	–	
Post revascularization											
• CABG (CP+)	–	–	–	–	–	–	–	–	–	–	–
• PCI (CP+) abrupt closure? ST?	–	–	–	–	–	–	–	–	U(6)	I(2)	Class IIb
• CABG (no CP)	–	–	–	–	–	–	–	–	U(5)	I(1)	Class I
• PCI (no CP) ISR	–	–	–	–	–	–	–	–	I(2)	–	Class IIb
• PCI <9 months	–	Y	–	–	–	–	–	–	I(2–3)	–	Class IIb
CABG (CP+)/constant angina (CP)	–	Y	–	–	–	–	–	–	–	–	Class I
no ischemia	–	–	–	–	–	–	–	–	–	–	Class IIb
	–	–	–	–	–	–	–	–	–	–	Class III

(Continued)

Table 18.2 (Continued) CTA/MRCA appropriateness criteria

	CAD PT	HRF NIT	ECG	Exercise	ECG changes	Cardiac markers	Prior CTA	Ris	CTA	MRCA	SCA
Non-specific CP	–	Y									
Recurrent hospitalization	–	–	–	–	–	–	–	–	–	–	Class I
Equivocal findings NIT	–	–	–	–	–	–	–	–	–	–	Class IIb
After QWMI or NQWMI											
• Active ischemia	–	–	–	–	–	–	–	–	–	–	Class I
• Presurgical therapy (MRCA, VSD)	–	–	–	–	–	–	–	–	–	–	Class I
• Hemodynamic instability	–	–	–	–	–	–	–	–	–	–	Class IIa
• MI due to embolism, arthritis,	–	–	–	–	–	–	–	–	–	–	Class IIa
trauma, metabolic disease,	–	–	–	–	–	–	–	–	–	–	Class IIb
spasm	–	–	–	–	–	–	–	–	–	–	Class IIb
• MI survivors (EF <40%, CHF, PCI,	–	–	–	–	–	–	–	–	–	–	Class IIb
CABG, arrhythmia)								–			
• Delayed PCI for IRA											
• LM or 3VD											
• Recurrent VT or all NQWMIs											

Source: Adapted from Otsuka, M., et al., *Int. J. Cardiovasc. Imaging,* 24(2), 201–210, 2008.

Note: 3VD, three-vessel disease; A, appropriate; Ca, calcium; SCA, standard coronary angiography; CABG, coronary artery bypass graft; CAD, coronary artery disease; CHD, congenital heart disease; CHF, congestive heart failure; CTA, computed tomography angiography; ECG, electrocardiogram; ETT, exercise treadmill test; HRF, high-risk features on non-invasive testing; I, inappropriate; Interm, intermediate; Interp, interpretable; IRA, infarct-related artery; ISR, in-stent restenosis; LM, left main; MI, myocardial infarction; MRCA, magnetic resonance coronary angiography; MT, medical therapy; N, no; NCS, non-cardiac surgery; Neg, negative; NIT, non-invasive testing; NOD, non-obstructive disease; NQWMI, non-Q-wave myocardial infarction; NSTEMI, non-ST segment elevation myocardial infarction; PCI, percutaneous coronary intervention; Pos, positive; PTP, pre-test probability; QWMI, Q-wave myocardial infarction; ST, stent thrombosis; U, uncertain; USA, unstable angina; VSD, ventricular septal defect; VT, ventricular tachycardia; y, years; Y, yes.

Contraindications

There are no absolute contraindications for coronary angiography other than an individual who is not willing to consent to the study. Several conditions, however, do present a relative contraindication to angiography. Active bleeding, severe anemia (hemoglobin < 8 gm/dL), unexplained fever, active or untreated infections, severe electrolyte imbalance, digitalis toxicity, uncontrolled systemic hypertension, previous serious contrast reaction, severe agitation, and acute renal failure are relative contraindications. Others include ongoing stroke, decompensated congestive heart failure (CHF), intrinsic or iatrogenic coagulopathy (International Normalized Ratio [INR >2]), and active endocarditis.[2,11] Individuals at risk for developing serious complications from coronary angiography are also important to recognize before the procedure.

Coronary angiography in vulnerable populations

There is an increased risk of complications in general among individuals that exceed 70 years of age, have congenital heart disease (CHD), obesity, cachexia, uncontrolled glucose, arterial oxygen desaturation, severe chronic obstructive lung disease, and renal insufficiency with creatinine greater than 1.5 mg/dL.[2,11] There is an increased risk of cardiac complications among patients with three vessel CAD, left main lesions, New York Heart Association (NYHA) class IV, significant mitral or aortic valve disease, ejection fraction (EF) < 35%, high-risk exercise treadmill test (ETT), pulmonary hypertension, and pulmonary artery wedge pressure (PCWP) in excess of 25 mmHg.[2,11] Another group of patients who are at risk of vascular complications include those with anticoagulation or bleeding diathesis, uncontrolled systemic hypertension, severe PVD, recent stroke, and severe aortic insufficiency.[2,11]

Fundamentals

Accurate diagnosis of CAD requires multiple injections in various views to produce clinically useful images of all coronary segments by minimizing overlap and foreshortening.[10] Traditionally, invasive coronary angiography has been performed with radiographic equipment that provides a simplistic, 2D representation of a patient's more complicated 3D anatomy. This "flattening" of a 3D image results in the generation of a final image that may be limited and inaccurate. To minimize these limitations, invasive cardiologists typically acquire 6–10 diagnostic views of the coronary arteries. In addition to the limitations of intravenous (IV) contrast, ionizing radiation, and procedural time, each angiographic view is subjectively chosen to best display an individual patient's coronary arteries. As it has been previously demonstrated, the combination of 2D imaging limitations and this trial-and-error technique can result in inherent and unrecognized imaging inaccuracies (Table 18.1).[12–15] Nonetheless, SCA remains a gold standard in the diagnosis of CAD.

Traditional coronary angiographic views

Not all of the many potential views of a patient's coronary tree are necessary for an adequate study; rather a reasonable combination of views must be acquired that adequately display the patient's coronary tree and abnormalities. The easy positioning of the gantry allows for a wide variety of combinations of rotation and angulation. Rotation is defined as the ability of the flat panel or II to come near the right side of the chest (RAO) or the left side of the chest (LAO). Angulation refers to the ability of the flat panel or II to come near the head of the patient (cranial) or toward the legs (caudal) (Figure 18.2). The rotation (LAO vs. RAO) may be recognized by the position of tip the catheter in relation to the spine or based on the shape of the catheter (Figures 18.2 and 18.3). In LAO, the catheter shape is that of an inverted "U" (Figures 18.2 and 18.3a through 18.3c), while the shape of the catheter in RAO shows it overlapped on itself (Figure 18.3e through 18.3h). The tip of the catheter to the right of the spine on the screen suggests RAO (Figure 18.3e through 18.3i). The tip of the catheter to the left of the spine on the screen suggests LAO (Figure 118.3a through 18.3c, k, l). The presence of the diaphragm on the image is usually seen in cranial shots (Figure 18.3h through 18.3l).

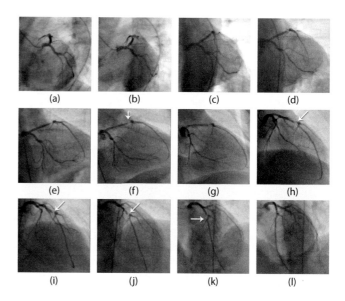

Figure 18.2 Dual-axis rotational coronary angiography of the left coronary artery. Note the different views and the lesion characterization of the mid-LAD obtained by a single injection. Several different views of the mid-LAD lesion are shown with an arrow. This set of views also shows the relationship of the spine and the diaphragm based on angulation and rotation of the gantry. Note the eccentricity of the plaque shown by the arrows. (a, b) LAO caudal, (c) posteroanterior caudal, (d, e) RAO caudal, (h, i) RAO cranial, and (k, l) LAO cranial. LAD, left anterior descending artery; LAO, left anterior oblique; RAO, right anterior oblique.

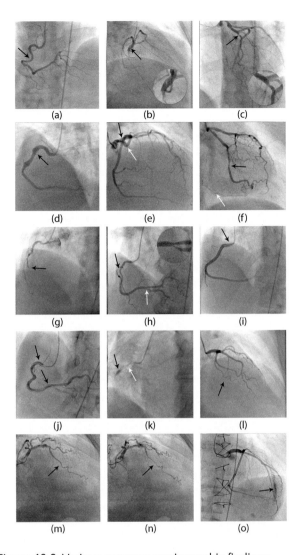

Figure 18.3 Various common angiographic findings.
(a) RCA vessel tortuosity (*black arrow*); **(b)** left main coronary dissection and zoomed image (*arrow* shows oblique line to the right of the catheter); **(c)** eccentric mid-LAD lesion (*arrow*) and zoomed image; **(d)** RCA proximal ectasia (*arrow*); **(e)** overlap of the proximal LAD (*black arrow*), angulation and foreshortening of the mid-Cx (*white arrow*); **(f)** concentric distal Cx lesion (*black arrow*) and RCA collaterals (*white arrow*); **(g)** complete occlusion of the mid-RCA (*black arrow*); **(h)** severe ostial right ventricular marginal lesion (*black arrow*) and moderate posterior descending artery ostial lesion (*white arrow*). There is also a mild RCA atrioventricular continuation lesion that then constitutes a bifurcation lesion (*in circle*); **(i)** ostial RCA catheter induced spasm (*black arrow*); **(j)** RCA contrast streaming simulating dissection that normalized with appropriate injection flow and volume (*black arrow*); **(k)** mid-RCA thrombus (*black arrow* points to contrast hang out). Please note that the white arrow points toward mild calcification of the vessel wall; **(l)** tortuous distal vessels (*black arrow* points to the distal Cx mild tortuosity); **(m)** black arrow points to mid-LAD in diastole with an obvious myocardial bridge during systole **(n)**; **(o)** distal LAD fistula to LV chamber (*black arrow*). Cx, circumflex artery; LAD, left anterior descending artery; LV, left ventricle; RCA, right coronary artery.

The technique used to acquire images impacts the accuracy and reproducibility of traditional angiography. To minimize imaging artifacts introduced by 2D acquisitions, traditional angiography depends on at least two views, which are orthogonal to the vessel segment of interest. Ideally, the acquired images are "triple" orthogonal views in which each projection pair is perpendicular to the other and to the vessel segment of interest. This principle led to the development and widespread use of biplane angiographic equipment.

Traditionally, a series of screening views have been used by operators. These screening views are ultimately complemented by additional views based on real-time interpretation of the angiogram. Any change in gantry angulation or rotation is reflected by a change in the image. Operators are required to be very proficient in real-time image interpretation and in the creation of a mental imprint of the 3D image while acquiring only 2D information. Over time, the use of coronary angiography has resulted in the recognition of views that are usually adequate to display certain coronary segments. While this "expert recommended" approach has evolved from the practice of angiography, no scientifically based analysis of these recommended views has been performed. It is important to recognize that the variability in anatomy from patient to patient makes the recommended views only a guide and the cardiologist must individualize the views acquired to produce a clinically adequate angiographic study. A detailed description of the coronary anatomy is the focus of Chapter 16. Detailed knowledge of the coronary anatomy is mandatory to perform optimal coronary image acquisitions.

RAO caudal views are used to visualize the LM, proximal left anterior descending (LAD) artery, and proximal circumflex (Figure 18.3e through 18.3g). RAO cranial views visualize the mid and distal LAD, without overlap of septal or diagonal branches, and the distal postero-lateral (PL) branches (Figure 18.3h through 18.3j). The LAO cranial views visualize the mid and distal LAD in an orthogonal projection (Figure 18.3k through 18.3l). LAO caudal views visualize the left main, ramus intermedius, and the proximal circumflex (Figure 18.3a through 18.3c). If uncertainty remains, supplemental views include posteroanterior (PA), lateral 60°–90° with cranial, or caudal angulation. The right coronary artery (RCA) views include the LAO to visualize the proximal portion, RAO cranial for the posterior-descending artery (PDA) and PL branches, RAO 30°, and lateral for the mid-segment.[2,10,16,17]

Universal optimal view map

Recognizing views that target specific vessel segments has evolved with the practice of angiography. An approach to scientifically validate optimal views has been studied using an in-depth analysis of a large patient population.[18] A database of vessel reconstructions segment by segment results in the creation of an optimal view map—that is, a graphic representation of gantry position and the quantification of a key visualization measurement to be optimized, such as vessel foreshortening and overlap with surrounding vessels. This scientifically based evaluation validated current coronary angiographic knowledge and clinical practice but also allows extension into challenges of optimizing bifurcation regions (Figure 18.4a and b).

Limitations of standard coronary angiography

Errors in image acquisition, evaluation, and interpretation can have a significant impact on the management strategy of CAD.[2,19] Ideally, a systematic approach aims at minimizing these inaccuracies and potentially avoids impacting clinical outcomes. Technical issues are generally mastered with experience. Inadequate vessel opacification due to conditions like aortic insufficiency, streaming, diluted contrast, competitive flow, anemia, and noncoaxial catheters can result in image interpretation limitations. Coronary angiography outlines the lumen of the vessel but is unable to provide wall thickness information.[12] The proper vessel information is highly dependent on the ability of the operator to compare to a "normal vessel" reference segment. Even experienced operators are subject to some interpretation limitations and variability.[1,19] These limitations have opened the door for technologies that evaluate the vessel lumen via ultrasound or perform pressure differential evaluation of the coronary segments.[1] While unrecognized occlusions, eccentric stenoses, myocardial bridging, and vessel recanalization are also considered pitfalls of coronary angiography, overlap and foreshortening remain the most common and important imaging shortcoming phenomena.[2] Radiation exposure and contrast use with the subsequent risk of nephropathy remain significant limitations of current X-ray–based angiographic practices as well.[20–22]

Vessel overlap, foreshortening, and ostial lesions

The tortuosity of coronary artery segments presents specific challenges in minimizing vessel foreshortening and angiographically separating adjacent structures. Historically, the LM coronary artery is difficult to image because of foreshortening and vessel overlap from the circumflex and LAD arteries.[6,23,24]

The clinical implications of unrecognized foreshortening include missed lesions, errors in lesion length assessment, incomplete coverage of lesions by stents, underestimation of stenosis severity, and inaccurate quantitative coronary angiography calculations. In an era of complex and expensive interventions with drug-eluting stents (DES) and other devices, precise length measurements and accurate device placement are critical to minimize the need for additional interventions resulting from inaccurate or incomplete imaging. Recognition of these limitations has resulted in the development of imaging techniques designed to specifically address the weaknesses of traditional angiographic techniques. Technologies capable of minimizing the shortcomings of traditional angiography have been developed and are now in clinical use.[6,15,18,25–27]

Ostial lesions are traditionally difficult to image due to challenges in avoiding the ostium of the vessel to be covered by the main branch or a contiguous vessel (Figure 18.1). Screening angiographic evaluations are often limited in providing a complete ostial vessel survey requiring multiple subsequent angiograms.

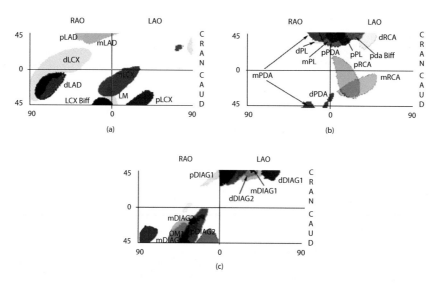

(a)

(b)

(c)

Figure 18.4 Optimal view map for each coronary vessel segment. Note that the quadrants represent the angulation and rotation of the gantry. Biff, bifurcation; CAUD, caudal; CRAN, cranial; d, distal; DIAG, diagonal; LAD, left anterior descending artery; LAO, left anterior oblique; LCX, left circumflex artery; LM, left main; m, mid; OM, obtuse marginal; p, proximal; PDA, posterior descending artery; PL, posterolateral; RAO, right anterior oblique; RCA, right coronary artery.

Complications of standard coronary angiography

The early days of coronary angiography relied on larger catheters and high-osmolar iodine-containing contrast media. Several adverse effects to coronary angiography have been described but have significantly decreased over time as catheters, techniques, and contrast have evolved. Once the coronary vessel was engaged, the replacement of blood with contrast media resulted in several signs and symptoms. Transient hypotension, elevation of left ventricular end diastolic pressure, *T*-wave inversion, sinus slowing, sinus arrest, PR segment prolongation, QRS prolongation, and QT interval prolongation were effects seen in response to high-osmolar contrast media. Arrhythmias that included ventricular tachycardia/ventricular fibrillation, myocardial ischemia due to decreased oxygen delivery, allergic reaction, and renal toxicity were also seen.[10,20,28–30] Some of these adverse effects have been reduced with the use of low-osmolar contrast media. Contrast agents are the focus of Chapter 4.

Constant hemodynamic monitoring is therefore necessary during coronary angiography. Major complications in contemporary practices are uncommon (<1%). They include death (0.10%–0.14%), myocardial infarction (MI) (0.06%–0.07%), contrast agent reaction (0.23%), and local vascular complications (0.8%–1.8%).[31–33] Vascular access and complications are the focus of Chapter 8. The risk of death is accentuated in vulnerable patients like those with left main disease (0.55%), EF <30% (0.30%), and those who are NYHA functional class IV (0.29%). Clinical stroke is uncommon (<0.1%) during coronary angiography,[2,34] but may develop due to cholesterol, atherosclerotic, or clot embolization.[35,36] The results of an embolic stroke during routine angiography are generally reversible. Embolization of air is also a potential complication but can be easily prevented with newer injectors designed to minimize its risk and also following basic, but necessary, precautions when using a manifold. Cholesterol embolization has been reported in several vascular beds as a result of angiography.[37, 38] Nerve damage and/or pain have been also described.[39] The once widely publicized risk of lactic acidosis with metformin has decreased by avoiding the medication before and after the procedure until renal function is known to be recovered.[40]

Severe allergic reactions are uncommon and avoidable with the premedication of those at risk 18–24 hours before the procedure. Prednisone 20–40 mg, cimetidine 300 mg every 6 hours, diphenhydramine, and the use of nonionic contrast minimize risk. A dose of steroids prior to the coronary angiography has also been successful in decreasing the risk of a reaction.[10] A severe in-lab reaction can be treated with the use of IV epinephrine (0.1 mg = 1 mL of the 1:10,000 solution) every 2 minutes until the systemic blood pressure and the effected airways respond favorably. (See Chapter 6 for more information on pharmacology.).

Contrast-associated nephropathy is a well-established and not uncommon complication of coronary angiography.

Measures like early hydration (pre- and postprocedure) and the use of low-osmolar contrast agent are of clear benefit. Other agents like *N*-acetyl-L-cysteine and sodium bicarbonate have been used to decrease the risk of renal failure in vulnerable patients with conflicting results.[20,29] Despite the fact that more complicated and morbidly compromised patients are being referred for coronary angiography, the rates of complications have not significantly changed.[31,34,41] Although radiation safety is the focus of Chapter 3, it is worth mentioning that the widespread usage and availability of angiography have allowed for patients to have multiple radiation-exposing procedures (angiographic and otherwise). This repeated exposure increases the risk of cumulative radiation injury.[42,43]

SINGLE- AND DUAL-AXIS ROTATIONAL CORONARY ANGIOGRAPHY

Fundamentals of rotational coronary angiography

Single-axis rotational angiography (Figure 18.2) is a novel image acquisition technique that was designed and developed to address some of the limitations of traditional angiography.[25,27,44,45] The justification for rotational acquisition is straightforward: coronary arteries and other vascular structures must be visualized from multiple projection angles to adequately appreciate their structure in the resultant 2D X-ray projection images (Figure 18.5). Rotational angiography acquires the same images as traditional angiography but is automated, can be standardized, and provides an extensive panoramic view of key anatomic features for diagnostic and interventional purposes (Figure 18.5).

Both standard and rotational angiography acquire runs of projection images, but the imaging perspective is fundamentally different. Coronary angiography has traditionally employed acquisitions with a fixed projection during each injection. The gantry is moved to multiple positions and additional imaging runs are acquired with different degrees of RAO and LAO rotation and different degrees of cranial and caudal angulation.

Single-axis dual-motion rotational angiography requires a cranial (Figure 18.2) and a caudal acquisition for the left coronary artery (LCA) and a cranial acquisition for the RCA. The preset acquisition arc rotates from the beginning position to the end position producing a set of trajectories that maximize coronary visualization. A complete study will therefore have three total acquisitions (one cranial for the LCA, one caudal for the LCA, and a cranial for the RCA). Single-axis rotational angiography has now evolved into a single acquisition that rotates from LAO caudal to RAO caudal subsequently breaking the "x" axis (dual axis) and angulating toward RAO cranial and ending at LAO cranial (Figure 18.3). A prolonged single-axis 180° rotation with no angulation that extends from LAO 120° to RAO 60° has been the driving imaging

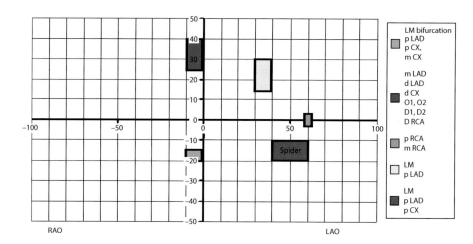

Figure 18.5 Basic representation of several coronary segment views. Please note the similarities in views when compared with the universal optimal view map. CX, circumflex; D, diagonal; LAD, left anterior descending artery; LAO, left anterior oblique; LM, left main; m, mid; O, obtuse marginal; p, proximal; RAO, right anterior oblique; RCA, right coronary artery.

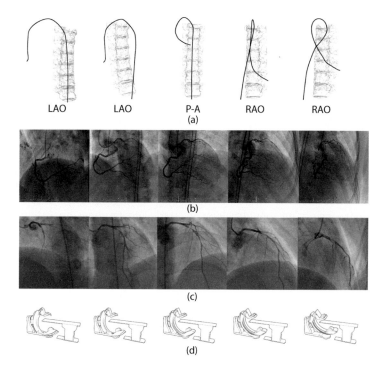

Figure 18.6 Rotational angiographic images. **(a)** Catheter position in relation to the spine. The tip of the catheter to the left of the spine and the catheter in the form of an inverted "U" shape suggest LAO rotation. The tip of the catheter to the right of the spine and the catheter shape in an overlapped form suggest RAO rotation. The tip of the catheter on top of the spine suggests no significant RAO or LAO rotation. This concept also applies to the RCA injection as shown on the dual injection performed in **(b)**. **(b)** RA (cranial) of a dual injection in the LCA and the RCA. **(c)** RA of the LCA. Note the relationship between the angiographic image obtained for both vessels and the position of the gantry below **(d)**. From left to right the angiographic images and the gantry representations rotate from LAO to RAO with 25° of cranial angulation. The presence of the diaphragm on all images suggests that they are cranial in angulation. LAO, left anterior oblique; LCA, left coronary artery; RA, rotational angiography; RAO, right anterior oblique; RCA, right coronary artery.

technique for newer and promising manual and automatic gated vessel reconstructions from actual volumetric data (Figure 18.6).[25] Different angiographic techniques, including standard angiography, single-axis rotational angiography, and dual-axis rotational angiography are further described in Figure 18.7.

ADVANTAGES OF ROTATIONAL ANGIOGRAPHY

The rotational representation of the coronary tree also allows for a better 3D understanding of the spatial relationships of the coronary tree branches by virtue of the rotating

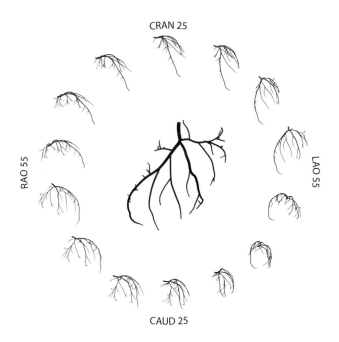

Figure 18.7 Single-axis rotational coronary angiography representation of trajectory images. Note how with two rotational acquisitions a complete survey of the anatomy is delivered. The cranial rotation goes from RAO 55° to LAO 55°. The caudal rotation goes from RAO 55° to LAO 55°. CAUD, caudal; CRAN, cranial; LAO, left anterior oblique; RAO, right anterior oblique.

2D image. Rotational angiography protocols can provide up to 360 projections of the arterial tree from different angles during a single coronary injection as opposed to the limited views provided by standard angiography. The safety of diagnostic rotational angiography has been well established and has shown a significant reduction in contrast and radiation exposure while maintaining similar or lower procedural times. The data show that rotational angiography has a 30%–40% reduction on contrast exposure and at least a 15% reduction in radiation exposure when compared to standard angiography.[27,44,45] Other studies show a similar contrast exposure reduction but fail to show a significant reduction in radiation exposure.[44] This is in part related to the different protocols used and the inherent difference in the imaging systems (flat X-ray detector vs. an image intensifier with or without cardiac optimization). Finally, the fact that rotational angiography uses a larger field of view is an important factor in the reduction of total radiation, although prior studies do show that the reduction is mostly driven by the acquisition of less images.[27] While all the studies have been with the single-axis rotational angiography platform, newer studies with the dual-axis rotational angiography promise to deliver lower radiation exposure and total contrast volume use.

Last but not least, rotational angiography provides the perfect platform for several advanced imaging applications, like online 3D modeling with optimal view map creation (Figure 18.1c), rapid 3D modeling, and manual or automated gated vessel reconstructions (Figure 18.6).

Rotational angiography provides the datasets that can be converted into 3D information via 3D volumetric reconstructions. As with the coronary circulation, 3D vascular angiography has the potential to provide optimal imaging, increase diagnostic accuracy, simulate complex procedures, and potentially improve patient outcomes.

LIMITATIONS OF ROTATIONAL ANGIOGRAPHY

Despite the visual appeal, better safety, and the standardized acquisition technique of rotational angiography, the inherent limitations of 2D projection imaging remain. While rotational angiography may improve the ability to visualize a lesion, the accurate selection of the optimal projection is still dependent on the operator's visual skills. Furthermore, rotational angiography cannot simulate views based on acquired images and provides no quantification of important 3D vessel features and, hence, the need for angiographic 3D image reconstructions. A list of attributes and limitations of all imaging technologies discussed in this Chapter are provided in Table 18.3.

3D CORONARY MODELING AND RECONSTRUCTIONS

Two techniques have been developed for the 3D representation of vascular structures, including the coronary anatomy (Table 18.4).

Coronary modeling

The 3D modeling technique uses 3D centerline data and shaded or rendered surfaces; the diameter and 3D morphologic structure of the vessel is subsequently derived with a computer algorithm (Figure 18.8). The 3D "modeling" technique uses two or more angiographic projections to extract features of the vessel and create a 3D representation (Figure 18.1c). A 3D modeling algorithm using single plane angiography that does not require a calibration object has been developed and prospectively validated.[8,46,47,49,50] The accuracy of the 3D modeling method is dependent on a computer-based, four-step algorithm that integrates 2D projections into a 3D image. Modeling is useful in the sense that it only requires orthogonal views of a given structure. Given the lack of volumetric data, it is not as precise as a reconstruction, but it allows 3D imaging of traditionally difficult to reconstruct structures, like the coronary arteries. This is mostly important in standard angiography laboratories without rotational capabilities. Rotational angiography provides the perfect platform for 3D modeling techniques (Table 18.5).

Coronary reconstruction

3D reconstructed images can be generated from techniques that acquire volumetric data points, such as rotational

Table 18.3 Comparison of coronary angiographic imaging technologies

| | | Invasive angiography | | Non-invasive angiography | |
	SCA	180° P–A rotational angiography	Single- and dual-axis rotational angiography	CTA	MRCA
Contrast exposure	+/++	++	+++	+/++	*Gadolinium*
Radiation exposure	++	+++	+++	+	*n/a*
Procedural time	++	++	+++	++	+
Invasiveness	+	+	+	+++	+++
Image quality	+++	++	+++	+++	++
Minimizes imaging inaccuracies	+	+++	++	+++	+++
Provides volumetric data	[a]+	+++	[b]++	+++	+++
Allows for pre-procedural planning	+	++	+	+++	+++
Applicability in unstable patients	+++	++	+++	*+ Elev. HR=+ Low BP=+*	*+ Elev. HR=+++ Low BP=+*
Applicability in obese patients	+++	+/++	+/++	+	+
Compatibility with implanted devices	+++	+++	+++	+	+
Applicability to calcified vessels	+++	+++	+++	+/++	+/++
Applicability to COPD patients	+++	+++	+/++	+	+

Note: +++, very favorable; ++, moderately favorable; +, least favorable. 3D, three-dimensional; 4D, four-dimensional; BP, blood pressure; COPD, chronic obstructive pulmonary disease; CTA, computed tomography angiography; HR, heart rate; MRCA, magnetic resonance coronary angiography; n/a, not applicable; P–A, posteroanterior; SCA, standard coronary angiography.
[a] Requires 3D vessel modeling.
[b] Requires 3D modeling or 3D/4D vessel reconstruction.

Table 18.4 Coronary angiographic data processing techniques

	3D modeling—3D representation	3D reconstruction
Image input	>2 orthogonal views (>30°)	Multiple images required
Image source	3D centerline based	True shape reconstruction
Vessel measurements	Size and diameter are derived from a computer algorithm	Uses actual volumetric data
Surface rendering	n/a	3D surface appearance is the product of shading
Volume rendering and maximum intensity projection (MIP)	n/a	Incorporates entire data set in image; intravascular details, spatial relationship, and structures are preserved

Note: 3D, three-dimensional; n/a, not applicable.

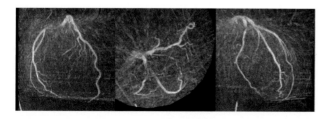

Figure 18.8 Three-dimensional reconstruction of the left coronary artery based on 180° rotational angiography.

angiography, computed tomography (CT), or magnetic resonance imaging (MRI) (Table 18.5). Several methods that are capable of generating 3D images have been described and, in general, can be divided into surface-rendering or volume-rendering techniques. The surface-rendering method relies on a computer algorithm to reconstruct intensity values that are above a specific defined threshold and represent volumetric surfaces within the data set; all values below the set threshold are discarded and not used for image generation. The resultant image is a representation of the surface contour and appears 3D through

Table 18.5 Comparison between 3D modeling and 3D reconstruction

	3D modeling	3D reconstruction
Ease of use	+++	++
Coronary measurements reliability	Size +, Length +++	+++
Image acquisition requirements (# views)	+++	+ (requires rotational angiography)
SCA compatible	Yes	No
RA compatible	Yes	Yes (requires 180° rotation)
CTA based	n/a	Yes
MRCA based	n/a	Yes

Note: +++, very favorable; ++, moderately favorable; +, least favorable; 3D, three-dimensional; CTA, computed tomography angiography; MRCA, magnetic resonance coronary angiography; RA, rotational angiography; SCA, standard coronary angiography. Newer algorithms are now fully automated·

computer-generated shading. While surface rendering is fast, it uses only a small portion of the acquired data and is less reliable during imaging of structures smaller than 2–3 mm. The maximum intensity projection (MIP) algorithm is another commonly used surface-rendering technique. 3D imaging using volume rendering is a more powerful technique that incorporates the entire dataset into the 3D image. In contrast to surface-rendering techniques, intravascular details and spatial relationships between adjacent structures are preserved.[51–55]

The 3D "reconstruction" technique is dependent upon multiple image projections for the creation of a volumetric representation of the vessel (Figure 18.6). In contrast, the 3D reconstruction technique refers to a computer-generated representation of the true shape and size of the imaged vessel using actual volumetric data obtained from rotational angiography, CTA (Figure 18.9), or magnetic resonance (Figure 18.6).[44,51,56] Interest in improving patient outcomes by optimizing the imaging of complex visual structures has been paramount in the design and creation of 3D imaging techniques. Over the last decade, significant progress has been made in the development of new invasive and noninvasive imaging techniques that permit accurate, real-time, 3D displays of structures.

Coronary optimal view map

3D modeling and 3D reconstructions are able to provide the datasets that allow for the development of an optimal view map. This optimal view map can be generated for each coronary segment and provides foreshortening and overlap for all segments.[18] The use of these 3D modeling techniques and view maps in the contemporary laboratory has been tested (Figures 18.1c and 18.8).[13,18,50,57]

Advantages of 3D imaging

Quantifying 3D vessel properties and characteristics of a given vessel are necessary in contemporary interventional cardiology. The ACC and AHA outline specific vessel properties that define the risk of a given lesion (Table 18.6).[58] It is important to note that these vessel characteristics are inherently 3D in nature; therefore, a complete analysis requires a 3D evaluation. Traditionally, the cardiologist has been unable to quantify some of these important variables, relying on visual estimation of given characteristics like tortuosity, flexion, torsion, and displacement of a vessel. Standardization of these vessel characteristics will lead to a more comprehensive evaluation of the vasculature that will subsequently improve procedural outcomes.

3D images via optimal view maps or simple direct evaluation can provide information on images with minimal foreshortening and minimal overlap.[9,13,14,25] In addition, recent X-ray–based advancements have allowed for the direct visualization of *in vivo* stents with 3D reconstructions.[59] Future research may allow a complete volumetric reconstruction based on a standard acquisition.

LESION CHARACTERISTICS

There is still controversy as to what diameter stenosis defines significant CAD. It is well known that typically a 70% lesion can provoke ischemia.[58] The Coronary Artery Surgery Study (CASS) criteria for defining significant disease was diameter stenosis >50% in the left main or diameter stenosis >70% in any other major epicardial vessel or branch. Lesion morphology and lesion characteristics are equally important when defining CAD (Table 18.6). This lesion classification allows the estimation of PCI procedural risk. Type A are simple lesions, Type B are moderately complex lesions divided into B1 (lesions with only one B characteristic), and B2 (lesions with more than 2 B characteristics), and C are high risk.[58–62] Further angiographic lesion characteristics are shown in Table 18.7.

CORONARY COMPUTED TOMOGRAPHY ANGIOGRAPHY

Fundamentals

The cardiac applications of CT are a rapidly growing diagnostic area because of the ability to visualize plaque

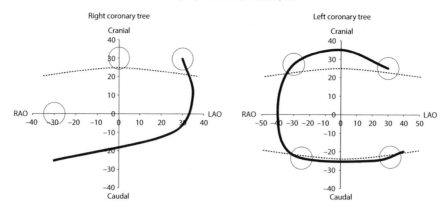

Figure 18.9 Representation of the imaging trajectories or sites of standard coronary angiography (*circled*), rotational coronary angiography (*dotted lines*), and DARCA (*solid lines*) for each coronary vessel. DARCA, dual-motion rotational coronary angiography; LAO, left anterior oblique; RAO, right anterior oblique.

Table 18.6 Type B1 lesions have one characteristic of Type B lesions, whereas Type B2 lesions have two or more of the Type B lesion characteristics

	Type A	Type B	Type C
Length	< 10 mm	10-20 mm	>20 mm
Lesion morphology	Concentric	Eccentric	Excessive tortuosity
Pathway to lesion	Easy access	Moderate tortuosity	Extreme angulation >90°
Angulation	<45 °	>45 ° but <90 °	>90°
Lesion contour	Smooth	Irregular	-
Calcium in vessel	Little or none	Moderate to heavy	-
% Stenosis	Not occluded	Occlusion <3 months	-
Location	Not ostial	Ostial	-
Side branch (SB)	No major SB	True bifurcation lesion	Unable to protect SB
Thrombus presence	None	Some	Degenerative vein graft

Source: Modified from Ellis, S.G., et al., *Circulation*, 82(4), 1193–1202, 1990. With permission.

burden, artery calcification, and luminal obstruction noninvasively.[63,64] Several studies have shown the indications that could aid physicians in the management of symptomatic and asymptomatic patients. A symptomatic patient who has no calcification is associated with both a lower risk of an abnormal nuclear study and angiographic obstruction. The invasive nature, expense, and risk resulting from invasive angiography have been instrumental in encouraging the development of new diagnostic methods that allow the coronary arteries to be visualized noninvasively.[64] Electron beam tomography and multidetector spiral computed tomography (MDCT) have been used in an effort to visualize the coronary arteries after the administration of IV contrast. Both have high spatial and temporal resolutions as well as excellent signal-to-noise ratios, which allows major branches of the coronary tree to be depicted.[65] The axial images are then used by the software to generate a volume rendering or reconstruction (Figure 18.9). Although reconstructions are used for the diagnosis of CAD because the images are visually appealing, the most reliable images come from the MIP of the vessels (Figure 18.10).

3D reconstructions have no added diagnostic value other than the documentation of the overall findings.[2]

Currently, there is much interest in the assessment of CAD using MDCT. Recent advances in MDCT have provided the opportunity to noninvasively and three-dimensionally evaluate the coronary vasculature in a safe and efficient manner. Newer CT imaging technology with faster gantry rotations, dual-source X-ray scanners, multidetector 64-, 128-, 256-, and recently 320-row acquisitions and electrocardiogram (ECG) gating has substantially improved both temporal and spatial resolutions to adequately visualize the moving coronary vasculature. Current generation MDCT scanners are able to achieve a spatial resolution of 0.4 mm with a temporal resolution as low as 83 m/sec during a less than 15 second cardiac acquisition. Initial relatively small studies evaluating the diagnostic accuracy of 64 slice-MDCT compared with diagnostic cardiac catheterization have demonstrated sensitivities ranging from 80% to 94% and specificities ranging from 95% to 97%.[66,67]

Table 18.7 Coronary angiographic lesions and their respective description

Angiographic lesion	Description
Angulated lesion	Angle from the vessel to the proximal lesion
Collaterals (Fig 18.3f)	Networks of tiny anastamotic branches interconnect the major coronary arteries
Contrast streaming (Fig 18.3j)	Inadequate vessel opacification results in uneven contrast lining of the vessel suggesting pseudolesions
Coronary aneurysm (Fig 18.3d)	Focal dilation of a coronary segment that includes all elements of the vessel wall.
Coronary artery fistula (Fig 18.3o)	Communication between a coronary and the PA, aorta, a cardiac vein, and another artery or a chamber
Coronary ectasia (Fig 18.3d)	Enlargement or increase of the size of a coronary artery
Coronary spasm (Fig 18.3i)	Transient vessel contraction (can be catheter induced)
Coronary thrombus (Fig 18.3k)	Filling defects consistent with clot within the arterial lumen
Diffuse disease (Fig 18.3n)	Long segments with varying degrees of stenosis
Eccentric lesion (Fig 18.3h)	Vessel lesion characterized by an uneven distribution of the plaque in relation to vessel wall
Foreshortening (Fig 18.10)	Imaging phenomenon that occurs based on perpendicularity of the vessel to X-ray beam
Muscle bridge (Fig 18.3n)	A dip in the coronary artery below the epicardial surface under small strips of myocardium
Ostial lesion and bifurcation lesion (Fig 18.3h)	Ostial is a lesion located 3 mm of the origin of the vessel. Bifurcation disease is that of the main branch and the side branch
Total occlusion (Fig 18.3g)	A complete lack of flow into a closed segment
Vessel calcification (Fig 18.3k)	Presence of calcium in the vessel
Vessel dissection (Fig 18.3b and 18.3k)	Creation of a false lumen between the intima and the media
Vessel overlap (Fig 18.3e)	Imaging phenomenon that occurs when vessels or coronary segments are one on top of the other
Vessel tortuosity (Fig 18.3a)	Refers to the lack of longitudinal path of the coronary. Frequent turns are of the vessel are seen

Note: PA, pulmonary artery.

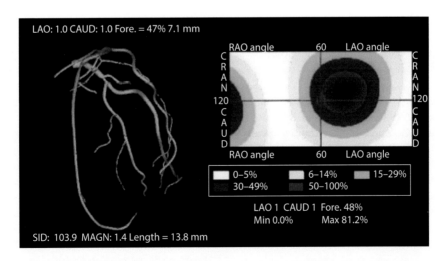

Figure 18.10 Three-dimensional representation of a "modeled" coronary tree with the subsequent optimal view map generation of the proximal left anterior descending artery. Please note the potential angiographic views on the map with the respective color representing foreshortening. White represents least amount of foreshortening, whereas red represents the most amount of foreshortening. The current LAO 1 CAUD 1 view angiographically has a 47% degree of foreshortening visually and on the optimal view map. CAUD, caudal; CRAN, cranial; Fore, foreshortening; LAO, left anterior oblique; MAGN, magnification; Max, maximum; Min, minimum; RAO, right anterior oblique.

Routine evaluation of coronary MDCT involves segmentation of the individual visualized coronary vessels. From the resulting coronary tree, determinations are easily made regarding vessel length, curvature, branching angles, stenosis length, location, and severity (Figure 18.10). Additionally, atherosclerotic plaque composition can be easily assessed. Due to high CT attenuation of calcified lesions, they are differentiated from fibrous or lipid-rich lesions. These angiographic features are easily displayed on MDCT-derived 3D volumetric and anatomic representations.[68–71]

Imaging of coronary stents with CTA is also possible. Newer algorithms do allow for the evaluation of postintervention patients, although the image quality of the stented segment lacks reliability. The evaluation of the in-stent restenosis is therefore possible but limited in certain patients. The visualization of the patency or occlusion of bypass grafts is also possible, but limitations do exist when accurately and completely evaluating the anastomosis sites.

Indications

The visualization of plaque is paramount in the diagnosis of CAD. The ability of CT to evaluate plaque has been the product of a significant amount of research. The detection, quantification, and characterization of coronary plaque do play a significant role in risk assessment. Under the assumption that lipid-rich, thin fibrous cap plaques are at risk of rupture with subsequent thrombosis more so than fibrotic plaque, researchers have tried to use CT attenuation values to differentiate plaque types.[72–74] The implications and clinical value of stenting vulnerable plaques have not been established. While one of the strongest indications for CT relies on its ability for risk stratification based on plaque presence evaluation, very few clinical guidelines exist in the United States for this imaging technology and MR. The appropriate use and indications for coronary angiography with CT are shown in Table 18.2. It is based on the ACCF/ACR/SCMR/ASNC/NASCI/SCAI/SIR 2006 Appropriateness criteria for Cardiac Computed Tomography and Cardiac Magnetic Resonance Imaging: A Report of the American College of Cardiology Foundation Quality Strategic Directions Committee Appropriateness Criteria Working Group, American College of Radiology, Society of Cardiovascular Computed Tomography, Society for Cardiovascular Magnetic Resonance, American Society of Nuclear Cardiology, North American Society for Cardiac Imaging, Society for Cardiovascular Angiography and Interventions, and Society of Interventional Radiology and the 2010 focused update.[75]

Contraindications

A list of appropriate/uncertain/inappropriate indications for CT is shown in Table 18.2. There are no absolute contraindications to perform CTA other than a patient unwilling to consent. Risks, such as radiation exposure and contrast adverse effects, should be considered. It is expected that patients being evaluated can achieve a breath hold that is required for the acquisition, are under the weight limit of the table, and have no significant heart rate variability. For the most part, it is expected that patients not present with any of the following:

1. Irregular heart rhythm (e.g., atrial fibrillation/flutter, frequent irregular premature ventricular contractions, or premature atrial contractions, and high-grade heart block)
2. Obesity (Body mass index > 40 kg/m²)
3. Renal insufficiency, creatinine greater than 1.8 mg/dL
4. Heart rate greater than 70 beats/minute refractory to heart-rate-lowering agents (e.g., a combination of beta-blocker and calcium-channel blocker)
5. Metallic interference (e.g., surgical clips, pacemakers, and/or defibrillator wires, coils, or tissue expander)[76]

For CT angiography, patients should be able to

1. Hold still
2. Follow breathing instructions
3. Take nitroglycerin (for performing coronary CT angiography only)
4. Take iodine in spite of steroid prep for contrast allergy
5. Lift both arms above the shoulders[76]

Advantages

Although patients are still exposed to radiation and contrast, CTA delivers a noninvasive coronary angiographic evaluation without the added risk of the more invasive SCA. Furthermore, some studies support the use of CTA as a safe and effective noninvasive imaging modality for defining coronary arterial anomalies in an appropriate clinical setting, providing detailed 3D anatomic information that may be difficult to obtain with invasive angiography.[77]

The use of CTA in the risk stratification, triage, and evaluation of patients continues to be evaluated with very promising results (Table 18.2).

Having the CTA images available for evaluation in planned PCI has now introduced the concept of preplanning. Operators are able to evaluate a myriad of coronary features that help in preparation for the case. Lesion characteristics (e.g., occlusion, calcification, side branch), pathway to the lesion (e.g., angulation, tortuosity), and even the shape of the aorta can be evaluated before an actual procedure. Potential equipment selection (e.g., stent size, stent length, guide catheter) is now a decision that the operator can make even before the procedure starts. The usefulness of this approach is formally being evaluated by several groups.[78,79]

3D imaging using volume rendering is a powerful technique that incorporates the entire dataset into the 3D image. In contrast to surface-rendering techniques, intravascular details and spatial relationships between adjacent structures are preserved (Tables 18.4 and 18.5). The vascular model can be refined further if data from the heart structures and vessel wall are available from the primary imaging modality, as with CTA, or after fusion of two modalities, such as intravascular ultrasound (IVUS) and the 3D coronary lumen

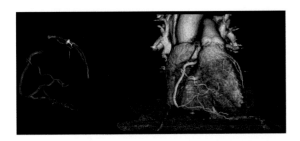

Figure 18.11 Computed tomography angiography rendering with subsequent image reconstruction.

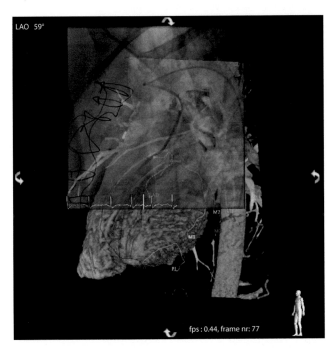

Figure 18.12 CTA and angiography image fusion. Note the overlay of the real-time angiographic data (*small square*) on the CTA data. The catheter is visualized in real time under X-ray guidance with an overlay of the CTA showing the position of an otherwise difficult to cannulate saphenous vein graft to the left anterior descending artery. Note the location of the rest of the coronary anatomy highlighted and labeled on the CTA image. CTA, computed tomography angiography; LAO, left anterior oblique; M1, obtuse marginal one; M2, obtuse marginal two; M3, obtuse marginal three; PL, posterolateral; RCA, right coronary artery.

from X-ray image–based reconstruction as an example. This new multimodality fusion concept that incorporates imaging technologies like CTA and X-ray–based images during a procedure holds the future of image guidance (Figures 18.11 and 18.12).[80,81]

Limitations

Impaired image quality, due to dense calcifications and multiple image artifacts, including coronary artery motion and breathing artifacts, limits the clinical utility of noninvasive coronary angiography. Due to several reasons as outlined above, some patients become less than ideal candidates for CTA as the images may be uninterpretable.

Patients may receive a considerable amount of radiation from X-ray–based studies and this includes CTA. A patient's exposure (effective dose equivalent) from a routine chest X-ray is 0.02–0.04 mSv. Although this is equipment and operator dependent, an average diagnostic catheterization is <8 mSv, while a coronary intervention is around 15 mSv. Multidetector CTA is around 20 mSv with a Thallium perfusion test just above that at 22–24 mSv.

The presence of any metallic interference (e.g., surgical clips, pacemakers, and/or defibrillator wires, coils, or tissue expander) is a limitation but not a contraindication to the imaging capabilities of CTA.[76]

MAGNETIC RESONANCE CORONARY ANGIOGRAPHY

Cardiac magnetic resonance imaging is a rapidly evolving noninvasive imaging modality that will further advance the goal of providing 3D imaging (Figure 18.13). Cardiac magnetic resonance has become an established imaging modality for the assessment of various cardiac disorders, including myocardial viability, infiltrative cardiomyopathies, CHD, anomalous coronary arteries, bypass grafts, cardiac masses, and aortic and pericardial diseases.[82–86]

MRCA is a technique that allows for a noninvasive visualization of the coronary arteries. MRCA has gained considerable importance as a noninvasive method to diagnose coronary artery stenosis and is an area of active research.[87–89] The benefit of MRCA is to not only visualize the coronary arteries, but also to evaluate cardiac morphology and function in one setting.[85,86]

Current techniques with 3D navigator MRCA imaging can obtain a coronary artery dataset in approximately 10–15 minutes. Analogous to MDCT, from a MRCA volumetric dataset, 3D vessel features, including vessel tortuosity, lesion lengths, and bifurcation angles can be evaluated, quantified, and translated to the interventional cardiologist.

Fundamentals

Since the concept of ionizing radiation has been discussed in Chapters 1 and 3, an abbreviated understanding of magnetic resonance is required. The physical interaction required for magnetic resonance is related to the atomic nucleus. The frequency of the radiowave absorption depends on the strength of the external magnetic field. Because magnetic resonance therefore does not interfere with the atomic shell, which is responsible for chemical binding, it is fundamentally safe, unlike ionizing radiation, which may interact with electrobinding, damaging molecules such as DNA. Magnetic resonance only interacts with unpaired spin atomic nuclei, which are basically seen in water and fat (hydrogen-1 abundant tissues).[2] Since these tissues are abundant in the body, images with a high signal-to-noise ratio can be easily obtained. The nuclei, when exposed to a magnetic field, will behave as

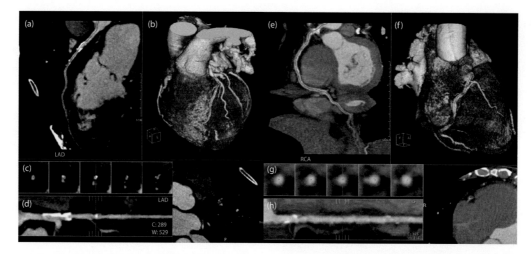

Figure 18.13 Computed tomography angiography of the LAD **(a–d)** and the RCA **(e–h)**. The initial image on the left **(a)** shows a MIP image of the LAD followed by a volume rendering **(b)** contiguous to it. The same applies for the RCA on the right panel that has a MIP image of the RCA **(e)** followed by its respective volume rendering **(f)**. The lower panel shows for each vessel a stretched MIP image displaying each vessel lumen **(d, h)** in a longitudinal fashion with its respective "intravascular ultrasound" like cut of the lumen **(c, g)**. The LAD shows moderate calcification in the proximal segment **(a, d)** with a moderate to severe obstruction that was also seen on standard angiography. The RCA has very mild proximal calcification **(e, h)** followed by a widely patent lumen with no significant disease on the regular MIP **(e)** image or the stretched MIP **(h)**. LAD, left anterior descending artery; MIP, maximum intensity projection; RCA, right coronary artery.

a magnet. The nuclei precess randomly about 1.5 T magnetic field at a resonance frequency of 63 MHz, which is in the radiowave range. When excited by radiowaves, the nuclei will rotate away from the direction of the main magnetic field and precess in a coordinated manner, which causes a net magnetization. In its relaxation form, this signal is then captured as radio wave echo by the scanner in a form that can be subsequently transformed into an image by the receiver antenna.[2]

The cardiac magnetic resonance scanner consists of several pieces: (1) the superconducting magnet that produces the static magnetic field; (2) the radiofrequency amplifier that generates the pulses; (3) the radiofrequency antenna or receiver that captures them; and (4) the computer hardware and software that allow for the management of the data with subsequent image creation. The gating of the images based on the electrocardiographic R-R is what allows for the system to minimize the movement through the changes of the cardiac cycle and respiratory motion. The acquisition sequence is composed of the following block components: (1) cardiac triggering to suppress cardiac motion; (2) respiratory motion suppression; (3) prepulses to enhance contrast-to-noise ratio (CNR) of the coronary blood; and (4) image acquisition enhancement. Multiple methods for coronary evaluation exist and include conventional spin-echo coronary MRI (very limited), 2D segmented k space gradient echo coronary MRI, 3D coronary MRI methods (the predominant approach for the past decade), the more advanced spiral and radial coronary MRI method, and 3T coronary MRI method.

MRCA is still technically challenging and relatively expensive but several studies have shown its value.[82,90] Although the imaging limitations of cardiac magnetic resonance related to its spatial resolution challenge its ability

to evaluate CAD with confidence, it is very useful in the diagnosis and recognition of anomalous coronary origins.[91] Cardiac magnetic resonance has also been used in the evaluation of coronary flow (adenosine stress related evaluation) reserve and the subsequent diagnosis of a significant coronary lesion and on saphenous vein graft evaluations.[92,93]

Indications

There is no formal guideline for use of MRCA, but Table 18.2 does include the appropriateness criteria from the ACCF/ACR/SCMR/ASNC/NASCI/SCAI/SIR 2006 Appropriateness criteria for Cardiac Computed Tomography and Cardiac Magnetic Resonance Imaging: A Report of the American College of Cardiology Foundation Quality Strategic Directions Committee Appropriateness Criteria Working Group, American College of Radiology, Society of Cardiovascular Computed Tomography, Society for Cardiovascular Magnetic Resonance, American Society of Nuclear Cardiology, North American Society for Cardiac Imaging, Society for Cardiovascular Angiography and Interventions, and Society of Interventional Radiology and 2010 focused update.[75]

Contraindications

Unlike CTA, there are currently several contraindications to the use of MRCA. Patients are assumed not to present with

1. Severe claustrophobia
2. Specific metallic devices that are contraindicated such as pacemakers, defibrillators, and certain aneurysm clips

Although studies are ongoing and have evaluated the safety of pacemakers and defibrillators when exposed to MR, the appropriateness criteria document from ACCF/ACR/SCMR/ASNC/NASCI/SCAI/SIR 2006 and 2010 focused update still does not reflect those changes.[75,76] In April 2005, the U.S. Food and Drug Administration (FDA) approved MRI studies immediately after implantation of sirolimus and paclitaxel-eluting stents.[75,76]

Although in the past gadolinium-based contrast for magnetic resonance was used in all patient populations, appropriate patient selection and caution should be exercised when using gadolinium in patients with renal failure due to the risk of nephrogenic fibrosing dermopathy.[94–96]

Advantages

MRCA without its requirement for more nephrotoxic contrast agents or exposure to ionizing radiation is an ideal noninvasive imaging modality to help plan and execute PCI. It allows for the evaluation of the coronary anatomy, pathway to the lesion, shape of the aorta, aneurysms, bypass patency, anomalous coronary origin, vessel wall characteristics, lesion characteristics, coronary flow reserve, and most importantly, can couple that with myocardial viability and potentially function. Due to its specificity, a normal coronary MRI suggests the absence of severe multivessel disease.

Limitations

Although the safety of MRI is well described, the full implications of magnetic field exposure have not been as well established as they have been for ionizing radiation. It is certainly reasonable that in the modern climate of safety priority, radiowave technology shares with echocardiography a sizable advantage over ionizing radiation.

The challenges for coronary MRCA include compensation for cardiac and respiratory motion, spatial resolution and coverage, high level of tortuosity of the coronary vessel, and signal-to-noise limitations due to adjacent epicardial fat and myocardium. Another limitation is that provided by the bare metal nature of stents (not so much tantalum). MRI has a sizable problem when evaluating coronary stents due to signal/voids artifacts at the site of the stent. Bypass graft imaging is limited by local signal loss/artifact caused by implanted metallic objects (hemostatic clips, ostial stainless steel graft markers, sternal wires, prosthetic valves, struts, rings, and graft stents). The technical aspects of MRCA are, however, quickly evolving, and multiple methods have been used to improve imaging (cardiac and respiratory motion compensation, breath-hold method, free-breathing methods, MR navigators-triggering alone, MR navigators-gating and slice tracking, electrocardiographic timing, and respiratory suppression methodology). Similar to cardiac CTA, ECG triggering is mandatory to prevent vessel blurring due to intrinsic cardiac motion. To suppress the effects of respiration, MRCA using respiratory gating (navigator echo technique) is performed to monitor diaphragmatic motion.

Current isotropic fast 3D techniques provide thinner slices, superior signal-to-noise ratios, and total coverage of coronary arteries over 2D MRCA techniques. Introduction of new intravascular contrast agents, novel data (k-space) sampling strategies, and higher field strength (3 Tesla) imaging will further enhance MRCA.[97]

A serious disadvantage of magnetic resonance is related to its inability to image patients with metallic implants. Although it is safe on valve prosthesis, vascular stents, and orthopedic implants, it has a serious limitation with pacemakers and defibrillators as the programming may change. There are, however, new FDA MRI approved devices and leads. Flying projectiles in the magnetic field have the potential to strike the patient or a staff member when the magnet is activated. Caution to avoid any metallic objects should be constantly exercised.

Magnetic resonance coronary angiography versus computed tomography angiography

In a meta-analysis of 39 studies published from 1991 to 2004,[98] the sensitivity and specificity of MRCA for the detection of CAD were 75% and 85% in per-vessel analyses, and 88% and 56% in per-patient analyses, respectively. In another meta-analysis in which 20 studies through 2009 were assessed,[99] the mean sensitivity and specificity of MRCA were 87% and 70%, respectively. The sensitivity and specificity of MRCA varied considerably between the studies, owing to heterogeneity of pulse sequences and analytic methods that were used. Higher magnetic field strength may improve the detection of CAD with coronary MRCA.

As for the difficulty in interpretation, there is no substantial difference between MRCA and CTA if the reader has sufficient experience in reading images obtained with both modalities. However, the number of hospitals performing CTA is much larger than is the number of those performing MRCA. Insufficient numbers of cardiac imaging practitioners with expertise in MRCA is one of the current major limitations of its assessment of the coronary arteries.[100]

CONCLUSION

Contemporary medicine has a diverse armamentarium of invasive and noninvasive imaging technologies to evaluate the coronary anatomy. The risk and benefits of each available imaging technique should be taken into consideration and tailored to the individual need of the clinical situation. This diversity allows the clinician the luxury of choosing an imaging evaluation that minimizes patient risk while delivering superior results.

DISCLOSURES

John D. Carroll is co-inventor of patented 3D vascular reconstruction and analysis software. The patents have been assigned to the University of Chicago and the University of Colorado. He has also received research grants from Philips Medical Systems.

REFERENCES

1. Runge MS, Ohman ME. *Netter's cardiology.* 1st edn. Teterboro, NJ: Icon learning systems LLC; 2004.
2. Zipes DP, et al. *Heart disease: A textbook of cardiovascular medicine.* 7th edn. Philadelphia, PA: Elsevier Saunders; 2005.
3. Mueller RL, Sanborn TA. The history of interventional cardiology: Cardiac catheterization, angioplasty, and related interventions. *Am Heart J.* 1995;129(1):146–172.
4. Schwartz JN, et al. Comparison of angiographic and postmortem findings in patients with coronary artery disease. *Am J Cardiol.* 1975;36(2):174–178.
5. Spears JR, et al. The minimum error in estimating coronary luminal cross-sectional area from cineangiographic diameter measurements. *Cathet Cardiovasc Diagn.* 1983;9(2):119–128.
6. Chen SJ, Carroll JD. 3-D reconstruction of coronary arterial tree to optimize angiographic visualization. *IEEE Trans Med Imaging.* 2000;19(4):318–336.
7. Chen SJ, et al. Three-dimensional reconstruction of coronary arterial tree based on biplane angiograms. *SPIE Med Imaging.* 1996;2710:103–114.
8. Chen SY, Metz CE. Improved determination of biplane imaging geometry from two projection images and its application to three-dimensional reconstruction of coronary arterial trees. *Med Phys.* 1997;24(5):633–654.
9. Garcia JA, et al. Initial clinical experience of selective coronary angiography using one prolonged injection and a 180 degrees rotational trajectory. *Catheter Cardiovasc Interv.* 2007;70(2):190–196.
10. Baim DS, Grossman W. *Grossman's cardiac catheterization, angiography, and intervention.* 6th edn. Philadelphia, PA: Lippincott Williams & Wilkins; 2000.
11. Scanlon PJ, et al. ACC/AHA guidelines for coronary angiography. A report of the American College of Cardiology/American Heart Association Task Force on practice guidelines (Committee on Coronary Angiography). Developed in collaboration with the Society for Cardiac Angiography and Interventions. *J Am Coll Cardiol.* 1999;33(6):1756–1824.
12. Topol EJ, Nissen SE. Our preoccupation with coronary luminology. The dissociation between clinical and angiographic findings in ischemic heart disease. *Circulation.* 1995;92(8):2333–42.
13. Green NE, et al. Angiographic views used for percutaneous coronary interventions: A three-dimensional analysis of physician-determined vs. computer-generated views. *Catheter Cardiovasc Interv.* 2005;64(4):451–459.
14. Green NE, et al. Three-dimensional vascular angiography. *Curr Probl Cardiol.* 2004;29(3):104–142.
15. Messenger JC, et al. 3D coronary reconstruction from routine single-plane coronary angiograms: Clinical validation and quantitative analysis of the right coronary artery in 100 patients. *Int J Card Imaging.* 2000;16(6):413–427.
16. Vetrovec G, Goudreau E. *Coronary angiography for the interventionalist.* 1st edn. New York: Chapman and Hall; 1994.
17. Kern MJ, editor. *The cardiac catheterization handbook.* 4th edn. Philadelphia, PA: Mosby; 2003.
18. Garcia JA. Optimal angiographic views based on 3D reconstructed models. *JACC.* 2007;49 Supplement B:(9):296A.
19. Galbraith JE, et al. Coronary angiogram interpretation. Interobserver variability. *JAMA.* 1978;240(19):2053–2056.
20. Mehran R, Nikolsky E. Contrast-induced nephropathy: Definition, epidemiology, and patients at risk. *Kidney Int Suppl.* 2006;100:S11–S15.
21. Mehran R, et al. A simple risk score for prediction of contrast-induced nephropathy after percutaneous coronary intervention: Development and initial validation. *J Am Coll Cardiol.* 2004;44(7):1393–1399.
22. Jorgensen NP, et al. Safety and tolerability of iodixanol in healthy volunteers with reference to two monomeric x-ray contrast media. *Eur J Radiol.* 1992;15(3):252–257.
23. Chen SY, Carroll JD. Kinematic and deformation analysis of 4-D coronary arterial trees reconstructed from cine angiograms. *IEEE Trans Med Imaging.* 2003;22(6):710–721.
24. Chen SY, et al. Quantitative analysis of reconstructed 3-D coronary arterial tree and intracoronary devices. *IEEE Trans Med Imaging.* 2002;21(7):724–740.
25. Garcia JA, et al. Rotational angiography (RA) and three-dimensional imaging (3-DRA): An available clinical tool. *Int J Cardiovasc Imaging.* 2007;23(1):9–13.
26. Leber AW, et al. Accuracy of 64-slice computed tomography to classify and quantify plaque volumes in the proximal coronary system: A comparative study using intravascular ultrasound. *J Am Coll Cardiol.* 2006;47(3):672–677.
27. Maddux JT, et al. Randomized study of the safety and clinical utility of rotational angiography versus standard angiography in the diagnosis of coronary artery disease. *Catheter Cardiovasc Interv.* 2004;62(2):167–174.
28. Pedersen HK, et al. Contrast-medium-induced ventricular fibrillation: Arrhythmogenic mechanisms and the role of antiarrhythmic drugs in dogs. *Acad Radiol.* 1995;2(12):1082–1088.
29. Nikolsky E, et al. Radiocontrast nephropathy: Identifying the high-risk patient and the implications of exacerbating renal function. *Rev Cardiovasc Med.* 2003;4 Suppl 1:S7–S14.
30. Bertrand ME, et al. Influence of a nonionic, iso-osmolar contrast medium (iodixanol) versus an ionic, low-osmolar contrast medium (ioxaglate) on major adverse cardiac events in patients undergoing percutaneous transluminal coronary angioplasty: A multicenter, randomized, double-blind study. Visipaque in Percutaneous Transluminal Coronary Angioplasty [VIP] Trial Investigators. *Circulation.* 2000;101(2):131–136.
31. Ammann P, et al. Procedural complications following diagnostic coronary angiography are related to the operator's experience and the catheter size. *Catheter Cardiovasc Interv.* 2003;59(1):13–18.
32. Samal AK, White CJ. Percutaneous management of access site complications. *Catheter Cardiovasc Interv.* 2002;57(1):12–23.
33. Witz M, et al. Retroperitoneal haematoma—a serious vascular complication of cardiac catheterisation. *Eur J Vasc Endovasc Surg.* 1999;18(4):364–365.
34. Segal AZ, et al. Stroke as a complication of cardiac catheterization: Risk factors and clinical features. *Neurology.* 2001;56(7):975–977.
35. Hinchey J, Sweeney PJ. Transient cortical blindness after coronary angiography. *Lancet.* 1998;351(9114):1513–1514.

36. Jackson JL, et al. Complications from cardiac catheterization: Analysis of a military database. *Mil Med.* 2000;165(4):298–301.

37. Blanco VR, et al. Retinal cholesterol emboli during diagnostic cardiac catheterization. *Catheter Cardiovasc Interv.* 2000;51(3):323–325.

38. Fukumoto Y, et al. The incidence and risk factors of cholesterol embolization syndrome, a complication of cardiac catheterization: A prospective study. *J Am Coll Cardiol.* 2003;42(2):211–216.

39. Kuruvilla A, et al. Femoral neuropathy following cardiac catheterization for balloon mitral valvotomy. *Int J Cardiol.* 1999;71(2):197–198.

40. Heupler FA, Jr. Guidelines for performing angiography in patients taking metformin. Members of the Laboratory Performance Standards Committee of the Society for Cardiac Angiography and Interventions. *Cathet Cardiovasc Diagn.* 1998;43(2):121–123.

41. Chandrasekar B, et al. Complications of cardiac catheterization in the current era: A single-center experience. *Catheter Cardiovasc Interv.* 2001;52(3):289–295.

42. Dehen L, et al. Chronic radiodermatitis following cardiac catheterisation: A report of two cases and a brief review of the literature. *Heart.* 1999;81(3):308–312.

43. Shechter G, et al. Three-dimensional motion tracking of coronary arteries in biplane cineangiograms. *IEEE Trans Med Imaging.* 2003;22(4):493–503.

44. Akhtar M, et al. Randomized study of the safety and clinical utility of rotational vs. standard coronary angiography using a flat-panel detector. *Catheter Cardiovasc Interv.* 2005;66(1):43–49.

45. Tommasini G, et al. Panoramic coronary angiography. *J Am Coll Cardiol.* 1998;31(4):871–877.

46. Chen SYJ, Carroll JD. 3-D reconstruction of coronary arterial tree to optimize angiographic visualization. *IEEE Trans Med Imag.* 2000;19:318–336.

47. Chen SYJ, et al. Quantitative analysis of reconstructed 3-D coronary arterial tree and intracoronary devices. *IEEE Trans Med Imag.* 2002;21(7):724–740.

48. Chen SYJ, et al. Three-dimensional reconstruction of coronary arterial tree based on biplane angiograms. *Proc SPIE Med Imag: Image Processing.* 1996;2710:103.

49. Gradaus R, et al. Clinical assessment of a new real time 3D quantitative coronary angiography system: Evaluation in stented vessel segments. *Catheter Cardiovasc Interv.* 2006;68(1):44–49.

50. Gollapudi RR, et al. Utility of three-dimensional reconstruction of coronary angiography to guide percutaneous coronary intervention. *Catheter Cardiovasc Interv.* 2007;69(4):479–482.

51. Budoff MJ, et al. Intravenous three-dimensional coronary angiography using contrast enhanced electron beam computed tomography. *Am J Cardiol.* 1999;83(6):840–845.

52. Kapouleas I, et al. Registration of three-dimensional MR and PET images of the human brain without markers. *Radiology.* 1991;181(3):731–739.

53. Rasche V, et al. *ECG-gated 3D-rotational coronary angiography (3DRCA).* In Lemke HU, Vannier MW, Inamura K, Farman AG, Doi K, Reiber JHC, editors. *CARS 2002 Computer Assisted Radiology and Surgery.* Paris: Springer; 2002. 827–831.

54. Schaffter T, et al. Motion compensated projection reconstruction. *Magn Reson Med.* 1999;41(5):954–963.

55. Hoffmann KR, et al. Determination of 3D imaging geometry and object configurations from two biplane views: An enhancement of the Metz-Fencil technique. *Med Phys.* 1995;22(8):1219–1227.

56. Makela T, et al. A 3-D model-based registration approach for the PET, MR and MCG cardiac data fusion. *Med Image Anal.* 2003;7(3):377–389.

57. Agostoni P, et al. Comparison of assessment of native coronary arteries by standard versus three-dimensional coronary angiography. *Am J Cardiol.* 2008;102(3):272–279.

58. Kern MJ, editor. *SCAI Interventional Cardiology review Book.* 1st edn. Philadelphia, PA: Lippincott Williams & Wilkins; 2007.

59. Movassaghi B, et al. 3D reconstruction of coronary stents in vivo based on motion compensated X-ray angiograms. *Med Image Comput Comput Assist Interv.* 2006;9(Pt 2):177–184.

60. Krone RJ, et al. Evaluation of the American College of Cardiology/American Heart Association and the Society for Coronary Angiography and Interventions lesion classification system in the current "stent era" of coronary interventions (from the ACC-National Cardiovascular Data Registry). *Am J Cardiol.* 2003;92(4):389–394.

61. Ellis SG, et al. Coronary morphologic and clinical determinants of procedural outcome with angioplasty for multivessel coronary disease. Implications for patient selection. Multivessel Angioplasty Prognosis Study Group. *Circulation.* 1990;82(4):1193–1202.

62. Kastrati A, et al. Prognostic value of the modified American College of Cardiology/American Heart Association Stenosis Morphology Classification for long-term angiographic and clinical outcome after coronary stent placement. *Circulation.* 1999;100(12):1285–1290.

63. Budoff MJ, Gul K. Computed tomographic cardiovascular imaging. *Semin Ultrasound CT MR.* 2006;27(1):32–41.

64. Budoff MJ, et al. Cardiac computed tomography: Diagnostic utility and integration in clinical practice. *Clin Cardiol.* 2006;29(9 Suppl 1):I4–14.

65. Budoff MJ. Noninvasive coronary angiography using computed tomography. *Expert Rev Cardiovasc Ther.* 2005;3(1):123–132.

66. Budoff MJ, et al. Prevalence of obstructive coronary artery disease in an outpatient cardiac CT angiography environment. *Int J Cardiol.* 2008;129(1):32–36.

67. Budoff MJ. Can non-invasive CT angiography effectively and safely triage patients? *Acad Radiol.* 2007;14(8):899–900.

68. De Feyter P, et al. MS-CT coronary imaging. *J Interv Cardiol.* 2003;16(6):465–468.

69. Nieman K, et al. Three-dimensional coronary anatomy in contrast-enhanced multislice computed tomography. *Prev Cardiol.* 2002;5(2):79–83.

70. Shapiro MD, et al. Utility of cardiovascular magnetic resonance to predict left ventricular recovery after primary percutaneous coronary intervention for patients presenting with acute ST-segment elevation myocardial infarction. *Am J Cardiol.* 2007;100(2):211–216.

71. Mueller D, Maeder A. Robust semi-automated path extraction for visualising stenosis of the coronary arteries. *Comput Med Imaging Graph.* 2008;32(6):463–475.

72. Kopp AF, et al. Non-invasive characterisation of coronary lesion morphology and composition by multislice CT: First results in comparison with intracoronary ultrasound. *Eur Radiol.* 2001;11(9):1607–1611.

73. Schroeder S, et al. Noninvasive plaque imaging using multislice detector spiral computed tomography. *Semin Thromb Hemost.* 2007;33(2):203–209.

74. Schuijf JD, et al. Differences in plaque composition and distribution in stable coronary artery disease versus acute coronary syndromes; non-invasive evaluation with multi-slice computed tomography. *Acute Card Care.* 2007;9(1):48–53.

75. Taylor AJ, et al. ACCF/SCCT/ACR/AHA/ASE/ASNC/NASCI/SCAI/SCMR 2010 appropriate use criteria for cardiac computed tomography. A report of the American College of Cardiology Foundation Appropriate Use Criteria Task Force, the Society of Cardiovascular Computed Tomography, the American College of Radiology, the American Heart Association, the American Society of Echocardiography, the American Society of Nuclear Cardiology, the North American Society for Cardiovascular Imaging, the Society for Cardiovascular Angiography and Interventions, and the Society for Cardiovascular Magnetic Resonance. *Circulation.* 2010;122(21):e525–555.

76. Hendel RC, et al. ACCF/ACR/SCCT/SCMR/ASNC/NASCI/SCAI/SIR 2006 appropriateness criteria for cardiac computed tomography and cardiac magnetic resonance imaging: a report of the American College of Cardiology Foundation Quality Strategic Directions Committee Appropriateness Criteria Working Group, American College of Radiology, Society of Cardiovascular Computed Tomography, Society for Cardiovascular Magnetic Resonance, American Society of Nuclear Cardiology, North American Society for Cardiac Imaging, Society for Cardiovascular Angiography and Interventions, and Society of Interventional Radiology. *J Am Coll Cardiol.* 2006;48(7):1475–1497.

77. Budoff MJ, et al. Coronary anomalies by cardiac computed tomographic angiography. *Clin Cardiol.* 2006;29(11):489–493.

78. Hecht HS. Applications of multislice coronary computed tomographic angiography to percutaneous coronary intervention: How did we ever do without it? *Catheter Cardiovasc Interv.* 2008;71(4):490–503.

79. Otsuka M, et al. Utility of multislice computed tomography as a strategic tool for complex percutaneous coronary intervention. *Int J Cardiovasc Imaging.* 2008;24(2):201–210.

80. Garcia JA, et al. On-line multi-slice computed tomography interactive overlay with conventional x-ray: A new and advanced imaging fusion concept. *Int J Cardiol.* 2009;133(3):e101–e105

81. Garcia JA, et al. Image guidance of percutaneous coronary and structural heart disease interventions using a CT and fluoroscopy integration. *Vasc Dis Manage.* 2007;4(3):89–97.

82. Nieman K, et al. Noninvasive coronary imaging in the new millennium: A comparison of computed tomography and magnetic resonance techniques. *Rev Cardiovasc Med.* 2002;3(2):77–84.

83. De Feyter PJ, et al. Non-invasive coronary artery imaging with electron beam computed tomography and magnetic resonance imaging. *Heart.* 2000;84(4):442–448.

84. Sakuma H. [Cardiac MRI: Current status and future prospective]. *Nihpon Igaku Hoshasen Gakkai Zasshi.* 2003;63(1):21–25.

85. Sakuma H. Cardiac magnetic resonance imaging. *Kyobu Geka.* 2007;60(8 Suppl):635–641.

86. Sakuma H, et al. Detection of coronary artery stenosis with whole-heart coronary magnetic resonance angiography. *J Am Coll Cardiol.* 2006;48(10):1946–1950.

87. Appelbaum E, et al. Coronary magnetic resonance imaging: Current state-of-the-art. *Coron Artery Dis.* 2005;16(6):345–353.

88. Maintz D, et al. Coronary magnetic resonance angiography for assessment of the stent lumen: A phantom study. *J Cardiovasc Magn Reson.* 2002;4(3):359–367.

89. Manning WJ, et al. Coronary magnetic resonance imaging. *Cardiol Clin.* 2007;25(1):141–70, vi.

90. Kim WY, et al. Cardiovascular magnetic resonance imaging of coronary atherothrombosis. *J Nucl Cardiol.* 2005;12(3):337–344.

91. Taylor AM, et al. Coronary artery imaging in grown up congenital heart disease: complementary role of magnetic resonance and x-ray coronary angiography. *Circulation.* 2000;101(14):1670–1678.

92. Langerak SE, et al. Value of magnetic resonance imaging for the noninvasive detection of stenosis in coronary artery bypass grafts and recipient coronary arteries. *Circulation.* 2003;107(11):1502–1508.

93. Salm LP, et al. Evaluation of saphenous vein coronary artery bypass graft flow by cardiovascular magnetic resonance. *J Cardiovasc Magn Reson.* 2005;7(4):631–637.

94. Artunc F, et al. [Nephrogenic systemic fibrosis] *Dtsch Med Wochenschr.* 2008;133 Suppl:F1.

95. Kintossou R, et al. Nephrogenic fibrosing dermopathy treated with extracorporeal photopheresis: Role of gadolinium?. *Ann Dermatol Venereol.* 2007;134(8–9):667–671.

96. Prchal D, et al. Nephrogenic systemic fibrosis: The story unfolds. *Kidney Int.* 2008;73(12):1335–1337.

97. Nassenstein K, et al. Magnetic resonance coronary angiography with vasovist: In-vivo T1 estimation to improve image quality of navigator and breath-hold techniques. Eur Radiol. 2008;18(1):103–109.

98. Danias PG, et al. Diagnostic performance of coronary magnetic resonance angiography as compared against conventional x-ray angiography: A meta-analysis. *J Am Coll Cardiol.* 2004;44(9):1867–1876.

99. Schuetz GM, et al. Meta-analysis: Noninvasive coronary angiography using computed tomography versus magnetic resonance imaging. *Ann Intern Med.* 2010;152(3):167–177.

100. Sakuma H, et al. Cardiovascular MR imaging. *Nippon Naika Gakkai Zasshi.* 2005;94(8):1625–1631.

PART 4

Catheterization in Special Circumstances

19

Cardiac catheterization for pediatric patients

ALBERT P. ROCCHINI

INTRODUCTION

Cardiac catheterization is an important diagnostic and therapeutic procedure in the pediatric patient with congenital heart disease. The four commonly used indications for cardiac catheterization in the pediatric patient are to make an anatomic diagnosis, to obtain a hemodynamic assessment, to perform a pharmacologic or catheter-based intervention, and to make an electrophysiological diagnosis and/or perform an electrophysiological intervention. With improvements in noninvasive imaging (echocardiography and magnetic resonance imaging), the use of cardiac catheterization to make an anatomic diagnosis has been significantly reduced. Today, the decision to catheterize a child with congenital heart disease is based on whether the anatomic diagnosis by noninvasive methods is incomplete or inconsistent with the clinical findings. In the preoperative patient, the surgeon's judgment as to the adequacy of the noninvasive imaging also is a major factor in determining whether or not a cardiac catheterization should be performed. This chapter deals only with diagnostic cardiac catheterization in the child with congenital cardiac disease. However, in actual clinical practice, the catheterization laboratory requires that the physician recognize unanticipated indications for intervention that may become evident during the course of a diagnostic catheterization and that he or she can perform these interventions when necessary. Therefore, this chapter also discusses the following areas that are important when performing a cardiac catheterization in a pediatric patient: sedation for the procedure, vascular access, hemodynamic assessment, and angiography.

CATHETERIZATION LABORATORY SEDATION FOR THE PEDIATRIC PATIENT

The approach to premedication and sedation varies widely among institutions. In some institutions, all catheterizations are performed under general anesthesia, and in many others, conscious sedation is performed and supervised by the pediatric cardiologist or by a pediatric anesthesiologist. The goals of sedation are to ensure patient comfort without airway compromise, to promote amnesia, and to facilitate performance of the procedure so it may be undertaken in a safe and efficient manner.

Indication for general anesthesia

The decision to use general anesthesia is determined by both patient and procedural factors. In the following circumstances, general anesthesia is necessary: airway issues, such as having either paralysis of a diaphragm or vocal cord, and/or obstructive sleep apnea; when hemodynamic compromise is likely to occur during an intervention, such as placement of a ventricular septal defect (VSD) device; if the child is very uncooperative or likely to become very agitated with sedation (e.g., a child or young adult with severe developmental disabilities); and if the child must remain absolutely still during a critical phase of an intervention, such as a device or stent placement. Not all interventions require general anesthesia; for example, conscious sedation works well for most individuals who require pulmonary or aortic valvuloplasties and patent ductus arteriosus (PDA) closure and coil occlusion of venous or arterial collaterals.

Appropriate conscious sedation protocols will enable the majority of diagnostic catheterizations to be managed by nurses trained in both pediatric sedation and the catheterization laboratory setting.

Pharmacologic agents

The drugs and doses commonly used to sedate children in the catheterization laboratory are shown in Table 19.1. These agents have minimal hemodynamic effects in a well-compensated patient and the main consideration is airway maintenance and avoidance of respiratory depression.[1]

Choral hydrate is commonly used to sedate infants. The onset of action is 15–30 minutes and duration of action is 2–4 hours. About 10%–20% of children will become excitable and uncooperative with choral hydrate. It is also important to remember that choral hydrate is metabolized to trichloroethanol and trichloroacetic acid, both of which are pharmacologically active with a long half-life of over 24 hours.[2]

Midazolam is a short-acting benzodiazepine commonly used in pediatric catheterization laboratories. If oral midazolam is used as a premedication, its onset of action is 15–30 minutes with duration of action of 2–4 hours. In addition, if cardiac output and splanchnic perfusion is reduced, hepatic metabolism of midazolam will be reduced and the drug will accumulate. Intravenous (IV) midazolam can cause significant hypotension in patients with poorly compensated cardiac failure.

Opioids provide excellent analgesia, and commonly used opioids in the catheterization laboratory are morphine and fentanyl. Unlike the synthetic opioid fentanyl, morphine has sedative properties in addition to providing analgesia. However, fentanyl has a shorter duration of action and generates much less histamine release and resultant vasodilation and hypotension than morphine. Chest wall rigidity may occur with a rapid bolus of fentanyl, although this is an idiosyncratic and dose-related reaction.[3]

Ketamine is a phencyclidine derivative that effectively dissociates the thalamic and limbic systems and provides intense analgesia. It provides hemodynamic stability through sympathomimetic actions resulting from central stimulation and diminished postganglionic catecholamine uptake that results in an increase in both heart rate and blood pressure. Ketamine will dilate cerebral vessels and should be

Table 19.1 Drugs and dosages of commonly used agents for conscious sedation or anesthesia in the pediatric catheterization laboratory

Drug	Route of administration	Dose
Analgesics		
Morphine	IV bolus	0.1–0.2 mg/kg
	IV infusion	25–50 mcg/kg/h
Fentanyl	IV bolus	0.5–1 mcg/kg (max 4–5 mcg/kg)
		2–5 mcg/kg/h
	IV infusion	
Ketamine	IV bolus	1–2 mg/kg
	IM bolus	5–10 mg/kg
Sedatives		
Chloral hydrate	PO	50–80 mg/kg (max 1 g)
Midazolam	IV	0.1 mg/kg q 10 min
	Intranasal	0.1 mL/kg (max 1 cc)
Benadryl	PO	1 mg/kg
	IV	1 mg/kg drip over 20 min
Anesthetics		
Propofol	IV bolus	1.5–3 mg/kg
	IV infusion	50–150 mcg/kg/min
Etomidate	IV bolus	0.2–0.3 mg/kg
Dexmedetomidine	IV infusion	0.5–1.14 mcg/kg/h (loading 0.15–1 mcg/kg)

Note: IV, intravenous; PO, oral.

avoided in patients with intracranial hypertension. There are conflicting reports about the effect of ketamine on pulmonary vascular resistance. On balance, it appears that the increase in pulmonary artery (PA) pressure with ketamine is minimal and should not prevent its use in individuals with pulmonary hypertension.[4] Although respiratory depression with ketamine can occur, children continue to breathe spontaneously; however, airway secretions are increased and aspiration and/or laryngospasm can result. The major side effects of ketamine are delirium, hallucinations, and nightmares; however, these can be minimized by pretreatment with benzodiazepines.

Propofol is a phenol derivative supplied in a soy emulsion and egg phospholipid to make an injectable emulsion. In most institutions, it is only used by anesthesiologists. It has a short duration of action and rapid clearance and is administered by infusion or repeated bolus doses. Side effects include pain on injection and hypotension secondary to a decrease in systemic vascular resistance and direct myocardial depression. The hypotension and the myocardial depression have limited its use as the sole anesthetic agent during cardiac catheterization; however, the combination of propofol and ketamine produces hemodynamic stability and excellent analgesia.[5]

Sevoflurane is the most commonly used inhalation agent. Sevoflurane has a rapid onset and a relatively safe hemodynamic profile. Sevoflurane can cause hypotension secondary to direct myocardial depression, and bradycardia and atrioventricular conduction blockade have also been reported.

Dexmedetomidine is being used as an adjunctive agent for sedation and analgesia in the pediatric cardiac catheterization laboratory. It also is frequently combined with ketamine. Adverse hemodynamic and respiratory effects are minimal.

VASCULAR ACCESS

Vascular access can be one of the more difficult parts of a pediatric cardiac catheterization. Access can be obtained from the femoral or umbilical vessels, from the subclavian, internal jugular, or hepatic veins, from the carotid arteries, or even via transthoracic puncture.

Umbilical access

For infants, the umbilical artery and vein are frequently used to perform diagnostic and therapeutic catheterizations. If umbilical catheters are in place when the infant arrives in the cardiac catheterization laboratory, they are prepared with a chlorhexidine gluconate solution, cut near the skin, and exchanged over a guidewire for the appropriate catheter or sheath. For the umbilical vein, a 5- or 6-Fr sheath—long enough to cross the ductus venosus—is positioned in the inferior vena cava (IVC) or right atrium (RA). For the umbilical artery, no sheath is necessary; usually a catheter can be advanced over the wire into the aorta.

If catheters have not been placed in the umbilicus, umbilical tape is tied to the base of the umbilicus, the umbilical cord is cut horizontally near the skin, and the artery and vein are cannulated with umbilical catheters. Once the umbilical catheters are positioned in the aorta and/or RA, they are exchanged over guidewires as previously described. If the umbilical venous catheter cannot be advanced into the RA, one can use fluoroscopic guidance and small hand injections of contrast to demonstrate patency of the ductus venous. A torque-controlled wire can then be manipulated into the RA and the catheter can be advanced over the wire, through the ductus venous into the IVC and RA.

A disadvantage of using the umbilical vessels is that the umbilical vein directs the catheter posteriorly in the RA toward the foramen ovale and left atrium (LA); therefore, it is ideal for advancing the catheter into the LA and ventricle and undesirable for advancing the catheter into the right ventricle (RV) and PA. Another disadvantage is that the umbilical arteries enter the internal iliac artery and add an additional curve to the catheter that makes it difficult to maneuver.

Femoral access

The Seldinger technique is used to obtain percutaneous entry into the femoral vessels in the vast majority of cases.[6,7] The child should be positioned with the hips elevated, and the leg should be straightened with slight outward rotation. The landmarks for determining site of vessel entry are the anterior superior iliac spine, the pubic tubercle, the inguinal ligament, and the femoral pulse. The vessel should be entered below the inguinal ligament to ensure the ability to obtain hemostasis at the end of the procedure. The area is prepped with a chlorhexidine gluconate solution and the skin and subcutaneous tissue anesthetized with lidocaine. Venous access is usually obtained first, but this is not mandatory. In infants, the vessel should be entered about 1 cm below the inguinal ligament. The vein is medial to the artery and will be quite close, within 2 mm of the artery in infants. In older patients it may be a centimeter away from the artery. The angle between the needle and the skin should be 45° or less. The needle should be advanced almost to bone and then slowly withdrawn with or without gentle aspiration with a syringe. Once blood is seen, the needle is stabilized and the soft end of a wire is advanced into the femoral vein. If any resistance is felt while advancing the wire, the wire should be withdrawn and the needle readjusted. After using fluoroscopy to confirm that the wire is in the correct vessel, a small skin incision is made, the needle is removed, and a sheath and dilator are advanced over the wire. If the wire cannot be advanced despite having excellent blood return, contrast should be injected into the vein to ensure that the common iliac vein is not occluded. A plexus of collateral will be seen if the vessel is occluded or stenotic. If collaterals fill the contralateral iliac vein, it is likely that the contralateral femoral vein is patent. A similar technique is used for obtaining femoral artery access.

The most common complications of femoral access are hematomas, arteriovenous fistulae, pseudoaneurysms, retroperitoneal hemorrhages, venous thrombosis, and loss of the arterial pulse. Absence of the arterial pulse is not uncommon in young infants immediately following removal of the arterial sheath. If the pulse has not returned within 2 hours, the infant should be heparinized with 100 units/kg, followed by an infusion of 20 units/kg/h for up to 12–24 hours or until the pulse returns. If the pulse is still absent at 24 hours, streptokinase or tissue plasminogen activator can be started.[8,9] Surgical thrombectomy may be required in rare cases.[10] A pseudoaneurysm of the femoral artery can frequently be treated with ultrasound-guided compression and thrombin injection.[11]

Subclavian access

The subclavian vein is routinely used in individuals with a Glenn anastomosis after a hemi-Fontan procedure, or if the femoral vessels are occluded. The major disadvantage with subclavian access is difficulty in crossing a patent foramen ovale (PFO) and the inability to perform a transseptal puncture.

The patient is positioned with the arm down at the side, with a small roll under the spine, and the head turned to the opposite side. The landmarks are the depression in the lateral third of the clavicle and the suprasternal notch. The skin and subcutaneous tissues and clavicular periosteum are infiltrated with lidocaine. A needle with a syringe attached is inserted at the junction of the medial and middle third of the clavicle (at the depression) and is advanced gently until it contacts the clavicle. It is then advanced under the clavicle and then advanced parallel to the floor and toward the suprasternal notch. Care must be taken to avoid passing the needle through the periosteum as this will make it nearly impossible to introduce the sheath. Once blood is freely being aspirated from the needle, the syringe can be removed and the soft end of a wire advanced under fluoroscopic guidance into the RA or cavopulmonary anastomosis. If access is not obtained after several attempts, contrast injection through an IV in the hand or arm should be performed to document vessel patency and location. Complications include pneumothorax, hemothorax, and subclavian artery or aortic puncture.

Internal jugular access

The internal jugular approach is frequently used for right heart endomyocardial biopsies to access the pulmonary arteries in children with a cavopulmonary connection, and when the femoral vessels are occluded. An advantage of the internal jugular approach over the subclavian approach is that the vessel is entered well outside the thorax, making pneumothorax an unlikely complication. As with subclavian access, the internal jugular approach is not well-suited to cross a PFO or to perform a transseptal puncture. The other disadvantage in an infant with the internal jugular approach is that it is difficult to immobilize uncooperative patients and more sedation or general anesthesia may be required.

The right internal jugular is preferred as it offers a more direct route to the RA. The patient is positioned with the neck hyperextended by placing a roll under the shoulders and the head turned to the opposite side. Always use ultrasound guidance to enter the internal jugular vein. The vein is imaged in short axis and the needle can be visualized as it enters the vein. Once the needle appears to be in the vein and is confirmed by free return of blood into a syringe, the soft end of a guidewire is passed through the needle and entry into the RA or pulmonary is confirmed by fluoroscopy. A hemostatic sheath should then be positioned into the vein. Complications include hemothorax, pneumothorax, carotid artery puncture, and tracheal puncture.

Hepatic access

Percutaneous transhepatic venous access is an excellent alternative to the femoral vein, especially in cases where it is necessary to cross an atrial septal defect (ASD) or perform a transseptal puncture.[12]

A Chiba needle is introduced into the skin at the costal margin near the anterior axillary line. The needle is advanced cephalad and posteriorly toward the intrahepatic IVC. The needle is usually advanced to within a few centimeters of the right border of the spine and the obturator is removed and a syringe with contrast is attached. As the needle is slowly withdrawn, contrast is simultaneously injected until contrast is observed to freely fill the hepatic vein. The syringe is removed and a guidewire inserted. The desired sheath is then advanced over the guidewire into the hepatic vein. At the end of the case, hemostasis is achieved with a Gianturco coil placed in the hepatic tract. This is accomplished by placing the dilator of the sheath into the hepatic vein. The dilator and sheath are slowly withdrawn while injecting contrast into the dilator. Once it is determined that the dilator is out of the hepatic vein and into the tract, an appropriately sized coil is placed in the tract.

Abdominal pain is frequent following transhepatic access, but a significant peritoneal hematoma is rare.[12]

Percutaneous transthoracic puncture

Percutaneous transthoracic puncture can be used to obtain access to the ventricles in a patient with a mechanical valve in the aortic and mitral, or tricuspid position.[13] It can also be used to puncture a surgically isolated LA in individuals following the Fontan procedure.[14]

The procedure should be performed under general anesthesia and requires either transesophageal or transthoracic echocardiographic guidance. A modified tri-axial system can be used with an 18-gauge lumbar needle inserted in a dilator/sheath combination. The subxiphoid position is used for RV puncture and LA puncture after the Fontan procedure, whereas an apical position is used for left ventricular (LV) puncture. Initially, a 4- to 6-Fr sheath is placed for diagnostic hemodynamics and angiography, and this sheath can be up-sized to facilitate an intervention. Following completion of the procedure, the sheath is removed and a purse-string suture is placed in the superficial skin wound.

Complications can include pericardial effusion and hemothorax. The procedure should only be done in individuals who have had previous cardiac surgery, since a surgically scarred pericardium is important for hemostasis especially after a ventricular puncture.

HEMODYNAMICS

Four important areas in the hemodynamic evaluation of an individual with congenital heart disease include measurement of pressures, measurement of blood oxygen content, measurement of cardiac output, and measurement of shunt size, vascular resistance, intracardiac pressure gradients, and valve areas.

Pressure measurement

In both adult and pediatric catheterization laboratories, pressures are usually measured with fluid-filled catheters. Six common errors can lead to inaccurate measurement of pressure:

1. Air in the system, which usually leads to a damped (artificially lower) pressure; however, occasionally air results in amplification of the pressure wave, leading to overshoot of fling (artificially high pressure) (Figure 19.1).

2. Loose connection in the system usually results in overdamping of the waveform.
3. Partial catheter obstruction leads to a damped pressure tracing. (This is especially common when using small, thin-walled catheters.)
4. Catheter fling resulting from the catheter being in a turbulent jet or if the catheter is struck by a cardiac structure, such as the anterior leaflet of the mitral valve, will result in an artificially high pressure.
5. Inaccurate calibration can result from either movement of the patient and/or the transducer during the study.
6. Catheter entrapment occurs when an endhole catheter is placed in a small or heavily trabeculated chamber and traps a small volume of fluid that results in an exaggerated systolic pressure elevation.

Another way to measure pressure, especially in neonates following the hybrid procedure for hypoplastic left heart syndrome or during fetal interventions (prenatal intrauterine interventions for structural congenital heart disease), is to use a pressure wire (RADI wire, RADI Medical Systems, Uppsala, Sweden, or PRIMEWIRE Prestige, Volcano, San Diego, CA).

Table 19.2 summarizes the normal hemodynamics for a child.

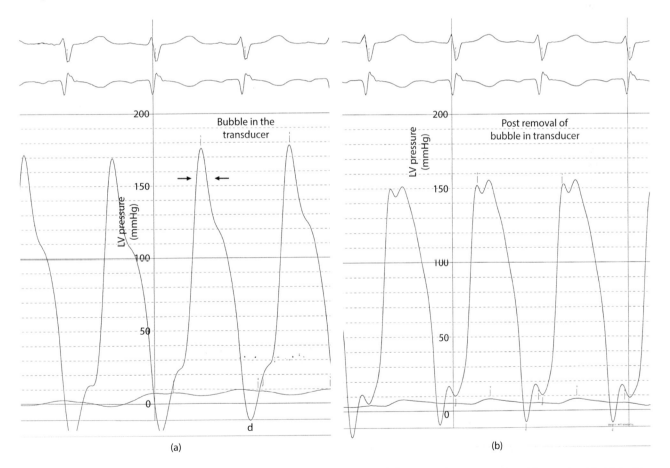

Figure 19.1 The effect of an air bubble in the pressure transducer. **(a)** The left ventricular pressure in a 10-month-old child with valvar aortic stenosis. This pressure was recorded with a small bubble in the transducer. The arrows depict the overshoot ("fling") produced by the air bubble. If one used this pressure tracing to measure LV pressure, the systolic pressure of 177 mmHg would have markedly overestimated the pressure. **(b)** The LV pressure after the air bubble was removed from the transducer. Notice the now normal LV pressure waveform without the fling. The true LV pressure is 150 mmHg, not 177 mmHg. LV, left ventricle.

Table 19.2 Normal hemodynamics for a child

Cardiac chamber	Normal pressures
Right atrium	Mean pressure of 3–5 mmHg
Right ventricle	20–25/3–5 mmHg
Pulmonary artery	Mean pressure of 13–15 mmHg
Pulmonary artery wedge	Mean pressure of 8–10 mmHg
Left ventricle	96–100/5–10 mmHg
Systemic artery	90–110/60–70 mmHg

Blood oxygen measurements

Oxygen is carried in the blood either dissolved in plasma or attached to hemoglobin. The amount of oxygen dissolved in the plasma at 378°C is about 0.03 mL/mmHg/L (or 3 mL of dissolved oxygen per liter, for every 100 mmHg partial pressure of oxygen). This amount of oxygen is quite small in comparison with the amount of oxygen bound to hemoglobin and is therefore usually ignored. However, if the child is in supplemental oxygen, with a $PO_2 > 100$ mmHg, then dissolved oxygen must be considered in the calculation of total oxygen content.

Most of the oxygen in blood is bound to hemoglobin. The amount is dependent on the type of hemoglobin, temperature, partial pressure of oxygen and carbon dioxide, and the level of 2,3-diphosphoglycerate (DPG). The maximum amount of oxygen that can be taken up by hemoglobin in blood is referred to as the oxygen capacity. Oxygen capacity can be directly measured by the method of Van Slyke[15]; however, in current practice it is assumed that the maximal oxygen capacity is 1.36 mL/g of hemoglobin; thus,

$$O_2 \text{ capacity (mLO}_2\text{/mL)} = \text{Hb (g/dL)} \times 1.36 \times 10$$

The oxygen content is the amount of oxygen present in a sample of blood, and this includes both dissolved oxygen and oxygen bound to hemoglobin:

$$O_2 \text{ content} = (\text{Hb (g/dL)} \times 1.36 \times O_2 \text{ saturation}) + (pO_2 \text{ (mmHg)} \times 0.03)$$

When the child is breathing room air, this can be simplified to

$$O_2 \text{ content} = (\text{Hb (g/dL)} \times 1.36\ O_2 \text{ saturation})$$

Oxygen saturation is usually measured using the spectrophotometric method. Measuring oxygen saturation directly rather than calculating it from the oxygen–hemoglobin dissociation curve makes the measurement independent of factors that may increase (alkalosis, hypothermia, fetal hemoglobin) or decrease (acidosis, fever) hemoglobin/oxygen affinity.

Measurement of cardiac output

The most common methods for measuring cardiac output use the indicator dilution technique first described by Fick.[16] The indicators most commonly used in congenital heart disease are oxygen and cold saline (thermodilution).[17] The basic principles of the indicator dilutions method are that an indicator is present in the fluid in a measurable concentration, and the indicator is added or removed at a known rate. If, for example, oxygen is the indicator, the equation to measure cardiac output is as follows:

$$Q_s = \frac{VO_2}{(AO\ O_2 \text{ content} - MV\ O_2 \text{ content})}$$

$$Q_p = \frac{VO_2}{(PV\ O_2 \text{ content} - PA\ O_2 \text{ content})}$$

where Q is systemic blood flow, AO is aortic, MV is mixed venous, PV is pulmonary venous, PA is pulmonary artery, Q_p is pulmonary blood flow, and VO_2 is oxygen consumption.

Using oxygen as the indicator, the most difficult parameter to measure is oxygen consumption. This is either measured directly using a flow-through method[18] or using an assumed value based on the formulas of Lafarge and Miettinen.[19]

In the thermodilution method, the indicator is temperature. A double-lumen catheter is used, and saline is injected in the proximal port usually in the RA. The thermistor for measuring temperature is positioned on the distal end of the catheter, usually in the PA.

The thermal dilution method is inaccurate in the following circumstances: significant pulmonary or tricuspid regurgitation, the presence of significant intracardiac shunts, and if the baseline temperature is unstable (i.e., patient has a fever or at the end of strenuous exercise).

Measure of shunt size, vascular resistance, valve areas, and intracardiac pressures.

Shunt detection and quantification

An increase in oxygen saturation between different sites on the right side of the heart is used to detect the presence of a left-to-right shunt; whereas a decrease in saturations between different sites on the left side of the heart is used to detect the presence of a right-to-left shunt. Since the oxygen saturations of blood in the superior vena cava (SVC), IVC, RA, RV, and PA are not the same even in individuals with no intracardiac shunting, it is important to be able to define the minimum change in blood oxygen saturation that is needed to reliably demonstrate an intracardiac shunt. In adults, it has been reported that an interchamber oxygen saturation difference as small as 3% (RV to PA) or as large as 9% (SVC to PA) can reliably detect a left-to-right shunt.[20] Table 19.3 lists the minimum saturation difference to detect a shunt at the 99% confidence limit for children.[21] If more than one set of

Table 19.3 Minimum saturation difference to detect a shunt at the 99% confidence limit

Chambers sampled	Minimum saturation difference (%)	Multiple samples difference (%)
Superior vena cava–right atrium	8.7	7
Right atrium–right ventricle	5.2	4
Right ventricle–pulmonary artery	5.6	4

saturations is obtained, the minimum saturation difference is reduced.[22]

If the aortic saturation is <94% or there is a 2% or greater step-down from LA or LV to aorta then a right-to-left shunt is suspected.

The Fick principle is used to calculate pulmonary and system blood flows. To calculate right-to-left and left-to-right shunts, the concept of effective pulmonary blood flow must be used. Effective pulmonary blood flow (Q_{ep}) is defined as the desaturated blood that flows to the lungs. In the absence of a right-to-left shunt, effective blood flow equals pulmonary blood flow. The equation to calculate effective pulmonary blood flow is

$$Q_{ep} = \frac{V_{O_2}}{(PV\ O_2\ content - MV\ O_2\ content)}$$

When intracardiac shunts are present, the SVC is probably the best estimate of mixed venous blood. The three situations where this may not be the case are individuals under general anesthesia, the presence of supracardiac partial or total anomalous pulmonary venous return, and in many individuals with an ASD in which atrial blood refluxes into the proximal portion of the SVC.

The volume of left-to-right shunt is equal to the difference between pulmonary blood flow and effective blood flow:

$$Q_{left\ to\ right} = Q_p - Q_{ep}$$

Q_{ep} is effective pulmonary blood flow

The volume of a right-to-left shunt is equal to the difference between systemic blood flow and effective blood flow:

$$Q_{right\ to\ left} = Q_s - Q_{ep}$$

Q_{ep} is effective pulmonary blood flow

The important exception to this definition is in an infant with D-transposition of the great arteries who has parallel circulations. In these infants, the Q_{ep} is the amount of blood that is mixing between the pulmonary and systemic circuits (i.e., the left-to-right and right-to-left shunting).

The ratio of pulmonary to systemic blood flow (Q_p/Q_s) is a useful estimate of the magnitude of left-to-right shunting. Small left-to-right shunts are defined as Q_p/Q_s of <1.5, moderate 1.5 to 2, and large >2. The formula to calculate Q_p/Q_s is

$$\frac{Q_p}{Q_s} = \frac{(MV\ saturation - AO\ saturation)}{(PV\ saturation - PA\ saturation)}$$

If the patient is on oxygen, then dissolved oxygen must also be taken into account. The formula then becomes

$$\frac{Q_p}{Q_s} = \frac{(MV\ O_2\ content - AO\ O_2\ content)}{(PV\ O_2\ content - PA\ O_2\ content)}$$

Vascular resistance

One of the most common reasons for performing a diagnostic cardiac catheterization is to assess pulmonary vascular resistance. This is especially important in the following situations:

- To determine if an individual can have his or her cardiac defect repaired—that is, a child with a VSD device and pulmonary artery hypertension (Table 19.4)
- To determine if the child is a candidate for cardiac transplantation
- To determine the hemodynamic response of a child with PA hypertension who is or may have to be treated with PA vasodilators

The calculation of vascular resistance is based in part on Poiseuille's law, which states that flow in a tube is directly related to pressure and cross-sectional area of the tube and inversely to the length of the tube and the viscosity of the fluid flowing in the tube. In the vascular system, the length of the tube and the viscosity of the fluid are assumed to be constant so that the pressure gradient across a vascular bed divided by the flow through the bed is equal to the resistance of the bed. Therefore, the formulas for pulmonary and systemic vascular resistance are as follows:

$$R_p = \frac{(PA\ mean\ pressure - LA\ mean\ pressure)}{Q_p}$$

$$R_s = \frac{(AO\ mean\ pressure - RA\ mean\ pressure)}{Q_s}$$

There are two different types of pulmonary resistance. Arteriolar resistance is resistance calculated across the vascular bed:

$$\left[\frac{(PA\ mean\ pressure - LA\ mean\ pressure)}{Q_p}\right]$$

Table 19.4 Example of pulmonary vasodilator testing in a 12-month-old infant with a large VSD

Site[a]	Saturation (%)	Pressure	PO$_2$ (mmHg)
SVC	60	Mean = 5 mmHg	42
PA	65	88/50 (63) mmHg	47
LA/PV	97	Mean = 12 mmHg	88
AO	93	88/55 (66) mmHg	69
Site[b]	Saturation (%)	Pressure	PO$_2$ (mmHg)
SVC	70	Mean = 5 mmHg	45
PA	92	90/30 (49) mmHg	68
LA/PV	100	Mean = 17 mmHg	425
AO	100	90/60 (70) mmHg	425
Site[c]	Saturation (%)	Pressure	PO$_2$ (mmHg)
SVC	70	Mean = 5 mmHg	45
PA	99	88/25 (46) mmHg	108
LA/PV	100	Mean = 17 mmHg	400
AO	100	88/65 (72) mmHg	400

Note: In this child, the combination of O$_2$ and NO normalized R$_p$ by increasing pulmonary blood flow while only slightly decreasing pulmonary artery pressure.

[a] The following hemodynamic measurements were made on diagnostic cardiac catheterization:
Hb = 13 g/dL and VO$_2$ measured at 188 mL/min·m^2
Q_p = 188 mL/min·m^2/(13*1.36*10)*(0.97−0.65) = 3.3 L/min·m^2
Q_s = 188 mL/min·m^2/(13*1.36*10)*(0.93−0.60) = 3.2 L/min·m^2
Q_{ef} = 188 mL/min·m^2/(13*1.36*10)*(0.97−0.60) = 2.9 L/min·m^2
Q_p/Q_s = 1.03 R_p = (63−12)/3.3 = 15.4 Wood's units·m^2

[b] The following hemodynamics were present after the child was in 100% O$_2$ for 10 min:
Q_p = 188 mL/min·m^2/(((13*1.36*10*1)+(0.03*425))−((13*1.36*10*0.92)+(0.03*68))) = 7.5 L/min·m^2
Q_s = 188 mL/min·m^2/(((13*1.36*10*1)+(0.03*425))−((13*1.36*10*0.70)+(0.03*45))) = 2.9 L/min·m^2
Q_p/Q_s = 2.6; Q_{ef} = Q_s R_p = (49−17)/7.5 = 4.2 Wood's units·m^2

[c] The following hemodynamics were present after the child was on O$_2$ and 50 ppm NO for 10 min:
Q_p = 188 mL/min·m^2/(((13*1.36*10*1)+(0.03*400))−((13*1.36*10*0.99)+(0.03*108))) = 17 L/min·m^2
Q_s = 188 mL/min·m^2/(((13*1.36*10*1)+(0.03*400))−((13*1.36*10*0.70)+(0.03*45))) = 2.9 L/min·m^2
Q_p/Q_s = 5.9; Q_{ef} = Q_s R_p = (46−17)/17 = 1.8 Wood's units·m^2

AO, aorta; LA, left atrium; PA, pulmonary artery; PV, pulmonary vein; SVC, superior vena cava; VSD, ventricular septal defect.

Where O$_2$ is oxygen, NO is nitric oxide, Q_{ef} is effective flow, Q_p is pulmonary blood flow, Q_s is systemic blood flow, R_p is pulmonary vascular resistance, and VO$_2$ is oxygen consumption.

and total resistance of the lungs $\left(\dfrac{\text{mean PA pressure}}{Q_p} \right)$. In the clinical setting, we are usually only interested in arteriolar resistance.

The units for this expression of vascular resistance are called Wood's units (named after Paul Wood) and are in mmHg/L/min. To convert this to metric units, the Wood's unit is multiplied by 80 to yield the units of dyne·s·cm^{-5}. Because of the considerable size range of pediatric patients, most cardiologists index the Wood's units to body surface area (Wood's unit m^2). The normal values for systemic and pulmonary resistance are <20 units for systemic and <3 Wood's units for pulmonary.

Pulmonary vasodilator testing

In patients with pulmonary hypertension in whom it is important to determine if their hypertension is fixed or reactive, pulmonary vasodilator testing is performed at the time of a diagnostic catheterization.

The two pulmonary vasodilators that are used are oxygen and nitric oxide (NO).[23,24] The usual protocol is to initially obtain PA, pulmonary venous wedge, and aortic pressures; saturations; and blood gases, along with a measurement of pulmonary blood flow (either using the Fick procedure or thermodilution if other cardiac lesions are not present). Following these baseline measurements, the individual is placed in 100% oxygen for 10 minutes and repeat measurements are made. If oxygen does not result in normalization of pulmonary vascular resistance, then the individual receives oxygen along with nitric oxide either at 50 ppm through a nasal cannula or at 20 ppm through an endotracheal tube. After 10 minutes of the nitric oxide, repeat hemodynamic measurements are made. Combination testing with NO + O$_2$ provides additional pulmonary vasodilation in patients with a reactive pulmonary vascular bed in a selective, safe, and expeditious fashion during cardiac catheterization.[25] Pulmonary vasoreactivity can also be assessed by using aerosolized iloprost (a stable carbacyclin derivative of prostacyclin, intravenous epoprostenol, and/or intravenous adenosine).[26] These agents are comparable to

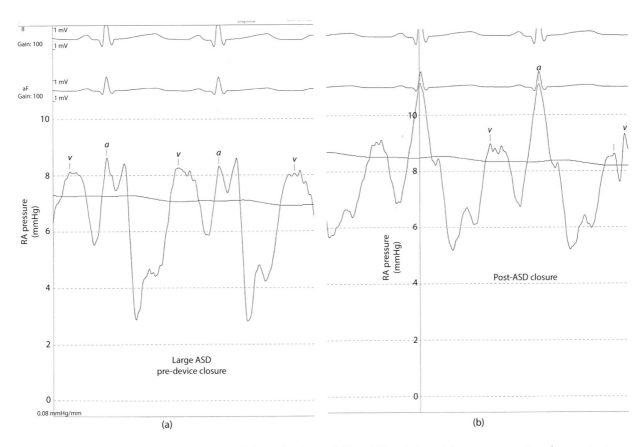

Figure 19.2 Right atrial pressure tracing in a child with a large ASD. **(a)** The right atrial pressure tracing demonstrates equal *a* and *v* waves. This tracing is characteristic of the atrial pressure tracing in a patient with a large ASD. **(b)** The right atrial pressure tracing in the same child after the ASD has been closed with a 22 mm Amplatzer ASD Septal Occluder. After the ASD has been closed, the right atrial pressure tracing has normalized with a much larger *a* wave than *v* wave. ASD, atrial septal defect; RA, right atrium.

inhaled NO in their ability to induce pulmonary vasodilatation, and since they do not require a special delivery system, they may even be more cost effective. A reactive pulmonary bed is defined by a drop in pulmonary vascular resistance. This can be due to an increase in pulmonary blood flow with little or no change in PA pressure (i.e., the child with a large VSD and pulmonary hypertension), a decrease in PA pressure without a change in pulmonary blood flow (i.e., the child with idiopathic pulmonary artery hypertension), or a combination of both. An example of the calculations associated with pulmonary vasodilatory testing is depicted in Table 19.4.

Valve areas

Valve areas are infrequently used in the management of children with congenital heart disease. Most decisions as to whether or not to perform surgery or balloon angioplasty are based on peak-to-peak pressure gradients at the time of a heart catheterization. When valve areas are calculated, either the Gorlin formula[27] or Bache's modification of the Gorlin formula[28] is used.

In addition to measuring absolute systolic, diastolic, and mean pressures, analyses of the intracardiac pressure waveforms and pressure gradients between chambers are very important in performing a diagnostic cardiac catheterization in a patient with congenital heart disease. For example, the dominant pressure waveform in the RA is the *a* wave, whereas the *v* wave is the dominant pressure wave in the LA; however, with an ASD, the *a* and *v* are nearly the same in both atria (Figure 19.2).

The pressure waveforms are critical for making the diagnosis of both cardiac tamponade and pericardial constriction. In tamponade, the pericardial fluid causes equalization of all diastolic pressures. The atrial pressures increase with inspiration rather than decrease, and there is a marked fall in arterial pressure (>10 mmHg) with inspiration. In individuals with chronic pericardial constriction, a fluid bolus (10–20 cc/kg of warm saline) uniformly increases all pressures; whereas, if the individual has chronic myocardial constriction, the fluid bolus will increase pressure to a greater degree in the cardiac chamber most severely affected.[29]

Pressure pullbacks with endhole catheters are very useful in identifying the precise site of obstruction—that is, a patient with multiple sites of left ventricular outflow tract (LVOT) obstruction.

Table 19.5 Commonly used angiographic projections and cardiac lesions best imaged with these projections

View	Frontal plane angle	Lateral plane angle	Cardiac lesion best imaged using these planes
Posteroanterior and lateral	0°	90°	Posteroanterior projection for complex heart disease, RV in most conditions, and pulmonary veins, lateral for coarctation, PS, and PDA
RAO and LAO	30° RAO	60° LAO	RAO useful for mitral valve, RPA, PDA, and anterior VSDs, RAO with 30° cranial angulation useful to see RPA after a hemi-Fontan. LAO for coarctation, aortic valve abnormalities
Long-axial oblique	30° RAO	60° LAO and 20° cranial	Membranous, outlet, mid-muscular, and some apical VSD's, LVOT obstruction, and the LPA
Hepatoclavicular	40° LAO and 40° cranial	120° LAO and 15° cranial	AV septal defects, apical and mid-muscular VSD's, truncus. With a little less LAO on frontal projection good to see ASD
Cranial–caudal	20° RAO and 40° cranial	90° and 20–30° caudal	Frontal plane: RPA and MPA in TOF, Lateral for PA bifurcation in TOF and after hemi-Fontan or bicaval shunt
Laid-back	0° and 45° caudal	90°	Coronary arteries in DTGA or DORV

Note: ASD, atrial septal defect; AV, atrioventricular; DTGA, D-transposition of the great arteries; DORV, double outlet right ventricle; LAO, lateral anterior oblique; LPA, left pulmonary artery; LVOT, left ventricular outflow tract; MPA, main pulmonary artery; PA, pulmonary artery; PDA, patent ductus arteriosis; PS, pulmonary stenosis; RAO, right anterior oblique; RPA, right pulmonary artery; RV, right ventricle; TOF, tetralogy of Fallot; VSD, ventricular septal defect.

ANGIOGRAPHY

Angiography remains an essential component of the diagnostic evaluation of the patient with congenital heart disease. The selection of the appropriate angiographic projection is critical for obtaining diagnostic images.[30,31] The standard angiographic projections currently used in individuals with congenital heart disease are frontal (posteroanterior), lateral, right anterior oblique (RAO), left anterior oblique (LAO), long-axial oblique, hepatoclavicular (four-chamber view), and the caudal views. All congenital heart disease angiography is performed using biplane angiography to reduce the amount of contrast agent given to the individual. Table 19.5 lists the commonly used angiographic projections.

In addition to selecting the appropriate angiographic view, it is important to remember that the anatomy of any chamber is best delineated when the chamber is selectively filled with the appropriate amount of contrast at the appropriate rate. For the best anatomic definition, contrast should be injected in 1 second or less. The volume of contrast should be modified according to both the size and flow rates of the chamber or vessel being imaged. For example, higher volumes and flow rates are required to define the ventricular anatomy of a child with a large intracardiac shunt than a child with ventricular outflow obstruction. In general, most angiograms in patients with congenital heart disease use 1–1.5 cc/kg of contrast.

Clinical aspects (angiography in specific lesions)

VENTRICULAR SEPTAL DEFECTS

Membranous defects are best visualized in the long-axial oblique projection (lateral tube at 60-70° LAO with 30° cranial angulation). This view elongates the LVOT. This view also is useful in evaluating the LVOT for possible outflow tract obstruction produced by a subaortic membrane and/or possible prolapse of the aortic valve into the VSD. The companion RAO projection is useful in identifying potential RV outflow tract obstruction and for making the diagnosis of associated LV–RA shunts.

Muscular VSDs require multiple views depending on the exact location of the defect or defects. The RAO projection is helpful in profiling the infundibular septum and defects in the anterior conal septum (subpulmonary defects). The long-axial oblique projection is useful for malalignment defects and defects in the midtrabecular portion and some defects in the apical portion of the ventricular septum (Figure 19.3). The hepatoclavicular (four-chamber view) projection is helpful to evaluate defects in the posterior trabecular septum, apical septum, and around the atrioventricular valves.

Atrioventricular septal defects

The RAO and companion long-axial oblique views are useful in assessing the degree of atrioventricular valve regurgitation and the status of the LVOT.

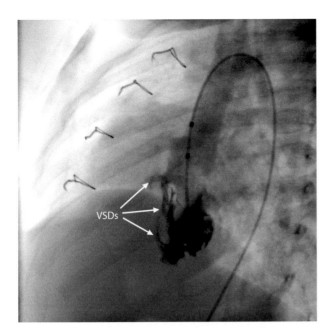

Figure 19.3 Left ventricular angiogram in a 12-month-old child with multiple VSDs. The angiogram was performed in the long-axial oblique projection left anterior oblique 65° with 30° cranial angulation. In this projection, one can demonstrate at least three VSDs. The lower defect is in the apical portion of the ventricular septum, the middle defect is in the midtrabecular portion of the septum, and the upper defect is in the outlet portion of the septum. The long-axial oblique projection profiles these portions of the atrial septum well. VSDs, ventricular septal defects.

The hepatoclavicular view is excellent for evaluation of the inlet (posterior interventricular) septum. This view is also well-suited to evaluate abnormal position of the atrioventricular valve attachments and the size of the ventricles. It is also useful in assessing the type and severity of atrioventricular valve regurgitation. The companion cranially-angled RAO projection is useful to evaluate the infundibular septum and the possibility of RV outflow tract obstruction.

Tetralogy of Fallot

The RV infundibular narrowing is best visualized by performing a RV angiogram in a slightly RAO projection with 30° of cranial angulation with the companion projection being a straight lateral (Figure 19.4). These views provide excellent visualization of the anterior deviation of the infundibular septum. The pulmonary arteries are best imaged with the frontal plane in an RAO projection with cranial angulation and with the lateral plane in a LAO projection with 30° to 40° of cranial angulation. The RAO projection defines the right pulmonary artery (RPA), and the LAO projection delineates the left pulmonary artery (LPA). The coronary arteries should always be visualized in any preoperative patient with tetralogy of Fallot who is undergoing a heart catheterization. An aortogram positioned in the RAO and long-axial oblique positions usually results in adequate delineation of the coronary anatomy.

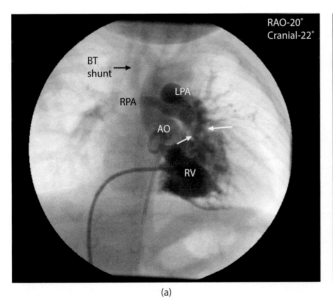

(a)

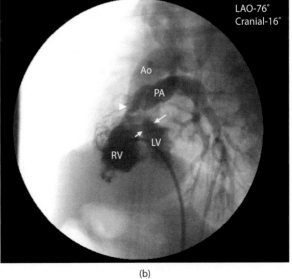

(b)

Figure 19.4 RV angiogram from a 4-month-old child with tetralogy of Fallot who has had a previous right BT shunt. **(a)** The frontal camera projection in the RAO cranial projection. The RV infundibular narrowing is marked by the two white arrows; the main, right, and left pulmonary arteries are visualized. One can note stenosis and hypoplasia of the proximal RPA at the site of the BT shunt. The fact that the AO is opacified on the RV injections suggests the presence of a VSD with right-to-left shunting. **(b)** The companion LAO cranial projection in the same patient. This projection again demonstrates the infundibular narrowing (*solid white arrowhead*) and the outlet malalignment VSD (*two smaller white arrows*). One can also note that the AO overrides this VSD. AO, aorta; BT, Blalock Taussig; LAO, left anterior oblique; LPA, left pulmonary artery; LV, left ventricle; PA, pulmonary artery; RAO, right anterior oblique; RPA, right pulmonary artery; RV, right ventricle.

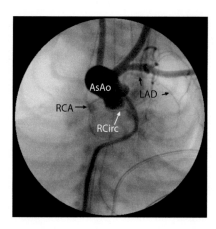

Figure 19.5 A laid-back aortogram in a newborn with DTGA. The frontal camera was positioned with 10° right anterior oblique and 40° caudal angulation. The LAD arises from the left-facing sinus and the RCA and RCirc arise from the right-facing sinus. This is a common coronary anomaly observed in transposition. Only the AsAo is visualized because the balloon of the antegrade angiographic catheter is inflated. One can also note that this child has a right aortic arch since the first branch is a left innominate artery. AsAo, ascending aorta; DTGA, d-transposition of the great arteries; LAD, left anterior descending coronary artery; RCA, right coronary artery; Rcirc, right circumflex coronary artery.

D-Transposition of the great arteries

A left ventricular angiogram in the long-axial oblique projection is useful to assess the size of the LV, status of the ventricular septum, and the LVOT anatomy. The RAO projection of the left ventricular angiogram is helpful to evaluate the mitral valve and anterior ventricular septum. The origins of the coronary arteries are best evaluated by performing an aortogram with marked caudal angulation and with a balloon angiographic catheter positioned antegrade across the aortic valve and with the balloon inflated (Figure 19.5).[32]

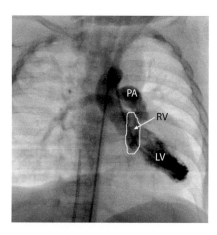

Figure 19.6 Left ventricular angiogram of a child with tricuspid atresia. The angiogram was performed in the posteroanterior projection. The LV opacifies the hypoplastic RV infundibular chamber (a line outlines the chamber) and PA. There is no apical portion of the right ventricle identified. LV, left ventricle; PA, pulmonary artery; RV, right ventricle.

Complex congenital defects

The standard posteroanterior and lateral projections are the initial views for evaluating a child with complex congenital heart disease (Figure 19.6). Other views can then be performed to define any structures that need better anatomic evaluation. The echocardiogram can be used to help determine the best angiographic view. An angiographic view that is perpendicular to the transducer position and provides the best echocardiographic definition of the anatomy is usually a good starting point.

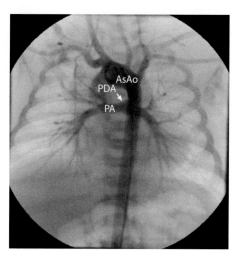

Figure 19.7 Aortogram in an infant with pulmonary atresia with VSD. The angiogram was filmed in the posteroanterior projection. The PA are filled by a PDA. AsAo, ascending aorta; PA, pulmonary arteries; PDA, patent ductus arteriosis.

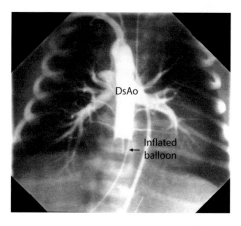

Figure 19.8 Balloon occlusion descending aortogram for documentation of the source of pulmonary blood flow in a neonate with pulmonary atresia with ventricular septal defect. The balloon-tipped angiographic catheter has been advanced from the right ventricle into the ascending and then the DsAo. Contrast injected behind the inflated balloon (arrow) produces dense opacification of single large collateral arising from the midthoracic aorta that opacifies confluent right and left pulmonary arteries. One should also note that the infant has a right aortic arch. DsAo, descending aorta.

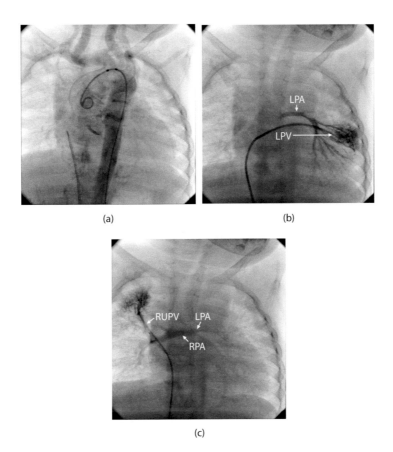

Figure 19.9 Series of angiograms performed to identify the pulmonary artery anatomy in a neonate with pulmonary atresia with ventricular septal defect. **(a)** An aortogram that fails to identify the pulmonary arteries. **(b)** A wedge pulmonary vein injection. The catheter is wedged in the LPV, contrast injected refluxes into the LPA. Although the LPA is well visualized, there is only a hint of a confluence and the RPA is not visualized. **(c)** A second wedge pulmonary vein injection. The catheter is wedged in the RUPV, contrast injected refluxes into RPA, outlining a confluence as well as the LPA. LPA, left pulmonary artery; LPV, left middle pulmonary vein; RPA, right pulmonary artery; RUPV, right upper pulmonary vein.

Peripheral pulmonary artery anatomy

In patients with pulmonary atresia, the first angiogram is usually an aortic angiogram in the posteroanterior and lateral projections (Figure 19.7). Once the source of pulmonary blood flow is identified, selective angiograms in the aortopulmonary collaterals can be performed.

In the neonate, balloon occlusion angiography is useful (Figure 19.8).[33] To perform balloon occlusion aortogram, the aorta is catheterized antegrade with a balloon-tipped angiocatheter. The balloon is inflated immediately prior to contrast injection and is then rapidly deflated.

Finally, if pulmonary arteries or segments of the pulmonary arteries are not visualized on the aortic angiogram, selective pulmonary venous wedge angiograms can be performed (Figure 19.9). The technique involves advancing an endhole catheter across the atrial septum into the pulmonary vein that is best for delineating the portion of the pulmonary tree that could not previously be visualized. The catheter should then be advanced until it is wedged in the pulmonary vein. If the catheter has a balloon tip, the balloon can be inflated and wedge position confirmed by the injection of a small amount of contrast. A 10 cc syringe in which contrast and saline have been layered, such that the saline is drawn up first and contrast second, is used for the injection. The catheter is then wedged, and the contrast/saline is injected by hand as fast as possible. Serious complications from this technique have been reported with the use of a non-balloon endhole catheter.[34]

CONCLUSION

Although advances in noninvasive imaging have reduced the role of diagnostic cardiac catheterization in the patient with congenital heart disease, recent developments in transcatheter interventions—as well as marked advancements in surgical management of many forms of extremely complex congenital heart disease—have resulted in diagnostic cardiac catheterization remaining a critical component in the evaluation and treatment of children with congenital heart disease. This chapter summarized four of the areas that are critical when performing a cardiac catheterization in a pediatric patient: sedation for the procedure, vascular access, hemodynamic assessment, and angiography.

REFERENCES

1. Cote CJ, Wilson S. Guidelines for monitoring and management of pediatric patients during and after sedation for diagnostic and therapeutic procedures: An update. *Pediatrics* 2006; 118:2587–2602.
2. American Academy of Pediatrics Committee on Drugs and Committee on Environmental Health. Use of chloral hydrate for sedation in children. *Pediatrics* 1993; 92:471–473.
3. Meretoja OA, Rautiainen P. Alfentanil and fentanyl sedation in infants and small children during cardiac catheterization. *Can J Anaesth* 1990; 37:624–628.
4. Berman W Jr., et al. Hemodynamic effects of ketamine in children undergoing cardiac catheterization. *Pediatr Cardiol* 1990; 11:72–76.
5. Tosun Z, et al. Dexmedetomidine-ketamine and propofol-ketamine combinations for anesthesia in spontaneously breathing pediatric patients undergoing cardiac catheterization. *J Cardiothorac Vasc Anesth* 2006; 20:515–519.
6. Seldinger SI. Catheter replacement of the needle in percutaneous arteriography; a new technique. *Acta Radiol* 1953; 39:368–376.
7. Takahashi M, et al. Percutaneous heart catheterization in infants and children. I. Catheter placement and manipulation with guide wires. *Circulation* 1970; 42:1037–1048.
8. Carlson KM, et al. Use of tissue plasminogen activator for femoral artery thrombosis following transcatheter coil occlusion of patent ductus arteriosus. *Pediatr Cardiol* 2005; 26:83–86.
9. Ino T, et al. Thrombolytic therapy for femoral artery thrombosis after pediatric cardiac catheterization. *Am Heart J* 1988; 115:633–639.
10. Vitiello R, et al. Complications associated with pediatric cardiac catheterization. *J Am Coll Cardiol* 1998; 32:1433–1440.
11. Luedde M, et al. Treatment of iatrogenic femoral pseudoaneurysm by ultrasound-guided compression therapy and thrombin injection. *Angiology* 2007; 58:435–439.
12. Shim D, et al. Transhepatic therapeutic cardiac catheterization: A new option for the pediatric interventionalist. *Catheter Cardiovasc Interv* 1999; 47:41–45.
13. Lim DS, et al. Percutaneous transthoracic ventricular puncture for diagnostic and interventional catheterization. *Catheter Cardiovasc Interv* 2008; 71:915–918.
14. Maher KO, et al. Transthoracic access for cardiac catheterization. *Catheter Cardiovasc Interv* 2004; 63:72–77.
15. Van Slyke DD, Neill JM. Blood gases I. *J Biol Chem* 1924; 61:524–584.
16. Fick A. Uber die messung des blutquantums in den herzventrikeln. *Sits der Physik-Med ges Wurtzberg* 1870; 2:16.
17. Freed MD, Keane JF. Cardiac output measured by thermodilution in infants and children. *J Pediatr* 1978; 92:39–42.
18. Lister G, et al. Oxygen uptake in infants and children: A simple method for measurement. *Pediatrics* 1974; 53:656–662.
19. LaFarge CG, Miettinen OS. The estimation of oxygen consumption. *Cardiovasc Res* 1970; 4:23–30.
20. Barratt-Boyes BG, Wood EH. The oxygen saturation of blood in the venae cavae, right-heart chambers, and pulmonary vessels of healthy subjects. *J Lab Clin Med* 1957; 50:93–106.
21. Freed MD, et al. Oximetric detection of intracardiac left-to-right shunts. *Br Heart J* 1979; 42:690–694.
22. Dexter L, et al. Studies of congenital heart disease. II. The pressure and oxygen content of blood in the right auricle, right ventricle, and pulmonary artery in control patients, with observations on the oxygen saturation and source of pulmonary "capillary" blood. *J Clin Invest* 1947; 26:554–560.
23. Cannon BC, et al. Nitric oxide in the evaluation of congenital heart disease with pulmonary hypertension: Factors related to nitric oxide response. *Pediatr Cardiol* 2005; 26:565–569.
24. Scheurer M, et al. Simplified pulmonary vasodilatory testing in the cardiac catheterization laboratory with nasal cannula nitric oxide. *Pediatr Cardiol* 2006; 27:84–86.
25. Atz AM, et al. Combined effects of nitric oxide and oxygen during acute pulmonary vasodilator testing. *J Am Coll Cardiol* 1999; 33:813–819.
26. Rosenzweig EB, et al. Pulmonary arterial hypertension in children. *Pediatr Pulmonol* 2004; 38:2–22.
27. Gorlin R, Gorlin SG. Hydraulic formula for calculation of the area of the stenotic mitral valve, other cardiac valves, and central circulatory shunts. I. *Am Heart J* 1951; 41:1–29.
28. Bache RJ, et al. Hemodynamic effects of exercise in isolated valvular aortic stenosis. *Circulation* 1971; 44:1003–1013.
29. Chun PK, Rocchini AP. Occult constrictive pericarditis in infancy. Documentation by rapid volume expansion. *Chest* 1980; 78:648–650.
30. Bargeron LM Jr., et al. Axial cineangiography in congenital heart disease. Section I. Concept, technical and anatomic considerations. *Circulation* 1977; 56:1075–1083.
31. Elliott LP, et al. Axial cineangiography in congenital heart disease. Section II. Specific lesions. *Circulation* 1977; 56:1048–1093.
32. Mandell VS, et al. The "laid-back" aortogram: An improved angiographic view for demonstration of coronary arteries in transposition of the great arteries. *Am J Cardiol* 1990; 65:1379–1383.
33. Keane JF, et al. Balloon occlusion angiography in infancy: Methods, uses and limitations. *Am J Cardiol* 1985; 56:495–497.
34. Alpert BS, Culham JA. A severe complication of pulmonary vein angiography. *Br Heart J* 1979; 41:727–729.

20

Cardiac catheterization for the adult with complex congenital heart disease

SUBRATA KAR AND JORGE R. ALEGRIA

INTRODUCTION

The incidence of congenital heart disease is 0.8% (8/1000) of live births in patients with cardiovascular abnormality from altered embryonic development.[1] Such patients develop abnormal shunting, which impairs the structure and function of the cardiovascular system. Currently, more patients are progressing into adulthood with congenital heart disease, and there are more adults than children in the United States with congenital heart disease.[2] Many of these patients with adult congenital heart disease (ACHD) will require either diagnostics or interventional catheter-based procedures for therapeutic benefit. The utilization of real-time three-dimensional (3D) echocardiography, cardiac magnetic resonance imaging (cMRI), and cardiac computed tomography (cCT) has expanded the realm of congenital interventions. The objective of this chapter is to provide the cardiologist with a general overview of complex ACHD and its management options in the cardiac catheterization laboratory.

ANATOMIC AND PRECATHETERIZATION CONSIDERATIONS

Congenital cardiac catheterization is performed with either general anesthesia or moderate sedation with a combination of opiates and benzodiazepines. Percutaneous access using the standard Seldinger technique in the femoral artery and/or vein is performed and alternative venous access could include the internal jugular, subclavian, or transhepatic approaches. Arterial access may also be obtained from the femoral and radial arteries. Hemodynamic measurements are obtained initially on room air always, precluding the need for a pulmonary vein partial pressure of oxygen (PO_2). For therapeutic procedures, a catheter is passed across the target area, such as a stenosis or abnormal shunt. A guidewire is then passed through the catheter to provide a track over which therapeutic devices are delivered. Balloon catheters are threaded directly, whereas stents and occlusion devices are protected or constrained within a long delivery sheath. Anticoagulation is managed with heparin, 100 units per kilogram of body weight (maximum 5,000–7,000 units), for a goal activated clotting time of 200–250 seconds. Antibiotics are also administered to patients receiving an implanted device.

CONGENITAL CARDIAC CATHETERIZATION

Hemodynamic assessment: Oxygen saturations obtained in room air

Oximetry can detect shunts and be utilized in the calculation of cardiac output. It is critical to avoid obtaining the data with the patient on oxygen via nasal cannula. The oxygen saturation should be obtained from the patient on room air, and it should be drawn from a location distal to the shunt lesion. *Oxygen saturation* is the percentage of hemoglobin that is present as oxyhemoglobin and is measured by reflectance. *Oxygen content* is the total amount of oxygen present in the blood. This includes the oxyhemoglobin plus the oxygen dissolved in the plasma. The oxygen content is calculated with the following formula:

$$O_2 \text{ content} = \left(O_2 \text{ saturation} \times 1.36 \times 10 \times \text{Hgb concentration}\right)$$

In this formula, 1.36 represents the amount of O_2 1 gram of hemoglobin carries when fully saturated. A left-to-right shunt is diagnosed when significant oxygen step-up is found. Specifically, a step-up of >11% from the superior vena cava (SVC) to right atrium (RA) indicates a left-to-right shunt at the atrial level, >7% from the RA to the right ventricle (RV) is consistent with a shunt at the RV level, >5% from the RV to the pulmonary artery indicates a systemic to pulmonary artery shunt, and 2.9% from the SVC to the pulmonary artery has a high predictive accuracy to detect a 2:1 left-to-right shunt.

To calculate blood flows, oxygen contents and oxygen consumption are used:

$$Systemic \; blood \; flow \left(Q_s\right) = \frac{V_{O_2}(mL/min)}{SA \; O_2 \; content - MV \; O_2 \; content}$$

$$Pulmonary \; blood \; flow \left(Q_P\right) = \frac{V_{O_2}(mL/min)}{PV \; O_2 content - PA \; O_2 \; content}$$

where SA is systemic arterial saturation, MV is mixed venous, PV is pulmonary vein, and PA is pulmonary artery saturation.

The mixed venous saturation is calculated with the following formula:

$$Mixed \; venous \; saturation \left(MV\right) = \frac{(2SVC + 1IVC)}{3}$$

Effective flow (Q_e) is the quantity of systemically mixed venous blood that circulates and is oxygenated in the lungs and then circulates through the systemic capillaries. On the basis of this, the effective flow is calculated using the pulmonary vein and mixed venous saturations, and in the absence of shunts equals $Q_p = Q_s = Q_e$:

$$Effective \; pulmonary \; flow = \frac{O_2 \; consumption}{PV \; O_2 \; content - MV \; O_2 \; content}$$

In the absence of shunting, the mixed venous saturation is equal to the pulmonary artery saturation. The left-to-right shunt (flow) is obtained by subtracting the effective pulmonary blood flow from the total pulmonary blood flow: left-to-right shunt = $Q_p - Q_e$.

Hemodynamic assessment: Intracardiac and intravascular shunts

Shunts allow the intermixing of saturated blood with unsaturated blood. Shunts can be either cardiac or vascular and are classified as left-to-right, right-to-left, and bidirectional. Left-to-right shunting results in increased pulmonary blood flow. Right-to-left shunt results in a lower arterial saturation, generally less than 95%. In bidirectional shunts, left-to-right shunting is calculated as $Q_p - Q_e$ and the right-to-left shunting as $Q_s - Q_e$. In patients with residual shunts and pacemaker leads there is a greater than two-fold increase in thromboembolic events.[3]

Hemodynamic assessment: Pressure data (room air)

Normally, in the right atrial pressure tracing, the *a* wave is dominant, and in the left atrial pressure tracing, the *v* wave is dominant. In the secundum atrial septal defect (ASD), there is a larger *v* wave in the right atrial pressure. Elevation of the *a* wave can be seen in pulmonary stenosis (PS). Large *cV* waves are seen in tricuspid insufficiency. A rise in right ventricular pressure is seen in outflow tract obstruction or pulmonary hypertension. Ventricular septal defects (VSDs) occasionally are associated with anomalous and hypertrophied muscle bands, creating the so-called double-chamber RV, which results in a proximal chamber with elevated pressure and a distal one with low pressure in the RV. Abnormal aortic tracings can be the result of abnormal gradients such as in coarctation of the aorta or supravalvular stenosis. A wide pulse pressure is seen in aortic insufficiency, aortopulmonary shunts, or systemic arteriovenous (AV) malformation.

Hemodynamic assessment: Angiography

In ACHD patients, angiography and oxygen saturations are performed at various cardiac locations, and

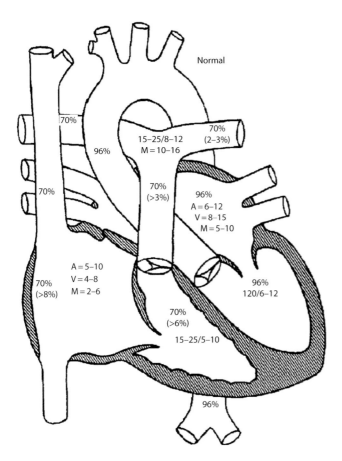

Figure 20.1 Normal anatomy and hemodynamics. The saturations show no step-up to suggest a shunt. In parentheses are the percent steps that would be necessary for a shunt to be considered beyond measurement error.

each structure is evaluated for anatomy, function, and connections (Figure 20.1). Contrast injection of the innominate vein is performed to exclude a persistent left SVC or other anomaly. Inferior vena cava (IVC) venograms are necessary in patients with Fontan circulation to assess for inferior baffle obstruction and shunts resulting in systemic hypoxemia. Right ventriculogram is frequently performed for either function or anatomy. In evaluation of function, the injection rate can be decreased to evaluate the systolic function over several heartbeats. In cases of anatomy, the injection should be approximately 0.5–1 cc/kg over a single heartbeat with 30–40 cc of contrast at 30–40 cc/sec when the heart rate is 60 beats per minute. Pulmonary angiography is used to evaluate pulmonary valve regurgitation or branch pulmonary stenoses. When performing such angiograms, the levophase angiogram is useful to identify the pulmonary vein drainage and additional left-sided structures and function. Pulmonary wedge angiogram is occasionally used to assess the pulmonary vascular anatomy and its changes when there is important pulmonary vascular obstructive disease. Biplane imaging is very useful in congenital heart disease. To visualize the atrial septum, a cranial 45° with a left anterior oblique (LAO) 45° view is useful. To visualize the transverse arch and the area of aortic coarctation, a direct lateral view using biplane imaging and a steep caudal/LAO view is utilized (Figure 20.2).

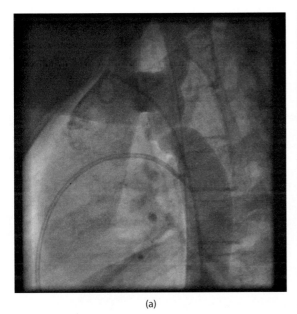

(a)

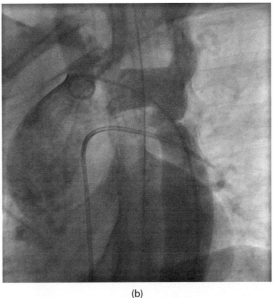

(b)

Figure 20.2 (a) The transverse arch and isthmus are best imaged by positioning the lateral camera in a direct lateral view and (b) the anteroposterior camera in a steep caudal and left anterior oblique view.

CATHETERIZATION FOR COMPLEX CONGENITAL HEART DEFECTS

Patent ductus arteriosus

Patent ductus arteriosus (PDA) is usually detected early in life and occasionally during adulthood. An audible PDA is generally an indication for treatment since such patients typically have a shortened life expectancy and potential increased risk for endarteritis.[4] Survival with an audible PDA to an advanced age is unusual without significant morbidity.[5] However, with a small or restrictive PDA, clinical findings, such as murmur and clinical symptoms, are uncommon except for a potentially higher risk of endarteritis. Historically, over half of the mortalities from PDA in the preantibiotic era were from endarteritis rather than heart failure.[6] In the presence of significant shunting, initially congestive heart failure (CHF) may occur followed by pulmonary hypertension. By 40 years of age, nearly one-third of patients with an unrepaired PDA develop heart failure, pulmonary hypertension, or endarteritis. Two-thirds of such patients do not survive beyond the fifth decade.[7] Therefore, the current standard of care is surgical or interventional PDA closure.[8] In the ACHD patient, coexistent pathologies, such as dilation of the aorta secondary to the chronic left-to-right shunt, calcified atheromatous lesions, and aneurysm of the ductus may result in surgical correction requiring cardiopulmonary bypass.[9] Consequently, percutaneous occlusion of the PDA is an excellent lower risk alternative and precludes the need for a potentially high-risk cardiopulmonary bypass procedure (Figure 20.3).[10]

In percutaneous PDA closure, a femoral venous and arterial sheath are inserted under local anesthesia, moderate sedation, and heparin. If possible, the PDA is crossed retrograde from the pulmonary artery into the aorta for the purpose of coil or device delivery. When the ductus can only be crossed antegrade (from the aorta), either a coil may be deployed or the delivery catheter may be advanced retrograde by using a snare and rail technique.[11] A biplane aortogram in the 40° right anterior oblique and direct lateral is preferred, but if the lab is single plane, the lateral projection or steep LAO is utilized. This angiogram is used to delineate the location, anatomy, and narrowest diameter of the PDA. A single or multiple 0.038-in Gianturco coil can be deployed in the PDA using a tapered catheter for enhanced control as previously described.[12] The goal is to deploy a 1:1 loop of the coil in the main pulmonary artery and the remaining loops in the ductal ampulla. Currently, many centers are using the Amplatzer duct occluder (AGA Medical Corporation, Golden Valley, MN) almost exclusively for adults.[13] A repeat aortogram is performed to evaluate for coil or device position and for residual shunts. The goal is to achieve complete closure of the ductus by angiography prior to leaving the catheterization laboratory. If a residual shunt, other than slow filtration through the device is seen on angiography, the PDA is crossed again and additional coils can be deployed in the same fashion. Prophylactic antibiotics are administered at the time of coil delivery and for 24 hours thereafter. The risk for adverse events is low with reported complications including coil or device embolization, hemolysis from high-velocity residual shunting, and infection. Adult patients can present with a calcified PDA and are at higher risk for surgical closure when calcification is present.

Chest X-ray and transthoracic echocardiography (TTE) are performed the following morning before discharge. Postclosure, standard endarteritis prophylaxis is recommended for 6 months to allow for coil or device endothelialization. Echocardiography is also obtained to confirm complete closure.

Persistent left superior vena cava with hypoxemia

This is a common congenital anomaly of the venous system. It is relevant for pacemaker lead placement from the left subclavian vein approach. The most common anatomy is absence or hypoplasia of the left innominate vein and a direct connection of the left internal jugular vein and left subclavian vein to either the left atrial appendage (LAA) to the left atrium (LA), or through the coronary sinus to the RA. This coronary sinus anatomy should be suspected when a prominent coronary sinus ostia is seen by echocardiography or MRI. The direct connection to the LA (Figure 20.4) should be suspected when patients present with resulting systemic hypoxemia or a history of brain abscess after dental procedures.

Interrupted inferior vena cava

This anomaly is commonly associated with complex congenital heart diseases or heterotaxy. The IVC below the

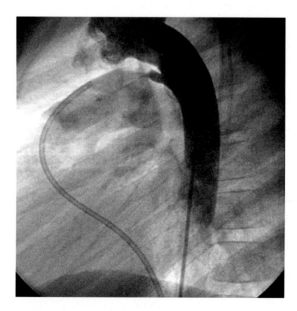

Figure 20.3 Lateral projection of a patent ductus arteriosus.

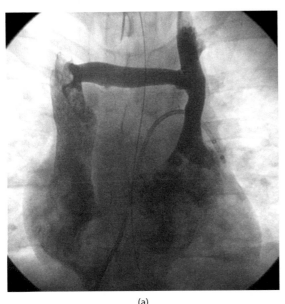
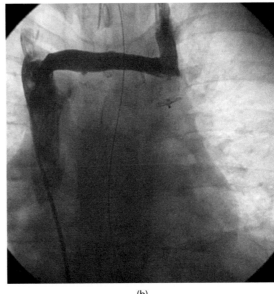

(a)   (b)

Figure 20.4 **(a)** Cineangiogram in the direct anteroposterior projection demonstrating a persistent left superior vena cava to the left atrium with a persistent left innominate vein. **(b)** The same projections after percutaneous closure from the left internal jugular vein using an Amplatzer vascular plug II.

hepatic veins, but above the renal veins, is absent. Thus, the venous return is interrupted with subsequent systemic venous drainage via the azygous vein into the SVC (Figure 20.5). The hepatic veins enter the RA directly.

Myocardial bridging

This intramural course of a coronary artery is a very common congenital coronary anomaly, although its clinical significance remains to be determined. In selected cases, percutaneous or surgical intervention is warranted (generally in severe bridging with evidence of ischemia). However, with adequate antegrade flow during diastole, the majority of cases do not warrant intervention (Figure 20.6),

Anomalous coronary arteries

These can occur isolated or in conjunction with other structural heart disease abnormalities. The recognition and evaluation of coronary anomalies have become a very important part of the evaluation of congenital heart disease. The left coronary artery arises from the left sinus of Valsalva, while the right coronary artery rises from the right sinus of Valsalva. The right or left coronary artery may arise from inappropriate sinus of Valsalva; the most common one is when the left circumflex artery arises from the right coronary sinus. Other types include anomalous right coronary artery from the left coronary sinus, single coronary artery, and anomalous left coronary artery from the pulmonary artery (ALCAPA), which is also called Bland-White-Garland syndrome. ALCAPA is

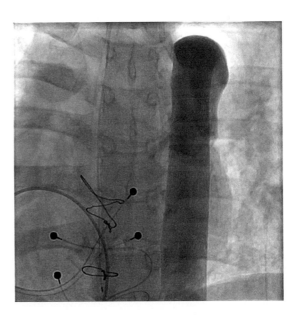

Figure 20.5 The inferior vena cava below the hepatic veins is interrupted with subsequent systemic venous drainage via the azygous vein to the left-sided superior vena cava.

characterized by pathologic q waves in leads I, aVL, and precordial leads V4 to V6. It is possible to find a small left-to-right shunt at the pulmonary level. The left ventriculogram demonstrates left ventricular dysfunction (anterolateral wall) and mitral valve regurgitation. The aortogram will demonstrate a large right coronary artery and filling of the left coronary by collaterals from the right coronary artery, with passage of contrast from the left main to the pulmonary artery.

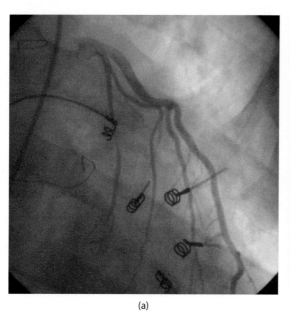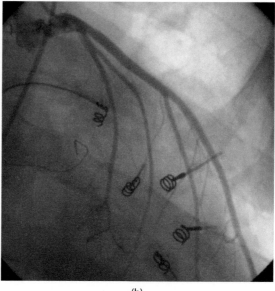

(a)   (b)

Figure 20.6 Myocardial bridging of the left circumflex coronary artery **(a)** during systole and **(b)** during diastole.

Coronary fistulae

Coronary fistulae commonly arise from the proximal portion of the native coronary artery and enter either the pulmonary artery or the atria. Coronary fistulae can produce ischemia secondary to coronary steal phenomenon. If the fistula is large, it can produce a left-to-right shunt. Percutaneous closure is indicated for symptomatic patients with coronary steal (Figure 20.7).

Coarctation of the aorta

Coarctation of the aorta has been estimated to occur with a frequency of 7%–9%.[14] It is usually diagnosed in infancy or early childhood but may go undetected into adulthood. The natural history suggests that isolated coarctation may represent one aspect of more diffuse arteriopathy. Complications can include aneurysm formation and dissection of the ascending aorta rather than the region of prior repair or intervention. Cerebrovascular events from rupture of berry aneurysms may occur before or after surgical repair of coarctation, so a brain screening MRI may be considered during evaluation. Persistent hypertension has been reported despite resolution of the obstruction either surgically or by angioplasty. Life expectancy beyond the sixth decade is unusual if the coarctation is not repaired with a mean survival of approximately 35 years.[15] The coarctation site is typically just beyond the origin of the left subclavian artery, across from the ampulla of the ductus arteriosus. In older patients, collateral circulation is often present to bypass the coarctation and provide blood flow to the lower extremities. The most common origins of these vessels are from the subclavian arteries through the internal thoracic arteries and the thyrocervical and costocervical branches.

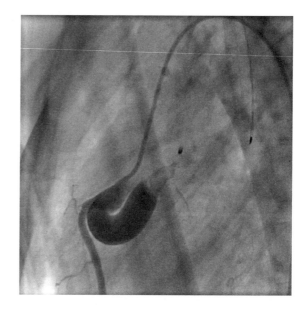

Figure 20.7 Lateral projection of a coronary fistula from the proximal right coronary artery to the superior vena cava resulting after transcatheter intervention with an Amplatzer vascular plug II.

These vessels communicate with the intercostal arteries, which then perfuse the descending aorta distal to the coarctation. This can produce diminished but palpable lower extremity pulses and mask substantial coarctation. MRI is particularly helpful in the evaluation of coarctation among adult patients. Meticulous hemodynamic assessment across the coarctation is essential to elucidate the peak systolic gradient. Intervention is typically indicated when the peak gradient is greater than 20 mmHg, but other clinical factors must also be considered (CHF, left ventricular hypertrophy, abnormal stress test result, uncontrolled upper extremity hypertension). Also, the gradient may be artificially decreased in the presence of collateral vessels.

Coarctation can be a recurrent or native obstruction. Recurrent coarctation is treated with angioplasty or stenting. Native coarctation should still be approached cautiously. For selected teenage to adult patients, stent placement may be considered as the primary intervention for native coarctation. However, the eventual growth of the aorta from adolescence into adulthood and risk for aneurysm formation should be considered to optimize results. The long-term outcome into late adulthood after stent placement remains undetermined (Figure 20.8).

Tetralogy of Fallot

Tetralogy of Fallot (TOF) occurs in approximately 6% of newborns with congenital heart disease. It is the most common form of cyanotic heart disease among adults with congenital heart disease.[16] TOF consists of a large ventricular septal defect (VSD), overriding aorta, PS (infundibular or valvular), and right ventricular hypertrophy.

Current surgical practice warrants early repair, usually within the first year of life. Without surgical intervention, only about 10% of patients survive beyond the age of 20 years. Adults with repaired TOF usually have undergone at least one surgical procedure, but sometimes two to three procedures before their twenties. The repair involves patch closure of the VSD, variable degrees of RV outflow tract resection and reconstruction, pulmonary valvotomy, or placement of an RV to pulmonary artery conduit—either bioprosthetic or homograft. Distal branch pulmonary arterial stenosis may have been repaired, or residual lesions may be present. Examination focuses on the detection of residual lesions. Cardiac catheterization can be used for diagnostic and

therapeutic interventions. Residual shunts are actively sought at the atrial, ventricular, and pulmonary arterial levels. RV pressure is systemic in a patient who has not undergone surgical repair. After surgical repair, elevated RV pressure supports the presence of residual obstructive lesions, the levels of which are documented. Careful pullback recordings are performed from the branch pulmonary arteries to the RV because stenosis at each level is possible. The presence of stenosis at a prior shunt site is expected. RV end diastolic pressures may be elevated in the setting of pulmonary insufficiency. Left heart catheterization is performed if noninvasive studies suggest residual VSDs. Angiography includes a cranialized right ventriculography and possibly, selective pulmonary arterial injections if hemodynamic findings suggest stenosis. Left ventriculography better demonstrates residual VSDs in the presence of subsystemic RV pressures. Aortic root injection demonstrates the presence of aortic insufficiency, confirms the presence of grossly abnormal coronary artery origins or branching patterns, and reveals prior surgical shunts or aortopulmonary collateral vessels. If present, shunts and collateral vessels are best visualized in the posteroanterior and lateral projections. Coronary arteriography is recommended in adults to exclude coronary artery disease before surgical reintervention. In a small proportion of patients, the left anterior descending coronary artery can arise from the right coronary cusp. This is important because a valved-RV to pulmonary artery conduit should be used since right ventriculotomy entails the risk of injuring the left anterior descending. Long-term follow-up studies have demonstrated that patients with TOF will have right ventricular enlargement and dysfunction due to chronic volume overload secondary to severe pulmonary valve regurgitation. Percutaneous pulmonary valve replacement is often indicated for patients with pulmonary regurgitation.

Percutaneous/transcatheter pulmonary valve replacement

The Melody valve (Medtronic, Minneapolis, MN) is used for percutaneous pulmonary valve replacement in patients who develop pulmonary regurgitation from ACHD including TOF, dysfunctional right ventricular outflow tract conduits, prior pediatric congenital heart surgery, transposition of the great arteries, truncus arteriosus, or PS. The Melody valve is a bovine jugular venous valve sutured within 8-zig, 28 mm covered Cheatham platinum stents.[17] It received approval from the U.S. Food and Drug Administration's Humanitarian Device Exemption in January 2010. The 22-Fr ensemble delivery system is used for valve deployment on an 18, 20, or 22 mm balloon in balloon (BiB) catheter. However, the Melody valve can only be expanded to 20, 22, or 24 mm diameters for implantation.[17] Thus, the Edwards Sapien valve (Edwards Lifescience, Irvine, CA) may be used off-label for pulmonary valve replacement in patients who have large right ventricular outflow tract or pulmonary annulus not suitable for the Melody valve (Figure 20.9).[17,18]

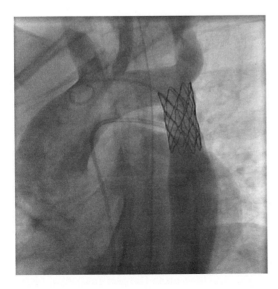

Figure 20.8 Stent angioplasty for native coarctation of the aorta.

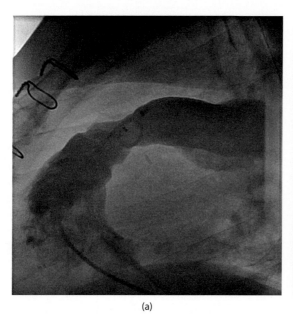
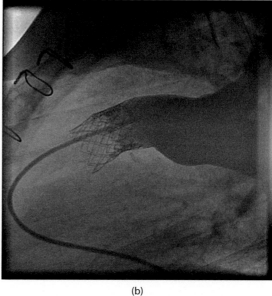

(a)   (b)

Figure 20.9 Percutaneous pulmonary stent valve placement for severe insufficiency of a surgically placed homograft **(a)** prior to intervention and **(b)** after placement of the Edwards stent valve.

The Sapien valve is composed of bovine pericardial tissue mounted on a stainless steel stent in diameters of 23 and 26 mm. The next-generation Sapien XT valve consists of 23, 26, and 29 mm diameters. The retroflex catheter for the Sapien valve requires a 22- to 24-Fr introducer, while the Sapien XT requires an 18- to 19-Fr introducer that is mounted on a stainless steel stent. Prestenting of the native right ventricular outflow tract is required to reduce the incidence of stent fracture in the Melody valve and to provide a landing zone for the Sapien valve.[17,18]

Indication for pulmonary valve replacement, which is commonly performed via femoral access, includes a host of clinical and imaging findings. These factors include clinical symptoms, exercise capacity (measured via cardiopulmonary exercise stress test), right ventricular end diastolic volume index of $\geq$150 mm/m^2 (cMRI assessment), right ventricular end systolic volume index of $\geq$80 mm/m^2 (cMRI), pulmonary regurgitant fraction of $\geq$40%, right ventricular ejection fraction of <40%, and the presence of arrhythmias.[17] Coronary compression testing with balloon inflation is routinely performed prior to valve implantation to confirm the absence of coronary artery compression during valve implantation, which may occur in 5% of patients.[17] The common major complications include pulmonary hemorrhage from stiff guidewires, malposition of the valve, or valve migration. Melody valve endocarditis may also occur in 5.8% of patients.[19]

In the U.S. Melody Valve Investigational Device Exemption Trial[20] for transcatheter pulmonary valve replacement, the long-term clinical outcomes of 171 adult and pediatric patients (median age 19) with right ventricular outflow tract obstruction or regurgitation were evaluated. In a mean follow-up of 4.5 years (range, 0.4–7 years), the Melody valve provided good 7-year hemodynamic and clinical outcomes.

Rare cases of primary valve failure include right ventricular outflow tract reintervention for obstruction ($n = 27$), stent fracture ($n = 22$), or endocarditis ($n = 3$). Fourteen patients overall had definite or presumed endocarditis. Once prestenting of the conduit with a bare metal stent was routinely performed, the incidence of stent fracture declined. The current operator and institutional requirements for transcatheter pulmonary valve repair and replacement are outlined in an expert consensus document.[21]

Right ventricular outflow tract obstruction: Native or postoperative

In severe cases, a large *a* wave will be seen in the right atrial tracing because of decreased compliance of the RV. A gradient will be found in the right ventricular outflow tract. Right ventricular angiography should be performed with anteroposterior (AP) and lateral views. The valve will be thickened and have restricted motion (doming). Usually, infundibular hypertrophy is present. On the basis of the peak gradient, it can be classified as mild (<30 mmHg), moderate (30–49 mmHg), and severe (>50 mmHg).

In valvular pulmonary stenosis, percutaneous balloon valvuloplasty is advised for asymptomatic patients with a domed pulmonary valve and a peak instantaneous Doppler gradient of >60 mmHg or mean Doppler gradient of >40 mmHg (concomitant pulmonary regurgitation must be less than moderate) (Class I recommendation, Level of Evidence: B).[22]

In symptomatic patients with a domed pulmonary valve, valvuloplasty is advised for a peak instantaneous Doppler gradient of >50 mmHg or mean Doppler gradient of >30 mmHg (concomitant pulmonary regurgitation must be less than moderate) (Class I recommendation, Level of Evidence: C).[22]

Otherwise, surgery is recommended for severe pulmonary stenosis with severe pulmonary regurgitation, subvalvular pulmonary stenosis, supravalvular pulmonary stenosis, dysplastic valve, or associated severe tricuspid regurgitation (Class I recommendation, Level of Evidence: C).[22]

The pulmonary valve can be dysplastic, such as in Noonan's syndrome. In nondysplastic valves, the treatment of choice is percutaneous pulmonary balloon valvuloplasty. Because of infundibular hypertrophy, immediately postvalvuloplasty, the gradient can increase (dynamic obstruction). In rare cases, a severe increase in the gradient occurs immediately postvalvuloplasty, with hypotension and hypoxemia ("suicide RV"). Infundibular contraction can be decreased with beta-blocker therapy, which is the treatment of choice, along with intravenous fluids as clinically indicated. Conversely, vasopressors may worsen the hemodynamic compromise, so they should be avoided.

Branch pulmonary stenoses or distortion

Transcatheter therapy in adults with TOF is limited to patients who have undergone surgical treatment with attention to residual obstructive lesions in the main pulmonary artery, RV to pulmonary artery conduit, or distal pulmonary arteries. Prior shunt sites may eventually become stenotic and necessitate balloon angioplasty with possible stent placement. Hypoplasia or stenosis of branch pulmonary arteries will result in an increased afterload to the RV and hypoperfusion to one lung or segment, with subsequent overcirculation to other segments. Branch PS can be congenital in origin or acquired as a complication of surgical interventions. In adults, the treatment involves stenting.

Sinus of Valsalva aneurysms

The sinus of Valsalva aneurysm can potentially rupture and produce a left-to-right shunt and right-sided volume overload. Also, postoperative adverse events with the right coronary artery can result in severe systemic hypoxemia in the presence of a patent foramen ovale (PFO) or atrial level shunt because of sudden compliance change within the RV.

Dextrotransposition of the great arteries

Dextro-transposition of the great arteries (D-TGA) is a malalignment of the great vessels with the pulmonary artery arising from the morphologic left ventricle (LV) and the aorta arising from the morphologic RV. It causes cyanotic congenital heart disease. Currently, all newborns and many teenagers have been treated for this with the arterial switch operation, the Jatene procedure, described by Dr. Adib Jatene.[23] Unfortunately, most young adults were previously treated with an atrial rather than arterial switch, such as a Mustard or Senning operation, depending on if the atrial baffle was made of pericardial tissue or Dacron material.[24] The main hemodynamic concerns in adulthood are the function of the RV as the systemic ventricle (it is

unable to support such increased workload); baffle leaks predominately within the connection of the SVC baffle to the RA, resulting in a right-to-left shunt; systemic hypoxemia or systemic embolic events; and baffle obstruction resulting in SVC syndrome or enlargement of the azygous vein as it "pops" off to the IVC and arrhythmias, especially sick sinus syndrome and the need for a pacemaker insertion. Diagnostic catheterization is primarily reserved for hemodynamic interpretation of the failing systemic RV to obtain an end diastolic pressure, filling pressures, and pulmonary vascular resistance. These data are critical prior to proceeding for possible heart transplantation.

The patient with multiple baffle leaks is often the most difficult intervention to undertake because of the irregular and abnormal connections within the baffle and the morphologic RA and right atrial appendage (RAA). Possible resolution of the baffle leaks[25] includes Gianturco coils (Cook, Bloomington, IN), Amplatzer vascular plugs (AGA Medical, Minneapolis, MN), and Amplatzer ASD and PDA devices (AGA Medical, Minneapolis, MN). Another option used by a few centers is the Gore cuffed "covered" stents (WL Gore, Flagstaff, AR) within the SVC baffle to essentially exclude the baffle leak.[26]

The patient with SVC baffle obstruction will require intervention with a balloon expandable peripheral diameter stent (12–18 mm). The position of the stent is important to avoid too much overlap of the inferior baffle, but it must be long enough to include the more distal SVC. Often, a second stent more distal may be necessary. The lesion may often be either scarred and resistant to the balloon, or compliant and consist of a kink in the baffle. Therefore, we often use a soft, noncompliant balloon to "test" the lesion resistance, measuring in the AP and lateral projections and then choosing a balloon and stent that will be large enough to adhere to the walls and not dislodge toward the atrioventricular (AV) valves. If a patient already has pacing wires across the baffle, a temporary wire is placed from the lower extremity and the pacing wires are then removed allowing the stent to be placed. Once the stent is fully dilated, the pacing wires are replaced across the SVC, and the lower extremity temporary wire is subsequently removed.

Baffle obstruction may also occur in the pulmonary venous baffle. This obstruction is quite difficult to diagnose and is often within the midpulmonary venous baffle, between the entrance of the pulmonary veins to the morphologic LA and the tricuspid valve apparatus. Multiple imaging modalities including MRI, CT angiography, or cardiac catheterization with pulmonary artery wedge pressures and angiograms are utilized to delineate the anatomy. Nevertheless, it remains difficult to image if the wedge pressures (PAWP) are elevated compared with the RV end diastolic pressures. Thus, we place a pigtail and floppy wire to position a hemodynamic catheter retrograde from the aorta to the RV across the tricuspid valve and into the morphologic LA. Precaution is taken to ensure the catheter is positioned near the pulmonary veins and across the midpulmonary baffle obstruction. Once the hemodynamic data are obtained, this catheter is exchanged for an angiographic catheter to perform a power injection directly in the morphologic LA. The main importance of these maneuvers is that long-standing pulmonary venous obstructions can result in pulmonary hypertension or elevated pulmonary vascular resistance, and subsequently, the patient may become a poor candidate for heart transplant.

Congenitally corrected transposition of the great arteries (levotransposition of the great arteries)

This defect is characterized by AV discordance and ventriculoarterial discordance. The aorta and pulmonary artery are transposed so that the aorta is anterior and to the left of the pulmonary artery. The morphological right and LV are transposed with their corresponding AV valves. The RV is the systemic ventricle and with time will develop left ventricular dysfunction. The tricuspid valve is the systemic AV valve and can develop significant regurgitation. Cardiac catheterization is indicated to assess the severity of systemic AV valve regurgitation, to rule out pulmonary hypertension, and to assess the systemic right ventricular function prior to consideration for heart transplantation later in life.[27]

Ebstein's anomaly

This rare congenital heart defect is associated with displaced tricuspid valve leaflets into the RV. It occurs due to a lack of delamination of the tricuspid valve, resulting in different degrees of tricuspid regurgitation. There is a portion of the RV that is "atrialized." Associated lesions include PFO, ASD, VSD, and pulmonary stenosis.[28] Furthermore, patients may develop right ventricular dysfunction and arrhythmias, including atrial fibrillation, atrial flutter, AV block, ventricular tachycardia, or ventricular fibrillation.

In cases of mild Ebstein's anomaly, patients may survive a lifetime without surgery.[29] In a recent single-center retrospective study by Kim et al.,[29] 60 patients (median age 37, range of 18–71) with Ebstein's anomaly were treated with either nonoperative treatment (Group 1, $n = 23$), immediate operative treatment (Group 2, $n = 27$), and delayed operative treatment (Group 3, $n = 10$) to assess their early and long-term clinical outcomes. The primary outcomes were major adverse cardiac and cerebrovascular events (MACCEs), including death, repeat surgery, rehospitalization from heart failure, myocardial infarction (MI), stroke, or major arrhythmias requiring treatment with a median follow-up of 38.9 months (range of 0–229.4 months). Group 1 patients (nonoperative) had better, event-free survival compared with operative groups 2 and 3 (90.9% versus 58.7%, $P = 0.007$). Also, patients who underwent surgical ablation ($n = 20$, Groups 2 and 3) compared with no ablation (Group 1) had more frequent recurrent arrhythmias

(50% versus 20%, $P = 0.034$). Thus, patients should still remain on medical therapy even after ablation. Also, immediate surgery in the presence of an ASD or PFO (even without significant right to left shunt) was an independent predictor of MACCE ($P = .047$).

Single-ventricle physiology: Postoperative physiology

A patient with a functional single ventricle typically proceeds with palliation, including the systemic shunt (Norwood operation, Potts shunt, Waterston shunt, or other central shunts), followed by the SVC shunt or Glenn operation, and ultimately, the completion of the caval pulmonary shunt with the Fontan operation (Figure 20.10). Congenital defects that may necessitate such palliation include hypoplastic left heart, tricuspid atresia, pulmonary atresia with intact ventricular septum, or unbalanced complete AV canal. The ACHD patient with single-ventricle physiology is usually palliated with a Fontan, but few patients remain with a single lung supplied by a SVC to the pulmonary artery shunt (Glenn) or a systemic artery to pulmonary artery shunt. The Fontan procedure represents the final palliative procedure for single-ventricle physiologic status. This procedure completes the direction of the remaining systemic venous blood from the IVC and hepatic veins to the pulmonary arteries. This is accomplished in most cases by either an external conduit or an intraatrial lateral tunnel, which courses from the lateral and inferior aspect of the RA.[30] The atrial appendage or superior vena caval stump transected during the Glenn procedure is directed to the pulmonary artery, effectively "septating" the circulation. Pulmonary blood flow is achieved passively without the assistance of a ventricular pumping chamber. For this reason, it is imperative to have low pulmonary pressures and vascular resistance.

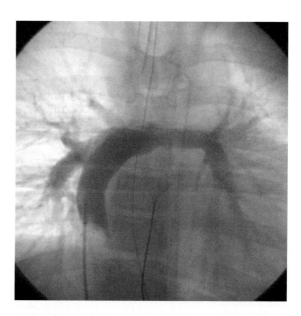

Figure 20.10 Anteroposterior projection demonstrating an external conduit Fontan pathway around the right atrium and directly connecting to the pulmonary arteries.

Important derangements include Fontan pathway obstruction, persistent fenestration, or venovenous fistulae, both of the latter resulting in systemic hypoxemia and increased risk of cerebrovascular events.

FONTAN PATHWAY OBSTRUCTION

There are multiple locations for Fontan pathway obstruction. These include the distal Fontan anastomosis along the hepatic veins, the proximal anastomosis at the pulmonary arteries due to the Fontan pathway, or the SVC anastomosis, and bilateral branch pulmonary artery stenoses. Also, the left innominate vein can become narrowed especially if there is a history of upper extremity central line placement during previous procedures. All of these locations are amendable to stent intervention using peripheral size 10–22 mm diameter stents. Hemodynamic derangements are assessed using mean pressures and careful pullbacks, as only 2–3 mmHg gradient can be significant, especially if there are venovenous "pop-off" routes for the blood flow.

PERSISTENT FENESTRATION

Persistent fenestration is fairly unusual in the adult population, but many younger teenagers and the rare adult may require transcatheter closure of a fenestration if there is concern regarding systemic hypoxemia with or without exercise, and if there is a concern regarding possible or previous cerebrovascular events. Multiple different septal occluder devices have been successfully used to close the Fontan fenestration, and few data exist using the covered stent technology to essentially isolate the fenestration within the Fontan baffle (Figure 20.11).

Venovenous fistula

Venovenous fistulae will manifest with systemic hypoxemia, with or without exercise, or a route for systemic embolic events. The standard angiograms to assess the Fontan circuit for these malformations are a biplane cineangiogram in the IVC distal to the hepatic veins, a biplane cineangiogram at the proximal anastomosis of the Fontan, a biplane cineangiogram in the left innominate vein for the patient with a right-sided Glenn shunt, and angiograms in both SVC in those patients with bilateral Glenn shunts. If these angiograms do not demonstrate the explanation for the patient's systemic hypoxemia or embolic events, we recommend agitated saline injections in the proximal right and left pulmonary arteries with simultaneous transesophageal echocardiography (TEE) or chest wall echocardiography to assess for tiny AV malformations in either lung. The lung with the least or no blood from including the hepatic veins is most likely to have the malformations. Transcatheter closure[31] of the venovenous fistulae or larger AV malformations can be performed using Gianturco coils, Amplatzer vascular plugs, or the Amplatzer PDA occluder (Figure 20.12). Final angiography or agitated saline injections can be utilized to assess for immediate closure and systemic oxygen saturations at rest or during follow-up exercise testing to confirm improvement and future risk for embolic events.

Aortopulmonary collaterals

Significantly decreased pulmonary blood flow is a stimulus for the development of collateral vessels from the

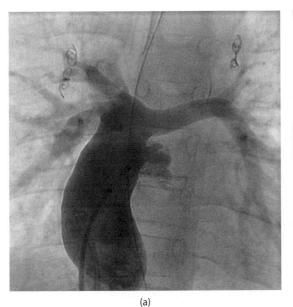
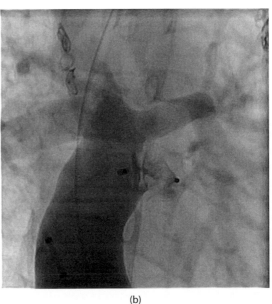

(a)   (b)

Figure 20.11 Fenestration within the Fontan baffle **(a)** before and **(b)** after percutaneous closure with a 4 mm Amplatzer vascular plug II.

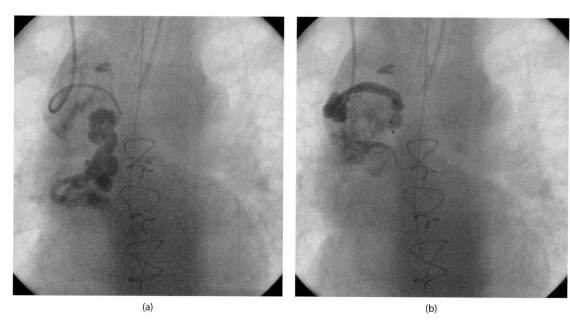

(a)   (b)

Figure 20.12 A patient after the Fontan operation with a venovenous fistula from the superior vena cava to the right pulmonary veins **(a)** prior to intervention and **(b)** after percutaneous placement of an Amplatzer vascular plug II.

systemic circulation. Major aortopulmonary collaterals are present in patients with pulmonary atresia and ventricular septal defect.

SPECIAL ISSUES

Pulmonary hypertension in congenital heart disease

Changes in the pulmonary vasculature are common in patients with congenital heart disease. It can be related to increased blood flow secondary to left-to-right shunting or distortion of the pulmonary arteries due to the shunts[32] Pulmonary angiography is frequently performed to exclude pulmonary branch stenosis (proximal, distal, bilateral, or unilateral), assess pulmonary capillary wedge pressure (PCWP), and evaluate the response of vasodilators on pulmonary pressures. Catheterization will also enable selection for heart or heart and lung transplantation.

Secundum ASDs with elevated pulmonary vascular resistance or left ventricular diastolic dysfunction should be carefully evaluated before proceeding with device closure. Transient balloon occlusion of the defect can be performed to assess the changes in cardiac output and left atrial pressure.

In patients with D-TGA with atrial switch procedures (Mustard or Senning) and pulmonary hypertension, pulmonary venous baffle obstruction must be ruled out.

When a catheter is wedged in a pulmonary vein, the pressure may reflect the pulmonary artery pressure. In cases that the pulmonary artery pressure cannot be measured, for example, in a patient with pulmonary valve atresia, pulmonary vein wedge pressure is used.

Eisenmenger syndrome

In untreated patients, the increased pulmonary blood flow from a left-to-right shunt will produce progressive structural changes in the pulmonary vasculature.[32] Such changes consist of medial thickening and hypertrophy, endothelial damage, and *in situ* thrombosis, resulting in an increase in the pulmonary vascular resistance secondary to the decrease in the cross-sectional area of the pulmonary circulation and vasoconstriction. As the pulmonary pressure continue to increase, the degree of left-to-right shunt will diminish, and eventually there will be right-to-left shunting, resulting in cyanosis. Eisenmenger syndrome refers to reversal of a left-to-right shunt to a right-to-left shunt due to the development of pulmonary vascular disease. Patients can present with syncope, cyanosis, palpitation, hyperviscosity symptoms, hemoptysis, stroke, or a brain abscess.

The diagnosis is based on physical examination, which reveals clubbing, cyanosis, a right parasternal heave, and loud P2 with a high-pitch decrescendo diastolic murmur of pulmonary valve regurgitation. If the RV fails, signs of right-sided heart failure will be evident, with worsening tricuspid valve regurgitation.

Patients are advised to avoid dehydration, heavy exertion, or systemic vasodilators that can increase the right-to-left shunting. If a surgical procedure is planned, meticulous anesthetic management should be available, and mandatory air filters should be used in all intravenous lines to avoid paradoxical air embolism.

Avoidance of hypotension is important; otherwise, the degree of right-to-left shunting will increase and progressive hypoxemia will develop, with the risk of death. If coronary angiography is needed, minimal contrast should be used to minimize contrast-induced nephropathy. Cyanotic patients are more susceptible to developing nephropathy with the use of contrast, nonsteroidal anti-inflammatory drugs, or other nephrotoxic drugs such as aminoglycosides.[33]

CONCLUSIONS

ACHD is a growing specialty with improved recognition, treatment, and survival of pediatric patients into adulthood. Such patients require specialized care as they transition into adulthood, so collaboration between pediatric and adult cardiologists facilitates this transition. Such integration of care is optimally attained in regional ACHD centers of excellence. Furthermore, with the burgeoning field of congenital interventions, it is an exciting time for a multidisciplinary team of physicians and, ultimately, patients who may benefit from a less invasive treatment alternative.

REFERENCES

1. Miyague NI, et al. Epidemiological study of congenital heart defects in children and adolescents. Analysis of 4,538 cases. *Arq Bras Cardiol* 2003;80(3):269–78.
2. Inglessis I, Landzberg MJ. Interventional catheterization in adult congenital heart disease. *Circulation* 2007;115(12):1622–33.
3. Khairy P, et al. Implantable cardioverter-defibrillators in tetralogy of Fallot. *Circulation* 2008;117(3):363–70.
4. Campbell M. Natural history of persistent ductus arteriosus. *Br Heart J* 1968;30(1):4–13.
5. Mesia CI, Moskowitz WB. Coil occlusion of elderly ductus arteriosus. *Am J Geriatr Cardiol* 1999;8(3):131–2.
6. Latson LA, et al. Endocarditis risk of the USCI PDA umbrella for transcatheter closure of patent ductus arteriosus. *Circulation* 1994;90(5):2525–8.
7. Connelly MS, et al. Canadian consensus conference on adult congenital heart disease 1996. *Can J Cardiol* 1998;14(3):395–452.
8. Brickner ME, et al. Congenital heart disease in adults. First of two parts. *N Engl J Med* 2000;342(4):256–63.
9. Fisher RG, et al. Patent ductus arteriosus in adults—Long term follow-up: Nonsurgical versus surgical treatment. *J Am Coll Cardiol* 1986;8(2):280–4.
10. Vita JA, et al. Transcatheter closure of a calcified patent ductus arteriosus in an elderly man. *J Am Coll Cardiol* 1988;12(5):1382–5.
11. Latson LA. Nonsurgical treatment of a neonate with pulmonary atresia and intact ventricular septum by transcatheter puncture and balloon dilation of the atretic valve membrane. *Am J Cardiol* 1991;68(2):277–9.
12. Kuhn MA, Latson LA. Transcatheter embolization coil closure of patent ductus arteriosus—Modified delivery for enhanced control during coil positioning. *Catheter Cardiovasc Diagn* 1995;36(3):288–90.
13. Schenck MH, et al. Transcatheter occlusion of patent ductus arteriosus in adults. *Am J Cardiol* 1993;72(7):591–5.
14. Bashore TM, Lieberman EB. Aortic/mitral obstruction and coarctation of the aorta. *Cardiol Clin* 1993;11(4):617–41.
15. de Divitiis M, et al. Ambulatory blood pressure, left ventricular mass, and conduit artery function late after successful repair of coarctation of the aorta. *J Am Coll Cardiol* 2003;41(12):2259–65.
16. Hokanson JS, Moller JH. Adults with tetralogy of Fallot: Long-term follow-up. *Cardiol Rev* 1999;7(3):149–55.
17. Holzer RJ, Hijazi ZM. Transcatheter pulmonary valve replacement: State of the art. *Catheter Cardiovasc Interv* 2016;87(1):117–28.
18. Levi DS, et al. Transcatheter native pulmonary valve and tricuspid valve replacement with the sapien XT: Initial experience and development of a new delivery platform. *Catheter Cardiovasc Interv* 2016;88(3):434–43.
19. Malekzadeh-Milani S, et al. Incidence and predictors of Melody(R) valve endocarditis: A prospective study. *Arch Cardiovasc Dis* 2015;108(2):97–106.
20. Cheatham JP, et al. Clinical and hemodynamic outcomes up to 7 years after transcatheter pulmonary valve replacement in the US melody valve investigational device exemption trial. *Circulation* 2015;131(22):1960–70.
21. Hijazi ZM, et al. SCAI/AATS/ACC/STS Operator and institutional requirements for transcatheter valve repair and replacement, Part III: Pulmonic valve. *J Am Coll Cardiol* 2015;65(23):2556–63.
22. Warnes CA, et al. ACC/AHA 2008 Guidelines for the Management of Adults with Congenital Heart Disease: Executive Summary: A report of the American College of Cardiology/American Heart Association Task Force on Practice Guidelines (writing committee to develop guidelines for the management of adults with congenital heart disease). *Circulation* 2008;118(23):2395–451.
23. Van Praagh R, Jung WK. The arterial switch operation in transposition of the great arteries: Anatomic indications and contraindications. *Thorac Cardiovasc Surg* 1991;39 Suppl 2:138–50.
24. Warnes CA. Transposition of the great arteries. *Circulation* 2006;114(24):2699–709.
25. Lock JE. The adult with congenital heart disease: Cardiac catheterization as a therapeutic intervention. *J Am Coll Cardiol* 1991;18(2):330–1.
26. Dragulescu A, et al. Successful use of covered stent to treat superior systemic baffle obstruction and leak after atrial switch procedure. *Pediatr Cardiol* 2000;29(5):954–6.
27. Graham TP, Jr., et al. Long-term outcome in congenitally corrected transposition of the great arteries: A multi-institutional study. *J Am Coll Cardiol* 2000;36(1):255–61.
28. Brown ML, et al. Functional status after operation for Ebstein anomaly: The Mayo Clinic experience. *J Am Coll Cardiol* 2008;52(6):460–6.
29. Kim HY, et al. Natural Course of Adult Ebstein Anomaly When Treated according to Current Recommendation. *J Korean Med Sci* 2016;31(11):1749–1754.
30. Fiore AC, et al. Fontan operation: A comparison of lateral tunnel with extracardiac conduit. *Ann Thorac Surg* 2007;83(2):622–9; discussion 629–30.
31. Beekman RH, et al. Embolization therapy in pediatric cardiology. *J Interv Cardiol* 1995;8(5):543–56.
32. Deanfield J, et al. Management of grown up congenital heart disease. *Eur Heart J* 2003;24(11):1035–84.
33. Berman EB, Barst RJ. Eisenmenger's syndrome: Current management. *Prog Cardiovasc Dis* 2002;45(2):129–38.

PART 5

Non-Coronary Angiographic Assessment

21

Ventriculography and aortography

JOSÉ G. DÍEZ AND JAMES M. WILSON

VENTRICULOGRAPHY

Introduction

Reliance on radiographic cardiac-chamber imaging has substantially declined in recent years because of the success of echocardiography and, more recently, magnetic resonance imaging (MRI). In 1980, left ventriculography was recommended as a routine part of the evaluation of patients undergoing cardiac catheterization.[1] More recently, other methods of accurately assessing left ventricular (LV) function or the aortic anatomy have supplanted cavity angiography to such a degree that the techniques and technical details necessary to optimize diagnostic images with ventriculography are being lost.

Nonetheless, ventriculography remains important because it allows efficient, timely diagnosis and guides intervention, particularly for structural heart disease. The LV ejection fraction (LVEF) provides diagnostic and prognostic information in patients with known or suspected heart disease. In clinical practice, the LVEF can be determined with any of five currently available imaging techniques: contrast angiography, echocardiography, radionuclide blood-pool and first-pass imaging, electron-beam computed tomography (CT), and MRI.[2]

In studies comparing different imaging techniques, the results have suggested that LVEF measurements are not interchangeable.[3] Therefore, conclusions and recommendations based on these studies should be interpreted in the context of locally available techniques. In addition, there are wide variances among different techniques in the estimation of volumes and LVEF, especially when echocardiography is used. The principal reason for this variance is the method used to convert two-dimensional (2D) images to three-dimensional (3D) information. Ventriculography typically uses the equations of Sandler and Dodge, which are based on the assumption that the heart is symmetrical and shaped like a prolate spheroid. However, this assumption is valid only for the normal heart. Similarly, echocardiographic methods are encumbered by geometric assumptions, which may result in estimates that differ substantially from those of ventriculography. Nuclear methods that are add-ons to perfusion imaging reconstruct the ventricular walls and measure the volume and LVEF with Simpson's rule. Unfortunately, these methods are hampered by poor spatial resolution (implying a larger error range) and difficulty in assessing transmural myocardial infarction (MI) (if the LV wall is not visible, the result must be imputed—that is, the location of the infarcted wall during systole must be inferred).

Count-determinant, multigated acquisition (MUGA) scanning provides an accurate LVEF but is not reliable for determining wall motion. Improvements in the efficiency of medical diagnosis have virtually excluded MUGA from the evaluation sequence except when other imaging methods are contraindicated or unsuccessful. In essence, the only available technique that can provide accurate spatial and temporal resolution without relying on geometric assumptions is cardiovascular MRI. Therefore, MRI is to be considered the new, true gold standard for measuring LV systolic function.

Left ventriculography can also be performed with digital subtraction angiography (DSA), which uses either an intravenous (IV) or a low-dose intraventricular contrast agent (Figure 21.1). Advantages over standard radiography include less use of radiation and contrast media, an ability to visualize with very low concentrations of contrast medium, and an image format that can be directly analyzed by means of quantitative techniques.[4] By enhancing the contrast-to-background signal, DSA allows angiography to be done with reduced doses of contrast medium. Nichols and coauthors performed a validation study that measured LV volume and segmental contraction, while also comparing the hemodynamic effects of low- and high-dose contrast injections in 28 patients.[5] The group that received the low-dose contrast injections underwent digital left ventriculography and received an intraventricular injection of 7 mL of contrast medium diluted in saline solution. This step was followed by conventional cineangiography of the LV using 45 mL of undiluted contrast medium. After injection of the diluted contrast medium, LV systolic and end-diastolic pressures did not change significantly, and patients had no discomfort. The LV volumes calculated from digital ventriculograms correlated well with the volumes calculated from conventional ventriculograms. Thus,

DSA eliminates the hemodynamic effects that result from injecting conventional doses of contrast medium, thereby markedly reducing the dose of contrast medium necessary for left ventriculography.

To determine the validity of intravenous DSA-left ventriculography (IVDSA-LVG) in evaluating the LVEF and regional wall motion, Kuribayashi and coauthors compared IVDSA-LVG using 30 mL of contrast medium with direct left ventriculography in 18 patients.[6] There was a good correlation between the two methods ($r = 0.877$) in determining the LVEF, and 90% of the interpretations of regional wall motion were in agreement between the two. IV DSA-LVG was useful and accurate in evaluating the LVEF and regional wall motion. The results of this study suggest that this method may be used in patients with impaired LV function to avoid hemodynamic derangement induced by conventional, direct left ventriculography using large doses of contrast medium.

The above-described ventriculography methods and techniques are experimental. They use contrast media, and the radiation doses are actually higher than those used in standard angiography. As these diagnostic imaging methods have evolved, improvements in standard angiography have kept pace. Currently, ventriculography allows clinicians to draw upon angiographic data, on which they base most of their decisions in the cardiac catheterization laboratory. In 2015, a consensus document from the Society for Cardiovascular Angiography and Interventions provided useful guidance for the optimal use of left ventriculography (Table 21.1).[7]

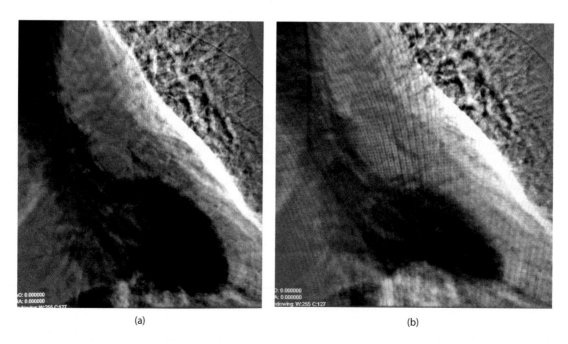

(a) (b)

Figure 21.1 Digital subtraction angiography (DSA) images in diastole **(a)** and systole **(b)** obtained in a patient with acute systolic heart failure due to tachycardia-induced cardiomyopathy. During the study, left ventricular end-diastolic pressure was elevated, which precluded the administration of a large load of contrast volume. When performed with the use of an iodinated contrast agent (10 mL in 20 mL of saline solution, injected at 800 psi), DSA ventriculography showed a severely depressed ejection fraction.

Table 21.1 Recommendations for use of left ventriculography[7]

1. Consider left ventriculography when left ventricular function or wall motion is unknown or mechanical disruption is suspected, and results of the study will help determine therapy. (Examples include acute coronary syndromes without prior noninvasive imaging, or an acute change in clinical status that suggests that left ventricular function has recently changed.)
2. Perform left ventriculography selectively. Avoid it when an adequate alternative left ventricular imaging study has been performed.
3. Avoid left ventriculography in patients for whom it poses significant risk. Examples include patients with renal insufficiency (for whom left ventriculography could increase the risk of contrast-induced nephropathy), elevated end-diastolic pressure (for whom left ventriculography could increase the risk of acute respiratory decompensation), known or suspected left ventricular mural thrombus, aortic valvular vegetation, and previous exposure to high levels of radiation.
4. Develop local criteria for performing left ventriculography, and work to decrease variation in its performance among operators within individual catheterization laboratories.
5. Perform left ventriculography with a multi-side-hole catheter by using a power injector.
6. Include left ventriculography technique and indications in random case reviews as part of a comprehensive catheterization laboratory quality assurance program.

Anatomic considerations and fundamentals

In imaging any cardiac cavity, the following variables must be considered: anatomy, systolic function, regurgitant fraction (RF), shunting, cavity size, cavity output, heart rate, the maximum flow rate of the diagnostic system chosen, and the catheter position and injection technique. For standard ventriculography, mid-cavity positioning of the catheter just below the inflow of the mitral valve is crucial. This position allows mitral inflow to carry the injected contrast material forward, opacifying the apex of the LV. The preferred angiographic view is usually the 30° right anterior oblique (RAO) projection. To evaluate ventricular septal defects (VSDs) or obstructions of the LV outflow tract, a 30°–60° left anterior oblique (LAO) projection with 20° cranial angulation is necessary (Table 21.2).

An underlying principle of ventriculography is that the contrast volume of the chamber being imaged should reach at least 10% of the total contrast volume for the period of imaging in question. Because of the volume of contrast needed for aortography and ventriculography, a power injector is typically used. Power-injection parameters include the volume of contrast medium to be infused, maximum injection pressure, injection rate, and timing of the pressure increase used to minimize catheter movement. The settings for adequate cavity imaging are condition-dependent. For example, a single-beat stroke volume (SV) of 70 mL would be expected in a patient with no cardiac murmur and with presumed normal LV function. Therefore, to achieve the 10% threshold over the target of three to five heartbeats, a volume infusion of 30 mL is more than sufficient. Assuming that the heart rate is 60–70 beats per minute (BPM), this volume can be infused over a period of 3 seconds. The maximum allowed pressure will be influenced by the necessary injection rate and the size of the catheter used. For example, power injection with a 4-Fr catheter system mandates the use of higher maximum allowed pressures and relatively low infusion rates (7 mL/s), as well as longer infusion periods (4 s) to provide diagnostic-quality images.

Consider a patient with suspected severe aortic valve insufficiency. Upon injecting the ascending thoracic aorta with contrast medium, one should be able to quantify the severity of aortic valve insufficiency and, if it is severe, properly opacify the LV, measure its volume, and quantify its function. Accomplishing this goal requires rapidly injecting a large volume of contrast material over a period of

Table 21.2 Anatomic areas of interest, catheter position, and angulation views

Evaluation	Catheter position	Angiographic view
LVEF	Mid-LV	30° RAO, 30° LAO
Mitral regurgitation	Mid-LV	30° RAO
Left ventricular outflow tract	Mid-LV	30° LAO, 30–60° cranial
Ventricular septal defect	Mid-LV	30° LAO, 30° cranial
Aortic valve/ascending aorta	3–20 cm above aortic valve	30° LAO
Aortic arch	Proximal to right subclavian (innominate) artery	45° LAO
Left atrium (ASD)	Right upper pulmonary vein	45° LAO, 45° cranial
Right ventricle	Mid-RV	AP, lateral

Note: AP, anteroposterior; ASD, atrial septal defect; LAO, left anterior oblique; LV, left ventricle; LVEF, left ventricular ejection fraction; RV, right ventricle; RAO, right anterior oblique.

three heartbeats, which is the threshold for distinguishing moderate from severe aortic valve insufficiency. It may not be possible to complete an adequate study with small-diameter catheters. To meet the above-mentioned threshold, let us assume that the LV end-diastolic volume (LVEDV) is 300 mL, the SV is 200 mL, and the LVEF is 66%. When the regurgitant volume is 140 mL, the contrast injection flow rate should exceed 20 mL/s so that the aorta and LV are opacified. Any catheter smaller than 6 Fr would not be able to achieve the flow rate necessary for opacifying both chambers at a normal heart rate. At a maximum pressure of 1,000 pounds per square inch (PSI) (for which most systems are rated) in patients with a normal resting heart rate, a 7-Fr diagnostic system would be necessary to inject more than 60 mL of contrast material over the required 3 second period. However, many catheterization laboratories do not have 7-Fr diagnostic catheters anymore.

Planimetry is more objective than ventriculography for quantifying LV function. With planimetry, the projection image of the chamber in question is outlined and the area measured. By means of a series of geometric assumptions, this area is used to derive the LV volume. The first and most important of these assumptions is that a ventricle that appears somewhat triangular in the RAO view is an ellipsoid. In a 2D view, something that looks like a football is an ellipse. In 3D, such a structure is referred to as an ellipsoid. To be precise, a football is a prolate spheroid. This assumption is not uniformly valid and is clearly violated in patients with previous MI (the population for whom estimating ejection fraction accurately is most important) and other patient populations whose diastolic or systolic anatomy deviates from normal. This is the principal reason why echocardiography and MRI are preferred for measuring LV function.

The volume of an ellipsoid is calculated with the following formula:

$$V = \frac{4}{3}\pi \times \frac{D_1}{2} \times \frac{D_2}{2} \times \frac{L}{2}$$

In the 2D representation, the ellipsoid is an ellipse. Therefore, one may measure the area of the ventricle and the length of its long axis. This allows one to calculate the short-axis diameter of the imaginary ellipse with the following formulas: RAO, $D_1 = 4A_1/\pi L_1$ and LAO, $D_2 = 4A_2/\pi L_2$.

After the axes are derived, these formulas can be used to calculate the ventricular volume. Because the ventricle is some distance from the detector, it will be magnified. Unless an object of a known size is present within the ventricle when the image is being captured, some means of correcting for the magnification is required. The correction factor can be calculated with the formula $CF = (H - P)/H$, where H is the distance from the tube to the detector and P is the distance from the object to the detector. Alternatively, an object of a known size may be placed in the field of view and used for calibration. If the object is placed on or behind the patient, the correction factor must be used (Figure 21.2).

The single-plane method of measuring the ventricular volume assumes that the long-axis diameter and the calculated short-axis diameter are the same in both the RAO and LAO projections. This assumption is acceptable. However, in patient populations with abnormal LV anatomy, this assumption is unreliable and may lead to errors in the calculation of the LV volume or function, regardless of whether the data were obtained in systole or diastole.

Automated edge-detection algorithms may be used to outline the borders of the LV cavity, thereby decreasing intraobserver and interobserver variability and the analysis time.[8] In addition, new modalities using 180° rotational LV injections and a series of projection images may be used for 3D reconstructions and potentially for four-dimensional (4D) reconstructions.[9]

Indications

Left ventriculography is indicated for the assessment of global LV systolic function and regional wall-motion abnormalities (Figure 21.3). Assessing regional wall-motion abnormality may at times be helpful to identify the culprit vessel in acute coronary syndromes. Ventriculography can also be used to assess the severity of mitral regurgitation and to identify and assess muscular and membranous VSDs. Other indications include proper positioning of the CardioKinetix Ventricular Partitioning Device (CardioKinetix, Redwood, CA), a nitinol-based intracavitary device that, when deployed and expanded at the apex of the LV, excludes the akinetic apex and reduces the LV dimensions. This allows for better

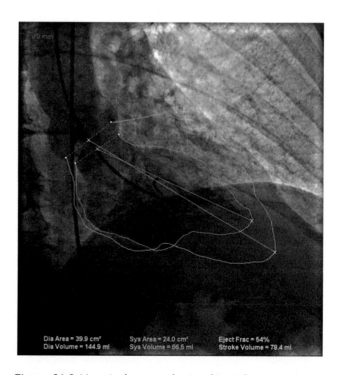

Figure 21.2 Ventriculogram obtained in right anterior oblique 30° view. LV measurements obtained with available software from commercial workstations. LV, left ventricular.

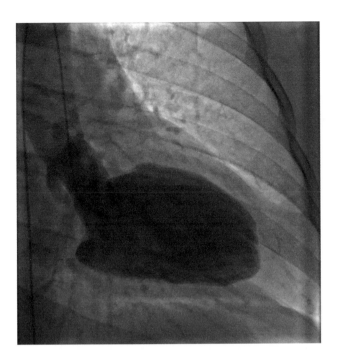

Figure 21.3 Ventriculogram obtained in right anterior oblique 30° view showing a dilated LV chamber in diastole. LV, left ventricular.

efficiency and improves ejection fraction. When properly positioned, this device isolates the malfunctioning portion of the LV in patients with symptoms of heart failure due to ischemic heart disease.

Equipment

Ventriculography is best performed with an angled pigtail catheter, which avoids some of the pitfalls of endhole catheters, such as inadequate opacification, ectopy, myocardial staining, and catheter movement (recoil). The straight pigtail catheter frequently becomes oriented beneath the posterior leaflet of the mitral valve, resulting in poor opacification of the LV or apically produced premature ventricular complexes (PVCs). The angled catheter is more appropriately located within the LV; this position reduces the incidence of PVCs. Pigtail catheters have an end loop that keeps the endhole (required for wire advancement) away from the endocardium, and the other holes along the distal shaft provide offset jets that help stabilize the catheter and reduce recoil.[10]

Alternative catheters include those with multiple sideholes (e.g., the NIH and Eppendorf catheters). As mentioned above, in obtaining measurements from angiographic data, a structure of a known size may be placed within the ventricle. This is most effectively done by using a pigtail catheter with radiopaque markers (1 cm from front edge to front edge). The Langston catheter (Vascular Solutions, Inc., Minneapolis, MN) is a dual-lumen 6- to 8-Fr device with endholes or sideholes that are 8 cm apart. It is available in angled pigtail, multipurpose, and straight configurations. With this catheter, aortic and LV pressures can be measured precisely and simultaneously. However, the lumen size limits the maximum contrast infusion rate, and the pigtail catheter often creates a spurious gradient. The multipurpose version of this dual-lumen catheter is much easier to use for hemodynamic measurements.

Smaller catheter diameters have been used in recent years to reduce the probability of groin-access complications (through either femoral or radial arterial access). However, very small catheter diameters may limit maximum injection rates, impairing the evaluation of the severity of regurgitant lesions. Small catheter diameters (4- and 5-Fr) are usually sufficient for performing coronary angiography, left ventriculography, and aortography in patients whose LV size and function and aortic diameter are normal. However, for the evaluation of dilated chambers or regurgitant lesions, larger catheter diameters (6- and 7-Fr) may be necessary.

In most instances, a standard 0.035-in J-wire is sufficient for positioning the catheter and crossing the aortic valve. In the setting of aortic valve stenosis, a smaller, soft-tipped, 0.032-in straight wire is frequently used. If multiple exchanges are necessary after the valve is crossed, a stiff exchange-length wire is highly useful. Examples include the J-tipped Amplatz device (Cook Medical, Bloomington, IN).

Clinical aspects

Once an indication for performing ventriculography has been established, the first step is to cross the aortic valve. As in several other invasive procedures, crossing the aortic valve in patients without significant aortic stenosis is regarded as straightforward. The presence of significant aortic stenosis necessitates a modified technique (see later in text). Although bioprosthetic valves may be crossed with catheters, it is not advisable for any catheter or wire to be placed across a tilting-disc valve prosthesis because the equipment can become entrapped. In addition, crossing a mechanical prosthetic valve may cause sudden, severe aortic regurgitation, leading to hemodynamic complications.

The classic approach to crossing the aortic valve in patients without stenosis requires the use of a 0.035-in J-tipped wire, which is placed inside the pigtail catheter and positioned slightly back from the tip. The catheter is inserted above the valve and is advanced until it prolapses above the valve and forms a loop resembling a reverse J-shape or the number 6. The loop is then pulled back and rotated slightly in a clockwise direction. During systolic opening of the aortic valve, the catheter will fall into the LV outflow tract, after which it can be advanced into the LV cavity. On occasion, the body of the catheter prolapses across the valve, but the tip stays in the aortic root. In this event, advancing the 0.035-in wire will usually cause the catheter to prolapse into the ventricle. This can result in severe ventricular ectopy and may even damage the valve leaflets. Having the patient take a breath while the pigtail catheter is advanced into the ventricle during systole can sometimes facilitate entry.

Aortic valve stenosis poses a more complex situation. Because this condition may necessitate multiple attempts, thereby prolonging the procedure, it poses a risk of embolization from the valve or from thrombus that may form on the wire or catheters. In these cases, anticoagulation with heparin (3000–5000 units bolus) is recommended. Because of the heightened risk, the valve should be crossed only if noninvasive assessment is inconclusive or interventions (e.g., valvuloplasty or percutaneous prosthetic valve deployment) are planned.

In patients with aortic stenosis, a preliminary aortic root angiogram will allow visualization of the valve opening. Fluoroscopic and cineangiographic guidance of the wire through the calcified opening can also be done in both the RAO and LAO projections. Once the opening has been identified, a straight-tipped 0.032-in wire is inserted through an Amplatz left 1 catheter or a similarly configured device such as an Amplatz left 2, an Amplatz right 1 modified, a multipurpose 1, or a Feldman catheter. In cases of a very horizontal aortic root, a Judkins right 4 curve may be helpful.

Once the wire crosses the valve, the diagnostic catheter is advanced, and pressures are recorded. If an angiography catheter or other catheter is required, it is exchanged over an exchange-length wire (usually a soft-tipped, shaped wire, to reduce the risk of inducing ventricular ectopy). With a 6-Fr dual-lumen pigtail catheter, one can simultaneously measure pressures in the LV and the ascending aorta. Although the proximal connector tubing allows angiography, we have found that it tends to rupture at high pressures.

VENTRICULOGRAPHY TECHNIQUE

Hemodynamic measurements should be performed before ventriculography to obtain baseline information. With single-plane equipment, ventriculography will provide only a 2D projection of the ventricle, and individual images will not include all the LV segments. The standard views for ventriculography are the RAO (30°), which shows the anterolateral, anterior, apical, and inferior ventricular walls, and the LAO 60° or 20° cranial view, which allows better imaging of the lateral, posterior, and septal ventricular walls (Figure 21.4). The LAO views are particularly useful in patients with lateral ischemia (especially circumflex ischemia), suspected VSD,

and mitral regurgitation (Figure 21.5). Some operators prefer to use biplane ventriculography, which correlates better with cardiac MRI than monoplane ventriculography does for the evaluation of function, volumes, and wall motion.[11]

The LV cavity is usually visualized with 30–50 mL of contrast material. Some clinical scenarios call for a modification of this volume; for example, in patients with known or suspected mitral regurgitation, 50–60 mL of contrast material is needed to completely opacify the left atrium (LA). In elderly

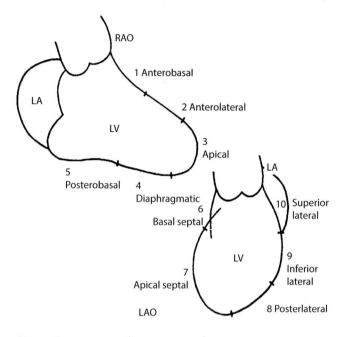

Figure 21.4 RAO and LAO views of the LV obtained during contrast angiography showing division of the LV wall into 10 numbered segments. LAO, left anterior oblique; LA, left atrium; LV, left ventricle; RAO, right anterior oblique. (From Hendel RC, et al., ACC/AHA/ACR/ASE/ASNC/HRS/NASCI/RSNA/SAIP/SCAI/SCCT/SCMR/SIR 2008 key data elements and definitions for cardiac imaging: A report of the American College of Cardiology/American Heart Association Task Force on Clinical Data Standards (Writing Committee to Develop Clinical Data Standards for Cardiac Imaging), *J Am Coll Cardiol* 2009;53(1):91–124. With permission.)

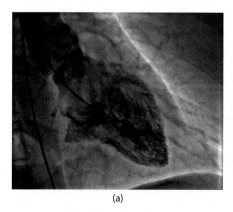
(a)

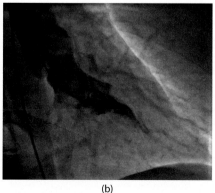
(b)

Figure 21.5 Ventriculogram obtained in right anterior oblique 30° view with an angled pigtail catheter. **(a)** Left ventricle in diastole, **(b)** left ventricle in systole.

patients with hypertensive disease and a small LV cavity, smaller volumes (30–36 mL) are adequate. If the patient has severe valvular disease, LV dysfunction, or an elevated end-diastolic pressure, use of a nonionic contrast agent is recommended. In patients with severely elevated LV end-diastolic pressure (LVEDP), ventriculography should be performed only after pharmacologic interventions (e.g., nitroglycerin or furosemide administration) have been carried out to prevent subsequent pulmonary edema (Figure 21.6).

Once advanced into the LV, the pigtail catheter should be positioned in the midventricular cavity over the region of mitral inflow. Apical positioning of the catheter might lead to excessive ectopy, which could interfere with the interpretation of wall-motion abnormalities. A position that is too basal can interfere with the mitral apparatus, leading to an overestimation of mitral regurgitation. A catheter that is difficult to manipulate, ectopically positioned, or visibly entangled may indicate that the mitral apparatus is involved. When this occurs, proper catheter positioning usually requires catheter withdrawal (preferably over a wire) and replacement in the LV. Repositioning the catheter usually requires countering and pulling it (ideally over the wire) and then advancing it once the tip is free (Figure 21.7).

If the patient is in unstable condition and DSA is available, manual injection can be attempted while the patient holds his or her breath (or by putting the ventilator in stand-by mode if the patient is intubated). This method should be used only for a quick estimate because important abnormalities, such as a VSD, may be missed because of incomplete opacification.

Settings

Optimal ventriculography is performed with a power injector so as to fill the LV cavity. Adjustable settings on the power injector include pressure and flow rates, volume, and the rate of pressure increase. In each case, the settings will vary slightly with patient sex, ventricular size, and catheter type and size. Generally, injection of 30–40 mL at a flow rate of 10–15 mL/s is sufficient for imaging a normal ventricle at a normal heart rate. A rate of pressure rise of 0.5–1 second is needed to prevent lunging of the catheter, which can lead to increased ectopy. The pressure rate settings are typically 400–600 psi, 600–900 psi, and 800–1200 psi for a 6-Fr, 5-Fr, and 4-Fr system, respectively. However, in our experience, adequate visualization can be obtained with a 5-Fr catheter at 400 psi and with a 4-Fr catheter at 600 psi. It is useful to test the integrity of the system when using high pressures and a 4-Fr system. Although most manifolds can tolerate these high pressures, short connectors might rupture. To prevent air embolism during ventriculography, one should pay careful attention to the connections and remove all air from the injector system and the catheter before using them.

During injection, the operator's left hand should be kept on the catheter to change its position as required during the procedure. If the catheter is too far into the cardiac apex, the operator should pull it back and reposition it in the mid-cavity. This is particularly useful to decrease the

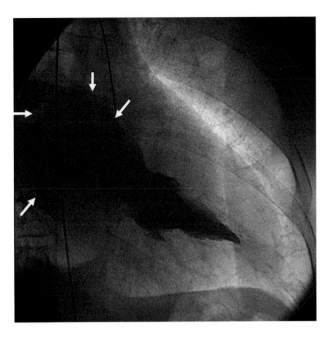

Figure 21.6 Ventriculogram showing severe mitral regurgitation, which was classified as 4+ on angiographic assessment. Arrows indicate the left atrium.

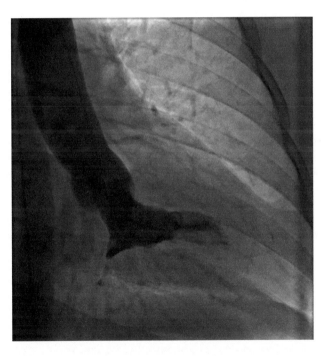

Figure 21.7 Ventriculogram from a patient with known left ventricular hypertrophy. The angled pigtail catheter was maintained in the mid-cavity without compromising the mitral valve apparatus (no mitral regurgitation).

patient's risk of arrhythmia. Conversely, if the catheter tends to go back into the aorta, it should be advanced.

Ventricular arrhythmias or inadequate opacification of the ventricular cavity during contrast-cineangiographic left ventriculography frequently interferes with evaluation of regional wall motion, the LVEF, or mitral regurgitation. In a prospective, randomized study of 95 patients, Deligonul and associates[12] compared a traditional (straight) pigtail catheter to a large-loop pigtail catheter (both 6-Fr devices with a large lumen) with respect to the quality of the resulting cine left ventriculograms. Ventricular tachycardia and couplets occurred at similar frequencies with the two devices. The frequency of catheter-induced mitral regurgitation was significantly higher with the angled pigtail than with the large-loop pigtail. Nevertheless, the intergroup opacification and overall quality of the left ventriculograms were similar. The patients with marginal opacification were significantly heavier ($P = 0.004$) and had larger LVEDVs ($P = 0.019$) and smaller contrast volumes per EDV ($P = 0.005$). The patients with excellent left ventriculograms were significantly younger ($P = 0.019$), were more frequently female ($P = 0.036$), and tended to be less heavy ($P = 0.09$). Ventricular tachycardia was the most common cause of unsatisfactory left ventriculograms. In the RAO view, deeper (more apical) placement of the catheter was associated with a heightened incidence of ventricular tachycardia (53%). The most "silent" area in terms of catheter-induced arrhythmias was the posterobasal region. With 6-Fr high-flow pigtail catheters and nonionic contrast agents, using a more basal catheter position and a higher contrast volume will increase the quality of the left ventriculograms.

Low-volume ventriculography has been shown to be similar to standard, larger-volume ventriculography for the estimation of LV systolic function. In 102 patients, Hodges and coworkers[13] compared low-volume ventriculography to standard-volume ventriculography by using standard (15 mL/s for 3 s) and low-volume (15 mL/s for 1 s) contrast agents. Each patient served as his or her own control. Of the 204 ventriculograms, 27% were not interpretable because of ectopy. Ectopy involving 2:3 beats was more common with standard-volume angiograms (41% vs. 14%; $P < 0.001$). With both methods of contrast-agent injection, the LVEDP increased from baseline levels ($P < 0.001$). In patients for whom both angiograms could be interpreted ($n = 58$), no differences were noted between LVEFs measured with planimetry (low-volume method = $61 \pm 20\%$ vs. standard-volume method = $62 \pm 20\%$; $r = 0.87$; $P < 0.001$). Therefore, low-volume ventriculography reduces the contrast load and ectopy, while providing estimates of the LVEF similar to those obtained with standard volumes.

Quantification of ventricular function

Depending on the angiographic projection, specific ventricular wall-motion abnormalities may be identified. These include hypokinesia (decreased but not absent motion of a ventricular segment); akinesia (a complete absence of wall motion); tardokinesia (delayed contraction of a ventricular segment); and dyskinesia (paradoxical expansion or wall motion, usually due to tethering from the adjacent segments). The LVEF calculated with ventriculography will usually be slightly higher than that calculated with echocardiography.

The American College of Cardiology (ACC), American Heart Association (AHA), and other cardiovascular organizations recognize the importance of having clinical data standards that define and standardize platforms and conditions. These elements are described in the ACC/AHA's 2008 publication titled "Key Elements and Definitions for Cardiac Imaging."[14] The authors acknowledge that each imaging modality uses a unique range of values for quantitatively determining the LVEF and that, even within a single modality, different quantitative methods may yield disparate results. The consensus is that systolic function should be classified into four categories: normal, mildly reduced, moderately reduced, and severely reduced. The quantitative value may be reported as a specific value (e.g., 64%) or as a 5% range (e.g., 30%–35%). The midpoint of the range would be used for data collection and storage. Regional function of myocardial segments assessed by means of contrast LV angiography should be described as normal, hypokinetic, akinetic, dyskinetic, or not visualized. The authors also suggest the use of a 10-segment division in the RAO or LAO views. In the RAO view, the segments should be described as anterobasal, anterolateral, apical, diaphragmatic, and posterobasal. In the LAO view, they should be described as basal septal, apical septal, posterolateral, inferolateral, and superior lateral (Figure 21.4).

Quantification of mitral regurgitation

Valvular regurgitation affects the cardiac chambers upstream or downstream from the leaking valve. The ability of these chambers to accommodate the excess workload is highly variable and at least partly related to the time span over which the regurgitation has developed. For example, if the LA has had insufficient time to dilate after rupture of a chorda tendinea, that chamber's compliance produces striking increases in the left atrial pressure in response to the volume introduced from the LV. Conversely, in chronic, slowly progressive regurgitation, the compliance characteristics of the LA are altered so that the volume of blood ejected into the LA may be accommodated with little change in pressure. As a result, the pressure measured within the accepting chamber may be a poor measure of the severity of regurgitation. Moreover, regurgitation severity may not be the sole determinant of the hemodynamic effect of valvular failure.

Angiographic quantification of valvular regurgitation severity requires opacifying the proximal chamber during contrast injection. Therefore, the visual measures that are commonly used depend on the severity of regurgitation, as well as the volume of the accepting chamber and the volume of flow through the affected chamber. High-volume flow may limit opacification and result in rapid clearance, and low-volume flow may do the opposite. A severely dilated chamber may be relatively difficult to opacify sufficiently to reach a threshold for diagnosing maximal severity. Thus, angiographic methods are accurately characterized as "semiquantitative." Valvular regurgitation may be readily visualized angiographically.

This requires sufficient contrast administration for excellent opacification of the distal chamber and relies on the degree of opacification of the proximal chamber and the time required for the contrast agent to clear. Administration of 40–60 mL of contrast agent over 3 seconds is generally necessary.

Both the RAO and the LAO cranial projections can be used to identify significant mitral regurgitation. The amount of regurgitation is graded according to the degree of opacification of the atrium and ventricle, as well as the size of the atrium and the number of cycles required for maximum opacification (Table 21.3). Both elevation of the left atrial pressure in acute regurgitation and dilation of the LA in chronic regurgitation can interfere with the use of this grading system.

Regurgitant fraction

Perhaps the most valuable indicator of regurgitation severity is the RF. The regurgitant volume is the amount of ejected blood that is returned to the chamber in question during the period of preparation for the next beat. The RF is the regurgitant volume divided by the SV. The effect of regurgitation may be estimated by combining the RF and LVEF with the LVEDV, which gives an idea of the effective forward flow (EFF). The following formula can be used to calculate the EFF:

$$EFF = (1 - RF) \times LVEF \times EDV$$

The same formula may be used to quantify the regurgitant volume if the SV and net cardiac output are known. As a general rule, when the EFF begins to decrease because the chamber has enlarged and cannot accommodate the excess load, the valve needs to be repaired.

The difference between the angiographic SV and the forward SV is the regurgitant volume. The angiographic SV is computed from the left ventriculogram, and the forward SV is derived from the cardiac output, as determined by the Fick or thermodilution method and the heart rate. The RF is the portion of the angiographic SV that does not contribute to the net cardiac output. It is computed as the regurgitant SV divided by the angiographic SV (Table 21.4).

LIMITATIONS

Ventriculography has been compared with other methods and technologies for assessing LV function and morphology. In 65 consecutive patients, Takenaka and associates[15] compared 2D echocardiography, thermodilution techniques, and biplane cineventriculography with respect to LVEDV, LV end-systolic volume (LVESV), SV, and LVEF (calculated with the modified Simpson rule). Two-dimensional echocardiography was performed within 3 days of cardiac catheterization. The results were compared with those obtained by means of the thermodilution technique and biplane cineventriculography. The heart rate and SV were

Table 21.3 Angiographic assessment of mitral regurgitation

Grade	Explanation
1+	Brief and incomplete atrial opacification over several cycles. Clears rapidly. No atrial enlargement.
2+	Moderate opacification of the atria with each cycle. Never greater than LV opacification. No significant LA enlargement.
3+	Atrial opacification equal to ventricular opacification. Delayed clearing of atria over several cycles. Significant enlargement of the LA.
4+	Atrial opacification immediate and greater than that of the ventricle. Severe enlargement of the LA. Opacification of the pulmonary veins.

Note: LA, left atrium; LV, left ventricle.

Table 21.4 Regurgitant fraction estimation in mitral regurgitation

Regurgitant fraction (%)	Equivalent
20	Grade 1+ regurgitation described visually
21–40	Grade 2+ regurgitation
41–60	Grade 3+ regurgitation
>60	Grade 4+ regurgitation

significantly different among the three techniques, and ventriculography yielded the highest values. These findings suggest that patients may have been in a hyperadrenergic state caused by anxiety during invasive cineventriculography and thermodilution examinations. The interobserver and intraobserver variabilities for echocardiography differed little from the variability for ventriculography. Although there were good correlations between the echocardiographic and cineventriculographic findings for the LVEDV ($r = 0.67$), LVESV ($r = 0.80$), and LVEF ($r = 0.78$) as assessed by two independent observers, there was a lack of agreement for the LVEDV, LVESV, and LVEF. The echocardiographic LVEDV values were significantly lower than the cineventriculographic values.

Three-dimensional echocardiography, being exempt from the need for geometric assumptions, correlates highly with ventriculography for estimating ventricular volumes. The 3D technique has approximately half the variability of 2D echocardiography in making these measurements.[16]

Radionuclide ventriculography is a valuable tool in the risk stratification of postinfarct patients,[17] but in this patient population, LVEF correlates poorly with radiographic ventriculography ($r = 0.42$). Therefore, in such patients, an alternative method is warranted. Nonfluoroscopic electromechanical mapping of the LV is feasible and safe. The LVESVs obtained with this method strongly correlate with those measured by means of ventriculography, but the LVEF does not.[18]

The utility of ventriculography in providing an estimation of the LVEF that is reproducible and correlated with survival has been well-demonstrated. Many LVEF calculations used for prognosis in the literature are, in fact, made from angiographic data. However, it should be clear that LVEF values obtained with alternative methods are not necessarily comparable with values obtained by means of ventriculography.

Contraindications

Cardiac catheterization and angiography share several relative contraindications: severe uncontrolled hypertension, ventricular arrhythmias, acute stroke, severe anemia, active gastrointestinal bleeding, allergy to radiographic contrast agents, acute renal failure, decompensated congestive heart failure (because the patient cannot lie flat), unexplained febrile illness, untreated active infection, electrolyte abnormalities (e.g., hypokalemia), and severe coagulopathy. Some of these factors can be corrected before the procedure, thereby mitigating the risk they pose.

In patients with cardiogenic shock who are undergoing percutaneous revascularization, contrast ventriculography either is deferred until after coronary angiography has been performed,[19] or is avoided to prevent further hemodynamic compromise resulting from arrhythmias or increases in ventricular pressure and renal failure. Contrast medium–induced hypotension and bradycardia were once serious concerns in patients with severe aortic stenosis and left main or severe three-vessel coronary artery disease, but the rates of these complications have been decreased by the use of low-osmolar or nonionic media.[20] In cases of severe coronary artery disease (including left main disease), it is uncertain whether the risks posed by a left ventriculogram are outweighed by its benefits.[21] However, as discussed above, ventriculography can be safely performed with less than 40 mL of a low-osmolar contrast agent. Proper access techniques and careful manipulation of the catheter are required because a catheter-induced arrhythmia or vasovagal response can cause hemodynamic instability.

Left ventriculography should be performed only in patients for whom the benefits from the information obtained are likely to be greater than the risks related to the procedure. Otherwise, noninvasive assessment of ventricular function and mitral regurgitation by means of echocardiography and nuclear or MRI techniques is more appropriate.[22]

Absolute contraindications for left ventriculography include critical left main disease, a tilting-disc aortic prosthesis (the catheter can cause acute aortic regurgitation, become entrapped, or damage the tilting mechanism), decompensated heart or renal failure, left-sided endocarditis, and a recently diagnosed (freshly formed) intracardiac thrombus. Because thrombi more than 6 months old may have a lower risk of dislodgement, some operators may proceed with ventriculography in their presence. However, because of the uncertainty involved in appropriately estimating the age of an intracavitary thrombus, we suggest deferring ventriculography and proceeding with noninvasive evaluation.

Complications

Among the complications that have been encountered during ventriculography are ventricular arrhythmias, conduction anomalies including atrioventricular block (especially in patients with preexisting right bundle branch block, in whom manipulation of the catheter near the septum may cause transient left bundle branch block and, as a consequence, complete atrioventricular block), embolization of air or thrombus, contrast agent–related complications, worsening of hemodynamic values in patients with decompensated heart failure, and myocardial staining or "tattooing."

Air or thrombus embolization has been observed during ventriculography and left-sided heart catheterization. Transcranial Doppler (TCD) imaging has shown that these complications commonly occur when patients are evaluated with ventriculography. To assess the prevalence, timing, and potential significance of microembolic signals (MESs) detected with TCD during left-heart catheterization, Leclercq and coworkers[23] monitored the right and left middle cerebral artery in 51 consecutive patients (36 men, 15 women) and detected MESs in all but two of them (mean number of signals, 17.1 ± 12.8 per patient), mainly during left ventriculography. The MESs were asymptomatic and probably of gaseous origin because they occurred predominantly during contrast media injection and were not related to the patients' cardiovascular history or to atheroma risk factors. No neurologic events occurred within 24 hours after ventriculography in the 49 patients who had MESs.

An unusual but potentially dangerous complication of left-sided heart catheterization is massive air embolization.[24,25] Therefore, the system should be meticulously checked for air before the injection is performed. If air bubbles embolize to the brain or coronary arteries, they can cause transient or permanent neurologic complications and hemodynamic collapse, respectively. The operator should be alerted if a sensory deficit is noted after a contrast medium has been injected for left ventriculography. Theoretically, the preferred treatment for cerebral air embolization is hyperbaric oxygen, but this is rarely done in clinical practice.

Left atrial angiography

The left atrial anatomy is complex, and the chamber borders are poorly defined, making assessment of left atrial function and volume somewhat difficult. However, opacifying the LA can be useful for the anatomic evaluation of an atrial septal defect (ASD) or a patent foramen ovale (PFO). Similarly, it may be important to evaluate the left atrial anatomy before and after radiofrequency ablation procedures. In most instances, the anatomy can be assessed quite well with noninvasive means. In fact, because of the complex and highly variable anatomy of the pulmonary veins, MRI and CT are superior to angiographic projection imaging. However, angiographic guidance is necessary for placing ASD, PFO, or left atrial occluder devices. Left atrial angiography is best performed with the NIH catheter, which is placed in the right upper pulmonary vein. This allows contrast material to "wash" along the interatrial septum. A 45° LAO imaging plane with 45° cranial angulation best outlines the septum to show ASDs and PFOs. Injection parameters for left atrial angiography are similar to those for ventriculography, except that lower maximum pressures may be used in the low-pressure LA.

Right ventriculography

The right ventricle's (RV) shape is poorly conducive to evaluation by means of projection imaging. It is both triangular in the anteroposterior projection and discoid in the lateral projection. Therefore, the use of angiographic imaging for volume estimates is fraught with error, and the geometric assumptions used in imaging the RV are of little value. However, RV angiography may be useful for evaluating tricuspid regurgitation, global RV function, suspected RV cardiomyopathy, or arrhythmogenic RV dysplasia, and for planning a pulmonary valvuloplasty. The severity of tricuspid regurgitation is evaluated qualitatively, and the grading system is similar to that used for mitral regurgitation: 1+, trivial; 2+, mild; 3+, moderate; and 4+, severe. Given that access to the RV requires crossing the tricuspid valve, evaluating tricuspid insufficiency is as potentially erroneous as imaging the RV.

Ideally, right ventriculography is best performed with a biplane system. When performed with a single-plane system, it is usually done in the AP projection. With a biplane system, the 60° LAO projection is added. The contrast volume ranges from 20 to 40 mL, injected over 2 seconds. In general, lower maximum pressures can be used when RV pressures are low.

An angled pigtail catheter, a variant of the angled pigtail catheter known as the Grollman catheter, or the NIH catheter can be used for this procedure. Some operators prefer the NIH catheter because it is easily maneuverable in patients who have difficult anatomy, and it can be concurrently used for subselective pulmonary artery (PA) angiography. The catheter is placed in the mid-cavity position, and injection parameters similar to those of left ventriculography are used.

When RV pressures are elevated, PA catheterization should be performed before right ventriculography (Figure 21.8). In patients with severe pulmonary hypertension, main pulmonary angiography or right ventriculography may result in hemodynamic compromise, so alternative methods for assessing RV anatomy and function should be chosen.

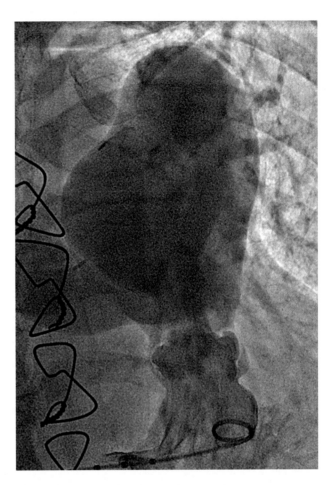

Figure 21.8 Right ventriculogram of the right ventricular outflow tract documenting large pulmonary artery aneurysm.

Left ventriculography conclusion

Catheterization of the LV to obtain hemodynamic measurements and to visualize the LV with contrast ventriculography is an important component of a complete angiographic study because it provides essential anatomic and functional information. Although noninvasive testing techniques continue to improve and become more accurate, cardiac catheterization remains the standard for evaluating hemodynamic parameters. In some instances, catheterization is preferred (e.g., when patients present acutely with a MI). By assessing myocardial and valvular function with ventriculography, the clinician may quickly gain information vital to making sound decisions about a patient's immediate care. In obese patients who have suboptimal echocardiographic windows, ventriculography may provide information not obtainable from the echocardiogram.

As new technologies and interventions such as percutaneous aortic valve replacement become available, it is important that cardiologists become skilled at crossing the aortic valve and appropriately assessing LV function and morphology. Meanwhile, ventriculography remains an important tool for diagnostic evaluation and for planning interventional procedures. Its principles are straightforward, but close attention to detail is necessary to obtain diagnostic-quality images.

AORTOGRAPHY

Introduction

Aortography is the radiographic technique used to opacify the lumen of the aorta, the superior aspect of the aortic valve leaflets, and all of the vessels that arise from the aorta.[26] Noninvasive radiographic evaluation of the aorta and its branches has evolved rapidly because of advancements in imaging techniques such as computed tomography angiography (CTA) and magnetic resonance angiography (MRA). Nevertheless, catheter-based angiographic evaluation remains an integral part of the diagnostic process and the main guide to choosing an intervention (either endovascular or surgical). An ascending aortogram allows one to determine the competency of the aortic valve, the anatomy and diameter of the ascending thoracic aorta, and the presence of aortic dissection or of patent aortocoronary bypass grafts. When the catheter is positioned proximal to the innominate artery, the examiner may evaluate the anatomy of the aortic arch and its major arterial branches (e.g., to guide percutaneous revascularization of the subclavian or the carotid arteries), detect the presence of a persistent ductus arteriosus or coarctation, and gain information about the descending thoracic aorta. When the catheter is positioned more distally, one may evaluate aneurysms, dissections, and abnormalities of the abdominal aorta and its arterial branches (Figure 21.9).

ANATOMIC CONSIDERATIONS AND FUNDAMENTALS

During aortography, variants in the anatomy may be identified. To understand and appropriately identify these variants, some basic concepts need to be reviewed. In the earliest stages of embryogenesis, the vessels are plexiform. As the fetus grows, the vessels become recognizable as conduits. The adult aorta and the aortic arch system result from the regression and fusion of six pairs of aortic arches (Table 21.5). Normal regression of the right dorsal aortic root results in the normal left aortic arch. Aortic arch branch variants can be identified in 30%–35% of individuals. The most frequent variant (20%) is a common origin of the innominate and left common carotid arteries (bovine arch). Other variants include a left vertebral artery arising from the arch (5%); an aberrant right subclavian artery or lusoria (1%); and, less frequently, a right-sided aortic arch, double aortic arch, or cervical aortic arch (Figure 21.10).

The abdominal aorta is formed from the right and left dorsal aortas. The numerous splanchnic branches that supply the primitive digestive tract are reduced to become the celiac, superior, and inferior mesenteric arteries. Anomalies of the abdominal aorta itself are rare, but they are common in the primary branches (Figure 21.11).[27]

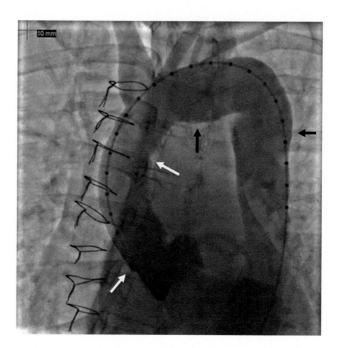

Figure 21.9 Aortogram in 60° left anterior oblique projection from a patient who had previously undergone repair of an ascending aortic aneurysm with a Dacron graft (white arrows indicate the beginning and end of the graft). Aortic dilatation distal to the graft compromises the arch and descending aorta (black arrows).

Table 21.5 Anatomic result of aortic arch regression and fusion during embryogenesis

Vessel	Origin
Proximal ascending aorta	Truncus arteriosus
Distal ascending aorta, innominate artery, and arch until left common carotid artery	Aortic sac
Right subclavian artery	Fourth aortic arch
Common carotid arteries	Third aortic arch
Aortic arch between the left common carotid artery and the left subclavian artery	Fourth aortic arch
Left subclavian artery	Left intersegmental artery
Ductus arteriosus	Sixth aortic arch
Descending aorta	Left dorsal aorta

Approximately one-third of patients have multiple renal arteries. Approximately 2%–7% of patients have bilateral accessory renal arteries. Persistence of the ventral connection results in the rare condition known as celiacomesenteric trunk. In addition, the hepatic, left hypogastric, or splenic arteries may have separate origins from the aorta. The presence of multiple branches accounts for the parietal collateral systems that can be identified in occlusive diseases of the aorta. Intercostal, subcostal, and lumbar

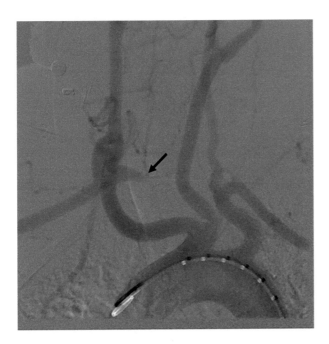

Figure 21.10 Digital subtraction angiogram from a woman with a history of dysphagia who presented with right-arm claudication. The occluded, aberrant right subclavian artery originates distal to the left subclavian artery. Collateral flow is reconstituting the aberrant vessel (arrow).

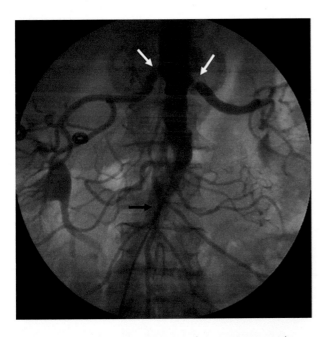

Figure 21.11 Abdominal aortogram from a patient with diffuse atherosclerosis, dyslipidemia, and hypertension who presented with claudication. This image, obtained in the anteroposterior view, shows bilateral renal artery stenosis (white arrows) and severe distal aortic stenosis (black arrow).

arteries can provide collaterals to the iliolumbar and superior gluteal branches of the internal iliac artery and to the circumflex branches of the external iliac artery. The visceral pathways for collaterals arise from the superior and inferior mesenteric arteries.

Even in healthy humans, the aorta lengthens with age, primarily because the ascending aorta elongates over time.[28] This elongation is also a function of blood pressure. At the same time, an increase in collagen augments aortic wall stiffness. Because these changes are balanced by changes in body morphology, the changes in the physical characteristics of the aorta cannot be detected by measuring the pulse wave velocity. Aged, hypertensive patients will frequently have a tortuous aorta that challenges the interventionalist with regard to catheter passage, catheter placement, and proper angiographic imaging. Because of the difficulties that the abdominal aorta may present when it is severely diseased (e.g., with an aneurysm, a dissection, a luminal thrombus, or tortuosity), a radial or brachial approach may be needed during aortography to obtain adequate images and avoid complications.

Optimal aortography requires using a power injector to opacify the vessel adequately. Settings must be varied slightly according to the size of the aortic root, presence of aneurysms, degree of aortic valve insufficiency, diameter of the catheter lumen, and patient size. The catheters used for aortography are similar in shape to those used for ventriculography (pigtail catheters), but because diameter measurements are required, a marker pigtail catheter is preferred. Alternatively, other angiographic catheters can be used, such as the Omniflush or the tennis racket.

Indications

Although aortography has been supplanted by transesophageal echocardiography (TEE), CTA, and MRA for many disorders of the aorta, angiographic imaging may be useful to exclude aortic dissection (Figure 21.12) in patients referred for urgent coronary angiography. This technique is also useful for measuring the aortic diameter—preferably with a marker pigtail—when other studies have rendered conflicting information for measuring the severity of aortic insufficiency, for delineating the aortic and coronary anatomy before surgical repair of an aneurysm, and for verifying the presence of an aortoenteric fistula.[29,30]

Perhaps the most important advance in aortography in recent years has been the use of digital subtraction, which allows anatomic details to be accurately delineated with relatively small quantities of contrast media. DSA is superior to standard imaging for evaluating congenital and acquired lesions of the arch and great vessel origins.[31] Contrast aortography has gained a central role in guiding aortic endovascular aneurysm repair (EVAR) and other percutaneous interventional procedures at the level of the aorta (Figure 21.13) and the supra-aortic vessels.

EQUIPMENT

For contrast aortography, angiographic equipment is required that provides a spatial resolution of at least 3–4 lines/mm. Ideally, large image intensifiers up to 16 inches (40.6 cm) in diameter should be used to provide a field of view large enough to show the entire arch and its branches or the entire abdominal aorta at the same time. Current technologies include postprocessing and image-reformatting modalities, which allow for diameter analysis, 3D rendering, and rotational 3D rendering. Flat-panel technology has significantly increased image resolution.

For arterial access, 4- to 7-Fr systems can be used. Dedicated radial sheaths or micropuncture devices (usually 4- to 6-Fr) are used for radial or brachial access. The length of the guidewire is determined by its intended use and varies

from 145 to 175 cm. However, if multiple catheter exchanges are required, or if maintaining position is important (i.e., in the presence of aortic dissections, complex aneurysms, severe tortuosity, or a large atherothrombotic burden), a long (260–350 cm) exchange wire is preferred. Although guidewire diameter may range from 0.014 to 0.038 inches, a 0.035-in guidewire is most often used.

Angiographic catheters are usually pigtail, marker pigtail, Omniflush or tennis racket devices, or catheters with multiple sideholes. A power injector is required for optimal opacification. Low-osmolar or iso-osmolar contrast agents are preferred because they cause less intravascular volume augmentation, fewer side effects, and possibly, less contrast-induced nephropathy.

Clinical aspects

In general, careful planning for the procedure is required. The access site must be selected first. Choosing the appropriate access site for peripheral arteriography is a most important procedural decision that is analogous with planning a surgical incision.[32] The site of access is determined by using anatomic information from previous noninvasive studies (if available), the patient's clinical history (including ascending or abdominal aortic pathology), and physical examination (including the presence of pulses). In our practice, the most common sites of access are the common femoral (70%) (Figure 21.14) and radial (30%) (Figure 21.15) arteries. With the aid of fluoroscopic guidance, access via the common femoral artery is usually obtained with a micropuncture system, which is later exchanged for a catheter with a larger French size.

In most of our angiographic studies, a 5-Fr system is used. Also, we most commonly use 0.035-in exchange-length wires, including the Wholey Hi-Torque model (Mallinckrodt Inc., St. Louis, MO), the Bentsen model

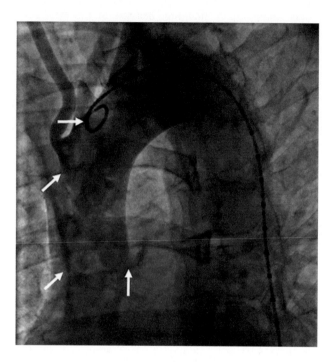

Figure 21.12 Aortogram in left anterior oblique demonstrating an ascending aortic dissection. The dissection extends from the sinuses of Valsalva to the origin of the innominate artery (arrows).

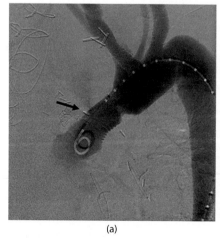
(a)

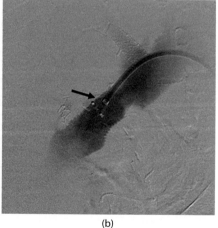
(b)

Figure 21.13 Aortogram from a critically ill patient with multiple comorbidities who presented with a large pseudoaneurysm several months after undergoing surgical repair of an ascending aortic aneurysm. (a) Evidence of a perforation at the level of the distal suture in the Dacron graft (arrow). (b) Successful closure of the graft perforation with an Amplatzer Cribriform Occluder (diameter, 18 mm [AGA Medical Corporation, Plymouth, MN]) (off-label indication) (arrow).

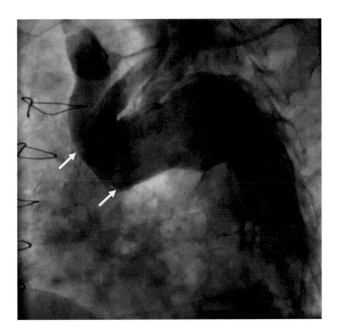

Figure 21.14 Angiogram obtained via common femoral access in a man with a history of ascending thoracic aortic aneurysm. The complex dissection flap (arrows) prohibited passage of the wires or catheters into the ascending aorta. Subsequent ascending aortic angiography and coronary angiography were performed via the right radial approach.

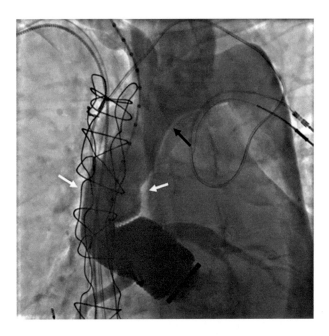

Figure 21.15 Angiogram performed via the right radial route with a marked pigtail showing an ascending aortic aneurysm (white arrows). Note the dissection flap at the level of the aortic arch (black arrow). A Dacron graft extends from the prosthetic aortic valve to the mid-segment of the ascending aorta, distal to which the dissection can be visualized.

(Cook, Inc., Bloomington, IN), and the hydrophilic Glidewire (Terumo, Somerset, NJ). If diameter measurements are important, a marker pigtail catheter is used.

When we are dealing with complex anatomy (involving an aortic dissection, previous aneurysm repair with a Dacron graft, or severe tortuosity) and are uncertain about reaching the aortic root via the femoral approach, we usually obtain access with a micropuncture system. We advance a 0.035-in Wholey wire until it reaches the ascending aorta. After establishing that the wire is in the true lumen (by verifying that the wire moves freely, responds to flow from the aortic valve, and loops easily at the sinuses), we exchange the micropuncture system for a 5-Fr system (including a long sheath, if necessary) and then advance the angiographic catheters. Severe aortic tortuosity can cause difficulties in advancing and manipulating the catheter. In such cases, a long access sheath may help when one is working from a femoral approach (Figure 21.16). However, one should carefully consider using a radial or brachial approach. With the radial approach (Figure 21.17), we prefer to use a dedicated radial sheath (Terumo) and to perform exchanges over a hydrophilic wire (e.g., Glidewire). At all times, careful manipulation of wires and catheters is essential to prevent traumatic disruption of intraluminal thrombus or wall atheromas.

ASCENDING AORTOGRAPHY

Dissections of the ascending aorta, anomalous coronary origins, and some saphenous vein grafts (SVGs) are best revealed by visualizing the ascending aorta in the 30° LAO

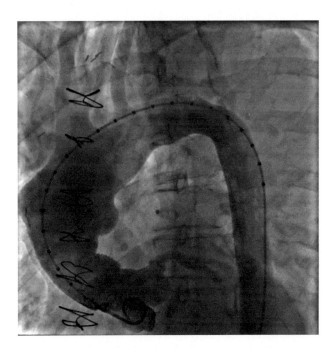

Figure 21.16 Aortogram performed via a common femoral approach, showing an ascending aortic aneurysm that extends into the arch.

projection with 30° cranial angulation (Figure 21.18). In contrast, the aortic arch and branch origins are best displayed in the 45° LAO projection with no cranial angulation. The catheter (preferably a regular or marker pigtail) is placed in the ascending thoracic aorta at the level of the sinotubular

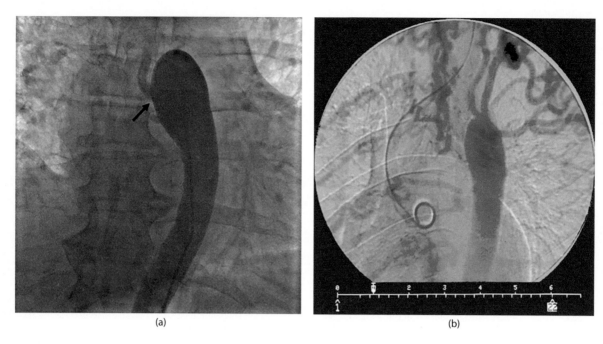

(a)   (b)

Figure 21.17 **(a)** Aortograms in anteroposterior projection from a 65-year-old man with a history of hypertension. The descending aorta was completely interrupted below the level of the left subclavian artery. A small collateral vessel is seen (arrow). **(b)** Aortogram obtained via the left radial approach showing aortic coarctation, with collaterals reconstituting the descending aorta.

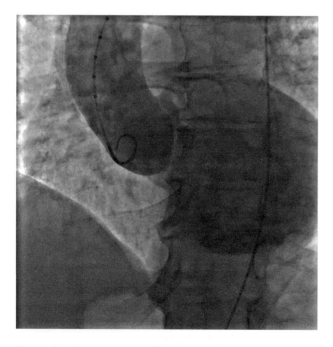

Figure 21.18 Aortogram of the ascending aorta (left anterior oblique 30° view with cranial angulation) showing a bicuspid aortic valve and immediate filling of the left ventricle allowing the diagnosis of severe aortic insufficiency (grade 4+).

ridge (2–3 cm above the aortic valve). This allows the catheter to stiffen and lengthen during power injection without encountering the aortic valve. Unintentional contact with the aortic valve may either produce iatrogenic aortic valve insufficiency or result in poor opacification of two of the

three sinuses of Valsalva. If the catheter is positioned just proximal to the right innominate branch, the aortic arch and the origin of the great vessels can be seen. The 30° RAO projection is best reserved for visualizing SVGs, but it may also be used to show aortic insufficiency.

TECHNIQUE

A 4- to 7-Fr pigtail catheter is generally used to perform aortography. The size is critically dependent on the specific situation. To assess the aortic anatomy, the injection velocity from a 4-Fr catheter is sufficient with the assistance of DSA. For aortic insufficiency, a catheter with a larger diameter (7 Fr) will allow rapid contrast injection. However, any catheter without endholes may be used. With endhole catheters, there may be a risk of aortic dissection or aortic valve damage during power injection (Figures 21.19 and 21.20).

SETTINGS

During injection, the high-viscosity contrast agent encounters resistance along the length of the catheter lumen. This resistance produces a force within the catheter, making the device as straight as possible within the constraints placed on it by the anatomy of the aorta. To reduce this "kick" during injection, the rate of pressure rise during power injection is modulated. A period of pressure rise of 0.5–1 second is often used, the rise time being a function of the size of the catheter lumen. The pressure settings are typically 600, 900, and 1200 psi for 6-Fr, 5-Fr, and 4-Fr systems, respectively. Generally, injecting 40–50 mL at 20–25 mL/s is sufficient for imaging a normal aorta. When DSA is used, contrast agent can be administered in lower volumes, such as 30 mL at a rate

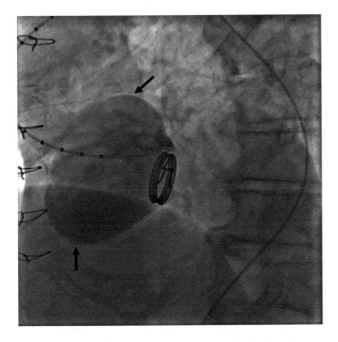

Figure 21.19 Aortogram from a patient who had undergone aortic valve replacement with a single-tilt disc valve and repair of an ascending aortic aneurysm with a Dacron graft several years earlier. Note the severe dilatation of the aortic root (arrows).

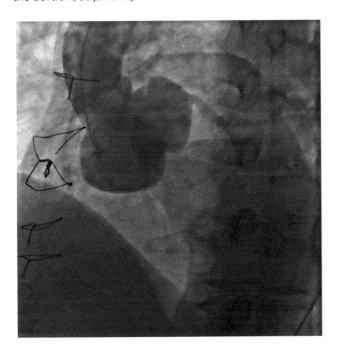

Figure 21.20 Aortogram showing dilatation of the sinuses of Valsalva and the presence of aortic regurgitation (grade 2+).

of 15 mL/s. A period of pressure rise of 1 second is recommended to avoid abrupt catheter movement. Pressure settings depend on catheter size as described above. To prevent air embolism during aortography—particularly if performed at the level of the ascending aorta or aortic arch—careful attention must be paid to removing air from the injector system before it is used. According to case reports, injecting 50 mL of air into the ascending aorta is fatal.

Quantification of aortic insufficiency

Quantifying aortic valve regurgitation requires injecting a sufficient volume of contrast material (about 40–60 mL) into the aorta via a catheter that is near, but not in contact with, the aortic valve. The severity of regurgitation is rated according to a semiquantitative scale similar to the one used for mitral regurgitation (Table 21.6). Although aortography is useful to guide the deployment of a transcatheter aortic valve prosthesis (because it provides valuable data on positioning, coronary artery patency, and aortic root and arch anatomy), the primary imaging method recommended for assessing prosthetic valve function is echocardiography (Figure 21.21).[33]

ABDOMINAL AORTOGRAPHY

Settings similar to those used in thoracic aortography can be used for abdominal studies (both conventional acquisition and DSA), as previously described. Abdominal aortography is usually performed by the common femoral approach with a multi-side-hole catheter (4- to 6-Fr). Depending on the patient's history and physical findings, radial or brachial access may be preferred. Once access has been obtained, a soft-tip wire is placed across the area of interest with the aid of fluoroscopy, and the angiographic catheter is advanced so that its tip is at the level of the T12 or L1 vertebra. If available, a biplane system allows the visceral branches to be visualized with only one injection of contrast material. The celiac (level T12–L1), superior mesenteric (L1–L2), and inferior mesenteric (L3–L4) arteries have an anterior origin, whereas the renal arteries originate laterally, just below the origin of the superior mesenteric artery. The required settings are similar to those used to image the ascending aorta and arch. The abdominal aorta bifurcates into the common iliac arteries at about the L4 level (Figure 21.22).

Table 21.6 Angiographic assessment of aortic insufficiency

Grade	Explanation
1+	Brief and incomplete ventricular opacification. Clears rapidly.
2+	Moderate opacification of the ventricle that clears in less than two cycles. Not greater than aortic root opacification.
3+	Opacification of the ventricle equal to aortic root opacification in more than three cycles. Delayed clearing of ventricle over several cycles.
4+	Opacification of the ventricle almost immediately or in less than three cycles that is equal to or greater than that of the aortic root, with delayed clearing of the ventricle.

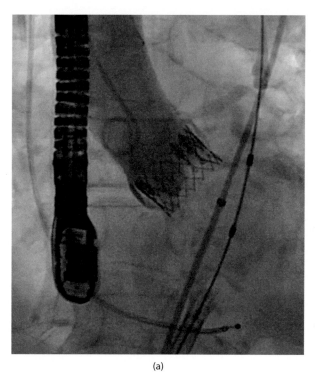
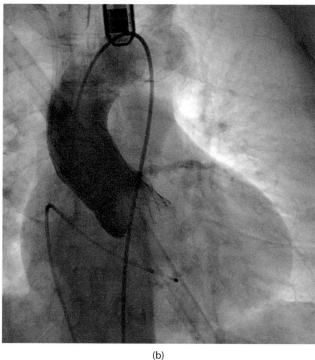

(a) (b)

Figure 21.21 Aortograms showing transcatheter aortic valve deployment. **(a)** Sapien valve (Edwards Lifesciences Corporation, Irvine, CA) and **(b)** CoreValve (Medtronic, Minneapolis, MN).

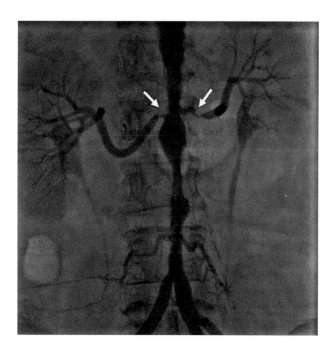

Figure 21.22 Abdominal aortogram from a 68-year-old woman with a history of Takayasu arteritis showing bilateral renal artery stenosis (arrows) and a significant decrease in the diameter of the distal abdominal aorta.

LIMITATIONS

The limitations of aortography include the fact that evaluation of the vessel is limited to the lumen and its branches; unlike TEE, CTA, and MRA, aortography does not provide information about the wall. This may be of importance in assessing pathologies, such as intramural hematoma and aortic dissection, and in the precise measurement of aortic aneurysms in the presence of laminar thrombus. Other limitations include the use of contrast agents, which can result in nephrotoxicity; the use of radiation, which can be harmful, especially to younger patients; and arterial access, which can lead to complications such as embolization of atherothrombi. Avoiding nephrotoxic contrast agents during diagnostic aortography or endovascular aneurysm repair (EVAR) may reduce the patient's risk of renal dysfunction after the procedure.[34] Carbon dioxide angiography, when conducted through the endograft delivery sheath, is not only reliable for endograft deployment but also is safe, nontoxic, and inexpensive. In addition, it may expedite EVAR by eliminating the need for multiple angiographic catheter placements and exchanges during the procedure. Despite these advantages, carbon dioxide angiography is vastly underused.

Conventional angiography is widely regarded as the gold standard for classifying endoleaks. Recently, with the advent of time-resolved MRA (TR MRA), faster magnetic resonance gradients have allowed rapid data acquisition and review of vascular data on a real-time continuous angiogram.[35] The initial results show that TR MRA is an effective noninvasive method for classifying endoleaks. It may allow screening of patients with endoleaks to identify leaks that require urgent repair.

In peripheral arterial disease, 3D dynamic contrast-enhanced subtraction MRA has high sensitivity and specificity. In segments with more than mild stenosis, MRA is 97.1%

sensitive and 99.2% specific.[36] This technique is a noninvasive alternative to conventional angiography for screening patients suspected of having lower-extremity ischemia.

CTA reveals mural changes in addition to luminal abnormalities.[37] Those abnormalities are high-attenuation wall in precontrast transverse CT images, circumferential wall thickening with or without enhancement, a concentric low-attenuation ring inside the aortic wall, and mural enhancement in delayed phase. In addition, CTA can provide valuable information regarding disease activity and progression.

Special issues

A severely diseased aorta can present multiple technical difficulties during angiography, resulting in potential complications. A difficult anatomy may necessitate excessive manipulation of catheters, causing distal embolization of atherothrombotic debris. In patients with aortic wall dissection, the operator may not realize that the catheter is in the false lumen; these dissections can be extended by the catheter, causing organ perfusion compromise and perforations.

During the procedure, wires, catheters, and other devices may penetrate the aortic wall, initiating dissection and/or rupture. The International Registry of Aortic Dissection[38] indicates that up to 5% of acute aortic dissections are iatrogenic (27% being due to percutaneous procedures). Patients with iatrogenic dissection are more likely to have myocardial ischemia (36% vs. 5%; $P < 0.001$) or a MI (15% versus 3%; $P < 0.001$) than patients with noniatrogenic dissection. In addition, patients with iatrogenic dissection have higher mortality (35% vs. 24%). In addition, when the ascending aorta and arch are manipulated, stroke can occur with devastating consequences.[39,40]

Atheroembolism can also lead to renal insufficiency, which develops slowly over several weeks. Other systemic manifestations of atheroembolism include livedo reticularis, abdominal or foot pain, and purple toes associated with systemic eosinophilia (blue toe syndrome).[41] Systemic complications can also occur. They are related to allergic and anaphylactoid reactions in 3% of cases (<1% of which involve hospitalization).[42]

Aortography conclusion

The multiple noninvasive imaging modalities that have evolved for evaluating the aorta and its branches include MRA, CTA, and duplex ultrasonography. These methods allow clinicians to appropriately diagnose patients, follow-up their conditions, and plan appropriate therapeutic strategies while avoiding the complications inherent in invasive percutaneous procedures. Aortography still plays an important role in the invasive evaluation of aortic disorders (valvular, traumatic, aneurysmal, and atherothrombotic). Before elective surgical repair of thoracic aortic aneurysms, aortography and coronary angiography provide important information about the relationship of nearby vessels to the aneurysm and about coronary artery locations and patency. Aortography is also fundamental in guiding therapeutic endovascular interventions. Careful procedural technique is required to maximize benefits and minimize the risk of complications.

REFERENCES

1. Hood WP, et al. Cardiac ventriculography. In: Grossman W, ed. *Cardiac Catheterization and Angiography*. 2nd edn. Philadelphia, PA: Lea & Febiger; 1980:170–184.
2. Rumberger JA, et al. Determination of ventricular ejection fraction: A comparison of available imaging methods. The Cardiovascular Imaging Working Group. *Mayo Clin Proc* 1997;72(9):860–870.
3. Bellenger NG, et al. Comparison of left ventricular ejection fraction and volumes in heart failure by echocardiography, radionuclide ventriculography and cardiovascular magnetic resonance; are they interchangeable? *Eur Heart J* 2000;21(16):1387–1396.
4. Vogel RA. Left ventricular imaging by digital subtraction angiography. *Int J Card Imaging* 1988;3(1):29–38.
5. Nichols AB, et al. Validation of the angiographic accuracy of digital left ventriculography. *Am J Cardiol* 1983;51(1):224–230.
6. Kuribayashi S, et al. [Evaluation of left ventricular function by digital subtraction angiography: Effect of dose and administration mode of contrast medium, and comparison with direct ventriculography]. *J Cardiogr* 1985;15(3):575–584.
7. Gigliotti OS, et al. Optimal use of left ventriculography at the time of cardiac catheterization: A consensus statement from the Society for Cardiovascular Angiography and Interventions. *Catheter Cardiovasc Interv* 2015;85(2):181–191.
8. Oost E, et al. Automated left ventricular delineation in X-ray angiograms: A validation study. *Catheter Cardiovasc Interv* 2009;73(2):231–240.
9. Manzke R, et al. Intra-operative volume imaging of the left atrium and pulmonary veins with rotational X-ray angiography. *Med Image Comput Comput Assist Interv* 2006;9(Pt 1):604–611.
10. Baim DS. Cardiac ventriculography. In: Baim DS, ed. *Grossman's Cardiac Catheterization, Angiography and Intervention*. 7th edn. Philadelphia, PA: Lippincott, Williams & Wilkins; 2006:222–226.
11. Grebe O, et al. Assessment of left ventricular function with steady-state-free-precession magnetic resonance imaging. Reference values and a comparison to left ventriculography. *Z Kardiol* 2004;93(9):686–695.
12. Deligonul U, et al. Contrast cine left ventriculography: Comparison of two pigtail catheter shapes and analysis of factors determining the final quality. *Catheter Cardiovasc Diagn* 1996;37(4):428–433.
13. Hodges MC, et al. Comparison of low-volume versus standard-volume left ventriculography. *Catheter Cardiovasc Interv* 2001;52(3):314–319.
14. Hendel RC, et al. ACC/AHA/ACR/ASE/ASNC/HRS/NASCI/RSNA/SAIP/SCAI/SCCT/SCMR/SIR 2008 key data elements and definitions for cardiac imaging: A report of the American College of Cardiology/American Heart

Association Task Force on Clinical Data Standards (Writing Committee to Develop Clinical Data Standards for Cardiac Imaging). *J Am Coll Cardiol* 2009;53(1):91–124.

15. Takenaka A, et al. The discrepancy between echocardiography, cineventriculography and thermodilution. Evaluation of left ventricular volume and ejection fraction. *Int J Card Imaging* 1995;11(4):255–262.

16. Sapin PM, et al. Comparison of two- and three-dimensional echocardiography with cineventriculography for measurement of left ventricular volume in patients. *J Am Coll Cardiol* 1994;24(4):1054–1063.

17. Urena PE, et al. Ejection fraction by radionuclide ventriculography and contrast left ventriculogram. A tale of two techniques. *J Am Coll Cardiol* 1999;33(1):180–185.

18. Van Langenhove G, et al. Evaluation of left ventricular volumes and ejection fraction with a nonfluoroscopic endoventricular three-dimensional mapping technique. *Am Heart J* 2000;140(4):596–602.

19. O'Neill WW. Interventional therapy of cardiogenic shock. In: Stack RS, Roubin SR, O'Neill WW, eds. *Interventional Cardiovascular Medicine, Principles and Practice*. 2nd edn. Philadelphia, PA: Churchill Livingstone; 2002:363–379.

20. Barrett BJ, et al. A comparison of nonionic, low-osmolality radiocontrast agents with ionic, high-osmolality agents during cardiac catheterization. *N Engl J Med* 1992;326(7):431–436.

21. Bergelson BA, Tommaso CL. Left main coronary artery disease: Assessment, diagnosis, and therapy. *Am Heart J* 1995;129(2):350–359.

22. Keeley EC, et al. Left main coronary interventions. In: Stack RS, Roubin SR, O'Neill WW, eds. *Interventional Cardiovascular Medicine, Principles and Practice*. 2nd edn. Philadelphia, PA: Churchill Livingstone; 2002:635–646.

23. Leclercq F, et al. Transcranial Doppler detection of cerebral microemboli during left heart catheterization. *Cerebrovasc Dis* 2001;12(1):59–65.

24. Goldenberg I, et al. Left ventriculography complicated by cerebral air embolism. *Catheter Cardiovasc Diagn* 1995;35(4):331–334.

25. Kearney KR, et al. Massive air embolus to the left ventricle: Diagnosis and monitoring by serial echocardiography. *J Am Soc Echocardiogr* 1997;10(9):982–987.

26. Delany DJ. Aortography. In: Grossman W, ed. *Cardiac Catheterization and Angiography*. 2nd edn. Philadelphia, PA: Lea & Febiger; 1980:197–211.

27. Valji K. Abdominal aorta. In: Valji K, ed. *Vascular and Interventional Radiology*. Philadelphia, PA: W B Saunders; 1999:102–126.

28. Sugawara J, et al. Age-associated elongation of the ascending aorta in adults. *JACC Cardiovasc Imaging* 2008;1(6):739–748.

29. Gundry SR, et al. Indications for aortography in blunt thoracic trauma: A reassessment. *J Trauma* 1982;22(8):664–671.

30. Kram HB, et al. Clinical and radiographic indications for aortography in blunt chest trauma. *J Vasc Surg* 1987;6(2):168–176.

31. Chernin MM, et al. Digital subtraction angiography of the aortic arch. *Cardiovasc Intervent Radiol* 1984;7(5):196–203.

32. Jaff MR, et al. Angiography of the aorta and peripheral arteries. In: Baim DS, ed. *Grossman's Cardiac Catheterization*. 7th edn. Philadelphia, PA: Lippincott, Williams, & Wilkins; 2006:254–282.

33. Kappetein AP, et al. Updated standardized endpoint definitions for transcatheter aortic valve implantation: The Valve Academic Research Consortium-2 consensus document. *J Thorac Cardiovasc Surg* 2013;145(1):6–23.

34. Criado E, et al. Catheter-less angiography for endovascular aortic aneurysm repair: A new application of carbon dioxide as a contrast agent. *J Vasc Surg* 2008;48(3):527–534.

35. Lookstein RA, et al. Time-resolved magnetic resonance angiography as a noninvasive method to characterize endoleaks: Initial results compared with conventional angiography. *J Vasc Surg* 2004;39(1):27–33.

36. Sueyoshi E, et al. Aortoiliac and lower extremity arteries: Comparison of three-dimensional dynamic contrast-enhanced subtraction MR angiography and conventional angiography. *Radiology* 1999;210(3):683–688.

37. Park JH. Conventional and CT angiographic diagnosis of Takayasu arteritis. *Int J Cardiol* 1996;54 Suppl:S135–S141.

38. Januzzi JL, et al. Iatrogenic aortic dissection. *Am J Cardiol* 2002;89(5):623–626.

39. Armstrong PJ, et al. Complication rates of percutaneous brachial artery access in peripheral vascular angiography. *Ann Vasc Surg* 2003;17(1):107–110.

40. Fayed AM, et al. Carotid and cerebral angiography performed by cardiologists: Cerebrovascular complications. *Catheter Cardiovasc Interv* 2002;55(3):277–280.

41. Rosman HS, et al. Cholesterol embolization: Clinical findings and implications. *J Am Coll Cardiol* 1990;15(6):1296–1299.

42. Bettmann MA, et al. Adverse events with radiographic contrast agents: Results of the SCVIR Contrast Agent Registry. *Radiology* 1997;203(3):611–620.

22

Pulmonary angiography

HONG JUN YUN, SYED SOHAIL ALI, AND PAUL MICHAEL GROSSMAN

INTRODUCTION

Even though diagnostic imaging modalities for the evaluation of pulmonary vasculature have made considerable advancements over the past couple of decades, pulmonary angiography historically remains the gold standard technique for the diagnosis of pulmonary embolism (PE). However, because of more widely available noninvasive imaging techniques, such as multislice computed tomography (CT) and magnetic resonance imaging (MRI), that offer similar diagnostic accuracy, the utilization of pulmonary angiography as a primary diagnostic modality has declined considerably. Catheter angiography is now more commonly used for various endovascular interventions on pulmonary circulation, such as mechanical embolectomy, embolization for tumors or retrieval of foreign bodies, as well as for the diagnosis and treatment of a variety of congenital heart diseases (CHDs).

ANATOMIC CONSIDERATIONS

Pulmonary circulation anatomy

The main pulmonary artery (PA) originates from the right ventricle (RV), travels anteriorly on the left side of the aorta, and then follows a posterior course, bifurcating into the right and left pulmonary arteries (Figure 22.1). The right PA gives rise to a right upper-lobe branch during its course in the mediastinum that further divides into three upper-lobe

segmental arteries. The right PA continues and then divides into middle-lobe and lower-lobe segmental arteries. The left PA continues in the mediastinum and gives rise to a variable number of small segmental arteries to the upper lobe. It then bifurcates into interlobaris and basalis branches that give rise to two lingular and four lower-lobe segmental arteries, respectively. Further branching of these vessels is remarkably variable. The segmental pulmonary veins are also variable; however, they form the superior and inferior veins on each side before draining into the left atrium (LA).

FUNDAMENTALS

Patients referred for pulmonary angiography almost invariably have acutely or chronically elevated right heart pressures and may be hemodynamically unstable. Therefore, pulmonary angiograms should be performed by experienced operators in laboratories with staff and equipment capable of invasive hemodynamic monitoring.

INDICATIONS

Pulmonary embolism

PE is one of the most important causes of cardiovascular morbidity and mortality with an annual incidence of 1 per 1,000 in the general adult population.[1,2] The main cause of death in the acute setting is right ventricular failure. Patients may present with a wide range

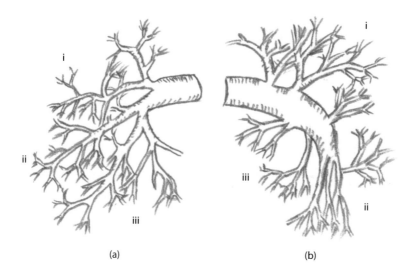

Figure 22.1 Pulmonary arteries. Right pulmonary artery **(a)**: (*i*) right upper-lobe segmental arteries, (*ii*) middle-lobe segmental arteries, (*iii*) lower-lobe segmental arteries. Left pulmonary artery **(b)**: (*i*) left upper-lobe segmental arteries, (*ii*) lower-lobe segmental arteries, (*iii*) lingular segmental arteries.

of symptoms; therefore, a high index of suspicion is necessary for prompt diagnosis. Symptoms may include dyspnea, hemoptysis, cough, and pleuritic chest pain. Syncope indicates hemodynamic compromise. Clinical signs include elevated jugular venous pressure, decreased pulmonic component of second heart sound, right ventricular heave, and tachycardia—all indicating right ventricular dysfunction. Wells and coworkers have described clinical means to estimate the probability of deep venous thrombosis and PE.[3,4]

Electrocardiography in acute PE usually shows sinus tachycardia. The presence of the classic S1Q3T3 pattern may help in making the diagnosis; however, this is not commonly seen. Other findings may include incomplete or complete right bundle branch block and right axis deviation. The presence of a Qr pattern in lead V1 and inverted T-waves in the anterior precordial leads indicates increased risk of poor clinical outcomes.[5] A negative D-dimer has a high negative predictive value (>90%) and low specificity (45%) for PE.[6–8] Therefore, the test is useful only as a "rule-out" modality in the office setting or emergency room. Arterial blood gas analysis should not be used for screening purposes because of its low specificity in PE, but may help direct therapy. The presence of hypoxemia, hypocapnia, respiratory alkalosis, and increased alveolar-arterial gradient is usually seen.[9]

Chest CT is now considered the initial imaging test for the diagnosis of PE. Chest radiographs and ventilation perfusion lung scanning should precede pulmonary angiography and serve as a planning aid. The ventilation perfusion scan is very useful for the diagnosis of PE when the chest radiograph is normal and chest CT with intravenous (IV) contrast cannot be performed.[10] A high-probability lung scan is diagnostic of PE. To interpret low or intermediate probability scans, clinical history should be considered to help direct any further use of diagnostic modalities and management.

The sensitivity of multidetector CT ranges from 70% to 90%.[11,12] Positive results on CT, in combination with a high or intermediate probability of PE based on clinical assessment, or normal findings on CT with a low clinical probability have a predictive value (positive or negative) of 92%–96%.[13] MRI can also be utilized for diagnosis of PE and can reach sensitivity and specificity as high as pulmonary angiography. MR angiography is more time consuming and less available in the acute setting than CT angiography. In addition, highly symptomatic patients may not comply sufficiently to have adequate quality images with MR. Venous ultrasonography can be performed in patients with symptoms of deep venous thrombosis, and if a thrombosis is confirmed, the finding is sufficient to diagnose PE if the patient has a suggestive clinical presentation. Contrast venography is rarely performed except when catheter-directed thrombolysis or other percutaneous interventions are planned, or an inferior vena cava (IVC) filter is to be inserted. Transthoracic echocardiography is an important tool for risk stratification in PE. Accordingly, RV dysfunction is associated with increased mortality and in the presence of hemodynamic instability warrants systemic thrombolysis, catheter intervention, or surgical embolectomy.

Predictors of a positive angiogram include the following:

1. Presence of one or more risk factors for pulmonary thromboembolism (bed rest, surgery or trauma within 6 weeks, previous history of deep vein thrombosis or PE, malignancy, or congestive heart failure)
2. Chest radiograph showing infiltrates, pleural effusion, or atelectasis
3. Ventilation perfusion scan interpreted as indeterminate or high probability

When only one of the three predictors is present, the likelihood of angiographically demonstrable PE is <5%, with two of three predictors positive, about 20%, and with all three predictors being positive, the likelihood is >70%.

The natural history of pulmonary thromboembolism suggests that most patients will have identifiable emboli for at least 1 week following the acute episode. However, the number of false-negative studies will increase after 48 hours, and the performance of angiography after 7 days may not be advisable.

Other indications

Pulmonary angiography and right heart catheterization can be utilized to both confirm the diagnosis and evaluate the possibility of surgical or endovascular treatment in a patient with pulmonary hypertension secondary to chronic thromboembolic disease. The characteristic angiographic findings of chronic thromboemboli include pouching of contrast in organized thrombus with obstruction of the distal artery and the presence of thin or thick webs or bands that appear as radiolucencies in lobar or segmental vessels that can cause stenosis with or without poststenotic dilatation. In this condition, luminal irregularities are common and characterized by vessel tapering of large pulmonary arteries and obstruction of lobar arteries, usually at their origin. Such findings were confirmed surgically in one study of 250 patients.[14] In addition to chronic anticoagulation, placement of an IVC filter should be considered. Patients with proximal pulmonary artery emboli should be considered for surgical pulmonary thromboembolectomy. Pulmonary hypertension may persist after thromboembolectomy and identifies patients with poor outcomes. Lung transplantation may be an option in patients with extensive chronic embolic disease. The percutaneous treatment (balloon angioplasty) of pulmonary hypertension secondary to chronic thromboembolic disease is being explored.[15,16]

Primary pulmonary hypertension is a disease of unknown etiology. Angiography in such patients shows nonspecific dilatation of the proximal arteries with smooth, rapid tapering of distal vessels and a corkscrew appearance of the distal arteries. If untreated, the RV fails secondary to gradual increase in pulmonary vascular resistance. Vasodilator challenge with IV adenosine or inhaled nitric oxide is often performed before initiation of vasodilator therapies. Reduction of ≥20% in pulmonary vascular resistance with a decrease in mean PA pressure ≥20% is considered a positive response. A vasodilator challenge may also be performed to document reversibility in pulmonary vascular resistance in a patient being considered for heart transplantation.

Pulmonary arteriovenous malformations are usually asymptomatic. However, patients may present with dyspnea, hemoptysis, cyanosis, and clubbing. Polycythemia and paradoxical embolism may occur due to extracardiac right-to-left shunting. A contrast-enhanced spiral chest CT can be utilized to establish the diagnosis, and pulmonary angiography is usually performed only to guide percutaneous embolization.

PA stenosis is usually seen in patients who survive repair of CHDs, such as tetralogy of Fallot, truncus arteriosus, pulmonary valvular stenosis, patent ductus arteriosus, aortic stenosis, ventricular septal defects, or transposition of great vessels during childhood. Pulmonary angiography is both diagnostic and part of therapeutic procedures in which such lesions can be treated with angioplasty and stents.

PA aneurysms—usually secondary to pulmonary hypertension—are seen in patients who underwent corrective surgery for CHD; in infectious diseases like tuberculosis and syphilis; and in rheumatologic processes such as Behcet disease. Percutaneous embolization can be performed after pulmonary angiography.

Partial anomalous pulmonary venous return can be diagnosed by pulmonary angiography with an oxygen saturation run and delayed filming to identify the venous phase and to quantify left-to-right shunting.

EQUIPMENT AND PROCEDURE

Venous access

The right common femoral vein is the most often utilized access site for pulmonary angiography due to the ease in cannulation and compression, and its relatively straight course into the right side of the heart through the IVC. The left common femoral vein is used if the right side is not accessible for reasons such as proximal deep venous thrombosis, fibrosis, infection, or recent hematoma. If iliac or IVC thrombosis is suspected at the time of the procedure, 15 mL of contrast can be injected into the femoral vein to confirm or rule out the presumptive diagnosis.

The internal jugular vein can be utilized if no femoral approach is possible. The basilic vein at the antecubital fossa is preferred over the internal jugular vein if thrombolytic therapy is being considered because it allows for a better hemostasis at the puncture site. The cephalic vein may not be a good choice due to its relatively smaller size and the presence of an acute angle when it joins the axillary vein.

Choice of contrast and injection rates

Traditionally, low-osmolar contrast agents are used for pulmonary angiography. The advantage of such agents includes less frequent side effects of flushing, hypotension, nausea, or cough reflex. Currently, there is limited data regarding iso-osmolar, nonionic agents for use in pulmonary angiography. The determinants of contrast injection rates include the rate of blood flow in the catheterized vessel, PA pressure, the type of catheter used for angiography, and the imaging mode. Digital imaging techniques require less contrast to be injected for adequate opacification of selected arteries. The injection rate and volume should be less if more subselective catheterization is performed in smaller vessels. This should also be considered in patients with pulmonary hypertension and right ventricular overload to avoid hemodynamic side effects.[17] Right ventricular end-diastolic pressure of 20 mmHg is usually considered the upper limit for safe use of contrast media in chronic pulmonary hypertension.[18] If available, biplane angiography may also be used to further reduce both total contrast volume and catheter dwell time.

Imaging modes

Digital subtraction angiography (DSA) is equivalent to conventional angiography in image quality and diagnostic performance.[19] In one study, comparable accurate detection of PE was noted by use of DSA as compared to conventional angiography.[20] There are many advantages of DSA as the imaging mode. It allows the use of less contrast media, which is particularly important in patients with pulmonary hypertension or renal insufficiency. The images are acquired rapidly in a flexible display format, in which images can be viewed individually or in cine format for both DSA and conventional angiography.

The main disadvantage of DSA is requirement of image acquisition without motion that may be suboptimal in patients with severe cardiac or pulmonary symptoms, and in patients who are unable to hold their breath. Motion artifacts can be reduced by mask-shifting techniques that may improve cardiac motion; however, it is less helpful in respiratory motion artifacts. For that reason, DSA is usually not possible in patients undergoing urgent angiography for massive PE other than if the patient is intubated, a situation in which DSA should be performed after induction of apnea.

The two standard views that have been validated in a large clinical trial are the anteroposterior and the 45° ipsilateral oblique view.[21] Lateral views are not useful because the frequently observed reflux of the contrast into the opposite lung may hinder interpretation.

Technique

Pulmonary angiography is usually performed in the acute setting for evaluation and catheter-directed treatment of massive or submassive PE. Close invasive blood pressure and ECG monitoring are required for early detection of hypotension, brady- or tachyarrhythmias, and atrioventricular (AV) block during the procedure. Angiography is initiated by performing complete right heart catheterization. Special considerations are made depending on the measured PA and right ventricular end-diastolic pressures. In the presence of a properly placed IVC filter, safe transfilter angiography using the transfemoral approach can be applied by carefully passing a J-tipped wire followed by the catheter through the filter. A long sheath with its tip beyond the filter may be inserted to prevent filter dislodgement.

The catheters usually used for diagnostic pulmonary angiography range in sheath size from 5- to 7-Fr. However, a lower-size 4-Fr nylon pulmonary catheter that allows flow rates of 20 mL/s can be used to reduce access site complications. The pigtail catheter has

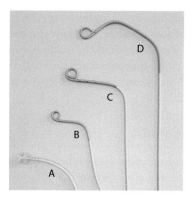

Figure 22.2 Catheters used in pulmonary angiography. **(A)** Berman angiographic balloon catheter (Arrow International, Inc., Reading, PA); **(B)** Grollman GPC pulmonary pigtail catheter (Cook, Inc., Bloomington, IN); **(C)** Van Aman APC pulmonary pigtail catheter (Cook, Inc., Bloomington, IN); **(D)** Montefiore MONT-1 catheter (Cook, Inc., Bloomington, IN).

multiple sideholes with a curled tip that provides safety during right heart catheterization as well as easy access to any segmental artery (Figure 22.2). The retrieval of such catheters should, however, always be made after straightening with a guidewire under direct fluoroscopic visualization to avoid entrapment in the tricuspid valve or subvalvular apparatus. The balloon-tipped catheters have sideholes in the shaft of the catheter proximal to the balloon and power injection after balloon occlusion allows for selective high-quality injections. After deflation of the balloon, the catheter can be removed without the use of fluoroscopy.

The approaches for PA catheterization using the pigtail and balloon-tipped catheters are shown in Figure 22.3. The most commonly used pigtail catheter is the Grollman PA catheter (Cook, Inc., Bloomington, IN), which has a gentle rightward curve with a 90° reversed secondary curve 3 cm proximal to the pigtail to allow easy manipulation into the right heart chambers and pulmonary arteries. In patients with right atrial enlargement, access into the RV may be difficult with the standard Grollman catheter, and a tip-deflecting wire may be needed to advance the catheter into the RV. One approach is to enlarge the secondary curve by introducing a manual curve to the proximal end of the tip-deflecting wire. Alternatively, the Van Aman catheter (Cook, Inc., Bloomington, IN), a modified Grollman catheter with a 90° reversed secondary curve 6 cm proximal to the pigtail, can be used in patients with dilated right heart chambers. Modified C-shaped catheters have been successfully used for PA catheterization using the brachiocephalic vein approach.[22]

In general, contrast medium is injected separately into the right and left PAs rather than the main PA, with an injection rate per artery of approximately 20 mL/s for a total of 30–40 mL depending on patient size at a maximum pressure of 600 pounds per square inch (psi). The regions that are suspected to be abnormal are examined first in

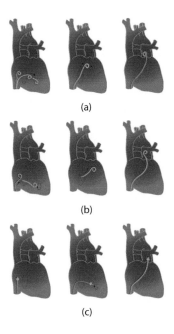

Figure 22.3 Approaches for pulmonary artery catheterization. **(a)** Straight pigtail catheter and deflecting wire. After placing the pigtail catheter into the right atrium, a wire deflecting wire is used to point and advance the catheter into the right ventricle. The deflection is released and the catheter is rotated and advanced into the main pulmonary artery. Further advancement usually directs it into the left main pulmonary artery. To engage the right main pulmonary artery, a deflecting wire can be used to direct the catheter downward and to the right into the right main pulmonary artery. **(b)** Grollman (or Van Aman or Montefiore) catheter. The catheter is advanced into the right atrium and the anteromedial portion is probed to direct the catheter through the tricuspid valve and into the right ventricle. The catheter is slightly withdrawn, rotated to facilitate entry into the right ventricular outflow tract, and advanced into the main pulmonary artery. **(c)** Balloon-tipped catheter. Under fluoroscopy, the balloon is inflated in the common iliac vein and advanced into the right atrium. The catheter is rotated anteromedially to gain entry into the right ventricle and further rotated clockwise to flip the balloon tip cranially toward the right ventricular outflow tract before advancing into the main pulmonary artery.

anteroposterior or oblique planes or with biplane angiography. Further injections may be required to better define the anatomy.

CLINICAL ASPECTS

A normal pulmonary angiogram is demonstrated in Figure 22.4. Often selective or superselective injections with magnification are required when suspicious areas require closer examination (Figures 22.5 and 22.6). These may be performed with balloon-tipped catheters following balloon occlusion. The findings depend on the size and number of emboli, on the location of the lesion—central or peripheral—and if the lesion results in partial or complete

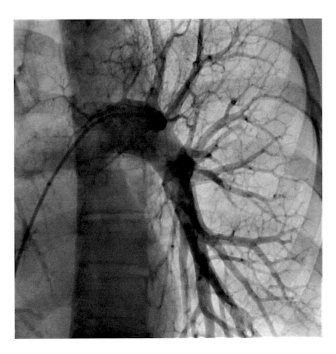

Figure 22.4 Normal left pulmonary artery angiogram.

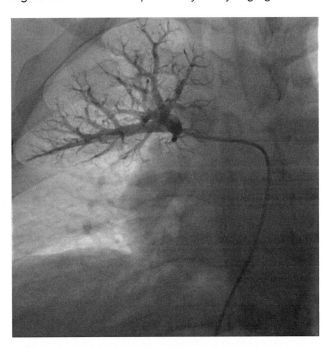

Figure 22.5 Selective right upper-lobe pulmonary artery angiography performed through a balloon-tipped catheter.

flow obstruction. Angiography may detect intraluminal filling defects of various sizes, shapes, and locations; abrupt arterial cutoffs; and localized pruning or lack of branching (Figure 22.7). The extent of these findings correlates with the severity of pulmonary arterial occlusion. As a correlate of hemodynamic compromise, cardiogenic shock patients may have, in addition, oligemia, asymmetrical filling, prolongation of the arterial phases, and bilateral lower-zone filling delay.

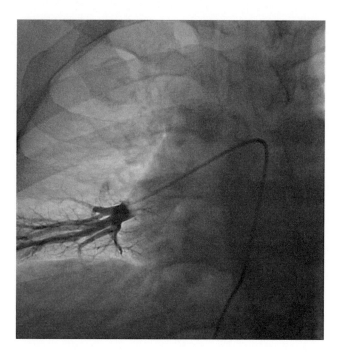

Figure 22.6 Selective left upper-lobe pulmonary artery angiography performed through a balloon-tipped catheter.

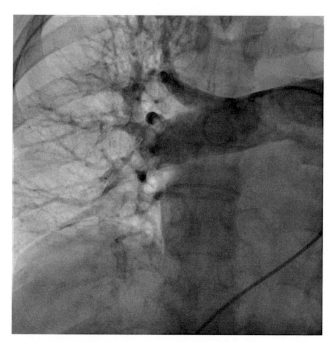

Figure 22.7 Right pulmonary artery nonselective angiography. Note the presence of embolus in the proximal middle- and lower-lobe branches.

LIMITATIONS

Pulmonary angiography studies are challenging to interpret. The reading physician, therefore, should give some estimate of the degree of certainty of the diagnosis—though arbitrary—based on a judgment of the completeness of visualization of pulmonary circulation.

COMPLICATIONS

Pulmonary angiography is a remarkably safe procedure in experienced hands. Reported major complications are approximately 1.5% and include death, respiratory distress requiring cardiopulmonary resuscitation or intubation, renal failure requiring dialysis, or access site complications requiring transfusion.[21] Patients with PA hypertension are at higher risk of having acute right heart failure.[23] However, in the Prospective Investigation of Pulmonary Embolism Diagnosis (PIOPED) study, increased mortality was not observed among 755 patients who underwent pulmonary angiography.[10] Nevertheless, due to this potential risk, PA and right ventricular end-diastolic pressures are usually measured directly at the time of the procedure. If considerable elevation in pressure is found (right ventricular end-diastolic pressure above 20 mmHg), the volume and rate of contrast injection can be modified, or in stable patients, the study deferred. Other minor complications include arrhythmias related to the catheter position; right bundle branch block; nausea, vomiting, hypotension, and respiratory distress related to sedation and narcotics; and itching, urticaria, or other allergic reactions due to contrast use.[18] Critically ill and/or elderly are at higher risk of

renal dysfunction.[24] As opposed to prior large retrospective series, no cardiac tamponade was observed or myocardial perforation in the PIOPED study. This finding is likely related to the catheter choice in PIOPED study, namely, catheters of pigtail type instead of straight catheters.

CONTRAINDICATIONS AND CONSIDERATIONS

There is no absolute contraindication to pulmonary angiography. However, minimization of contrast and special care should apply for high-risk patients, such as those with severe pulmonary hypertension, known allergic reaction to iodine-based contrast media, renal insufficiency, left bundle branch block, and right heart or biventricular congestive heart failure.[17] Patients with a history of severe allergic reactions should be pretreated with corticosteroids and antihistamines and use of nonionic low-osmolar contrast agents should be considered as conventional ionic monomer contrast media transiently increase PA and right ventricular pressures.

SPECIAL ISSUES

Catheter-directed therapy for acute pulmonary embolism

Acute PE is a potentially life-threatening condition. In-hospital mortality for patients with massive or high-risk PE—defined as sustained systemic arterial hypotension, cardiogenic shock, or need for cardiopulmonary resuscitation—can exceed 50%.[25] In hemodynamically stable patients with submassive or intermediate-risk PE, short-term mortality can range from 3% to 15% if there is imaging or biomarker evidence of right ventricular dysfunction.[26] Systemic thrombolysis improves hemodynamic parameters and reverses right ventricular dilation and dysfunction but is associated with high rates of major bleeding complications. Catheter-based interventions with or without local thrombolysis have been shown to be effective in reversing right ventricular dysfunction and reducing adverse clinical events without causing an increase in the complication rate compared with anticoagulation alone. Such therapies include aspiration thrombectomy, thrombus fragmentation, rheolytic thrombectomy, rotational embolectomy, catheter-directed thrombolysis, and ultrasound-assisted catheter-directed thrombolysis (USAT) (Table 22.1).

Recent randomized clinical trial data have shown that USATs using the EkoSonic MACH4e Endovascular Systems (EKOS Corporation, Bothell, WA) are effective at reversing right ventricular dilation. The Ultrasound Accelerated Thrombolysis of Pulmonary Embolism (ULTIMA) trial randomized 59 patients presenting with acute main or lower lobe PE and echocardiographic evidence of right ventricular dilation to standardized fixed-dose USAT and anticoagulation or anticoagulation with heparin alone. USAT plus anticoagulation was superior in reversing right ventricular dilatation at 24 hours (mean difference in RV/left ventricle [LV] ratio 0.30 ± 0.20 vs. 0.03 ± 0.16 [$P < 0.001$]), without an increase in bleeding complications.[27] Similarly, in the SEATTLE II trial—a single-arm prospective cohort study of 150 patients with massive and submassive PE—USAT was associated with a decrease in RV dilation, reduced pulmonary hypertension, and decreased anatomic thrombus burden, while no patient experienced intracranial hemorrhage.[28]

At our institution, we use the EkoSonic Endovascular system with or without adjunctive thrombus fragmentation or aspiration for the treatment of massive and submassive PE confirmed by CT pulmonary angiography. The EkoSonic Endovascular System consists of three components: an Intelligent Drug Delivery Catheter (IDDC); a removable MicroSonic Device containing multiple small ultrasound transducers distributed over the treatment zone; and the EkoSonic control unit. Venous access is obtained via the right femoral vein or right internal jugular vein (if the femoral vein approach is not feasible) using the modified Seldinger technique under ultrasound guidance. A 7-Fr introducer sheath or 10-Fr double-lumen introducer sheath is inserted depending on the need for a unilateral or bilateral EkoSonic device placement. The embolic occlusion is crossed using a 0.035-in guidewire and standard diagnostic angiographic catheter (either a 7-Fr Van Aman APC or 7-Fr Montefiore MONT-1 catheter). With the guidewire tip in a safe position, the angiographic catheter is exchanged for the IDDC. The guidewire is then removed and the MicroSonic Device inserted into the IDDC. A fixed-dose regimen of tissue-plasminogen activator (t-PA) of 24 mg is administered at 1 mg/h with saline coolant at 35 mL/h for both unilateral and bilateral PEs for 12–24 hours. Baseline right heart pressures are measured before and following infusion of fibrinolytic therapy. This procedure may be preceded by use of a mechanical thrombectomy device to debulk clot in patients with massive PE.

Table 22.1 Catheter-directed intervention techniques and devices

Method	Device name
Aspiration thrombectomy	Greenfield suction embolectomy catheter (Boston Scientific, Natick, MA)
	Sheath with detachable hemostatic valve 8- to 9-Fr (Argon Medical Devices, Athens, TX) + multipurpose guide catheter (8- to 9-Fr) + aspiration syringe (60 mL)
Thrombus fragmentation	Pigtail catheter fragmentation
	Peripheral balloon catheters
	Fogarty arterial balloon embolectomy catheter (Edwards Lifesciences, Irvine, CA)
	Amplatz thrombectomy device (Microvena, White Bear Lake, MN)
Rheolytic thrombectomy	AngioJet (Medrad, Warrendale, PA)
	Hydrolyser (Cordis, Miami, FL)
	Oasis (Boston Scientific, Natick, MA)
Rotational thrombectomy	Rotarex (Straub Medical, Wangs, Switzerland)
	Aspirex (Straub Medical, Wangs, Switzerland)
	Cleaner (Rex medical, Athens, TX)
Catheter-directed thrombolysis	UniFuse (AngioDynamics, Latham, NY)
	Cragg-McNamara (ev3 Endovascular, Plymouth, MN)
	ClearWay RX Infusion Catheter (Atrium Medical Corporation, Hudson, NH)
Ultrasound-assisted catheter-directed thrombolysis	EkoSonic (EKOS, Bothell, WA)

CONCLUSIONS

Although rarely needed for diagnostic purposes, pulmonary angiography remains the gold standard imaging modality for acute and chronic PE. In addition, angiography may, on occasion, be indicated in the evaluation of pulmonary hypertension, CHD, pulmonary arteriovenous malformations, and pulmonary aneurysms. Finally, angiography guides all catheter-based interventions in the pulmonary circulation. Pulmonary angiographic studies should be performed by experienced operators in catheterization laboratories capable of invasive hemodynamic monitoring. Pulmonary angiography requires venous access, passage of the angiographic catheter under fluoroscopic guidance, and contrast injection during cineangiography. Moreover, current evidence suggests that catheter-directed therapies are an effective and safe alternative to systemic thrombolytic therapy in the contemporary management of patients with acute massive or submassive PE, though more robust, clinical outcomes studies are warranted. Ideally, such diagnostic and interventional procedures should be performed in experienced centers with expertise in catheter-based interventions and the capability of managing procedural complications.

REFERENCES

1. Silverstein MD, et al. Trends in the incidence of deep vein thrombosis and pulmonary embolism: A 25-year population-based study. *Arch Intern Med* 1998;158(6):585–593.
2. Tapson VF. Acute pulmonary embolism. *N Engl J Med* 2008;358(10):1037–1052.
3. Wells PS, et al. Accuracy of clinical assessment of deep-vein thrombosis. *Lancet* 1995;345(8961):1326–1330.
4. Ginsberg JS. Management of venous thromboembolism. *N Engl J Med* 1996;335(24):1816–1828.
5. Kucher N, et al. QR in V1—An ECG sign associated with right ventricular strain and adverse clinical outcome in pulmonary embolism. *Eur Heart J* 2003;24(12):1113–1119.
6. Brown MD, et al. The accuracy of the enzyme-linked immunosorbent assay D-dimer test in the diagnosis of pulmonary embolism: A meta-analysis. *Ann Emerg Med* 2002;40(2):133–144.
7. Dunn KL, et al. Normal D-dimer levels in emergency department patients suspected of acute pulmonary embolism. *J Am Coll Cardiol* 2002;40(8):1475–1478.
8. Goldhaber SZ, et al. Quantitative plasma D-dimer levels among patients undergoing pulmonary angiography for suspected pulmonary embolism. *JAMA* 1993;270(23):2819–2822.
9. Stein PD, et al. Arterial blood gas analysis in the assessment of suspected acute pulmonary embolism. *Chest* 1996;109(1):78–81.
10. PIOPED Investigators. Value of the ventilation/perfusion scan in acute pulmonary embolism. Results of the prospective investigation of pulmonary embolism diagnosis (PIOPED). *JAMA* 263(20):2753–2759.
11. Schoepf UJ, et al. Subsegmental pulmonary emboli: Improved detection with thin-collimation multi-detector row spiral CT. *Radiology* 2002;222(2):483–490.
12. Rathbun SW, et al. Sensitivity and specificity of helical computed tomography in the diagnosis of pulmonary embolism: A systematic review. *Ann Intern Med* 2000;132(3):227–232.
13. Stein PD, et al. Multidetector computed tomography for acute pulmonary embolism. *N Engl J Med* 2006;354(22):2317–2327.
14. Auger WR, et al. Chronic major-vessel thromboembolic pulmonary artery obstruction: Appearance at angiography. *Radiology* 1992;182(2):393–398.
15. Landzberg MJ. Balloon pulmonary angioplasty for chronic thromboembolic pulmonary hypertension: A need for further dialogue, development, and collaborative study. *Circ Cardiovasc Interv* 2012;5(6):744–745.
16. Andreassen AK, et al. Balloon pulmonary angioplasty in patients with inoperable chronic thromboembolic pulmonary hypertension. *Heart* 2013;99:1415–1420.
17. van Loveren M, et al. Pulmonary angiography: Technique, indications and complications. In Edwin J. R. van Beek, Harry R. Büller, Matthijs Oudkerk, eds., *Deep Vein Thrombosis and Pulmonary Embolism* 2009;221-246, Chichester, West Sussex, UK: John Wiley & Sons.
18. Mills SR, et al. The incidence, etiologies, and avoidance of complications of pulmonary angiography in a large series. *Radiology* 1980;136(2):295–299.
19. Hagspiel KD, et al. Pulmonary embolism: Comparison of cut-film and digital pulmonary angiography. *Radiology* 1998;207(1):139–145.
20. Johnson MS, et al. Possible pulmonary embolus: Evaluation with digital subtraction versus cut-film angiography—Prospective study in 80 patients. *Radiology* 1998;207(1):131–138.
21. Stein PD, et al. Complications and validity of pulmonary angiography in acute pulmonary embolism. *Circulation* 1992;85(2):462–468.
22. Rosen G, et al. The Hunter pulmonary angiography catheter for a brachiocephalic vein approach. *Cardiovasc Intervent Radiol* 2006;29(6):997–1002.
23. Perlmutt LM, et al. Pulmonary arteriography in the high-risk patient. *Radiology* 1987;162(1 Pt 1):187–189.
24. Stein PD, et al. Diagnosis of acute pulmonary embolism in the elderly. *J Am Coll Cardiol* 1991;18(6):1452–1457.
25. Kucher N, et al. Massive pulmonary embolism. *Circulation* 2006;113(4):577–582.
26. Konstantinides SV, et al. 2014 ESC guidelines on the diagnosis and management of acute pulmonary embolism. *Eur Heart J* 2014;35(43):3033–3080.
27. Kucher N, et al. Randomized, controlled trial of ultrasound-assisted catheter-directed thrombolysis for acute intermediate-risk pulmonary embolism. *Circulation* 2014;129(4):479–486.
28. Piazza G, et al. A prospective, single-arm, multicenter trial of ultrasound-facilitated, catheter-directed, low-dose fibrinolysis for acute massive and submassive pulmonary embolism. *JACC Cardiovasc Interv* 2015;8(10):1382–1392.

23

Transseptal catheterization

ZOLTAN G. TURI

INTRODUCTION

Left atrial access has been a challenge in cardiac catheterization since the earliest cardiac surgical procedures mandated accurate assessment of left atrial pressure in the 1940s. The occasional direct measurement was by a number of hazardous routes, including transbronchial and direct left atrial puncture. Modern left atrial catheterization by puncture of the interatrial septum is a half-century old. It resulted from the pioneering efforts of a young medical resident named Constantine Cope at the East Orange, New Jersey Veteran's Administration Hospital. Cope developed an apparatus working with the Becton Dickinson Company.[1] This led to animal and clinical investigation at Hahnemann Hospital in Philadelphia, in conjunction with Charles Bailey, the pioneering cardiac surgeon who performed the first successful mitral commissurotomy in 1948.[2] Ross and colleagues at the National Institutes of Health subsequently described a similar approach.[3] The technique was inherently dangerous,[4] and was used primarily for pressure measurement and angiography. Several factors contributed to its near disappearance from clinical practice. First, right heart catheterization, developed in the 1940s, allowed for indirect left atrial pressure measurement through the pulmonary arterial wedge pressure.[5] Second, the introduction of balloon flotation catheters simplified and enhanced the safety of right heart catheterization.[6] Finally, the availability of echocardiography further decreased the need for a highly invasive means of assessing hemodynamics. As a result, there was a dramatic decrease in the use of transseptal puncture, and by the late 1970s, most adult catheterizers had either stopped doing the procedure or had never been trained to perform it. Occasional transseptal puncture was still mandated by prosthetic aortic valves that were inherently dangerous to cross-retrograde, in particular, the Bjork–Shiley tilting disc valve. However, the declining emphasis on structural heart disease in favor of coronary angiography and the introduction of ever more sophisticated cardiac ultrasound in lieu of hemodynamic studies resulted in fewer operators with training, experience, or maintenance of transseptal puncture skills.[7]

Although the technique continued to have adherents for high-fidelity hemodynamic measurements and for antegrade access in patients with aortic stenosis[8] or hypertrophic obstructive cardiomyopathy,[9] the reappearance of transseptal catheterization owed much to the introduction

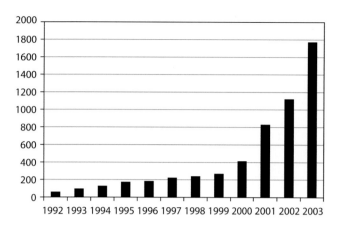

Figure 23.1 Growth of transseptal puncture in a survey of 33 hospitals in Italy over a 12-year period. This exponential growth was driven primarily by atrial fibrillation ablation procedures. (From De Ponti, R., et al., *J. Am. Coll. Cardiol.*, 47(5), 1037–1042, 2006. With permission.)

of percutaneous balloon mitral valvuloplasty in the 1980s, a procedure that requires primarily antegrade left atrial access. The real stimulus for the rebirth of transseptal catheterization, however, has been the electrophysiology laboratory, where left-sided ablations have resulted in exponential growth (Figure 23.1).[10] Further utilization is related to the expansion of structural heart disease interventions in the past decade, and a substantial number of relatively new or experimental technologies will likely continue the trend. A list of procedures for which transseptal catheterization is required is provided in Table 23.1.

Transseptal technology was relatively stagnant for the first 30 years after its introduction. In 1979, Mullins introduced a dilator and sheath combination that provided a platform for the advancement of a variety of catheters into the left atrium (LA), and enhanced the safety of the procedure overall.[11] The primary tools for left atrial access have remained the Mullins sheath, along with the Brockenbrough needle, a combination with origins that are 30 and 50 years old, respectively. More recently, however, with increasing utilization of transseptal puncture, a number of novel technologies have appeared and are discussed later in this chapter.[12]

ANATOMY OF THE INTERATRIAL SEPTUM

The interatrial septum is embryologically derived from growth of the septum primum and secundum toward the endocardial cushions (Figure 23.2a). During prenatal development, a circular opening, the foramen ovale, develops in the inferior–posterior portion of the septum secundum. As the septum primum resorbs, it continues to overlap the foramen ovale, forming a flap that functionally acts as a valve. Because of high pulmonary vascular resistance during gestation, right atrial pressure drives the valve to open and allow blood to flow from the right atrium (RA) to the LA. After birth, pulmonary vascular resistance decreases, right atrial pressure falls below left atrial pressure, and the valve fuses to the septum secundum. Because the septum

Table 23.1 Indications for transseptal puncture

1. Diagnostic studies
   a. Hemodynamic assessment where noninvasive data are equivocal
      i. Aortic outflow obstruction
         A. Tilting disc prosthetic aortic valve dysfunction
         B. Hypertrophic obstructive cardiomyopathy
         C. Inability to cross a stenotic native aortic valve
      ii. Mitral stenosis—particularly prosthetic valve obstruction
   b. Arterial angiography when access can only be obtained by antegrade access through the aortic valve
2. Interventions
   a. Electrophysiology mapping and ablation
      i. Atrial fibrillation
      ii. Left atrial tachyarrhythmias (left atrial tachycardia/left atrial flutter)
      iii. Left-sided accessory pathways
      iv. Left ventricular arrhythmias**
   b. Structural heart interventions
      i. Balloon mitral valvuloplasty
      ii. Left atrial appendage occlusion
      iii. Percutaneous mitral valve repair
      iv. Prosthetic paravalvular leak closure*
      v. Pulmonary vein stenosis dilatation and stenting*
      vi. Percutaneous aortic valve implantation**
      vii. Patent foramen ovale closure
      viii. Left atrial pressure monitor placement
      ix. Atrial septostomy
   c. Percutaneous cardiac assist

* procedure off-label, experimental, or pending U.S. Food and Drug Administration approval;
** transseptal approach used when aortic stenosis, peripheral vascular disease, or mechanical prosthetic valve prevents retrograde access to the left ventricle.

primum is thin and membranous compared to the thicker and more muscular septum secundum, the fossa ovalis is only approximately 2 mm thick and is recessed unless the left atrial pressure is high. It averages less than 2.5 cm² in diameter, making for a relatively small target (Figure 23.2b). A patent foramen ovale, present in approximately one-quarter of the population, allows for easy transseptal access but may not be the ideal entry route to the LA as discussed subsequently. Important anatomic variants include a prominent Eustachian valve, which can limit access to the septum from the inferior vena cava (IVC), and left superior vena cava (SVC), which may result in a markedly enlarged adjacent coronary sinus ostium.

EQUIPMENT FOR TRANSSEPTAL PUNCTURE

The standard Mullins technique calls for use of the Brockenbrough needle, a dilator, and sheath as shown in Figure 23.3. The needle is curved to allow access to the fossa

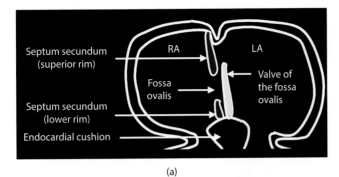

(a)

(b)

Figure 23.2 **(a)** Anatomy of the interatrial septum. The fossa ovalis is formed by the valve created in utero between the foramen ovale and the portion of the septum primum that does not resorb. The latter functions as a flap, or valve, and allows right to left flow to bypass the lungs during gestation. The fusion of the valve with the septum secundum takes place within 3 months after birth, with patency of foramen continuing into adulthood in approximately one-quarter of the population. Because the septum primum is thin and membranous, the fossa is typically the thinnest portion of the septal wall. **(b)** Anatomy of the interatrial septum, right atrial view. Note the proximity of the coronary sinus, immediately inferior to the fossa, and the location of the torus aorticus (the prominence at the level of the aortic cusps). (Courtesy of Dr. Kalyanam Shivkumar, University of California, Los Angeles, CA.) LA, left atrium; RA, right atrium.

ovalis; several curvatures are available, with typical ones ranging from a relatively shallow 19° angle to a steeper 53° angle (Figure 23.4a). We prefer the steeper angle for easier access to the septum in the average patient. Some operators gently bend the needle (with the stylet in place) to provide a custom configuration, in particular, to provide a steeper angle to access the septum when the RA is large or the anatomy is distorted, such as when a prominent Eustachian valve interferes with access. Patients with high left atrial pressure, where the entire septum protrudes toward the RA, may require a less angled approach. An example of the latter

is mitral stenosis, where the fossa is both enlarged as well as more horizontally aligned.[13] Needles are typically 71 cm in length and taper from a proximal 18 gauge to 21 gauge at the distal tip. A number of needle modifications exist, including a 16-gauge needle that does not taper. The Mullins sheath is typically 59 cm, with a 67 cm dilator, and is available in a wide range of diameters. Typically, 6- to 8-Fr are used for routine diagnostic procedures, but 14- to 21-Fr are used with interventions requiring large-diameter devices.

Transseptal sheaths with a wide range of shapes are available (Figure 23.4b) and are primarily designed for electrophysiology access to various structures within or originating from the LA. A transseptal sheath that allows the operator to vary the distal curvatures (Figure 23.4c) is widely used in ablations[14] and some specialized left atrial interventions, such as percutaneous closure of prosthetic mitral paravalvular leaks (Agilis, St. Jude Medical).[15] The Agilis can be used in the initial transseptal puncture (in which case a longer needle is required to accommodate the additional length added by the control handle) or introduced by an exchange technique after access to the LA is already achieved.

INDICATIONS

Indications are discussed as follows and in Table 23.1.

Diagnostic studies

The initial use of transseptal puncture for direct hemodynamic assessment of left heart pressures has become uncommon given the small but significant risk associated with the procedure, the low risk of pulmonary wedge pressure measurement, and the availability of noninvasive alternatives in most cases. Nevertheless, in settings where echocardiographic data are equivocal, transseptal catheterization remains an important alternative means of access to the LA and the left ventricle (LV).

MITRAL VALVE HEMODYNAMICS: WEDGE VERSUS LEFT ATRIAL PRESSURE

Pulmonary artery wedge pressure differs from left atrial pressure measured directly in several clinically important ways. First, the additional resistance in the pulmonary vascular bed dampens the phasic excursion of the wedge-derived a and v waves. Second, a substantial phase delay is introduced. Thus, as shown in Figure 23.5a, although the mean wedge and left atrial pressures are usually identical (barring the still uncommon but no longer rare phenomenon of pulmonary veno-occlusive disease[16] typically secondary to radiofrequency ablation in the pulmonary vein[17]), the height of the a and v waves is prone to significant underestimation when pulmonary wedge pressures are recorded (Figure 23.5b). Since the rate of fall in left atrial pressure (negative dP/dt) is substantially diminished by recording across the pulmonary vascular bed, the gradient between pulmonary wedge and left ventricular pressure is artifactually higher than

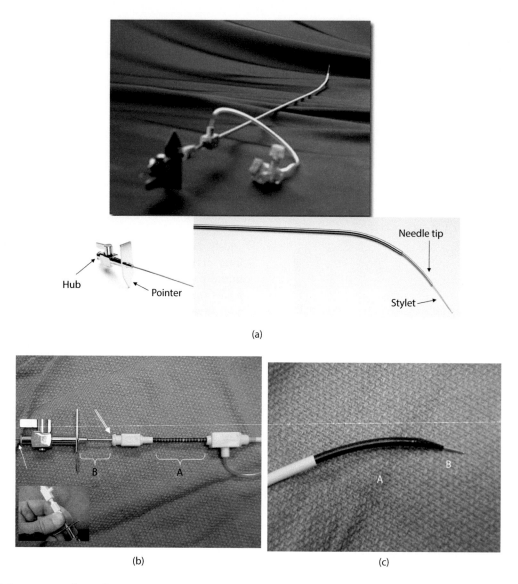

Figure 23.3 **(a)** Transseptal needle, stylet, sheath, and dilator. Note the parallel orientation of the needle arrow, sheath sidearm, dilator, and needle tip. The pointer allows for orientation of the needle and the rest of the Mullins assembly as it is withdrawn from the superior vena cava and maneuvered against the fossa ovalis. (Images courtesy of Medtronic, Inc., Minneapolis, MN and St. Jude Medical, Saint Paul, MN.) **(b)** The transseptal needle, dilator, and sheath showing the distance markers that identify the length of the dilator protruding from the sheath (A) and the relative distance between the position arrow of the transseptal needle and the dilator hub when the needle tip is just inside the end of the dilator (B). The Bing stylet is seen to protrude from the needle hub at the extreme left (arrow). The double arrow points to the site of entry of the needle into the dilator; finger compression of the space adjacent to the needle (inset) is necessary to prevent air from being sucked into the assembly during careful drawback of blood through the needle to establish an air-free fluid column for pressure recording and dye injection. **(c)** The sheath with the dilator (A) and needle (B) both fully inserted into the hub. Since there are several commonly available lengths of the Brockenbrough needle, it is essential to confirm that the needle and sheath sizes are matched.

that noted between left atrial and left ventricular pressure. An example is shown in Figure 23.6. This, in turn, leads to substantial overestimation of the severity of mitral stenosis, especially when any degree of mitral insufficiency is superimposed on preexisting valve obstruction. This phenomenon has led to overestimation of prosthetic mitral valve stenosis and unnecessary repeat mitral valve surgery when wedge pressure, rather than left atrial pressure, has been relied on to assess prosthetic valve dysfunction.[18]

AORTIC OUTFLOW OBSTRUCTION

Technical failure to cross the aortic valve retrograde should be quite rare and is usually associated with severe calcification and an eccentric orifice; this can be addressed by the alternative of transseptal antegrade access.[8] In addition, some mechanical valves should not be crossed retrograde because of the risk of catheter entrapment and potential difficulties with extracting the catheter.[19] Furthermore, entrapment of the catheter in a mechanical

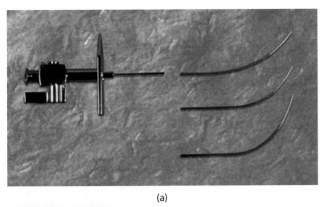

(a)

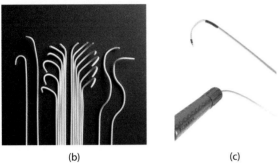

(b)   (c)

Figure 23.4 Gallery of **(a)** transseptal needles, **(b)** pre-formed, and **(c)** steerable sheaths. (Images courtesy of St. Jude Medical, Saint Paul, MN.)

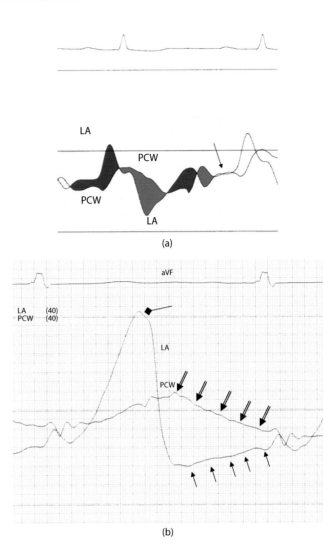

(a)

(b)

Figure 23.5 **(a)** Left atrial and simultaneous pulmonary artery wedge pressures, 40 mmHg scale. Note that the height of the a-wave in this patient is higher on the left atrial pressure tracing, while the v-wave is similar. An arrow points to diastasis between the pressure waveforms; the mean pressures are typically identical, with the exception of patients with pulmonary venous outflow obstruction. **(b)** Simultaneous left atrial and pulmonary artery wedge pressures at 40 mmHg scale in a patient with severe prosthetic mitral perivalvular regurgitation. Although the mean pressures are the same, note that the peak left atrial pressure (diamond-shaped arrow) is 42 mmHg, while the peak wedge pressure is 24 mmHg, with a significant phase delay. The gradient between wedge pressure (double arrows) and left atrial pressure (single arrows) is substantial, but entirely artifactual, induced by measuring the wedge pressure indirectly across a high resistance system: the pulmonary capillary bed. LA, left atrial; PCW, pulmonary capillary wedge.

aortic valve will distort hemodynamics since a leaflet is pinned in an open position resulting in artifactual aortic insufficiency. Simultaneous measurement of left ventricular pressure via antegrade access to the LV and retrograde access to the central aorta does address two concerns: artifact induced by measurement of left ventricular pressure against femoral artery sheath sidearm pressure and the potential for a small reduction in systemic pressure created by the obstruction of the aortic valve by the catheter itself[20] (Carabello's sign); the latter is uncommon with 6-Fr catheters. Using the femoral artery rather than central aortic pressure does result in underestimation of the transvalvular gradient regardless of whether the left ventricular pressure is measured via transseptal access[21] or by retrograde left ventricular entry (Figure 23.7).[22] There is also a concern that retrograde passage of catheters across the aortic valve is associated with cerebral emboli[23] in over 20% of patients, although most are not clinically apparent. Furthermore, the frequency of these initial findings has not been confirmed.[24] Importantly, left ventricular and central aortic pressures can be measured simultaneously using several techniques that avoid transseptal puncture, including use of a catheter designed for simultaneous measurement using a retrograde technique (Langston, VascularSolutions, Minneapolis, MN),[25] a simultaneous catheter and pressure wire method,[26] and dual arterial punctures. Overall, routine transseptal puncture for hemodynamic evaluation of aortic stenosis is not warranted.

A second setting for use of transseptal puncture to assess left ventricular hemodynamics via an antegrade approach has been in patients with hypertrophic cardiomyopathy with obstruction. The transseptal route can avoid catheter entrapment and artifact;[27] pullback to the mitral valve allows differentiation between apical or mid-cavitary obliteration and true outflow obstruction (Figure 23.8).

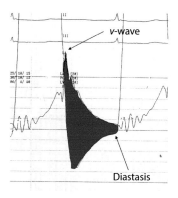
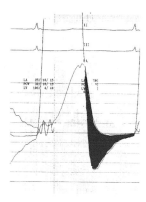

Figure 23.6 The patient whose hemodynamics are presented in this figure was initially misdiagnosed as having severe mitral stenosis and referred for balloon mitral valvuloplasty. The tracing at left demonstrates a substantial gradient measured using a pulmonary arterial wedge pressure against left ventricular diastolic pressure (40 mmHg scale). Two clues to the true nature of the actual diagnosis are present: first, note the v-wave peak is more than twice the mean wedge pressure; second, note the presence of diastasis at end-diastole. In contrast, a simultaneous left atrial and left ventricular pressure measured in the same patient clarifies the hemodynamics: the gradient is primarily due to the sizeable v-wave, with decompression of left atrial pressure only slightly delayed by the presence of mild mitral stenosis; diastasis can now be seen to occur much earlier in diastole. (From Turi, Z.G., Percutaneous balloon valvuloplasty, in Kern, M.J. (Ed.), *Hemodynamic Rounds: Interpretation of Cardiac Pathophysiology from Pressure Waveform Analysis*, Wiley-Liss, New York, NY, 2009:173–196. With permission.)

TRANSSEPTAL ACCESS TO THE ARTERIAL CIRCULATION

In selected patients, access to the arterial circulation cannot be obtained by any practical means. These patients typically have obstructions of the subclavian arteries and aorta, and limited approaches such as carotid or lumbar transaortic access are almost always high risk. An alternative has been transseptal access, typically for aortography. Coronary angiography is technically difficult but has been described.[28] In addition, carotid stenting has been performed via the transseptal route in Takayasu's arteritis,[29] as well as in the setting of a type III aortic arch, where neither femoral nor arm access was deemed suitable.[30]

INTERVENTIONS

Electrophysiology

Ablation for atrial fibrillation and other left-sided electrophysiologic interventions have accounted for the largest segment of the growth of transseptal puncture in the past two decades (Figure 23.1). Treatment of preexcitation syndromes transitioned from medical therapy to an investigational retrograde left ventricular approach to a transseptal access-based procedure as the first-line therapy.[31] The

advantages of the transseptal approach include avoidance of several potential complications associated with retrograde left atrial access. These include large femoral artery puncture-related adverse events, potential damage to the aortic valve or submitral apparatus from extensive catheter manipulation, and perforation, dissection, or embolization from catheter manipulations in the LV and aorta. In addition, some patients are not suitable for retrograde ablations, such as those with severe peripheral vascular disease and those with mechanical aortic valves. Treatment of atrial fibrillation and other atrial arrhythmias by catheter ablation in the LA and the pulmonary vein ostia is now widely performed.[32] Dual transseptal access to the LA is required for some procedures and is achieved either by performing two separate transseptal punctures or by placing two catheters across a single puncture site; the safety implications are discussed subsequently.

Structural heart interventions

Since the introduction of percutaneous balloon valvuloplasty with a device originally designed for atrial septostomy,[33] transseptal catheterization has been utilized for a variety of structural heart interventions. In patients with rheumatic mitral stenosis with favorable anatomy, balloon dilatation is the procedure of choice.[34] Several innovative technologies require left atrial access, including percutaneous mitral valve repair,[35] left atrial appendage occlusion,[36] implantation of a left atrial pressure monitoring device,[37] and closure of prosthetic paravalvular leaks.[15] PFO closure, in the setting of a long foramen tunnel, is sometimes performed by placing a closure device through a transseptal puncture placed *across* rather than *through* the tunnel.[38] Scarring of the pulmonary veins, a consequence of ablation procedures, can result in pulmonary venous obstruction that can be treated by balloon dilatation and stenting,[16] also by transseptal approach. Percutaneous balloon valvuloplasty of the aortic valve via the antegrade approach has a few adherents, in particular because of superior immediate hemodynamic results with the Inoue balloon compared with cylindrical balloons;[39] it is also an option for patients with limited arterial access. The Inoue balloon is typically not long enough for retrograde access to the aortic valve but is of sufficient length to place transseptally. However, long-term benefit of this technique compared with the conventional retrograde approach has not been shown.[40] Finally, percutaneous aortic valve implantation was initially performed antegrade via the transseptal route.[41] This approach has been abandoned because of complexity and associated morbidity, in particular, trauma to the submitral apparatus[42] caused by shortening of the catheter loop in the LV that effectively "filleted" the chordae and papillary muscles.

Cardiac assist

Transseptal access is required for a percutaneous cardiac assist device that provides extracorporeal circulation

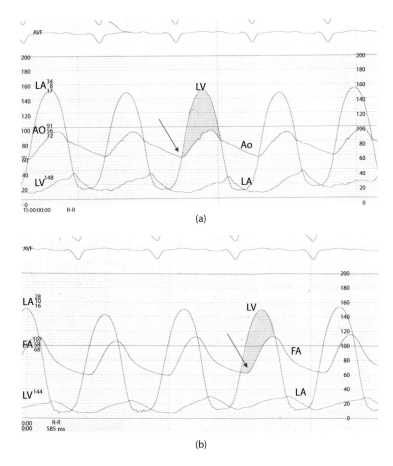

Figure 23.7 **(a)** Severe aortic valve stenosis with left ventricular, central aortic, and left atrial pressure on 200 mmHg scale. The left ventricular pressure was obtained by antegrade introduction of a pigtail catheter into the left atrium through a Mullins sheath. Aortic pressure was measured through a pigtail catheter in the central aorta. The peak-to-peak gradient is approximately 60 mmHg. The arterial pressure upslope (dP/dt) is markedly blunted. The red arrow points to the start of the upstroke of central aortic pressure coincident with opening of the aortic valve. **(b)** Left ventricular, femoral artery, and left atrial pressure on 200 mmHg scale in the same patient obtained moments after the tracing in 23.7A. The gradient is underestimated and the arterial pressure upslope (dP/dt) appears relatively well preserved, both the result of recruitment of harmonics as the pulse waveform travels distally through the arterial tree. The red arrow points to the substantial delay in pressure upstroke seen when femoral artery rather than central aortic pressure is compared to the left ventricular pressure. Although left ventricular-femoral artery gradient measurement is the most commonly used, it leads to inaccurate estimation of aortic valve area.[24] Several less invasive means of obtaining the gradient are discussed in the text. Ao, central aorta; FA, femoral artery; LA, left atrium; LV, left ventricle. (From Turi, Z.G., Percutaneous balloon valvuloplasty, in Kern, M.J. (Ed.), *Hemodynamic Rounds: Interpretation of Cardiac Pathophysiology from Pressure Waveform Analysis*, Wiley-Liss, New York, NY, 2009:173–196. With permission.)

by shunting oxygenated blood from the LA using a 21-Fr transseptal cannula that needs stable positioning in the LA (TandemHeart, CardiacAssist, Pittsburgh, PA).[43] Blood is then pumped into a large femoral arterial cannula. The technology provides circulatory support during high-risk percutaneous interventions, perioperatively during cardiac surgery, and temporarily augments cardiac output in a variety of settings.

CONTRAINDICATIONS

Uncorrected anticoagulation as well as significant coagulopathy were considered a relative or absolute contraindication to transseptal puncture until the past decade; this

has changed dramatically and most electrophysiologists puncture with the patient fully anticoagulated as discussed subsequently.[44] Thrombus in either the RA or LA does remain a contraindication. Anatomic abnormalities that alter landmarks and interfere with septal access are a challenge; these include severe kyphoscoliosis, giant LA, prominent Eustachian valve, left SVC, vena caval interruption, and an azygous continuation of the IVC. While transseptal puncture has been described in most of these settings, the risks are augmented. Some other features that make transseptal puncture technically more complex include a thickened or fibrotic septum and atrial septal aneurysm (which increases risk of perforating the left atrial free wall). Repeat transseptal puncture has been reported as more difficult, in

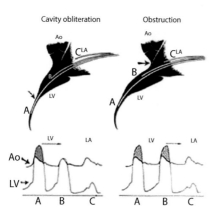

Figure 23.8 The benefit of transseptal access for invasive assessment of left ventricular outflow track obstruction. In the figure at the left, the gradient is caused by catheter entrapment in a hypertrophic apex with cavitary obliteration in systole. As the catheter is pulled back from the apex toward the outflow track, the gradient disappears. In the tracing at right, the outflow track narrows, and the gradient persists until the catheter is pulled back into the left atrium. (From Ref. 27. With permission.) Ao, aorta; LA, left atrium; LV, left ventricle.

part because of increased atrial septal thickness.[45] Finally, the presence of a prior atrial septal defect (ASD) closure, either by surgery or percutaneously placed device, has been addressed using intracardiac (ICE) or transesophageal (TEE) echocardiographic guidance. Limited experience in these settings has suggested that transseptal puncture can be performed with reasonably high success and low complication rates.[46]

TECHNIQUE

Preprocedure Evaluation

Knowledge of the anatomy of the septum, the LA and its appendage, and the RA can be extremely helpful prior to transseptal puncture. This is particularly true in patients predisposed to thrombus. Although most clots occur in the left atrial appendage, they occur with much higher frequency in the rest of the LA in the setting of atrial fibrillation and rheumatic heart disease.[47] Thrombus along the septum, on prosthetic valves, and on pacemaker wires adds substantial risk, and most operators consider these absolute contraindications to transseptal puncture. However, safe performance of procedures such as balloon mitral valvuloplasty despite the presence of appendage thrombus has been described; nevertheless, most operators would consider this an absolute contraindication as well.[48] The relative thickness of the septum, aneurysmal excursion, deviation into the RA (more common with left atrial hypertension such as is seen with mitral valve stenosis[49]), and presence of a PFO are all potentially important variables to know prior to attempting transseptal puncture.

Imaging

The most common techniques for adjunctive imaging are ICE[49] and TEE,[50] both of which can blunt the learning curve for transseptal puncture, and provide for a margin of safety even for highly experienced operators. Transthoracic echo alone has been used as an adjunct when transseptal puncture with fluoroscopic guidance alone was difficult,[51] but this technique has largely been supplanted. TEE preprocedure in patients at high risk of left atrial thrombus is a class I indication,[34] and both TEE and computed tomography (CT) angiography have been used to assess for thrombus.[53,54] The consensus statement published by the Heart Rhythm Society lists TEE as the "gold standard," with a recommendation that all patients with atrial fibrillation at the time of ablation should be screened with TEE.[54] More recently, real-time three-dimensional (3D) echo guidance has been utilized to facilitate transseptal puncture (Figure 23.9).[55] Preprocedure CT angiography, in conjunction with electroanatomic mapping,[56] has been used as an adjunct to transseptal puncture, and an animal model using intraprocedural magnetic resonance imaging (MRI) to guide laser-driven transseptal puncture has been described as well.[57]

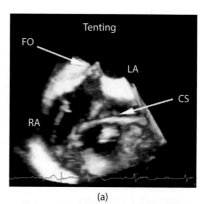

(a)

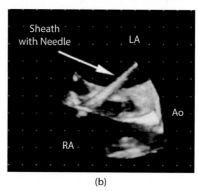

(b)

Figure 23.9 (a) Three-dimensional echocardiography to demonstrate apposition of the transseptal apparatus with tenting of the septum, (b) and the appearance after needle and sheath entry into the left atrium. Intracardiac or transesophageal echo is used for echo guidance by most operators. Ao, aorta; CS, coronary sinus; FO, foramen ovale; LA, left atrium; RA, right atrium. (From Ref. 55. With permission.)

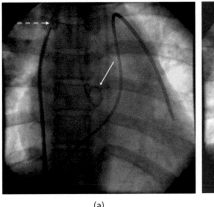 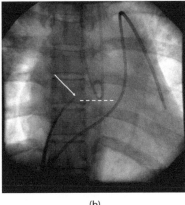

(a)   (b)

Figure 23.10 **(a)** The Mullins assembly has been advanced into the superior vena cava (dashed arrow), a pigtail catheter (white arrow) is in the aortic cusp, and a pulmonary artery catheter is in the left pulmonary artery (the pulmonary artery catheter was placed from the left femoral vein). **(b)** The Mullins assembly has been withdrawn from the superior vena cava into the right atrium. The tip (white arrow) is above the bottom of the pigtail catheter (broken white line), and may be too high to attempt puncture. If the needle is advanced in this position, there is an increased chance of inadvertent entry into the aorta. Both images are in anterior–posterior view.

In certain settings, such as pregnant patients where the operator has deemed fluoroscopy to be hazardous, the procedure has been done with echo guidance alone,[58] or with fluoroscopy plus echo designed to minimize radiation.[59] Since minimal radiation is required for a transseptal, most operators continue to use fluoroscopy in pregnant patients to minimize procedure duration and for the added margin of safety provided by the additional imaging guidance.[60]

TRANSSEPTAL PROCEDURE

Preparation

Although transseptal puncture has been performed by venous access from a variety of approaches, including the internal jugular, subclavian, and even hepatic veins, the standard remains the right femoral route. Left femoral venous access requires negotiating the additional curvature of the left iliac vein, particularly as it enters the IVC, and provides technically more difficult access to the interatrial septum; it is nevertheless quite feasible. We place a short 7-Fr sheath in the right femoral vein, and perform right heart catheterization if clinically warranted. This helps identify hemodynamics *before* transseptal puncture, including the pressure to expect when the needle enters the LA, and establishes the baseline hemodynamics should a subsequent suspicion of tamponade occur. We also fluoroscope the left heart border in the anteroposterior view to note the degree of motion seen before puncture. At this point, we advance a pigtail catheter retrograde to the aortic valve, usually from the femoral artery, although a radial approach can also be used. Because the fossa is usually below the level of the aortic cusps, placement of the pigtail at the aortic valve is an important adjunct to prevent entry

into the aorta or perforation of the RA secondary to a high puncture (Figure 23.10).[61] Electrophysiologists performing transseptal puncture will frequently place a catheter in the coronary sinus to provide an alternative or additional anatomic landmark (Figure 23.2b).[62,63] The pigtail catheter is connected to a pressure manifold, and systemic pressure is continuously displayed during the procedure, from pretransseptal puncture to at least 5 minutes after withdrawal of the transseptal sheath, to ensure that sheath withdrawal does not unmask a stitch perforation (discussed subsequently) or other errant puncture that may result in early tamponade.

Maneuvering to the septum

After withdrawal of the right heart catheter, the venous sheath is carefully flushed. The Mullins assembly is potentially quite thrombogenic and should not be introduced into the vein until *all* the equipment is completely prepared and the operator is ready to perform the puncture. A 0.032-in J-tipped guidewire is then advanced through the femoral venous sheath (some Mullins assemblies will accept a 0.035-in wire); when advanced from the femoral vein directly (rather than inside a catheter), the wire tends to enter the SVC easily. If introduced through the Mullins dilator, the curvature tends to steer the wire away from the ostium of the SVC, and more manipulation is typically required. Once the wire is in place in the SVC, the venous sheath is removed and the Mullins dilator and sheath are advanced; some operators place the assembly into the left subclavian vein. The dilator is flushed, taking care to make sure there is venous return, since aggressive flushing of the dilator buried in the vessel wall can cause local dissection. The Brockenbrough needle and Bing stylet (Figure 23.3a) are advanced through the dilator with care taken to allow the needle to rotate freely as it traverses toward the SVC. If the needle is held rigidly during advancement and prevented from rotating freely, there is a small risk of perforation; in addition, it places pressure against structures that abut the vena cava, particularly Glissen's capsule of the liver, and can cause considerable discomfort. The Bing stylet helps prevent perforation of the sheath and dilator as the needle is advanced. Once the needle and stylet enter the RA, the needle can be turned to face toward the patient's left (3 o'clock) as it is advanced up into the SVC, and the stylet withdrawn when the needle is a few centimeters from the tip of the dilator. The needle is then connected to extension tubing attached to the manifold. Flushing the needle requires some care while drawing back on the column of fluid in the needle and should be done slowly with the operator using his fingers pressed against the point where the needle enters the dilator hub to prevent air from entering around the needle (Figure 23.3b). The needle should be kept at least a few millimeters proximal to the dilator tip. If it is too proximal, there is a risk of the dilator kinking when the assembly is pressed against the septum and can result in perforation of the dilator when the needle is advanced. If it is too distal, there is a risk of inadvertent needle deployment and perforation of the SVC or RA. The operator should maintain his or her fingers in the space between the needle arrow and the dilator hub to prevent inadvertent movement of the needle proximally or distally. The alignment of the Mullins sheath, dilator, and needle should be parallel (Figure 23.3a). Care should be taken to maintain this alignment throughout the subsequent movement of the Mullins assembly.

Once properly flushed and an undamped pressure tracing is seen on the monitor, the entire assembly is pulled down into the RA with the needle pointer aimed in a posterior medial direction (approximately 4 to 5 o'clock, with 6 o'clock being straight posterior). The tip of the dilator can usually be seen to deflect off the SVC–right atrial junction, and then to fall below the limbus. We typically pull it back an additional centimeter and advance into the fossa. At this point, unless the fossa is displaced toward the RA by elevated left atrial pressure, resistance should be felt.

Localization at the fossa ovalis

Several maneuvers can confirm appropriate location of the dilator prior to attempted puncture. Fluoroscopy may demonstrate that the tip of the Mullins assembly is below the pigtail that was placed in the aortic root; the relevant relationship of the dilator to the pigtail catheter and anatomic structures can be seen in different views in Figures 23.10 and 23.11. Although puncture can also be performed in the 20° right anterior oblique (RAO) view[64] (Figure 23.12) or the anteroposterior view as well, in our experience, the best guidance to avoiding the left atrial free wall is the 90° lateral (Figure 23.13). When ICE or TEE are done, the echo equipment frequently prevents the gantry from being moved into this position. (Adequate imaging in this view requires that

the patient's arms be raised out of the field; if the procedure is done under anesthesia, the arms should be moved prior to induction or with great care afterward, since brachial plexus injury can result if inadvertent traction is placed on the arms.) The relationship of the fossa ovalis to the aortic cusps and posterior LA is most likely to be fixed in the center of a line drawn at a 45° angle between the aortic valve and the left atrial posterior wall. If the catheter is low, it can be moved into position with a gentle to-and-fro "windshield wiper" maneuver: clockwise turns the assembly posteriorly and counterclockwise anteriorly. Aggressive manipulation should be avoided; besides trauma to the RA, patients in sinus rhythm predisposed to atrial arrhythmias, such as those with mitral stenosis and dilated LA, are prone to develop atrial fibrillation. With normal anatomy, the dilator tip will be tented against the fossa; contrast injection to "tag" the septum is benign and can assist visualization but is not ordinarily necessary (Figures 23.11 and 23.13). If the operator is uncertain of location, however, this is a useful maneuver.

If ICE[49] or TEE is performed as an adjunct to the procedure, tenting of the fossa (Figure 23.9) should be seen. The advantages of intraprocedural echocardiographic guidance have been extensively demonstrated,[65] although operators should be sufficiently versed in transseptal anatomy so that they are not unduly dependent on echo guidance. Echocardiographic guidance is now almost universal; however, ICE catheters are expensive, and TEE guidance requires general anesthesia in the opinion of most operators, since sedation alone is usually associated with substantial patient discomfort. Hence angiography only is still done by some operators; rotational angiography can add substantial additional anatomic information for non-echo-guided punctures,[66] as can 3D augmented fluoroscopy.[67] However, there are additional benefits of ICE beyond anatomic guidance for transseptal puncture, including early warning of pericardial effusion. A review of tamponades during ablation procedures revealed echocardiographically apparent pericardial effusion before hemodynamic compromise in 11–13 patients.[68] A characteristic electrogram recorded through the Brockenbrough needle and associated with the fossa ovalis has been described,[69] although this technique is rarely if ever used. A number of other schemes (Figure 23.14) for assessing location of the septum and the fossa have been described and include right atrial angiography in a variety of views, including visualization of the LA in the levo phase of the injection.

At this point, with pressure applied by the dilator tip against the fossa ovalis, and without deployment of the needle, it is possible to advance into the LA through the foramen ovale in a significant percent of patients, variably described as 25%–90%.[70] Although a classic PFO may not be present, prolonged gentle pressure may allow "peeling" apart the overlapping layers of septum secundum and residual septum primum when the foramen does not ordinarily open with the usual maneuvers. Catheter passage through a PFO is suitable for diagnostic catheterization but

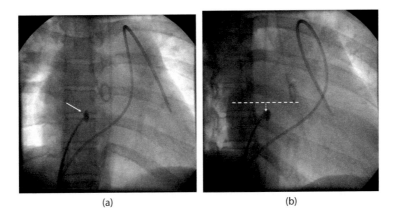

Figure 23.11 The typical correct position for transseptal puncture in the **(a)** anteroposterior and **(b)** 20° right anterior oblique planes. The fossa ovalis has been stained (white arrow), and the Mullins assembly can be seen to have entered the fossa. Note that the target for transseptal puncture is approximately 1–2 cm below the bottom of the aortic cusp (as demarcated by the location of the pigtail catheter in the aorta). In the 20° right anterior oblique view, the fossa is typically located below the center of a line drawn from the right anterior free wall to the bottom of the aortic cusp.

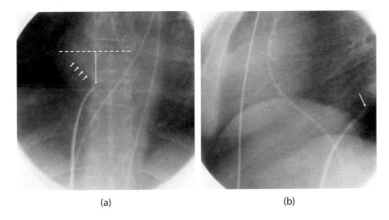

Figure 23.12 The Mullins assembly in simultaneous **(a)** anteroposterior and **(b)** 90° left lateral views; the needle is too low and too posterior to consider attempted transseptal puncture. In the image on the left, the tip of the catheter can be seen to be well below the aortic cusps; in the image on the right, the catheter tip abuts the posterior free wall of the right atrium. Needle advancement in this position would lead to pericardial entry and likely tamponade. This patient had severe mitral stenosis and was undergoing transseptal puncture for mitral valvuloplasty; note the double density caused by the enlarged left atrium (short arrows).

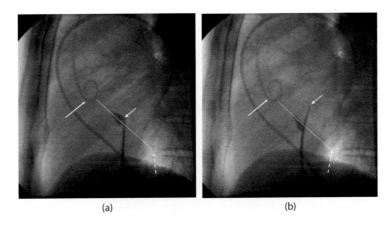

Figure 23.13 The correct position for transseptal puncture in the left lateral view. **(a)** The tip of the transseptal assembly (double arrow) is tenting the stained fossa, which is located halfway along a dotted line drawn at a 45° angle from the pigtail in the aortic root (solid white arrow) to the free wall of the left atrium (dashed arrow). The fossa is tented. **(b)** The needle has been advanced into the left atrium. Left atrial entry was confirmed by pressure measurement and dye injection, and the tip of the dilator can be seen to have advanced through the fossa as well.

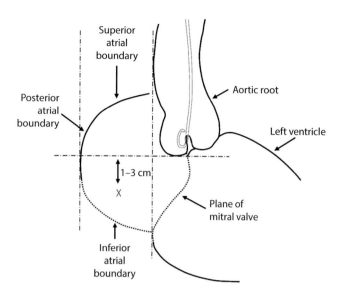

Figure 23.14 One scheme for transseptal puncture in the 40° right anterior oblique view. The fossa is typically located 1–3 cm below the horizontal line drawn from the wall of the aorta to the posterior free wall. A number of different schemes to identify the location of the fossa have been published. (After from Hung, J.S., *Catheter Cardiovasc. Diag.*, 26(4), 275–284, 1992. With permission.)

causes problems for many interventional procedures, since the foramen tunnel restricts pivoting of the sheath, and the orientation is relatively superior and anterior. In some cases, passage without needle deployment is not through the foramen tunnel but directly across an extremely thin fossa, the latter in keeping with the membranous nature of the septum primum that forms the embryonic fossa valve.

Although transseptal puncture at the center of the fossa is usually ideal, some interventions require high or low puncture. The adjunctive use of ICE or TEE has allowed customization of the location of puncture with relative accuracy (Figure 23.15). High fossa puncture is desirable when a relatively perpendicular plane of access is required toward the mitral valve, such as for percutaneous mitral valve repair with a clip device,[71] where a high and posterior approach is helpful for primary or degenerative mitral regurgitation. For left atrial appendage occlusion,[72] low and posterior puncture is generally best. Low puncture is desirable when a relatively shallow entry to the mitral valve is ideal; such was the case for percutaneous metallic mitral commissurotomy.[73]

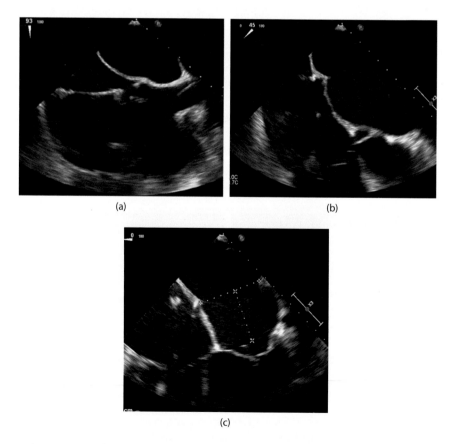

Figure 23.15 Transseptal puncture with transesophageal echo guidance in a patient undergoing percutaneous mitral valve repair. In the bicaval view **(a)**, initial needle placement is high in the fossa, and in short axis view **(b)**, the needle can be seen to be posterior. The location of puncture is critical to allowing a suitably orthogonal access to the mitral valve once the transseptal apparatus has been introduced **(c)**.

Puncture and device advancement

STANDARD PUNCTURE

Once the operator has ascertained that the location is suitable, it is essential that only the needle and not the rest of the assembly perforate the septum (Figure 23.13b). A video demonstrating transseptal entry using a 90° lateral view can be downloaded from an article by Cheng and colleagues.[74] The technique shown features combined entry of the dilator and needle into the LA, a technique best avoided because needle entry alone is usually benign, while errant entry of both needle and dilator is much more likely to lead to tamponade.

The operator has several means of confirming left atrial entry. A tactile sensation of the catheter popping through the septum is usually felt. Entry of the needle into the LA should be immediately apparent when a distinctive left atrial pressure is seen on the monitor (Figure 23.16). When the fossa is thickened, or the operator advances into the thick septal wall outside of the fossa, a damped pressure is usually seen; in older patients, the septal wall can be fibrosed or calcified, in which case the waveform may occasionally appear to be a reflection of a slightly damped left ventricular pressure. In some cases, a higher velocity of needle entry will allow for penetration of the thickened or fibrosed septum; it is occasionally necessary to pass the needle and dilator together in this setting. It is essential that the operator be reasonably certain of the needle's location against the fossa before committing to such combined entry. In addition to tactile sensation and pressure monitoring, contrast injection will confirm needle location in the LA. Oxygen saturation can also be obtained through the transseptal needle. If ICE or TEE is being performed, the needle and catheter are usually visualized in the LA (Figure 23.9), the tenting of the septum resolves, and saline or contrast injection appears as "bubbles" in the LA on echo. Some operators use a coronary guidewire immediately after needle puncture to confirm entry into the LA (Figure 23.17).[75]

At this point, we rotate the image intensifier to visualize catheter advancement in an anteroposterior plane. If the septum is thin, it may be possible to advance the dilator and sheath without further advancement of the needle. If the septum is thick, it may be necessary to advance the entire assembly in order to have enough support to prevent the sheath from buckling as it advances against the septum. Care needs to be taken at this point since it is possible to have the entire assembly prolapse back into the RA if the septum offers resistance. Of greater concern is the risk of perforating the LA as the assembly is advanced. Continuous pressure monitoring through the needle with immediate cessation of advancement if pressure damping is noted, as well as small puffs of contrast to identify if the assembly is near to the left atrial wall, will protect the LA (Figure 23.18). If the septum is relatively soft, it may be possible to withdraw the needle completely once the dilator has crossed the septum, in which case a J-tipped guidewire can be placed through the dilator to allow safe advancement of the sheath and dilator assembly. Alternatively, if support from the shaft of the needle is required, a 0.014-in coronary guidewire can be advanced through the needle into the LA or a pulmonary vein to visualize approach to the left atrial wall, and provide some protection from perforation (Figure 23.17).[76] A significant risk for perforation occurs during blind advancement of needle or dilator (with no guidewire of any kind used), and an abrupt forward movement frequently occurs as the sheath penetrates the septum over the dilator, especially if the sheath is overcoming resistance caused by a thickened septal wall. For certain procedures, such as percutaneous

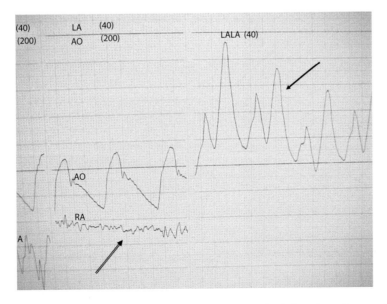

Figure 23.16 One of several modalities for confirming catheter entry into the left atrium. Damped right atrial pressure (RA, double arrow) was recorded while the dilator tip was against the fossa. Immediately after transseptal puncture, the phasic waveform characteristic of left atrial pressure is seen (LA, black arrow). Right and left atrial pressures, 40 mmHg scale; aortic pressure (Ao), 200 mmHg scale.

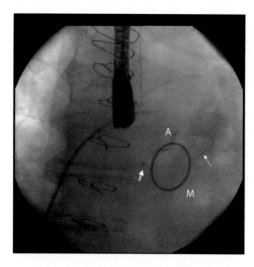

Figure 23.17 Transseptal assembly advanced into the left atrium over a 0.014-in coronary angioplasty guide-wire (white arrow). The needle was advanced only to a point just across the septum, and left in place to support advancement of the dilator and sheath. This patient has prosthetic bi-leaflet aortic (A) and mitral (M) valves, and a patent ductus arteriosus plug (double arrow) adjacent to the mitral annulus used to treat a prosthetic paravalvular leak. A TEE probe and endotracheal tube can also be seen in the image. The coronary guidewire was introduced through the Brockenbrough needle, and provides visual clues as to distance of the dilator tip from adjacent cardiac structures. The image was recorded at the beginning of a procedure where a second paravalvular leak was closed.

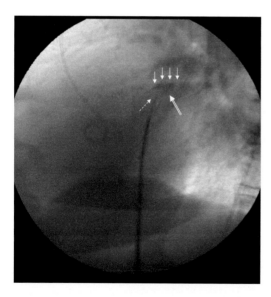

Figure 23.18 The transseptal needle (dashed arrow) is seen to approach the roof of the left atrium. Contrast pools (double arrow) along the curved wall of the left atrial roof (small arrows). Even a few millimeters of further advancement would have resulted in perforation and possible tamponade or hemothorax.

balloon mitral valvuloplasty, sheath entry is optional, since the Inoue guidewire can be advanced through the dilator alone.

FACILITATED PUNCTURE

Several new technologies provide alternatives to the Brockenbrough needle and are designed to require less force to cross the septum, avoiding the typical high-velocity movement with a rigid needle and attendant risks associated with uncontrolled advance of both needle and Mullins assembly. The techniques are particularly appealing when there is a thick or fibrosed septum that may be difficult or impossible to penetrate. One of the technologies uses radiofrequency (RF) energy to puncture the septum and includes a catheter system[77] that is approved by the U.S. Food and Drug Administration (FDA) (Baylis Medical, Montreal, Canada). The system has a curved and flexible tip designed to decrease the risk of trauma to the LA, and sideholes to facilitate dye injection; its tip is closed, which potentially eliminates the issue of tissue coring and its associated risk of debris embolization.[78] RF has been compared to standard puncture in a 1,550 patient comparison that demonstrated fewer tamponades and faster left atrial access with RF.[79] In a similar comparison of smaller cohorts, RF was associated with shorter procedure times and less septal tenting (the latter is a marker for amount of force needed).[80] Accuracy of puncture location, a theoretical benefit of RF, which limits the "sliding" of the needle along the septum during puncture, was not demonstrated in this study but may have been a type II error related to small cohorts. Using a similar approach, but without the cost of a dedicated catheter, electrocautery or RF can be applied directly through a transseptal needle to facilitate transseptal puncture.[81]

Another technique to minimize the force required to cross the septum and decrease perforation risk is a 0.014-in nitinol wire with a needle-like tip that assumes a J-shape once free in the LA and functions as a guidewire to facilitate dilator access[82] (SafeSept, Pressure Products, San Pedro, CA). In a study reviewing the outcomes of 251 patients undergoing transseptal puncture who had multiple prior transseptal punctures, prior surgical or percutaneous ASD closure, the SafeSept, RF, cautery via the transseptal needle, or in many cases standard needle puncture, resulted in successful and safe transseptal passage.[83]

Anticoagulation

There has been a dramatic change in the approach to anticoagulation for transseptal puncture in the last decade. This represents a dichotomy between interventional cardiologists performing structural heart disease interventions who have been concerned predominantly with tamponade, and electrophysiologists performing ablations whose primary focus has been the avoidance of thrombus formation and stroke. Ablations tend to be of longer duration and have several features that increase the predisposition to clotting, including platelet activation by the catheters themselves and char formation that triggers thrombus formation. An increasing number of operators, including many electrophysiologists, give at least a small amount of heparin before the puncture[84] based on data suggesting a lower rate of intraprocedural left atrial thrombus, while others perform transseptal puncture with patients fully heparinized[74] or maintained on therapeutic oral anticoagulation.[44] A comparison of warfarin discontinuation plus bridging of anticoagulation with enoxaparin, versus maintenance of therapeutic range oral anticoagulation during the periprocedure period, did not demonstrate a difference in complication rates.[85]

In contrast, interventional cardiologists have focused on avoidance of tamponade, with most deferring transseptal puncture if the international normalized ratio is greater than 1.6 or if patients are heparinized. However, stroke secondary to thrombus formation is an important source of morbidity and mortality during prolonged structural heart disease interventions as well, an example being closure of prosthetic paravalvular leaks.[86] And while aggressive anticoagulation may help prevent thrombus formation, it is important to note that the most common single cause of peritransseptal mortality with structural heart disease interventions, *as well as* ablation procedures, remains pericardial tamponade.[87] Importantly, even when anticoagulation is deferred until after puncture, the tamponade rate is higher than 1%.[88] The exact peri- and postprocedure anticoagulation management of these patients remains a focus of investigation.[89]

If patients are not anticoagulated at the time of needle entry into the LA, transseptal puncture should be performed expeditiously to allow anticoagulation as soon as the LA has been entered to prevent thrombus formation on the catheter tip or guidewire. The target for activated clotting time (ACT) has increased in the recent literature to a range of 300–400 seconds;[90] comparison of two groups with ACTs of 250–300 seconds versus ACT greater than 300 seconds demonstrated a reduction of catheter-associated thrombus from 11% to 3%.[91] The consensus statement by the Heart Rhythm Society recommends continuous heparin infusion at 10 units/kg/hour with ACT checked every 10–15 minutes until therapeutic anticoagulation is achieved, and then every 30 minutes thereafter.[54,92] Despite the relatively aggressive anticoagulation regimen, stroke continues to be a factor after transseptal puncture; in the ablation literature, transient ischemic events and stroke continue to occur in the 0.5% range.[88] However, transcranial Doppler does demonstrate that a significant portion of microembolic signals are unrelated to the puncture itself.[93]

Sheath management

Handling of the transseptal sheath for the rest of the procedure needs to follow certain basic principles. Wires and catheters should be withdrawn from the Mullins sheath slowly, since abrupt negative pressure caused by rapid catheter or wire withdrawal can induce air to enter the sheath. Similarly, flushing should be performed with care to avoid sucking air in through the sheath diaphragm; we prefer to allow back bleeding through the sheath sidearm and not putting negative pressure on the sheath since the diaphragm can leak air into the fluid column when negative pressure is applied. Passive air embolization due to the gradient between atmospheric pressure and low left atrial pressure, a phenomenon most common in the setting of sedation and exacerbated by placement of a guidewire through a sheath hemostatic valve, is an important and relatively common occurrence, and requires careful technique to avoid.[94] If the left atrial pressure is low, it may be necessary to suspend the end of the Mullins sheath below the patient to ensure that pressure at the open side arm is lower than left atrial pressure. Some operators keep the proximal end of the sheath inside a large bowl of saline or other solution. Introduction of air during introduction of devices through the Mullins sheath is a common occurrence. We maintain a column of diluted contrast in the sheath so that as a device is introduced, bubbles in the column are readily detected under fluoroscopy, in which case the device can be withdrawn and the sheath reprepped as necessary. The Mullins sheath needs to be flushed regularly, or a drip maintained with a system designed to prevent air from entering the column of fluid.

COMPLICATIONS

Complications of transseptal puncture are significant and potentially life-threatening (Table 23.2). The event rates are quite variable and are influenced by several important factors, including level of anticoagulation, duration of the procedure, size of catheter used, intracavitary pressure, status of pericardium (intact or removed), use of echocardiographic guidance, and most importantly, the operator

Table 23.2 Complications of transseptal puncture

1. Mechanical
a. Perforation
i. Pericardial tamponade
ii. Hemothorax
b. Persistent atrial septal defect
c. Right-to-left shunting
d. Aorto-right atrial fistula
2. Embolization—peripheral or central nervous system
a. Thrombus
b. Air
3. Arrhythmias
a. Atrial fibrillation
b. Supraventricular tachycardia
c. Inferior ST segment elevation
d. Bezold–Jarisch reflex
e. Sinus node dysfunction
4. Death

learning curve.[95] The major complication rate is far lower in diagnostic (1%)[96] than interventional procedures (4%),[97] likely because of less aggressive anticoagulation in most diagnostic studies, shorter duration of diagnostic procedures, and the addition of morbidity associated with the interventions themselves. In the era before ablation procedures were common, the incidence of tamponade was more than 10-fold higher (1.2%) than the incidence of stroke (0.1%).[96] While the profile of complications seen after transseptal puncture for structural heart disease interventions may be significantly different than that seen with electrophysiology procedures, as the complexity and duration of the former increase, these differences may be muted.

Tamponade

As discussed, the most dreaded complications of transseptal puncture remain pericardial tamponade and clot or air embolization. The incidence of tamponade is highly variable but remains a significant concern in a wide variety of procedures associated with transseptal puncture,[98] and has been described to range from 0.5% to 4% in patients undergoing percutaneous balloon mitral valvuloplasty.[99] In patients undergoing ablation, tamponade has been described as occurring in up to 6% of cases[54] associated with the type (linear) and energy of ablation[100] and therefore presumably, but not necessarily, related to the transseptal puncture itself. The occurrence of tamponade underestimates the frequency of pericardial effusion secondary to small iatrogenic effusions; in one study of 1,150 patients with left atrial access preparatory to planned atrial fibrillation ablation, effusion occurred in 2.7% while tamponade requiring pericardiocentesis occurred in approximately one-third of these patients (1%).[101] An uncommon but important cause of tamponade is stitch perforation.[102] In this scenario, the needle exits the RA and enters the LA

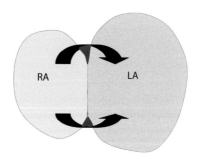

Figure 23.19 Mechanism of a stitch perforation. The transseptal puncture enters the left atrium passing outside the septal wall into extracardiac space, typically adipose tissue. The Mullins assembly and any catheters subsequently placed across the fenestration may prevent tamponade until the catheters are removed at the end of the case. Some operators leave a guidewire across the septum after sheath withdrawal to confirm absence of fluid accumulation for a few minutes prior to sheath withdrawal. LA, left atrium; RA, right atrium.

while traversing tissue folds or periadventitial fat (Figure 23.19). The separation between the chamber walls is limited, and the operator is typically unaware of extracardiac passage of the needle. During most of the subsequent procedure, tamponade may not occur because the fenestration is sealed by catheters or sheaths; when these are removed at the end of the case, effusion and tamponade may occur. The phenomenon is most likely to occur with a low stick. Some operators address this possibility by leaving a guidewire in place prior to withdrawal of all hardware from the septum and observing for a few minutes to detect any new pericardial effusion. If, in fact, this occurs, the guidewire can provide access for placing a sheath to tamponade the hole temporarily while anticoagulation is reversed.[98]

Embolization

Once the Mullins sheath has been placed, maintenance of adequate anticoagulation, proper flushing, and avoidance of introduction of air are integral to the safety of the procedure. Air as well as clot embolization remain important sources of morbidity;[103] setting up a continuous flush through the sheath during extended procedures has been described as preventing air and clot embolization, and the stroke risk appears to be lower when a high flow state is maintained through the transseptal sheath.[104] If bolus flushing of the sheath is performed, consideration should be given to using a high heparin concentration, since there is evidence that thrombus formation is inversely related to the concentration.[105] Stroke and transient ischemic attack, secondary to transseptal catheterization, have been widely reported to occur in the range of approximately 1% with values as high as 5% in patients with ablation procedures for atrial fibrillation.[106] A phenomenon of migraines has been described in approximately 0.5% of patients, and may occur up to 1 week after transseptal puncture.[107]

Persistent atrial septal communication

The creation of a communication between left and right atria commonly results in postprocedure shunting.[108] A number of factors predict the occurrence and persistence of an iatrogenic ASD.[109] The size of the transseptal catheter or sheath is a major factor; thus for arrhythmia ablation, percutaneous balloon mitral valvuloplasty, left atrial appendage occlusion, TandemHeart, and percutaneous mitral valve repair, respectively, the sizes are 8-Fr, 14-Fr, 14-Fr, 21-Fr, and 24-Fr, respectively.[110] Use of balloon dilatation to allow larger sheaths to enter the septum increases the risk of persistent ASD,[111] as well as tamponade. Some transseptal flow after the procedure is almost always seen on TEE, and correlates with size of the puncture as well as driving pressure determined by disparity between left and right atrial pressures. Thus, early in the era of percutaneous balloon mitral valvuloplasty, when the septum was routinely dilated with peripheral angioplasty balloons

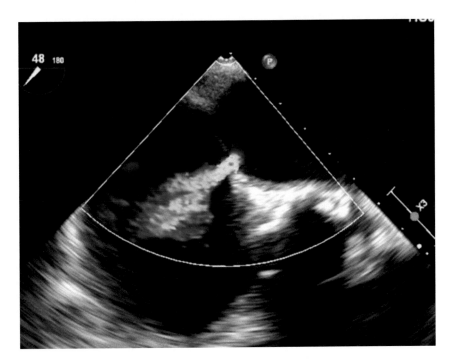

Figure 23.20 Persistent iatrogenic atrial septal defect in a patient who had a 24-Fr sheath placed across the septum for a percutaneous mitral valve repair procedure 9 months earlier. This left the patient with significant mitral stenosis and in essence an iatrogenic Lutembacher syndrome.

ranging in size from 5 to 10 mm, and two transseptal sheaths were usually placed, left to right flow was detected by TEE in 87% of patients, although the majority of these resolved within 6 months.[112] These patients usually had a degree of residual mitral stenosis; thus, a 10 mmHg or more driving pressure across an iatrogenic 5–10 mm defect in the septum would result in a significant-sized, permanent ASD; this essentially constitutes a form of Lutembacher syndrome (Figure 23.20). In addition, balloon dilatation of the septum can cause ripping rather than stretching of the septal opening. At present, dilators are typically used to create a sufficient size fenestration; transseptal flow is almost always seen immediately after sheath removal but typically resolves within a few months to 1 year. Similarly, persistent ASD after electrophysiology procedures, particularly when two catheters are placed across the septum, is also seen in approximately 87% of patients, with resolution in all except 4% by 1 year.[113] Using two transseptal punctures rather than placing two catheters across a single fenestration appears to decrease the risk of a persistent shunt.[114] Because the left-to-right gradient is smaller in electrophysiology procedures, the presence of a residual shunt remains more common with mitral valvuloplasty.[97]

Transseptal puncture in patients with high right-sided pressures increases the risk of right-to-left shunting and systemic arterial desaturation. One scenario is the use of a transseptally placed percutaneous ventricular assist device (TandemHeart) in the setting of right heart failure or right ventricular infarction when a PFO is also present. The simultaneous decompression of the LA has been demonstrated to result in substantial cyanosis because the iatrogenic pressure gradient drives large amounts of blood across the PFO from right to left.[115] For similar reasons, in the rare case of percutaneous dilatation of both tricuspid and mitral stenosis, the tricuspid valve should be dilated first to prevent a setting in which left atrial pressure is substantially lower than right atrial pressure after mitral valve dilatation results in right-to-left shunting.[116]

Bezold–Jarisch Reflex

ST segment elevation, accompanied by chest pain, hypotension, bradycardia, and diaphoresis, has been reported by a number of operators to occur during or immediately after transseptal access. While the phenomenon resembles a Bezold–Jarisch reflex, the mechanism is unclear. It occurs in slightly less than 1% of cases.[101] Although introduction of air with consequent right coronary embolization has been postulated,[117] coronary angiography during such episodes has failed to confirm this,[118] and a neurally mediated mechanism remains the likely etiology. The phenomenon is typically transient and may respond to atropine.

TREATMENT OF COMPLICATIONS

Tamponade

Prompt recognition of tamponade is essential for a successful outcome. If ICE or TEE is performed during the procedure, it can provide early recognition of pericardial effusion in over 80% of cases prior to the onset of hemodynamic compromise.[68] Hypotension is commonly the first sign, although early in tamponade, hypertension and tachycardia may occur, likely secondary to catecholamine stimulation.[98] In some patients, there is an abrupt slowing of heart rate, likely a vasovagal response, to sudden pericardial stretch. Knowledge of the patient's baseline hemodynamics is helpful; incipient or actual tamponade should be accompanied by familiar hemodynamic findings, including a narrow pulse pressure with pulsus paradoxus, near-obliteration during inspiration, and elevation with equalization, in most cases, of right and left heart filling pressures. Early diagnosis of tamponade is greatly facilitated by continuous arterial pressure display during the procedure. One of the earliest and most specific findings in the catheterization laboratory is straightening and immobility of the left heart border that is readily seen on fluoroscopy in the anteroposterior view. This reflects the profile of the tense pericardium along with the markedly diminished stroke volume that accompanies tamponade. Although ICE or TEE can provide immediate confirmation of the diagnosis, if the procedure is done without continuous echo guidance, a transthoracic echo can be obtained. However, if the echocardiographic equipment is not already in the cardiac catheterization laboratory, waiting for its arrival prior to performance of pericardiocentesis may be fatal, and the operator needs to proceed promptly in the setting of critical hemodynamic compromise. Once the pericardium has been tapped, a catheter should be left in place for drainage; the average withdrawn after tamponade in anticoagulated patients was greater than 800 mL in one study of 15 peri-ablation tamponades.[69] Reversal of anticoagulation is helpful in this setting and is one reason that we routinely use heparin rather than bivalirudin in patients undergoing transseptal puncture. Surgical evacuation of the pericardium is usually not necessary, frequently results in the surgeon finding no obvious locus of perforation, and may expose the patient to substantial, unnecessary morbidity and some mortality. Nevertheless, in certain scenarios, such as inadvertent laceration of a coronary artery, there may be no alternative to surgery.[68] If the patient is in extremis, transthoracic pericardiocentesis is unsuccessful, and the delay to surgical evacuation is likely to be fatal, one other alternative has been described: access to the pericardium using an intracardiac approach with the transseptal apparatus purposely utilized to perforate the heart and enter the pericardial space.[119]

Air or clot embolism

Treatment of air embolization is variably successful. Aggressive oxygenation, particularly in a hyperbaric chamber, and especially if performed promptly, is the procedure of choice.[103] Infusion of volume to maintain cerebral perfusion and administration of lidocaine to protect cerebral tissue may also be beneficial. Aggressive transcatheter suctioning of air if trapped in a cardiac chamber has occasionally prevented clinically significant embolism.

Treatment of clot embolization is more complex. Iatrogenic embolization of thrombus has been treated by intravenous[120] and intraarterial[121] thrombolysis, as well as a variety of clot disruption[122] and extraction techniques,[121] although the evidence base remains minimal.[123] We have had successful experience with thrombus embolization from a transseptal sheath to the left main coronary artery treated successfully with aspiration using techniques primarily employed for primary coronary intervention in acute myocardial infraction.[124]

TRAINING CONSIDERATIONS

In order to facilitate safe transseptal puncture and modernize the Mullins apparatus, a transseptal access device, ACross (St. Jude Medical, Saint Paul, MN), has been developed (Figure 23.21). The device prevents inadvertent advancement of the needle while still inside the dilator, a concept that had been described previously using a safety stop.[125]

Training to perform transseptal punctures has been challenging. There is no consensus on the number of procedures required to achieve or maintain competence, despite the significant learning curve and periprocedural risks associated with the procedure. Training with a minimum of 20 transseptals[126] and proficiency at emergency pericardiocentesis have been proposed[127] as minimal requirements. Transseptal puncture meets the criteria for procedures where simulator training is appealing: high risk, relatively low volumes of procedures to which trainees are exposed, and potential for additive risk to the patient when the procedure is done under supervision rather than entirely by an experienced primary operator. Accordingly, several simulation systems have been developed. A small, prospective randomized study compared the effect of simulator training on training time and composite performance and found substantial advantages when simulator training was incorporated in the teaching process.[128]

CONCLUSIONS

Transseptal puncture, the gateway to the LA for a growing variety of structural heart disease and electrophysiologic procedures, is of increasing importance in invasive cardiology. The significant benefits of proficiency in performing transseptals are somewhat offset by the substantial learning curve and complication profile associated with the procedure. However, the dramatic rise in overall performance of transseptals has been accompanied by an expanding evidence base in the literature addressing issues such as optimal periprocedure management, in particular, anticoagulation. A number of technologies, including adjunctive imaging and, more recently, equipment to facilitate the transseptal puncture itself, may improve the overall success rate and safety of this now nearly 60-year-old procedure.

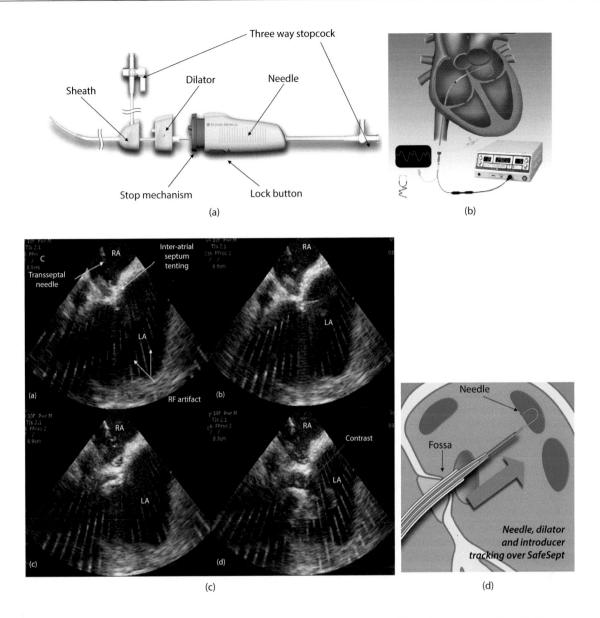

Figure 23.21 A gallery of alternative technologies for transseptal puncture: **(a)** The ACross device is a Mullins apparatus with needle and safety lock (St. Jude); **(b)** the Toronto catheter is designed to allow controlled radiofrequency entry, contrast injection, and sheath introduction (Baylis Medical);[77] **(c)** radiofrequency applied through a transseptal needle, from Bidart et al.;[81] **(d)** a nitinol needle system (SafeSept).[82] (Images [a], [b], and [d] are by permission of the manufacturers; [c] by permission of the publishers; see text for manufacturer name and location.)

REFERENCES

1. Cope C. Technique for transseptal catheterization of the left atrium; preliminary report. *J Thorac Surg* 1959;37(4):482–486.
2. Bailey CP. The surgical treatment of mitral stenosis (mitral commissurotomy). *Dis Chest* 1949;15(4):377–396.
3. Ross J, Jr., et al. Transseptal left atrial puncture; new technique for the measurement of left atrial pressure in man. *Am J Cardiol* 1959;3(5):653–655.
4. Russell RO, Jr., et al. Cardiac tamponade: A complication of the transseptal technic of left heart catheterization resulting in a fatality. *Am J Cardiol* 1964;13:558–563.
5. Dexter L, et al. Studies of congenital heart disease. II. The pressure and oxygen content of blood in the right auricle, right ventricle, and pulmonary artery in control patients, with observations on the oxygen saturation and source of pulmonary "capillary" blood. *J Clin Invest* 1947;26(3):554–560.
6. Swan HJ, et al. Catheterization of the heart in man with use of a flow-directed balloon-tipped catheter. *N Engl J Med* 1970;283(9):447–451.
7. Schoonmaker FW, et al. Left atrial and ventricular transseptal catheterization review: Losing skills. *Catheter Cardiovasc Diagn* 1987;13(4):233–238.
8. O'Keefe JH, Jr., et al. Revival of the transseptal approach for catheterization of the left atrium and ventricle. *Mayo Clin Proc* 1985;60(11):790–795.
9. Geske JB, et al. Left ventricular outflow tract gradient variability in hypertrophic cardiomyopathy. *Clin Cardiol* 2009;32(7):397–402.

10. De Ponti R, et al. Trans-septal catheterization in the electrophysiology laboratory: Data from a multicenter survey spanning 12 years. *J Am Coll Cardiol* 2006;47(5):1037–1042.

11. Mullins CE. Transseptal left heart catheterization: Experience with a new technique in 520 pediatric and adult patients. *Pediatr Cardiol* 1983;4(3):239–245.

12. Babaliaros VC, et al. Emerging applications for transseptal left heart catheterization old techniques for new procedures. *J Am Coll Cardiol* 2008;51(22):2116–2122.

13. Chaudhari RG, et al. Morphometric analysis of fossa ovalis in rheumatic heart disease. *Indian Heart J* 2005;57(6):662–665.

14. Arya A, et al. Long-term results and the predictors of outcome of catheter ablation of atrial fibrillation using steerable sheath catheter navigation after single procedure in 674 patients. *Europace* 2010;12(2):173–180.

15. Eleid MF, et al. Techniques and outcomes for the treatment of paravalvular leak. *Circ Cardiovasc Interv* 2015;8(8):e001945.

16. Holmes DR, Jr., et al. Pulmonary vein stenosis complicating ablation for atrial fibrillation: Clinical spectrum and interventional considerations. *JACC Cardiovasc Interv* 2009;2(4):267–276.

17. Edriss H, et al. Pulmonary vein stenosis complicating radiofrequency catheter ablation for atrial fibrillation: A literature review. *Respir Med* 2016;117:215–222.

18. Schoenfeld MH, et al. Underestimation of prosthetic mitral valve areas: Role of transseptal catheterization in avoiding unnecessary repeat mitral valve surgery. *J Am Coll Cardiol* 1985;(6):1387–1392.

19. Kober G, Hilgermann R. Catheter entrapment in a Bjork-Shiley prosthesis in aortic position. *Catheter Cardiovasc Diagn* 1987;13(4):262–265.

20. Carabello BA, et al. Changes in arterial pressure during left heart pullback in patients with aortic stenosis: A sign of severe aortic stenosis. *Am J Cardiol* 1979;44(3):424–427.

21. Gordon JB, Folland ED. Analysis of aortic valve gradients by transseptal technique: Implications for noninvasive evaluation. *Catheter Cardiovasc Diagn* 1989;17(3):144–151.

22. Carabello BA. Advances in the hemodynamic assessment of stenotic cardiac valves. *J Am Coll Cardiol* 1987;10(4):912–919.

23. Omran H, et al. Silent and apparent cerebral embolism after retrograde catheterisation of the aortic valve in valvular stenosis: A prospective, randomised study. *Lancet* 2003;361(9365):1241–1246.

24. Hamon M, et al. Cerebral microembolism during cardiac catheterization and risk of acute brain injury: A prospective diffusion-weighted magnetic resonance imaging study. *Stroke* 2006;37(8):2035–2038.

25. Jayne JE, et al. Double-lumen catheter assessment of aortic stenosis: Comparison with separate catheter technique. *Catheter Cardiovasc Diagn* 1993;29(2):157–160.

26. Bae JH, et al. Feasibility of a pressure wire and single arterial puncture for assessing aortic valve area in patients with aortic stenosis. *J Invasive Cardiol* 2006;18(8):359–362.

27. Ross J, Jr. Transseptal left heart catheterization a 50-year odyssey. *J Am Coll Cardiol* 2008;51(22):2107–2115.

28. Pearce AC, et al. Antegrade selective coronary angiography via the transseptal approach in a patient with severe vascular disease. *Catheter Cardiovasc Diagn* 1992;26(4):300–303.

29. Joseph G, et al. Transseptal approach to aortography and carotid artery stenting in pulseless disease. *Catheter Cardiovasc Diagn* 1997;40(4):416–420.

30. Yoon YS, Shim WH. Transseptal approach for stent implantation in right internal carotid artery stenosis. *J Invasive Cardiol* 2000;12(1):70–74.

31. Montenero AS, et al. Catheter ablation of left accessory atrioventricular connections: The transseptal approach. *J Interv Cardiol* 1995;8(6 Suppl):806–812.

32. Bonanno C, et al. Efficacy and safety of catheter ablation versus antiarrhythmic drugs for atrial fibrillation: A meta-analysis of randomized trials. *J Cardiovasc Med (Hagerstown)* 2010;11(6):408–418.

33. Inoue K, et al. Atrial septostomy by a new balloon catheter. *Jpn Circ J* 1981;45:730–738.

34. Nishimura RA, et al. 2014 AHA/ACC guideline for the management of patients with valvular heart disease: A report of the American College of Cardiology/American Heart Association Task Force on Practice Guidelines. *J Am Coll Cardiol* 2014;63(22):e57–e185.

35. Feldman T, et al. Randomized comparison of percutaneous repair and surgery for mitral regurgitation: 5-year results of EVEREST II. *J Am Coll Cardiol* 2015;66(25):2844–2854.

36. Reddy VY, et al. Percutaneous left atrial appendage closure vs. warfarin for atrial fibrillation: A randomized clinical trial. *JAMA* 2014;312(19):1988–1998.

37. Ritzema J, et al. Direct left atrial pressure monitoring in ambulatory heart failure patients: Initial experience with a new permanent implantable device. *Circulation* 2007;116(25):2952–2959.

38. Moon J, et al. Comparison of outcomes after device closure with transseptal puncture and standard technique in patients with patent foramen ovale and ischemic events. *J Interv Cardiol* 2016;29(4):400–405.

39. Eisenhauer AC, et al. Balloon aortic valvuloplasty revisited: The role of the inoue balloon and transseptal antegrade approach. *Catheter Cardiovasc Interv* 2000;50(4):484–491.

40. Sakata Y, et al. Percutaneous balloon aortic valvuloplasty: Antegrade transseptal vs. conventional retrograde transarterial approach. *Catheter Cardiovasc Interv* 2005;64(3):314–321.

41. Cribier A, et al. Early experience with percutaneous transcatheter implantation of heart valve prosthesis for the treatment of end-stage inoperable patients with calcific aortic stenosis. *J Am Coll Cardiol* 2004;43(4):698–703.

42. Hanzel GS, et al. Retrograde percutaneous aortic valve implantation for critical aortic stenosis. *Catheter Cardiovasc Interv* 2005;64(3):322–326.

43. Aragon J, et al. Percutaneous left ventricular assist device: "TandemHeart" for high-risk coronary intervention. *Catheter Cardiovasc Interv* 2005;65(3):346–352.

44. Hussein AA, et al. Radiofrequency ablation of atrial fibrillation under therapeutic international normalized ratio: A safe and efficacious periprocedural anticoagulation strategy. *Heart Rhythm* 2009;6(1):1425–1429.

45. Marcus GM, et al. Repeat transseptal catheterization after ablation for atrial fibrillation. *J Cardiovasc Electrophysiol* 2007;18(1):55–59.

46. Lakkireddy D, et al. Intracardiac echo-guided radiofrequency catheter ablation of atrial fibrillation in patients with atrial septal defect or patent foramen ovale repair: A feasibility, safety, and efficacy study. *J Cardiovasc Electrophysiol* 2008;19(11):1137–1142.

47. Blackshear JL, Odell JA. Appendage obliteration to reduce stroke in cardiac surgical patients with atrial fibrillation. *Ann Thorac Surg* 1996;61(2):755–759.

48. Chen WJ, et al. Safety of percutaneous transvenous balloon mitral commissurotomy in patients with mitral stenosis and thrombus in the left atrial appendage. *Am J Cardiol* 1992;70(1):117–119.

49. Cafri C, et al. Transseptal puncture guided by intracardiac echocardiography during percutaneous transvenous mitral commissurotomy in patients with distorted anatomy of the fossa ovalis. *Catheter Cardiovasc Interv* 2000;50(4):463–467.

50. Hung JS, et al. Usefulness of intracardiac echocardiography in complex transseptal catheterization during percutaneous transvenous mitral commissurotomy. *Mayo Clin Proc* 1996;71(2):134–140.

51. Hurrell DG, et al. Echocardiography in the invasive laboratory: Utility of two-dimensional echocardiography in performing transseptal catheterization. *Mayo Clin Proc* 1998;73(2):126–131.

52. Patel A, et al. Multidetector row computed tomography for identification of left atrial appendage filling defects in patients undergoing pulmonary vein isolation for treatment of atrial fibrillation: Comparison with transesophageal echocardiography. *Heart Rhythm* 2008;5(2):253–260.

53. Knight BP. Transesophageal echocardiography before atrial fibrillation ablation: Looking before cooking. *J Am Coll Cardiol* 2009;54(22):2040–2042.

54. Calkins H, et al. HRS/EHRA/ECAS expert consensus statement on catheter and surgical ablation of atrial fibrillation: Recommendations for personnel, policy, procedures and follow-up. A report of the Heart Rhythm Society (HRS) Task Force on catheter and surgical ablation of atrial fibrillation. *Heart Rhythm* 2007;4(6):816–861.

55. Chierchia GB, et al. First experience with real-time three-dimensional transoesophageal echocardiography-guided transseptal in patients undergoing atrial fibrillation ablation. *Europace* 2008;10(11):1325–1328.

56. Graham LN, et al. Value of CT localization of the fossa ovalis prior to transseptal left heart catheterization for left atrial ablation. *Europace* 2007;9(6):417–423.

57. Elagha AA, et al. Real-time MR imaging-guided laser atrial septal puncture in swine. *J Vasc Interv Radiol* 2008;19(9):1347–1353.

58. Kultursay H, et al. Mitral balloon valvuloplasty with transesophageal echocardiography without using fluoroscopy. *Catheter Cardiovasc Diagn* 1992;27(4):317–321.

59. Poirier P, et al. Mitral balloon valvuloplasty in pregnancy: Limiting radiation and procedure time by using transesophageal echocardiography. *Can J Cardiol* 1997;13(9):843–845.

60. Mishra S, et al. Percutaneous transseptal mitral commissurotomy in pregnant women with critical mitral stenosis. *Indian Heart J* 2001;53(2):192–196.

61. Doorey AJ, Goldenberg EM. Transseptal catheterization in adults: Enhanced efficacy and safety by low-volume operators using a "non-standard" technique. *Catheter Cardiovasc Diagn* 1991;22(4):239–243.

62. Tzeis S, et al. Transseptal catheterization: Considerations and caveats. *Pacing Clin Electrophysiol* 2010;33(2):231–241.

63. Yao Y, et al. The training and learning process of transseptal puncture using a modified technique. *Europace* 2013;15(12):1784–1790.

64. Kong XQ, et al. A new approach for transseptal catheterization in patients undergoing percutaneous balloon mitral valvuloplasty. *Cardiology* 2002;98(1–2):46–49.

65. Park SH, et al. The advantages of On-line transesophageal echocardiography guide during percutaneous balloon mitral valvuloplasty. *J Am Soc Echocardiogr* 2000;13(1):26–34.

66. Koektuerk B, et al. Rotational angiography based three-dimensional left atrial reconstruction: A new approach for transseptal puncture. *Cardiovasc Ther* 2016;34(1):49–56.

67. Bourier F, et al. Transseptal puncture guided by CT-derived 3D-augmented fluoroscopy. *J Cardiovasc Electrophysiol* 2016;27(3):369–372.

68. Bunch TJ, et al. Outcomes after cardiac perforation during radiofrequency ablation of the atrium. *J Cardiovasc Electrophysiol* 2005;16(11):1172–1179.

69. Bidoggia H, et al. Transseptal left heart catheterization: Usefulness of the intracavitary electrocardiogram in the localization of the fossa ovalis. *Catheter Cardiovasc Diagn* 1991;24(3):221–225.

70. Krishnamoorthy KM, Dash PK. Transseptal catheterization without needle puncture. *Scand Cardiovasc J* 2001;35(3):199–200.

71. Feldman T, et al. Percutaneous mitral repair with the MitraClip system: Safety and midterm durability in the initial EVEREST (Endovascular Valve Edge-to-Edge REpair Study) cohort. *J Am Coll Cardiol* 2009;54(8):686–694.

72. Holmes DR, et al. Percutaneous closure of the left atrial appendage versus warfarin therapy for prevention of stroke in patients with atrial fibrillation: A randomised non-inferiority trial. *Lancet* 2009;374(9689):534–542.

73. Cribier A, et al. Percutaneous mechanical mitral commissurotomy with a newly designed metallic valvulotome: Immediate results of the initial experience in 153 patients. *Circulation* 1999;99(6):793–799.

74. Cheng A, Calkins H. A conservative approach to performing transseptal punctures without the use of intracardiac echocardiography: Stepwise approach with real-time video clips. *J Cardiovasc Electrophysiol* 2007;18(6):686–689.

75. Haruta S, et al. The guidewire technique for transseptal puncture. *J Invasive Cardiol* 2005;17(2):68–70.

76. Hildick-Smith D, et al. Transseptal puncture: Use of an angioplasty guidewire for enhanced safety. *Catheter Cardiovasc Interv* 2007;69(4):519–521.

77. Sakata Y, Feldman T. Transcatheter creation of atrial septal perforation using a radiofrequency transseptal system: Novel approach as an alternative to transseptal needle puncture. *Catheter Cardiovasc Interv* 2005;64(3):327–332.

78. Greenstein E, et al. Incidence of tissue coring during transseptal catheterization when using electrocautery and a standard transseptal needle. *Circ Arrhythm Electrophysiol* 2012;5(2):341–344.

79. Winkle RA, et al. The use of a radiofrequency needle improves the safety and efficacy of transseptal puncture for atrial fibrillation ablation. *Heart Rhythm* 2011;8(9):1411–1415.

80. Sharma G, et al. Accuracy and procedural characteristics of standard needle compared with radiofrequency needle transseptal puncture for structural heart interventions. *Catheter Cardiovasc Interv* 2016. doi:10.1002/ccd.26608.

81. Bidart C, et al. Radiofrequency current delivery via transseptal needle to facilitate septal puncture. *Heart Rhythm* 2007;4(12):1573–1576.

82. de Asmundis C, et al. Novel trans-septal approach using a safe sept J-shaped guidewire in difficult left atrial access during atrial fibrillation ablation. *Europace* 2009;11(5):657–659.

83. Arkles J, et al. Feasibility of transseptal access in patients with previously scarred or repaired interatrial septum. *J Cardiovasc Electrophysiol* 2015. doi:10.1111/jce.12730.

84. Bruce CJ, et al. Early heparinization decreases the incidence of left atrial thrombi detected by intracardiac echocardiography during radiofrequency ablation for atrial fibrillation. *J Interv Card Electrophysiol* 2008;22(3):211–219.

85. Wazni OM, et al. Atrial fibrillation ablation in patients with therapeutic international normalized ratio: Comparison of strategies of anticoagulation management in the periprocedural period. *Circulation* 2007;116(22):2531–2534.

86. Cortes M, et al. Usefulness of transesophageal echocardiography in percutaneous transcatheter repairs of paravalvular mitral regurgitation. *Am J Cardiol* 2008;101(3):382–386.

87. Cappato R, et al. Prevalence and causes of fatal outcome in catheter ablation of atrial fibrillation. *J Am Coll Cardiol* 2009;53(19):1798–1803.

88. Dagres N, et al. Complications of atrial fibrillation ablation in a high-volume center in 1,000 procedures: Still cause for concern? *J Cardiovasc Electrophysiol* 2009;20(9):1014–1019.

89. Okumura Y. Which is the optimal therapy to prevent thromboembolism after atrial fibrillation ablation procedures in low stroke risk patients, anticoagulation or antiplatelet therapy? *J Cardiovasc Electrophysiol* 2009;20(9):994–996.

90. Cha YM, et al. Prevention of thromboembolic stroke in patients undergoing catheter-based ablation for atrial fibrillation: Has it been optimized? *J Cardiovasc Electrophysiol* 2009;20(12):1364–1365.

91. Ren JF, et al. Increased intensity of anticoagulation may reduce risk of thrombus during atrial fibrillation ablation procedures in patients with spontaneous echo contrast. *J Cardiovasc Electrophysiol* 2005;16(5):474–477.

92. Calkins H, et al. 2012 HRS/EHRA/ECAS expert consensus statement on catheter and surgical ablation of atrial fibrillation: Recommendations for patient selection, procedural techniques, patient management and follow-up, definitions, endpoints, and research trial design: A report of the Heart Rhythm Society (HRS) Task Force on Catheter and Surgical Ablation of Atrial Fibrillation. Developed in partnership with the European Heart Rhythm Association (EHRA), a registered branch of the European Society of Cardiology (ESC) and the European Cardiac Arrhythmia Society (ECAS); and in collaboration with the American College of Cardiology (ACC), American Heart Association (AHA), the Asia Pacific Heart Rhythm Society (APHRS), and the Society of Thoracic Surgeons (STS). Endorsed by the governing bodies of the American College of Cardiology Foundation, the American Heart Association, the European Cardiac Arrhythmia Society, the European Heart Rhythm Association, the Society of Thoracic Surgeons, the Asia Pacific Heart Rhythm Society, and the Heart Rhythm Society. *Heart Rhythm* 2012;9(4):632–696.

93. Kilicaslan F, et al. Transcranial Doppler detection of microembolic signals during pulmonary vein antrum isolation: Implications for titration of radiofrequency energy. *J Cardiovasc Electrophysiol* 2006;17(5):495–501.

94. Franzen OW, et al. Mechanisms underlying air aspiration in patients undergoing left atrial catheterization. *Catheter Cardiovasc Interv* 2008;71(4):553–558.

95. Rihal CS, et al. Percutaneous balloon mitral valvuloplasty: The learning curve. *Am Heart J* 1991;122(6):1750–1756.

96. Roelke M, et al. The technique and safety of transseptal left heart catheterization: The Massachusetts General Hospital experience with 1,279 procedures. *Catheter Cardiovasc Diagn* 1994;32(4):332–339.

97. Liu TJ, et al. Immediate and late outcomes of patients undergoing transseptal left-sided heart catheterization for symptomatic valvular and arrhythmic diseases. *Am Heart J* 2006;151(1):235–241.

98. Holmes DR, Jr., et al. Iatrogenic pericardial effusion and tamponade in the percutaneous intracardiac intervention era. *JACC Cardiovasc Interv* 2009;2(8):705–717.

99. Glazier JJ, Turi ZG. Percutaneous balloon mitral valvuloplasty. *Prog Cardiovasc Dis* 1997;40(1):5–26.

100. Hsu LF, et al. Incidence and prevention of cardiac tamponade complicating ablation for atrial fibrillation. *Pacing Clin Electrophysiol* 2005;28(Suppl 1):S106–S109.

101. Fagundes RL, et al. Safety of single transseptal puncture for ablation of atrial fibrillation: Retrospective study from a large cohort of patients. *J Cardiovasc Electrophysiol* 2007;18(12):1277–1281.

102. Deshpande J, et al. Balloon mitral valvotomy: An autopsy study. *Int J Cardiol* 1995;52(1):67–76.

103. Mofrad P, et al. Case report: Cerebral air embolization in the electrophysiology laboratory during transseptal catheterization: Curative treatment of acute left hemiparesis with prompt hyperbaric oxygen therapy. *J Interv Card Electrophysiol* 2006;16(2):105–109.

104. Cauchemez B, et al. High-flow perfusion of sheaths for prevention of thromboembolic complications during complex catheter ablation in the left atrium. *J Cardiovasc Electrophysiol* 2004;15(3):276–283.

105. Maleki K, et al. Intracardiac ultrasound detection of thrombus on transseptal sheath: Incidence, treatment, and prevention. *J Cardiovasc Electrophysiol* 2005;16(6):561–565.

106. Kok LC, et al. Cerebrovascular complication associated with pulmonary vein ablation. *J Cardiovasc Electrophysiol* 2002;13(8):764–767.

107. Chilukuri K, et al. Association of transseptal punctures with isolated migraine aura in patients undergoing catheter ablation of cardiac arrhythmias. *J Cardiovasc Electrophysiol* 2009;20(11):1227–1230.

108. Kessler DJ, et al. Intracardiac shunts resulting from transseptal catheterization for ablation of accessory pathways in otherwise normal hearts. *Am J Cardiol* 1998;82(3):391–392.

109. Alkhouli M, et al. Iatrogenic atrial septal defect following transseptal cardiac interventions. *Int J Cardiol* 2016;209:142–148.

110. McGinty PM, et al. Transseptal left heart catheterization and the incidence of persistent iatrogenic atrial septal defects. *J Interv Cardiol* 2011;24(3):254–263.

111. Thomas MR, et al. Residual atrial septal defects following balloon mitral valvuloplasty using different techniques. A transthoracic and transoesophageal echocardiography study demonstrating an advantage of the Inoue balloon. *Eur Heart J* 1992;13(4):496–502.

112. Yoshida K, et al. Assessment of left-to-right atrial shunting after percutaneous mitral valvuloplasty by transesophageal color Doppler flow-mapping. *Circulation* 1989;80(6):1521–1526.

113. Rillig A, et al. Persistent iatrogenic atrial septal defect after pulmonary vein isolation : Incidence and clinical implications. *J Interv Card Electrophysiol* 2008;22(3):177–181.

114. Hammerstingl C, et al. Persistence of iatrogenic atrial septal defect after pulmonary vein isolation—An underestimated risk? *Am Heart J* 2006; 152(2):362.e1–e5.

115. Loyalka P, et al. Percutaneous left ventricular assist device complicated by a patent foramen ovale: Importance of identification and management. *Catheter Cardiovasc Interv* 2007;70(3):383–386.

116. Sharma S, et al. Percutaneous double-valve balloon valvotomy for multivalve stenosis: Immediate results and intermediate-term follow-up. *Am Heart J* 1997;133(1):64–70.

117. Turi ZG. Puncturing the septum: Resurgent technique with inherent risk. *J Invasive Cardiol* 2004;16(1):3–4.

118. Hildick-Smith DJ, et al. Inferior ST-segment elevation following transseptal puncture for balloon mitral valvuloplasty is atropine-responsive. *J Invasive Cardiol* 2004;16(1):1–2.

119. Hsu LF, et al. Transcardiac pericardiocentesis: An emergency life-saving technique for cardiac tamponade. *J Cardiovasc Electrophysiol* 2003;14(9):1001–1003.

120. Serry R, et al. Treatment of ischemic stroke complicating cardiac catheterization with systemic thrombolytic therapy. *Catheter Cardiovasc Interv* 2005;66(3)364–368.

121. Al Mubarak N, et al. Immediate catheter-based neurovascular rescue for acute stroke complicating coronary procedures. *Am J Cardiol* 2002;90(2):173–176.

122. Chan AW, Henderson MA. Immediate catheter-directed reperfusion for acute stroke occurring during diagnostic cardiac catheterization. *Catheter Cardiovasc Interv* 2006;67(2):314–318.

123. Sankaranarayanan R, et al. Stroke complicating cardiac catheterization—A preventable and treatable complication. *J Invasive Cardiol* 2007;19(1):40–45.

124. Svilaas T, et al. Thrombus aspiration during primary percutaneous coronary intervention. *N Engl J Med* 2008;358(6):557–567.

125. Bloomfield DA. Transseptal catheterization technique: A simple safety procedure. *Catheter Cardiovasc Diagn* 1991;22(2):153–155.

126. Linker NJ, Fitzpatrick AP. The transseptal approach for ablation of cardiac arrhythmias: Experience of 104 procedures. *Heart* 1998;79(4):379–382.

127. Tracy CM, et al. American College of Cardiology/American Heart Association 2006 update of the clinical competence statement on invasive electrophysiology studies,catheter ablation, and cardioversion: A report of the American College of Cardiology/American Heart Association/American College of Physicians Task Force on Clinical Competence and Training developed in collaboration with the Heart Rhythm Society. *J Am Coll Cardiol* 2006;48(7):1503–1517.

128. De Ponti R, et al. Superiority of simulator-based training compared with conventional training methodologies in the performance of transseptal catheterization. *J Am Coll Cardiol* 2011;58(4):359–363.

24

Mesenteric and renal angiography

RONY LAHOUD AND LESLIE CHO

INTRODUCTION

Catheter-based contrast angiography remains the "gold standard" in the diagnosis of mesenteric and renal artery disease and usually follows a high index of clinical suspicion and corroborative noninvasive testing. Duplex ultrasonography, computed tomography angiography (CTA), and magnetic resonance angiography (MRA) have become extremely helpful in the initial assessment of patients with suspected disease, but invasive angiography is often required for definitive diagnosis. Catheter-based angiography has the added benefit of providing simultaneous interventional therapy if required. This chapter reviews the vascular anatomy and equipment essential to conducting a proper mesenteric and renal angiographic examination and highlights the proper indications for invasive testing of these vessel territories. Percutaneous mesenteric and renal interventions are addressed in separate chapters.

ANATOMIC CONSIDERATIONS

Mesenteric circulation

The mesenteric arteries arise from the anterior aspect of the lower thoracic and abdominal aorta. These vessels—the celiac trunk, superior mesenteric artery (SMA), and inferior mesenteric artery (IMA)—are responsible for the blood supply to all organs located within the abdominal cavity. The celiac trunk is the first major branch of the abdominal aorta and is an essential source of blood supply to the liver, stomach, and parts of the esophagus, spleen, duodenum, and pancreas. Its origin from the anterior aorta is typically midline at the level of the T12 vertebral body, and it courses inferiorly for 1–2 cm before branching into the left gastric, common hepatic, and splenic arteries (Figure 24.1). The common hepatic artery divides into the proper hepatic artery and, typically, also the gastroduodenal artery. The proper hepatic gives off the right gastric artery before branching into the right and left hepatic arteries. The gastroduodenal artery then goes on to divide into the right gastroepiploic artery and the anterior and posterior superior pancreaticoduodenal arteries. The right gastroepiploic artery and the left gastroepiploic artery (from the splenic artery) join together along the greater curvature of the stomach. The right gastric artery and the left gastric artery join together to run along the lesser curvature of the stomach. Because of the redundant blood supply to the stomach, gastric ischemia is uncommon.

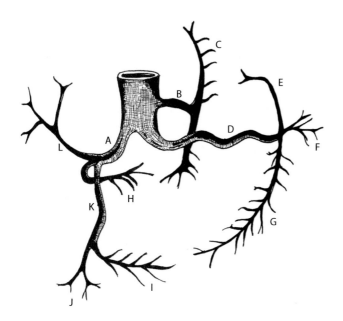

Figure 24.1 Normal anatomy of the celiac artery. **(A)** Common hepatic artery, **(B)** left gastric artery, **(C)** esophageal branches, **(D)** splenic artery, **(E)** short gastric branches, **(F)** splenic branches, **(G)** left gastroepiploic artery, **(H)** right gastric artery, **(I)** right gastroepiploic artery, **(J)** superior pancreaticoduodenal artery, **(K)** gastroduodenal artery, **(L)** hepatic artery. (From Rajaopalan, S., et al., (Eds.), *Manual of Vascular Diseases*, Lippincott Williams & Wilkins, Philadelphia, PA, 2005, pp. 202–204. With permission.)

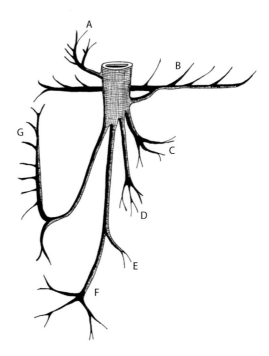

Figure 24.2 Normal anatomy of the superior mesenteric artery. **(A)** Inferior pancreaticoduodenal (anterior and posterior branches), **(B)** middle colic artery, **(C)** jejunal artery, **(D)** ileal artery, **(E)** ileal artery, **(F)** ileocolic artery, **(G)** right colic. (From Rajaopalan, S., et al., (Eds.), *Manual of Vascular Diseases*, Lippincott Williams & Wilkins, Philadelphia, PA, 2005, pp. 202–204. With permission.)

The SMA usually originates 1 cm lower than the celiac trunk and anterior to the L1 vertebral body.[1] The SMA travels inferiorly and slightly rightward to supply the duodenum and pancreas. In its course, the SMA passes beneath the pancreas and divides into the inferior pancreaticoduodenal, middle colic, right colic, ileocolic, and intestinal branches (Figure 24.2). In general, the middle colic artery provides blood supply to the proximal and midtransverse colon. In some individuals, the middle colic may provide the main source of blood to the splenic flexure. The right colic artery provides the blood supply to the middle and distal ascending colon, while the ileocolic artery supplies the distal ileum, cecum, and proximal ascending colon. The middle, right, and ileocecal branches join together with the left colic artery (from the inferior mesenteric) forming the marginal artery or artery of Drummond that courses along the inside border of the colon. Multiple anatomic variations of the colic arteries exist.

The IMA is the smallest of the mesenteric vessels. It originates below the level of the renal arteries and approximately 6–7 cm below the SMA. The IMA courses inferiorly and leftward, giving off the left colic artery and several sigmoid branches before terminating in the superior rectal artery (Figure 24.3). The IMA is responsible for providing the blood supply to the distal transverse colon, descending colon, and the rectum. The left and middle colic branches may join together, effectively anastomosing the SMA and IMA circulations in what is known as the arc of Riolan.

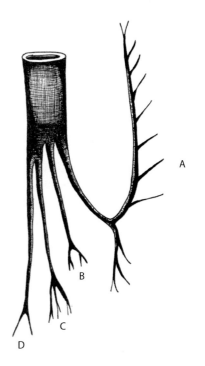

Figure 24.3 Normal anatomy of the inferior mesenteric artery. **(A)** Left colic artery (superior and inferior branches), **(B)** lower left colic artery, **(C)** sigmoid artery, **(D)** superior rectal artery. (From Rajaopalan, S., et al., (Eds.), *Manual of Vascular Diseases*, Lippincott Williams & Wilkins, Philadelphia, PA, 2005,pp. 202–204. With permission.)

Renal arteries

The renal arteries originate from the lateral abdominal aorta immediately below the SMA at the level of the lower border of the L1 vertebral body. There are slight anatomic differences between the two renal arteries. In one study of 100 patients who underwent spiral CTA, the right and left renal arteries originated at the same level in 50% of patients.[2] In the other 50% of cases, the right renal artery arose higher than the left. The right renal artery also typically courses downward to supply the more inferiorly located right kidney; the left renal artery typically has a horizontal course. The right renal artery has an anterolateral origin from the aorta, while the left renal artery has a posterolateral origin. Both renal arteries typically give off small inferior suprarenal branches before dividing into segmental branches. These segmental branches subsequently divide into arcuate and multiple interlobular branches terminating within the renal cortex and medulla. Accessory renal arteries are the most common vascular variant.[3] These accessory vessels may be of similar or smaller caliber and typically originate lower than the main artery, supplying the inferior pole of the kidney (Figure 24.4). Another variant occurs when the main artery divides early in its course into segmental branches. Finally, it should be noted that the renal arteries can be surgically bypassed or reimplanted in the pelvis ("autotransplant").

FUNDAMENTALS

Catheter selection

For abdominal aortography, a pigtail or an Omni Flush catheter (AngioDynamics Inc., Queensbury, NY) placed at the T12-L1 intervertebral space is commonly used. For selective mesenteric angiography obtained from a femoral access site, a reverse angulation catheter like a Sos catheter is preferred, or alternatively a Judkins Right (JR) 4, internal mammary artery (IMA), or left coronary bypass (LCB) catheter could be used. For selective mesenteric angiography obtained from a brachial or radial approach, a multipurpose catheter is preferred. For renal angiography, femoral access is most commonly used and a JR 4 catheter is our workhorse catheter. An IMA catheter or renal double curve catheter could be used, or in the case of excessive tortuosity, a Cobra C2, Sos, or Simmons catheter could be used. In some instances, brachial or radial artery cannulation can be useful for very downward take off of renal arteries using Multipurpose A or B catheters.

Contrast selection

Ionic tri-iodinated contrast agents are typically used for obtaining these studies. For most studies, the contrast should be diluted as 70% dye and 30% heparinized saline.

Angiography projections

For abdominal aortography, the first view is typically a standard posteroanterior (PA) projection using digital substraction. The second view typically consists of a lateral projection if the mesenteric arteries are the focus of the study (given their anterior origin), or a 15° left anterior oblique (LAO) view if the renal arteries are the focus of the study. Contrast is typically injected with a power injector at a rate of 10 cc/s for 1–2 s with the patient holding his/her breath and not moving. For selective mesenteric angiography, digital substraction angiography is also recommended. A 15°–30° LAO angulation is ideal for visualization of the celiac trunk and SMA, while a 15°–30° right anterior oblique (RAO) is ideal for visualization of the IMA. For selective renal angiography, right and left renal angiography is usually obtained with a 10°–20° LAO angulation. Slight cranial or caudal angulation may be required for optimal visualization.

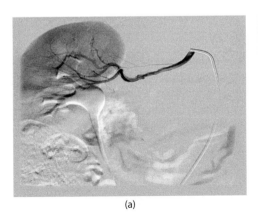
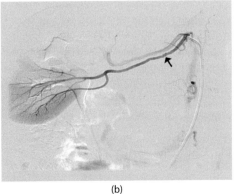

(a) (b)

Figure 24.4 Accessory renal artery. Accessory renal arteries typically originate lower than the main artery and supply the inferior pole of the kidney. In this angiogram, selective contrast injection of the main renal artery does not perfuse the inferior renal pole (a) as this segment is instead perfused by an accessory artery (b). Fibromuscular dysplasia of the accessory artery is indicated by the arrow.

Frame rate

A frame rate of 2–4 frames/sec is typically recommended for renal and mesenteric angiography obtained under digital substraction. A higher frame rate for cineangiography without digital subtraction is typically required.

Visualization of nephrogram

When obtaining a nephrogram, it is important to adjust the field of view to incorporate the entire kidney, and prolong the limit of cineangiogram runtime if necessary to ensure adequate capture of the influx of contrast into the renal cortical zone. It supplements the renal angiogram with information regarding the size of the kidney and its regional function.

INDICATIONS

Mesenteric angiography

The principal indication for mesenteric angiography is evaluation of intestinal ischemia when the CT scan is not conclusive and the level of clinical suspicion is high.[4] Classically, patients with acute intestinal ischemia present with sudden or recent onset of pain and little or no findings on abdominal physical exam. These patients often have a history of coronary artery disease, peripheral arterial disease, atrial fibrillation, or other cardiovascular risk factors (Table 24.1). Acute intestinal ischemia should also be suspected in patients with severe abdominal pain following endovascular procedures that involve catheter traversal in the abdominal aorta. The decision to perform angiography on patients with suspected acute intestinal ischemia needs to be individualized. For instance, patients presenting with acute abdominal pain due to suspected arterial occlusion with intestinal infarction should be referred for immediate laparotomy instead of angiography. Alternatively, patients with nonocclusive disease may benefit from a strategy that incorporates initial angiography.

As in those with acute ischemia, patients with chronic mesenteric ischemia often have coexisting atherosclerotic disease (Table 24.2). In cases of suspected chronic intestinal ischemia, there is often time for initial assessment with noninvasive testing, including duplex ultrasound, CTA, or MRA. Angiographic evaluation should be performed in patients with abnormal or indeterminate noninvasive testing. Alternatively, diagnostic mesenteric angiography may be performed as an initial diagnostic tool if these noninvasive testing modalities are not available.

Renal angiography

Renal angiography is indicated in patients in whom renal artery stenosis (RAS) is clinically suspected and who have also corroborative noninvasive testing, suggesting significant disease. Renal arterial disease is prevalent in patients with other forms of atherosclerotic disease, such as multivessel coronary artery disease and peripheral arterial disease. The clinical clues suggesting the diagnosis of RAS are detailed in Table 24.3. Of these, the strongest clinical indicators are early onset of hypertension prior to age of 30 years (in case of fibromuscular dysplasia [FMD]); multidrug-resistant hypertension; development of renal failure or declining renal function after institution of angiotensin-converting enzyme inhibitor (ACE-I) or angiotensin receptor blocker (ARB); atrophic kidney or 1.5 cm size discrepancy between kidneys; flash pulmonary edema; and unexplained renal failure. When renal arterial disease is suspected, noninvasive imaging with duplex ultrasound, MRA with gadolinium enhancement, or CTA is recommended to first establish the diagnosis of RAS.

Table 24.1 Risk factors for the development of acute mesenteric ischemia

- Advanced age
- Low cardiac output
- Cardiac arrhythmia (e.g., atrial fibrillation)
- Valvular heart disease
- Recent myocardial infarction
- Malignancy
- Hypercoagulable states
- Critical illness or prolonged intensive care unit stay
- Trauma

Table 24.2 Risk factors for the development of chronic mesenteric ischemia

- Peripheral arterial disease
- Coronary artery disease
- Advanced age
- Diabetes mellitus
- Smoking
- Obesity
- Hyperlipidemia
- Sedentary lifestyle

Table 24.3 Clinical clues to the diagnosis of renal artery stenosis

- Early onset of hypertension before the age of 30 years
- Onset of severe hypertension after the age of 55 years
- Multidrug resistant hypertension
- Development of new renal failure or worsening renal function following initiation of ACE (angiotensin-converting enzyme) inhibitor or ARB (angiotensin receptor blocker) therapy
- Size difference between kidneys of more than 1.5 cm or unexplained atrophic kidney
- Systolic–diastolic epigastric bruit
- Unexplained renal failure
- Multivessel coronary artery disease
- Unexplained or recurrent pulmonary edema
- Angina refractory to medical management

EQUIPMENT

Abdominal aortography

Prior to selective engagement, initial abdominal aortic angiography should be performed with a pigtail or Omni Flush catheter (AngioDynamics Inc., Queensbury, NY) (Table 24.4). The Omni Flush catheter is designed to minimize the amount of upward-refluxed contrast and thus may result in more contrast concentrated at the level of the renal and mesenteric vessels. Usually, the aortogram is adequate to demonstrate patency but often is insufficient to adequately assess degree of stenosis of the mesenteric and renal vessels. The aortogram does, however, provide important adjunctive information regarding the presence of aortic calcification, aneurysmal dilatation, and anatomical anomalies (e.g., number of accessory renal arteries), as well as the location of the renal and mesenteric ostia (Figure 24.5). The catheter should be placed with its sideholes at the T12-L1 intervertebral space (i.e., above the origin of the renal arteries). For optimal imaging, the field of view should be maximized, the

table elevated to its highest setting, and the table positioned such that the catheter tip is at top of the screen. If a recent prior abdominal aortogram is available for review, repeat study is not necessary and the operator should proceed to selective assessment of the arteries of interest.

The abdominal aortogram is first performed in a standard PA projection using digital subtraction. Our practice is to use a 5-Fr system with a total volume of 10–20 mL of contrast at a rate of 10 mL/sec. Patients should be instructed not to breathe or move prior to angiography. Lateral projection aortography may then be performed to visualize the mesenteric arteries since these vessels arise anteriorly (Figure 24.6). This should also be done with digital subtraction, and similar settings may be used. If the renal arteries are the sole focus of the study, a 15° LAO projection is recommended and can be performed using a smaller amount of contrast (10 mL/sec for 10 mL total). For these studies, the contrast may be diluted as 70% dye and 30% heparinized saline. This dilution technique reduces the total contrast exposure and still results in acceptable image quality.

Selective mesenteric angiography

A 5-Fr system is usually adequate for diagnostic mesenteric angiography (Table 24.5). Femoral access is commonly used; but in general, a brachial or radial artery approach is easier for the selective engagement of the mesenteric vessels.[5] From a femoral access, our preference is to use a reverse angulation catheter such as a Sos (AngioDynamics) catheter that allows easy access to the inferiorly directed ostia of the celiac trunk, SMA, and IMA (Figures 24.7 through 24.10). A JR 4 diagnostic, IMA or LCB catheter can also be used to engage these vessels. Reverse angulation catheters should be positioned by moving them caudally with a generous amount of wire extending from the tip that allows for

Table 24.4 Equipment for abdominal aortic angiography

- **Sheath**
  - 4- or 5-Fr
- **Catheters**
  - Pigtail
  - Straight Flush (AngioDynamics, Queensbury, NY)
  - Omniflush (AngioDynamics, Queensbury, NY)
- **Wires (0.035-in)**
  - Standard J-wire (Cook Medical, Bloomington, IN)
  - Glidewire (Terumo, Tokyo)
  - Wholey (Tyco Healthcare, Mallinckrodt, St. Louis, MO)
  - Rosen (Cook Medical, Bloomington, IN)

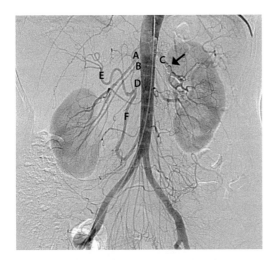

Figure 24.5 Posteroanterior (PA) abdominal aortogram. **(A)** Right renal artery, **(B)** accessory right renal artery, **(C)** left renal artery, **(D)** celiac trunk, **(E)** proper hepatic artery, **(F)** gastroduodenal artery. The left renal artery has changes consistent with fibromuscular dysplasia (arrow).

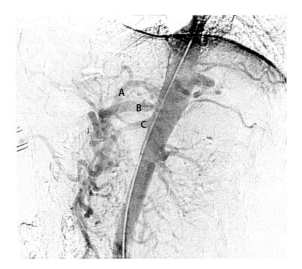

Figure 24.6 Lateral abdominal aortogram demonstrating the anterior origins of the celiac artery **(A)** and superior mesenteric artery **(B)**. Nonobstructive narrowing of the proximal celiac artery **(C)** is present.

Table 24.5 Equipment for selective mesenteric angiography

- **Sheath**
  - 5- or 6-Fr
- **Catheters**
  - JR 4
  - IMA
  - Sos
  - Simmons 1, 2, 3
  - Cobra C2
  - Hockey Stick
  - Multipurpose (arm approach)
- **Wires (0.035-in)**
  - Standard J-wire
  - Glidewire
  - Wholey
  - Rosen

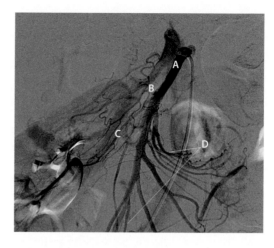

Figure 24.8 Selective angiography of the superior mesenteric artery (SMA). The SMA **(A)** travels inferiorly and slightly rightward to supply the duodenum and pancreas. In its course, the SMA gives off the inferior pancreaticoduodenal arteries **(B)**, the middle colic artery **(C)**, and several intestinal arteries **(D)**.

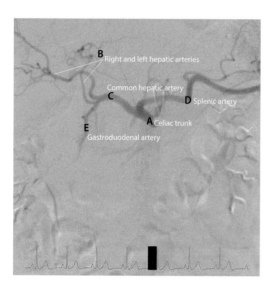

Figure 24.7 Selective angiography of the celiac trunk. As the first major branch of the abdominal aorta, the celiac trunk **(A)** originates from the anterior aorta at the level of the T12 vertebral body and branches into the left gastric **(B)**, common hepatic **(C)**, and splenic **(D)** arteries. The common hepatic artery further divides into the proper hepatic and gastroduodenal **(E)** arteries. This angiogram demonstrates an anomalous left hepatic artery arising from the gastroduodenal artery.

a relatively atraumatic bend of wire over which the catheter can pass. Once the catheter is positioned superiorly to the vessel ostia, its curve is formed by the slow withdrawal of the wire. If kept in an anterior orientation and walked down the aorta, such reverse angle catheters should readily find the mesenteric ostia, but care should be taken as these catheters also will readily catch onto sidewall atheroma.

Alternatively, many operators prefer a brachial artery approach in selective mesenteric studies. From the brachial artery approach, the mesenteric arteries can usually be easily engaged using a multipurpose diagnostic catheter. In most cases, catheters that are 125 cm in length are

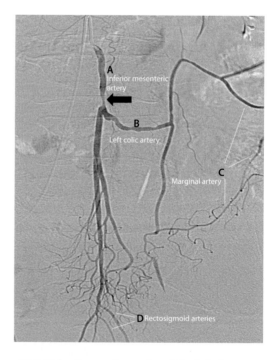

Figure 24.9 Selective angiography of the inferior mesenteric artery (IMA). The IMA **(A)** courses inferiorly and leftward giving off the left colic artery **(B)**, which, in part, supplies the marginal artery **(C)**. In its terminal segment, the IMA supplies the sigmoid colon and rectum **(D)**. The arrow indicates an IMA stenosis prior to the origin of the left colic branch.

necessary with the (right) radial approach. Arm access is particularly helpful in patients with severe aortoiliac tortuosity and highly angulated vessel origins. Arm access should also be used in patients with known abdominal aortic aneurysms and in patients with severe aortoiliac disease.

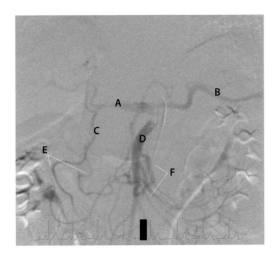

Figure 24.10 Selective angiography of the superior mesenteric artery. The SMA and celiac vessels normally communicate via the anterior and posterior pancreaticoduodenal arteries such that selective contrast injection of the SMA fills both vessels. **(A)** Common aortic artery, **(B)** splenic artery, **(C)** gastroduodenal artery, **(D)** superior mesenteric artery, **(E)** posterior and anterior pancreaticoduodenal arteries, **(F)** intestinal arteries.

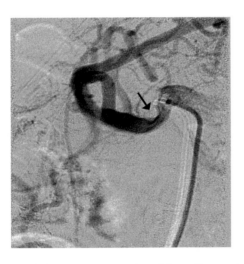

Figure 24.11 Selective angiography of the celiac trunk with respiratory maneuver. In cases of suspected celiac artery compression, comparative selective views should be obtained at end-inspiration and end-expiration. Expiration causes the aorta and its major branches to move cephalad, thus exacerbating vessel compression of the celiac artery by a median arcuate ligament. This angiogram demonstrates moderate stenosis of the celiac trunk with expiration (*arrow*).

Selective angiography of the celiac trunk is performed with a 15°–30° LAO angulation to demonstrate the celiac axis origin and trifurcation into the left gastric, common hepatic, and splenic arteries. In cases of suspected celiac artery compression, comparative, selective views should be obtained at end-inspiration and end-expiration as expiration may exacerbate vessel compression (Figure 24.11). Given its course to the rightward pelvis, angiography of the SMA should be performed in a 15°–30° LAO. In comparison,

the IMA has a leftward course; thus, selective angiography of this vessel should be performed in a 15°–30° RAO projection. As with abdominal aortography, digital subtraction angiography is recommended. The field of view should be adequate to visualize the mesenteric vessel of interest, as well as all potential collateral networks in cases of occlusion.

Selective renal angiography

When performing renal angiography, we predominately use femoral access with a 5-Fr system (Table 24.6). Arm access is reserved for those patients with severe aortoiliac disease or known abdominal aortic aneurysm. The JR 4 catheter is our workhorse catheter for selectively engaging the renal arteries. Alternatively, an internal mammary or renal double-curve catheter can also be used. In cases of aortoiliac tortuosity, a Cobra C2 (Terumo, Somerset, NJ), Sos, or Simmons catheter may be necessary to reach the ostia (Figure 24.12). Regardless of the equipment chosen, the catheter must never be advanced to the renal ostia without the use of a wire. Such manipulation can result in

Table 24.6 Equipment for selective renal angiography

- **Sheath**
  - 5- or 6-Fr
- **Catheters**
  - JR 4
  - IMA
  - Renal Double Curve
  - Cobra C2
  - Multipurpose (arm approach)
- **Wires (0.035-in)**
  - Standard J-wire
  - Glidewire
  - Wholey
  - Rosen

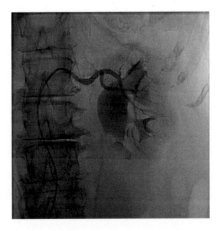

Figure 24.12 Selective angiography of the left renal artery using a Cobra (C2) catheter. In cases of aortoiliac tortuosity, a C2 or Simmons catheter is sometimes necessary to reach the renal ostia. This angiogram demonstrates mild to moderate narrowing of the left renal artery.

advancement of atheromatous debris into the renal ostium ("snowplow effect"). Using a 0.035-in wire, the catheter should be positioned anteriorly at the L1 level. Gentle retraction with clockwise (left renal artery) or counterclockwise (right renal artery) manipulation of the catheter allows for selective engagement.

Aortic calcifications and prior placed renal artery stents serve as important landmarks indicating the renal ostia (Figure 24.13). Importantly, the renal arteries do not originate directly from the lateral aorta. The right renal artery originates about 20°–30° anteriorly, and the left originates only slightly posteriorly. Therefore, PA projection angiography may not adequately illustrate the renal ostium. Accordingly, one study demonstrated optimal visualization of the right renal ostia in only 26% of cases and of the left in 38% of cases.[1] Our practice is to perform selective right and left renal angiography with a 10°–20° LAO angulation. Occasionally, additional slight (10°) cranial or caudal angulation may be necessary for optimal visualization. Since the right renal artery travels down below the inferior vena cava, additional RAO projections may be necessary to adequately visualize the entire course of this vessel. Care should be taken to visualize any accessory renal arteries given their common occurrence.

Prior to injection, the catheter must be aspirated well and the pressure waveform should reflect a crisp arterial tracing. The field of view should be large enough to incorporate the kidney, and the cineangiogram run should also be long enough to visualize the influx of contrast into the renal cortex. This nephrogram yields important insight into renal size and regional function. Such adjunctive information becomes particularly important in individuals with suboptimal or equivocal noninvasive studies.

With selective renal angiography, a few additional technical points should be mentioned. The operator should be careful to avoid unnecessary trauma to the renal ostia with engagement as this may lead to showering of aorto-ostial

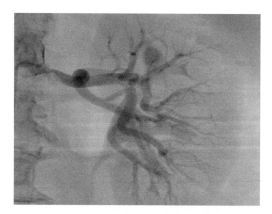

Figure 24.13 Selective left renal angiogram. Renal artery stenosis is an aorto-ostial disease process, and calcification can serve as an important landmark indicating the location of the renal ostia. This indicates the presence of circumferential calcium in the proximal vessel.

atherosclerotic debris. Care should also be taken not to deep-seat the catheter past the renal ostium as this may lead to underestimation of the lesion severity due to insufficient opacification of the ostium. Damping of the pressure waveform on selective engagement may indicate significant ostial stenosis.

CLINICAL ASPECTS

Acute mesenteric ischemia

Although relatively infrequent, acute mesenteric ischemia is a life-threatening condition caused by a sudden decrease in blood flow to the intestines. Prolonged intestinal hypoperfusion can culminate in bowel necrosis and death, and mesenteric ischemia is associated with mortality ranging from 60% to 100%.[6–9] While the early use of angiography has resulted in a decline in mortality rates over the past 30 years, patient outcome is highly dependent on prompt recognition and early treatment of this disease process.[10–12]

Acute mesenteric ischemia is characterized with duration of hours to days and may be caused by embolic (50%), thrombotic (20%), nonocclusive mesenteric ischemia (20%), or acute mesenteric venous thrombosis etiologies (10%).[13–15] Classically, patients present with sudden severe abdominal pain out of proportion to the findings on clinical exam and may have fever and bloody stool. With occlusive acute mesenteric ischemia, patients often have coexisting atherosclerotic disease or risk factors that predispose them to embolism or thrombus formation. Most often, occlusive acute mesenteric ischemia involves the proximal SMA either by thrombosis of preexisting plaque or by embolism to this site.[16] In the case of arterial embolism, the source of embolus is usually cardiac (left atrial appendix thrombus, most commonly in atrial fibrillation, left ventricular mural thrombus, or valvular sources less commonly),[15] and the branch most commonly affected is the SMA because of its high basal flow rate and "favorable" anatomic angle of its origin.[13] In thrombotic ischemia, the presentation is usually an acute-on-chronic mesenteric, with a low flow event precipitating acute ischemia superimposed on symptoms of chronic ischemia. In nonocclusive mesenteric ischemia, intestinal hypoperfusion results from a low-flow state in the splanchnic circulation caused by a sudden drop in systemic blood pressure, for example, from septic shock,[4] severe arterial vasospasm (e.g., from cocaine use,[17] digoxin toxicity,[18] ergot treatment,[19] or prolonged treatment with vasopressin or norepinephrine), or cardiogenic shock.[6,14,20] The splenic flexure, a watershed area supplied by the SMA and IMA, is particularly susceptible to ischemia in low-flow states. The least common cause of acute ischemia is mesenteric venous thrombosis, which is usually secondary to a systemic illness such as neoplastic or hypercoagulable syndromes.[21] Overall, the incidence of acute mesenteric ischemia is rising.[7] The etiology is unclear but may, in part, be due to a growing elderly population with atherosclerotic disease and an increased proportion of patients with shock states requiring vasoactive medications.[7]

Chronic mesenteric ischemia

In comparison to acute mesenteric ischemia, chronic mesenteric ischemia is more indolent in nature, with duration of onset over weeks to months. Patients are most commonly female and present with postprandial abdominal pain and weight loss in the setting of a lack of an alternative explanation. The abdominal discomfort is variable in character and may have associated bloating; it typically occurs 30 minutes to 3 hours after food ingestion. Recurrent intestinal angina causes sitophobia (*fear of food*). Patients suffering from chronic intestinal ischemia often reduce their food intake and on an average lose 10–20 kg prior to diagnosis.

The patients are typically smokers and have additional cardiovascular risk factors or evidence of systemic atherosclerosis (Table 24.2). Indeed, progressive atherosclerotic disease causes the vast majority of chronic mesenteric ischemia.[22] Less common etiologies include vasculitis, FMD, and aortic dissection. The classical teaching has been that chronic mesenteric ischemia is nearly always caused by narrowing of two or more mesenteric vessels. The mesenteric vessels—celiac trunk, SMA, and IMA—can develop collaterals at multiple levels such that a high-grade stenosis of any single vessel is generally well-tolerated. In fact, while significant SMA and celiac stenosis are relatively common (30% and 50%, respectively), chronic mesenteric ischemia remains relatively rare.[23] Patients who have had surgical interruption of these splanchnic collateral networks are more likely to be symptomatic from single-vessel mesenteric disease.[24,25] Additionally, single-vessel disease involving the SMA has been reported to cause chronic mesenteric ischemia. Chronic mesenteric ischemia can also result from mesenteric vein thrombosis, most often involving the superior mesenteric vein. While the mortality rate in chronic mesenteric ischemia is far lower than that of acute mesenteric ischemia, the natural history of chronic mesenteric ischemia is less well-defined and some patients with chronic ischemia progress to acute mesenteric ischemia.[26]

Median arcuate ligament syndrome

Median arcuate ligament syndrome (also known as celiac artery compression syndrome, celiac axis syndrome, and Dunbar syndrome) is a rare clinical entity thought to be caused by the compression of the celiac axis by anomalous fibrous diaphragmatic bands. It is characterized by postprandial abdominal discomfort and weight loss and is occasionally associated with an abdominal bruit.[27] While the pathophysiology of this disorder is not clearly understood, some have suggested a congenital origin.[28] Since the SMA and the IMA remain widely patent in these cases, there should, in theory, still be ample blood supply to the bowel.

As such, the diagnosis of median arcuate ligament syndrome remains controversial and is often one of exclusion.[29–31] Expiration may accentuate regional structure in patients with median arcuate ligament syndrome, and catheter angiography during respiratory maneuvers is often helpful in evaluating these patients.

Visceral artery aneurysms

Aneurysms of the mesenteric vessels are uncommon. The majority of patients with these visceral aneurysms are asymptomatic, and these aneurysms are found incidentally during unrelated abdominal imaging.[32,33] However, these aneurysms do carry a risk of rupture and hemorrhage that can be fatal. Splenic artery aneurysms are the most common, occurring in 60% of cases. In a Mayo Clinic series of 217 patients, only 6.4% of patients with splenic artery aneurysms presented with abdominal pain or rupture.[34] The mortality rate for nonpregnant patients with splenic artery aneurysms ranges between 10% and 25% but may be as high as 70% for pregnant females.[35] In general, splenic aneurysms greater than 2 cm in diameter are thought to be of sufficient risk of rupture to warrant treatment. Aneurysms involving the hepatic artery are increasingly common and presently make up 20% of cases. This is probably due to an increase in percutaneous biliary procedures being performed today, as well as increased recognition from incidental imaging.[36] Aneurysms of the SMA are less common, accounting for only 6% of total cases. Aneurysms of the renal arteries are most commonly associated with FMD, which is discussed in the following section. Vasculitis and trauma have also been associated with renal artery aneurysms.[37]

Renal artery stenosis

Renovascular disease is well-recognized as a potentially reversible cause of hypertension and renal failure. RAS has been associated with coronary artery disease and congestive heart failure, and patients with RAS have a markedly reduced survival rate. RAS by ultrasound is also prevalent in patients with other forms of atherosclerotic disease, such as peripheral arterial or coronary artery disease. Population-based studies have demonstrated that approximately 20% to 60% of patients with peripheral arterial disease also have RAS.[38] In a study of patients who underwent screening aortography at the time of coronary angiography, 4.8% had significant renal stenosis of >75% narrowing.[39]

Clinically, RAS may present as uncontrolled hypertension, flash pulmonary edema, intolerance to ACE-I or ARB treatment, progressive renal deterioration, or refractory angina. The presence of renal arterial disease does not necessarily indicate that the patient's hypertension or renal failure is caused by RAS, and outcomes in renal revascularization studies have been discordant.[40–42] When hypertension is attributed to RAS, the term *renovascular hypertension* is commonly used. Flash pulmonary edema or renal failure following administration of ACE-I or ARB

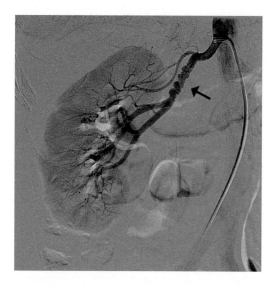

Figure 24.14 Selective right renal angiogram demonstrating fibromuscular dysplasia (FMD). Degenerative changes lead to fibroplasia and arterial wall weakening, resulting in fibrous, band-like stenoses often interposed with aneurysmal dilatations. The angiographic appearance of FMD has thus been characterized as "beads on a string" (arrow).

could indicate significant bilateral renal arterial disease or significant disease in a solitary kidney.

RAS is most commonly due to either atherosclerotic disease or FMD.[43] Atherosclerosis is the main mechanism of RAS in patients older than 55 years. Atherosclerotic renal arterial lesions are most often aorto-ostial in location, involving the ostial and proximal segment of the vessel; distal or branch vessel involvement is uncommon.[42] Progression in atherosclerotic RAS occurs in more than 40% of patients.[44] FMD is a nonatherosclerotic, noninflammatory disease of medium-sized arteries that is seen predominately among young female patients. It could affect a variety of vascular beds including carotid, vertebral, renal, coronary, mesenteric, coronary, celiac, or iliac arteries.[45] The etiology of FMD is unknown, but a genetic predisposition has been suggested.[46] Degenerative changes lead to fibroplasia and arterial wall weakening, resulting in fibrous band-like stenosis often interposed with aneurysmal dilatations. The angiographic appearance of FMD has thus been characterized as "beads on a string" (Figure 24.14). Unlike in atherosclerotic RAS, distal or branch vessel involvement in FMD may occur. Disease progression occurs in more than 30% of patients in FMD.[44] Once renal artery FMD is diagnosed, clinicians should consider assessing for extrarenal involvement (especially cerebrovascular arteries) in this population.

LIMITATIONS

All invasive angiography is limited by access site complications, such as access site bleeding, hematoma, arteriovenous fistulas, median nerve injury (for brachial artery access), and arterial spasms and thrombosis (for radial approach).

Iatrogenic dissections of the aortic branches could occur with selective or nonselective engagement with the diagnostic catheters. Air embolization or injection of thrombotic material could occur and lead to distal infarction in the injected territory. Cholesterol embolization could occur, especially in patients with advanced atherosclerotic disease. Furthermore, the use of iodinated contrast could lead to contrast-induced nephropathy (CIN), especially in patients receiving larger doses or patients with chronic or acute renal disease. Last, the use of X-ray radiation is obviously required to obtain mesenteric and renal angiography, and the minimization of exposure to radiation should always be practiced.

SPECIAL ISSUES/CONSIDERATIONS/ CONTRAINDICATIONS

Contrast selection and renal insufficiency

An optimal diagnostic angiography should allow for complete examination of the arterial bed with the least amount of contrast used. In patients with renal insufficiency, it is critical to minimize the amount of contrast used during the angiographic study. Low-osmolar contrast agents are preferred as they minimize patient discomfort and reduce both the risk of CIN and allergic reactions. The only available iso-osmolal contrast agent, iodixinol, may be associated with a lower risk of nephropathy than low-osmolal agents, particularly among patients at high risk for contrast nephropathy.[47] Despite the lower risk of complications with these agents, the possibility of CIN and allergic reaction remain. Carbon dioxide (CO_2) angiographic imaging is an alternative in patients who remain at high risk for these complications. CO_2 is a very dissolvable gas that is nontoxic to the kidneys and does not induce allergic reactions.[48,49] It works by displacing blood cells inside the vessel, effectively reducing the radiographic density within the lumen.

There are certain limitations to this form of imaging that should be noted. Importantly, contrast resolution with CO_2 angiography, while often adequate, is inferior to that with traditional iodinated contrast agents.[50] CO_2 angiography must also be performed in a controlled fashion with carefully administered gas volumes to avoid gas trapping in the pulmonary circulation.[51] Gadolinium has also been studied as a possible alternative agent in patients at risk for CIN. However, this agent has not been proven to have any significant advantage over low-osmolar agents in reducing CIN and has been largely abandoned.[52]

Difficulty in visualizing renal ostia

Renal artery ostial disease may be missed by standard angiography. If clinical suspicion of RAS is high, nontraditional views with added cranial or caudal angulation should be attained. Intravascular ultrasound is an alternative modality that can be used for better visualization of the renal arteries and to determine the presence of renal artery ostial disease. The operator should pay attention to hemodynamic clues, such as catheter damping, that may indicate a significant ostial lesion. Finally, measurement of fractional flow reserve (FFR) across intermediate lesions has emerged as an attractive technique to assess indeterminate lesions, with an FFR less or equal to 0.8 being a determinant parameter for significant hemodynamic severity. Maximal vessel hyperemia could be achieved with administration of papaverine or dobutamine. A resting translesional pressure gradient larger than 10 mmHg or a hyperemic translesional pressure gradient greater than 20 mmHg is generally considered indicative of a hemodynamically significant stenosis.

Difficulty using arm approach

As discussed above, an arm approach for mesenteric and renal angiography can be very helpful in certain circumstances. However, in cases of subclavian stenosis, innominate stenosis, or tortuous aortic arch, the passage of diagnostic catheters and equipment from an arm approach can be challenging. In these cases, a long sheath should be used and advanced into the descending aorta and placed above the level of the mesenteric vessels. For right radial approach, catheters that are 125 cm in length must be used. However, for very tall patients, even 125 cm may not be long enough to reach the renal arteries. A stiff 0.035-in wire, such as a Rosen or a stiff Glidewire, may also facilitate catheter and sheath placement in this circumstance.

CONCLUSIONS

The invasive assessment of patients with suspected mesenteric or renal vascular disease needs to be performed cautiously and meticulously. These patients, particularly those with preexisting renal insufficiency and advanced atherosclerosis, can have a high risk of procedure-related complications. However, if careful technique is observed and minimal contrast used, such angiographic assessment can yield critical clinical information and potentially set the stage for important interventional therapies.

REFERENCES

1. Rajagopalan S, et al. *Manual of Vascular Diseases.* Philadelphia, PA: Lippincott Diseases & Wilkins; 2005.
2. Beregi JP, et al. Anatomic variation in the origin of the main renal arteries: Spiral CTA evaluation. *Eur Radiol* 1999;9(7):1330–1334.
3. Kadir S. *Angiography of the Kidneys.* Philadelphia, PA: Saunders; 1986.
4. Hirsch AT, et al. ACC/AHA 2005 Practice Guidelines for the management of patients with peripheral arterial disease (lower extremity, renal, mesenteric, and abdominal aortic): A collaborative report from the American Association for Vascular Surgery/Society for Vascular Surgery, Society for Cardiovascular Angiography and Interventions, Society for Vascular Medicine and Biology, Society of Interventional Radiology, and the ACC/AHA Task Force on Practice Guidelines (Writing Committee to Develop Guidelines for the Management of Patients With Peripheral Arterial Disease): Endorsed by the American Association of Cardiovascular and Pulmonary Rehabilitation; National Heart, Lung, and Blood Institute; Society for Vascular Nursing; TransAtlantic Inter-Society Consensus; and Vascular Disease Foundation. *Circulation* 2006;113(11):e463–e654.
5. Lorenzoni R, Roffi M. Transradial access for peripheral and cerebrovascular interventions. *J Invasive Cardiol* 2013;25(10):529–536.
6. McKinsey JF, Gewertz BL. Acute mesenteric ischemia. *Surg Clin N Am* 1997;77(2):307–318.
7. Bradbury AW, et al. Mesenteric ischaemia: A multidisciplinary approach. *Br J Surg* 1995;82(11):1446–1459.
8. Sachs SM, et al. Acute mesenteric ischemia. *Surgery* 1982;92(4):646–653.
9. Bergan JJ, et al. Nontraumatic mesenteric vascular emergencies. *J Vasc Surg* 1987;5(6):903–909.
10. Boley SJ, et al. History of mesenteric ischemia. The evolution of a diagnosis and management. *Surg Clin North Am* 1997;77(2):275–288.
11. Bobadilla JL. Mesenteric ischemia. *Surg Clin North Am* 2013;93(4):925–940, ix.
12. Chang RW, et al. Update in management of mesenteric ischemia. *World J Gastroenterol* 2006;12(20):3243–3247.
13. Cappell MS. Intestinal (mesenteric) vasculopathy. I. Acute superior mesenteric arteriopathy and venopathy. *Gastroenterol Clin North Am* 1998;27(4):783–825, vi.
14. Reinus JF, et al. Ischemic diseases of the bowel. *Gastroenterol Clin North Am* 1990;19(2):319–343.
15. Vokurka J, et al. Acute mesenteric ischemia. *Hepatogastroenterology* 2008;55(85):1349–1352.
16. Brandt LJ, Boley SJ. AGA technical review on intestinal ischemia. American Gastrointestinal Association. *Gastroenterology* 2000;118(5):954–968.
17. Sudhakar CB, et al. Mesenteric ischemia secondary to cocaine abuse: Case reports and literature review. *Am J Gastroenterol* 1997;92(6):1053–1054.
18. Guglielminotti J, et al. Fatal non-occlusive mesenteric infarction following digoxin intoxication. *Intensive Care Med* 2000;26(6):829.
19. Liu JJ, Ardolf JC. Sumatriptan-associated mesenteric ischemia. *Ann Intern Med* 2000;132(7):597.
20. Wilcox MG, et al. Current theories of pathogenesis and treatment of nonocclusive mesenteric ischemia. *Dig Dis Sci* 1995;40(4):709–716.
21. Rhee RY, et al. Mesenteric venous thrombosis: Still a lethal disease in the 1990s. *J Vasc Surg* 1994;20(5):688–697.
22. Fisher DF, Jr., Fry WJ. Collateral mesenteric circulation. *Surg Gynecol Obstet* 1987;164(5):487–492.
23. Reiner L, et al. Atherosclerosis in the mesenteric circulation. Observations and correlations with aortic and coronary atherosclerosis. *Am Heart J* 1963;66:200–209.
24. Buchardt Hansen HJ. Abdominal angina. Results of arterial reconstruction in 12 patients. *Acta Chir Scand* 1976;142(4):319–325.
25. Mikkelsen WP. Intestinal angina: Its surgical significance. *Am J Surg* 1957;94(2):262–267; discussion, 7–9.
26. Korotinski S, et al. Chronic ischaemic bowel diseases in the aged—Go with the flow. *Age Ageing* 2005;34(1):10–6.
27. Dunbar JD, et al. Compression of the celiac trunk and abdominal angina. *Am J Roentgenol Radium Ther Nucl Med* 1965;95(3):731–744.

28. Bech F, et al. Median arcuate ligament compression syndrome in monozygotic twins. *J Vasc Surg* 1994;19(5):934–938.

29. Holland AJ, Ibach EG. Long-term review of coeliac axis compression syndrome. *Ann R Coll Surg Engl* 1996;78(5):470–472.

30. Horton KM, et al. Median arcuate ligament syndrome: Evaluation with CT angiography. *Radiographics* 2005;25(5):1177–1182.

31. Karahan OI, et al. Celiac artery compression syndrome: Diagnosis with multislice CT. *Diagn Interv Radiol* 2007;13(2):90–93.

32. Messina LM, Shanley CJ. Visceral artery aneurysms. *Surg Clin North Am* 1997;77(2):425–442.

33. Shanley CJ, et al. Uncommon splanchnic artery aneurysms: Pancreaticoduodenal, gastroduodenal, superior mesenteric, inferior mesenteric, and colic. *Ann Vasc Surg* 1996;10(5):506–515.

34. Abbas MA, et al. Splenic artery aneurysms: Two decades experience at Mayo clinic. *Ann Vasc Surg* 2002;16(4):442–449.

35. Kasirajan K, et al. Endovascular management of visceral artery aneurysm. *J Endovasc Ther* 2001;8(2):150–155.

36. Nosher JL, et al. Visceral and renal artery aneurysms: A pictorial essay on endovascular therapy. *Radiographics* 2006;26(6):1687–1704; quiz 1687.

37. Henke PK, et al. Renal artery aneurysms: A 35-year clinical experience with 252 aneurysms in 168 patients. *Ann Surg* 2001;234(4):454–462; discussion 62–63.

38. Streather C, et al. Progression of occlusive renal vascular disease and axillofemoral bypass grafts. *Nephrol Dial Transplant* 1993;8(10):1186–1187.

39. Conlon PJ, et al. Severity of renal vascular disease predicts mortality in patients undergoing coronary angiography. *Kidney Int* 2001;60(4):1490–1497.

40. Rihal CS, et al. Incidental renal artery stenosis among a prospective cohort of hypertensive patients undergoing coronary angiography. *Mayo Clin Proc* 2002;77(4):309–316.

41. Leertouwer TC, et al. Stent placement for renal arterial stenosis: Where do we stand? A meta-analysis. *Radiology* 2000;216(1):78–85.

42. Novick AC, et al. Trends in surgical revascularization for renal artery disease. Ten years' experience. *JAMA.* 1987;257(4):498–501.

43. Safian RD, Textor SC. Renal-artery stenosis. *N Engl J Med* 2001;344(6):431–442.

44. Schreiber MJ, et al. The natural history of atherosclerotic and fibrous renal artery disease. *Urol Clin North Am* 1984;11(3):383–392.

45. Shivapour DM, et al. Epidemiology of fibromuscular dysplasia: A review of the literature. *Vasc Med* 2016;21(4):376–381.

46. Perdu J, et al. Inheritance of arterial lesions in renal fibromuscular dysplasia. *J Hum Hypertens* 2007;21(5):393–400.

47. Aspelin P, et al. Nephrotoxic effects in high-risk patients undergoing angiography. *N Engl J Med* 2003;348(6):491–499.

48. Shaw DR, Kessel DO. The current status of the use of carbon dioxide in diagnostic and interventional angiographic procedures. *Cardiovasc Intervent Radiol* 2006;29(3):323–331.

49. Liss P, et al. Renal effects of CO2 and iodinated contrast media in patients undergoing renovascular intervention: A prospective, randomized study. *J Vasc Interv Radiol* 2005;16(1):57–65.

50. Huang SG, et al. A prospective study of carbon dioxide digital subtraction versus standard contrast arteriography in the detection of endoleaks in endovascular abdominal aortic aneurysm repairs. *Ann Vasc Surg* 2013;27(1):38–44.

51. Kessel DO, et al. Carbon-dioxide-guided vascular interventions: Technique and pitfalls. *Cardiovasc Intervent Radiol* 2002;25(6):476–483.

52. Boyden TF, Gurm HS. Does gadolinium-based angiography protect against contrast-induced nephropathy?: A systematic review of the literature. *Catheter Cardiovasc Interv* 2008;71(5):687–693.

25

Peripheral vascular angiography

FADI A. SAAB

INTRODUCTION

Peripheral arterial disease (PAD) is a condition that describes atherosclerosis involving major vascular beds. These vessels include the aorta, aortic arch vessels, mesenteric, upper extremity, iliacs, femoral, popliteal, and tibio-plantar circulation. The prevalence of PAD has been increasing worldwide and the number of patients suffering from PAD is expected to increase by 15% in Western countries and 30% in developing countries.[1] This increase is a reflection of other comorbidities driving the rise in numbers. Patients with PAD suffer from higher morbidity and mortality.[2,3] There are multiple modalities to evaluate patients with PAD. Endovascular revascularization of patients with PAD is becoming a front-line strategy. This has been adopted by multiple disciplines, including vascular surgery, radiology, and cardiology. Bypass surgery is an excellent procedure in appropriately selected patients.[4,5] However, many PAD patients may not be adequate candidates for surgical bypass. Endovascular therapy has been fueled by continuous innovation in techniques and devices.[6] Prior to revascularization, patients need to be adequately assessed by noninvasive and physiological testing. However, there are some limitations in applying these tests. Peripheral vascular angiography may be argued as the gold standard when it comes to assessing vessel patency. This chapter focuses on evaluation of vessel patency from an endovascular revascularization perspective.

GENERAL CONSIDERATIONS

The goal of peripheral angiography is to confirm clinical examination and noninvasive test findings to pave the way for revascularization. However, there are significant limitations. For example, diabetic patients may have falsely elevated ankle-brachial index values, suggesting normal results where the patient, in fact, has significant arterial disease. Other imaging modalities may also not offer adequate information. Computed tomography angiography can be limited in evaluating small-caliber vessels, especially in the below-the-knee (BTK) circulation (and in the presence of severe calcification). Magnetic resonance (MR) angiography may not be used in patients with advanced renal disease secondary to concerns regarding systemic nephrogenic calcinosis.[7]

With peripheral angiography, the use of digital subtraction offers superior images in comparison to nonsubtracted images. The use of automated injector systems can be helpful (e.g., ACIST contrast delivery system). These systems allow the operator to monitor pressure in a closed hemodynamic circuit and to control the amount of contrast delivered, as well as the pressure and rise times of administration. In addition, there are safety checks included in the system, such as autodetection of the presence of air.

Patients with diabetes and chronic kidney disease (CKD) are at a higher risk of PAD. In our practice, most patients undergo a detailed diagnostic angiogram prior to delivering endovascular therapy. This staged approach decreases the amount of contrast a patient is exposed to. Contrast-induced nephropathy remains a major concern in PAD patients and particularly CKD patients. Carbon dioxide (CO_2) is a nontoxic compressible gas that has been used as a contrast agent for a long time.[8] As a contrast agent, CO_2 does not appear to carry the risks of either contrast nephropathy or allergic reaction.[9] CO_2 angiography offers limited accuracy with imaging in the popliteal artery and below. However, using CO_2 in the aorto-iliac and femoral segments can dramatically decrease patients' exposure to contrast. At our institution, patients with CKD receive CO_2 angiography to evaluate the aorto-iliac vessels (Figure 25.1a). The superficial femoral artery (SFA) can still be adequately visualized (Figure 25.1b). Selective angiography with a catheter placed in the popliteal artery allows selective angiography with diluted contrast. In the example shown in Figure 25.2, we were able to perform a detailed diagnostic angiogram with less than 30 cc of contrast. Note the difference in the quality of visualization of the peroneal artery between CO_2 angiography and diluted contrast (50% saline, 50% contrast). A typical diagnostic angiogram will require 150–200 cc of contrast. Patients with multilevel and multivessel disease need to be fully assessed. It is for that reason that we stage all of our interventions. It also depends on the disease evaluated.

It is the opinion of this author that a diagnostic angiogram without intervention is required in certain conditions like carotid artery disease and critical limb ischemia (CLI). In CLI, patients have a high likelihood of CKD that limits their ability to tolerate large amounts of contrast. In addition, the use of alternative access like antegrade and tibial access may

be necessary. There are multiple catheters and wires that can be utilized in performing peripheral nonselective and selective angiography. Table 25.1 lists some of the common catheters and wires in use for peripheral angiography.

Upper extremity anatomy and peripheral angiography

The arterial inflow to the right and left upper extremities is provided by the right and left subclavian arteries. The left subclavian artery arises directly from the aortic arch as the third vessel (Figure 25.3). The right subclavian arises from the bifurcation of the brachiocephalic artery. The aortic arch vessels have multiple patterns describing their takeoff. Anatomical variation in the upper extremity may occur. For example, the right subclavian artery may rise directly from the aorta in less than 1% of cases.

The subclavian artery extends to the lateral border of the first rib. Its course is divided into three segments based on the relationship of the artery to the scalenus anterior muscle. The first segment provides the most important branches of the subclavian artery, the vertebral, internal mummeries, and the thyrocervical trunk. The vertebral artery rises from the proximal subclavian artery. Typically, there is one dominant vertebral artery. It may be the right or the left one. In rare cases, the left vertebral artery may arise directly from the aortic arch (less than 5%). The subclavian artery continues into the axillary artery. The axillary artery borders extend from the lateral aspect of the first rib into the head of the humorous (Figure 25.4). The vessel beyond this point will be defined as the brachial artery. The brachial artery used to be a common access point for a variety of procedures, including left heart catheterization. This access has been widely replaced for coronary angiography and revascularization and is being used increasingly also for peripheral procedures. The brachial artery provides two major vessels with the radial and ulnar arteries (Figure 25.5). Contrary to lower extremity anatomy, the profunda brachii artery splits from the brachial artery and tends to have no significant clinical impact on the arm muscles (Figure 25.6). The ulnar artery bifurcates medially from the brachial artery. The ulnar artery tends to be the more dominant vessel. The bifurcation starts at the neck of the radius. It provides the intraosseous artery that runs more laterally supplying the intraosseous membrane with the forearm muscles. The ulnar artery carries on through the pisiform carpal bone. It eventually reaches the hand and is the major supplier of the superficial arch. The radial artery is a smaller vessel. After it bifurcates from the brachial artery, it runs as the most lateral vessel toward the styloid process of the radius. The ulnar artery supplies the deep palmar arch and the superficial palmar arch is supplied by the radial artery. The common digital arteries arise from the superficial and deep arches and supply the interdigital space. These vessels are usually spared from atherosclerosis. However, some patients with advanced renal disease and diabetes may have significant obstructions and/or calcifications (Figure 25.7).

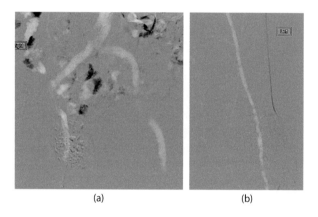

(a)   (b)

Figure 25.1 CO_2 angiography. **(a)** Nonselective CO_2 angiography of the aorta. **(b)** Selective CO_2 angiography of the left superficial femoral artery.

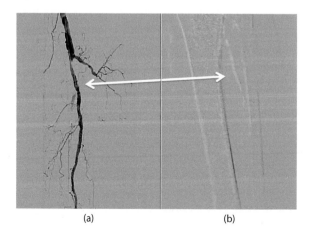

(a)   (b)

Figure 25.2 The difference between selective angiography on the popliteal/tibial vessels using diluted contrast **(a)** and CO_2 angiography **(b)**.

Table 25.1 Common catheters and wires used in peripheral angiography

Catheters	Upper extremity	Lower extremity	Non-selective angiography	Selective angiography
Omni Flush	X	X	X	X
Pigtail	X	X	X	X
Rim	X	X	X	X
Judkins right	X	X		X
Left internal mammary	X	X		X
SIMS	X	X		X
Vitek (Cook)	X	X		X
Dav	X	X		X
Bernstein (Cordis)	X	X		X
Glide Catheter	X	X		X
Trailblazer	X	X		X
Navicross (Terumo)				X
CXI (Cook)				
0.035-in wires				
J-tipped wire	X	X	X	X
Magic Torque (Boston Scientific)	X	X	X	X
Glidewire	X	X	X	X
Glide Advantage	X	X	X	X
Wholey	X	X	X	
Supercore	X	X	X	
Amplatz	X	X	X	
0.018-in wires				
SV-5	X	X	X	X
V-18	X	X		X
Gladius (Asahi)	X	X		X
Glide Advantage	X	X		X
Glide		X		X
Gold-tip Glidewire		X		X

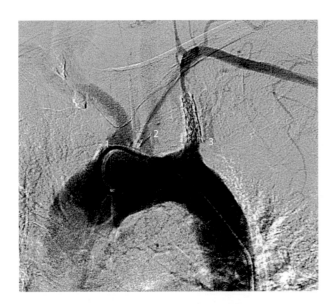

Figure 25.3 An aortic arch angiogram showing the take-off of the three major vessels. Brachiocephalic (1), left common carotid (2), and the left subclavian artery (3).

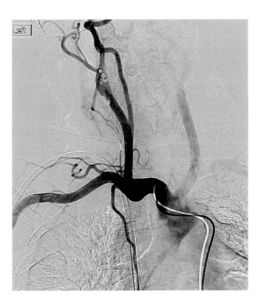

Figure 25.4 Selective angiography of the right subclavian artery extending into the axillary artery. Note the right vertebral artery (1) and the right internal mammary artery (2).

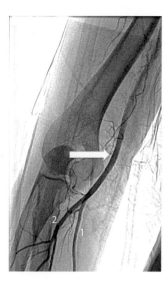

Figure 25.5 Nonsubtracted selective angiography of the right brachial artery (arrow). Note the takeoff of the radial artery (1) and the ulnar artery (2).

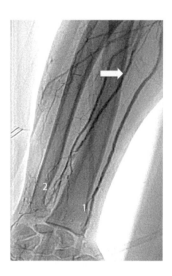

Figure 25.6 The right radial (1) and right ulnar arteries (2) with the profunda brachii branch (arrow).

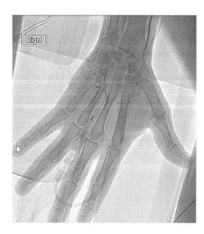

Figure 25.7 Nonsubtracted image of diseased palmar arch vessels in a patient with end-stage renal disease.

Peripheral upper extremity angiography assessment

GENERAL CONSIDERATION

An endovascular specialist must recognize all major vessels and branches. This knowledge extends to recognizing disease patterns. We discuss common femoral artery (CFA) access in the next section. Below are the common steps when performing upper extremity angiography.

ACCESS

Typically, an upper extremity access is reserved for planned intervention. After obtaining lower CFA ultrasound-guided access, the operator will perform an aortic arch angiogram (Figure 25.3).

NONSELECTIVE AORTIC ARCH ANGIOGRAPHY

Using digital subtraction will eliminate any bony interference. This, however, will require a cooperative patient who is not moving and able to hold his or her breath. Despite following that recommendation, artifact movement may occur simply because of cardiac contraction. Overall, adequate images can be obtained. We recommend a left anterior oblique (LAO) view of 25°–30°. This will allow adequate visualization of the major vessels takeoff. We prefer to inject contrast at a rate of 15 cc for 2 seconds (a total of 30 cc). Aortic arch angiography should be performed with a closed catheter (e.g., pigtail). We typically advise to maintain a closed system where hemodynamic monitoring is constant. The ACIST system is an automatic contrast injection device that will allow continuous hemodynamic monitoring and different variation in contrast injection volumes and pressures. The pounds per square inch (PSI) pressure preferred in an aortogram is between 800 and 1,000.

SELECTIVE VESSEL ANGIOGRAPHY

Selective angiography allows the operator to better define the degree of disease. It will save on the amount of contrast and, in addition, may allow the operator to measure arterial pressures in different segments of the vessel. Visual assessment of what appears to be an intermediate lesion tends to overestimate the degree of stenosis. Having a hemodynamic measurement before and after the stenosis can offer more conclusive evidence regarding the significance of the disease. We typically will use the cut-off point of 20 mmHg pressure differences as a significant drop. There are different catheters that have been utilized for selective angiography. They range anywhere from simple catheters with a mild bend at the tip (Judkins Right, Dav, Vertebral) to more complex catheters that will engage complex anatomy and difficult aortic arches (SIMS, Vitek catheters). The volume injected may range from 6 to 12 cc. Again, making sure that there is adequate waveform offers reassurance that the open-end catheter is not embedded against the arterial wall. Injecting contrast against the arterial wall can create significant complications, such as dissection, distal embolization, and in some cases, even perforation. A right anterior oblique projection of 30°–45° is best suited to visualize the takeoff of the left and right vertebral arteries. In addition, it is the best orientation to visualize internal mammary arteries.

Disease patterns

When talking about upper extremity peripheral angiography, the operator should recognize areas more likely to contain disease. A common area of disease is the ostial left subclavian artery. In some patients it may be occluded (Figure 25.8). The subclavian artery usually reconstitutes via collaterals. The true length of the chronic total occlusion (CTO) is poorly defined. In this case, obtaining a retrograde angiogram via a radial artery access will define the true borders of the CTO by showing the distal edge (Figure 25.9). In the same clinical scenario, having dual angiogram injection from the CFA (aortic arch) and the radial artery will better define the degree of stenosis or the length of the CTO (Figure 25.10). Another less common pattern of illness is end-stage renal disease in patients who have radial and ulnar occlusion causing digital ischemia and possible limb loss. Heavy calcification within the vessels is noted on fluoroscopy and some patients may

be treated with endovascular therapy (Figure 25.11). This is in contrast to patients with Raynaud's disease or vasculitis, where the disease is limited to digital branches and no endovascular therapy is feasible.

Lower extremity anatomy and peripheral angiography

The distal abdominal aorta typically bifurcates at the level of third or fourth lumbar vertebra into right and left common iliac arteries (CIA) (Figure 25.12).[10] Performing an aortogram with the catheter in the supra- and infrarenal position identifies major mesenteric vessels and renal arteries. Depending on the indication of the angiogram, selective engagement of

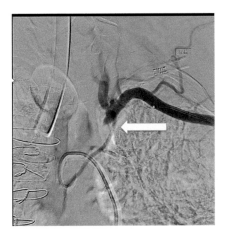

Figure 25.10 Nonsubtracted dual-injection angiogram from the aortic arch and the retrograde radial artery showing the true length of the left subclavian artery chronic total occlusion.

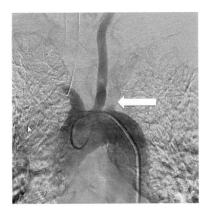

Figure 25.8 Nonselective aortic arch angiography showing an occluded left subclavian artery at the take off point (arrow).

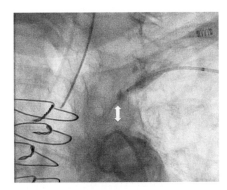

Figure 25.9 Retrograde angiogram via radial artery access showing the distal reconstitution of the left ostial subclavian artery chronic total occlusion.

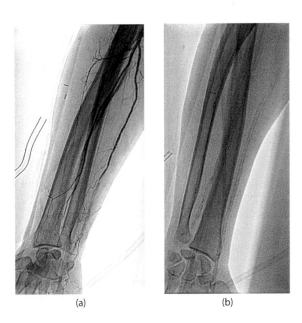

(a)   (b)

Figure 25.11 Selective angiography of the right arm with (a) and without (b) contrast. Note the heavy calcification impacting the radial and ulnar arteries.

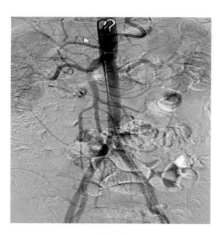

Figure 25.12 Abdominal aortogram with the catheter placed in the suprarenal position.

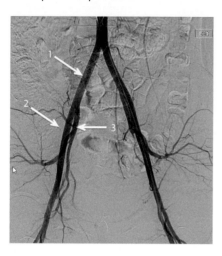

Figure 25.13 Anterior posterior aortogram with the catheter placed in the infrarenal position. The CIA (1) bifurcates into the EIA (2) and the IIA (3). Note the difficulty in distinguishing the takeoff of the IIA. CIA, common iliac artery; EIA, external iliac artery; IIA, internal iliac artery.

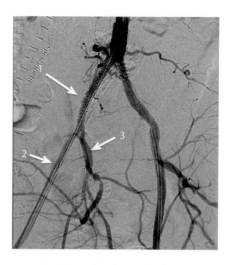

Figure 25.14 Same aortogram to prior image, with the catheter placed in the infrarenal position. The detector is placed in a contralateral left anterior oblique position at 30° with 15° caudal orientation. Note the clear separation of the right IIA (3) takeoff from the right EIA (2) and the right CIA (1). CIA, common iliac artery; EIA, external iliac artery; IIA, internal iliac artery.

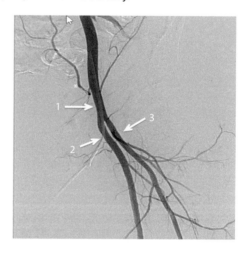

Figure 25.15 The common femoral artery (1) separating into the superficial femoral artery (2) and the profunda (3). (*Inferior epigastric artery.)

the mesenteric or renal arteries may be warranted. Generally speaking, it is not performed unless there is a clear indication. After the aorta splits, each CIA passes in an anterior direction in the pelvis before bifurcating into external (EIA) and internal (IIA) iliac artery branches. The IIA divides into two branches in the majority of patients. The IIA supplies the pelvic organs (i.e., bladder, rectum, female and male reproductive organs) (Figures 25.13 and 25.14). Occlusion of the IIA may be responsible for gluteal claudication and in some instances erectile dysfunction. The IIA provides the superior and inferior gluteal branches. These branches serve as an important source of collaterals to the ipsilateral and contralateral limb in the presence of iliac occlusive disease.

The EIA continues with an anterior trajectory, becoming the CFA at the level of the inguinal ligament (Figure 25.15). There is some variability in the location of the CFA bifurcation into the SFA and profunda (PFA) branches. In 98% of the cases, the separation happens below the mid-femoral head.[11,12] There are still some cases where the separation

occurs above the femoral head. This has important consequences especially in cases where you have to perform antegrade access. The operator wants to avoid above the inguinal ligament/inferior epigastric artery access because it is generally a noncompressible site. Arterial access within a noncompressible site may lead to retroperitoneal bleeding (Figure 25.16). Arising from the proximal portion of the PFA are the medial and lateral circumflex femoral branches. The PFA continues laterally into the thigh supplying the perforator branches to the muscles of the thigh. The PFA is the lifeline of the leg and should be protected at all cost. It provides important collaterals to the lower extremity when the SFA is occluded (Figure 25.17). The ostium of the PFA tends to be involved in diseases affecting the CFA, but the rest of the vessel generally remains intact.

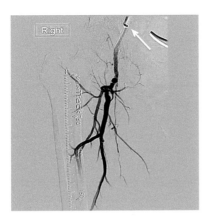

Figure 25.16 Antegrade angiogram showing the sheath (arrow) inserted above the femoral head into the external iliac artery. This patient suffered from a retroperitoneal bleed.

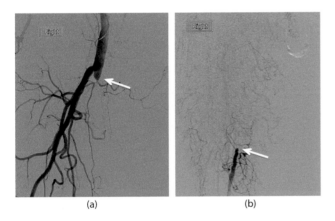

(a)   (b)

Figure 25.17 Chronic total occlusion of the right superficial femoral artery with reconstitution with the proximal popliteal artery (arrow).

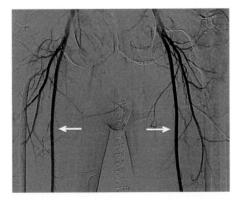

Figure 25.18 Bilateral superficial femoral artery traveling through the thigh muscles (arrow).

The SFA provides arterial flow to the knee, leg, and foot. As the SFA passes through the muscular adductor canal, it becomes the popliteal artery (Figure 25.18). This junction area is commonly the most affected with atherosclerosis. The majority of SFA occlusions reconstitute below that segment (Figure 25.17). This area is under constant mechanical

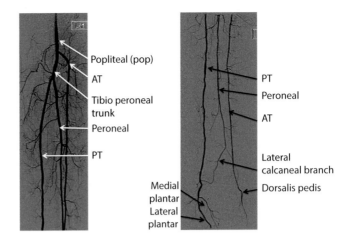

Figure 25.19 Proximal, mid, and distal tibial-plantar vessels with collaterals. AT, anterior tibial; PT, posterior tibial.

pressure with stretching, torsion, and twisting. The popliteal artery runs in the popliteal fossa posterior to the distal third of the femur, and subsequently along the posterior surface of the tibial plateau, providing branches that supply the calf muscles. The popliteal artery bifurcates into an anterior tibial (AT) artery and tibioperoneal trunk. The AT passes anteriorly through the interosseous membrane between the tibia and fibula; the AT reaches the anterior compartment of the leg and travels inferiorly toward the foot. At the ankle level, it becomes the dorsalis pedis (DP) artery. The tibioperoneal trunk divides into the posterior tibial (PT) and peroneal arteries. Both of these arteries continue inferiorly in the posterior compartment of the leg. The peroneal artery connects distally to the AT and PT via the anterior communicating artery and the posterior communicating artery, respectively. These are important branches especially in CLI patients where the AT and PT become occluded. The PT passes posterior to the medial malleolus before dividing into medial and lateral plantar branches (Figure 25.19). Before the plantar branches, it gives rise to the medial calcaneal branch, supplying the medial aspect of the heel. The peroneal artery typically terminates above the level of the ankle joint. The peroneal artery is responsible to supply the lateral calcaneal branch of the ankle. This in turn supplies the lateral aspect of the heel. All three tibial branches provide the major arterial supply to the calf muscles. Within the foot, the plantar branches of the PT, and the dorsalis pedis branch of the AT create the pedal loop. Typically the DP connects with the lateral plantar artery through the tarsal branch. The metatarsal branches arise from this loop and provide the digital branches to the toes (Figures 25.20 and 25.21).

Peripheral lower extremity angiography assessment

GENERAL CONSIDERATION

While the use of upper extremity access has been advocated for the evaluation and in some cases treatment of PAD, CFA access remains the preferred method. Selective angiography with a catheter placed as distal as possible within the limb requiring therapy is essential to creating an adequate treatment plan and minimizing dye administration. Our group conducted a trial comparing noninvasive arterial duplex imaging to selective versus nonselective angiography. The results confirmed what is commonly advocated with better correlation between noninvasive arterial duplex assessment and selective angiography.[13] Limitations related to upper extremity access will be discussed in other chapters. We

discuss details related to variable access points within the lower extremity in the following section.

ACCESS

Retrograde traditional CFA is the preferred modality for evaluating and treating PAD. This access point affords the operator the ability to navigate difficult anatomy and treat areas necessary to relieve symptoms. Most catheters, atherectomy devices, balloons, and stents are designed for use via traditional retrograde CFA. We teach our fellows to image the access wire through the needle (Figure 25.22). This image offers important information with respect to the entry site and the relationship with the femoral bifurcation. All modalities advocated to gaining access into the CFA revolve around obtaining access within a compressible site, but at the same time, without involving the CFA bifurcation or its branches, as the risk of complications increases and the use of closure devices may be precluded. In the example shown in Figure 25.22, despite the correct entry point, the vessel accessed was the SFA. In fact this patient had an anomalous high takeoff of the SFA. For 5- or 6-Fr catheters, the access remains adequate, if the vessel is not diseased, since the area punctured is compressible. However, the introduction of a larger sheath (e.g., 14–18 Fr for abdominal aortic aneurysm repair) would be problematic and associated with an increased risk of complications. We also always advocate performing an angiogram of the access site to assess the puncture site (i.e., high puncture may be associated with retroperitoneal bleeding and manual compression may be challenging; puncture at the level or below the femoral bifurcation may be associated with higher rate of vascular complications and may preclude the use of vascular closure devices) and rule out any complications related to vessel puncture (Figure 25.15). The use of the needle fluoro techniques takes away any confusion regarding the access site. Figure 25.23 shows an example of antegrade access via

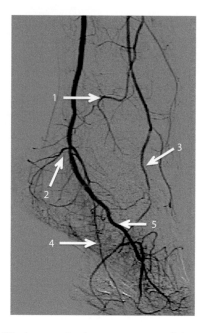

Figure 25.20 An anterior/posterior view of the pedal loop with cranial orientation. This shows the lateral calcaneal branch of the peroneal artery (1), the medial calcaneal branch of the posterior tibial (2), the dorsalis pedis (3), the medial plantar artery (4), and the lateral plantar artery (5).

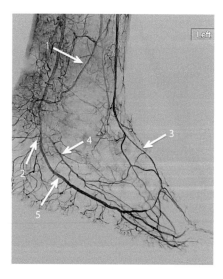

Figure 25.21 A lateral view of the pedal loop. This shows the calcaneal branch of the peroneal artery (1), the calcaneal branch of the posterior tibial (2), the dorsalis pedis (3), the medial plantar artery (4), and the lateral plantar artery (5).

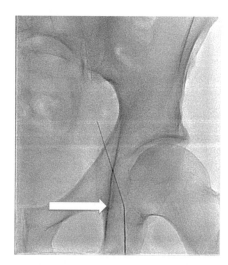

Figure 25.22 Fluoroscopic image showing the tip of the access needle with the access wire through the common femoral artery into the external iliac artery.

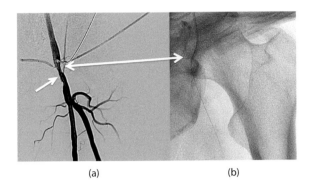

Figure 25.23 Antegrade access of the common femoral artery. Note the appearance of high access based on angiographic images **(a)**. **(b)** Our access site against the mid-femoral head. Note the low take of the inferior epigastric artery (small arrow).

angiography; it appears that the access is in the external iliac artery. However, the needle fluoro image clearly shows the access point against the mid-femoral head. The operator should obtain the fluoro image in an ipsilateral view to the access site at 30° without any caudal or cranial orientation (Figures 25.22 and 25.23).

ALTERNATIVE ACCESS

Since more and more complex and distal peripheral vascular disease is approached by endovascular means, the use of alternative access (in case of recanalization failure using a retrograde femoral access) is becoming a critical skill. Antegrade femoral access is becoming a preferred modality for evaluation and treatment of femoropopliteal disease in patients with challenging aorto-iliac anatomy or prior surgeries like an aorto-iliac bypass. In addition, it may be the preferred access for Bruton tyrosine kinase (BTK) disease. The use of ultrasound in guiding arterial access is becoming a common and preferred strategy. It is the opinion of this author that ultrasound guidance should be the gold standard in gaining access to any vascular conduit. Figure 25.24 shows an example of

arterial access gained in a retrograde and antegrade fashion under ultrasound guidance. Tibio-pedal access is utilized in patients with advanced PAD and CLI in case of failure of antegrade revascularization. Using tibio-pedal access for diagnostic purposes is not advocated. However, in cases where it is required, a low-profile sheath should be placed. Performing a retrograde angiogram via tibio-pedal access requires the operator to inject slowly with no more than 4–6 cc of contrast. Tibial contrast injection tends to cause discomfort for the patient. Figure 25.25 shows an example of retrograde tibial access in a patient who was informed there was no tibial vessel runoff. This example demonstrates the importance of selective angiography. The patient had multilevel disease from the aorta into the SFA/Profunda systems. This prohibits an adequate amount of contrast to opacity of the tibial vessels. This patient presented with a nonhealing wound.

Nonselective angiography

After gaining access, the catheter is placed in the suprarenal position in anteroposterior (AP) view. If the takeoff of the renal arteries is of particular importance, that of 20°–30° in the LAO projection is chosen, as it better defines the ostia of the renal arteries. Catheters used include the pigtail, Omni Flush, and RIM catheters, to name a few. Using a closed catheter system is usually preferred. There are important vertebral braches that may be injured if a large contrast volume with high PSI pressure was injected directly into the vessel. We generally recommend a total of 30 cc of contrast with a rate of 15 cc/s for 2 seconds with digital subtraction angiography at 1–2 frames/s. PSI pressure recommended is between 800 and 1,000. The same positions apply with CO_2 angiography. For iliac imaging, the catheter is pulled down to the infrarenal position. Identifying the separation between the internal and external iliac is necessary in cases where exclusion of the ostium of the internal iliac is important. Generally, we find that a contralateral projection to the vessel of interest at 20°–25° with a 15° caudal orientation shows the separation between the external iliac and

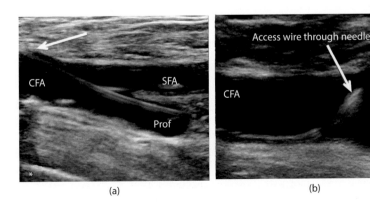

Figure 25.24 Longitudinal ultrasound-guided access of the CFA in an antegrade fashion. Note the wire in the SFA and profunda **(Prof, a)**. **(b)** Longitudinal ultrasound-guided access of the CFA in a retrograde fashion. Note the wire through the needle. (*Femoral head. Arrow shows the access point in antegrade access.) CFA, common femoral artery; SFA, superficial femoral artery.

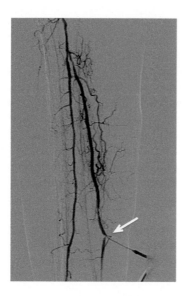

Figure 25.25 Retrograde angiography with a sheath (arrow) placed in the distal right posterior tibial artery.

the internal iliac (Figure 25.14). The next step is imaging the proximal SFAs (Figure 25.18). The catheter will be maintained in the same position. There are other strategies with using a single bolus chase with cine-angiography and following the contrast from the aorta to the popliteal arteries. Generally, we would use 15 cc for a total of 90 cc. With this protocol, you will image the vessels from the aorta to the proximal tibials in some cases. The bolus protocol is effective when there is no significant or multilevel disease. We generally prefer the static images as they offer more details, especially in cases with multilevel disease

Selective angiography

The idea of selective angiography revolves around advancing a catheter to the limb in question. We generally create a road map to advance the catheter over a wire (Figure 25.26). Catheters utilized may include the Omni, Rim, Judkins right, Multipurpose, Navicross, Glide, and Traiblazer, to name a few. As an open-end catheter, we recommend making sure that the waveform with pressure is assessed. We usually recommend 12 cc contrast injection with 6 cc/s for 2 seconds. An AP projection is adequate for the SFA and popliteal. To image the tibial vessels, we recommend an ipsilateral view at 30° (Figure 25.19). For plantar vessels, a lateral view will identify the anterior and posterior circulation vessels. If an AP view is necessary, the foot is maintained in a natural orientation with slight dorsiflexion. The detector will be rotated with a cranial angle at 30°–40°. This view will show the distal DP artery as it connects into the tarsal branch (Figure 25.20). A lateral view of the foot will allow the operator to see the connection between the anterior circulation (i.e., dorsalis pedis) and the posterior circulation (i.e., lateral plantar artery) (Figure 25.21). This image is obtained by placing the detector in a parallel plane against the medial surface of the foot.

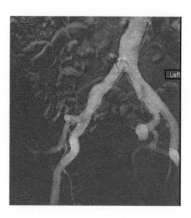

Figure 25.26 Road map feature allowing the operator to manipulate the wire and catheter to the desired location. The catheter shown is the Omni Flush catheter engaged in the right common iliac artery.

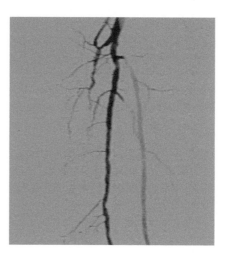

Figure 25.27 A common pattern of occlusion within the anterior tibial artery. It tends to occlude after its takeoff from the popliteal artery.

Disease patterns

There are few common disease patterns the operator must be ready to recognize. We will not be able to describe all disease patterns, but we focus on the most common ones. CIA disease tends to impact both ostia, requiring both vessels to be treated in the same setting. SFA's occlusion generally occurs after the takeoff of the profunda (Figure 25.17). The vessel usually reconstitutes at the proximal popliteal artery after the adducer's canal. Tibial vessels have significant variations in their disease patterns. A few are worth mentioning. Generally, the peroneal artery remains patent and supplies flow to the distal AT and PT through the anterior and posterior communicating arteries. The AT usually occludes after its takeoff. After the AT crosses the intraosseous membrane, it occludes after heading down in the anterior compartment. A common collateral that originates at the occlusion site is the posterior lateral branch. It tends to follow the trajectory of the native AT and can be mistaken as the AT proper (Figure 25.27).

CONCLUSION

Peripheral angiography remains the gold standard in defining peripheral anatomy and locating disease levels. The operator must be able to utilize the information obtained in junction with the clinical presentation. Establishing a uniform protocol that all providers follow will ensure the same quality of images obtained. Considering alternative access to perform angiography may offer valuable information that will aid the clinician in deciding the best course of therapy.

REFERENCES

1. Fowkes FG, et al. Comparison of global estimates of prevalence and risk factors for peripheral artery disease in 2000 and 2010: A systematic review and analysis. *Lancet* 2013;382(9901):1329–1340.

2. Patel MR, et al. Evaluation and treatment of patients with lower extremity peripheral artery disease: Consensus definitions from Peripheral Academic Research Consortium (PARC). *J Am Coll Cardiol* 2015;65(9):931–941.

3. Rooke TW, et al. Management of patients with peripheral artery disease (compilation of 2005 and 2011 ACCF/AHA Guideline Recommendations): A report of the American College of Cardiology Foundation/American Heart Association Task Force on Practice Guidelines. *J Am Coll Cardiol* 2013;61(14):1555–1570.

4. Leather RP, et al. Resurrection of the in situ saphenous vein bypass. 1000 cases later. *Ann Surg* 1988;208(4):435–442.

5. Taylor LM, Jr., et al. Present status of reversed vein bypass grafting: Five-year results of a modern series. *J Vasc Surg* 1990;11(2):193–205; discussion 205–206.

6. Jaff MR, et al. An update on methods for revascularization and expansion of the TASC lesion classification to include below-the-knee arteries: A supplement to the Inter-Society Consensus for the Management of Peripheral Arterial Disease (TASC II): The TASC Steering Committee. *Ann Vasc Dis* 2015;8(4):343–357.

7. Kurtkoti J, et al. Gadolinium and nephrogenic systemic fibrosis: Association or causation. *Nephrology (Carlton)* 2008;13(3):235–241.

8. Harvard BM, et al. Experimental studies in acute retroperitoneal carbon dioxide insufflation. *J Urol* 1959;81(3):481–485.

9. Hawkins IF, et al. Carbon dioxide in angiography to reduce the risk of contrast-induced nephropathy. *Radiol Clin North Am* 2009;47(5):813–825, v–vi.

10. Kadir S. Abdominal aorta and pelvis. In: Kadir S, editor, *Atlas of Normal and Variant Angiographic Anatomy*. Philadephia, PA: W.B. Saunders; 1991:123–160.

11. Spijkerboer AM, et al. Antegrade puncture of the femoral artery: Morphologic study. *Radiology* 1990;176(1):57–60.

12. Dauerman HL, et al. Vascular closure devices: The second decade. *J Am Coll Cardiol* 2007;50(17):1617–1626.

13. Mustapha JA, et al. Comparison between angiographic and arterial duplex ultrasound assessment of tibial arteries in patients with peripheral arterial disease: On behalf of the Joint Endovascular and Non-Invasive Assessment of LImb Perfusion (JENALI) Group. *J Invasive Cardiol* 2013;25(11):606–611.

26

Carotid and cerebral angiography

ROBERT D. SAFIAN

INTRODUCTION

Traditionally, cerebral angiography has been performed by neuroradiologists, but the application of percutaneous intervention for chronic brachiocephalic occlusive diseases and acute stroke has resulted in the increasing involvement of interventional cardiologists. Accordingly, cardiologists are expected to have an understanding of diseases that impact circulation to the brain, including diseases of the aortic arch, carotid artery, subclavian and vertebral artery, and intracranial diseases. This chapter discusses the purpose, specific goals, technique, and complications of catheter-based cerebral angiography. Subclavian artery (SCA) intervention, extracranial carotid and vertebral intervention, and intracranial and stroke intervention are covered in separate chapters.

PURPOSE OF ANGIOGRAPHY

Despite the availability of noninvasive techniques, such as duplex ultrasound, computerized tomography angiography (CTA), and magnetic resonance angiography (MRA), invasive angiography remains the gold standard for the diagnosis of extra- and intracranial arterial diseases because of superior spatial and temporal resolution. In general, invasive angiography may be recommended to clarify ambiguous results of noninvasive imaging, to obtain baseline angiographic evaluation prior to extra- or intracranial interventions, and to assess some patients with unusual diseases, such as vasculitis, fibromuscular dysplasia, dissection, and prior arterial bypass surgery.

While carotid duplex ultrasound is often used for the diagnosis of carotid and vertebral artery diseases, the quality of these studies is dependent on the acquisition technique and the skill of the physician interpreting the study. Some duplex studies are limited by vessel tortuosity, heavy calcification, or other difficult anatomy. Other noninvasive imaging procedures, such as CTA and MRA, provide excellent images of the extracranial circulation but can be limited by imaging artifacts. Overreliance on noninvasive imaging can result in misdiagnosis or the performance of unnecessary surgery.[1,2] It is not unusual for interventions scheduled purely on the basis of noninvasive imaging to be abandoned or modified once invasive angiographic images have been obtained.

Table 26.1 Specific goals of cerebral angiography

Aortic arch study
- Type of aortic arch (type 1, 2, and 3)
- Configuration of the great vessels (usual and anomalous)
- Extent of atherosclerosis

Extracranial circulation
- Intrathoracic segments
- Cervical segments
- Collaterals

Intracranial circulation
- Intracranial vertebral and carotid arteries
- Circle of Willis
- Intracranial branches
- Collaterals

SPECIFIC GOALS OF ANGIOGRAPHY

The specific goals of cerebral angiography are to provide a detailed assessment of the aortic arch, extracranial brachiocephalic vessels, intracranial circulation, and collaterals (Table 26.1).

Arch aortography

Every arch study must include an assessment of three key characteristics: the type of aortic arch, the configuration of the great vessels, and the extent of atherosclerosis. The aortic arch type depends on the relationship between the point of origin of the great vessels and the apex of the arch. Although several classifications are available, we rely on a modification of the Myla classification[3] (Figure 26.1): type 1, in which all three great vessels originate from the apex of the arch; type 2, in which the first two great vessels (usually the innominate artery [IA] and left common carotid artery [CCA]) originate below the apex of the arch; and type 3, in which all three great vessels originate below the apex of the arch. Regardless of which classification is used, the goal is to distinguish "simple" (type 1) from "complex" (type 2 or 3) arches. Simple arches are conducive to selective cannulation of the great vessels from a femoral approach, whereas complex arches make selective cannulation more difficult due to aortic uncoiling, tortuosity, and the angle of origin of the great vessels. Aging itself, as well as the long-term consequences of atherosclerosis and hypertension, lead to elongation of the aortic arch, superior displacement of the aortic knob, inferior and posterior displacement of the great vessels, and elongation and sharp angulation of the left CCA (Figure 26.1). Together, these morphological changes substantially increase the technical difficulties of selective cannulation and angiography, and may partially explain the increased risk of carotid interventions in octogenarians.

In contrast to the arch type, arch configuration refers to the usual or anomalous origin of the great vessels. In the usual configuration, the IA, left CCA, and the left SCA originate as the first, second, and third great vessels from the arch, respectively (65% of individuals) (Figure 26.1). Anomalous configurations

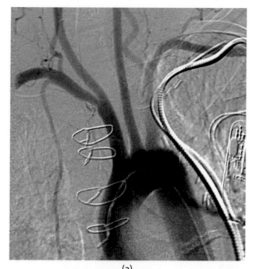

(a)

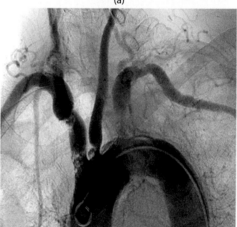

(b)

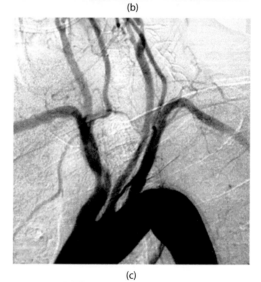

(c)

Figure 26.1 Classification of the types of aortic arch. Type 1, in which all three great vessels originate from the apex of the arch **(a)**. Type 2, in which the innominate artery and left common carotid artery originate below the apex of the arch. Note the extent of atherosclerosis, ulceration, and stenosis in the origin of all three great vessels **(b)**. Type 3, in which all three great vessels originate below the apex of the arch **(c)**.

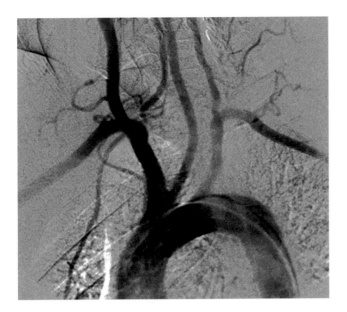

Figure 26.2 Bovine configuration of the aortic arch.

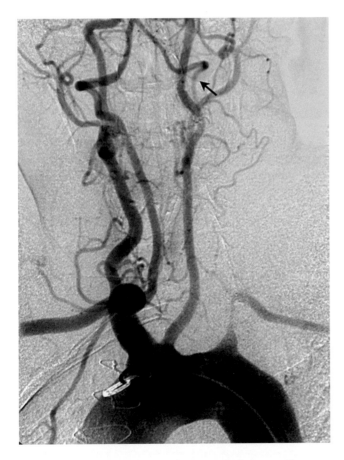

Figure 26.3 Anomalous configuration of the aortic arch in which the innominate artery and left common carotid artery share a common infundibulum (bovine configuration). Note the severe stenosis of the left subclavian artery and retrograde filling of the left vertebral artery (*arrow*) from the right vertebral artery (subclavian steal).

include common origin of the IA and left CCA (the so-called bovine configuration, 25%) (Figures 26.2 and 26.3), origin of the left CCA from the proximal IA (7%), separate origin of the left vertebral artery (VA) from the arch (0.5%), separate origin of the right SCA from the distal arch (arteria lusoria, 0.6%), and origin of the left CCA and left SCA from a left IA (1%). A true bovine configuration is extremely rare and consists of a single IA that trifurcates into a right SCA, a single CCA, and a left SCA; the single CCA divides into right and left CCA.

The extent of arch disease should be described in detail, including the presence of stenosis, degree of calcification, and tortuosity, as well as the presence of aneurysm or ulceration. In general, it is important to perform arch aortography prior to selective angiography, since the arch type, arch configuration, and degree of atherosclerosis will influence the need for catheter manipulation and catheter selection.

While arch aortography details the anatomy of the proximal intrathoracic brachiocephalic circulation (Figure 26.1), selective angiography is preferred for more detailed assessment of the intrathoracic, cervical, and intracranial segments (Table 26.2). The purpose of selective angiography is to assess the presence, location, severity, and length of stenosis; normal reference vessel dimensions; morphological features of the stenosis (calcification, thrombus, ulceration, angulation); vessel tortuosity proximal and distal to the stenosis; patency of the major branches; and the integrity of the intracranial circulation and collateral pathways. Clinically, selective SCA angiography is often performed to assess SCA or internal mammary artery (IMA) graft patency, symptoms of vertebrobasilar insufficiency, or arm claudication. Subclavian arteriography should be performed in all patients who require cardiac catheterization after IMA bypass surgery (Figure 26.4). Subclavian arteriography during coronary angiography prior to coronary artery bypass surgery is reasonable in patients with known occlusive disease of the brachiocephalic circulation, cervical or supraclavicular bruits, discrepant blood pressure between both arms, symptoms suggestive of vertebrobasilar insufficiency, or arm claudication.[4]

In most situations, selective SCA angiography provides sufficient images of the SCA and VA without selective VA angiography, particularly since most VA stenoses are located at the VA origin. In selected cases, particularly if VA intervention is

Table 26.2 Goals of selective cerebral angiography

Vessel assessment
- Proximal and distal tortuosity
- Patency of major branches

Stenosis assessment
- Stenosis severity
- Cause of stenosis (atherosclerosis, fibromuscular dysplasia, and dissection)
- Stenosis morphology
- Normal reference vessel dimensions

Integrity of intracranial circulation
- Circle of Willis
- Collateral pathways

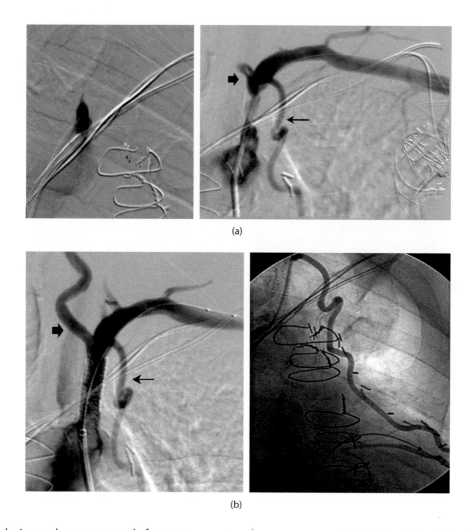

(a)

(b)

Figure 26.4 Subclavian and coronary steal after coronary artery bypass surgery. **(a)** Selective left subclavian arteriogram (30° RAO projection) demonstrates total occlusion of the left subclavian artery, and no antegrade filling of the left vertebral artery or the left internal mammary artery (LIMA) graft to the LAD (left). After initial angioplasty, there is high-grade residual stenosis extending up to the origin of the left vertebral artery (right). Note the lucency at the origin of the left vertebral artery (*arrowhead*), which represents bidirectional blood flow and should not be mistaken for thrombus. **(b)** After successful stenting, there is prompt antegrade flow in the left subclavian and vertebral arteries (left, *arrowhead*), as well as the internal mammary bypass graft (*arrow*). Selective angiography demonstrates patency of the LIMA graft to the LAD (right). LAD, left anterior descending; RAO, right anterior oblique.

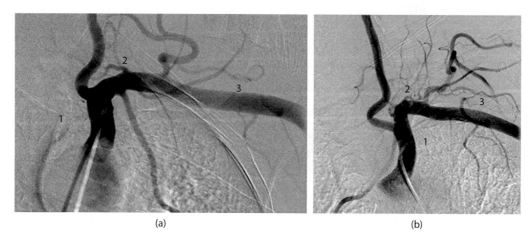

(a)   (b)

Figure 26.5 Selective angiography of the left subclavian artery. RAO projection **(a)**, LAO projection **(b)**. The proximal (1), mid (2), and distal segments (3) are evident; the axillary artery is not shown. LAO, left anterior oblique; RAO, right anterior oblique.

performed, selective VA angiography is required. The SCA is considered in four sections (Figure 26.5): proximal (origin of SCA to origin of VA), mid (segment of SCA involving the origin of the VA, IMA, and thyrocervical trunk), distal (segment of SCA distal to thyrocervical trunk and extending up to the axillary artery), and the axillary artery (Table 26.3). Although angiography of the brachial artery circulation is not routine during arch and cerebral angiography, it is important to have an understanding of the arterial circulation to the arm and hand. Selective carotid angiography is performed most often to assess symptomatic or asymptomatic carotid artery atherosclerosis (Figure 26.6). Less commonly, carotid angiography is performed to evaluate the patency of a carotid-SCA bypass, fibromuscular dysplasia, or spontaneous carotid dissection (Figure 26.7). The carotid artery is considered in four segments (Table 26.3): the CCA (intrathoracic and cervical regions), the

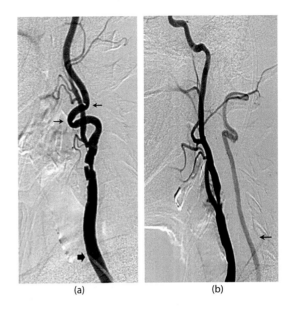

(a) (b)

Figure 26.6 Selective bilateral carotid artery angiography in a 68-year-old woman with right hemispheric transient ischemic attack. Results of a carotid duplex ultrasound study were ambiguous due to ischemic cardiomyopathy, low cardiac output, and aortic valve disease. Selective left carotid angiography **(a)** demonstrated an unexpected severe stenosis in the distal common carotid artery (CCA) with prominent ulceration and eccentricity. Note the catheter position in the mid-CCA (*arrowhead*), moderate disease, and prominent tortuosity of the cervical and petrous segments of the left internal carotid artery (ICA) (*arrows*). Selective right carotid angiography **(b)** demonstrated severe ulcerated stenosis of the ICA with calcification, later treated by successful carotid artery stenting with embolic protection. Note that the diagnostic catheter is in the proximal right CCA, resulting in reflux of contrast into the right subclavian and vertebral arteries (*arrow*).

Table 26.3 Sections of the carotid and subclavian arteries

Section of the subclavian artery
- Proximal (origin of SCA to origin of VA)
- Mid (SCA involving VA, IMA, and TCT)
- Distal (Distal to TCT to AA)
- Axillary (AA)

Sections of the carotid artery
- CCA (intrathoracic and cervical)
- ECA
- Cervical ICA
- Intracranial circulation (ICA, MCA, ACA, and PCOM)

Note: AA, axillary artery; ACA, anterior cerebral artery; CCA, common carotid artery; ECA, external carotid artery; ICA, internal carotid artery; IMA, internal mammary artery; MCA, middle cerebral artery; PCOM, posterior communicating artery; SCA, subclavian artery; TCT, thyrocervical trunk; VA, vertebral artery.

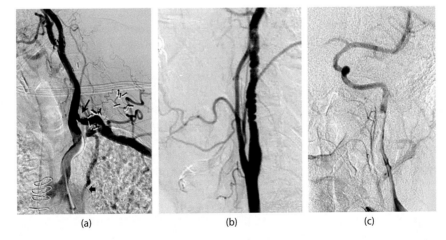

(a) (b) (c)

Figure 26.7 Selective left carotid artery angiogram **(a)** in a 72-year-old woman with severe stenosis in the proximal carotid-to-subclavian bypass (*arrow*), which explained a loud supraclavicular bruit, thrill, and discrepant blood pressures in both arms. Selective left carotid artery angiogram **(b)** in a young woman with fibromuscular dysplasia (FMD). Although the angiogram is highly reliable for identifying FMD, it is less reliable for assessing stenosis severity. Note the beaded aneurysms characteristic of medial fibroplasia. She did not have intracranial aneurysms. Selective left carotid artery angiogram **(c)** in a young woman who presented with severe neck pain and partial Horner's syndrome. Note the long spiral spontaneous dissection of the cervical and petrous segments of the internal carotid artery.

external carotid artery (ECA), the cervical internal carotid artery (ICA), and the intracranial circulation (intracranial ICA, middle cerebral artery [MCA], anterior cerebral artery [ACA], and posterior communicating artery [PCOM]).

SPECIFIC VASCULAR TERRITORIES

External carotid artery

After its intrathoracic origin, the CCA bifurcates into the ECA and ICA at the level of the C3–C5 interspaces. The ECA is important because it supplies blood flow to most extracranial structures in the head and neck (Figure 26.8), provides numerous anastomoses to the ICA and VA (Table 26.4), and may supply blood to intracranial neoplasms and vascular malformations. Some of these diseases may be outside the expertise of interventional cardiologists, but may be encountered during angiography for other reasons. For physicians interested in carotid artery stenting, the anatomy of the ECA is important for use of proximal embolic protection devices. Branches of the ECA include five anterior and three posterior arteries, which are visualized best in the lateral projection. Variations in the origin, size, and distribution of ECA branches are fairly common (Figure 26.9), but anomalies of the ECA are rare.

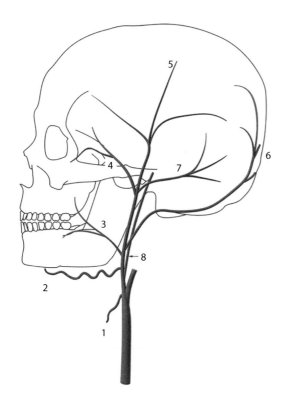

Figure 26.8 Branches of the external carotid artery. 1, superior thyroid artery; 2, lingual artery; 3, facial artery; 4, maxillary artery; 5, superior temporal artery; 6, occipital artery; 7, posterior auricular artery; 8, ascending pharyngeal artery. Note that the internal carotid artery has been cut away for clarity.

Table 26.4 Major anastomoses of the external carotid artery

ECA branch	Destination
Superior thyroid artery	SCA[a]
Ascending pharyngeal artery[b]	ICA, ECA, SCA, VA
Lingual artery	ECA
Facial artery	ICA[c], ECA
Occipital artery[b]	ECA, SCA, VA
Posterior auricular artery[b]	ECA
Superior temporal artery	ICA[c], ECA
Inferior maxillary artery	ICA, ECA

Note: ECA, external carotid artery; ICA, internal carotid artery; SCA, subclavian artery; VA, vertebral artery.
[a] Collateral to ipsilateral SCA via inferior thyroid artery and thyrocervical trunk, or to contralateral SCA via opposite superior thyroid artery.
[b] These branches usually have posterior origin from the ECA.
[c] Via ophthalmic artery.

Internal carotid artery

In most patients, the ICA has no extracranial branches and is longer than the ECA. Aberrant origin of the occipital artery or ascending pharyngeal artery from the ICA is rare. The ICA provides most of the blood flow to the cerebral hemispheres, and vascular diseases of the ICA and its branches are important causes of serious morbidity, disability, and mortality. There are several classifications of the segments of ICA (Table 26.5), but we prefer a simplified classification based on cervical (extracranial), petrous (intracranial but extradural), cavernous (within the cavernous sinus), and cerebral (intradural) segments (Figures 26.10 and 26.11). The cervical segment of the ICA is the most common site for carotid atherosclerosis and consists of the carotid bulb and the ascending ICA (Figure 26.12). The proximal cervical ICA is anatomically related to the cervical sympathetic ganglion, the vagus nerve, and the hypoglossal nerve, which may explain vasovagal and vasodepressor responses during ICA stimulation. The petrous segment of the ICA has a characteristic appearance that includes a vertical segment and a sharp horizontal segment (upside-down "L" or genu), whereas the cavernous segment has two sharp genus (short vertical segment, longer horizontal segment, and a short vertical segment) (Figures 26.10 and 26.11). Operators who perform carotid artery stenting will commonly position a distal embolic protection device in the upper cervical segment and the guidewire tip will often reside in the petrous segment, avoiding the cavernous and cerebral segments (Figure 26.12).

Circle of Willis

It is important to have an understanding of the normal anatomy, common anatomic variations, and vascular anomalies of the circle of Willis. The circle of Willis provides blood flow to the anterior, posterior, left, and right portions of the

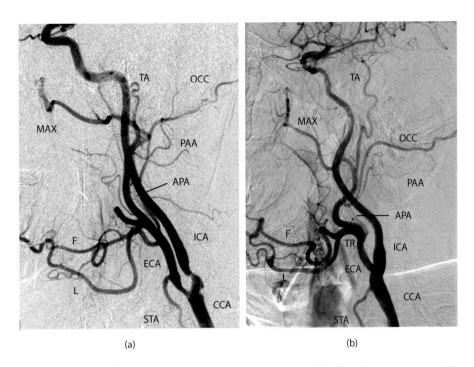

(a)　　　　　　　　　　　　(b)

Figure 26.9 Selective angiography of the left carotid artery demonstrating the distal common carotid artery (CCA), internal carotid artery (ICA), and branches of the external carotid artery (ECA). **(a)** Note the severe stenoses at the origin of the ICA and ECA. **(b)** Note the variation in the ECA in which the lingual and facial arteries originate from a common trunk (TR), rather than as separate branches from the ECA. APA, ascending pharyngeal artery; F, facial artery; L, lingual artery; MAX, maxillary artery; OCC, occipital artery; PAA, posterior auricular artery; STA, superior thyroid artery; TA, temporal artery.

Table 26.5 Cervical and intracranial segments of the internal carotid artery

Region	Segment	Description	Notable branches
Cervical	C1 Cervical	Carotid bulb and ascending cervical ICA (extracranial)	None
Petrous	C2 Petrous	ICA contained within petrous bone; characteristic genu	Vidian artery, carticotympanic artery
	C3 Lacerum	ICA travels above FL between petrous bone and PL ligament (extradural, intracranial)	None
Cavernous	C4 Cavernous[a]	Only artery that courses through a vein (cavernous sinus); characteristic genu (extradural, intracranial)	Posterior trunk,[b] lateral trunk, capsular arteries (medial)
	C5 Clinoid[a]	Short wedge of ICA in terminal cavernous sinus (interdural)	None
Cerebral	C6 Opthalmic[a]	ICA exits cavernous sinus (intradural)	Opthalmic artery, superior hypophyseal artery
	C7 Communicating	Origin of PCOM to ACA/MCA bifurcation	PCOM, anterior choroidal artery

Note: ACA, anterior cerebral artery; FL, foramen lacerum; ICA, internal carotid artery; MCA, middle cerebral artery; PL, petrolingual ligament; PCOM, posterior communicating artery.

[a] C4, C5, C6, carotid siphon.
[b] May cause a pituitary blush (meningohypophyseal artery).

brain, and is a key source of collateral blood flow in occlusive diseases of intra- and extracranial circulation. A complete circle of Willis is present in 50% of individuals and consists of a nine-sided polygon (nonagon) and the basilar artery (Figure 26.13). The complete "circle" includes the anterior communicating artery (ACOM), two precommunicating anterior cerebral arteries (A1), two intracranial ICAs, two precommunicating posterior cerebral arteries (P1), and two PCOMs (Table 26.6). The postcommunicating anterior (A2) and posterior (P2) cerebral arteries and the MCA are not part of the circle of Willis. The entire circle of Willis is rarely identified during a single-vessel angiogram, so visualization of the individual components depends on the extent of the cerebral angiogram.

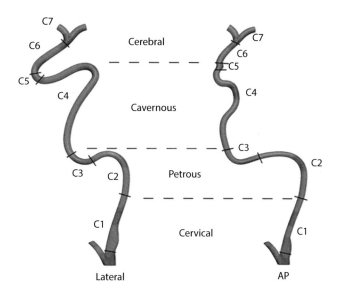

Figure 26.10 Classification of the segments of the internal carotid artery in the lateral and anteroposterior projections. The simplified classification designates four segments, including cervical (C1), petrous (C2, C3), cavernous (C4, C5), and cerebral (C6, C7) segments.

Anatomic variations in the circle of Willis are very common (found in approximately 50%), particularly aplasia or hypoplasia of the PCOM and P1 (Figure 26.14), and may impair potential collateral pathways. Individuals with ipsilateral aplasia or severe hypoplasia of A1 and P1 have an isolated cerebral hemisphere and cannot receive collateral flow from the vertebrobasilar system or from the contralateral ICA; these patients are especially prone to cerebral ischemia if they develop proximal occlusive disease. Anomalies of the circle of Willis and other intracranial arteries are uncommon. However, duplication and fenestration of intracranial vessels are associated with intracranial aneurysms and arteriovenous malformations (AVM) (Table 26.7).

Anterior cerebral artery

The ACA and its branches supply the majority of blood flow to the anterior, medial, and anterobasal portions of the brain (Figures 26.15 through 26.20). The most common classification of the ACA includes three segments (A1, A2, A3), which provide perforating and cortical branches to the brain (Table 26.8). Perforating branches usually arise from A1 and A2 (basal ganglia, internal capsule, corpus callosum) and cortical branches usually arise from A2 (ventral medial frontal lobe) and A3 (corpus callosum, medial cerebral hemisphere, cortical convexity) (Table 26.9). Most of the penetrating and cortical branches can be readily identified by selective ipsilateral carotid angiography in anteroposterior (AP)-cranial and lateral projections. The pericallosal artery represents the distal continuation of the main ACA (Figure 26.19). Aplasia or hypoplasia of A1 is observed in 12% of individuals, but

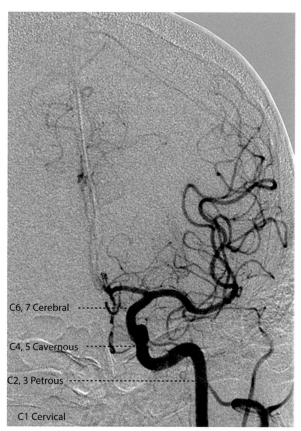

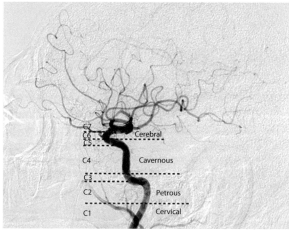

Figure 26.11 Selective angiography of the left internal carotid artery (ICA) in the anteroposterior (top) and lateral projection (bottom). Note that the segments of the ICA are easier to discern in the lateral projection due to less foreshortening of the cavernous segment.

other anatomic variations are rare. Two ACA anomalies—infraoptic origin and azygous ACA—are associated with intracranial aneurysms and AVM, but bihemispheric ACA is not (Table 26.7).

Middle cerebral artery

The MCA and its branches supply most of the blood flow to the superior, lateral, and central portions of the brain

(Figures 26.15 and 26.17 through 26.21). The most common classification of the MCA includes four segments (M1, M2, M3, M4); M2 and M3 are conduit segments between M1 and M4, and usually do not provide significant branches (Table 26.10). Perforating branches arise from M1 (lateral lenticulostriate branches to basal ganglia and internal capsule), and cortical branches arise from M1 (anterior temporal artery to anterior and inferior temporal lobe) and from M4 (supplying large sections of the temporal, frontal, parietal, and occipital lobes) (Tables 26.11 and 26.12; Figures 26.15 and 26.21). A common anatomic variation is early MCA bifurcation (20% of individuals), but other variations are rare. MCA anomalies such as fenestrations,

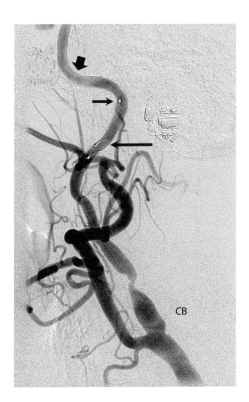

Figure 26.12 Selective angiography of the left carotid artery during carotid artery stenting. Note the severe stenosis in the proximal internal carotid artery (ICA) just distal to the carotid bulb (CB). A distal embolic protection device is positioned in the upper cervical segment (*large arrow*), and the guidewire tip is in the proximal petrous segment of the ICA (*short arrow*).

Table 26.6 Components of the complete circle of Willis[a]

Component	Number
ACOM	1[a]
A1	2[a]
ICA	2[a]
PCOM	2[a]
P1	2[a]
BA	1

Note: ACOM, anterior communicating artery; A1, precommunicating anterior cerebral artery; BA, basilar artery; ICA, distal intracranial internal carotid artery; PCOM, posterior communicating artery; P1, precommunicating posterior cerebral artery.

[a] Nine-sided polygon plus the BA.

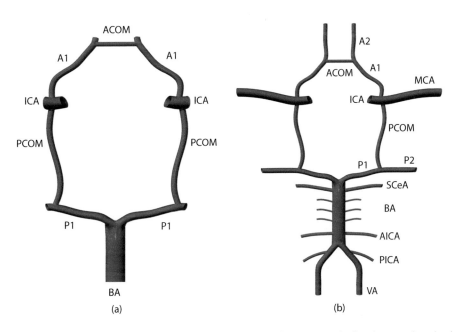

Figure 26.13 The circle of Willis. **(a)** A complete circle of Willis is actually a nine-sided polygon plus the basilar artery. **(b)** A complete circle of Willis with associated major branches. See text for details. ACA, anterior cerebral artery; ACOM, anterior communicating artery; AICA, anterior inferior cerebellar artery; A1, precommunicating ACA; A2, postcommunicating ACA; BA, basilar artery; ICA, internal carotid artery; MCA, middle cerebral artery; PCA, posterior cerebral artery; PCOM, posterior communicating artery; P1, precommunicating PCA; P2, postcommunicating PCA; PICA, posterior inferior cerebellar artery; SCeA, superior cerebellar artery; VA, vertebral artery.

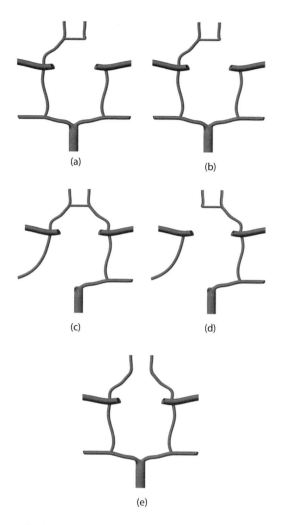

Figure 26.14 Common variations in the circle of Willis. **(a)** Aplasia or severe hypoplasia of P1 (precommunicating posterior cerebral artery [PCA]); **(b)** aplasia or severe hypoplasia of A1 (precommunicating anterior cerebral artery [ACA]); **(c)** aplasia or severe hypoplasia of P1 and persistent fetal PCA; **(d)** isolated cerebral hemisphere, due to aplasia or severe hypoplasia of A1 and P1 (with persistent fetal PCA); **(e)** aplasia or severe hypoplasia of the anterior communicating artery (ACOM).

duplications, and accessory MCA are associated with intracranial aneurysm and AVM (Table 26.7).

Vertebrobasilar circulation

The vertebrobasilar system provides virtually all of the blood flow to the posterior circulation, including the pons, medulla, midbrain, and cerebellum (Figures 26.15 through 26.17). The vertebrobasilar system consists of extracranial (vertebral arteries) and intracranial (vertebral arteries, basilar artery, and posterior cerebral arteries [PCAs]) components (Table 26.13). The most common classification of the VA includes four segments (V1, V2, V3, V4) depending on the relationship to the cervical transverse foramina and foramen magnum

(Table 26.14; Figures 26.22 and 26.23). Cervical branches originate from the V1 segment (branches to the spinal cord and skeletal muscles of the head and neck); meningeal branches originate from V2 and V3; and intracranial branches originate from V4 (branches to the cerebellum, pons, medulla, and spinal cord). Anatomic variations in the size of the VA are common; although the left VA is large and dominant in most individuals, the right VA is dominant in 25% of cases (Table 26.7). The most common VA anomaly directly originates from the arch rather than from the SCA, which occurs in 5% of individuals. Although anomalous origin of the VA is not associated with serious intracranial diseases, duplications and fenestrations of the VA are associated with fused vertebrae, intracranial aneurysms, and AVM (Table 26.7).

The basilar artery is a large midline artery that is formed by the merging of the left and right VA, and extends to the bifurcation of both PCAs (Figures 26.13, 26.16, 26.17, 26.22, and 26.23). Although only 3–4 mm in diameter and 30 mm in length, the basilar artery has several important branches, including pontine perforators and two of three major cerebellar arteries (the anterior inferior cerebellar artery [AICA], and the superior cerebellar artery) (Table 26.13; Figures 26.16, 26.17, and 26.23). The third major artery to the cerebellum (posterior inferior cerebellar artery [PICA]) is a branch of the VA. Anatomic variations of the basilar artery are not common, but a common AICA-PICA trunk occurs in 10% of individuals. Basilar artery fenestrations and duplications are associated with intracranial aneurysms (Table 26.7).

Posterior cerebral artery

The PCA and its branches supply most of the blood flow to the posterior and posterobasal portions of the brain and brainstem (Table 26.15; Figures 26.15 through 26.17 and 26.24). The most common classification of the PCA includes four segments (P1, P2, P3, P4), which provide perforating branches, branches to the choroid plexus and ventricles, and cortical branches to the brain (Table 26.16). Perforating branches usually arise from P1 and P2, providing blood flow to the internal capsule, basal ganglia, and midbrain; choroidal branches arise from P2 and provide blood flow to the choroid plexus and basal ganglia; and cortical branches arise from P2 (providing blood flow to the temporal lobe) and P4 (providing blood flow to the temporal, parietal, and occipital lobes) (Table 26.16; Figure 26.24). Normal variations of the PCA are quite common, including P1 hypoplasia in 20% of individuals, which is associated with persistent fetal origin of the PCA (Table 26.7; Figure 26.25). Anomalies of the PCA are quite rare.

Intracranial aneurysms and other conditions

Cardiologists are rarely involved in the angiographic evaluation and treatment of patients with intracranial aneurysms or tumors. However, aneurysms may be identified incidentally

Table 26.7 Normal variations and anomalies of the cerebral artery circulation

Vessel	Variation	Incidence (%)	Anomaly	Incidence (%)
VA	Right dominant	25	Aortic origin	5
	AICA–PICA trunk	10	Fenestration[a]	<1
			Duplication[a]	<1
			PICA from V_1	10
BA	–		Fenestration[a]	<1
			Duplication	<1
PCA	P1—hypoplasia/aplasia[b]	20	–	
MCA	Early bifurcation	20	Accessory MCA[a]	2
			Fenestration[a]	<1
ACA	A1—hypoplasia/aplasia	12	Duplication[a]	2
			Infraoptic origin[a]	<1
			Bihemispheric ACA	4
			Azygous ACA[a]	2
PCOM	Hypoplasia/aplasia	5	–	
ACOM	Hypoplasia/aplasia	5	–	

Note: ACA, anterior cerebral artery; ACOM, anterior communicating artery; AICA, anterior inferior cerebellar artery; AVM, arteriovenous malformation; BA, basilar artery; MCA, middle cerebral artery; PCA, posterior cerebral artery; PCOM, posterior communicating artery; PICA, posterior inferior cerebellar artery; VA, vertebral artery.

[a] Associated with intracranial aneurysm and AVM.
[b] Associated with persistent fetal origin of PCA.

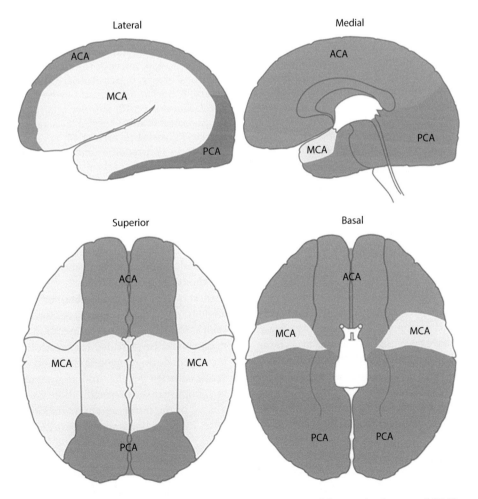

Figure 26.15 Vascular distributions of the anterior cerebral artery (ACA), middle cerebral artery (MCA), and posterior cerebral artery (PCA), shown in the lateral, medial, superior, and basal views.

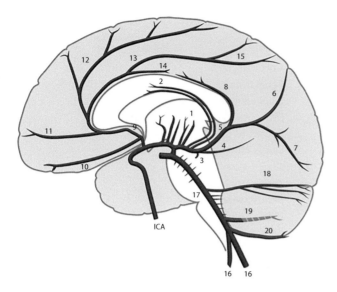

Figure 26.16 Intracranial circulation, medial view. Note that in this view, about one-third of blood flow is derived from the vertebrobasilar system, posterior cerebral artery (PCA), and their branches (1–8, 16–20), and two-thirds from the ACA and its branches (9–15). 1, Perforator branches; 2, choroidal and ventricular branches; 3, anterior temporal artery (cut away); 4, posterior temporal artery; 5, medical occipital artery; 6, parieto-occipital artery; 7, calcarine artery; 8, splenial artery; 9, postcommunicating ACA; 10, orbitofrontal artery; 11, frontopolar artery; 12, callosomarginal artery; 13, pericallosal artery; 14, splenial artery; 15, parietal artery; 16, vertebral artery; 17, basilar artery and perforators; 18, superior cerebellar artery; 19, anterior inferior cerebellar artery; 20, posterior inferior cerebellar artery. ACA, anterior cerebral artery; ICA, internal carotid artery.

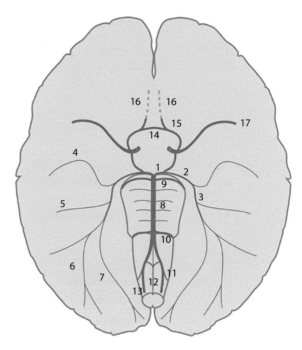

Figure 26.17 Intracranial circulation, basal view. Note that in this view, about 50% of blood flow is derived from the vertebrobasilar system, posterior cerebral artery, and their branches (1–13); 35% from the anterior cerebral artery and its branches (14–16); and 15% from the middle cerebral artery and its branches (17). 1, Precommunicating PCA; 2, postcommunicating PCA; 3, P4 (calcarine) segment of PCA; 4, anterior temporal artery; 5, posterior temporal artery; 6, parieto-occipital artery; 7, calcarine artery; 8, basilar artery and perforators; 9, superior cerebellar artery; 10, anterior inferior cerebellar artery; 11, posterior inferior cerebellar artery; 12, anterior spinal artery; 13, vertebral artery; 14, anterior communicating artery; 15, precommunicating ACA; 16, orbitofrontal artery; 17, middle cerebral artery.

during cerebral angiography for other reasons (Figure 26.20), so cardiologists should have an understanding of the incidence, distribution, and outcomes of intracranial aneurysms (Table 26.17). Other incidental findings might include neovascular tumor blush, an arteriovenous fistula (AVF), or an AVM.

ANGIOGRAPHIC TECHNIQUE

Arterial access

Cerebral angiography and intervention are generally performed from a femoral artery approach, but radial,[5] brachial,[6] and ulnar[7] approaches have been used when femoral access is difficult. Local anesthesia is achieved with 1% lidocaine, and light conscious sedation may be employed with midazolam (1 mg intravenously). We recommend a 5-Fr sheath and 5-Fr catheters for diagnostic angiography, and intra-arterial heparin (1,500–2,000 IU) in all patients (Table 26.18).

Pressure monitoring and imaging

As is true for left heart catheterization and coronary angiography, we recommend intra-arterial pressure monitoring from the catheter tip using a standard three- or four-port

manifold (Table 26.18). Meticulous attention must be paid to monitoring catheter tip pressure during cannulation of the great vessels. If a dampened pressure waveform is observed, the catheter should be repositioned. Catheters that cannot be aspirated should never be flushed in the arch or great vessels, but should be removed and reflushed outside the patient. The highest quality images are obtained with digital subtraction angiography (DSA), a power injector, and isosmolar contrast such as iodixanol. Patient cooperation is essential, so instructions should be provided on breath-hold and avoidance of movement during angiography. Hand injections are useful to verify catheter position and alignment, but generally result in suboptimal vessel opacification, contrast streaming, poor images of the intracranial circulation, and higher radiation doses to the angiographer (Figure 26.26).[8]

Arch study

A formal arch aortogram (40° left anterior oblique [LAO]) should be performed in all patients unless the arch type and configuration have been previously defined by noninvasive

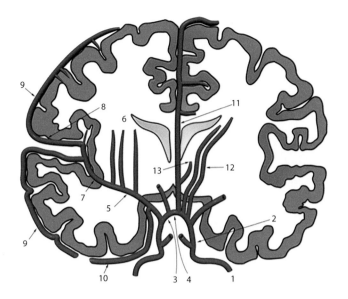

Figure 26.18 Intracranial circulation (anterior, coronal view), including a portion of the circle of Willis (1–4). The left side demonstrates the middle cerebral artery (MCA) and its branches (5–10), and the right side demonstrates the anterior cerebral artery (ACA) and its branches (3, 11–13). ACA is cut away on the left, MCA is cut away on the right. 1, Internal carotid artery; 2, posterior communicating artery; 3, precommunicating ACA; 4, anterior communicating artery; 5, M1 (horizontal) segment of MCA; 6, lateral lenticulostriate branches; 7, M2 (insular) segment of MCA; 8, M3 (opercular) segment of MCA; 9, M4 (cortical) segments of MCA; 10, anterior temporal artery; 11, postcommunicating ACA; 12, medial lenticulostriate branches; 13, recurrent artery of Heubner.

or invasive imaging (Table 26.18; Figures 26.1 through 26.3). For patients who require only left SCA arteriography to evaluate patency of an IMA graft, a formal arch study may not be necessary. Several catheters may be used for arch aortography, but the ones used most often are the pigtail and tennis racquet catheters (Figure 26.27). The sidehole arrangement on the tennis racquet catheter minimizes contrast in the ascending aorta and promotes contrast flow from the catheter shaft directly into the great vessels. High-quality DSA images can be obtained by instructing the patient to turn the head to the left, and by injecting 25–30 cc contrast over 2 s (600 pounds per square inch [psi]), with a field of view of 34–42 cm (Table 26.18).

Selective cannulation

Several catheters and techniques are available for selective cannulation of the great vessels, and it is useful to become familiar with more than one (Tables 26.19 and 26.20). The arch study serves as a road map before selective cannulation and minimizes the need for catheter manipulation in the arch. If an arch study is not available, the tracheal air stripe (40° LAO projection) is a useful landmark for the origin of the great vessels; in many patients, the IA is just proximal (left), the left CCA is in the middle, and the left SCA is just distal (right) to the air stripe (Figure 26.28). If rapid cannulation cannot be achieved, it is better to perform an arch study than to persist with prolonged catheter manipulation. The most common reasons for failed selective cannulation of a great vessel are complex arch configurations and anomalous origins; both are readily identified by an arch study.

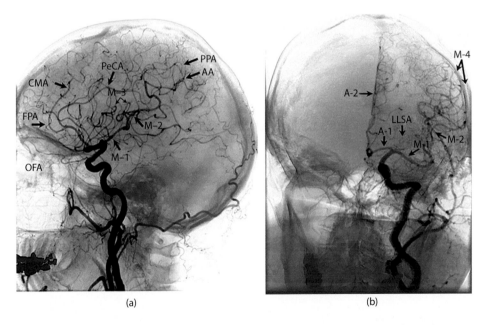

(a) (b)

Figure 26.19 Selective angiography of the left carotid artery, demonstrating the intracranial circulation in the lateral (a) and anteroposterior (b) projections. Note that the branches of the anterior cerebral artery (ACA) and middle cerebral artery (MCA) are superimposed in the lateral projection. A1, precommunicating ACA; A2, postcommunicating ACA; AA, angular artery (M4 segment of MCA); CMA, callosomarginal artery; FPA, frontopolar artery; LLSA, lateral lenticulostriate branches; M1, horizontal segment of MCA; M2, insular segment of MCA; M3, opercular segment of MCA; OFA, orbitofrontal artery; PeCA, pericallosal artery; PPA, posterior parietal artery (M4 segment of MCA).

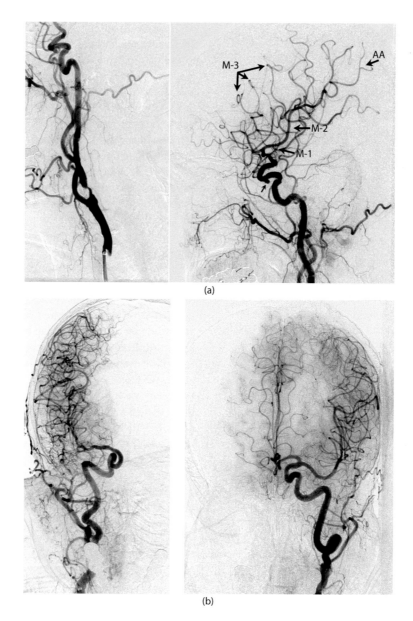

(a)

(b)

Figure 26.20 Selective angiography of both carotid arteries and intracranial circulation. **(a)** Selective right carotid angiography demonstrates the right internal carotid artery (ICA) (left 40° LAO projection) and right intracranial circulation (right, lateral projection). Note the severe stenosis in the ICA, tortuosity of the petrous and cavernous ICA, absence of opacification of the right anterior cerebral artery (ACA) and its branches (see Figure 26.19 for comparison), and a small aneurysm of the cavernous segment (*arrow*). **(b)** Composite of selective right (left) and left (right) intracranial circulation in the AP-cranial projection, confirms absence of opacification of the right ACA (see Figure 26.19 for comparison), and extensive left-to-right crossover via the ACA and anterior communicating artery. AA, angular artery; AP, anteroposterior; LAO, left anterior oblique; MCA, middle cerebral artery; M1, horizontal segment of MCA; M2, insular segment of MCA; M3, opercu-

Table 26.8 Classification of the anterior cerebral artery

Segment	Region	Branches	Projection
A_1	Horizontal (precommunicating; horizontal segment of ACA between ICA and ACOM)	Perforating	AP-C
A_2	Vertical (postcommunicating; vertical segment of ACA after ACOM)	Perforating and cortical	AP-C, LAT
A_3	Callosal (distal segment of ACA that extends around corpus callosum)	Cortical	LAT

Note: ACA, anterior cerebral artery; ACOM, anterior communicating artery; AP-C, anteroposterior with cranial angulation; ICA, internal carotid artery; LAT, lateral.

lar segment of MCA.

Table 26.9 Perforating and cortical branches of the anterior cerebral artery

Vessel	Perforating branch	Territory	Cortical branch	Territory
A_1[a]	MLSA RAH[b] Callosal	Basal ganglia, internal capsule, corpus callosum	–	–
A_2	RAH[a,b]	Basal ganglia, internal capsule	Orbitofrontal[c] Frontopolar[c]	Ventral, medial frontal lobe, and olfactory bulb
A_3[c]	–	–	Pericallosal Callosomarginal Parietal Splenial	Corpus callosum, 2/3 of medial cerebral hemisphere, strip of cortex over superior convexity

Note: ACA, anterior cerebral artery; AP-C, anteroposterior with cranial angulation; LAT, lateral; MLSA, medial lenticulostriate arteries; RAH, recurrent artery of Heubner.
[a] Best seen in AP-C projection.
[b] RAH originates from A_1 in 40% of patients, RAH from A_2 in 60% of patients.
[c] Best seen in LAT projection.

Table 26.10 Classification of the middle cerebral artery

Segment	Region	Branches	Projection
M_1	Horizontal (ICA bifurcation to genu)	Perforating and cortical	AP-C
M_2[a]	Insular (superior course after genu)	None	AP-C, LAT
M_3[a]	Opercular (top of insula to lateral end of Sylvian fissure)	None	AP-C, LAT
M_4	Cortical (lateral surface of Sylvian fissure to cortical surface of cerebral hemisphere)	Cortical	AP-C, LAT

Note: AP-C, anteroposterior with cranial angulation; ICA, internal carotid artery; LAT, lateral. M_2[a] and M_3[a] are conduit vessels between M_1 and M_4, and do not have major penetrating or cortical branches.

Table 26.11 Perforating and cortical branches of the middle cerebral artery

Vessel	Perforating branch	Territory	Cortical branch	Territory
M_1	LLSA[a]	Basal ganglia	ATA[a,b]	Anterior, medial, and inferior
M_4	–	–	See Table 26.12	See Table 26.12

Note: AP-C, anteroposterior with cranial angulations; ATA, anterior temporal artery; LAT, lateral; LLSA, lateral lenticulostriate arteries.
[a] Best seen in AP-C projection.
[b] Best seen in LAT projection.

Table 26.12 Cortical branches of M_4

Region	Location	Branch	Territory
Anterior	Frontotemporal	Anterior temporal Temporopolar	Anterior, medial, and inferior temporal lobe
		Orbitofrontal Prefrontal	Anterior frontal lobe
Central	Frontoparietal	Precentral sulcus	Posterior frontal, anterior parietal lobes
		Central sulcus	Superior parietal lobe
Posterior	Parieto-occipital-temporal	Posterior parietal	Posterior parietal lobe
		Angular[a]	Posterior parietal and occipital lobes
		Temporo-occipital	Posterior temporal and occipital lobes
		Posterior temporal	Middle temporal lobes

[a] Major terminal branch of the middle cerebral artery.

Catheter selection is largely based on operator preference, arch type, and the presence of anomalous origins (Table 26.19). Catheters for selective angiography are often classified as simple or complex, depending on the primary and secondary curves (Figure 26.29). Simple catheters include the Judkins right (JR), no torque right (NTR), Headhunter, jugular bulb, and vertebral catheters. In general, simple catheters have simple primary and secondary

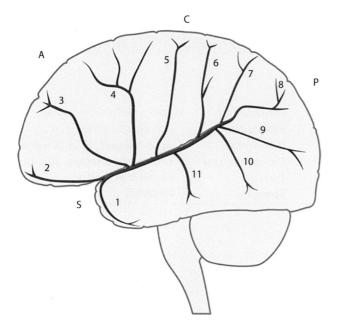

Figure 26.21 Middle cerebral artery (MCA) and branches of the M4 segment in the lateral view. In this view of the lateral surface of the brain, the MCA branches are considered anterior (A, 1–3), central (C, 4–6), or posterior (P, 7–11). The central sulcus (C) and Sylvian fissure (S) are important land marks for MCA branches. 1, Anterior temporal artery; 2, orbitofrontal artery; 3, prefrontal artery; 4, precentral sulcus artery; 5, central sulcus artery; 6, postcentral sulcus artery; 7, posterior parietal artery; 8, angular artery; 9, temporo-occipital artery; 10, posterior temporal artery; 11, middle temporal artery.

Table 26.13 Branches of the vertebrobasilar system

Vertebral artery[a]
- Cervical branches (originate from V1 segment)
  - Muscular branches
  - Spinal branches
- Meningeal branches (originate from distal V2 and V3 segments)
  - Anterior meningeal artery (small; originate from distal V2 segment)
  - Posterior meningeal artery (large; originate from V3 segment)
- Intracranial branches (originate from V4 segment)
  - Posterior spinal artery
  - Anterior spinal artery
  - Perforating branches
  - Posterior inferior cerebellar artery (PICA)

Basilar artery[b]
- Pontine perforators
- Anterior inferior cerebellar artery (AICA)
- Superior cerebellar artery (SCeA)
- Posterior cerebral artery (PCA)

[a] Supplies blood flow to spinal cord, medulla, inferior cerebellum, and pons.
[b] Supplies blood flow to brainstem, cerebellum, vermis, occipital lobe, temporal lobe, thalamus, midbrain, and internal capsule.

Table 26.14 Cervical and intracranial segments of the vertebral artery

Region	Segment	Description
Extraosseus	V$_1$	Subclavian artery to C6 transverse foramina
Foraminal	V$_2$	C6 to C1 transverse foramina
Extraspinal	V$_3$	C1 to foramen magnum
Intradural	V$_4$	Foramen magnum to basilar artery

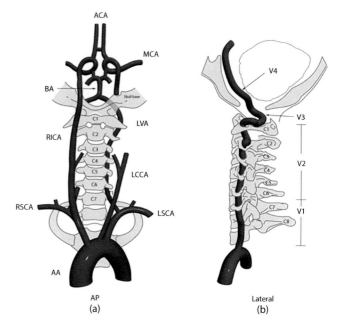

Figure 26.22 The vertebrobasilar system. The AP projection (a) demonstrates the anatomic relationship to the carotid arterial circulation (left internal carotid artery and right vertebral artery are cut away for clarity). The lateral projection (b) provides nice delineation of the segments of the vertebral artery and their relationship to the cervical transverse foramina and foramen magnum. AA, ascending aorta; ACA, anterior cerebral artery; AP, anteroposterior; BA, basilar artery; LCCA, left common carotid artery; LSCA, left subclavian artery; LVA, left vertebral artery; MCA, middle cerebral artery; RICA, right internal carotid artery; RSCA, right subclavian artery; VA, vertebral artery; V1, extraosseous segment of VA; V2, foraminal segment of VA; V3, extraspinal segment of VA; V4, intradural segment of VA.

curves, are easier to use, require less contact with the outer curvature of the arch, and are well suited for relatively simple arch configurations. Selective engagement with a simple catheter involves retraction of the catheter and counterclockwise rotation (Figure 26.30). If the tip is too long, a shorter curve may be used. In contrast, complex catheters, such as Simmons and Vitek (Cook, Inc., Bloomington, IN), have complex curves, require more manipulation and skill, result in more contact with the outer curvature of the arch, and are suited for many simple and complex arch

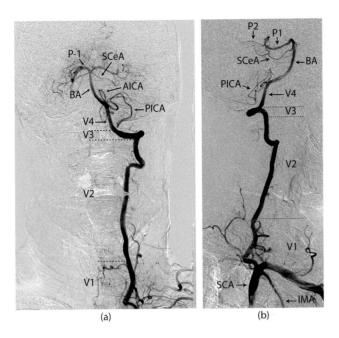

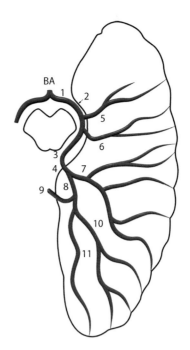

Figure 26.23 Selective angiogram of a dominant left vertebral artery (VA) in the AP **(a)** and RAO **(b)** projections. Note the clear delineation of the basilar artery, both precommunicating segments (P1) of the posterior cerebral artery (PCA), and left anterior and posterior inferior cerebellar arteries (AICA, PICA). There is faint opacification of the left posterior communicating artery (PCOM) and postcommunicating (P2) PCA. AP, anteroposterior; BA, basilar artery; IMA, internal mammary artery; RAO, right anterior oblique; SCA, subclavian artery; SCeA, superior cerebellar artery; V1, extraosseous segment of VA; V2, foraminal segment of VA; V3, extraspinal segment of VA; V4, intradural segment of VA.

Figure 26.24 Posterior cerebral artery (PCA) and its cortical branches in an axial view through brainstem, temporal lobe, and occipital lobe. Note that cortical branches arise from P2 (2) and P4 (4), and supply major portions of the temporal and occipital lobes. 1, Precommunicating (P1) segment of PCA; 2, postcommunicating (P2) segment of PCA; 3, quadrigeminal (P3) segment of PCA; 4, calcarine (P4) segment of PCA; 5, anterior temporal artery; 6, posterior temporal artery; 7, lateral occipital artery; 8, medial occipital artery; 9, splenial artery (cut); 10, parieto-occipital artery; 11, calcarine artery. BA, basilar artery.

Table 26.15 Classification of the posterior cerebral artery

Segment	Region	Description	Branches	Projection
P_1	Precommunicating	From BA to PCOM	Perforating	AP
P_2	Ambient	From PCOM to distal to PTA	Perforating, choroid plexus, cortical	AP, LAT
P_3	Quadrigeminal	Short medial segment	Usually none	AP
P_4	Calcarine	Termination of PCA in calcarine fissure	Cortical	AP, LAT

Note: AP, anteroposterior; BA, basilar artery; LAT, lateral; PCA, posterior cerebral artery; PCOM, posterior communicating artery; PTA, posterior temporal artery.

configurations. Among complex catheters, the Vitek is the easiest to use: selective engagement involves positioning the catheter distal to the left SCA then rotating and advancing it until the tip points superiorly. Each great vessel may be selectively engaged by advancing the Vitek catheter from the left SCA to the left CCA to the IA (Figure 26.30). The Simmons catheter requires more manipulation and must be formed first in either the left SCA or the ascending aorta (Figure 26.30). Most cardiologists will prefer the Vitek catheter, which handles in a fashion similar to a left Amplatz catheter; gentle retraction results in deeper seating, while advancement results in disengagement. In our experience, all great vessels have been successfully engaged with a simple curve catheter and/or a Vitek catheter. For a diagnostic

angiogram, the sequence of selective cannulation is generally proximal to distal with a simple curve catheter and distal to proximal with a Vitek catheter (Figure 26.30).

Once the great vessel has been selectively engaged and if the catheter provides good coaxial alignment without pressure damping, selective angiography may be performed with the same catheter, preferably using a power injector. If there is pressure damping, suboptimal position, or noncoaxial alignment that cannot be corrected by gentle catheter manipulation, the catheter may be exchanged over a guidewire for a multipurpose angiographic catheter (or modified tennis racquet [Meditech/Boston Scientific, Watertown, MA]), if necessary (Tables 26.19 and 26.20; Figures 26.27 and 26.29).

Table 26.16 Branches of the posterior cerebral artery

Branch	Segment	Territory	Projection
Perforating			
Thalamic (n ¼ 1-6)[a]	P^1	Thalamus, hypothalamus internal capsule, midbrain	LAT
Thalamogeniculate (n ¼ 2-12)[a]	P^2 (80%)	Putamen. geniculate, subthalamus	
	P^3 (20%)		
Peduncular (n ¼ 0-6)[a]	P^2	Midbrain	
Choroid plexus/ventricular			
Medial PChA	P^2	Choroid plexus	LAT
Lateral PChA	P^2	Caudate, thalamus	
Cortical			
Anterior temporal	P^2	Anterior temporal lobe	AP, LAT
Posterior temporal	P^2	Posterior temporal lobe	AP, LAT
Medial occipital	P^4	Parieto-occipital, corpus callosum	LAT
Parieto-occipital			
Calcarine			
Splenial			
Lateral occipital	P^4	Inferior temporal, occipital lobe	AP, LAT

Note: AP, anteroposterior; LAT, lateral; PChA, posterior choroidal artery.
[a] Numbers in parenthesis indicate the usual number of perforating branches.

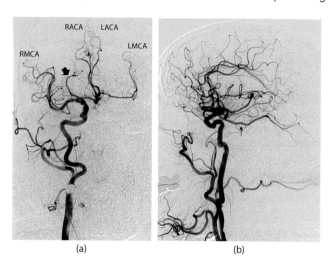

(a)   (b)

Figure 26.25 Selective right carotid angiogram in a patient with chronic total occlusion of the left internal carotid artery, anteroposterior (AP) cranial **(a)** and lateral **(b)**, projections. Note extensive right to left crossover via the right anterior cerebral artery (RACA) and the anterior communicating artery (ACOM), filling the left ACA (LACA) and middle cerebral artery (LMCA). There are two major intracranial arteries (LACA, LMCA) in the left hemisphere, but three major arteries in the right hemisphere. In the AP-cranial projection (a), the artery (*arrow*) between the RACA and right MCA (RMCA) is a persistent fetal posterior cerebral artery, which is also seen in the lateral projection (*arrow*) (see Figures 26.11, 26.19, and 26.20 for comparison).

Selective angiography of the innominate artery

The LAO arch study (Figures 26.1 through 26.3) provides nice images of the ostia and proximal IA, left CCA, and left SCA, but is less useful for visualizing the IA bifurcation into the right CCA and right SCA (Figure 26.31). Imaging the IA in the LAO

Table 26.17 Intracranial aneurysms

Incidence
- General population—1%
- Cerebral angiography—7%

Location
- Anterior circulation—90%
  - Anterior communicating artery—30%
  - Middle cerebral artery—30%
  - Internal carotid artery/posterior communicating artery—30%
- Posterior circulation—10%
- Multiple—20 to 30%

Rupture risk
- ≤6 mm—1% per year
- ≤7 mm—2.5% per year
- ≤25 mm (giant)—very high

and AP projections may result in overlap of the right VA and right CCA, making selective cannulation of the SCA and CCA more difficult. In contrast, selective angiography of the IA in a 30° right anterior oblique (RAO) projection will clearly demonstrate the IA bifurcation and separate the right VA from the CCA (Table 26.20; Figure 26.31). This angiogram may be performed by hand injection. The purpose of the IA angiogram is to provide a better road map for selective cannulation and angiography of the right SCA and right CCA and should not be used for images of the right VA, right ICA, and intracranial circulation due to vessel overlap and poor opacification.

Selective angiography of the right subclavian artery

Depending on the clinical circumstances, selective right SCA angiography may be performed after advancing the

Table 26.18 Sequence of diagnostic cerebral angiography

Patient preparation
- Hydration if eGFR < 60 cc/min/1.73 m²
- Light sedation if needed
- 2% lidocaine for local anesthesia

Arterial access
- Retrograde femoral arterial approach
- 5-Fr sheath
- 5-Fr catheters
- Heparin 1,500–2,000 IU
- 4-Port manifold
- Intra-arterial pressure monitoring

Arch study
- 40° LAO, pigtail, or TR catheter
- Iodixanol
- Power injection (25–30 cc over 2 s; 600 psi)
- FOV 34–42 cm

Selective cannulation
- 40° LAO guided by arch study (or tracheal air stripe)
- Simple arch: simple catheter (as described in Table 26.19) or Vitek
- Complex arch: Vitek
- DMA²

Selective angiography
- See Tables 26.19 and 26.20

Note: DMA², don't monkey around in the arch; eGFR, estimated glomerular filtration rate; FOV, field of view; Fr, French; LAO, left anterior oblique; TR, tennis racquet catheter.

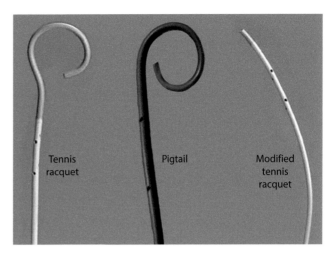

Figure 26.27 Catheters commonly employed for arch aortography. The modified tennis racquet (MTR) is created by amputating the head of the tennis racquet, retaining a few millimeters of the radiopaque shaft. The MTR (or any equivalent multipurpose catheter) may be useful for selective carotid angiography if coaxial alignment cannot be achieved with another simple or complex catheter.

IA catheter into the right SCA (Table 26.20). This may be accomplished by clockwise rotation and advancement of a simple catheter using fluoroscopy, pressure monitoring, and test injections by hand. If necessary, a J-tip guidewire may be positioned in the axillary artery, followed by advancement of any suitable coaxial catheter into the right SCA. To study the right IMA, an IMA or Bartorelli catheter may be used for selective cannulation and angiography. If the purpose is to image the VA and PCA, it is best to perform right SCA with a power injector or to selectively image the right VA with a vertebral or JR catheter. The best angiographic projections depend on the vessel of interest (Table 26.20); cine angiography rather than DSA is preferred for images of the IMA and coronary artery using a hand injection.

Selective angiography of the right common carotid artery

From the IA, selective right CCA angiography may be performed after advancing the IA catheter into the right CCA. This is most easily accomplished in the RAO projection by clockwise rotation (from the IA) and advancement of a simple catheter using fluoroscopy, pressure monitoring, and test injections (Figure 26.31). If a complex catheter was used to engage the IA, gentle retraction of the catheter and clockwise rotation will point the catheter tip into the right CCA. If these maneuvers do not work, a J-tip guidewire can be advanced into the mid-CCA followed by advancement of any suitable coaxial catheter. For images of the carotid bifurcation and intracranial circulation, hand injections usually result in contrast streaming and suboptimal image quality, so a power injector is preferred (Figure 26.26). If the catheter position is not ideal

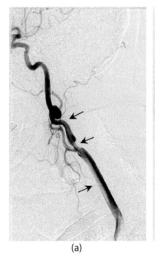
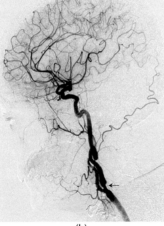

(a)   (b)

Figure 26.26 Selective left carotid artery angiogram using a 5-Fr Vitek catheter (lateral projection). Angiogram with hand injection **(a)** resulted in streaming of contrast (*arrows*), and poor opacification of the stenosis at the origin of the internal carotid artery (ICA) and of the intracranial circulation (not shown). Another angiogram was performed with a power injector **(b)**, resulting in excellent opacification of the ICA stenosis (*arrow*) and intracranial circulation.

Table 26.19 Catheter selection for selective cerebral angiography

Catheter configuration	Catheter type	Advantages	Disadvantages
Simple	JR, NTR, AR, VERT, BERN, HN, BEN, JB	Need minimal manipulation for simple arch type, minimal contact with aortic wall	Difficult to use for complex arch type
Complex	Vitek	Easy to use for simple and complex arch types: no need to form catheter in SCA or aortic root	More contact with aortic wall than simple catheter
Complex	SIM	Useful for complex arch configurations or if Vitek fails	More contact with aortic wall; need to form catheter in SCA or aortic root
Multipurpose	MP[a], Glide, MTR[a,b]	Excellent coaxial alignment for virtually all vessel configurations and arch types	Cannot be used to cannulate the great vessels; requires guidewire and catheter exchange

Note: Producer names are given in text.

AR, Amplatz right; BEN, Bentson; JB, jugular bulb; JR, Judkins right; HN, headhunter; MP, multipurpose; MTR, modified tennis racquet; NTR, no torque right; SCA, subclavian artery; SIM, Simmons; VERT, vertebral.

[a] Catheter with side holes; all others are end-hole catheters; PSI ¼ 500–550 psi for side-hole catheters, 400–450 psi for end-hole catheters.

[b] MTR is formed by amputating the head of the tennis racquet catheter, leaving 1–2 mm of the radiopaque shaft in place (Figure 26.27).

Table 26.20 Technique of selective cerebral angiography

Catheter position	Target vessel	Injection technique	Projection	Catheter
IA	IA	Hand	RAO	JR, Vitek
SCA	R-SCA	Hand	LAO, RAO	JR, Vitek
	R-VA	Power[a]	AP, RAO, LAT	
	R-PCA	Power[a]	AP, LAT	JR, Vitek
R-VA	R-VA	Hand/Power[b]	AP, RAO, LAT	JR, Vertebral
	R-PCA	Hand/Power[b]	AP-C, LAT	JR, Vertebral
R-CCA	R-CCA	Power[c]	AP, RAO	JR, Vitek, MP[d]
	R-ICA	Power[c]	AP, RAO, LAT	JR, Vitek, MP[d]
	R-ACA/MCA	Power[c]	AP-C, LAT	JR, Vitek, MP[d]
L-CCA	L-CCA	Power[c]	AP, LAO	JR, Vitek, MP[d]
	L-ICA	Power[c]	AP, LAO, LAT	JR, Vitek, MP[d]
	L-ACA, MCA	Power[c]	AP-C, LAT	JR, Vitek, MP[d]
L-SCA	L-SCA	Hand	LAO, RAO	JR, Vitek
	L-VA	Power[a]	AP, LAO, LAT	JR, Vitek
	L-PCA	Power[a]	AP, LAT	JR, Vitek
L-VA	L-VA	Hand/Power[b]	AP, LAO, LAT	JR, Vertebral
	L-PCA	Hand/Power[b]	AP-C, LAT	JR, Vertebral

Note: ACA, anterior cerebral artery; AP, anteroposterior; AP-C, anteroposterior with cranial angulation; CCA, common carotid artery; IA, innominate artery; ICA, internal carotid artery; JR, Judkins right; L, left; LAO, left anterior oblique; LAT, lateral; MCA, middle cerebral artery; MP, multipurpose; MTR, modified tennis racquet; PCA, posterior cerebral artery; R, right; RAO, right anterior oblique; SCA, subclavian artery; VA, vertebral artery.

[a] 8–10 total volume, 4–6 cc/s, 450–500 psi.

[b] 5–7 cc total volume, 3–5 cc/s, 450–500 psi.

[c] 8–12 cc total volume, 6–9 cc/s, 450–500 psi (end hole), 500 psi (side hole).

[d] Any multipurpose catheter, such as MP, glide catheter, or MTR.

or the catheter recoils into the arch, the catheter can be repositioned with a guidewire or exchanged for a more coaxial catheter, such as a modified tennis racquet, multipurpose, or glide catheter (Figures 26.27 and 26.29). In most patients, the best images of the right CCA and cervical ICA are obtained in AP, lateral, and ipsilateral oblique (RAO) projections (Figures 26.20 and 26.32). Depending on the individual patient, contralateral oblique (LAO) and cranial or caudal angulation may be useful to image highly eccentric stenoses, straighten bends, or eliminate overlying branches of the ECA. For the intracranial circulation, the best images are AP-cranial and lateral projections (Figures 26.20, 26.25, and 26.32). In some patients, highly angulated or tortuous sections of the cerebral ICA may appear aneurysmal, in which case an ipsilateral (RAO) caudal projection may prove very useful.

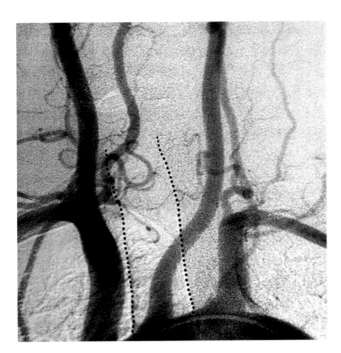

Figure 26.28 Relationship of the tracheal air stripe (dotted lines) to the origin of the great vessels. In the 40° LAO projection, the tracheal air stripe is a good landmark for selective cannulation of the innominate artery (proximal to the air stripe), left carotid artery (middle of the air stripe), and left subclavian artery (distal to the air stripe). LAO, left anterior oblique.

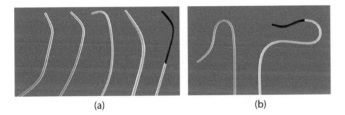

Figure 26.29 Catheters commonly employed for selective cannulation and angiography of the great vessels (see text for details). Simple catheters **(a)** have a simple primary curve and minimal secondary curve (from left to right: headhunter, JB-1, JR-4, MPA, vertebral). Note that the multipurpose (MPA), glide catheter (not shown), and modified tennis racquet (see Figure 26.27) are not readily suited for selective cannulation, but are useful for selective angiography when other catheters do not provide coaxial alignment. Complex catheters **(b)** have more complex relationships between the catheter tip and shaft (¼ Simmons, ¼ Vitek).

Selective angiography of the left common carotid artery

In the presence of simple or complex arch anatomy, the left CCA may be cannulated in a 40° LAO projection with the same catheter that was used to engage the IA. In some patients, the curve of a simple catheter is too long to engage the left CCA, and a catheter with a more horizontal orientation (shorter) may work better

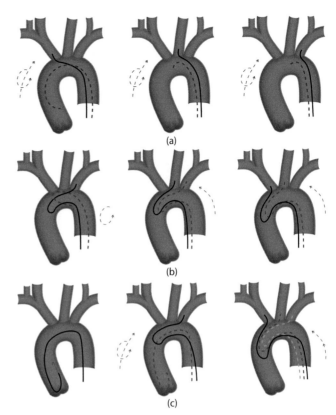

Figure 26.30 Manipulation of simple and complex catheters for selective angiography of great vessels. **(a)** Simple catheter manipulation involves placement of the catheter in the ascending aorta, followed by retraction and counterclockwise rotation to engage the innominate artery (IA). Retraction and counterclockwise rotation are repeated to engage the left common (CCA) and left subclavian arteries (SCA). **(b)** Vitek catheter manipulation involves positioning the catheter distal to the left SCA, followed by advancement and counterclockwise rotation into the left SCA. While retaining the curve of the catheter, the Vitek is advanced to the left CCA and IA. **(c)** Simmons catheter manipulation involves positioning the catheter in the ascending aorta (or left SCA), and forming a curve in the catheter by advancing it over a J-wire. After removing the J-wire, the Simmons can be retracted and rotated counterclockwise to engage the left SCA. While retaining the curve, the Simmons is advanced to the left CCA and IA, similar to the Vitek.

(Tables 26.19 and 26.20). For example, if a JR4 is used to engage the IA but is too long to engage the left CCA, greater success will be achieved with a JR3.5, NTR, or AR-1 catheter. A Vitek catheter will also successfully engage the left CCA in virtually all patients with simple or complex arch anatomy. Advancement of a simple catheter or retraction of a complex catheter and clockwise rotation will usually result in a more stable and deeper position. If the catheter tip is coaxial and there is no pressure clamping, DSA can be performed with a power injector. If the position is not ideal or the catheter recoils into the arch, the catheter can be repositioned with a guidewire or

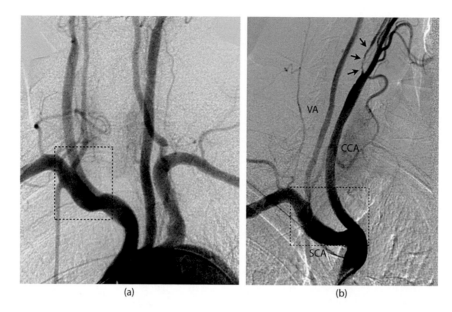

Figure 26.31 Angiography of the innominate artery (IA) and its bifurcation (*dotted box*) into right subclavian (SCA) and common carotid arteries (CCA). The arch aortogram (40° LAO) demonstrates a type 1 arch with the usual configuration of the great vessels **(a)**. This projection obscures the IA bifurcation into the right SCA and CCA, and results in close overlap of the right vertebral artery (VA) and CCA. Selective angiography of the IA (30° RAO) results in better separation of the right SCA and CCA **(b)**, and no overlap of the right VA and CCA. Note the "string sign" in the right internal carotid artery (*arrows*). LAO, left anterior oblique; RAO, right anterior oblique.

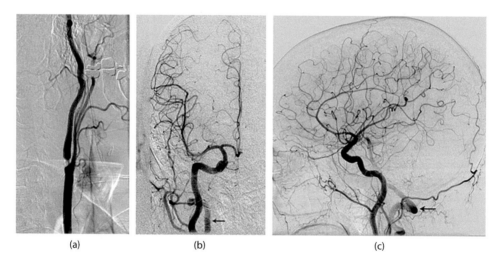

Figure 26.32 Selective right carotid artery angiography in a patient with asymptomatic carotid stenosis. Lateral projection demonstrates a focal, ulcerated, severe stenosis at the origin of the internal carotid artery (ICA) **(a)**. The intracranial circulation is normal in the AP **(b)** and lateral **(c)** projections. Note faint filling of the right vertebral artery from reflux of contrast during power injection (*arrow*).

exchanged for a more coaxial catheter, such as a modified tennis racquet, multipurpose, or glide catheter (Figures 26.27 and 26.29). In most patients, the best images of the left CCA and cervical ICA are observed in the AP, lateral, and ipsilateral oblique (LAO) projections (Figures 26.12, 26.19, and 26.33). The contralateral oblique (RAO) and cranial and caudal angulation may be useful in selected patients. The best images of the intracranial circulation are AP-cranial and lateral projections (Figures 26.11, 26.19, 26.26, and 26.33); LAO caudal may be useful to differentiate intracranial aneurysms from tortuous loops of intracranial arteries.

Selective angiography of the left subclavian artery

The 40° LAO projection is the best view for selective cannulation of the left SCA (Figures 26.1 and 26.3), and catheter selection is identical to the IA and left CCA. For complex arch configurations, the Vitek catheter will work for virtually

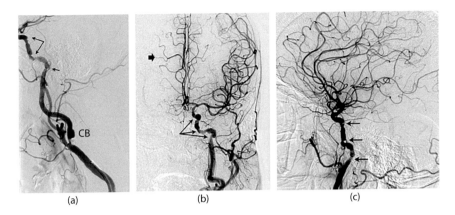

(a)   (b)   (c)

Figure 26.33 Selective left carotid artery angiogram in an elderly patient with symptomatic left carotid stenosis. There is eccentric severe stenosis at the origin of the left internal carotid artery (ICA) at the level of the carotid bulb (CB) and multiple sequential moderate stenosis (*arrows*) in the petrous segment of the ICA (**a**, 40° left anterior oblique projection). Images of the intracranial circulation in the AP-cranial **(b)** and lateral **(c)** projection demonstrate normal antegrade filling of the left anterior (ACA) and middle (MCA) cerebral arteries. Note left to right crossover via the anterior communicating artery (*arrowhead*), associated with asymptomatic severe stenosis of the right ICA (not shown), and considerable atherosclerosis in the petrous and cavernous left common carotid artery (*arrows*).

all patients. Hand injections usually suffice for imaging the left SCA, and the 30° RAO projection usually provides ideal separation of the VA, left IMA, and thyrocervical trunk (Figures 26.4 and 26.5). When it is necessary to image the VA and PCA, a power injector provides the best images when the catheter is in the left SCA; alternatively, hand or power injections can be used for selective VA angiography using a JR or vertebral catheter. If the purpose is to image the left IMA graft, the left SCA catheter can be exchanged for an IMA or Bartorelli for selective IMA angiography.

Intracranial circulation

Angiographic views of the intracranial circulation are an essential part of the cerebral angiogram. AP-cranial (Towne's) projections are used to characterize the ACA, MCA, PCA, circle of Willis, and their branches (Table 26.20; Figures 26.11, 26.19, 26.20, 26.23, 26.25, 26.26, 26.32, and 26.33). It is useful to have an understanding of intracranial collaterals and crossover, particularly in patients with carotid stenosis, and the location of common intracranial aneurysms (Figure 26.34). Ipsilateral caudal views are valuable for differentiating tortuous intracranial vessels from aneurysms. When using a power injector, intra-arterial contrast injection is divided into an early arterial phase (the artery being injected and its major branches are opacified), a late arterial phase (reveals smaller, more distal arterial branches), a capillary phase (resulting in a "brain blush" or "brainogram"), and a venous phase (filling of the cerebral veins and sinuses). By adjusting the window settings during the capillary phase, it is possible to create a distinct brainogram. Some patients may develop focal neurological impairment after carotid intervention that is not associated with embolic cutoff of a visible intracranial artery. A postintervention brainogram may demonstrate a wedge-shaped cortical perfusion defect consistent with distal embolization.

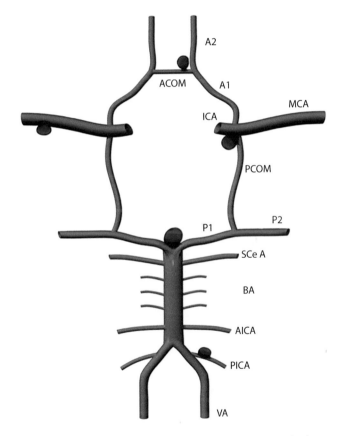

Figure 26.34 The circle of Willis demonstrating typical locations of intracranial aneurysms (see Table 26.20). ACA, anterior cerebral artery; ACOM, anterior communicating artery; AICA, anterior inferior cerebellar artery; A1, precommunicating ACA; A2, postcommunicating ACA; BA, basilar artery; ICA, internal carotid artery; MCA, middle cerebral artery; PCA, posterior cerebral artery; PCOM, posterior communicating artery; PICA, posterior inferior cerebellar artery; P1, precommunicating PCA; P2, postcommunicating PCA; SCeA, superior cerebellar artery; VA, vertebral artery.

OTHER ANGIOGRAPHIC TECHNIQUES

Quantitative angiography

Visual estimates are notoriously unreliable for quantitative assessment of vessel dimensions and stenosis severity. Virtually all angiographic systems have software that allows for rapid digital quantitative angiography, which can be useful for sizing balloons and other interventional devices. NASCET (North American Symptomatic Carotid Endarterectomy Trial) is the most widely used method for assessment of carotid stenosis severity, using the ICA distal to the carotid bulb as the diameter of the normal reference segment. In contrast, the ECST (European Carotid Surgery Trial) method uses the carotid bulb as the normal reference diameter and consistently yields higher percent stenoses than the NASCET method (Figure 26.35).[9]

Gradient assessment and intravascular ultrasound

Measurement of translesional pressure gradient is useful for assessing the functional significance of stenoses and may be measured at rest and after intra-arterial nitroglycerin (200–400 mg). A peak-to-peak pressure gradient, 2:20 mmHg, is considered hemodynamically significant. From a practical standpoint, translesional pressure gradients are useful for assessment of SCA stenoses but are rarely necessary (and may increase the risk of stroke) in patients with ICA stenosis. In addition, the established benefit of carotid revascularization in terms of stroke prevention has been based on stenosis severity and not translesional gradient. Intravascular ultrasound is feasible in the brachiocephalic circulation but has not been widely adopted.

COMPLICATIONS

In addition to complications associated with other invasive angiographic procedures, cerebral angiography has unique complications related to the central nervous system. Access site complications (i.e., hematoma, dissection, AVF, pseudoaneurysm, or hemorrhage) and systemic complications (i.e., contrast reactions, contrast nephropathy, or cholesterol embolization) are encountered in <5% of patients undergoing invasive angiographic procedures, including cerebral angiography.

Neurological complications are the most feared complications of cerebral angiography. Causes of neurological events during cerebral angiography include embolism (plaque, thrombus, air) and direct arterial injury (vasospasm, dissection, perforation) (Figure 26.36). Although older series reported death, stroke, and transient ischemic attacks (TIAs) in 0.06%, 0.14%, and 2% of patients undergoing cerebral angiography, respectively,[10] the incidence of neurologic complications appears to have decreased substantially. In a recent series from 2001 to 2006, procedure-related TIAs occurred in 0.34%, none of which resulted in permanent neurologic deficit.[11] Factors accounting for the decrease in complications have not been precisely defined but may include the use of intra-arterial pressure monitoring,

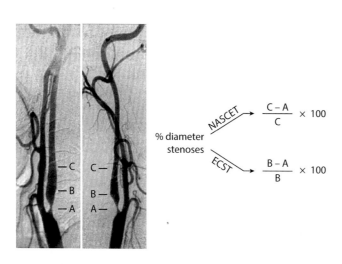

Figure 26.35 Methodology for quantitative carotid artery angiography. Calculations for percent diameter stenosis vary depending on the site of the normal reference segment. (**A**) is the target lesion. The NASCET method utilizes the proximal internal carotid artery (**C**) as the reference segment, whereas the ECST method utilizes the carotid bulb (**B**) as the reference segment. ECST, European Carotid Surgery Trial; NASCET, North American Symptomatic Carotid Endarterectomy Trial.

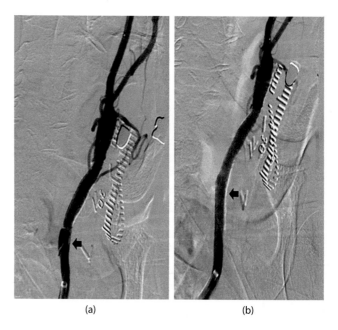

Figure 26.36 Catheter-induced dissection (*arrowhead*) of the left common carotid artery (55° RAO). Severe asymptomatic eccentric dissection (**a**) was treated by successful direct carotid stenting using embolic protection (**b**). RAO, right anterior oblique.

heparin anticoagulation, isosmolar contrast, and better catheter designs requiring less catheter manipulation.

The potential for complications mandates that neurologic surveillance be performed during and after the procedure. Light conscious sedation is reasonable, but deep sedation should be avoided. Angiography and recovery room staff should be trained to evaluate changes in consciousness, cognitive and language deficits, visual complaints, headache, gait and vestibular symptoms, and focal motor and sensory deficits. Physicians performing cerebral angiography must be competent in performing a thorough neurological examination, be familiar with the National Institutes of Health Stroke Scale (NIHSS),[12,13] and recognize criteria for immediate stroke intervention.

REFERENCES

1. Collins P, et al. Is carotid duplex scanning sufficient as the sole investigation prior to carotid endarterectomy? *Br J Radiol* 2005;78(935):1034–1037.
2. Khaw KT. Does carotid duplex imaging render angiography redundant before carotid endarterectomy? *Br J Radiol* 1997;70:235–238.
3. Casserly IP, Yadav JS. Carotid Intervention. In: Casserly IP, Sachar R, Yadav JS, eds. *Manual of Peripheral Vascular Intervention.* Philadelphia, PA: Lippincott Williams & Wilkins, 2005:83–109.
4. Patel P, et al. Routine visualization of the left internal mammary artery before bypass surgery: Is it necessary? *J Invasive Cardiol* 2005;17(9):479–481.
5. Matsumoto Y, et al. Transradial approach for diagnostic selective cerebral angiography: Results of a consecutive series of 166 cases. *AJNR Am J Neuroradiol* 2001;22(4):704–708.
6. Layton KF, et al. Use of the ulnar artery as an alternative access site for cerebral angiography. *AJNR Am J Neuroradiol* 2006;27(10):2073–2074.
7. Sievert H, et al. Brachial artery approach for transluminal angioplasty of the internal carotid artery. *Catheter Cardiovasc Diagn* 1996;39(4):421–423.
8. Hayashi N, et al. Radiation exposure to interventional radiologists during manual-injection digital subtraction angiography. *Cardiovasc Interv Radiol* 1998;21(3):240–243.
9. Osborn AG, ed. *Diagnostic Cerebral Angiography.* 2nd edn. Philadelphia, PA: Lippincott Williams & Wilkins, 1999:373.
10. Kaufmann TJ, et al. Complications of diagnostic cerebral angiography: Evaluation of 19,826 consecutive patients. *Radiology* 2007;243(3):812–819.
11. Dawkins AA, et al. Complications of cerebral angiography: A prospective analysis of 2,924 consecutive procedures. *Neuroradiology* 2007;49(9):753–759.
12. Howard G, et al. Statistical and experimental design issues in the evaluation of carotid artery stenting. In: Al-Mubarak N, Roubin GS, Iyer SS, et al., eds. *Carotid Artery Stenting: Current Practice and Technique.* Philadelphia, PA: Lippincott Williams & Wilkins, 2004:313–326.
13. Stroke Scales and Clinical Assessment Tools. NIH Stroke Scale (NIHSS). Available at: http://www.strokecenter.org/trials/scales/nihss.html (accessed December 1, 2016).

PART 6

Intracoronary and Intracardiac Assessment

27

Application of intracoronary physiology: Use of pressure and flow measurements

MORTON J. KERN AND ARNOLD H. SETO

INTRODUCTION

The goal of coronary revascularization with either coronary stenting or bypass surgery is the relief of ischemia and restoration of coronary blood flow. Coronary stenting improves exercise tolerance and reduces use of anti-ischemic medications but does not improve survival, except in patients with ST-segment elevation myocardial infarction (STEMI). Moreover, stent placement is of no benefit and, in fact, can be detrimental to patients with angiographic stenosis that is not producing myocardial ischemia and associated symptoms.

For four decades, the use of angiography to guide percutaneous coronary intervention (PCI) has been used with variable results for coronary artery disease (CAD). The first introduction of physiology for the characterization of stenosis severity by Lance Gould in 1974[1] demonstrated that coronary flow was predictably reduced for increasing severity of coronary narrowing in an animal model. Unfortunately, in man, this relationship does not hold, except at the extremes of stenosis (minimal and severe), because the angiogram is not a true representation of the flow-limiting potential of any given stenosis. The modern use of translesional pressure and flow

for lesion assessment is for a singular purpose—to overcome the inaccuracy of angiography in identifying those lesions best treated with coronary revascularization. Coronary angiography produces two-dimensional (2D) "lumenograms," a silhouette image of the three-dimensional (3D) vascular lumen in a given projection (Figure 27.1). The contrast-filled coronary artery does not permit imaging of the atherosclerotic accumulation of plaque within the vessel wall.[2] It instead provides a "shadow" without intraluminal detail.

Furthermore, the eccentric shape of a stenosis does not reflect the true limitation of flow and thus prevents even the astute observer from determining whether such a stenosis is reducing coronary blood flow. Equally confusing is the inability of angiography to accurately distinguish "normal" and "diseased" vessel segments, which complicates the assessment of lesion significance, especially in the setting of diffuse CAD. In addition, routine angiography must overcome a number of artifacts, including contrast streaming, branch overlap, vessel foreshortening, calcifications, and ostial origins, further making the interpretation of some luminal narrowings unreliable. Despite numerous attempts to improve the angiographic technique, stenosis imaging

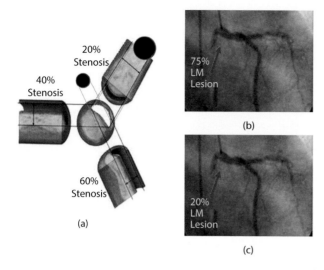

Figure 27.1 **(a)** Cross section of coronary stenosis viewed from different radiographic projections. The eccentric lumen produces an image with uncertainty related to true lumen size and its impact on coronary blood flow. The same lesion may appear significant in one radiographic view **(b)** and nonsignificant in another **(c)**.

remains a dilemma that cannot be resolved with even multiple views. For these reasons, coronary physiology directly obtained in the catheterization laboratory has become critical to making the best clinical decisions regarding CAD revascularization.

ANATOMICAL CONSIDERATIONS

Determinants of myocardial blood flow

Epicardial arteries consist of three layers—the intima, media, and the adventitia. The endothelial cell of the intima constitutes the barrier with blood and plays an important role in the regulation of hemostasis and vascular tone. The strategic location of the endothelium allows it to sense changes in hemodynamic forces and blood-borne signals and to respond by releasing vasoactive substances. A balance between endothelium-derived relaxing (e.g., nitric oxide) and contracting factors (e.g., endothelin) maintains vascular homeostasis. When this balance is disrupted (i.e., in atherosclerosis), it predisposes the vasculature to vasoconstriction and, thus, to a disturbance in coronary blood flow.[3]

Atherosclerosis predominately involves the large epicardial arteries producing variable resistance to blood flow to the myocardium. The resistance is related to severity of luminal reduction and several additional morphologic features (Figure 27.2), as well as the extent of disease in the artery involved.

Size of the arteries is proportional to myocardial mass

In normal individuals, there is a close correlation between the luminal cross-sectional area of a coronary artery and

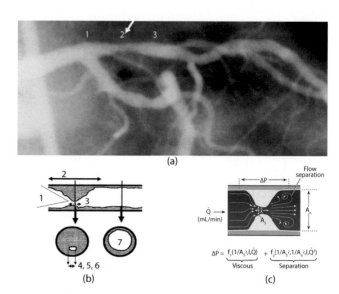

Figure 27.2 **(a)** Cineangiographic frame with an intermediate stenosis. **(b)** Diagram of coronary stenosis showing seven factors producing resistance to flow: 1 is entrance angle; 2 is disease segment length; 3 is stenosis length; 4, 5, and 6 are shape factors of lumen area; and 7 is the reference vessel size. **(c)** Total pressure loss across a stenosis (ΔP) is derived from two sources: (1) frictional losses along the leading edge of the stenosis and (2) inertial losses stemming from the sudden expansion, which causes flow separation and eddies (exit losses). Frictional losses are linearly related to flow by the law of Poiseuille, and exit losses increase with the square of the flow (law of Bernoulli). The total change in pressure gradient (ΔP) is the sum of the two. The loss coefficients, f1 and f2, are functions of stenosis geometry and rheologic properties of blood (viscosity and density). The graphic representation of this equation results in a quadratic relationship, in which the curvilinear shape demonstrates the presence of nonlinear exit losses. If no stenosis is present, the second term is zero, and the graphical curve becomes a straight line (with a positive slope that depends on the diameter of the vessel, based on the law of Poiseuille). A_n, area of the normal segment; A_s, area of the stenosis; L, length; Q, flow. (Redrawn from Kern, M.J., *Circulation*, 101, 1344–1351, 2000.)

the subtended myocardial mass. In contrast, in patients with coronary atherosclerosis, measured coronary artery lumen area is diffusely 30%–50% too small for the distal myocardial bed size compared with normal subjects.[4] This relationship between vessel size and myocardial mass as it relates to blood flow is important when considering a stenosis in a large artery (i.e., left anterior descending [LAD]) compared with a smaller branch.

Fundamentals of flow, pressure, and resistance

The main parameters of the circulatory function are flow, pressure, and resistance:

$$Q/DP = R$$

where Q is flow, DP is diastolic pressure, and R is resistance.

Because flow and, therefore, resistance both depend on the myocardial mass perfused, there is no unequivocal normal value for coronary flow and resistance. In contrast, because the large epicardial artery without disease has negligible resistance under normal conditions, coronary pressure equals central aortic pressure over the entire length of the epicardial arteries, even during hyperemia. This unique characteristic of coronary pressure establishes an unequivocal reference value: whatever the myocardial mass, the size of the artery, the systemic hemodynamics, the age of the patient, and the status of the microvasculature, the pressure in the distal part of an epicardial artery will be identical to central aortic pressure, unless the resistance of the epicardial artery becomes abnormal (most often due to atherosclerosis).

Coronary flow and myocardial contractions

Because of ventricular contraction, coronary blood flow occurs mainly during diastole. Phasic coronary blood flow is, thus, more pronounced in diastolic compared with systolic flow, and the diastolic predominance is greater in the left than the right coronary artery. In case of an epicardial stenosis, translesional pressure loss (i.e., the aortic-coronary gradient) will initially be evident in diastole.

Control of myocardial flow

The regulation of myocardial blood flow is multifactorial, involving the interaction of the neurohumoral, endothelial, endocrine, paracrine, and metabolic systems with physical factors acting in a largely nonlinear fashion. This makes the study of individual factors difficult, if not impossible, in the intact animal model.

Coronary circulation can be considered a two-compartment model. The first compartment consists of epicardial vessels, which are also referred to as "conductance vessels" because they do not offer resistance to blood flow in the normal state. The second compartment consists of arteries that are <400 microns in diameter, or "resistive vessels" (Figure 27.3). When no stenosis is present in the epicardial vessel, myocardial flow is primarily controlled by resistive vessels,[5] as they are able to vasodilate (or constrict) under physiological and pharmacological stress. At coronary angiography, microvascular vessels are not clearly delineated but appear as a myocardial blush of contrast medium. During exercise or any other form of increased oxygen demand, the resistance of the microvasculature decreases, allowing for an increased blood flow. Similarly, an epicardial stenosis increases epicardial resistance, which is compensated by an equivalent decrease in microvascular resistance. This results in a maintained total resistance to blood flow and a preserved resting flow, with residual—albeit reduced—coronary flow reserve (CFR). This maintenance of constant resting coronary blood flow is referred to as autoregulation. As the epicardial stenosis progresses further, its relative

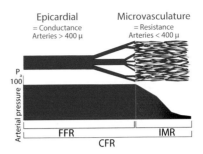

Figure 27.3 Since the epicardial vessels contribute only a minimal fraction of the total vascular resistance, there is no significant pressure drop along the conductance vessels. In contrast, passage through the resistive vessels produces a large drop in pressure. CFR, coronary flow reserve; FFR, fractional flow reserve; IMR, microvascular resistance.

contribution to total resistance increases. When the stenosis becomes "critical," the compensation capacity of the microvasculature (i.e., CFR) is exhausted. Any additional increase in epicardial resistance will result in an increase in total resistance, a decrease in resting myocardial flow, and a loss of autoregulation.

PHYSIOLOGICAL INDICES OF THE CORONARY CIRCULATION

Since the seminal work of Gould,[1] several indices of coronary physiology have been proposed to guide clinical decision-making. Fractional flow reserve (FFR) is the best-validated index. A recent review by Gould and Johnson[6] provides an examination of current available indices. Although extensive, this chapter devotes most discussion to those in common use, FFR, CFR, and potentially the resting instantaneous wave-free pressure ratio (iFR). A discussion of resting and hyperemic indices will follow (Table 27.1).

Coronary flow and flow reserve

CFR is defined as the ratio of maximal hyperemic blood flow (Q_{max}) to resting myocardial blood flow (Q_{rest}):

$$CFR = Q_{max} / Q_{rest}$$

CFR measures the response of the two major resistance components (the epicardial coronary artery and the supplied vascular bed) to stimuli producing maximal blood flow. Although there is no true "normal CFR," a higher CFR implies that both epicardial and microvascular bed resistances are low (normal) (Figure 27.3). However, a lower CFR (<2 in adults) suggests that one or both of the components are impaired—that is, either the epicardial resistance is very high or the microvascular resistance is abnormal. A low CFR does not indicate which component is affected, preventing applicability for lesion assessment. Furthermore, since CFR

Table 27.1 Coronary physiologic measurements in the catheterization lab

Fractional flow reserve, FFR

Derivation: $FFR = Q_{sten}/Q_{normal}$ at maximal hyperemia. (Where Q is flow, sten is stenotic artery, and normal is theoretic same artery without stenosis.)

$$Q_{sten} = P_{sten}/Resistance_{sten}$$

$$Q_{normal} = P_{aorta}/Resistance_{sten} \text{ then } Q_{sten}/Q_{normal} = P_{sten}/P_{aorta}$$

Hence, $FFR = P_{distal\ to\ stenosis}/P_{aorta,}$

[complete derivation includes venous pressure Pv as $FFR = P_{distal\ to\ stenosis} - Pv/P_{aorta} - Pv$, see reference 2]

Features: Nonischemic threshold range >(0.75–0.80); normal value of 1.0 for every artery and every patient; epicardial lesion-specific linear relation with relative maximum blood flow, independent of hemodynamic alterations, value that accounts for total myocardial blood flow, including collaterals, highly reproducible, high spatial resolution (pressure pullback recording).

Coronary flow velocity reserve, CFVR

Derivation: $CFVR = Q_{hyperemia}/Q_{base}$. Q = Velocity if cross-sectional area unchanged during hyperemia.

Features: Nonischemic threshold range of CFR>2.0; coronary flow reserve in non-obstructed vessels assesses microvascular integrity, useful for studies of coronary endothelial function, accurate estimation of volumetric flow when vessel cross-sectional area available.

Combined pressure and flow velocity measurements (e.g., hyperemic stenoses resistance [HSR])

Derivation: $HSR = P_{aorta} - P_{distal\ to\ stenosis}/Q_{hyperemic}$

Features: Separate assessment of stenosis and microvascular resistances allows construction of pressure-flow curves (assessment of compliant lesions and hemodynamic gain after PCI).

For stenosis resistance index: Nonischemic threshold values <0.8 mmHg/cm/s; normal value of 0; lesion specific, highly reproducible, high sensitivity; useful in cases of discordance between CFR and FFR.

Source: Modified from Kern M.J., Samady, H., *J. Am. Coll. Cardiol.,* 55, 173–185, 2010.

can be altered by changes in basal and hyperemic flows, both of which are influenced by hemodynamics, loading conditions, and contractility, reproducibility even in the short term may be questioned. For example, tachycardia increases basal flow and decreases hyperemic flow, thus reducing CFR by 10% for each 15-beat increase in heart rate. In clinical terms, CFR is best used to assess the microcirculation in the absence of epicardial artery narrowings.

Although early studies in animals and humans indicated a normal value for CFR of 3.5 to 5, the CFR in adult patients with chest pain syndromes and CAD risk factors undergoing cardiac catheterization with "angiographically normal" vessels was 2.7 ± 0.6, with some degree of patient variability and concomitant microvascular disease.[7] In patients with normal coronary arteries and reduced CFR, conditions that produce myocardial hypertrophy (e.g., hypertension, aortic stenosis, hypertrophic cardiomyopathy) are often associated with an abnormal microvasculature.

Regardless of technical signal acquisition aspects (which are a significant challenge), the concept of CFR has several limitations: (1) resting flow, which appears as the denominator, is highly variable; (2) hyperemic flow is directly dependent on systemic blood pressure; (3) the hyperemic and resting measurements are not performed simultaneously but successively; and (4) CFR is not specific for epicardial stenosis.

Stated another way, when CFR is too low, it is impossible to tell whether this abnormal value is related to a stenosis in the epicardial artery, to microvascular disease, or to a combination of both. For these reasons, CFR is of limited value for clinical decision-making (Figure 27.4).[8]

Translesional pressure measurements and fractional flow reserve

DEFINITION

FFR is the ratio of the maximal myocardial blood flow in the presence of a stenosis relative to the expected normal flow in the absence of a stenosis. It can be expressed as a fraction of its normal expected value in that artery if there were no lesions. FFR measurement using only translesional pressure signals is based on the relationship between pressure and flow during minimal resistance (i.e., maximal hyperemia), a point at which the slope of the pressure-flow curve is linear, relating pressure to flow (Figure 27.5).[9]

The FFR derivations arise from a theoretical model of the coronary circulation and have been validated experimentally in animals, and later in humans, by positron emission tomography (PET).[10] During maximal hyperemia (induced pharmacologically), coronary resistance is at a minimum

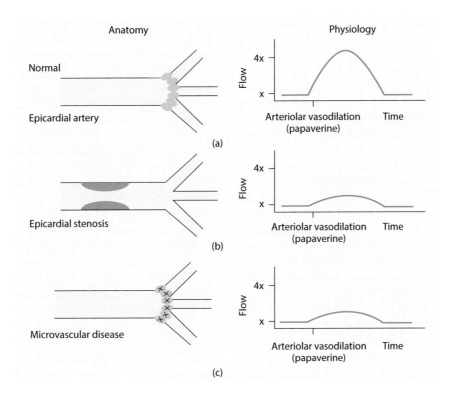

Figure 27.4 Coronary flow reserve findings. **(a)** A normal artery without any epicardial stenosis or microvascular disease demonstrates the ability to significantly increase coronary flow when a hyperemic agent is given. **(b)** An artery with a significant epicardial stenosis that blunts the ability to increase flow over baseline. **(c)** The same finding of an artery unable to increase its flow rate due to severe microvascular disease. (Redrawn from Wilson, R.F., and Lascon, D.D., *Cathet. Cardiovasc. Diagn.*, 29, 93–98, 1993.)

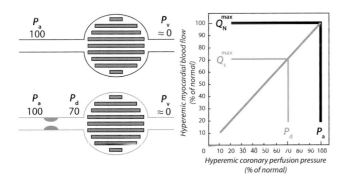

Figure 27.5 Simplified theoretical explanation illustrating how a ratio of two flows can be derived from a ratio of two pressures, provided these pressures are recorded during maximal hyperemia. (Right panel) Concept of FFR measurements. When no epicardial stenosis is present (black lines), the driving pressure (P_a) determines a normal (100%) maximal myocardial blood flow. In case of stenosis responsible for a hyperemic pressure gradient of 30 mmHg (*gray lines*), the driving pressure (P_d) will no longer be 100 mmHg but 70 mmHg. Since during maximal hyperemia the relationship between driving pressure and myocardial blood flow is linear, myocardial blood flow in the stenosed vessel (Q_s) will only reach 70% of its normal value. This numerical example shows how a ratio of two pressures (P_d/P_a) corresponds to a ratio of two flows (Q_S/Q_N). It also illustrates how important it is to induce maximal hyperemia.

and remains constant. Under this circumstance, flow is directly related to pressure in the epicardial artery.

The FFR derivation provides formulas for the determination of the percent of myocardial (FFR_{myo}), coronary (FFR_{cor}), and collateral (FFR_{collat}) blood flow relative to the normal values for that individual. The three FFR formulas are noted below:

Myocardial FFR (FFR_{myo}) = $1 - 'P/P_a - P_v = (P_d - P_v)/(P_a - P_v)$

Coronary FFR (FFR_{cor}) = $1 - 'P/(P_a - P_w) = (P_d - P_w)/(P_a - P_w)$

Collateral FFR (FFR_{collat}) = $FFR_{myo} - FFR_{cor}$

where P_a = mean aortic pressure; P_d = mean distal coronary pressure; $'P$ = mean translesional pressure gradient; P_v = mean right atrial pressure; and P_w = mean coronary wedge pressure or distal coronary pressure during balloon inflation.

FFR_{cor} is rarely measured, as it requires the use of a coronary balloon occlusion wedge pressure (P_w) during coronary angioplasty. FFR_{myo} differs from FFR_{cor} by including a term, the venous or, more precisely, the right atrial pressure to account for the collateral flow contribution to myocardial perfusion. Since FFR is measured during maximal hyperemia, resistance is the same minimal value in both the numerator and denominator, and P_v is assumed to be negligible relative to P_a. Thus, the FFR becomes

$$FFR_{myo} = (P_d - P_v)/(P_a - P_v)$$

However, for daily clinical use, the P_v is omitted as it is assumed to be negligible relative to P_a (right atrial pressure, 5–10 mmHg vs. aortic pressure, 80–100 mmHg). Thus, the FFR_{myo} is simplified to

$$FFR = P_d/P_a \text{ (during hyperemia)}$$

Because each myocardial territory and its resistance bed serves as its own control, FFR is a lesion-specific index. Furthermore, because FFR is measured only at maximal hyperemia, it is independent of microcirculation, heart rate, blood pressure, and other hemodynamic variables. Unlike most other physiologic indexes, FFR has a normal value of 1 for every patient and every coronary artery. FFR has high reproducibility and low intra-individual variability. Moreover, FFR, unlike CFR, is independent of gender or CAD risk factors, such as hypertension and diabetes, and has less variability with common doses of adenosine. De Bruyne and associates demonstrated that in humans, FFR was independent of hemodynamic conditions. Changes in heart rate by pacing, contractility by dobutamine infusion, and blood pressure by nitroprusside infusion did not alter FFR.[11] The coefficient of variation between two consecutive measurements was 4.2%, lower than the 17.7% for CFR measured with a Doppler wire.

FFR represents the extent to which maximal myocardial blood flow is limited by the presence of an epicardial stenosis. If FFR is 0.60, it means that maximal myocardial blood flow reaches only 60% of its normal value. Thus, FFR provides the interventionalist with knowledge of the extent to which optimal stenting of the epicardial stenosis will increase maximal myocardial blood flow. An FFR of 0.60 implies that stenting the focal stenosis responsible for this abnormal FFR should bring FFR to 1, which represents an increase in maximal myocardial blood flow of 67%.[12]

Technique of intracoronary sensor wire use

Intracoronary (IC) sensor wires are similar to standard 0.014-in angioplasty guidewires and are inserted and positioned using the identical technique as that used for routine PCI. FFR is often measured using 6-Fr guiding catheters, but 5-Fr guiding catheters and diagnostic catheters as small as 4-Fr have been successfully used. The smaller the catheter utilized, the greater the chance of poor signal transmission due to pressure damping. The operator must take care to flush and optimize the aortic pressure signal. Attention to detail is required in the measurement of FFR. A more complete description of the techniques and applications of coronary pressure measurements can be found elsewhere.[13]

Before the guidewire is advanced into the artery, guide catheter and guidewire pressures are balanced (i.e., "zeroed") to atmospheric pressure. For coronary pressure measurements, a pressure sensor wire is available from several companies (St. Jude Medical Inc., Minneapolis, MN; Volcano Therapeutics, Del Mar, CA; Opsens Inc., Quebec City, Canada; Boston Scientific Inc., Boston, MA) (Figure 27.6). The angioplasty sensor guidewires have mechanical properties similar to standard guidewires and, in addition, have a pressure sensor located 3 cm from the distal tip at the junction of the radiopaque and radiolucent portions of the wire. Recently, a novel 0.022-in pressure-sensing monorail microcatheter (The Navvus microcatheter, ACIST Medical Systems, Eden Prairie, MN) has been available to measure pressure over any 0.014-in standard guidewire of the operator's choice. The microcatheter has a pressure sensor that transmits its signal via a fiber-optic cable to the table-mounted analyzer (Figure 27.7).

For flow velocity, the Doppler sensor wire (Flowire or Combowire, Volcano Therapeutics, Inc.) has the crystal sensor located at the very distal guidewire tip (Figure 27.8). Before pressure or flow velocity signal acquisition, IC nitroglycerin (100–200 mcg) is given to minimize vasomotion. The sensor portion of the guidewire is advanced at least 5–10 artery-diameter lengths (>2 cm) beyond the stenosis. This distance is needed to make the measurement in a region of restored laminar flow (otherwise the turbulent flow close to the stenosis may underestimate true velocity). Resting flow pressure/velocity is recorded, and coronary hyperemia is then induced by IC or intravenous (IV) adenosine (or other suitable agents) with continuous recording of the flow velocity signals. Coronary vasodilatory reserve (CVR) is computed as the ratio of maximal hyperemic to basal average peak velocity (Figure 27.9). Because of the highly position-dependent signal, poor signal acquisition may occur in 10%–15% of patients even within normal arteries. As with transthoracic echo Doppler studies, the operator must adjust the guidewire position (sample volume) to optimize the velocity signal.

For FFR, after the guidewire is introduced into the guide catheter, the sensor is positioned at the tip of the guiding catheter, where the guiding catheter and wire pressures are equalized (or normalized). The sensor is then advanced across the stenosis several artery-diameters distal to the target lesion (or to the most distal part of the coronary artery for assessment of serial lesions or diffuse disease). The pharmacologic hyperemic stimulus (e.g., adenosine) is then administered as for CFR, either by IC (i.e., directly into the guide catheter) or by IV infusion. The mean and phasic pressure signals are continuously recorded, with the lowest P_d/P_a ratio after the onset of peak hyperemia being defined as the FFR, a parameter displayed on nearly all signal analyzers (Figure 27.10).

To identify a specific region of disease along a coronary artery (e.g., serial lesions or diffuse disease), the pressure sensor can be pulled back slowly during hyperemia, observing both the location of the wire by fluoroscopy and the pressure tracings to locate any hemodynamically

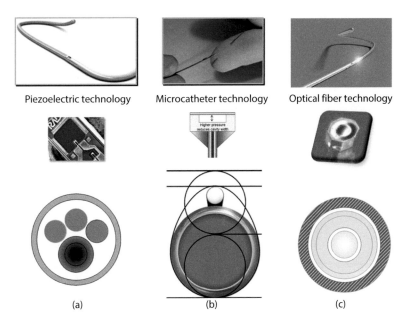

Figure 27.6 Pressure sensor wire and catheter technologies. From left to right: **(a)** piezoelectric sensors, microcatheter optical sensor, and optical fiber technology. Piezoelectric wires are specially constructed 0.014-in wires with a piezoelectric sensor incorporated 3 cm from the distal tip. (Courtesy of St. Jude Medical, St Paul, MN, Volcano Therapeutics Rancho Cordova, CA.) **(b)** Microcatheter over standard wire. A low-profile catheter with a fiber-optic pressure sensor incorporated into the distal end. (Courtesy of Acist Medical Eden Prairie, MN.) **(c)** Optical fiber guidewires. A specially constructed 0.014-in nitinol construction with fiberoptic sensor incorporated into the tip. (Courtesy of Opsens Inc., Quebec City, QC, Canada. Boston Scientific Marlborough, MA.)

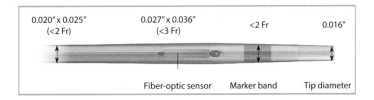

Figure 27.7 Navvus Rxi catheter. (Courtesy of Acist Medical, Eden Prairie, MN.)

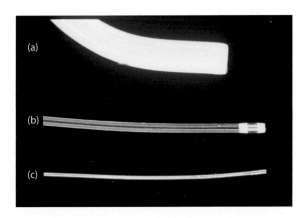

Figure 27.8 Evolution of Doppler flow sensors. **(a)** Doppler-tipped guide catheter. **(b)** 1-Fr pressure catheter. **(c)** 0.018-in Doppler-tipped guidewire.

significant atherosclerotic region. On retracting the wire, the pressure in a vessel with diffuse disease shows a gradual pressure recovery along the course of the vessel. In contrast, a vessel with a focal stenosis will demonstrate an abrupt increase in pressure proximal to the lesion. By moving the sensor back and forth, the exact location of a pressure drop representing a focal obstruction can be determined (Figure 27.11).

Pharmacologic hyperemia

The pharmacologic agents most often used to induce hyperemia are listed in Table 27.2. Maximal coronary hyperemia is required for an accurate FFR. The most widely used maximal vasodilator agent is adenosine administered either IC or IV. IC nitroprusside has similar hyperemic effects compared with IC adenosine but causes more hypotension. Papaverine is no longer used for IC hyperemic stimulation because of the potential of QT interval prolongation and associated ventricular tachycardia (VT) or fibrillation.

Submaximal hyperemia can be induced with iodinated contrast media as well as intracoronary nitroglycerine. Submaximal hyperemia may provide an estimate of the FFR that is sufficient for decision-making and, in many cases, without the use of adenosine. For example, when a submaximal hyperemic FFR value falls below the standard FFR ischemic threshold value (<0.80), a valid

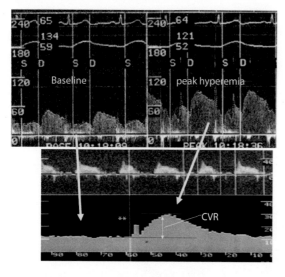

Figure 27.9 Measurement of coronary flow velocity with a Doppler guidewire. At baseline, the average peak velocity is approximately 10 cm/s. At peak hyperemia, the peak velocity is 30 cm/s, resulting in a coronary velocity reserve (CVR) of 3.

treatment decision can be rendered without further investigation. Nitrates increase volumetric flow, but because they also dilate the epicardial conductance vessels, the increase in coronary flow velocity is less predictable than with adenosine or papaverine. Table 27.3 lists FFR and FFR-like indices for clinical use.

Adenosine

Adenosine has a short half-life, with a return to basal flow within 30–60 seconds after cessation of infusion. IV and IC adenosines are very well tolerated with a ~10% drop in mean arterial pressure and may be accompanied by short-lived symptoms of dyspnea or chest burning. Although transient, AV block may rarely occur also producing a short-lived drop in mean arterial pressure.

IV adenosine uses weight-adjusted dosing (140 mcg/kg/min) and is required over IC administration for the evaluation of ostial lesions or for the assessment of diffuse disease during pullback recordings. Compared to IC, IV administration has a higher incidence of side effects such as flushing, chest tightness, bronchospasm, nausea, and transient AV block or bradycardia. IC adenosine bolus doses that produce maximal hyperemia equivalent to IV adenosine infusion are 50–100 mcg for the right coronary artery and 100–200 mcg for the left coronary artery (Figure 27.12).[14]

Regadenoson

Regadenoson is an α2A adenosine receptor agonist that induces coronary vasodilatation and increases myocardial blood flow in a manner reportedly equivalent to adenosine with fewer adverse effects. Regadenoson has a half-life of 2–3 minutes in the initial phase, 30 minutes in the

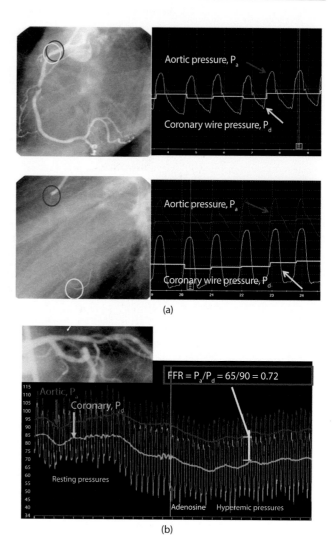

(a)

(b)

Figure 27.10 **(a)** Method of fractional flow reserve (FFR) measurement. The first step is to advance the pressure wire to the tip of the catheter (a, top left) to be certain the pressures are superimposed. Red and yellow circles depict the guidewire sensor and the guide catheter in the proximal right coronary artery with corresponding pressures (P_d and P_a, respectively) depicted on the right, showing "equalization" of pressures. (a, bottom left) The guidewire has been advanced across the right coronary artery lesion and now is in the distal vessel with corresponding pressure loss as depicted on the right. **(b)** FFR measurement across a proximal left anterior descending (LAD) lesion. The red pressure tracing is aortic guide catheter pressure (P_a) and the green tracing is coronary wire pressure (P_d). Adenosine infusion is started and the tracings from left to right reflect the pressure changes over time. The yellow bar reflects the lowest P_d/P_a at steady state, from which the FFR is computed. The nadir of distal pressure is used for the FFR calculation. FFR = P_d/P_a = 65/90 = 0.72.

intermediate phase, and 2 hours in the terminal phase. It is administered as single intravenous bolus (0.4 mg), and thus may be easier to use, but its cost and prolonged effect may complicate the measurement of multiple lesions or arteries.[15,16]

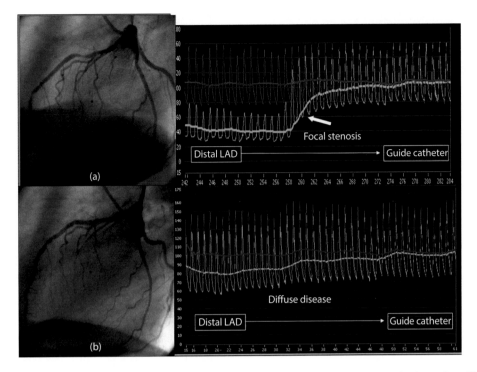

Figure 27.11 Fractional flow reserve pattern in focal stenosis **(a)** and diffuse disease **(b)**. Both show the effects of pressure wire pullback toward the coronary ostium. LAD, left anterior descending.

Table 27.2 Coronary physiologic indexes—Hyperemic agents used for coronary physiology assessment

Agent	Route	Dose	Comments
Adenosine	IV infusion	140 mcg/kg/min	Reference standard. Side effects include dyspnea and chest pain. Prolonged hyperemia allows pressure wire pullback.
Adenosine	IC bolus	>100 mcg	Easy to use, inexpensive, and no significant side effects. Transient heart block at high doses. Hyperemia lasts only 10–15 sec.
Adenosine	IC infusion	240–360 mcg/min	Inconvenient setup. Fewer side effects compared with IV infusion. Prolonged hyperemia allows pullback. Not well validated.
Regadenoson	IV bolus	400 mcg	Convenient, single IV bolus. Expensive. Side effects similar to IV adenosine but less severe and briefer. Hyperemia lasts 20 sec to 10 min.
Papaverine	IC bolus	10–20 mg	Easy to use, inexpensive. Rare, but significant side effects of polymorphic VT. Hyperemia lasts 30 sec, allowing pullback.
Nitroprusside	IC bolus	0.3–0.9 mcg/kg	Easy to use, inexpensive. Major side effect is hypotension. Hyperemia lasts 50 sec, allowing pullback. Not well validated.
Dobutamine	IV infusion	50 mcg/kg/min	Inconvenient as it takes time for onset and offset. Side effects include palpitations and hypotension. Not well validated for FFR.
Nicorandil	IC bolus	2 mg	Not available in the United States. Fewer side effects compared with IV adenosine. Hyperemia lasts 30 sec. Not well validated.

Source: Fearon, W.F., *Circ. Cardiovasc. Interv.*, 8(2), e001942, 2015.
Note: FFR, fractional flow reserve; IC, intracoronary; IV, intravenous; VT, ventricular tachycardia.

Sodium nitroprusside

IC nitroprusside can be an alternative to IC adenosine. Serial doses of IC nitroprusside (boluses of 0.3, 0.6, and 0.9 mcg/kg)[17] produce equivalent coronary hyperemia with a longer duration (about 25%) compared with IC adenosine. IC nitroprusside (0.9 mcg/kg) decreases systolic blood pressure by 20% with minimal change in heart rate, whereas IC adenosine has no effect on these parameters. FFR measurements with IC nitroprusside are identical to those obtained with IC adenosine. IC nitroprusside, in doses commonly used for the treatment of the no-reflow phenomenon, can produce coronary hyperemia suitable to measure FFR without detrimental systemic hemodynamics.

MEASUREMENTS OF MICROVASCULAR DISEASE

The ratio of distal coronary pressure to the inverse of the mean transit time during maximal hyperemia defines an index of microvascular resistance (IMR) (Figure 27.13).

Table 27.3 FFR and other FFR-like indices

Index	Normal value	Ischemic threshold	Comments
FFR	1.0	≤0.80	See Table 27.1
cFFR	1.0	≈0.83	Avoids adenosine by using contrast media; may correlate with FFR better than iFR and P_d/P_a
iFR	1.0	≈0.90	Avoids need for hyperemia; 80% accurate when compared with FFR
Rest P_d/P_a	1.0	≈0.92	Avoids need for hyperemia; 80% accurate when compared with FFR

Source: Fearon, W.F., *Circ. Cardiovasc. Interv.*, 8(2), e001942, 2015.
Note: cFFR, contrast FFR; FFR, fractional flow reserve; iFR, instantaneous wave-free pressure ratio; P_d/P_a, distal coronary pressure/proximal coronary pressure.

IMR is superior to CFR because it is not affected by resting hemodynamics, making it more reproducible, even after hemodynamic perturbations. It is also specific for the microvasculature, whereas CFR is affected by epicardial stenosis. IMR, when measured immediately after primary PCI for STEMI, predicts the amount of myocardial damage, as well as left ventricular recovery better than other indices, such as CFR, ST-segment resolution, or thrombolysis in myocardial infarction (TIMI) myocardial perfusion grade. IMR can also be useful for identifying microvascular dysfunction in patients with chest pain and no epicardial artery disease.

For determination of IMR, small bolus injections of 3 mL of saline in triplicate at maximal are given to the target artery as described by Fearon et al.[18] Mean transit time (T_{mn}) and P_d are measured simultaneously. IMR is calculated by multiplying the mean P_d by the hyperemic T_{mn}. IMR is taken as the average of the three consecutive measurements at hyperemia.

Clinical applications

FRACTIONAL FLOW RESERVE AND ISCHEMIA

Direct translesional pressure measurements correlate well with noninvasive assessment of CAD. The initial landmark study of Pijls et al.[19] established a FFR threshold of 0.75, below which ischemia was present (Figure 27.14). Applying this ischemic threshold to the clinical outcome of patients in whom PCI has been deferred because the FFR indicated no

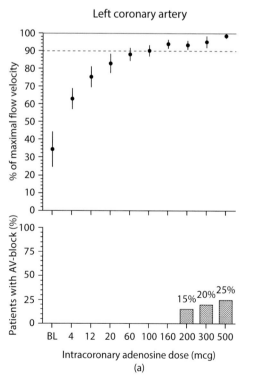
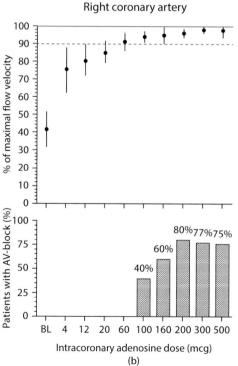

Figure 27.12 Intracoronary adenosine dose-flow relationship. **(a)** Dose-response data for the left coronary artery (left panel) and the right coronary artery (right panel). The data are expressed as the percent of maximum flow velocity for each patient at each dose of intracoronary adenosine. The error bars represent the 95% confidence intervals for each value. **(b)** The bars represent the percent of patients in whom high-grade atrioventricular (AV) block occurred with that dose of adenosine. BL = baseline. (From Adjedj, J., et al., *J. Am. Coll. Cardiol. Interv.*, 8, 1422–1430, 2015, with permission.)

hemodynamically significant stenosis (i.e., FFR >0.75), is associated with a low incidence of clinical events.[20] In this population, the risk of death or myocardial infarction (MI) is approximately 1% per year, and this risk is not decreased by PCI. Outcome studies (see below) strongly support the use of FFR measurements as a guide for decision-making about the need for revascularization in "intermediate" lesions.

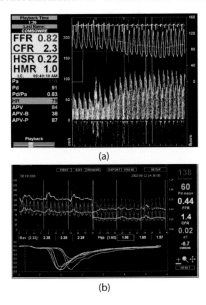

Figure 27.13 Characterizing the microcirculation. **(a)** Combined pressure and Doppler flow measurements during adenosine-induced hyperemia. **(b)** Combined fractional flow reserve and coronary flow reserve measurements using the thermodilution technique. Both techniques have been validated to measure coronary flow. Hyperemic Stenosis Resistance Index (HSR$_v$) = P$_a$ – P$_v$/ APV$_{hyper}$. IMR = P$_a$*T$_{mn}$ [(P$_d$ – P$_w$)/(P$_a$ – P$_w$)]. (From Ng, M.K., et al., *Circulation*, 113, 2054–2061, 2006. With permission.) APV, average peak velocity; IMR, index of microcirculatory resistance; P$_a$, aortic pressure; P$_d$, resting distal coronary artery pressure; P$_v$, coronary venous pressure; P$_w$, coronary occlusion wedge pressure; T$_{mn}$, mean transit time.

Percutaneous coronary intervention clinical outcomes and fractional flow reserve

Several prospective randomized trials have demonstrated the safety and efficacy of using FFR to guide PCI, forming supporting evidence to incorporate FFR as a routine tool to improve outcomes in the catheterization lab.

The DEFER Trial[20] asked the question: Is it safe and efficacious to not treat lesions with FFR >0.75? FFR was performed in 325 patients with stable ischemic heart disease and an intermediate angiographic lesion. Those patients having an FFR <0.75 were treated with PCI and those with an FFR >0.75 were randomized to either PCI or medical therapy (i.e., perform or defer angioplasty, respectively). After 15 years, the rate of death was not different between the three groups: 33% in the defer group, 31% in the perform group, and 36% in the reference group of FFR <0.75 where PCI was performed. The rate of MI was significantly lower in the defer group (2.2%) compared with the perform group (10%) ($P = 0.03$), primarily due to fewer target vessel MIs. There was no difference in subsequent revascularization, and thus no "late catch-up" of events in patients who had deferral of PCI in FFR-negative stenosis (Figure 27.15).

The FAME Trial[21] (Fractional Flow Reserve Versus Angiography for Guiding Coronary Intervention) was a prospective randomized trial that tested the hypothesis that FFR-guided PCI would be superior to standard angiographic-guided PCI. In this trial, 1,005 patients with multivessel CAD (at least two vessels with a >50% angiographic stenosis) were randomized to a strategy of FFR or angiographic-guided PCI. The angiographic-guided ($n = 500$) group had a drug-eluting stent placed in all prospectively identified lesions, and the FFR-guided group ($n = 500$) had a drug-eluting stent placed in only those lesions producing an FFR of ≤0.80. The primary composite endpoint of death, nonfatal MI, and repeat revascularization was significantly reduced by FFR-guided PCI at 1 year and was maintained out to 5 years (Figure 27.16).

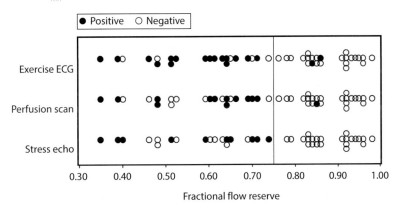

Figure 27.14 Relation between fractional flow reserve (FFR) and the results of three noninvasive tests. The test results for each patient are shown on one column according to that patient's FFR. The hollow circles represent negative tests. The black dots represent positive tests. The dashed line representing an FFR of 0.75 indicates the cutoff between the two groups assessed in this study. In all patients with an FFR <0.75, reversible myocardial ischemia was demonstrated on at least one noninvasive test. Coronary revascularization was performed in the 21 patients with myocardial ischemia, and all the positive noninvasive tests reverted to normal. (From Piljs, N., *N. Engl. J. Med.*, 334, 1703–1708, 1996, with permission.) ECG, electrocardiogram.

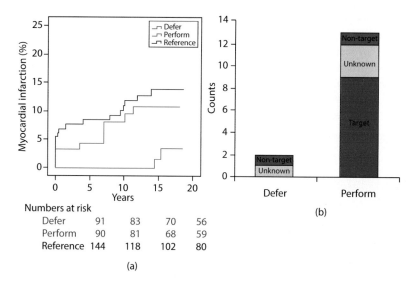

Figure 27.15 Kaplan–Meier curves of rate of myocardial infarction (MI) (a) and relationship to MI with vessel territory (b). Fifteen-year follow-up of patients in the DEFER trial. **(a)** The incidence of MI for patients with normal FFR in the defer group treated medically (blue), patients with normal FFR that were stented (red), and patients with abnormal FFR that were stented (black). **(b)** The number of patients in the defer and perform groups having events in the target vessel, other vessel, or unknown site. (From Zimmermann, F.M., et al., *Eur. Heart J.*, 36, 3182–3188, 2015, with permission.)

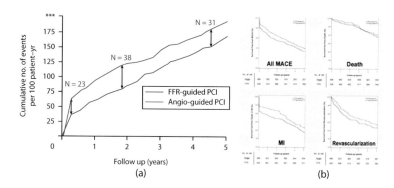

Figure 27.16 FAME 5-year follow-up event rates. **(a)** Cumulative event rates over 5 years comparing fractional flow reserve (FFR)-guided compared to angiographic-guided percutaneous coronary internvetion (PCI). **(b)** Kaplan Meier event curves over 5 years for major adverse cardiac events, death, myocardial infarction (MI), and revascularization. (Presented at European Society of Cardiology, August 2015, by Dr. Nico Pijls. Initial study: Tonino, P.A., et al., *N. Engl. J. Med.*, 360, 213–234, 2009, with permission.)

Interestingly, in the FAME trial, there were 513 lesions with a FFR >0.80 (i.e., deferred PCI) in 509 patients. In a 2-year follow-up, there was a 0.2% rate of late MI in FFR negative lesions not receiving a stent. There were 53 repeat revascularizations; 37 of those were performed for restenotic lesions; only 10 lesions were *de novo* stenosis needing revascularization—a rate of 1.9%, confirming a low risk of deferring PCI on patients with FFR >0.80.

An important recent study by Adjedj et al.[14] examined outcomes of 1,459 patients treated with FFR in the "gray zone" (i.e., FFR 0.76–0.80); 449 patients were revascularized and 1,010 patients were treated with medical therapy. The major adverse cardiovascular events rate was similar (37 [13.9%] vs. 21 [11.2%], respectively; P = 0.3) between medical therapy and revascularization groups, whereas a strong trend toward a higher rate of death or MI (25 [9.4%] vs. 9

[4.8]%, P = 0.06) and overall death (20 [7.5%] vs. 6 [3.2%], P = 0.059) was observed in the medical therapy group. A significant increase in the rate of major adverse cardiovascular events was observed with proximal lesion location for borderline FFR values. In revascularization patients, the major adverse cardiovascular events rate was not different across the FFR strata. The authors concluded that FFR, in and around the gray zone, has important prognostic value, especially in proximal lesions. The study confirms that FFR ≤0.80 is a valid guide to clinical decision-making.

The FAME 2 Trial[22] (Fractional Flow Reserve-Guided PCI Versus Medical Therapy in Stable Coronary Disease) compared the effectiveness of treating ischemic lesions (i.e., those with FFR ≤0.80) with optimal medical therapy (OMT) alone or with revascularization with PCI plus OMT. Accordingly, 1,220 patients with angiographic disease in one, two, or three vessels that were suitable for PCI underwent FFR. All patients with lesions having FFR ≤0.80 were randomized to either PCI or medical therapy. A composite of all-cause mortality, nonfatal MI, or unplanned hospitalization leading to urgent revascularization during a 2-year follow-up was the primary endpoint (Figure 27.17). As in prior studies, lesions that did not undergo PCI for FFR >0.80 were entered into a registry and followed. These patients had a low rate of death (0%), MI (1.8%), or urgent revascularization (2.4%) over the 12-month follow-up, thus reproducing the findings of the pre-DES era DEFER trial conducted before drug-e.

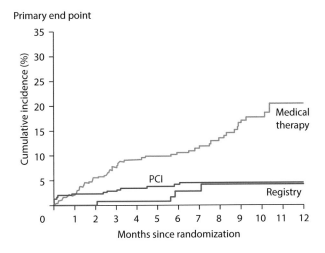

Figure 27.17 The FAME 2 study results. Kaplan–Meier curve for primary endpoint of death, myocardial infarction, or urgent revascularization at 12 months in the group assigned to percutaneous coronary intervention (PCI) and optimal medical therapy versus optimal medical therapy alone versus those who did not undergo revascularization. Patients with lesions who did not undergo PCI for fractional flow reserve (FFR) >0.80 were entered into a registry. (Modified from De Bruyne, B., et al., *N. Engl. J. Med.*, 367, 991–1001, 2012.)

Together, these data are the core source of FFR-related outcomes. They strongly support the concept that coronary stenosis with an FFR that is not physiologically significant (i.e., >0.80) have an exceptionally good prognosis without PCI and should be treated with OMT alone.

LEFT MAIN CORONARY ARTERY DISEASE

Numerous studies support FFR use for assessment of left main (LM) coronary stenosis (Table 27.4). In the largest of such studies, Hamilos et al.[23] examined 5-year outcomes in 213 patients with an angiographically equivocal LM coronary artery stenosis in which revascularization decisions were guided by FFR. When FFR was ≥0.80, patients were treated medically or another stenosis was treated by coronary angioplasty (nonsurgical group; $n = 138$). When FFR was <0.80, coronary artery bypass grafting (CABG) surgery was performed (surgical group; $n = 75$). The 5-year survival rates were similar for the nonsurgical (FFR >80) and surgical groups (FFR <0.80) (90% and 85%, respectively) as were the 5-year event-free survival rates (74% and 82%, respectively) ($P = 0.48$) (Figure 27.18). Noteworthy was that only 23% of patients with LM diameter stenosis >50% had a hemodynamically significant FFR.

SIMPLE AND COMPLEX LEFT MAIN LESION ASSESSMENT

Accurate FFR requires maximal flow to be achieved across the target vessel. The LM transmits flow to the majority of the left ventricle through both the LAD and left circumflex (LCX) branches in proportion to the size of their associated viable myocardial beds. The myocardial bed for the LM is then the sum of both the LAD and LCX territories (Figure 27.19). Simple or isolated LM disease can be assessed in the routine FFR fashion. Distal LM involving both LAD and LCX must be assessed with two measurements, one FFR with the wire in the LAD and one with the wire in the LCX.

Table 27.4 Left main revascularization outcomes and FFR—Summary of FFR-guided clinical outcomes trials involving assessment and treatment decision-making for left main coronary stenoses

First author (Ref. #)	Number of patients			Cutoff value	FU (months)	Overall survival (%)	
	Total no. pts	Defer group	Surgical group			Defer group	Surgical group
Bech (39)	54	24	30	0.75	29 ± 15	100	97
Jasti (40)	51	37	14	0.75	25 ± 11	100	100
Jimenez-Navarro (41)	27	20	7	0.75	26 ± 12	100	86
Legutko (42)	38	20	18	0.75	24 ± 12	100	89
Suemaru (43)	15	8	7	0.75	33 ± 10	100	100
Lindstaedt (44)	51	24	27	0.75	29 ± 16	100	81
Hamilos (23)	213	138	75	0.80	35 ± 12	90	85
Total or (mean)	449	271	178	–	(28 ± 13)	95*	89

Source: Puri, R., et al., *JACC Cardiovasc. Interv.*, 5(7), 697–707, 2012.
Note: FFR, fractional flow reserve; FU, mean duration of follow-up.
* = NS compared with surgical group.

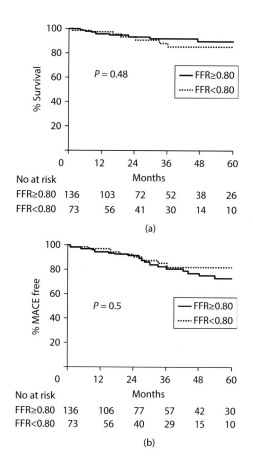

Figure 27.18 Outcomes in patients with intermediate left main coronary artery disease based on treatment guided by fractional flow reserve (FFR) assessment. (a) Survival curves for patients with medical therapy (FFR >0.80), and patients treated with coronary artery bypass grafting (CABG) (FFR <0.80) over 5 years. (b) Major adverse cardiac events in patients treated with medical therapy (FFR >0.80) and CABG (FFR <0.80) over 5 years. (From Hamilos, M., et al., *Circulation*, 120, 1505–1512, 2009, with permission.)

LM assessment in the presence of a significant downstream LAD stenosis is complicated. The LM stenosis can be assessed by FFR with the wire in the LCX, but the true LM FFR may be erroneously elevated since flow across the LAD may be reduced, possibly limiting maximal hyperemia and thus reducing total LM flow and FFR accuracy. The higher "apparent" LM FFR is not a concern if either the LAD or LCX are not hemodynamically significant. As Yong et al.[24] and Fearon[25] show (see below), the "apparent" and true LM FFR will be very close to one another.

When measuring FFR across serial lesions in the LM and LAD, first place the pressure transducer distal to the most distal lesion. If the FFR at that level is >0.80, neither lesion is physiologically significant. If the FFR is ≤0.80, a pressure pullback during hyperemia is performed, noting the largest pressure gradient (ΔP), and then the lesion (LAD or LM) with the largest ΔP is treated and FFR repeated on the remaining lesion. The downside of this approach is that once a significant LAD lesion is removed (i.e., stented), the LM FFR may become significant, mandating further revascularization by stenting

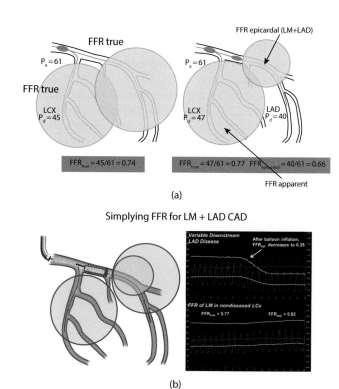

Simplying FFR for LM + LAD CAD

Figure 27.19 (a) Physiological measurements. Animal model of left main (LM) with and without left anterior descending (LAD) stenosis. Example of physiological measurements. True fractional flow reserve (FFR$_{true}$) of the LM coronary artery obtained during LM balloon inflation and no stenosis in the LAD artery (FFR$_{true}$ = distal pressure [P_d] in the left circumflex (LCX) artery divided by proximal arterial pressure (P_a). (B) FFR$_{app}$ obtained during balloon inflation in the LAD (FFR$_{app}$ = LCX P_d/P_a during downstream balloon inflation). FFR$_{epicardial}$ represents FFR of LM plus LAD (FFR$_{epicardial}$ = LAD P_d/P_a during LAD balloon inflation). (Modified from Yong, A.S., et al., *Circ. Cardiovasc. Interv.*, 6, 161–165, 2013.) (b) Cartoon of experimental layout to test relationship between left main (LM) and left anterior descending (LAD) lesions of increasing severity. There is a deflated ("winged") balloon in the LM coronary artery with a variably inflated balloon within the newly placed LAD stent, and pressure wires down the LAD and the LCX coronary artery. The green circle represents a smaller myocardial perfusion bed size when the LAD balloon is inflated. Only when the LAD lesion is very severe does the fractional flow reserve (FFR) apparent in the LCX rise. (From Fearon, W.F., et al., *J. Am. Coll. Cardiol. Intv.*, 8, 398–403, 2015, with permission.)

or CABG. Thus, performing a PCI of a downstream lesion solely to measure the LM FFR may not be the best option.

Fearon and colleagues[25] assessed the effect of downstream disease on FFR across an intermediate left main coronary artery (LMCA) stenosis in 25 patients with both LAD and LCX stenosis. After stenting of the LAD, the LCX, or both, an intermediate LMCA stenosis was created with a deflated balloon catheter. FFR was measured in the LAD and LCX coronary arteries before and after creation of a stenosis in these vessels by inflating an angioplasty balloon within the newly placed stent. The true FFR (FFR_{true}) of the LMCA, measured in the nondiseased downstream vessel in the absence of stenosis in the other vessel, was compared with the apparent FFR (FFR_{app}) measured in the presence of stenosis. LMCA FFR_{true} was significantly lower than (FFR_{app} (0.81 ± 0.08 vs. 0.83 ± 0.08, $P < 0.001$) (Figure 27.20), although the absolute numerical difference was small. This difference correlated with the severity of the downstream disease ($r = 0.35$, $P < 0.001$). In all cases in which FFR_{app} was >0.85, FFR_{true} was >0.80.

The data from *in vitro*, animal, and human studies of LM stenosis demonstrate that, in most cases, downstream disease does not have a clinically significant impact on the assessment of FFR across an intermediate LM stenosis. Downstream stenosis in the LAD or LCX has to be both severe (i.e., FFR <0.60) and proximal to have a marked effect on the LM FFR. In these situations, intravascular ultrasound (IVUS) assessment of the LM with a threshold minimal luminal area of <6 mm² is recommended.

TANDEM OR SERIAL LESIONS

In the setting of serial or sequential lesions, each stenosis will blunt the hyperemic effect of the other, making accurate FFR of individual lesions difficult, if not impossible, to determine. If the distance between two lesions is greater than six times the vessel diameter, the stenoses generally behave independently, and the overall pressure gradient is

the sum of the individual pressure losses at any given flow rate. For lesions in series, equations have been derived to mathematically predict the FFR (FFR_{pred}) of each stenosis separately (i.e., as if the other ones were removed), using arterial pressure (P_a), pressure between the two stenoses (P_m), distal coronary pressure (P_d), and coronary occlusive pressure (P_w).[26,27] In clinical practice, the use of the pressure pull-back recording is particularly well suited to identify the regions of the largest pressure gradients that may benefit from treatment. The stenosis with the largest gradient can be treated first, after which the FFR can be remeasured for the remaining stenosis to determine the need for further treatment (see case examples in Figure 27.21.)

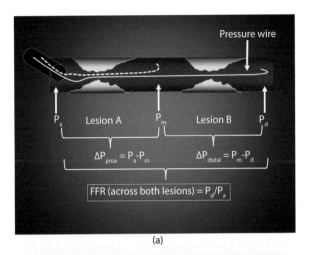

(a)

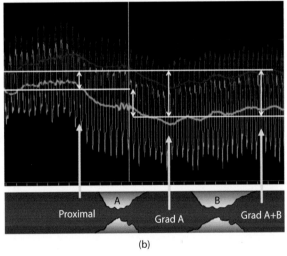

(b)

Figure 27.21 **(a)** Serial lesion assessment. Pressures and pressure gradients across lesions in series. FFR, fractional flow reserve; P_a, aortic pressure; P_d, distal pressure; P_m, mid-pressure between lesions; ΔP_{prox} and ΔP_{distal} are pressure gradients produced by each lesion. **(b)** Serial (multiple) lesions in a single vessel. When more than one discrete stenosis is present in the same vessel, the hyperemic flow and pressure through the first lesion will be attenuated by the second and vice versa. The FFR value recorded reflects the value across both lesions. Individual lesion FFR cannot be determined without a coronary occlusion wedge pressure.

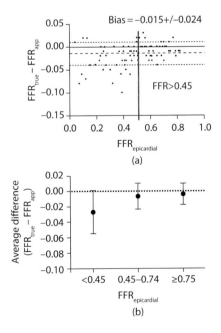

Figure 27.20 **(a)** Bland-Altman plot demonstrating the relationship between the difference in true (FFR_{true}) and apparent fractional flow reserve (FFR_{app}) based on the severity of downstream disease as assessed by FFR of the left main coronary and the downstream stenosis (FFR_{epi}). **(b)** Chart demonstrating the average difference between the FFR_{true} and FFR_{app} depending on the severity of the downstream stenosis (FFR_{epi}). (From Fearon, W.F., et al., *J. Am. Coll. Cardiol. Interv.*, 8(3), 398–403, 2015, with permission.)

DIFFUSE CORONARY DISEASE

Diffuse coronary atherosclerotic disease acts as a series of multiple mild stenoses with branches gradually distributing flow along the length of the conduit. As a function of gradually increasing resistance, the perfusion pressure also gradually diminishes over the diseased segment. FFR may be below the ischemic threshold of ≤0.80 but not clearly associated with a focal stenosis. A continuous pullback of the pressure wire from a distal location to a proximal location will identify any specific area of focal angiographic narrowing and confirm the presence of diffuse atherosclerosis. Diffuse atherosclerosis, as opposed to a focal narrowing, is characterized by a continuous and gradual pressure recovery during pullback without localized abrupt increase in pressure related to an isolated region.[28] In some cases, the gradual decline of pressure along the vessel occurs over a very long segment, such that interventional treatment is not feasible. Medical treatment (or bypass grafting) would be appropriate in these cases.

FRACTIONAL FLOW RESERVE IN ACUTE CORONARY SYNDROMES

Acute myocardial injury produces transient microvascular dysfunction to various degrees and impairs maximal coronary hyperemia, thereby reducing flow across a stenosis. After the patient recuperates, myocardial recovery may increase coronary flow across the stenosis, and higher flow would lower the FFR, perhaps below the ischemic threshold, thus changing a treatment decision from that made during the acute event. As a result, the FFR of a vessel (i.e., a lesion different from the culprit lesion, but in the same vessel) that is involved in a STEMI or large non-STEMI can result in a false-negative result. FFR has been demonstrated to be accurate after 4–6 days in most patients with unstable angina or a non-STEMI. Sels et al. reported that FFR was accurate and equally beneficial in the 328 patients in the FAME trial with positive troponin, but creatine kinase (CK) levels <1000 U/L, compared with the stable angina patients. They posit that the degree of microvascular dysfunction for such small myocardial injury is minimal, and the benefit of FFR applies equally to such patients.[29]

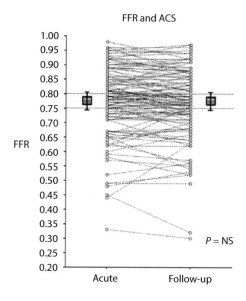

Figure 27.22 Fractional flow reserve (FFR) and acute coronary syndromes (ACS). FFR values are of nonculprit coronary artery stenosis during acute myocardial infarction and at follow-up. (From Ntalianis, A., et al., *J. Am. Coll. Cardiol. Cardiovasc. Interv.*, 3, 1274, 2010, with permission.)

In an acute STEMI, FFR of most nonculprit lesions at a distance from the infarct-related artery has also been shown to be accurate. Therefore, in this setting, a low FFR indicates hemodynamic significance of the nonculprit lesion, but a normal FFR may not be definitive. Ntalianis et al.[30] measured FFR of 112 nonculprit lesions during an acute MI (75 patients with STEMI, 26 patients with non-STEMI) and again 35 ± 24 days later. Only two lesions had a clinically meaningful change where FFR was >0.80 during the acute episode and <0.75 at follow-up (Figure 27.22).

De Bruyne et al.[31] and Samady et al.[32] obtained FFR measurements of culprit vessels 3 or more days after acute MI and compared them to subsequent single-photo emission computed tomography (SPECT) imaging to identify true positives and negatives. Both studies showed that an FFR <0.75 had high sensitivity, specificity, and overall accuracy for detecting reversible ischemia identified by SPECT imaging, and they both reached the same best cutoff value for FFR of 0.78. Trials that have evaluated the use of FFR in the setting of an acute coronary syndrome are summarized in Table 27.5.

Table 27.5 Fractional flow reserve and acute coronary syndrome trials

Setting	Culprit/ nonculprit	Validity	First author (Ref. #)	N	Comment
Acute MI	Culprit vessel	Unreliable	Tamita (45)	33 STEMI	Mean FFR after successful PCI was higher (0.95 ± 0.04) than in reference group of stable angina patients (0.90 ± 0.04, P = 0.002) despite identical IVUS parameters, likely reflecting microvascular stunning and dysfunction.

(Continued)

Table 27.5 (Continued) Fractional flow reserve and acute coronary syndrome trials

Setting	Culprit/ nonculprit	Validity	First author (Ref. #)	N	Comment
Acute MI	Nonculprit vessel	Reliable	Ntalianis (30)	75 STEMI, 26 NSTEMI	112 nonculprit lesions measured acutely and 35 ± 24 days later. Only two lesions had clinically meaningful change—FFR >0.80 during the acute episode and <0.75 at follow-up
Recent MI	Culprit vessel	Reliable	De Bruyne (31)	57 Acute MI with viable myocardium on left ventriculog-raphy	FFR after acute MI (≥6 days, mean 20 days) compared to SPECT before and after PCI. FFR <0.75 had high sensitivity (87%) and specificity (100%) for detecting ischemia on true positive/negative SPECT. BCV for FFR 0.78. Inverse correlation between FFR and LVEF—for a similar degree of stenosis, FFR depends on mass of viable myocardium.
Recent MI	Culprit vessel	Reliable	Samady (32)	36 STEMI, 12 NSTEMI	FFR after acute MI (STEMI ≥3 days, NSTEMI ≥2 days, mean 3.7 days) compared to SPECT at 11 weeks. FFR ≤0.75 had high sensitivity (88%), specificity (93%), and overall accuracy (91%) for detecting reversibility on true positive/negative SPECT. BCV for FFR 0.78.
Recent MI	Nonculprit vessel	FFR-guided PCI = good clinical outcomes	Potvin (46)	125 ACS, 60 SIHD, 16 atypical CP	201 consecutive pts (62% unstable angina, NSTEMI, or >24 h after STEMI) with ~50% stenosis in which PCI was deferred based on FFR ≥0.75. No difference in clinical outcomes between ACS and stable angina pts.
Recent MI		FFR-guided PCI = good clinical outcomes	Fischer (47)	35 ACS	FFR-guided PCI of intermediate lesions (50–70%). Deferring PCI for FFR ≥0.75 in pts with recent ACS. Similar MACE rates at 12 mo compared with pts without ACS.
UA/NSTEMI	Culprit vessel	FFR-guided PCI = good clinical outcomes	Leesar (48)	70 UA/ NSTEMI	Recent NSTE-ACS with intermediate single-vessel lesion randomized to immediate FFR-guided PCI versus post-angio SPECT. FFR-guided treatment reduced hospital stay and cost, with no increase in procedure time, radiation exposure, or clinical event rates at 1 year.
UA/NSTEMI	Culprit + nonculprit Vessel	FFR-guided PCI = good clinical outcomes	Sels (29)	326 UA/ NSTEMI	FAME study. FFR-guided PCI versus angiography-guided PCI for multivessel disease. In subset of pts with recent NSTE-ACS, significantly lower MACE rate with FFR-guided PCI.

Note: ACS, acute coronary syndrome; BCV, best cut-off value; CP, chest pain; FFR, fractional flow reserve; IVUS, intravascular ultrasound; LVEF, left ventricular ejection fraction; MACE, major adverse coronary event; MI, myocardial infarction; NSTE, non-ST-segment eleva-tion; PCI, percutaneous coronary intervention; pts, patients; SIHD, stable ischemic heart disease; SPECT, single-photon emission computed tomography; STEMI, ST-segment elevation myocardial infarction; NSTEMI, non-ST-segment elevation myocardial infarc-tion; UA, unstable angina.

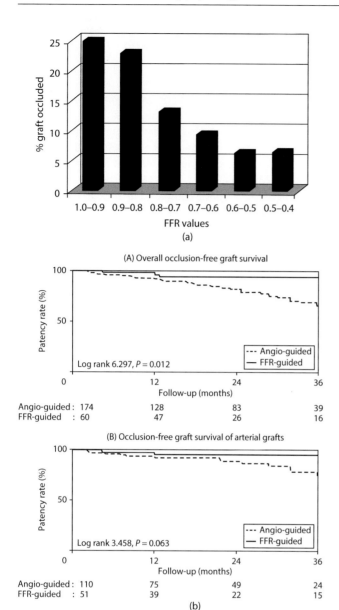

Figure 27.23 **(a)** The relation between functional stenosis severity established by fractional flow reserve (FFR) measurements and graft failure at angiographic follow-up after 1 year. (From Botman, C.J., et al., *Ann. Thorac. Surg.*, 83, 2093–2097, 2007, with permission.) **(b)** Occlusion-free survival of grafts with angiographic follow-up. (Top) Occlusion-free survival of all grafts. (Bottom) Occlusion-free survival of arterial grafts only. Angio, angiography; FFR, fractional flow reserve. (From Toth, G., et al., *Circulation*, 128, 1405–1411, 2013, with permission.)

Fractional flow reserve and coronary artery bypass graft lesions

Assessment of stenosis severity in coronary artery bypass grafts by FFR is technically very easy. In addition, all theoretical assumptions underlying the concept of FFR hold in cases of bypass grafts. There is no reason to believe that another threshold value should be found even though this has not been formally investigated in large series and no clinical outcome

data have been obtained from patients in whom decisions regarding revascularization have been based on FFR

Of note, Botman et al. investigated the relationship between graft patency after 6 months and stenosis severity in the bypassed native artery (Figure 27.23). The authors showed that the rate of graft occlusion was approximately three times higher when the bypass was placed on a native artery determined by FFR to have a hemodynamically non-significant stenosis as compared to a significant stenosis.[33] These results corroborate the data reported by Berger et al. who showed that internal mammary artery grafts placed on mildly diseased native arteries showed a high attrition rate.[34] Toth et al. also demonstrated improved CABG patency in coronaries with a hemodynamically significantly stenosis by FFR than those with angiographic-only guided surgery.[35]

NONHYPEREMIC INDICES OF CORONARY STENOSIS SIGNIFICANCE

The assessment of stenosis severity by FFR requires that coronary resistance is stable and minimal, usually achieved by the administration of adenosine. Utilization of an adenosine-free or adenosine independent pressure-derived index of coronary stenosis severity may facilitate the incorporation of physiology into the catheterization laboratory. Using wave intensity analysis, Sen et al.[36] identified a period of diastole in which equilibration or balance between pressure waves from the aorta and distal microcirculatory reflection was a "wave-free period" with a low and fixed resistance. During this period the resistance may be sufficiently low—compared with adenosine hyperemia—to assess translesional hemodynamic significance (Figure 27.24). The ratio of P_d/P_a during the wave-free period was called the instantaneous wave-free pressure ratio (iFR). In the ADVISE study, 157 stenoses were assessed with pressure and flow distal to the lesion, and another 118 stenoses were assessed using pressure alone. The intracoronary resistance at rest during the wave-free period was similar in variability and magnitude to that during FFR, and the iFR correlated closely with FFR, $r = 0.90$. However, there were limitations to this analysis despite having high sensitivity, specificity, negative and positive predictive values for iFR versus FFR. In particular, there is concern that the iFR at rest was different than the iFR during hyperemia, suggesting that the wave-free period does not have as low a resistance as a hyperemic period would.

Subsequently, Petraco et al.[37] demonstrated that at iFR cutpoints of >0.93 or <0.86, there was a strong correlation with normal and abnormal FFR values (using 0.80 as an FFR cutpoint). Thus, potentially 57% of the patients with intermediate stenosis could be assessed without the need for hyperemic stimulus.

The RESOLVE study[38] compared the diagnostic accuracy of iFR and resting pressure ratio P_d/P_a to FFR in a core laboratory. The IFR, P_d/P_a, and FFR were measured in 1,768 patients from 15 clinical sites. Core lab technicians were used to analyze the data. Thresholds corresponding

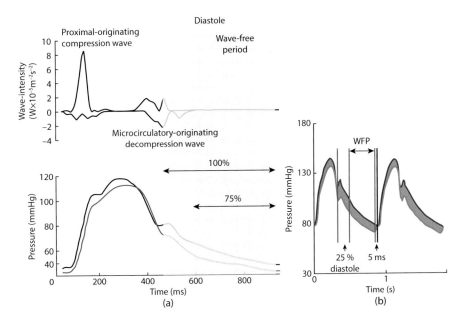

Figure 27.24 Wave-free instantaneous wave-free pressure ratio (iFR). **(a)** Wave-free period (WFP) is demonstrated by absence of reflected backward and forward traveling waves during diastole. **(b)** Using aortic (red line) and distal coronary pressure (green line) across a lesion to compute iFR. (Adapted from Sen, S., et al., *J. Am. Coll. Cardiol.*, 61(13), 1409–1420, 2013.)

to 90% accuracy in predicting ischemic versus nonischemic FFR were then identified. In 1,974 lesions, the optimal iFR to predict an FFR <0.8 was 0.90 with accuracy of 80%. For the resting P_d/P_a ratio, the cutpoint was 0.92 with an overall accuracy of 80% with no significant differences between iFR and P_d/P_a. Both measures have 90% accuracy to predict positive or negative FFR in 65% and 48% of lesions, respectively. These data suggest that the overall accuracy of iFR with FFR was about 80% which can be improved to 90% in a subset of lesions. Clinical outcome studies are in progress to determine whether the use of iFR or some variation thereof, might obviate the need for hyperemia in selected patients.

CONCLUSION

Invasive assessment of coronary hemodynamics is increasingly being integrated into modern laboratories. Strong outcome data exist to support this practice for management of in-patients with simple ambiguous CAD, as well as those with LMCA and multivessel disease. Future advances in coronary physiology will give practitioners the ability to evaluate the contribution of microvascular disease to a patient's symptoms and target therapies that can improve microvascular dysfunction. Conscientious operators should employ FFR and IVUS for appropriate decision-making and best outcomes in patients undergoing PCI.

REFERENCES

1. Gould KL, et al. Physiologic basis for assessing critical coronary stenosis. Instantaneous flow response and regional distribution during coronary hyperemia as measures of coronary flow reserve. *Am J Cardiol* 1974;33(1):87–94.

2. Topol EJ, Nissen SE, Our preoccupation with coronary luminology. The dissociation between clinical and angiographic findings in ischemic heart disease. *Circulation* 1995;92(8):2333–2342.

3. Verma S, Anderson TJ. Fundamentals of endothelial function for the clinical cardiologist. *Circulation* 2002;105(5):546–549.

4. Seiler C, et al. Basic structure-function relations of the epicardial coronary vascular tree. Basis of quantitative coronary arteriography for diffuse coronary artery disease. *Circulation* 1992;85(6):1987–2003.

5. Duncker DJ, Bache RJ. Regulation of coronary vasomotor tone under normal conditions and during acute myocardial hypoperfusion. *Pharmacol Ther* 2000;86(1):87–110.

6. Johnson NP, et al. History and development of coronary flow reserve and fractional flow reserve for clinical applications. *Intervent Cardiol Clin* 2015;4(4):397–410.

7. Kern MJ, et al. Variations in coronary vasodilatory reserve by artery, sex, status post transplantation, and remote coronary disease. *Circulation* 1994;90(4):I–154.

8. Kern MJ, et al. Physiological assessment of coronary artery disease in the cardiac catheterization laboratory: A scientific statement from the American Heart Association Committee on Diagnostic and Interventional Cardiac Catheterization, Council on Clinical Cardiology. *Circulation* 2006;114(12):1321–1341.

9. Pijls NH, et al. Experimental basis of determining maximum coronary, myocardial, and collateral blood flow by pressure measurements for assessing functional stenosis severity before and after percutaneous transluminal coronary angioplasty. *Circulation* 1993;87(4):1354–1367.

10. De Bruyne B, et al. Coronary flow reserve calculated from pressure measurements in humans. Validation with positron emission tomography. *Circulation* 1994;89(3):1013–1022.

11. De Bruyne B, et al. Simultaneous coronary pressure and flow velocity measurements in humans. Feasibility, reproducibility, and hemodynamic dependence of coronary flow velocity reserve, hyperemic flow versus pressure slope index, and fractional flow reserve. *Circulation* 1996;94(8):1842–1849.

12. Pijls NH, et al. Fractional flow reserve. A useful index to evaluate the influence of an epicardial coronary stenosis on myocardial blood flow. *Circulation* 1995;92(11):3183–3193.

13. Pijls, NH, et al. Practice and potential pitfalls of coronary pressure measurement. *Catheter Cardiovasc Interv* 2000;49(1):1–16.

14. Adjedj J, et al. Significance of intermediate values of fractional flow reserve in patients with coronary artery disease. *Circulation* 2016;133(5):502–508.

15. Prasad A, et al. Use of regadenoson for measurement of fractional flow reserve. *Catheter Cardiovasc Interv* 2014;83(3):369–374.

16. Arumugham P, et al. Comparison of intravenous adenosine and intravenous regadenoson for the measurement of pressure-derived coronary fractional flow reserve. *EuroIntervention* 2013;8(10):1166–1171.

17. Parham WA, et al. Coronary hyperemic dose responses of intracoronary sodium nitroprusside. *Circulation* 2004;109(10):1236–1243.

18. Fearon WF, et al. Novel index for invasively assessing the coronary microcirculation. *Circulation* 2003;107(25):3129–3132.

19. Pijls NH, et al. Measurement of fractional flow reserve to assess the functional severity of coronary-artery stenoses. *N Engl J Med* 1996;334(26):1703–1708.

20. Zimmermann FM, et al. Deferral vs. performance of percutaneous coronary intervention of functionally non-significant coronary stenosis: 15-year follow-up of the DEFER trial. *Eur Heart J* 2015;36(45):3182–3188.

21. Pijls NHJ, et al. Fractional flow reserve versus angiography for guiding percutaneous coronary intervention in patients with multivessel coronary artery disease: 2-year follow-up of the FAME (Fractional Flow Reserve Versus Angiography for Multivessel Evaluation) study. *J Am Coll Cardiol* 2010;56(3):177–184.

22. De Bruyne B, et al. Fractional flow reserve-guided PCI versus medical therapy in stable coronary disease. *N Engl J Med* 2012;67(11):991–1001.

23. Hamilos M, et al. Long-term clinical outcome after fractional flow reserve-guided treatment in patients with angiographically equivocal left main coronary artery stenosis. *Circulation* 2009;120(15):1505–1512.

24. Yong AS, et al. Fractional flow reserve assessment of left main stenosis in the presence of downstream coronary stenoses. *Circ Cardiovasc Interv* 2013;6(2):161–165.

25. Fearon WF, et al. The impact of downstream coronary stenosis on fractional flow reserve assessment of intermediate left main coronary artery disease: Human validation. *J Am Coll Cardiol Intv* 2015;8(3):398–403.

26. De Bruyne B, et al. Pressure-derived fractional flow reserve to assess serial epicardial stenoses: Theoretical basis and animal validation. *Circulation* 2000;101(15):1840–1847.

27. Pijls NH, et al. Coronary pressure measurement to assess the hemodynamic significance of serial stenoses within one coronary artery: Validation in humans. *Circulation* 2000;102(19):2371–2377.

28. De Bruyne B, et al. Abnormal epicardial coronary resistance in patients with diffuse atherosclerosis but "normal" coronary angiography. *Circulation* 2001;104(20):2401–2406.

29. Sels JW, et al. Fractional flow reserve in unstable angina and non-ST-segment elevation myocardial infarction experience from the FAME (Fractional flow reserve versus Angiography for Multivessel Evaluation) study. *JACC Cardiovasc Interv* 2011;4(11):1183–1189.

30. Ntalianis A, et al. Fractional flow reserve for the assessment of nonculprit coronary artery stenoses in patients with acute myocardial infarction. *JACC Cardiovasc Interv* 2010;3(12):1274–1281.

31. De Bruyne B, et al. Fractional flow reserve in patients with prior myocardial infarction. *Circulation* 2001;104(2):157–162.

32. Samady H, et al. Fractional flow reserve of infarct-related arteries identifies reversible defects on noninvasive myocardial perfusion imaging early after myocardial infarction. *J Am Coll Cardiol* 2006;47(11):2187–2193.

33. Botman CJ, et al. Does stenosis severity of native vessels influence bypass graft patency? A prospective fractional flow reserve-guided study. *Ann Thorac Surg* 2007;83(6):2093–2097.

34. Berger A, et al. Long-term patency of internal mammary artery bypass grafts: Relationship with preoperative severity of the native coronary artery stenosis. *Circulation* 2004;110(11 Suppl 1):II36–II40.

35. Toth G, et al. Fractional flow reserve-guided versus angiography-guided coronary artery bypass graft surgery. *Circulation* 2013;128(13):1405–1411.

36. Sen S, et al. Development and validation of a new adenosine-independent index of stenosis severity from coronary wave-intensity analysis: Results of the ADVISE (ADenosine Vasodilator Independent Stenosis Evaluation) study. *J Am Coll Cardiol* 2012;59(15):1392–1402.

37. Petraco R, et al. Hybrid iFR-FFR decision-making strategy: Implications for enhancing universal adoption of physiology-guided coronary revascularisation. *EuroIntervention* 2013;8(10):1157–1165.

38. Jeremias A, et al. Multicenter core laboratory comparison of the instantaneous wave-free ratio and resting Pd/Pa with fractional flow reserve: The RESOLVE study. *J Am Coll Cardiol* 2014;63(13):1253–1261.

28

Intravascular ultrasound and virtual histology

CHARIS COSTOPOULOS, ADAM J. BROWN, ADRIANO CAIXETA, AKIKO MAEHARA,
GARY S. MINTZ, AND MARTIN R. BENNETT

INTRODUCTION

Real-time ultrasound imaging originated in the late 1960s following the development of linear array transducers for visualizing cardiac chambers and valves.[1] The first transluminal images of human arteries were recorded by Yock and colleagues in 1988, when a miniaturized and single-transducer system was placed within the coronary arteries.[2] Ever since, intravascular ultrasound (IVUS) has become an increasingly important catheter-based imaging technology. In contemporary clinical practice, the major utility of IVUS is to guide and optimize stent implantation, especially in complex lesion subsets, including bifurcations and during left main coronary artery (LMCA) intervention.[3] IVUS can also inform management of lesions of intermediate angiographic stenosis, providing data as to when revascularization can be safely deferred.[4] As IVUS directly images the full thickness of the coronary arterial wall, its use allows measurement of plaque size, distribution, and composition.[5] Thus, IVUS has become established as the method of choice for the serial assessment of changes in atherosclerotic plaque burden in numerous progression-regression trials. Spectral analysis of the radiofrequency IVUS signals, termed virtual histology (VH)-IVUS, has led to a more detailed assessment of atherosclerotic plaque composition.[6] Although this remains principally a research tool, use of VH-IVUS has led

to important advances in the understanding of the natural history of atherosclerotic plaques.[7]

This chapter examines the rationale, technique, and interpretation of IVUS and VH-IVUS imaging in diagnostic, therapeutic, and research applications.

GRAYSCALE INTRAVASCULAR ULTRASOUND

Intravascular ultrasound imaging: definitions and basics

Ultrasound is acoustic energy with a frequency above human hearing. The upper limit of frequency that the human ear can detect is approximately 20,000 cycles per second (20 kHz). For medical diagnostic purposes, ultrasound imaging frequencies are much higher and typically range in the millions of cycles per second (MHz).

The IVUS transducer converts electrical energy into acoustic energy through a piezoelectric (pressure-electric) crystalline material that expands and contracts to produce sound waves when electrically excited. After reflection from tissue, part of the ultrasound energy returns to the transducer; the transducer then generates an electrical impulse that is converted into moving pictures.[5] All materials in the body reflect sound waves, but the waves are transmitted back to the transducer at various intervals depending on the type of material imaged and the distance from the source. It is the variation in reflective sound waves that creates the ultrasound image on the console. The intensity of the reflected (or backscattered) ultrasound depends on a number of variables including the intensity of the transmitted signal, the attenuation of the signal by the tissue, the density of the tissue, the distance from the transducer to the target, and the angle of the signal relative to the target.

Several clinically relevant properties of the ultrasound image, such as the resolution, depth of penetration, and attenuation of the acoustic signal, are dependent on the geometric and frequency properties of the transducer. The higher the center frequency, the better the axial resolution but the lower the depth of penetration. As the transducer is close to the arterial wall in coronary imaging, high ultrasound frequencies are used that range from 20 to 60 MHz. Axial and lateral resolution varies among catheters but is typically in the range of 70–120 μm (axial) and 100–250 μm (lateral), resulting in >5 mm penetration depth into the vessel wall.[8]

Equipment

Two different transducer designs are used: mechanically rotated and electronic solid-state phased array. Mechanical probes use a drive cable to rotate a single-element transducer at the catheter tip at high speed (around 1,800 revolutions per minute [rpm]). At approximately 18 increments, the transducer sends and receives ultrasound signals providing 256 individual radial scan lines for each image. In electronic phased-array systems, 64 tiny transducer elements in an annular array are activated sequentially to generate the cross-sectional image of the vessel.[5]

Imaging artifacts

The recognition of an artifact during IVUS acquisition is critical, as it may interfere with image interpretation and measurements. The most common imaging artifacts are (1) ring-down, (2) nonuniform rotational distortion (NURD), and (3) reverberations. Ring-down artifacts are usually observed as a series of parallel bright bands or halos of variable thickness surrounding the catheter and obscuring near-field imaging. Although ring-down can occur with any IVUS system, solid-state systems tend to be more affected. Ring-down artifact can be reduced by placing the IVUS catheter in a large vessel (e.g., LMCA) and adjusting the time gain control.[9] NURD is an artifact that is specific to motorized IVUS catheters and arises from frictional forces to the rotating elements. NURD creates stretched or compacted portions on the images. Because accurate reconstruction of IVUS two-dimensional (2D) images is dependent on uniform rotation of the catheter, NURD may create errors during IVUS measurements.[10] NURD artifacts can also occur because of bends in the catheter driveshaft or in the presence of acute bends in the artery. Reverberations are false repetitive echoes of the same structure that give the impression of second or various interfaces at fixed multiple distances from the transducer. Reverberation artifacts are more common from strong echo reflectors, such as stents, guidewires, guiding catheters, and calcium (especially after rotational atherectomy). There are a few other artifacts that can also interfere in IVUS interpretation, including side lobes and ghost artifacts, which are also generated from strong echo reflectors, such as calcium and stent metal. In longitudinal or L-mode display, catheter motion artifacts during the pullback may result in a "sawtooth" appearance.

Catheter position also plays an important role in image quality. Off-axis position of the catheter may alter vessel geometry in an elliptical fashion, misleading the operator to overestimate lumen and vessel area. Axial (antegrade-retrograde) movement of the IVUS probe during the cardiac cycle scrambles consecutive image slices that may have implications for three-dimensional (3D) reconstruction and attempts to assess coronary artery compliance.[11]

Image acquisition and presentation

Two important consensus documents have been published on image acquisition and reporting of IVUS data: (1) Standards for the Acquisition, Measurement, and Reporting of IVUS Studies: A Report of the American College of Cardiology (ACC) Task Force on Clinical Expert Consensus Documents[5] and (2) the Study Group on Intracoronary Imaging of the Working Group of Coronary Circulation and the Subgroup on Intravascular Ultrasound of the Working Group of Echocardiography of the European Society of Cardiology (ESC).[12]

IVUS supplements angiography by providing a tomographic perspective of lumen geometry and vessel wall structure. A longitudinal view can also be displayed, but this should be done only when using motorized transducer pullback. Longitudinal representation of IVUS images is useful for length measurements for interpolation of shadowed deep arterial structures (i.e., external elastic membrane [EEM] behind calcium or stent metal).[5] There are advantages and disadvantages of using manual or motorized pullback; however, motorized pullback is usually preferred. Using motorized transducer pullback allows assessment of lesion length, volumetric measurements, consistent and systematic IVUS image acquisition among different operators, and uniform and reproducible image acquisition for multicenter and serial studies.[13]

Standard IVUS image acquisition is performed after the administration of anticoagulation. The use of intracoronary nitroglycerin is recommended to minimize arterial spasm and to achieve maximum vasodilatation.[9] The catheter is then advanced over a 0.014-in coronary guidewire to a safe position distal to the segment of interest (ideally at least 10 mm of distal reference). Positioning the catheter and initiating pullback at a landmark, for example, a side branch, can be beneficial to aid co-localization with other imaging modalities. An automated, continuous, motorized pullback to the guide catheter or aorta should then be performed. The preferred pullback speed is 0.5 mm/s.

Normal coronary artery morphology

Validation studies have characterized the appearance of normal coronary arteries by IVUS, demonstrating three distinct tissue layers: the intima, media, and adventitia.[14] There are also two distinct tissue interfaces that can be observed, providing image acquisition is optimal. The first is the border between blood and the leading edge of the intima, and the second at the external elastic membrane, which is located at the media-adventitia border.[15] The innermost intima layer is typically more echogenic when compared with the lumen and media; it is displayed as a bright concentric ring on IVUS. Although debate continues on the normal value for intimal thickness, most investigators would use 300–500 μm as the upper limit of normal.[16] Indeed, in some cases, intima thickness may be <100 μm, a value lower than the resolution of IVUS, resulting in the vessel appearing "monolayered." The intima-media border in general is poorly defined and cannot be reliably used for measurements. The media itself is typically represented by a layer of low ultrasound reflectivity due to its homogeneous structure rich in smooth muscle cells. Histologically, media thickness is around 200 μm, but thinning can occur in the presence of atherosclerosis. The EEM can be accurately defined on IVUS due to a pronounced step-up in ultrasound reflectivity. The outermost layer, the adventitia, is composed of collagen and elastic tissue and is 300–500 μm thick. The outer border of the adventitia is also indistinct due to echo reflectivity similar to the surrounding periadventitial tissues.[17] Thus, the typical appearance of a normal coronary artery is "three layered," with a bright layer from the intima, a dark layer from the media, and a final bright outer layer from the adventitia and surroundings (Figure 28.1).

Quantitative analysis

IVUS imaging is able to identify two acoustic interfaces in the majority of cases, these being the blood-intima and media-adventitia (EEM) interfaces. Based on these two visual landmarks, two cross-sectional area (CSA) measurements can be defined: the lumen CSA and the media/adventitia CSA (or EEM CSA). The atheroma or plaque and media (P&M) complex is calculated as EEM CSA minus lumen CSA; the media cannot be measured as a distinct structure. Thus, complete quantification of a nonstented lesion is possible by tracing the EEM and lumen areas of the proximal reference, lesion, and distal reference; calculating derived measures, including minimum and maximum EEM and lumen diameters, P&M area and thickness, and plaque burden (P&M area divided by EEM); and measuring lesion length (distance between the proximal and distal reference segments) (Figure 28.2). If motorized pullback was performed at a constant rate, volumetric IVUS measures can be calculated using the Simpson rule[5] and can be reported as total volumes or normalized area (volume divided by length).[18]

In stented vessels, the stent forms a third measurable structure (stent CSA). Metallic stent struts appear as bright points along the circumference of the vessel. Complete quantification of a stented lesion is possible by tracing the EEM and lumen areas of the proximal and distal reference segments and the EEM, lumen, and stent areas of the stented lesion; calculating derived measures (minimum and maximum EEM, stent, and lumen diameters; persistent P&M area and thickness; and intrastent intimal hyperplasia [IH, area and %IH]); and measuring stent length.

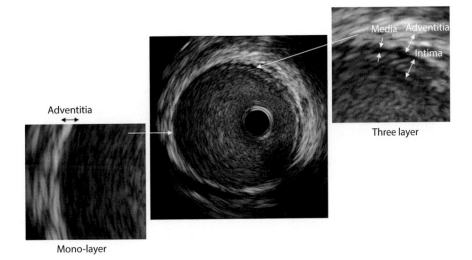

Figure 28.1 Normal coronary artery morphology in a cross-sectional view. In the magnified image on the left, only the outer bright adventitial layer is representative of the monolayered appearance. In the magnified image on the right, the bright inner layer (intima), middle echolucent zone (media), and outer bright layer (adventitia) are representative of the three-layered appearance of intravascular ultrasound.

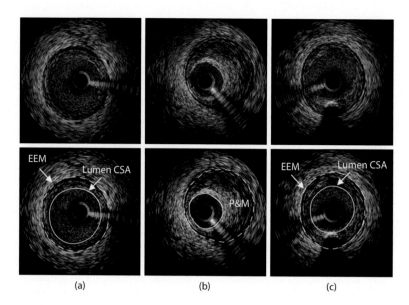

Figure 28.2 IVUS measurements in a nonstented artery. The proximal **(a)** and distal reference **(c)** and minimum lumen area **(b)** of the lesion are shown. The IVUS study is shown in duplicate: one unlabeled (top panels) and one highlighted with lines to illustrate quantitative analyses (bottom panels). The dashed line highlights each external elastic membrane cross-sectional area (EEM CSA), and the solid line indicates each lumen interface (lumen CSA). Between the EEM CSA and lumen CSA, the atheroma or plaque and media (P&M) complex is calculated. IVUS, intravascular ultrasound.

Plaque composition

Atherosclerotic plaques are heterogeneous and contain a mixture of plaque components with different echo-reflectivity. Grayscale IVUS imaging can categorize lesions into subtypes according to echo-density, typically by using the collagen-rich "bright" adventitia as a reference.[19] Four basic types of lesions are distinguished according to plaque echogenicity: (1) "soft" or hypoechoic plaque does not reflect much ultrasound and appears dark with less echo intensity compared to the adventitia; (2) "hard" or hyperechoic, composed primarily of fibrous tissue with echogenicity of equal or greater intensity than the adventitia; (3) calcific plaques, characterized by the presence of acoustic shadowing along with the brightest echoes and reverberations; and (4) mixed plaque, where no single acoustical subtype represents >80% of the plaque (Figure 28.3).[20] However, this methodology is based on qualitative visual interpretation of IVUS images and therefore has potential for interobserver variability.[21] To overcome this limitation, computational postprocessing methods have been developed to analyze the ultrasound backscatter signal. Although several platforms are commercially available, VH-IVUS has the most robust clinical data and will be discussed in detail later in this chapter.

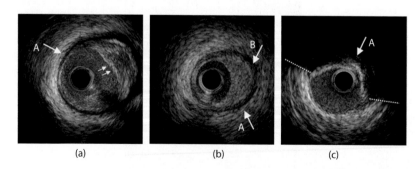

Figure 28.3 **(a)** An example of a predominantly soft plaque—a thin fibrous cap (*small arrows*) and lipid core underlying it; the plaque is less bright than the adventitia (A). In **(b)**, fibrous or hyperechoic plaque is as bright as or brighter than the adventitia (A) without shadowing. In this eccentric plaque, the thickness of the media behind the thickest part of the plaque (B) is an artifact caused by attenuation of the beam as it passes through the hyperechoic plaque. In reality, the media becomes thinner with increasing atherosclerosis. Note that the media behind the thinnest part of the plaque is also thinner—without artifacts. **(c)** Superficial calcium—defined as calcium (A) that is closer to the intima than it is to the adventitia. Calcium shadows the deeper arterial structures; in this case, the arc of calcification is <180° (*dashed line*).

CLINICAL ASPECTS

Assessment of coronary artery disease

EVALUATION OF INTERMEDIATE LESIONS IN THE NON-LEFT MAIN CORONARY ARTERIES

Management of angiographic intermediate lesions, defined as 30%–70% stenosis, often pose a challenge to the interventional cardiologist, especially when the patients' symptoms are difficult to ascertain. This becomes particularly challenging in cases of diffuse coronary disease, where it is difficult to determine healthy vessel size, and in areas of tortuosity where the lesion may not be well visualized. Although fractional flow reserve (FFR)[22,23] and more recently, instantaneous wave-free ratio (iFR)[24] are interventional tools of choice for the assessment of such lesions, IVUS imaging can also be of benefit. In particular, it allows the estimation of lesion length by accurately identifying lesion margins while also providing information on lesion morphology, thereby influencing procedural strategy and device selection. Furthermore, it identifies areas of arterial remodeling that have been shown to be associated with procedural and future events in the patient.[25,26] This is often expressed in the form of an index (remodeling index [RI]) commonly derived by dividing the EEM CSA at the minimum lumen area (MLA) over the average of the proximal and distal reference segment EEM CSAs.[26] "Positive," "outward," or "expansive" remodeling—defined as an increase in arterial dimensions in response to increasing plaque burden—has been associated with unstable symptoms, plaque rupture, periprocedural myocardial infarction (MI), and future adverse clinical events.[27–30] More recently, "negative," "inward," or "constrictive" remodeling (Figure 28.4)

has also been linked to subsequent events when defined as RI <0.88.[26]

Studies have also demonstrated a reasonable correlation between certain IVUS parameters and physiological measures of myocardial ischemia with a MLA cut-off of 2.4–3.6 mm^2 associated with hemodynamically significant lesions as assessed by FFR.[31–33] In the study of Stone et al. in which 544 lesions were examined, a MLA ≤2.9 mm^2 was found to best predict an FFR ≤0.80 with, however, an accuracy of only 66%.[34] Similar results were reported by the multicenter prospective FIRST (Fractional Flow Reserve and Intravascular Ultrasound Relationship Study) registry where an IVUS measured MLA <3.07 mm^2 had the best sensitivity and specificity (64% and 65%, respectively) for correlating with FFR <0.80.[35] A MLA >4 mm^2 in non-left main stem lesions on the other hand has been shown to be associated with a low risk of major adverse cardiovascular events (MACEs).[4] The relatively broad MLA range identified by these studies is a reflection of the fact that parameters other than MLA, such as location along the arterial tree, lesion length, and the amount of myocardial subtended by the vessel, are equally important in determining the hemodynamic significance of intermediate lesions. Therefore, these factors, along with plaque burden and the presence of collaterals, need to be considered when utilizing IVUS for the assessment of such lesions.

EVALUATION OF INTERMEDIATE LESIONS IN THE LEFT MAIN CORONARY ARTERY

Several studies have shown that a high percentage of patients with an angiographically normal LMCA demonstrate significant disease on IVUS. Positive remodeling, diffuse disease, and the absence of a reference vessel when the

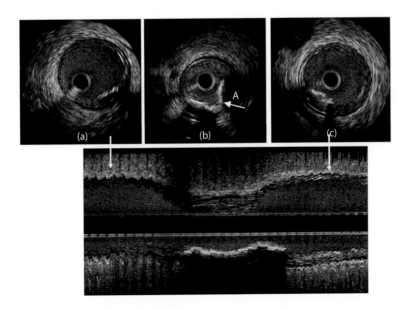

Figure 28.4 An eccentric, calcific, and small plaque accumulation (A) leading to negative remodeling. Proximal **(a)** and distal **(c)** vessel references and their respective longitudinal views (*white arrows*). In **(b)**, notice how the vessel cross-sectional area (or external elastic membrane) is smaller than both the proximal and distal vessels. The longitudinal view depicts clearly the artery shrinkage at the lesion site.

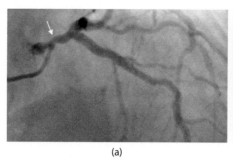
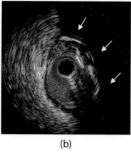

(a)   (b)

Figure 28.5 **(a)** Mildly diseased ostium in the left main coronary artery by angiography (*white arrow*). **(b)** Intravascular ultrasound diagnostic study showing an eccentric stenotic plaque with a minimum lumen area of 4.4 mm². Notice the superficial and deep calcium with shadowing (*arrows*).

LMCA is short are some of the reasons for the discrepancy between angiography and IVUS (Figure 28.5). Assessment of the LMCA ostium can be particularly challenging due to contrast streaming and the presence of calcification at the aortic cusp with vessel overlap between the left anterior descending, left circumflex, and ramus intermediate arteries (when present), making it difficult to assess the distal LMCA. IVUS overcomes all of these limitations, thereby becoming an invaluable tool for assessing disease severity in the LMCA and thus the need for further treatment. In the study by Jasti et al., an IVUS minimal lumen diameter (MLD) and MLA of <2.8 mm and <5.9 mm², respectively, strongly predicted the physiological significance of LMCA stenosis.[36] In agreement with this, a separate study of 354 intermediate LMCA lesions demonstrated a low risk of future events when a MLA <6 mm² was used as a cut-off for revascularization.[37] The study of Park et al. suggested that a lower cut-off might apply in Asian populations, with a MLA ≤4.5 mm² in left main ostial and shaft lesions found to correlate well with an FFR ≤0.80 (77% sensitivity, 82% specificity, 84% positive predictive value, 75% negative predictive value, area under the curve: 0.83, 95% CI: 0.76–0.96; $P <$ 0.001).[38] The aforementioned studies suggest that deferring revascularization in patients with a LMCA MLA >6 mm² is reasonably safe, particularly for lesions located at the ostial and middle segments. Further assessment with functional testing should nevertheless be considered in the patient subset where symptoms are incongruent with LMCA dimensions, especially when the MLA is between 6 and 7.5 mm².[22]

UNSTABLE LESIONS AND LESIONS WITH UNUSUAL MORPHOLOGY

Acute coronary syndrome (ACS) is often precipitated by plaque rupture, which is readily identified on IVUS as a ruptured capsule with an underlying cavity or plaque excavation by atheromatous extrusion with no visible capsule.[39] Culprit lesions usually exhibit positive remodeling, have a large plaque area, and tend to be more echo lucent compared to stable plaques; the latter property is a reflection of greater lipid accumulation.[40] They also tend to be less calcified, although small, focal, deep areas of calcification are not uncommon.[41]

IVUS also allows accurate characterization of lesions that are not well characterized on angiography, including ill-defined filling defects, aneurysms, and spontaneous dissections. Although most filling defects reflect true thrombi, a small percentage are due to highly calcified plaque or even calcified nodules, an unusual form of vulnerable plaque. In an IVUS analysis of 77 angiographically diagnosed aneurysms, only 27% were true aneurysms with 4% characterized as pseudoaneurysms, 16% as complex plaques, and 53% as normal arterial segments adjacent to stenoses.[42] By IVUS, a spontaneous dissection appears as a medial dissection with an intramural hematoma occupying some or all of the dissected false lumen without identifiable intimal tears and communication between the true and false lumens, typically in a nonatherosclerotic artery.

Intravascular ultrasound and percutaneous coronary intervention

STENT SIZING

IVUS can provide accurate information on vessel size and lesion length, especially in cases of significant remodeling and diffuse disease where angiography can be misleading. Stent undersizing can lead to strut malapposition, thereby increasing the possibility of stent thrombosis (ST),[43] whereas aggressive dilatation of an undersized stent can cause strut disruption, risking restenosis, and ST. Oversizing, on the other hand, can lead to diameter mismatch between stented and nonstented segments while also increasing the risk of coronary rupture and edge dissection. Selecting an appropriate stent size requires either measuring the maximum reference lumen diameter (proximal or distal to the lesion), or the "media-media" dimensions at plaque level, with the latter being particularly important in cases of extensive remodeling. Determining lesion length is also important. This can be identified through the longitudinal IVUS view, allowing for a stent length sufficient enough to cover the entire diseased segmented, thereby reducing the risk of plaque shift and geographical miss (i.e., inadequate coverage of the diseased segment)[44] and consequent potential for edge restenosis, which can require further stenting.

Information regarding side-branch location in relation to the intended-to-treat lesion can also be obtained from the longitudinal view. This helps to ensure that side branches are not covered unnecessarily as this can impinge on their ostia and, therefore, blood flow.

STENT EXPANSION AND MALAPPOSITION

IVUS studies have shown that lumen enlargement after stent implantation is a combination of vessel expansion and plaque redistribution/embolization rather than plaque compression.[45,46] Plaque reduction in patients with ACS is attributed to plaque or thrombus embolization.[47] Intrusion or prolapse of plaque through the stent mesh into the lumen is more common in ACS and in saphenous vein graft (SVG) lesions. Importantly, after stent implantation, there is a significant residual plaque burden behind the stent struts that almost always measures 50%–75% at the center of the lesion. Thus, the stent CSA always looks smaller than the EEM, even when the stent is fully expanded. IVUS can reliably identify stent underexpansion despite evidence of satisfactory deployment on angiography. This occurs when part of the stent is insufficiently expanded compared to the proximal and distal segments and is more likely to occur in calcific lesions, which have not been adequately predilated. In this setting, the use of IVUS can be very helpful not in only identifying underexpansion, but also in guiding postdilatation technique, which may require the use of ultra-high-pressure noncompliant balloons. Optimal expansion is particularly important with the recently introduced bioresorbable vascular scaffolds, which have been associated with a trend toward higher ST.[48] Inadequate expansion in this setting is more difficult to identify on angiography as these devices lack a metallic scaffold. Intravascular imaging has, therefore, been recommended following their implantation, especially when treating complex lesions.[49] Apposition refers to the contact between the stent struts and the arterial wall,[5] with incomplete stent apposition linked to future events and late ST.[50] On IVUS, malapposition is defined as one or more struts clearly separated from the vessel wall with evidence of blood speckles behind the strut (Figure 28.6). Once recognized, postdilatation can help to correct this with subsequent IVUS imaging always required to confirm resolution.

Whether this, however, has an impact on future clinical outcomes remains to be elucidated.

INTRAVASCULAR ULTRASOUND-GUIDED STENT IMPLANTATION

Although IVUS has a role to play in lesion stratification and assessment, its main purpose is to plan and guide stent implantation. Preintervention IVUS helps to assess vessel size and lesion length, thus determining stent selection. Information regarding lesion composition prior to stent implantation helps to decide whether more specialized tools, such as cutting or scoring balloons, are required for lesion preparation. Following stent deployment, IVUS can assess adequate stent expansion, which is an important risk factor for restenosis and ST.[51–53] Although ST is rare (annual risk $\approx 0.5\%$), it can be detrimental with mortality rates ranging between 10% and 30%.[54] IVUS studies have provided insights into the causes of ST with Fujii et al. being one of the first to identify underexpansion, smaller minimum stent area, and residual edge stenosis as important contributing factors in sirolimus-eluting ST.[52] Stent malapposition has also been linked with ST, although it is unclear whether this alone can determine ST.[55]

A range of studies has suggested that IVUS-guided percutaneous coronary intervention (PCI) can reduce future adverse events, especially in the context of drug-eluting stents (DES), with the meta-analysis of Zhang et al. demonstrating improved ST and mortality rates when this was utilized.[56,57] Hur et al. found similar results in a more recent observational study with IVUS-guided DES implantation associated with reduced mortality at 3 years (HR 0.46; 95% CI: 0.33–0.66, $P < 0.001$).[58] In the AVIO (Angiography Versus IVUS Optimization) trial, an IVUS-guided strategy was associated with larger postprocedural MLD although this did not translate to improved clinical outcomes at 9 months.[59] The IVUS criteria used in this study (Table 28.1) offer an easy guide for target lumen areas after stent implantation and balloon postdilatation.

Further supporting evidence comes from the large prospective, multicenter ADAPT-DES (Assessment of Dual AntiPlatelet Therapy With Drug Eluting Stents) registry in which 3,349 of 8,583 patients (39%) underwent IVUS-guided PCI (63% both pre- and postimplantation IVUS).

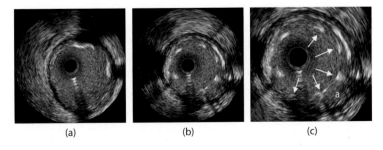

(a)   (b)   (c)

Figure 28.6 An example of acute stent malapposition. **(a)** The vessel before stent implantation; the intravascular ultrasound study in **(b)** and **(c)** shows the stent malapposition. In the magnified image in the right, notice the space between the stent strut and the intima and the blood speckle behind the stent struts labeled a. Five stent struts are malapposed (*white arrows*). Because of stent malapposition, the stent area (9.4 mm²) is smaller than the lumen area (14.4 mm²).

Table 28.1 AVIO (Angiography Versus IVUS Optimization) trial criteria for optimal stent implantation (balloon size refers to either stent or post dilatation balloon)

Balloon size, mm	Target area, mm²
2.5	4
3.0	6
3.5	8
4.0	10
4.5	12

Source: Chieffo, A., et al., Am. Heart J., 165(1), 65–72, 2013. With permission.
Note: IVUS, intravascular ultrasound.

In a propensity-adjusted multivariable analysis, IVUS guidance was associated with reduced rates of definite or probable ST (HR 0.40; 95% CI: 0.21–0.73; $P = 0.003$), MI (HR 0.66; 95% CI: 0.49–0.88; $P = 0.004$), and MACE (HR 0.70; 95% CI: 0.55–0.88; $P = 0.003$) at 1-year follow-up.[60] Although this was a nonrandomized study, these findings suggest that IVUS imaging should be considered in DES PCI, especially when dealing with complex lesions or when concerns exist regarding the final result. In agreement with this, the randomized study by Hong et al. demonstrated that implantation of everolimus-eluting stents (EES) in patients with long coronary lesions under IVUS guidance is associated with lower MACE at 1 year (2.9% vs. 5.8%; $P = 0.007$) and lower ischemia-driven target lesion revascularization (2.5% vs. 5%; $P = 0.02$) compared to angiographically guided implantation.[61] Similar results were observed in the recent meta-analysis of Elgendy et al. which included 3,192 patients with diffuse disease (mean lesion length of 32 mm). At 15-month mean follow-up, IVUS-guided PCI was associated with more favorable cardiovascular outcomes compared to angiographically determined PCI, especially with regard to target lesion revascularization (4.1% vs. 6.6%; $P = 0.003$) and ST (0.6% vs. 1.3%; $P = 0.04$).[62] The larger meta-analysis of Zhang et al. (29,068 patients) demonstrated improvements with IVUS-guided PCI not only in revascularization and ST rates but also in cardiovascular hard endpoints including death (OR: 0.62; 95% CI: 0.54–0.71; $P < 0.001$), a benefit that appeared more significant in the subgroup of patients with complex lesions or ACS.[63] IVUS-guided PCI may be particularly important with the LMCA as ST here is almost always fatal. In agreement with this, Park et al. demonstrated that IVUS-guided DES implantation in this lesion subset is also associated with reductions in mortality at long-term follow-up when compared with conventional angiography guidance (4.7% vs. 16%, log-rank $P = 0.048$; hazard ratio, 0.39; 95% CI: 0.15–1.02; $P = 0.055$).[38]

RECOGNITION OF COMPLICATIONS

IVUS has a higher sensitivity than angiography in identifying complications that occur during PCI with angiography underestimating the presence and extent of dissection. Edge dissections are more common when the stent ends in a coronary segment that contains both plaque and normal vessel wall or both calcific and soft plaque elements. An edge dissection may not be visible by IVUS when it results in significant lumen compromise, as the IVUS catheter may press the flap against the arterial wall, thus sealing the dissection. This can also be observed when the dissection occurs behind a calcified plaque that prevents accurate morphological definition. Management of coronary dissection following stent implantation depends on whether flow is compromised, the presence of signs or symptoms of ischemia, certain IVUS findings, and angiographic appearance. IVUS findings that suggest that further treatment is required include (1) reduced lumen dimensions below the threshold for an optimum result, (2) impingement of the dissection flap on the IVUS catheter, (3) increased mobility of the dissection flap, and (4) increased dissection length. In general, minor edge dissections do not require treatment unless there is lumen compromise, as these tend to heal spontaneously over time.

Intramural hematoma is another PCI complication readily identified on IVUS. With an intramural hematoma, blood accumulates in the medial space; the EEM expands outward and the internal elastic membrane is pushed inwards resulting in lumen compromise. On IVUS, an intramural hematoma is typically hyperechoic and crescent-shaped with straightening of the internal elastic membrane. In general, intramural hematomas need to be treated, as there is a significant risk of propagation and further lumen compromise.

Coronary perforation and rupture usually occurs with overaggressive and/or oversized balloon dilation, especially in lesions with extensive, nonuniform calcification (Figure 28.7). These are easily identified on angiography and tend to be more severe than the usually small guidewire perforations. On IVUS, coronary perforations after stent deployment show three distinct morphologic patterns: (1) free blood speckle outside the EEM, (2) extramural hematoma—an accumulation of blood outside the EEM, and (3) a new periadventitial echolucent interface representing contrast extravasation. Acute management includes simple monitoring, prolonged low-pressure balloon inflation, use of covered stents, and in severe cases, surgery.

Insights from serial intravascular ultrasound studies

RESTENOSIS AND ACQUIRED LATE-STENT MALAPPOSITION

Serial IVUS studies have shown that the main mechanism of restenosis following balloon angioplasty is negative remodeling (decrease in EEM area) with in-stent restenosis (ISR) primarily resulting from neo-intimal hyperplasia (IH) rather than chronic stent recoil. The introduction of DES has led to improvements in ISR and revascularization rates compared with bare-metal stents (BMS), with IVUS demonstrating that this is predominantly due to reductions in IH.[64,65]

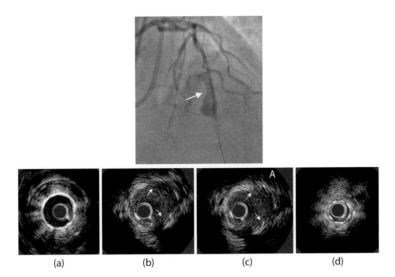

(a)   (b)   (c)   (d)

Figure 28.7 This patient presented with in-stent restenosis. After balloon dilation, coronary perforation with myocardial contrast extravasation occurred, as seen by angiography (*arrows*). On IVUS, notice the small vessel with stenting at a distal site **(d)** and the medial and adventitial discontinuation at the site of perforation (**b**, **c**, and *arrows*). Notice also an accumulation of blood outside the external elastic membrane (A). One stent graft was implanted prior to IVUS assessment **(a)**, followed by an additional stent graft after IVUS assessment. IVUS, intravascular ultrasound.

Despite these improvements, ISR continues to be encountered in routine clinical practice. It is often associated with stent under expansion, itself a result of inadequate expansion during implantation, usually in a poorly prepared lesion, rather than stent recoil. Other factors associated with restenosis include (1) incomplete lesion coverage, usually seen with aorto-ostial lesions; (2) stent crush; and (3) stent fracture (Figure 28.8).[66]

Serial IVUS analysis has also been particularly helpful when evaluating new stent technologies. Absorb BVS (Abbott Vascular, Santa Clara, CA), the first bioresorbable vascular scaffold to be used in routine clinical practice, has been extensively evaluated with intravascular imaging with studies demonstrating enlargements in mean lumen, scaffold, plaque, and vessel area up to 2 years following implantation (Figure 28.9).[67] IVUS has also provided information on the impact bioresorbable scaffold technology has on arterial remodeling as well as on the time it takes for these devices to be resorbed.[68]

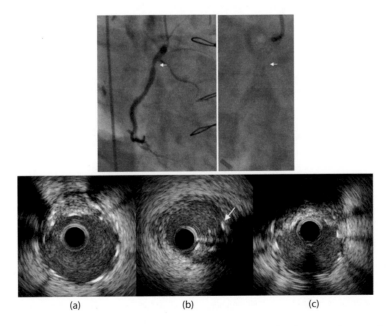

(a)   (b)   (c)

Figure 28.8 This patient presented with restenosis at follow-up after sirolimus-eluting stent implantation in the right coronary artery (*arrows* on angiogram). Note the stent fracture with acquired transection on fluoroscopy. On intravascular ultrasound, all stent struts were seen at proximal **(a)** and distal **(c)** reference segments, whereas at the fracture site (**b**; minimal lumen area of 4.8 mm^2), only one stent strut was seen (*arrow*).

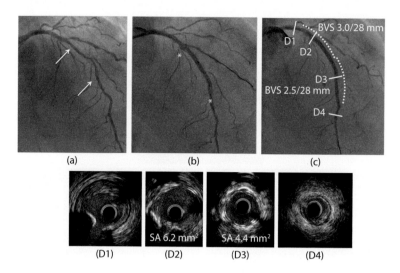

Figure 28.9 Angiographic and IVUS images of a calcified LAD lesion treated with Absorb BVS. **(a)** Baseline angiographic image of a long calcified LAD lesion (arrows). **(b)** Angiographic image following rotational atherectomy and balloon pre-dilatation with evidence of dissection (*). **(c)** Final angiographic image following Absorb BVS implantation and post-dilatation with corresponding final intravascular ultrasound images (D1–D4). BVS, bioresorbable vascular scaffold; IVUS, intravascular ultrasound; LAD, left anterior descending; SA, scaffold area.

IVUS has also played an important role in recognizing and assessing the importance of late stent malapposition. Late stent malapposition can be classified as late persistent when an inadequately apposed stent at the time of intervention remains incompletely apposed at follow-up, or labeled late-acquired stent malapposition when observed at follow-up despite the appropriate apposition of the stent during the index procedure.[69] The latter is usually due to positive remodeling after stent implantation (Figure 28.10),[70] although occasionally it can be seen after PCI for ST-segment elevation MI following thrombus dissolution behind the stent. The study by Cook et al. suggested

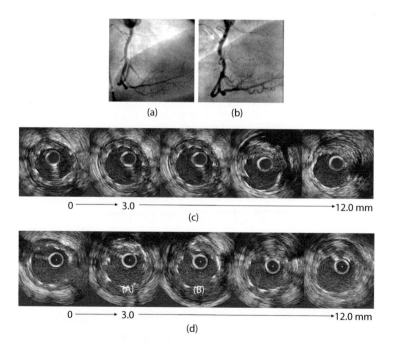

Figure 28.10 This patient underwent sirolimus-eluting stent implantation in a right coronary stenosis. The final angiogram is shown in **(a)**. At follow-up **(b)**, there was a proximal, focal aneurysm (*white arrows*). Final (poststent implantation) IVUS image is shown in **(c)**, and the follow-up IVUS image is shown in **(d)**. Note the late-acquired stent malapposition (A and B) in **(d)**. At the site of maximum stent malapposition (B), there has been an increase in external elastic membrane CSA from 17.8 to 28.9 mm². The stent CSA (8.8 mm²) and the persistent plaque and media (8.9 mm²) have not changed. CSA, cross-sectional area; IVUS, intravascular ultrasound.

that late stent malapposition could be a contributing factor to very late ST (VLST).[71] In this study, 13 patients presenting with VLST (>1 year) after DES implantation were compared with 144 control patients with no ST. Compared with DES controls, patients with VLST had longer lesions and stents, more stents per lesion, and more stent overlap. Vessel CSA was significantly larger for the in-stent segment (28.6 ± 11.9 vs. 20.1 ± 6.7 mm²; $P = 0.03$) in VLST patients compared with DES controls, suggesting the existence of positive arterial remodeling. Although IVUS was not performed at stent implantation in any patients of either group, incomplete stent apposition was more frequent (77% vs. 12%, $P = 0.001$), and maximal incomplete stent apposition area was larger (8.3 ± 7.5 vs. 4 ± 3.8 mm²; $P = 0.03$) in patients with VLST compared to controls. In contrast, the study by Steinberg et al. did not find any association between MACE and late-acquired stent malapposition irrespective of whether BMS or DES were used.[72] The conflicting results of these studies suggest that VLST is likely to be influenced by both patient and stent factors with malapposition a contributing factor in a subset of these patients as the recent optical coherence tomography study by Souteyrand et al. suggests.[43]

Impact of drug therapy on coronary atherosclerosis

The ability of IVUS to quantify plaque burden has been applied as a means of assessing plaque behavior *in vivo* following pharmacological intervention. In the REVERSAL (Reversing Atherosclerosis with Aggressive Lipid Lowering) trial, 18 months of moderate serum low-density lipoprotein cholesterol (LDL-C) reduction to a mean level of 110 mg/dL with pravastatin 40 mg was associated with significant disease progression, with plaque regression only observed when lower mean on-treatment LDL-C levels (61 mg/dL) were achieved.[73] In agreement with this, the SATURN (Study of Coronary Atheroma by Intravascular Ultrasound: Effect of Rosuvastatin Versus Atorvastatin) study that compared the efficacy of rosuvastatin 40 mg and atorvastatin 80 mg daily for 24 months demonstrated plaque burden reduction only when low on-treatment LDL-C levels were achieved (LDL-C 62 mg/dL vs. 70 mg/dL).[74] Grayscale IVUS studies have also examined the impact of lowering systemic blood pressure on atherosclerosis. The IVUS substudy of the CAMELOT (The Comparison of Amlodipine vs. Enalapril to Limit Occurrences of Thrombosis) trial demonstrated a correlation between the extent of blood pressure reduction and coronary plaque burden with a trend toward plaque regression in the cohort of patients that achieved a systolic blood pressure ≤120 mmHg.[75]

Cardiac allograft vasculopathy

Cardiac allograft vasculopathy has a more diffuse distribution than atherosclerotic disease, involving both the epicardial and more distal vessels.[76] It can be particularly difficult to diagnose, as it is often clinically silent due to the denervation of the transplanted heart. IVUS in this setting is a useful tool for the early diagnosis of intimal thickening and monitoring of disease progression. Serial IVUS studies have shown that intimal thickening primarily occurs during the first year post-transplantation with remodeling—first positive and then negative—predominating thereafter.[77,78] Such studies have helped to risk stratify allograft vasculopathy with intimal thickening <0.3 mm involving ≥180° or >0.3 mm involving <180° of vessel circumference associated with future events and the development of significant disease.[79,80] This offers the possibility to modify immunosuppressive and anti-atherosclerotic therapy early in the disease process, which can potentially prolong organ life.

VIRTUAL-HISTOLOGY INTRAVASCULAR ULTRASOUND

Although grayscale IVUS provides robust quantitative measures on luminal, vessel, and stent dimensions, studies have found that it has limited ability to identify individual atherosclerotic plaque components.[19] Furthermore, tissue characterization by grayscale IVUS is subjective and remains open to interobserver differences in image interpretation.[81] VH-IVUS attempts, somewhat, to overcome these issues. In standard grayscale IVUS, the image is created from differences in the reflected amplitude of the ultrasound signal. VH-IVUS differs in that it also utilizes changes in the frequency of the reflected ultrasound signal in an attempt to discriminate between tissue components.[6] The "raw" reflected signal first undergoes automatic calibration and is then analyzed using a spectral analysis and compared with a histological database. The algorithm computes eight spectral parameters (maximum power, frequency at maximum power, minimum power, frequency at minimal power, slope, intercept, mid-band fit, and integrated backscatter) and combines these in a statistical model to assess plaque composition.[82] VH-IVUS subsequently labels four major plaque components, namely, (1) fibrous, (2) fibrofatty, (3) necrotic core, and (4) dense calcium (Figure 28.11). Fibrous tissue on VH-IVUS is portrayed as dark green and consists of densely packed bundles of collagen fiber with no evidence of intrafiber lipid accumulation. Fibrofatty tissue is shown as light green and consists of loosely packed collagen fibers with lipid deposition. However, these regions remain cellular and have no evidence of necrosis or cholesterol crystal formation. Necrotic core on VH-IVUS is displayed as red and histologically represents a highly lipid region with evidence of foam cell and lymphocyte death. There is evidence of cholesterol crystal deposition and microcalcification with no collagen present, which implies a degree of mechanical instability. Finally, dense calcium is shown as white as it represents focal macrocalcification. Validation studies have shown that use of VH-IVUS increases the sensitivity and specificity of IVUS for plaque characterization, as compared with grayscale IVUS. Predictive accuracies for all four major tissue components are >93%, with VH-IVUS

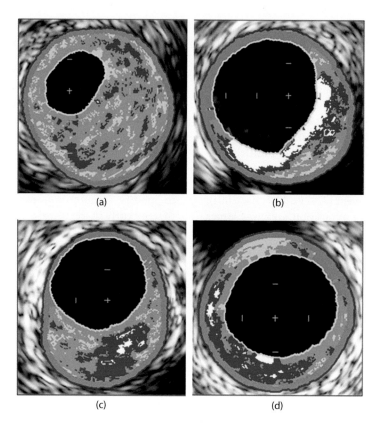

Figure 28.11 Plaque composition and classification using virtual-histology intravascular ultrasound (VH-IVUS). Plaque tissue components on VH-IVUS are color coded and displayed as dark green (fibrous), light green (fibrofatty), red (necrotic core), and white (dense calcium). Here, examples of four different plaque types, classified as pathological intimal thickening **(a)**, fibrocalcific plaque **(b)**, thick-cap fibroatheroma **(c)**, and thin-cap fibroatheroma **(d)**. (Reproduced from Brown, A.J., et al., *Circ. Cardiovasc. Imaging.*, 8, e003487, 2015. With permission.)

having a sensitivity of 92% and specificity of 97% for the identification of necrotic core.[82]

Plaque classification using virtual histology intravascular ultrasound

The majority of sudden ischemic cardiovascular events are due to rupture of an atheromatous coronary plaque. Plaques responsible for MI are known to have large, necrotic, lipid cores with thin overlying fibrous caps. A precursor lesion for rupture has been proposed, which shares many morphological features of a ruptured plaque but does not exhibit luminal thrombosis and is labeled as thin-cap fibroatheroma (TCFA).[83] VH-IVUS represents one imaging technology that may allow TCFA identification through application of a plaque classification algorithm based on the tissue characterization described above. On VH-IVUS, a fibroatheroma is first defined as a plaque (plaque burden >40% vessel CSA for three consecutive VH frames) with >10% confluent necrotic core maintained for three consecutive frames.[40] For a fibroatheroma to be labeled as TCFA, the confluent necrotic core should be in direct contact with the vessel lumen (Figure 28.11). The extent with which the necrotic core abuts the lumen varies between studies, but may be as little as "any" contact to contact extending >30°.[7,40]

Autopsy studies have shown that the diagnostic accuracy of VH-IVUS to classify TCFA correctly is around 76%, implying that advanced coronary plaques can be reliably identified.[84,85] However, false-positive TCFA identification can occur, especially around regions of calcification where the adjacent plaque composition is incorrectly shown as necrotic core.[86] Furthermore, VH-IVUS has limited axial resolution (around 200 μm) and is, therefore, unable to directly quantify the thickness of the overlying fibrous cap—an important criteria for histological TCFA classification.

Potential clinical applications of virtual histology intravascular ultrasound

The ability of VH-IVUS to identify TCFA has led to a number of prospective studies designed to assess whether VH-IVUS is capable of predicting MACE. In one of the first to be performed, the VH-IVUS in Vulnerable Atherosclerosis (VIVA) study assessed 170 patients with either stable angina or troponin-positive ACS undergoing PCI with three-vessel VH-IVUS. Of the 1,096 plaques identified, 19 resulted in subsequent nonrestenotic MACE defined as the composite of all-cause death, MI, and unplanned revascularization over a median follow-up of 625 days from enrollment. VH-TCFA was the only plaque subtype associated with MACE (HR: 7.53; 95% CI: 1.12–50.55; $P = 0.038$), along with plaque burden ≥70% (HR: 8.13; 95% CI: 1.63–40.56; $P = 0.01$).[40] Similar results were reported by the larger PROSPECT (A Prospective Natural-History Study of Coronary Atherosclerosis) study in which 697 patients with ACS also underwent three-vessel VH-IVUS. The cumulative MACE rate at 3 years, defined as the composite of cardiac death, cardiac arrest, MI, or rehospitalization due to unstable/progressive angina was 20.4%, with 11.6% of these events adjudicated to be attributable to nonculprit lesions. Plaque burden ≥70%, MLA ≤4 mm², and VH-TCFAs were all found to be independent predictors of nonculprit lesion MACE. In contrast, nonfibroatheroma lesions were found to be clinically stable and rarely associated with adverse clinical events over the same time period.[87] The results of PROSPECT and VIVA studies were reproduced in the recently published ATHEROREMO-IVUS (The European Collaborative Project on Inflammation and Vascular Wall Remodeling in Atherosclerosis-Intravascular Ultrasound Study) study, which recruited 581 patients to VH-IVUS imaging of a nonculprit artery, following a planned PCI procedure.[88] In this study, both VH-TCFA (HR: 1.98; 95% CI: 1.09–3.60; $P = 0.026$) and plaque burden ≥70% (HR: 2.90; 95% CI: 1.60–5.25; $P < 0.001$) were identified as independent plaque predictors of MACE at 1 year, particularly of death and ACS. The results of the aforementioned studies are in agreement with those from autopsy studies where TCFAs were identified as the plaque subtype

most prone to rupture and acute vessel thrombosis.[83] Despite these encouraging results, it is clear that VH-IVUS alone cannot accurately predict which plaques proceed to cause future events, as <10% of VH-TCFA lead to MACE at ≈3 years. Recently, in an attempt to improve VH-IVUS accuracy, biomechanical modeling using finite element analysis has been applied to VH-IVUS data. This allows for estimation of plaque structural stress (PSS), with plaque rupture thought to occur when PSS exceeds the material strength of the plaque. In the first study to evaluate this hypothesis, Teng et al. examined 4,429 VH-IVUS frames from 53 patients, 30 with stable angina and 23 with ACS. PSS was shown to be higher in noncalcified VH-TCFA as compared to thick-cap fibroatheroma (8.44 vs. 7.63; $P = 0.002$) and also higher in patients with an ACS as compared to those with stable angina, where MLA was ≤4 mm² (8.24 vs. 7.72; $P = 0.03$) and plaque burden ≥70% (9.18 vs. 7.93; $P = 0.02$). PSS was also found to increase the positive predictive value of VH-IVUS to identify clinical presentation, suggesting that integration of PSS with VH-IVUS may improve our ability to predict plaques at risk of rupture or rapid progression.[89] Examples of PSS calculations with their corresponding VH-IVUS images are shown in Figure 28.12.

VH-IVUS has also been used to assess the effect of anti-atherosclerotic therapy on plaque composition. In the VH-IVUS study by Hong et al., reductions in necrotic core with concomitant increases in fibrous tissue volumes were observed after a 12-month treatment period with either

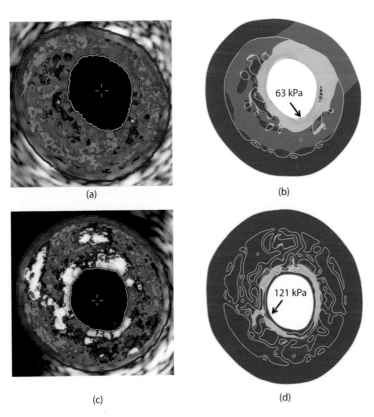

(a) (b) (c) (d)

Figure 28.12 An illustrative example of plaque structural stress (**a** and **c**) from virtual-histology intravascular ultrasound (**b** and **d**) through finite element analysis.

simvastatin or rosuvastin.[90] Plaque regression with high-intensity statin therapy was also observed in the recently published IBIS-4 (Integrated Biomarkers and Imaging Study-4) study, in which 103 ST-segment elevation MI patients were treated with rosuvastatin 40 mg for a period of 13 months. Despite reductions in nonculprit vessel plaque burden, necrotic core volume and VH-TCFA properties, however, remained unchanged in this particular cohort.[91] These studies suggest that VH-IVUS can be a helpful tool in investigating the impact of novel therapeutic agents on plaque composition and classification.[92]

CONCLUSIONS

Grayscale IVUS provides (1) high-quality, tomographic imaging of the lumen, atheroma, and vessel wall; (2) incremental and more detailed qualitative and quantitative information than coronary angiography; and (3) practical guidance during PCI. IVUS remains an important tool in helping to understand the mechanisms, effects, and complications of new stent technology. VH-IVUS, on the other hand, provides a reliable representation of plaque composition and architecture. TCFAs can reliably be identified with VH-IVUS and have been linked by a number of prospective studies with future adverse events. Newer technologies that utilize VH-IVUS data offer information beyond plaque anatomy and, thus, a more comprehensive plaque assessment that can potentially lead to the better identification of those plaques truly at risk of rupture and clinical events.

REFERENCES

1. Bom N, et al. Ultrasonic viewer for cross-sectional analyses of moving cardiac structures. *Biomed Eng* 1971;6(11):500–503.
2. Yock PG, et al. Intravascular ultrasound guidance for catheter-based coronary interventions. *J Am Coll Cardiol* 1991;17(6 Suppl B):39–45.
3. McDaniel MC, et al. Contemporary clinical applications of coronary intravascular ultrasound. *JACC Cardiovasc Interv* 2011;4(11):1155–1167.
4. Abizaid AS, et al. Long-term follow-up after percutaneous transluminal coronary angioplasty was not performed based on intravascular ultrasound findings: Importance of lumen dimensions. *Circulation* 1999;100(3):256–261.
5. Mintz GS, et al. American College of Cardiology Clinical Expert Consensus Document on Standards for acquisition, measurement and reporting of intravascular ultrasound tudies (IVUS). A report of the American College of Cardiology Task Force on Clinical Expert Consensus Documents. *J Am Coll Cardiol* 2001;37(5):1478–1492.
6. Nair A, et al. Coronary plaque classification with intravascular ultrasound radiofrequency data analysis. *Circulation* 2002;106(17):2200–2206.
7. Stone GW, et al. A prospective natural-history study of coronary atherosclerosis. *N Engl J Med* 2011;364(3):226–235.
8. Maehara A, et al. Advances in intravascular imaging. *Circ Cardiovasc Interv* 2009;2(5):482–490.
9. Bangalore S, Bhatt DL. Coronary intravascular ultrasound. *Circulation* 2013;127(25):e868–e874.
10. Kimura BJ, et al. Distortion of intravascular ultrasound images because of nonuniform angular velocity of mechanical-type transducers. *Am Heart J* 1996;132(2 Pt 1):328–336.
11. Arbab-Zadeh A, et al. Axial movement of the intravascular ultrasound probe during the cardiac cycle: Implications for three-dimensional reconstruction and measurements of coronary dimensions. *Am Heart J* 1999;138(5 Pt 1):865–872.
12. Di Mario C, et al. Clinical application and image interpretation in intracoronary ultrasound. Study Group on Intracoronary Imaging of the Working Group of Coronary Circulation and of the Subgroup on Intravascular Ultrasound of the Working Group of Echocardiography of the European Society of Cardiology. *Eur Heart J* 1998;19(2):207–229.
13. Mintz GS, et al. Clinical expert consensus document on standards for acquisition, measurement and reporting of intravascular ultrasound regression/progression studies. *EuroIntervention* 2011;6(9):1123–1130.
14. St Goar FG, et al. Intravascular ultrasound imaging of angiographically normal coronary arteries: An in vivo comparison with quantitative angiography. *J Am Coll Cardiol* 1991;18(4):952–958.
15. Nissen SE, Yock P. Intravascular ultrasound: Novel pathophysiological insights and current clinical applications. *Circulation* 2001;103(4):604–616.
16. Tuzcu EM, et al. High prevalence of coronary atherosclerosis in asymptomatic teenagers and young adults: Evidence from intravascular ultrasound. *Circulation* 2001;103(22):2705–2710.
17. Isner JM, et al. Attenuation of the media of coronary arteries in advanced atherosclerosis. *Am J Cardiol* 1986;58(10):937–939.
18. Maehara A, et al. Definitions and methodology for the grayscale and radiofrequency intravascular ultrasound and coronary angiographic analyses. *JACC Cardiovasc Imaging* 2012;5(3 Suppl):S1–S9.
19. Palmer ND, et al. In vitro analysis of coronary atheromatous lesions by intravascular ultrasound; reproducibility and histological correlation of lesion morphology. *Eur Heart J* 1999;20(23):1701–1706.
20. Garcia-Garcia HM, et al. IVUS-based imaging modalities for tissue characterization: Similarities and differences. *Int J Cardiovasc Imaging* 2011;27(2):215–224.
21. Gonzalo N, et al. Coronary plaque composition as assessed by greyscale intravascular ultrasound and radiofrequency spectral data analysis. *Int J Cardiovasc Imaging* 2008;24(8):811–818.
22. Kern MJ, Samady H. Current concepts of integrated coronary physiology in the catheterization laboratory. *J Am Coll Cardiol* 2010;55(3):173–185.
23. van Nunen LX, et al. Fractional flow reserve versus angiography for guidance of PCI in patients with multivessel coronary artery disease (FAME): 5-year follow-up of a randomised controlled trial. *Lancet* 2015;386(10006):1853–1860.
24. Sen S, et al. Diagnostic classification of the instantaneous wave-free ratio is equivalent to fractional flow reserve and is not improved with adenosine administration. Results of

CLARIFY (Classification Accuracy of Pressure-Only Ratios Against Indices Using Flow Study). *J Am Coll Cardiol* 2013;61(13):1409–1420.

25. Okura H, et al. Culprit lesion remodelling and long-term prognosis in patients with acute coronary syndrome: An intravascular ultrasound study. *Eur Heart J Cardiovasc Imaging* 2013;14(8):758–764.

26. Inaba S, et al. Impact of positive and negative lesion site remodeling on clinical outcomes: Insights from PROSPECT. *JACC Cardiovasc Imaging* 2014;7(1):70–78.

27. Nakamura M, et al. Impact of coronary artery remodeling on clinical presentation of coronary artery disease: An intravascular ultrasound study. *J Am Coll Cardiol* 2001;37(1):63–69.

28. Maehara A, et al. Morphologic and angiographic features of coronary plaque rupture detected by intravascular ultrasound. *J Am Coll Cardiol* 2002;40(5):904–910.

29. Mehran R, et al. Atherosclerotic plaque burden and CK-MB enzyme elevation after coronary interventions : Intravascular ultrasound study of 2256 patients. *Circulation* 2000;101(6):604–610.

30. Gyongyosi M, et al. Intravascular ultrasound predictors of major adverse cardiac events in patients with unstable angina. *Clin Cardiol* 2000;23(7):507–515.

31. Kang SJ, et al. Usefulness of minimal luminal coronary area determined by intravascular ultrasound to predict functional significance in stable and unstable angina pectoris. *Am J Cardiol* 2012;109(7):947–953.

32. Koo BK, et al. Optimal intravascular ultrasound criteria and their accuracy for defining the functional significance of intermediate coronary stenoses of different locations. *JACC Cardiovasc Interv* 2011;4(7):803–811.

33. Naganuma T, et al. The role of intravascular ultrasound and quantitative angiography in the functional assessment of intermediate coronary lesions: Correlation with fractional flow reserve. *Cardiovasc Revasc Med* 2014;15(1):3–7.

34. Mintz GS. Clinical utility of intravascular imaging and physiology in coronary artery disease. *J Am Coll Cardiol* 2014;64(2):207–222.

35. Waksman R, et al. FIRST: Fractional flow reserve and intravascular ultrasound relationship study. *J Am Coll Cardiol* 2013;61(9):917–923.

36. Jasti V, et al. Correlations between fractional flow reserve and intravascular ultrasound in patients with an ambiguous left main coronary artery stenosis. *Circulation* 2004;110(18):2831–2836.

37. Kim JS, et al. Impact of intravascular ultrasound guidance on long-term clinical outcomes in patients treated with drug-eluting stent for bifurcation lesions: Data from a Korean multicenter bifurcation registry. *Am Heart J* 2011;161(1):180–187.

38. Park SJ, et al. Impact of intravascular ultrasound guidance on long-term mortality in stenting for unprotected left main coronary artery stenosis. *Circ Cardiovasc Interv* 2009;2(3):167–177.

39. Ge J, et al. Screening of ruptured plaques in patients with coronary artery disease by intravascular ultrasound. *Heart* 1999;81(6):621–627.

40. Calvert PA, et al. Association between IVUS findings and adverse outcomes in patients with coronary artery disease: The VIVA (VH-IVUS in Vulnerable Atherosclerosis) Study. *JACC Cardiovasc Imaging* 2011;4(8):894–901.

41. Mintz GS, et al. Determinants and correlates of target lesion calcium in coronary artery disease: A clinical, angiographic and intravascular ultrasound study. *J Am Coll Cardiol* 1997;29(2):268–274.

42. Maehara A, et al. An intravascular ultrasound classification of angiographic coronary artery aneurysms. *Am J Cardiol* 2001;88(4):365–370.

43. Souteyrand G, et al. Mechanisms of stent thrombosis analysed by optical coherence tomography: Insights from the national PESTO French registry. *Eur Heart J* 2016;37(15):1208–1216.

44. Calvert PA, et al. Geographical miss is associated with vulnerable plaque and increased major adverse cardiovascular events in patients with myocardial infarction. *Catheter Cardiovasc Interv* 2016; 88(3):340–347.

45. Ahmed JM, et al. Mechanism of lumen enlargement during intracoronary stent implantation: An intravascular ultrasound study. *Circulation* 2000;102(1):7–10.

46. Maehara A, et al. Longitudinal plaque redistribution during stent expansion. *Am J Cardiol* 2000;86(10):1069–1072.

47. Prati F, et al. Stenting of culprit lesions in unstable angina leads to a marked reduction in plaque burden: A major role of plaque embolization? A serial intravascular ultrasound study. *Circulation* 2003;107(18):2320–2325.

48. Lipinski MJ, et al. Scaffold thrombosis after percutaneous coronary intervention with ABSORB bioresorbable vascular scaffold: A systematic review and meta-analysis. *JACC Cardiovasc Interv* 2016;9(1):12–24.

49. Costopoulos C, et al. Comparison of early clinical outcomes between absorb bioresorbable vascular scaffold and everolimus-eluting stent implantation in a real-world population. *Catheter Cardiovasc Interv* 2015;85(1):E10–E15.

50. Cook S, et al. Impact of incomplete stent apposition on long-term clinical outcome after drug-eluting stent implantation. *Eur Heart J* 2012;33(11):1334–1343.

51. Cheneau E, et al. Predictors of subacute stent thrombosis: Results of a systematic intravascular ultrasound study. *Circulation* 2003;108(1):43–47.

52. Fujii K, et al. Stent underexpansion and residual reference segment stenosis are related to stent thrombosis after sirolimus-eluting stent implantation: An intravascular ultrasound study. *J Am Coll Cardiol* 2005;45(7):995–998.

53. Okabe T, et al. Intravascular ultrasound parameters associated with stent thrombosis after drug-eluting stent deployment. *Am J Cardiol* 2007;100(4):615–620.

54. Serruys PW, Daemen J. Are drug-eluting stents associated with a higher rate of late thrombosis than bare metal stents? Late stent thrombosis: A nuisance in both bare metal and drug-eluting stents. *Circulation* 2007;115(11):1433–1439; discussion 1439.

55. Mori H, et al. Malapposition: Is it a major cause of stent thrombosis? *Eur Heart J* 2016; 37(15):1217–1219.

56. Zhang Y, et al. Comparison of intravascular ultrasound versus angiography-guided drug-eluting stent implantation: A meta-analysis of one randomised trial and ten observational studies involving 19,619 patients. *EuroIntervention* 2012;8(7):855–865.

57. Ahn JM, et al. Meta-analysis of outcomes after intravascular ultrasound-guided versus angiography-guided drug-eluting stent implantation in 26,503 patients enrolled in three randomized trials and 14 observational studies. *Am J Cardiol* 2014;113(8):1338–1347.

58. Hur SH, et al. Impact of intravascular ultrasound-guided percutaneous coronary intervention on long-term clinical outcomes in a real world population. *Catheter Cardiovasc Interv* 2013;81(3):407–416.

59. Chieffo A, et al. A prospective, randomized trial of intravascular-ultrasound guided compared to angiography guided stent implantation in complex coronary lesions: The AVIO trial. *Am Heart J* 2013;165(1):65–72.

60. Witzenbichler B, et al. Relationship between intravascular ultrasound guidance and clinical outcomes after drug-eluting stents: The assessment of dual antiplatelet therapy with drug-eluting stents (ADAPT-DES) study. *Circulation* 2014;129(4):463–470.

61. Hong SJ, et al. Effect of intravascular ultrasound-guided vs angiography-guided everolimus-eluting stent implantation: The IVUS-XPL randomized clinical trial. *JAMA* 2015;314(20):2155–2163.

62. Elgendy IY, et al. Outcomes with intravascular ultrasound-guided stent implantation: A meta-analysis of randomized trials in the era of drug-eluting stents. *Circ Cardiovasc Interv* 2016;9(4):e003700.

63. Zhang YJ, et al. Comparison of intravascular ultrasound guided versus angiography guided drug eluting stent implantation: A systematic review and meta-analysis. *BMC Cardiovasc Disord* 2015;15(1):153.

64. Moses JW, et al. Sirolimus-eluting stents versus standard stents in patients with stenosis in a native coronary artery. *N Engl J Med* 2003;349(14):1315–1323.

65. Stone GW, et al. Comparison of an everolimus-eluting stent and a paclitaxel-eluting stent in patients with coronary artery disease: A randomized trial. *JAMA* 2008;299(16):1903–1913.

66. Castagna MT, et al. The contribution of "mechanical" problems to in-stent restenosis: An intravascular ultrasonographic analysis of 1090 consecutive in-stent restenosis lesions. *Am Heart J* 2001;142(6):970–974.

67. Diletti R, et al. Clinical and intravascular imaging outcomes at 1 and 2 years after implantation of absorb everolimus eluting bioresorbable vascular scaffolds in small vessels. Late lumen enlargement: Does bioresorption matter with small vessel size? Insight from the ABSORB cohort B trial. *Heart* 2013;99(2):98–105.

68. Costopoulos C, et al. Looking into the future with bioresorbable vascular scaffolds. *Expert Rev Cardiovasc Ther* 2013;11(10):1407–1416.

69. Karalis I, et al. Late acquired stent malapposition: Why, when and how to handle? *Heart* 2012;98(20):1529–1536.

70. Mintz GS, Weissman NJ. Intravascular ultrasound in the drug-eluting stent era. *J Am Coll Cardiol* 2006;48(3):421–429.

71. Cook S, et al. Incomplete stent apposition and very late stent thrombosis after drug-eluting stent implantation. *Circulation* 2007;115(18):2426–2434.

72. Steinberg DH, et al. Long-term impact of routinely detected early and late incomplete stent apposition: An integrated intravascular ultrasound analysis of the TAXUS IV, V, and VI and TAXUS ATLAS workhorse, long lesion, and direct stent studies. *JACC Cardiovasc Interv* 2010;3(5):486–494.

73. Nissen SE, et al. Effect of intensive compared with moderate lipid-lowering therapy on progression of coronary atherosclerosis: A randomized controlled trial. *JAMA* 2004;291(9):1071–1080.

74. Nicholls SJ, et al. Effect of two intensive statin regimens on progression of coronary disease. *N Engl J Med* 2011;365(22):2078–2087.

75. Sipahi I, et al. Effects of normal, pre-hypertensive, and hypertensive blood pressure levels on progression of coronary atherosclerosis. *J Am Coll Cardiol* 2006;48(4):833–838.

76. Tuzcu EM, et al. Dichotomous pattern of coronary atherosclerosis 1 to 9 years after transplantation: Insights from systematic intravascular ultrasound imaging. *J Am Coll Cardiol* 1996;27(4):839–846.

77. Li H, et al. Vascular remodelling after cardiac transplantation: A 3-year serial intravascular ultrasound study. *Eur Heart J* 2006;27(14):1671–1677.

78. Tsutsui H, et al. Lumen loss in transplant coronary artery disease is a biphasic process involving early intimal thickening and late constrictive remodeling: Results from a 5-year serial intravascular ultrasound study. *Circulation* 2001;104(6):653–657.

79. Tuzcu EM, et al. Intravascular ultrasound evidence of angiographically silent progression in coronary atherosclerosis predicts long-term morbidity and mortality after cardiac transplantation. *J Am Coll Cardiol* 2005;45(9):1538–1542.

80. Rickenbacher PR, et al. Prognostic importance of intimal thickness as measured by intracoronary ultrasound after cardiac transplantation. *Circulation* 1995;92(12):3445–3452.

81. Obaid DR, et al. Identification of coronary plaque sub-types using virtual histology intravascular ultrasound is affected by inter-observer variability and differences in plaque definitions. *Circ Cardiovasc Imaging* 2012;5(1):86–93.

82. Nair A, et al. Automated coronary plaque characterisation with intravascular ultrasound backscatter: Ex vivo validation. *EuroIntervention* 2007;3(1):113–120.

83. Virmani R, et al. Lessons from sudden coronary death: A comprehensive morphological classification scheme for atherosclerotic lesions. *Arterioscler Thromb Vasc Biol* 2000;20(5):1262–1275.

84. Obaid DR, et al. Atherosclerotic plaque composition and classification identified by coronary computed tomography: Assessment of computed tomography-generated plaque maps compared with virtual histology intravascular ultrasound and histology. *Circ Cardiovasc Imaging* 2013;6(5):655–664.

85. Brown AJ, et al. Direct comparison of virtual-histology intravascular ultrasound and optical coherence tomography imaging for identification of thin-cap fibroatheroma. *Circ Cardiovasc Imaging* 2015;8(10):e003487.

86. Sales FJ, et al. Evaluation of plaque composition by intravascular ultrasound "virtual histology": The impact of dense calcium on the measurement of necrotic tissue. *EuroIntervention* 2010;6(3):394–399.

87. Dohi T, et al. Non-fibroatheroma lesion phenotype and long-term clinical outcomes: A substudy analysis from the PROSPECT study. *JACC Cardiovasc Imaging* 2013;6(8):908–16.

88. Cheng JM, et al. In vivo detection of high-risk coronary plaques by radiofrequency intravascular ultrasound and cardiovascular outcome: Results of the ATHEROREMO-IVUS study. *Eur Heart J* 2013;35(10):639–647.

89. Teng Z, et al. Coronary plaque structural stress is associated with plaque composition and subtype and higher in acute coronary syndrome: The BEACON I (Biomechanical Evaluation of Atheromatous Coronary Arteries) study. *Circ Cardiovasc Imaging* 2014;7(3):461–470.

90. Hong MK, et al. Effects of statin treatments on coronary plaques assessed by volumetric virtual histology intra-vascular ultrasound analysis. *JACC Cardiovasc Interv* 2009;2(7):679–688.

91. Raber L, et al. Effect of high-intensity statin therapy on atherosclerosis in non-infarct-related coronary arteries (IBIS-4): A serial intravascular ultrasonography study. *Eur Heart J* 2015;36(8):490–500.

92. Costopoulos C, et al. Intravascular ultrasound and optical coherence tomography imaging of coronary atherosclerosis. *Int J Cardiovasc Imaging* 2016;32(1):189–200.

29

Optical coherence tomography

MOHAMAD SOUD, GABRIEL TENSOL RODRIGUES PEREIRA, MARCO A. COSTA,
HIRAM G. BEZERRA, AND GUILHERME F. ATTIZZANI

INTRODUCTION

The introduction of optical coherence tomography (OCT) into the catheterization laboratory was received with great expectation, as this light-based imaging modality offers 10 times higher resolution and 40 times faster imaging acquisition compared to intravascular ultrasound (IVUS). However, the first-generation time-domain OCT (TD-OCT) (M2CV OCT Imaging System, LightLab Imaging, Westford, MA) was plagued with the requirement for proximal vessel occlusion to create a blood-free imaging environment. Today, the frequency-domain OCT (FD-OCT) has overcome the inherent technical limitations of TD-OCT while preserving and potentially improving image quality, thus allowing for a widespread clinical intracoronary application in research and patient care. Semi-automated imaging analyses of OCT systems permit accurate measurements of luminal architecture and provide insights regarding stent apposition, expansion, overlap, neointimal thickening, and, in the case of bioresorbable stents, information regarding the time course of stent dissolution. This chapter discusses these technical principles of intracoronary OCT, summarizes the preclinical and clinical research, discusses clinical applications, and explains the practical performance of OCT as a diagnostic and interventional tool in the catheterization laboratory.

FUNDAMENTALS

The coronary OCT light source uses a bandwidth in the near-infrared spectrum with central wavelengths ranging from 1250 to 1350 nm. Although longer wavelengths provide deeper tissue penetration, the optimal choice of wavelength in an arterial vessel is also defined by tissue absorption characteristics and the refractive index of the interface between the catheter and vessel wall.[1] The image is formed by the backscattering of light from the vessel wall or the time it takes for emitted light to travel between the target tissue and back to the lens, producing an "echo time delay" with a measurable signal intensity or "magnitude." Multiple axial scans (A-lines) are continuously acquired as the ImageWire (St. Jude Medical/LightLab Imaging Inc., Westford, MA) rotates and a full revolution creates a complete cross section of the vessel. The speed of light $(3 \times 10^8$ m/s) is much faster than that of sound (1500 m/s); therefore, interferometry techniques are necessary to measure the backscattered signal since a direct quantification cannot be achieved on such a time scale. Figure 29.1 shows the general scheme of an intravascular OCT system. Blood must be completely removed, as any amount of residual red blood cells causes significant signal attenuation.

The development from TD-OCD to FD-OCT led to faster image acquisition speeds with greater penetration depth

FD-OCT (OFDI)

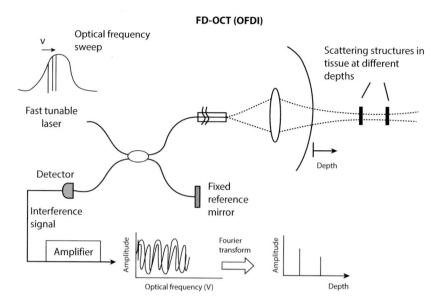

Figure 29.1 Characteristics of FD-OCT: light source with variable wavelength and fixed reference mirror. FD-OCT, frequency-domain optical coherence tomography; OFDI, optical frequency domain imaging.

without loss of vital detail or resolution, and represents a great advance, permitting imaging of coronary arteries within seconds and allowing for widespread clinical use in a broad range of patients and lesions.

Normal vessel wall appearance

Due to its high resolution, OCT is able to differentiate the three layers of coronary artery wall. The normal coronary vessel wall has a three-layer architecture with a signal-rich intima, a low backscattering, or signal poor media, and a heterogeneous and high backscattering adventitia (Figure 29.2).

Intravascular ultrasound versus optical coherence tomography

Both IVUS and OCT offer an anatomic assessment of the vasculature. However, they differ in several respects (Table 29.1).

IVUS-guided percutaneous coronary intervention (PCI) is essentially a poststent assessment/optimization tool. On this regard, the central parameter is lumen assessment, and this is translatable between the two methods. Not surprisingly, as documented on the Ilumien II trial, both methods achieved a similar percent of stent expansion when operators have the freedom to apply IVUS concepts to OCT.[2] We believe that OCT should position itself as a periprocedural tool to take full advantage of the superior plaque characterization, acute coronary syndrome (ACS) applications, stent planning, and volumetric lumen segmentation for stent optimization. This can be applied to virtually every coronary intervention, but it is apparently even more important with the upcoming Absorb bioresorbable vascular scaffold (BVS) (Abbott Vascular, Santa Clara, CA).[3]

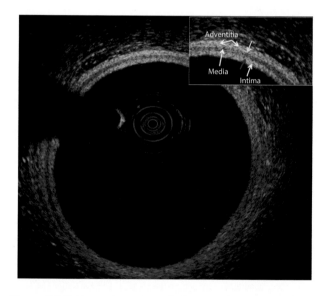

Figure 29.2 Normal artery wall shows a three-layered architecture, with external elastic membrane (yellow arrow) and internal elastic membrane (red arrow).

EQUIPMENT

The FD-OCT system (LightLab Imaging Inc./St. Jude Medical, Westford, MA) is equipped with a tunable laser light source with a sweep range of 1250–1370 nm. The optical fiber is encapsulated within a rotating torque wire built in a rapid exchange catheter compatible with a 6-Fr guide, connected to a rotary junction that utilizes a motor unit to rotate the optical fiber in the catheter. Rotation and translation of the fiber in the catheter, actuated by the rotary junction and pullback motor units, is transmitted to the distal imaging tip by the optical fiber itself, or by a flexible drive cable encapsulating the fiber. Figure 29.3 shows different OCT systems.

Table 29.1 Comparison of optical coherence tomography (OCT) and intravascular ultrasound (IVUS)

	OCT	IVUS
Image example		
Catheter size	0.8–1 mm	1.1 mm
Axial resolution	10–20 mm	100–150 mm
Lateral resolution	40–90 μm	250 μm
Penetration depth into tissue	2–3.5 mm	4–8 mm
Wavelength	1.3 μm	35–80 μm
Maximum frame rate	100–200 fps	30
Pullback speed	Up to 40 mm/s	1.0 mm/s
Blood removal needed	Yes	No
Plaque characterization	Yes	Yes
Fibrous cap measurement	Yes	No
Vessel remodeling	No	Yes

Note: fps, frames per second.

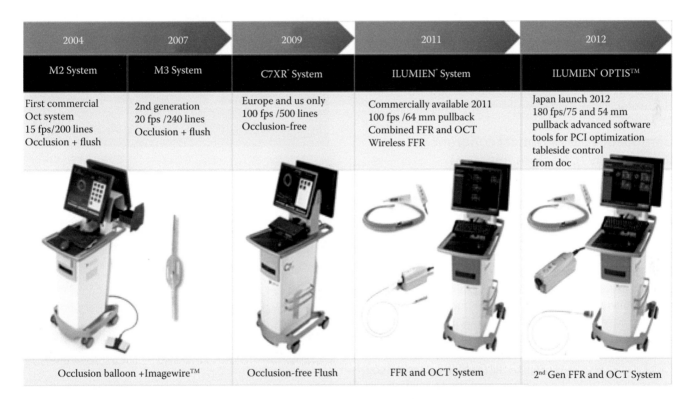

2004	2007	2009	2011	2012
M2 System	M3 System	C7XR System	ILUMIEN System	ILUMIEN OPTIS™
First commercial Oct system 15 fps/200 lines Occlusion + flush	2nd generation 20 fps /240 lines Occlusion + flush	Europe and us only 100 fps /500 lines Occlusion-free	Commercially available 2011 100 fps /64 mm pullback Combined FFR and OCT Wireless FFR	Japan launch 2012 180 fps/75 and 54 mm pullback advanced software tools for PCI optimization tableside control from doc
Occlusion balloon +Imagewire™		Occlusion-free Flush	FFR and OCT System	2nd Gen FFR and OCT System

Figure 29.3 Advances of OCT systems, including the first available commercial OCT and currently available system. OCT, optical coherence tomography.

Imaging technique

Because of its higher imaging speed, helical pullback image acquisition with FD-OCT is primarily conducted with nonocclusive flushing techniques for removing blood from the artery.

A 6-Fr or larger diameter guiding catheter is recommended for FD-OCT imaging (Figure 29.4).

Lactated Ringer's solution, viscous iso-osmolar contrast media, and mixtures of lactated Ringer's and contrast media, or low molecular weight dextrose, can be used for nonocclusive flushing, although higher viscosity solutions provide superior results. The OCT imaging catheter is advanced distally into the coronary artery via a standard angioplasty guide wire (0.014-in). Care should be taken to position the guide catheter coaxially and deeply into the coronary ostium. Correct guide catheter position can be confirmed by manual injection of a small flush bolus through the guide catheter prior to imaging, if needed. Automated OCT pullback is performed during contrast injection through the guide catheter, which is accomplished manually using a syringe or automatically using a power injector connected to the standard Y-piece of the guiding catheter.

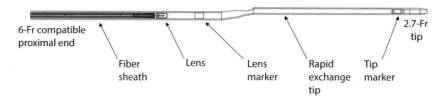

Figure 29.4 A 6-Fr optical coherence tomography guiding catheter.

Flushing should be terminated when the region of interest has been imaged, when blood reenters the image, or when the OCT catheter optics enter the guide catheter.

INDICATIONS

Coronary angiography is the standard invasive imaging method for diagnosis of coronary artery disease (CAD) and for guiding coronary interventional procedures.[4] OCT can add value to angiography as a diagnostic and/or intervention tool for PCI guidance.[5,6] When used systematically, it has been reported to alter procedural strategy in over 80% of cases.[7] The interest in the long-term stent strut and vessel wall interaction is manifold and includes the assessment of the stability of the acute result and the visualization of complex anatomy that is not accessible by angiography or IVUS.

Diagnostic role of optical coherence tomography (pre-stent imaging)

ASSESSMENT OF PLAQUE RUPTURE AND INTRACORONARY THROMBOSIS

Plaque rupture (Figure 29.5) with subsequent thrombosis is the most frequent cause of ACS. OCT has unique features that favor its utilization in the setting of ACS, having 100% sensitivity (versus 33% with IVUS) in detecting intraluminal thrombus when compared to coronary angioscopy, in addition to being able to differentiate white and red thrombus (Figure 29.6). The high sensitivity of the method in detecting thrombus can fulfill angiographic limitations in differentiating thrombus from calcium and other etiologies of ambiguous angiographic radiolucency. Several reports indicate the ability of the method to discern the underlying mechanism of the ACS, which can directly impact the management strategy.[8] This method is also very suitable for the detection of non-CAD-related ACS causes like spontaneous coronary artery dissection; in this particular clinical setting, OCT-derived information could defer unnecessary stenting. These characteristics make it the ideal method for identifying the etiology, defining anatomic location of the culprit vessel or segment, and ruling out ACS.

ATHEROSCLEROTIC PLAQUE COMPOSITION

The propensity of atherosclerotic lesions to destabilize and rupture is highly dependent on their composition. Due to its high spatial resolution, OCT has proved superior to other imaging modalities, including IVUS, in detecting and characterizing different atherosclerotic plaque components (Figure 29.7).[9]

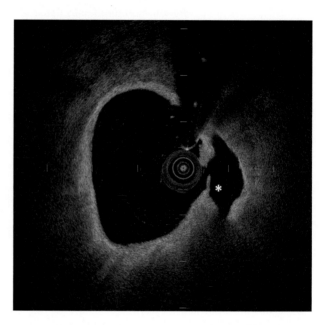

Figure 29.5 Optical coherence tomographic imaging showing plaque rupture (indicated by asterisk).

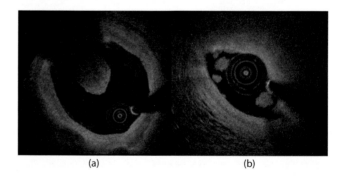

Figure 29.6 **(a)** Red thrombus protruding into the vessel lumen with high optical coherence tomography backscattering and attenuation. **(b)** White thrombus with homogeneous backscattering and low attenuation.

Yabushita et al.[10] performed an *in vitro* study of more than 300 human atherosclerotic artery segments. When compared with histological examination, OCT had a sensitivity ranging from 71% to 79% for fibrous plaques; 95% to 96% for fibrocalcific plaques; and 90% to 95% for lipid-rich plaques; and specificity ranging from 97% to 98% for fibrous plaques; 97% for fibrocalcific plaques; and 90% to 92% for lipid-rich plaques. Furthermore, the interobserver and intraobserver agreements of OCT measurements were high (k values of 0.88

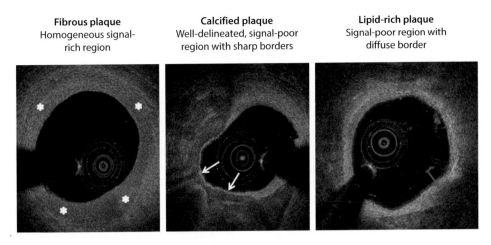

Fibrous plaque	Calcified plaque	Lipid-rich plaque
Homogeneous signal-rich region	Well-delineated, signal-poor region with sharp borders	Signal-poor region with diffuse border

Figure 29.7 Optical coherence tomographic images of three different types of atherosclerotic plaques.

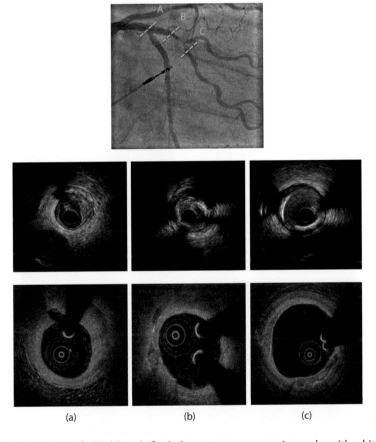

(a)   (b)   (c)

Figure 29.8 *In vivo* intravascular imaging of a highly calcified plaque—coronary angiography with white dashed lines **(a, b,** and **c)** corresponding to intravascular ultrasound (*top*) and optical coherence tomography (*bottom*) cross sections, respectively.

and 0.91, respectively). *Ex vivo* validations have also shown that OCT is superior to conventional and integrated backscatter IVUS for the characterization of coronary atherosclerotic plaque composition (Figure 29.8).[11–14] *In vivo*, OCT is able to identify most of the architectural features detected by IVUS and may be superior for the identification of lipid pools.[9] Several authors have evaluated the OCT appearance of coronary plaques in different groups of patients, reporting higher prevalence of lipid-rich plaques in ACS than in patients with stable angina[15] and no differences in the culprit plaque imaged by OCT between diabetic and nondiabetic patients.[16] Using OCT, investigators of the OCTAVIA (Optical Coherence Tomography Assessment of Gender diVersity in Primary Angioplasty) trial found no morphologic plaque differences between men and women with acute myocardial infarction (MI) undergoing primary PCI.[17]

Heavy calcification within coronary atherosclerotic plaque is considered a serious challenge in interventional cardiology and can adversely influence both clinical and procedural success after PCI. OCT has demonstrated accuracy in volumetric characterization of coronary calcium content.[18]

OCT has also been helpful in the characterization of carotid artery disease and investigating carotid plaque characteristics. Indeed, it could eventually have the potential of altering our understanding and treatment of carotid artery disease in several respects.[19]

VISUALIZATION OF MACROPHAGE ACCUMULATION

Intense infiltration by macrophages of the fibrous cap is another feature of the vulnerable plaques. An *ex vivo* study by Tearney et al. demonstrated that OCT can quantify macrophage within the fibrous cap.[20] *In vivo*, it has been demonstrated that patients with unstable CAD have a significantly higher macrophage density detected by OCT in the culprit lesion than patients with stable CAD. Furthermore, in the same population, the sites of plaque rupture had a greater macrophage density than nonruptured sites.[21] Raffel et al. reported that macrophage density in the fibrous cap detected by OCT correlated with the white blood cell count, and both parameters could be useful in predicting the presence of a fibroatheroma.[22] Tahara et al. also focused on the feasibility of OCT in macrophage quantification and demonstrated a high histological correlation.[23]

Figure 29.9 illustrates detailed OCT-based tissue characterization of a coronary segment, including the distribution of macrophages.

THICKNESS OF THE FIBROUS CAP

Autopsy studies of sudden cardiac death victims have shown that the most frequent cause of coronary occlusion is rupture of a thin-cap fibroatheroma (TCFA). Such lesions are characterized by a large necrotic core with a thin fibrous cap that is usually <65 μm in thickness. Conventional intracoronary imaging techniques such as virtual histology-IVUS lack the resolution to evaluate the fibrous cap in detail.

On the other hand, OCT has been shown to provide accurate measurements of the fibrous cap thickness overlying a lipid plaque, therefore enabling the detection of TCFA.[24,25] However, the current methodology for determining fibrous cap thickness is based on manual individual measurements of arbitrary points which could lead to high variability and decreased accuracy. A new computer-aided method for semi-automatic volumetric quantification of the fibrous cap is fast, highly accurate, and able to segment the boundaries and quantify the three-dimensional (3D) morphology of fibrous caps (Figure 29.10) with results more consistent

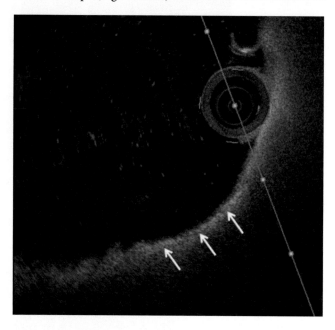

Figure 29.9 Optical coherence tomography image demonstrating a macrophage-rich region (*white arrows*).

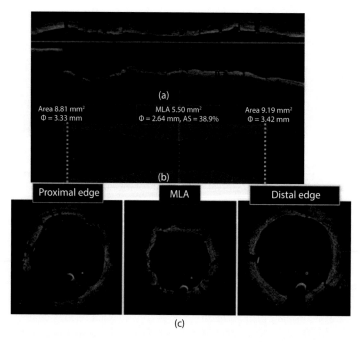

Figure 29.10 Optical coherence tomographic longitudinal **(a)** and cross-sectional views **(c)**. The corresponding lumen profile display **(b)** with automatic detection of minimal luminal area (MLA). AS, area stenosis.

than the manual method.[26,27] In a study of IVUS, OCT, and angioscopy in acute MI patients by Kubo et al., the incidence of TCFA was 83% and only OCT was able to estimate the fibrous cap thickness (mean 49 ± 21 mm).[28] Two studies have reported that the plaque color by angioscopy is related to the thickness of the fibrous cap as measured by OCT with yellow plaques often presenting with thin caps.[29,30]

CLINICAL ASPECTS

Optical coherence tomography's role in coronary artery intervention

PROCEDURE PLANNING

OCT helps with PCI procedure planning and facilitating the selection of the appropriate stent diameter and length.

LESION PREPARATION

Calcium plaque is one of the most important predictors of suboptimal stent expansion. Although both IVUS and OCT are sensitive for detecting calcium,[31] OCT has higher tissue penetration with calcium, which allows assessment of its thickness. Concentric but thin calcium may be fractured by regular or scoring balloons. In the setting of concentric and thicker calcium, however, atherectomy may be considered. Another strategy is to perform more aggressive predilatation with nominal vessel-size noncompliant balloons. Unfortunately, at the moment, there are no specific cutoff values to indicate the need for atherectomy or aggressive predilatation. But, as previously discussed, it is easier to achieve adequate stent expansion with plaque modification than to react to a grossly underexpanded stent. The need for careful lesion preparation seems to be even more important with the first generation of BVS, since these devices have thicker struts and mass compared to the metallic stents whose thinner struts can be considered scoring devices. The ability to embed BVS struts in the coronary arterial wall is reduced compared to metal stents; lesion preparation with calcium debulking or the creation of dissection planes in the plaque is key in order to achieve ideal expansion of the BVS.

STENT SELECTION

Current metallic stents can be expanded an average of 1.5 mm in diameter over their nominal size. Consequently, initial diameter selection can be extensively modified with postdilatation. This is not true for the first generation of BVS that generally should not be expanded 0.5 mm over their nominal value. Thus, appropriate diameter selection is particularly important with BVS. Diameter selection with OCT is dictated by the smallest reference vessel diameter, which is usually the distal reference. Depending on the "quality" (qualitative assessment) of the landing zone, different degrees of diameter oversizing can be applied. In "close to normal" vessels or concentric predominantly fibrotic lesions, we recommend 0.25–0.5 mm stent diameter

oversizing. When a stent/scaffold is oversized, it should be deployed at no more than the nominal pressure. While landing zones with eccentric calcified or lipid-rich plaque should usually be avoided, sometimes this is not possible due to the diffuse nature of CAD. In this setting, nominal 1:1 sizing is preferable in order to avoid edge dissections.[32] Stent length selection on OCT is determined mostly by volumetric assessment of the lumen area profile and adding a minimum of 3 mm to the total length. The quality of the landing zone may influence length selection. Avoiding landing in eccentric calcium or lipid-rich plaques may prevent edge dissection[32] and longitudinal geographic miss.[33] The very fast pullback acquisition obtained with OCT makes the method precise for length measurements, since it is less susceptible than IVUS to movement of the heart. Furthermore, the combination of fully automated volumetric lumen segmentation and features like angiographic co-registration facilitate stent length selection.

Stent optimization (post-stent implantation)

After adequate stent planning with OCT, poststent implantation imaging can determine the potential need for additional dilatation. There are a number of potential aspects to look for with OCT after stent implantation; the most important is stent expansion.

INCOMPLETE STRUT APPOSITION (STENT MALAPPOSITION)

Stent strut malapposition remains an important consideration. It is qualitatively defined as the lack of contact of stent struts with the vessel wall in nonbifurcated segments. The high-resolution nature of OCT reveals malapposition frequently. Incomplete strut apposition (ISA) is a morphological feature that is affected by multiple procedure-related elements and by stent-vessel interactions over time.[34] The nature of malapposition is an important concept. A 360° malapposed stent is always a consequence of stent and vessel size mismatch (Figure 29.11), while stent malapposition of a few degrees of arc or with a single strut is often the

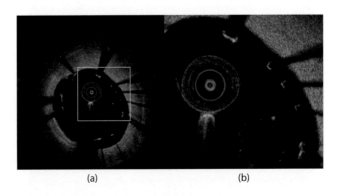

(a)   (b)

Figure 29.11 **(a)** Optical coherence tomographic image demonstrates malapposition of stent struts in all quadrants. **(b)** Magnification illustrates stent struts are not in contact with the vessel wall.

result of the inability of the stent to conform to irregularities in the lumen contour, which is typically calcium related (Figure 29.12).

Postulated causes for stent strut malapposition are various and include incomplete stent expansion, stent recoil or fracture, late outward vessel remodeling, and the dissolution of thrombus that was compressed during PCI between the stent strut and the vessel wall. Late-acquired malapposition is an epiphenomenon that results from tissue necrosis, inflammation (with positive remodeling), and thrombus dissolution; it has been reported frequently at sites of stent thrombosis.[35]

Regardless of the pathophysiological mechanism, there is a concern that strut malapposition might contribute to the prothrombotic vascular milieu. Although a clear cause-effect relationship with stent thrombosis is still unclear, the assumption is that the areas of strut malapposition cause nonlaminar and turbulent blood flow characteristics, which in turn trigger platelet activation and thrombosis. Adequate stent sizing, optimal techniques of implantation, and intravascular imaging guidance can effectively reduce the stent malapposition rate.[34]

Prospective, serial OCT observations immediately and at longer-term follow-up after stenting have improved our understanding of these complex mechanisms and shed light on the likely clinical significance of this phenomenon. Optical Coherence Tomography Following Paclitaxel Eluting Stent (PES) Implantation in Multivessel Coronary Artery Disease (OCTAXUS), a prospective OCT study on the completeness of strut coverage and vessel wall response after Taxus Liberte` stent implantation, evaluated vascular response to stent implantation by assessing the proportion of uncovered and/or malapposed struts at different time points after the implant. The study revealed the first 3 months after PES implantation to be the main period when the proliferative reaction takes place and malapposition resolves.[36]

STENT EXPANSION

Stent expansion is an important procedural variable that has been correlated with clinical outcomes. Different from malapposition, it should always be approached in a quantitative fashion. There are more similarities than differences between IVUS and OCT when assessing stent expansion. Both IVUS and OCT rely on lumen assessment quantification to optimize the expansion results. OCT has the advantage of automatically segmenting all frames and determining not only the reference vessel size but also the minimal lumen area (MLA) (Figure 29.10). Conversely, with IVUS, the operator should first qualitatively select the cross section in which the stent underexpansion is evident followed by measurements.

EDGE DISSECTIONS AND INTRAMURAL HEMATOMA

OCT has a very high sensitivity for edge dissections,[32] which is usually related to the presence of atherosclerosis at stent edges and to PCI technique. The vast majority of edge dissections observed by OCT (and usually not seen by angiogram) heal without clinical consequences; therefore, they do not need further intervention, such as bailout stenting.[32] Intramural hematoma, a variant of a dissection, is visible on OCT as an accumulation of flushing medium within the medial space (Figure 29.13). It requires further stenting to seal the dissection in order to avoid propagation of the hematoma with luminal compromise and vessel occlusion.[32]

TISSUE PROLAPSE

Tissue prolapse happens more often with lipid-rich plaque or in ACS with atherothrombotic material. Unfortunately,

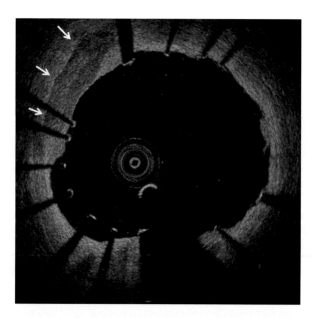

Figure 29.12 Malapposed stent struts in the left inferior quadrant. White arrows indicate calcium plaque distorting the lumen.

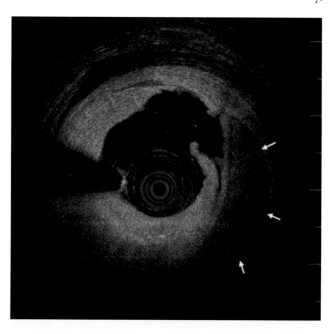

Figure 29.13 Flap dissection with intramural hematoma (*white arrows*).

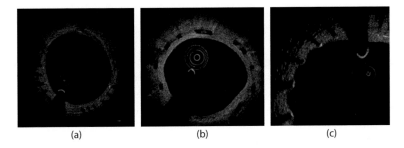

Figure 29.14 Stent coverage in different stent types: **(a)** metal stent, **(b)** absorb bioresorbable vascular scaffold (BVS) (Abbott Vascular, Santa Clara, CA), and **(c)** metal stent with well-apposed struts that protrude into the vessel's lumen.

there is no clear guidance on how to address this finding. Anecdotal data of prolonged nominal pressure balloon inflation for "stabilizing" the tissue have been reported.

Visualization and quantification of stent strut tissue coverage

OCT has been used extensively to assess neointimal hyperplasia and strut coverage with different types of stents and techniques (Figure 29.14) with or without adjunctive techniques, by providing various quantitative measurements (Figure 29.15).[37-41] Accuracy of quantitative measurements is better with OCT than with IVUS; both the completeness of individual strut coverage and the thickness of endothelial coverage can be assessed.[42] DES, designed to locally deliver antiproliferative agents to the vascular wall in a controlled manner,[43,44] reduce excessive neointimal tissue, restenosis, and repeat revascularization rates that are major limitations of bare-metal stents (BMS).[45] Many OCT studies were performed for the evaluation of strut coverage between different stent types (e.g., OCTDESI, OCTAMI)[46,47] or for single-arm studies with one stent type (e.g., the ongoing ABSORB III, ENDEAVOR).[48] Using the same stent type with assessment of coverage patterns between different target populations is also one of the strategies that provides useful information. Kubo et al.[49] evaluated long-term strut coverage of sirolimus-eluting stents (SES) for both stable angina and unstable angina populations and found that strut coverage was significantly delayed in the latter.

Assessment of stent failure

STENT THROMBOSIS

Late (i.e., between 1 month and 1 year after stent implantation) and very late (i.e., beyond 1 year) stent thrombosis (LST and VLST, respectively) is an infrequent (up to 0.6% per year) but potentially life-threatening complication that is poorly understood. It appears that this condition is multifactorial with risk factors including premature discontinuation of dual antiplatelet therapy (DAPT), neoatherosclerosis, stent under expansion, stent malapposition, and lack of endothelial tissue coverage all being implicated. The results

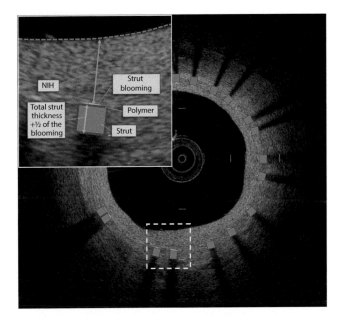

Figure 29.15 Example of stent details (morphology and metrics measurements). NIH, neointimal hyperplasia.

of small observational OCT studies are compatible with evidence from animal and human postmortem series showing that DES cause impairment in arterial healing, some with suggested incomplete re-endothelialization and persistence of fibrin, possibly triggering LST.[50,51] Pathological data in humans suggest that neointimal coverage of stent struts could be used as a surrogate marker of endothelialization due to the good correlation between strut coverage and endothelialization. OCT is the only imaging modality to date that offers the possibility to understand tissue coverage and neointima formation in DES over time.[52] Guagliumi et al. showed that the presence of uncovered stent struts as assessed by OCT and positive vessel remodeling by IVUS were associated with LST after DES.[35] Neoatherosclerosis rupture and stent malapposition were also identified as mechanisms of LST and VLST.[53,54] A recent study demonstrated that the leading associated findings in DES-VLST were stent malapposition, neoatherosclerosis, uncovered struts, and stent underexpansion with the longitudinal extension of malapposed stent being the most important correlate of thrombus formation.[55,56] Larger stent trials with

OCT performed at different time periods are needed to obtain a representative assessment of the true time course of endothelial coverage of these stents.

The Optical Coherence Tomography for Drug Eluting Stent Safety (ODESSA) study, on the other hand, investigated the number of uncovered and/or malapposed stent struts at overlapping versus nonoverlapping sites in DES versus BMS. The 6-month follow-up revealed higher rates of uncovered or malapposed stent struts with DES compared to BMS.[40]

IN-STENT RESTENOSIS

OCT is able to identify various patterns of in-stent restenosis tissue and can be very useful in the evaluation of the causes that contribute to restenosis after DES implantation.[57] Strut fracture (with subsequent defect of local drug delivery) has been associated with DES restenosis and can be detected with OCT.[58,59] A growing number of reports have demonstrated, using OCT in patients presenting with in-stent restenosis, the presence of in-stent neoatherosclerosis after stent implantation of both BMS and DES.[60,61]

Treating in-stent restenosis remains challenging. OCT may help in selecting the appropriate therapeutic modality (whether to use balloon angioplasty, cutting balloon, repeat stenting, or debulking techniques, such as laser and rotational atherectomy).[62]

Optical coherence tomography assessment of innovative stent designs and materials

Since OCT can precisely characterize *in vivo* stent apposition, strut coverage, tissue details (e.g., calcium plaques), (re)stenosis, thrombus, and stent details (morphology and metrics measurements) (Figure 29.16), it is becoming an integral tool to assess stent technologies, leading to a better understand of the mechanisms related to stent success

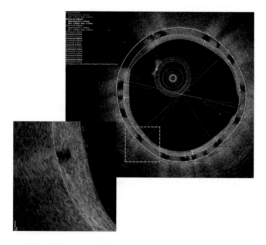

Figure 29.16 Representative frame depicts measurement and strut-level analysis. Strut-level analysis consists of a qualitative assessment for strut coverage and quantitative measurement from the surface of the blooming to the lumen contour.

or failure. Several trials designed to evaluate a "new generation" of bioabsorbable coronary stents (e.g., the ongoing ABSORB III study) are using OCT image technology. In an era when DES safety is the current challenge of interventional cardiology, the "strut-level analysis," with accurate assessment and quantification of neointimal coverage of stents (Figure 29.16), has been adopted as a surrogate endpoint in numerous clinical trials of DES and as an important parameter for the approval of new DES technologies by regulatory agencies.

Optical coherence tomography safety

OCT is a safe method that can be used on a daily basis in a heterogeneous population.[63] The applied energies in intravascular OCT are low and are not considered to cause functional or structural damage to the tissue. Several studies[64–67] have evaluated the safety and feasibility of OCT in the clinical setting and reported rare complications, the most frequent being the presence of transient events, such as chest discomfort, brady- or tachycardia, and ST-T wave changes on the electrocardiogram, all of which resolved immediately after the procedure.[63,64] There were no major complications, including MI, emergency revascularization, or death.

LIMITATIONS

OCT is considered a safe clinical tool. However, some considerations arise from the fact that OCT requires a blood-free environment. Consequently, caution should be exercised when performing OCT in patients with severely impaired left ventricular function or with severe hemodynamic compromise, as the image acquisition can induce brief ischemia. In patients with impaired renal function, operators should be attentive to the possibility of contrast-induced nephrotoxicity, a consequence inherent to the method. OCT should be performed with caution in patients with a single remaining coronary vessel, since guidewire or catheter insertion carries a small risk of dissection or arterial spasm. A technical drawback is that plaques located at the very ostium of the left or right coronaries cannot be addressed by OCT because of lack of blood clearance.[68]

Artifacts

Some OCT artifacts are common to both OCT and IVUS, and others are unique to OCT imaging systems. Most of these artifacts will not substantially compromise clinical interpretation of the image, if restricted to a few noncontinuous frames (Figure 29.17).

RESIDUAL BLOOD

Blood attenuates the OCT light beam and may defocus the beam if red cell density is high. This will reduce brightness of the vessel wall, especially at large radial distances

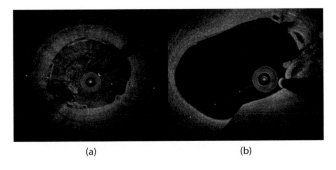

Figure 29.17 Most frequently observed artifacts: **(a)** incomplete blood displacement, resulting in light attenuation; and **(b)** sew-up artifact—the result of rapid wire or vessel movement along one frame formation, resulting in misalignment of the image.

from the imaging wire. If the lumen surface is still clearly defined, the presence of diluted blood does not appear to affect area measurements.

POOR CALIBRATION

A small change in the ideal calibration (e.g., 1%) can result in a much larger error (e.g., 12%–14%) in area measurements. Small changes in magnitude can also amplify contour distortion, which may result in misinterpretation of the image.

NONUNIFORM ROTATIONAL DISTORTION

Nonuniform rotational distortion is the result of variation in the rotational speed of the spinning optical fiber. It is usually produced by vessel tortuosity or by an imperfection in the torque wire or sheath that interferes with smooth rotation of the optical fiber, which can result in focal image loss or shape distortion.

SEW-UP ARTIFACT

This is the result of rapid artery or imaging wire movement in one frame's imaging formation, leading to single point misalignment of the lumen border.

SATURATION ARTIFACT

Artifact saturation occurs when light reflected from a highly specular surface (usually stent struts) produces signals with amplitudes that exceed the dynamic range of the data acquisition system. This should be kept in mind when defining the stent surface.

FOLD-OVER ARTIFACT

Fold-over artifact is the consequence of the "phase wrapping" or "alias" along the Fourier transformation when structure signals are reflected from outside the system's field of view. Typical examples are side-branch and large vessels.

CONCLUSIONS

OCT is a safe and versatile imaging technique that enables comprehensive evaluation of clinical and research parameters, leading to a better understanding of vessels, stents, and their underlying interactions. In daily practice at a catheterization laboratory, it may improve preprocedure and poststent implantation assessments, ultimately facilitating and customizing the decision-making process. In a research center, OCT is able to provide reliable qualitative and quantitative information regarding stent-vessel interactions, as consistently shown in clinical trials.

REFERENCES

1. Huang D, et al. Optical coherence tomography. *Science* 1991;254(5035):1178–1181.
2. Maehara A, et al. Comparison of stent expansion guided by optical coherence tomography versus intravascular ultrasound. The ILUMIEN II Study (Observational Study of Optical Coherence Tomography [OCT] in Patients Undergoing Fractional Flow Reserve [FFR] and Percutaneous Coronary Intervention), *JACC Cardiovasc Interv* 2015;8(13):1704–1714.
3. Ellis S, et al. Everolimus-eluting bioresorbable scaffolds for coronary artery disease. *N Engl J Med* 2015;373(20):1905–1915.
4. Garrone P, et al. Quantitative coronary angiography in the current era: Principles and applications. *J Interv Cardiol* 2009;22(6):527–536.
5. Ferrante G, et al. Current applications of optical coherence tomography for coronary intervention. *Int J Cardiol* 2013;165(1):7–16.
6. Lopez JJ, et al. Techniques and best practices for optical coherence tomography: A practical manual for interventional cardiologists. *Catheter Cardiovasc Interv* 2014;84(5):687–699.
7. Stefano G, et al. Unrestricted utilization of frequency domain optical coherence tomography in coronary interventions. *Int J Cardiovasc Imaging* 2012;29(4):741–752.
8. Refaat H, et al. Optical coherence tomography features of angiographic complex and smooth lesions in acute coronary syndromes. *Int J Cardiovasc Imaging* 2015;31(5):927–934.
9. Jang IK, et al. Visualization of coronary atherosclerotic plaques in patients using optical coherence tomography: Comparison with intravascular ultrasound. *J Am Coll Cardiol* 2002;39(4):604–609.
10. Yabushita H, et al. Characterization of human atherosclerosis by optical coherence tomography. *Circulation* 2002;106(13):1640–1645.
11. Rieber J, et al. Diagnostic accuracy of optical coherence tomography and intravascular ultrasound for the detection and characterization of atherosclerotic plaque com-position in ex-vivo coronary specimens: A comparison with histology. *Coron Artery Dis* 2006;17(5):425–430.
12. Patwari P, et al. Assessment of coronary plaque with optical coherence tomography and high-frequency ultrasound. *Am J Cardiol* 2000;85(5):641–644.
13. Kawasaki M, et al. Diagnostic accuracy of optical coherence tomography and integrated backscatter intravascular ultrasound images for tissue characterization of human coronary plaques. *J Am Coll Cardiol* 2006;48(1):81–88.
14. Kume T, et al. Assessment of coronary arterial plaque by optical coherence tomography. *Am J Cardiol* 2006;97(8):1172–1175.

15. Jang IK, et al. In vivo characterization of coronary atherosclerotic plaque by use of optical coherence tomography. *Circulation* 2005;111(12):1551–1555.

16. Chia S, et al. Comparison of coronary plaque characteristics between diabetic and non-diabetic subjects: An in vivo optical coherence tomography study. *Diabetes Res Clin Pract* 2008;81(2):155–160.

17. Guagliumi G, et al. Mechanisms of atherothrombosis and vascular response to primary percutaneous coronary intervention in women versus men with acute myocardial infarction: Results of the OCTAVIA study. *JACC Cardiovasc Interv* 2014;7(9):958–968.

18. Mehanna E, et al. Volumetric characterization of human coronary calcification by frequency-domain optical coherence tomography. *Circ J* 2013;77(9):2334–2340.

19. Jones M, et al. Intravascular frequency-domain optical coherence tomography assessment of carotid artery disease in symptomatic and asymptomatic patients. *JACC Cardiovasc Interv* 2014;7(6):674–684.

20. Tearney GJ, et al. Quantification of macrophage content in atherosclerotic plaques by optical coherence tomography. *Circulation* 2003;107(1):113–119.

21. MacNeill BD, et al. Focal and multi-focal plaque macrophage distributions in patients with acute and stable presentations of coronary artery disease. *J Am Coll Cardiol* 2004;44(5):972–979.

22. Raffel OC, et al. Relationship between a systemic inflammatory marker, plaque inflammation, and plaque characteristics determined by intravascular optical coherence tomography. *Arterioscler Thromb Vasc Biol* 2007;27(8):1820–1827.

23. Tahara S, et al. Intravascular optical coherence tomography detection of atherosclerosis and inflammation in murine aorta. *Arterioscler Thromb Vasc Biol* 2012;32(5):1150–1157.

24. Kume T, et al. Measurement of the thickness of the fibrous cap by optical coherence tomography. *Am Heart J* 2006;152(4):755.e1–e4.

25. Cilingiroglu M, et al. Detection of vulnerable plaque in a murine model of atherosclerosis with optical coherence tomography. *Catheter Cardiovasc Interv* 2006;67(6):915–923.

26. Wang Z, et al. Volumetric quantification of fibrous caps using intravascular optical coherence tomography. *Biomed Opt Express* 2012;3(6):1413–1426.

27. Bezerra HG, et al. Three-dimensional imaging of fibrous cap by frequency-domain optical coherence tomography. *Catheter Cardiovasc Interv* 2013;81(3):547–549.

28. Kubo T, et al. Assessment of culprit lesion morphology in acute myocardial infarction. *Journal of the American College of Cardiology* 2007;50(10):933–939.

29. Takano M, et al. In vivo comparison of optical coherence tomography and angioscopy for the evaluation of coronary plaque characteristics. *Am J Cardiol* 2008;101(4):471–476.

30. Kubo T, et al. Implication of plaque color classification for assessing plaque vulnerability. *JACC Cardiovasc Interv* 2008;1(1):74–80.

31. Mintz G. Intravascular imaging of coronary calcification and its clinical implications. *JACC Cardiovasc Imaging* 2015;8(4):461–471.

32. Chamié D, et al. Incidence, predictors, morphological characteristics, and clinical outcomes of stent edge dissections detected by optical coherence tomography. *JACC Cardiovasc Interv* 2013;6(8):800–813.

33. Costa MA, et al. Impact of stent deployment procedural factors on long-term effectiveness and safety of sirolimus-eluting stents (final results of the multicenter prospective STLLR trial). *Am J Cardiol* 2008;101(12):1704–1711.

34. Attizzani GF, et al. Mechanisms, pathophysiology, and clinical aspects of incomplete stent apposition. *J Am Coll Cardiol* 2014;63(14):1355–1367.

35. Guagliumi G, et al. Examination of the in vivo mechanisms of late drug-eluting stent thrombosis. *JACC Cardiovasc Interv* 2012;5(1):12–20.

36. Guagliumi G, et al. Serial assessment of coronary artery response to paclitaxel-eluting stents using optical coherence tomography. *Circ Cardiovasc Interv* 2012;5(1):30–38.

37. Toušek P, et al. Neointimal coverage and late apposition of everolimus-eluting bioresorbable scaffolds implanted in the acute phase of myocardial infarction: OCT data from the PRAGUE-19 study. *Heart Vessels* 2015; 31(6):841-84.

38. Picchi A, et al. Comparison of strut coverage at 6 months by optical coherence tomography with everolimus-eluting stenting of bare-metal stent restenosis versus stenosis of nonstented atherosclerotic narrowing (from the DESERT Study). *Am J Cardiol* 2015;115(10):1351–1356.

39. Kume T, et al. Assessment of coronary intima—media thickness by optical coherence tomography. *Circ J* 2005;69(8):903–907.

40. Guagliumi G, et al. Optical coherence tomography assessment of in vivo vascular response after implantation of overlapping bare-metal and drug-eluting stents. *JACC Cardiovasc Interv* 2010;3(5):531–539.

41. Girassolli A, et al. Utility of optical coherence tomography and intravascular ultrasound for the evaluation of coronary lesions. *Rev Port Cardiol* 2013;32(11):925–929.

42. Gonzalo N, et al. Reproducibility of quantitative optical coherence tomography for stent analysis. *EuroIntervention* 2009;5(2):224–232.

43. Morice MC, et al. A randomized comparison of a sirolimus-eluting stent with a standard stent for coronary revascularization. *N Engl J Med* 2002;346(23):1773–1780.

44. Stone GW, et al. A polymer based, paclitaxel-eluting stent in patients with coronary artery disease. *N Engl J Med* 2004;350(3):221–223.

45. Sousa JE, et al. Sirolimus eluting stent for the treatment of in-stent restenosis: A quantitative angiography and three-dimensional intravascular ultrasound study. *Circulation* 2003;107(1):24–27.

46. Guagliumi G, et al. Strut coverage and vessel wall response to a new-generation paclitaxel-eluting stent with an ultrathin biodegradable abluminal polymer: Optical coherence tomography drug-eluting stent investigation (OCTDESI). *Circulation Cardiovasc Interv* 2010;3(4):367–375.

47. Guagliumi G, et al. Strut coverage and vessel wall response to zotarolimus-eluting and bare-metal stents implanted in patients with ST-segment elevation myocardial infarction. *JACC Cardiovascular Interventions* 2010;3(6):680–687.

48. Kim J, et al. Evaluation in 3 months duration of neointimal coverage after zotarolimus-eluting stent implantation by optical coherence tomography. *JACC Cardiovasc Interv* 2009;2(12):1240–1247.

49. Kubo T, et al. Comparison of vascular response after sirolimus-eluting stent implantation between patients with unstable and stable angina pectoris: A serial optical coherence tomography study. *JACC Cardiovasc Imaging* 2008;1(4):475–484.

50. Finn AV, et al. Pathological correlates of late drug-eluting stent thrombosis: Strut coverage as a marker of endothelialization. *Circulation* 2007;115(18):2435–2441.

51. Finn AV, et al. Vascular responses to drug eluting stents: Importance of delayed healing. *Arterioscler Thromb Vasc Biol* 2007;27(7):1500–1510.

52. Barlis P, et al Novelties in cardiac imaging—optical coherence tomography (OCT). *EuroIntervention* 2008;4 Suppl C:C22–C26.

53. Higo T, et al. atherosclerotic and thrombogenic neointima formed over sirolimus drug-eluting stent. *JACC Cardiovasc Imaging* 2009;2(5):616–624.

54. Cook S, et al. incomplete stent apposition and very late stent thrombosis after drug-eluting stent implantation. *Circulation* 2007;115(18):2426–2434.

55. Souteyrand G, et al. Mechanisms of stent thrombosis analysed by optical coherence tomography: Insights from the national PESTO French registry. *Eur Heart J* 2016;37(15):1208–1216.

56. Taniwaki M, et al. Mechanisms of very late drug-eluting stent thrombosis assessed by optical coherence tomography. *Circulation* 2016;133(7):650–660.

57. Gonzalo N, et al. In vivo assessment of high-risk coronary plaques at bifurcations with combined intravascular ultrasound and optical coherence tomography. *JACC Cardiovasc Imaging* 2009;2(4):473–482.

58. Okamura T, Matsuzaki M. Sirolimus-eluting stent fracture detection by three-dimensional optical coherence tomography. *Catheter Cardiovasc Interv* 2011;79(4):628–632.

59. Shite J, et al. Sirolimus-eluting stent fracture with thrombus, visualization by optical coherence tomography. *Eur Heart J* 2006;27(12):1389.

60. Kang S, et al. Optical coherence tomographic analysis of in-stent neoatherosclerosis after drug-eluting stent implantation. *Circulation* 2011;123(25):2954–2963.

61. Habara M, et al. Difference of tissue characteristics between early and very late restenosis lesions after bare-metal stent implantation: An optical coherence tomography study. *Circ Cardiovasc Interv* 2011;4(3):232–238.

62. Alfonso F, et al. Current treatment of in-stent restenosis. *J Am Coll Cardiol* 2014;63(24):2659–2673.

63. van der Sijde J, et al. Safety of optical coherence tomography in daily practice: A comparison with intravascular ultrasound. *Eur Heart J Cardiovasc Imaging* 2016;pii:jew037.

64. Lehtinen T, et al. Feasibility and safety of frequency-domain optical coherence tomography for coronary artery evaluation: A single-center study. *Int J Cardiovasc Imaging* 2013;29(5):997–1005.

65. Setacci C, et al. Safety and feasibility of intravascular optical coherence tomography using a non-occlusive technique to evaluate carotid plaques before and after stent deployment. *J Endovasc Ther* 2012;19(3):303–311.

66. Yoon J, et al. Feasibility and safety of the second-generation, frequency domain optical coherence tomography (FD-OCT): A multi-center study. *J Invasive Cardiol* 201224(5):206–209.

67. Imola F, et al. Safety and feasibility of frequency domain optical coherence tomography to guide decision making in percutaneous coronary intervention. *EuroIntervention* 2010;6(5):575–581.

68. Fujino Y, et al. Frequency-domain optical coherence tomography assessment of unprotected left main coronary artery disease-a comparison with intravascular ultrasound. *Catheter Cardiovasc Interv* 2013;82(3):E173–E183.

PART 7

Interventional Cardiology

30

Percutaneous coronary intervention: General principles

JACK P. CHEN AND SPENCER B. KING

INTRODUCTION

Percutaneous coronary intervention (PCI) was made possible by the pioneering work of Andreas Gruentzig, who in 1977 performed the first angioplasty procedure. Gruentzig's first patient is still doing well almost 40 years later. Ongoing innovations in procedural techniques, interventional devices, and pharmacology continue to expand the indications and treatment options for PCI. In addition, advances in the management of thrombotic complications, vascular recoil, acute vessel closure, and restenosis have been dramatic. More than two million PCI procedures are performed annually, and PCI has significantly eclipsed coronary artery bypass surgery (CABG) as the leading revascularization method for coronary artery disease (CAD).

INDICATIONS FOR PERCUTANEOUS CORONARY INTERVENTION

In general, elective PCI may be indicated in patients with stable angina or ischemic stress tests, and suitable coronary anatomy. Primary PCI, when performed promptly, improves outcomes compared with fibrinolytic therapy in patients with ST-segment elevation myocardial infarction (STEMI). In non-ST elevation acute coronary syndromes (NSTE-ACS), an invasive approach is recommended by the American College of Cardiology (ACC)/American Heart Association (AHA) guidelines in patients with high-risk features (Figure 30.1).[1]

The Thrombolysis in Myocardial Infarction (TIMI) risk score is a prognostication tool for NSTE-ACS patients (Table 30.1).[2] Similarly, the Global Registry of Acute Coronary Events (GRACE) risk score includes eight variables: advanced age, Killip class, systolic blood pressure, ST-segment deviation, cardiac arrest during presentation, serum creatinine level, elevated cardiac markers, and heart rate.[3] A meta-analysis reported an 18% relative reduction in the combined endpoint of death or myocardial infarction (MI) in high-risk NSTE-ACS patients initially treated with an invasive compared with a medical strategy, despite a slight increase in early in-hospital mortality.[4] Not all studies have confirmed these findings, however. The Invasive versus Conservative Treatment in Unstable coronary Syndromes (ICTUS)[5] study randomized 1,200 NSTE-ACS patients to invasive versus medical therapy and found no difference in the composite endpoint at 1 year. Nonetheless, the majority of large randomized trials, including Fragmin and Fast Revascularisation during InStability in Coronary artery disease (FRISC)[6] and Treat Angina with Aggrastat and Determine Cost of Therapy with an Invasive or Conservative Strategy (TACTICS-TIMI 18),[7] support the invasive approach for this high-risk patient cohort.

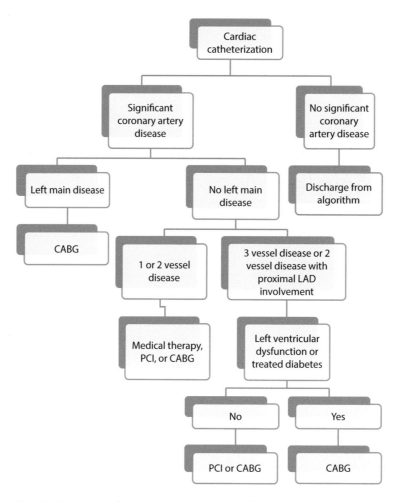

Figure 30.1 Proposed algorithm for invasive and conservative treatment of patients presenting with acute coronary syndromes. CABG, coronary artery bypass grafting; LAD, left anterior descending; PCI, percutaneous coronary intervention.

Table 30.1 Thrombolysis in myocardial infarction (TIMI) risk score for acute coronary syndrome (ACS)

TIMI risk variables

Age 65 or greater

Three or more CAD risk factors

Known coronary stenosis(es) of 50% or greater on previous angiography

ST-segment deviation ≥ 0.05 mV on initial ECG

At least 2 anginal episodes in prior 24 h

ASA use in prior 7 days

Elevated cardiac markers

Note: ASA, acetylsalicylic acid; CAD, coronary artery disease; ECG, electrocardiogram.

The ACC, the AHA, and the Society for Cardiovascular Angiography and Interventions (SCAI) have developed indications for PCI using evidence-based literature and expert consensus.[8] These guidelines have emphasized the importance of optimal medical therapy (OMT) before and after PCI. OMT consists of risk factor control, anti-ischemic therapy, antiplatelet therapy, and lifestyle modification. Additionally, the appropriate use criteria (AUC) aim "to improve patient care and health outcomes in a cost-effective manner while recognizing that some ambiguity and nuance is intrinsic to clinical decision-making."[9]

For patients with stable angina pectoris, PCI has not been shown to improve survival and should be reserved for unacceptable symptoms on OMT or significant ischemia on functional testing. Determination of risk on noninvasive functional testing is based on predicted annual mortality (Table 30.2).[10] Patients presenting with acute coronary syndrome (ACS) experience greater short-term morbidity and mortality. These patients are usually appropriate candidates for PCI.

LESION CLASSIFICATION

The ACC/AHA lesion classification scheme has been used to predict the success rate and risk of PCI for specific anatomic subsets (Table 30.3).[11] It incorporates angiographic characteristics including angulation (both proximal to and at the lesion site), location, existence and importance of side branches, length, calcification, and presence of chronic total occlusion (CTO). Type B lesions are further subcategorized as B1 or B2 if one or more than one B characteristic is present. Major technical and device advances during the ensuing years have greatly improved

Table 30.2 Risk stratification in non-invasive testing

High Risk (greater than 3% annual mortality rate)

1. Severe resting left ventricular dysfunction (LVEF less than 35%)
2. High-risk treadmill score (score less than or equal to 11)
3. Severe exercise left ventricular dysfunction (exercise LVEF less than 35%)
4. Stress-induced large perfusion defect (particularly if anterior)
5. Stress-induced multiple perfusion defects of moderate size
6. Large, fixed perfusion defect with LV dilation or increased lung uptake (thallium-201)
7. Stress-induced moderate perfusion defect with LV dilation or increased lung uptake (thallium-201)
8. Echocardiographic wall motion abnormality (involving greater than two segments) developing at low dose of dobutamine (less than or equal to 10 mg/kg/min) or at a low heart rate (less than 120 beats/min)
9. Stress echocardiographic evidence of extensive ischemia

Intermediate Risk (1% to 3% annual mortality rate)

1. Mild/moderate resting left ventricular dysfunction (LVEF equal to 35% to 49%)
2. Intermediate-risk treadmill score (−11 to <5)
3. Stress-induced moderate perfusion defect without LV dilation or increased lung intake (thallium-201)
4. Limited stress echocardiographic ischemia with a wall motion abnormality only at higher doses of dobutamine involving less than or equal to two segments

Low Risk (less than 1% annual mortality rate)

1. Low-risk treadmill score (score greater than or equal to 5)
2. Normal or small myocardial perfusion defect at rest or with stress
3. Normal stress echocardiographic wall motion or no change of limited resting wall motion abnormalities during stress.

Source: Modified from Patel, M.R., et al., *Cathet. Cardiovasc. Interv.*, 80(3), E50–E81, 2012.
Note: LV, left ventricle; LVEF, left ventricular ejection fraction.

Table 30.3 ACC/AHA lesion classifications

Type A: (High Success Rate > 85%; Low Risk)

Discrete (<10 mm in length)
Concentric
Easily accessible
Relatively straight (<45°)
Smooth contour
Minimal to no calcification
Non-occluded
Non-ostial in location
No major branch involvement
No thrombus

Type B (Moderate Success Rate = 60% to 85%; Moderate Risk)

Tubular (10–20 mm in length)
Eccentric
Moderate tortuosity of proximal segment
Moderate lesion angulation (45–90°)
Irregular contour
Moderate to heavy calcification
Ostial in location
Bifurcation location, necessitating double wires
Thrombus present
Total occlusion (<3 months)

(Continued)

Table 30.3 (Continued) ACC/AHA lesion classifications

Type C (Low Success Rate < 60%; High Risk)

Diffuse (>20 mm in length)
Severe tortuosity of proximal segment
Extreme lesion angulation (>90°)
Inability to protect major side-branch
Degenerated vein grafts, with friable lesions
Chronic total occlusion (>3 months)

Source: Krone, R.J., et al., *Am. J. Cardiol.*, 92(4), 389–394, 2003. With permission.
Note: ACC, American College of Cardiology; AHA, American Heart Association.

the success rate and safety for PCI and thus reduced the predictive accuracy of this classification system. One of the most predictive lesion features for PCI success is coronary patency.[12] Specifically, the success rate of a patent class B lesion was similar to that of any class A lesion; and the success rate of a patent class C lesion surpassed that of an occluded class B lesion. A simplified, updated system has thus been proposed (Table 30.4)[11,12] and has demonstrated enhanced predictive accuracy. Nevertheless, it is clearly recognized that no anatomic classification scheme can comprehensively assess the complexity of a specific lesion; indeed, the success and risk of any PCI is further dependent upon the patient's clinical status, the operator's expertise, as well as pharmacologic and device selections.

Table 30.4 New lesion classification

	Patent	Occluded
Non-C	Patent, non-C	Occluded, non-C
C	Patent, C	Occluded, C

EQUIPMENT

Guiding catheters

There is continued technological innovation to "down-size" interventional devices. Most contemporary PCI procedures, including final kissing balloon inflation (FKBI) and small burr rotational atherectomy (RA), can be performed with 5- or 6-Fr guiding catheters. On rare occasions, more complex techniques, such as simultaneous kissing stents (SKSs) or large burr RA, may require 7-Fr catheters; while 8-Fr catheters are essentially unnecessary. While seemingly simplistic in design when compared with other PCI equipment, the guiding catheter may be the most important determinant of procedural success. Stable guiding catheter backup support is crucial to ensure delivery of the interventional device to the lesion, especially in the presence of inhospitable anatomy such as severe calcification or tortuosity.

In general, it is preferred to select the smallest diameter (French size) and least aggressive guiding catheter shape necessary for the specific coronary anatomy. Conservative, atraumatic tip conformations, such as Judkins right and left curves, are generally selected for low-complexity cases. Gentle, shallow ostial engagement minimizes potential vessel trauma and risk of catheter-induced dissection. When faced with more challenging anatomy, enhanced backup support is required. The moderate support designs are commonly known as the "extra backup" group, while even deeper engagement can be achieved with the Amplatz catheters. Meticulous manipulation is required to avoid ostial left main or right coronary dissection, which not infrequently leads to distal spiraling dissection propagation. At the conclusion of the procedure, disengagement of Amplatz catheters should be performed under fluoroscopic observation and may require a slight forward push with rotation, as direct withdrawal may actually result in deep, forceful distal advancement.

At times, more backup support becomes necessary as the procedure progresses. Extension catheters are soft, atraumatic catheters inserted through the guiding catheters to provide enhanced backup support through which devices such as stents can be delivered. These "child-in-mother" catheters can be placed distally into the coronary and should be advanced over a balloon shaft to minimize vessel trauma and dissection. Additionally, distal balloon inflation, the "anchor balloon" technique, provides an enhanced rail to deliver the extension catheter further into difficult anatomy (Figure 30.2).

GUIDEWIRES

Structurally, guidewires are divided into spring-tip and plastic varieties. The former can either be constructed entirely from stainless steel or feature a nitinol tip. The spring-tip

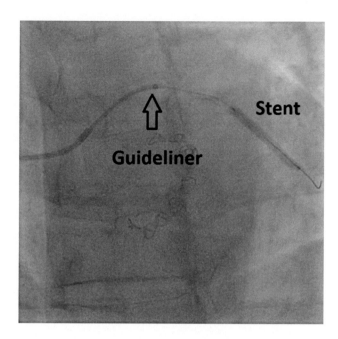

Figure 30.2 "Child-in-mother" catheter extension deployed with "anchor balloon" technique.

wires offer excellent steerability by enhanced torque transmission and are particularly useful in complex lesions such as CTOs. Plastic wires are hydrophilically coated and offer the advantage of reduced friction, facilitating advancement through tortuous or calcified anatomies. However, this same lubricious coating also promotes wire entry into false channels.[13] Short and long guidewires are designed for use with rapid-exchange and over-the-wire devices, respectively. (These systems are discussed in the section entitled Balloon Dilatation Catheters.)

Varying tip stiffness allows for penetration into hard lesion caps frequently associated with CTOs. Additionally, tapered tips may further improve penetration. Extreme caution must be exercised with these specialty wires, as vessel dissection or perforation can result.[13] Supportive shaft wires are used to straighten tortuous vessels to allow passage of higher-profile devices such as atherotomes or stents. Not infrequently, however, "pseudo-lesions" may result from vessel pleating and may be difficult to angiographically discern from iatrogenic vessel trauma. If intracoronary nitroglycerin fails to resolve this finding, an over-the-wire catheter can be exchanged for a stiff wire. This maneuver will resolve the pleating artifact, while maintaining distal access should further work be necessary.

BALLOON DILATATION CATHETERS

The original PCI device introduced by Gruentzig in 1977, the balloon catheter, remains the workhorse for today's interventionalist. In the modern era, balloons are predominately used for pre- and postdilatation of stents.

Compliant balloons, made of soft materials such as polyolefin copolymer which allow varying diametric expansion without exerting excessive pressure, are useful for predilatation to prepare the intended lesion for stent deployment.

Occasionally, small-caliber branches may be inappropriate for stent implantation and can be adequately treated with plain old balloon angioplasty (POBA). Noncompliant balloons, fashioned from stiff materials such as polyethylene terephthalate, maintain a near-constant diameter in the face of increasing inflation pressures, making them ideal devices for stent postdilatation to ensure full expansion. Additionally, noncompliant balloons can be used to expand hard, calcific, or fibro-calcific plaques. Semi-compliant balloons display hybrid features of both the compliant and noncompliant counterparts.[12] When inflated to the nominal pressure, the balloon achieves its prespecified diameter.

The monorail or rapid-exchange shaft design features a short wire lumen, with the wire exit opening near the distal tip. This system allows use of a short guidewire, often preferred by operators for simpler cases. Alternatively, the wire lumen for the over-the-wire balloon catheter runs the entire shaft length. While the required long guidewire may be more tedious, this system permits catheter exchange, as well as distal intracoronary drug administration through the central lumen.

PERFUSION BALLOON

Although perfusion balloons were initially developed to reduce ischemia during prolonged balloon inflations during the present era, they are now largely relegated to sealing vessel perforations. Proximal inflow and distal outflow lumens allow distal perfusion during protracted inflation of the rupture site. These devices are rarely used in contemporary practice.

THROMBECTOMY DEVICES

PCI of friable thrombotic and/or atherosclerotic lesions can result in plaque fragmentation and distal embolization. This can lead to diminished or absent distal perfusion known as "slow-flow" or "no-reflow." The perfusion adequacy of the distal vasculature and subtended myocardium are measured by the TIMI flow and myocardial blush scores, respectively. The clinical impact of pretreatment with certain aspiration devices to decrease the incidence of slow- and no-reflow remains controversial.

A mechanical thrombectomy catheter, the AngioJet (Possis Medical Corporation, Minneapolis, MN), utilizes an Archimedes screw mechanism to create a proximally directed high-pressure jet that generates a vacuum rheolytic action. The captured debris is then removed through the system. The catheter is advanced distal to the thrombus and withdrawn at a rate of 0.5 mm/s. Not infrequently, there is concomitant bradycardia (especially in the right coronary artery) and transient ST-segment elevation. Prophylactic temporary right ventricular pacemaker placement has been recommended; intravenous (IV) aminophylline infusion has been shown to prevent heart rate disturbances.[13]

Manual aspiration catheters are rapid-exchange catheters with a second central aspiration lumen attached to a syringe at the proximal end. Gentle manual aspiration is performed by the assistant while the distal tip traverses and is advanced beyond the stenosis. The attraction of these devices is ease of setup and use, as well as lack of associated bradyarrhythmias. However, their efficacy with large thrombus burden or late patient presentation remains unclear.[14,15] Recent disappointing trial results have failed to demonstrate a survival benefit and raised concern regarding increased stroke risk.[16] While routine use is discouraged, selective utilization of aspiration thrombectomy may be considered.

DISTAL PROTECTION DEVICES

Distal protection devices, including occlusion balloons or filters, trap and retrieve atheroemboli distal to the lesion. The GuardWire system (Medtronic Corporation, Minneapolis, MN) incorporates a wire-based distal occlusion balloon in combination with the Export aspiration catheter. The Saphenous Vein Graft Angioplasty Free of Emboli Randomized (SAFER) trial[17] randomized 801 patients with saphenous vein graft (SVG) disease to stent deployment with and without concomitant GuardWire protection. The investigators reported a 42% relative reduction in major adverse cardiac events (MACE) for the treatment arm; this benefit was mainly due to reductions in MI (8.6% vs. 14.7%, $P = 0.008$) and "no-reflow" (3% vs. 9%, $P = 0.02$).

Technically simpler to deploy, filter devices preserve perfusion during deployment, so their use is not limited by ischemic time. However, they do not trap small debris and nonparticulate vasoconstrictive compounds. The FilterWire EX distal filtration device (Boston Scientific, Natick, MA) is a guidewire that terminates in a loop net with 110 micron pores. The FilterWire EX Randomized Evaluation (FIRE) trial[18] demonstrated noninferiority of this device to the GuardWire during PCI in SVGs.

ATHERECTOMY DEVICES

Atherectomy or atheroablative devices are applicable in specific anatomic subsets such as calcified or thrombotic lesions, either as stand-alone therapy or, more commonly, as pretreatment to facilitate stent deployment. Although quite varied in mechanism and design, these tools may share a slightly higher risk of coronary perforation, compared with balloon angioplasty. Additionally, while a few trials have reported modest restenotic advantages, no atherectomy device has clearly demonstrated superior clinical outcomes compared with balloon angioplasty.[19]

ROTATIONAL ATHERECTOMY

The rotational atherectomy (Boston Scientific, Natick, MA, Figure 30.3) system consists of a rapidly rotating oval-shaped burr encrusted with tiny diamond chips. The mechanistic principle is that of differential cutting, whereby hard plaque is selectively ablated while the deflected soft vascular wall is left unharmed. The burr is welded on a drive shaft that is advanced over a proprietary 0.09-in guidewire. The recommended burr-to-artery ratio is 0.7. Through gentle pecking motions of 0.5 mm or less, the operator manipulates the burr with the advancer console at a typical rotational speed of approximately 140,000 rotations per minute (rpm).

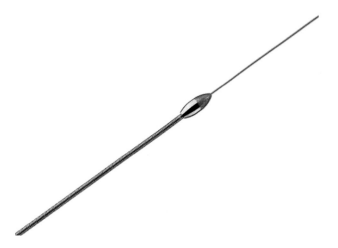

Figure 30.3 Rotational atherectomy burr. (Reprinted with permission from Boston Scientific Corporation.)

When encountering decelerations of greater than 5,000 rpm indicating extreme lesion resistance, operation should be paused. Further burring in this scenario may result in vascular trauma from dissection, excessive heat buildup, or embolization.[19]

Wire bias refers to the phenomenon whereby greater cutting force is exerted upon the inner curvature of a tortuous vessel. While this occurrence may be advantageous for eccentric lesions in this location, it can lead to excessive vessel trauma. Significant bradycardia may result from microembolization; hence, prophylactic temporary pacemaker placement is recommended, especially for right coronary interventions.

The Study to Determine Rotablator and Transluminal Angioplasty Strategy (STRATAS)[20] evaluated aggressive versus conservative rotational atherectomy strategies using burr-to-artery ratios of 0.7–0.9 versus 0.7, respectively. While overall success rates were similar, the aggressive arm demonstrated significantly higher restenotic (58% vs. 52%) and MI rates (11% vs. 7%). In the Angioplasty versus Rotational Atherectomy for Treatment of Diffuse In-stent Restenosis Trial (ARTIST),[21] the investigators compared rotational atherectomy with balloon angioplasty for treatment of in-stent restenosis (ISR) in 298 patients. Surprisingly, in-hospital complication and restenosis rates were higher with rotational atherectomy, and the 6-month event-free survival was lower (79.6% vs. 91.1%). Nonetheless, rotational ablation of calcific, resistant lesions remains a valuable tool in some complex cases.

The recently approved orbital atherectomy device (Diamondback 360°, CSI Systems, St. Paul, MN) is likewise indicated for debulking of calcified lesions. The centrifugal rotation action of the diamond-coated crown is useful in modification of calcified lesions prior to stent implantation. In the ORBIT I and ORBIT II trials, coronary orbital atherectomy was shown to facilitate stent delivery in this lesion subset and improved both acute and 30-day clinical outcomes, compared with historic controls.[22,23] The ongoing COAST trial will assess the efficacy of this device in lesions with intravascular ultrasound (IVUS) or optical coherence tomography (OCT) confirmed severe calcification.[24]

DIRECTIONAL ATHERECTOMY

Since its inception, versions of directional atherectomy devices have progressed through several iterations. The excised plaque debris is pushed into a distal nose-cone and subsequently retrieved when the compartment is filled. Selection of guiding catheters is crucial, as a gentle curve is necessary to allow smooth vessel entry. Under fluoroscopic visualization, the eccentrically located concave cutting window is directed toward the plaque. A counterfacing compliant balloon is inflated to low pressures to maximize atherotome-to-plaque contact. Early experience, however, revealed that some of the immediate luminal gain was secondary to balloon stretch and failed to result in long-term benefit.

In the stent era, the Atherectomy before Multi-link Improves Lumen Gain and Clinical Outcomes (AMIGO)[25] trial failed to demonstrate either angiographic or clinical benefit of directional atherectomy pretreatment prior to stenting versus stenting alone. Technical difficulties, as well as need for large-caliber guiding catheters, have essentially eliminated directional atherectomy from clinical use. Thus, despite initial enthusiasm, directional atherectomy is an essentially obsolete technology today.

LASER ATHERECTOMY

The XeCl excimer utilizes ultraviolet energy with a wavelength of 308 nm to ablate debris through photochemical dissociation. The subsequent photoacoustic effect and heat generation elicits formation of a vapor bubble, which ultimately implodes. Typically, the repetition rate is set at 40 Hz and energy or fluence set up to 60 mJ/mm^2. Initial issues with arterial dissection were largely attributed to excessive heat generation in the blood- or contrast-filled lumen. While the revised technique of constant saline infusion during activation has greatly reduced this complication,[26] coronary indications for this device are quite limited. The recommended catheter-to-artery ratio is 2:3. Technique-wise, the catheter is advanced at a slow rate of 0.5–1 mm/s, with simultaneous gentle intracoronary saline injection at 2–3 cc/s.

The Excimer Laser-Rotational Atherectomy-Balloon Angioplasty Comparison (ERBAC)[27] trial randomized 685 patients to PCI with these three therapeutic modalities. Slightly higher overall MACE and restenosis rates were observed for laser subjects. However, the Amsterdam-Rotterdam (AMRO)[28] trial found no significant differences in 6-month MACE between balloon and laser-treated patients. Laser atherectomy may be rarely considered for thrombotic, friable SVG, bifurcation, and moderately calcific lesions. Even moderately tortuous vessels should be avoided, however, as wire bias can result in perforation from asymmetric vessel wall contact with the vapor bubble. Like directional atherectomy, laser atherectomy is rarely used in modern interventional practice.

CUTTING BALLOON

The cutting balloon catheter (Flextome, Boston Scientific Corporation, Natick, MA) incorporates longitudinal stainless steel blades affixed to the balloon. When deployed, discrete cuts made in the atheroma may avoid large uncontrolled dissections, resulting in less vessel trauma. Utilizing a similar mechanistic principle, the AngioSculpt catheter (AngioScore Corporation, Fremont, CA) (Figure 30.4) features helical wires surrounding the balloon, thus enhancing its flexibility to access tortuous anatomies. Both devices have been used to treat ISR, bifurcation lesions, and moderately calcified plaques.

BARE-METAL STENTS

The advent of bare-metal stents (BMSs) has dramatically reduced the significant target lesion revascularization (TLR) rates previously associated with balloon angioplasty. Up to this point, no other nonballoon PCI device had clearly demonstrated a superior impact on restenosis.

By scaffolding the dilated segment, BMSs have eliminated the elastic recoil ubiquitously seen with balloons. Ironically, BMS implantation actually triggers greater neointimal proliferation than observed with balloon angioplasty. However, the significantly larger initial luminal gain, coupled with freedom from elastic recoil, results in a marked restenosis and TLR advantage over balloons.

Importantly, BMSs have greatly enhanced the procedural safety of PCI. Dissections can often be successfully treated, dramatically decreasing the need for emergent CABG. Nonetheless, the implantation of an intracoronary prosthesis is not without risk. Nonendothelialized stent struts, as well as gaps between the stent and vascular wall, are potent niduses for thrombosis. To ensure adequate stent expansion, meticulous high-pressure postdilatation is often performed with a noncompliant balloon. A minimum of 1 month of dual antiplatelet therapy (DAPT) is strongly recommended following BMS deployment.[29]

DRUG-ELUTING STENTS

To overcome the enhanced endothelial growth induced by BMS implantation, drug-eluting stents (DESs) were developed by incorporating antiproliferative coatings on stent

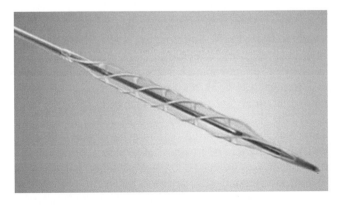

Figure 30.4 The Angioscore balloon catheter.

struts. The seminal Randomized Study with the Sirolimus-Coated Bx Velocity Balloon-Expandable Stent in the Treatment of Patients with *de novo* Native Coronary Artery Lesions (RAVEL),[30] Sirolimus-Eluting Stent in *De Novo* Native Coronary Lesions (SIRIUS),[31] and Treatment of *De Novo* Coronary Disease Using a Single Paclitaxel-Eluting Stent (TAXUS)[32] trials reported dramatically lower clinical restenosis rates with sirolimus-eluting stents (SESs, Cordis, Miami Lakes, FL) and paclitaxel-eluting stents (PES, Boston Scientific Corporation, Natick, MA) compared with BMS. Newer-generation zotarolimus-eluting stents (ZES, Medtronic Corporation, Minneapolis, MN) and everolimus-eluting stents (EES, Abbott Laboratories, Abbott Park, IL) are available for clinical use in the United States.

Indeed, DES may challenge the long-term patency superiority of CABG. The Arterial Revascularization Therapies Study (ARTS)-II investigators compared SES therapy for multivessel disease to historical data from patients assigned to the surgical arm of its randomized predecessor, the ARTS-I trial. The investigators found no differences in MACE, mortality, repeat revascularization, or stroke at 1 year.[33]

DRUG-ELUTING STENT SAFETY AND EFFICACY

To standardize definitions of stent thrombosis (ST), the Academic Research Consortium (ARC) has subclassified ST according to the relative certainty of the diagnosis. Definite thrombosis includes angiographic target vessel occlusion or intrastent thrombus. Probable thrombosis is defined as acute MI in the target vessel territory, while possible thrombosis represents any unexplained death in a patient with a previously implanted DES.[34] It appears that late ST risk with DES is counterbalanced by a reduction in TLR, resulting in equivalent (if not slightly superior) MI, mortality, and MACE rates compared with BMS. The Swedish Coronary Angiography and Angioplasty Registry (SCAAR)[35] observed equivalent long-term mortality risks for DES and BMS patients, despite a slight increase in late ST with DES.

Another large meta-analysis[36] documented persistent and continued TLR benefits of 50%–70% for up to 4 years, without notable differences in death or MI. They further found incidences of ARC-defined ST to be similar. Additionally, the use of SES was associated with lower risk of MI, compared with PES (HR, 0.83; $P = 0.045$) or BMS (HR, 0.81; $P = 0.030$). Consistent with previous findings, rates of ST were higher for BMS within 1 year and higher for DES beyond 1 year. Notably, the numbers needed to treat to prevent 1 MACE was 7 for SES and 8 for PES versus BMS; these benefits were similarly observed in diabetic subjects.

The safety and efficacy of DES in diabetic patients was further underscored in a meta-analysis of nine randomized DES trials involving 1,141 diabetic patients. DES utilization was associated with lower ISR (8% vs. 41%; OR, 0.13; 95% CI, 0.09–0.20; $P < 0.00001$) and TLR (8% vs. 27%; OR, 0.23; 95% CI, 0.16–0.33; $P < 0.00001$). Interestingly, while overall ST or death rates were similar between groups, subsequent MI was more frequent in BMS patients (7.2% vs.

3.5%, $P = 0.02$). The DES advantages prevailed regardless of insulin-dependency status.[37]

In a Korean-based registry involving 3,042 patients with multivessel disease, Park and others compared the clinical outcome of DES implantation versus CABG. After adjustment for baseline risks, the authors reported no significant mortality differences between groups, in concurrence with previous literature. However, through subgroup analysis, lower mortality was observed with PCI for patients with non-left anterior descending double-vessel disease (HR, 0.23; 95% CI, 0.01–0.78; $P = 0.016$).[38]

Multiple subsequent trials and meta-analyses have substantiated equivalent of death and MI rates. Furthermore, despite a slight increase in late ST for DES, *overall* thrombosis and MACE rates were similar for all stents. Some later studies involving later-generation DES have even suggested a nonsignificant decrease in ST risk versus BMS. Major contributing factors to ST include male gender, continued tobacco use, overlapping stents, and DAPT noncompliance.[39,40]

BIOABSORBABLE STENT PLATFORMS

The potential disadvantages of an intracoronary stent have prompted development of bioresorbable vascular scaffolds.[41] While initial results suggest noninferiority versus contemporary generation DES, long-term clinical data are yet unavailable. Nonetheless, the theoretical advantages of a completely bioresorbable vascular scaffold are potentially attractive. The Absorb vascular scaffold (Abbott Vascular, Abbott Park, IL) has been Conformité Européene (CE) marked for clinical use abroad but is not yet approved in the United States. The SYNERGY stent (Boston Scientific Corporation, Minneapolis, MN) is a domestically available stent system that features an absorbable polymer. In the EVOLVE trial, the SYNERGY stent was associated with 0% ARC definite/probable ST, with a 1.1% target lesion revascularization rate at 4 years.[42]

COVERED STENT

The covered stent (Jomed International AB, Helsingborg, Sweden) features a circumferential polytetrafluoroethylene membrane sandwiched between double stent layers and is approved for emergent bail-out treatment of coronary perforation. Given the device's high profile and relative rigidity, adequate catheter backup is crucial. As the need for this stent is rare, but invariably emergent, interventionalists should familiarize themselves with its deployment technique. Trials involving elective covered stent implantation have uniformly failed to demonstrate a restenosis advantage.[43]

Lesion assessment

INTRAVASCULAR ULTRASOUND

IVUS interrogation allows for intraluminal cross-sectional assessment of plaque calcification and severity, vessel size, stent apposition, dissection, and thrombus.

When angiographic findings are questionable, IVUS can often provide valuable additional information. Accepted minimal luminal cross-sectional areas of 4 mm^2 and 5 mm^2 are used to define critical non-left main and left main stenoses, respectively.[43] The decision regarding use of rotational atherectomy for an angiographically calcified lesion may be impacted by superficial versus deep location of calcium. Poststent evaluation of strut apposition, stent-to-vessel sizing, and stent symmetry may indicate the need for further treatment. Finally, IVUS assessment of in-stent restenosis may elucidate the mechanism of restenosis, such as inadequate stent sizing, plaque prolapse, dissection, or rarely stent fracture, thereby directing therapeutic strategies.

OPTICAL COHERENCE TOMOGRAPHY

Adopted from its original retinal applications, OCT (Dragonfly, St. Jude Medical Corporation, St. Paul, MN) uses light to capture high-resolution volumetric imaging of tissue morphology and composition from intravascular scattering media. The resolution of 1–20 microns surpasses that of IVUS; however, the depth of penetration is limited. At an imaging speed approaching 200 frames/s, the image acquisition time is typically shorter than that of IVUS. The imaging catheter retracts automatically inside a fully contained sheath at the predetermined rate. Critical to optimal imaging is constant clearance of the intravascular blood column with manual injection. The ILUMIEN I study demonstrated the safety and efficacy of this device.[44] OCT may provide enhanced plaque composition imaging and identification of thrombus and fibrous cap thickness, as well as stent strut coverage, edge dissection, malapposition, and tissue protrusion (Figure 30.5). Further studies, however, are needed to fully elucidate the long-term clinical implications of such, at times, subtle findings.

PRESSURE WIRE

The pressure wire features a distal pressure sensor to measure the hemodynamic significance of angiographically borderline stenoses. The ratio of pressures distal and proximal to the lesion at maximal hyperemia is known as the fractional flow reserve (FFR). Adenosine, administered by either IV infusion or intracoronary bolus, is often used to induce hyperemia. FFR above and below 0.80 have been validated to correlate with functionally benign and significant stenoses, respectively. Additionally, FFR > 0.90 correlates with adequate stent deployment.

The FFR offers comprehensive physiologic assessment and importantly accounts for both the size of the subtended territory and the oxygen demand of the myocardium. The same stenosis may result in either a normal or abnormal FFR depending on the adequacy of collateral flow in the subtended myocardial territory. Additionally, if perfusion requirement is low in a predominately scarred region, an anatomically "critical" lesion may be associated with a high FFR, indicating an adequate supply-to-demand relationship. FFR accuracy, however, may be limited in situations of high filling pressures (hypertension or left ventricular [LV] hypertrophy), cardiac transplantation, and SVGs.

ADJUNCT PHARMACOLOGY

Heparin versus bivalirudin

While unfractionated heparin (UFH) has been the traditional anticoagulant used during PCI procedures, recent studies involving more modern agents have challenged its role. Bivalirudin, a direct thrombin inhibitor, was assessed in the Intracoronary Stenting and Antithrombotic Regimen–Rapid Early Action for Coronary Treatment 3 (ISAR-REACT 3) trial.[45] In a double-blind study, 4,570 subjects with either stable or unstable angina were randomized to undergo PCI with UFH versus bivalirudin after a loading dose of clopidogrel 600 mg. At 30 days, no differences were reported for the primary composite endpoint of death, MI, urgent target vessel revascularization (TVR), or in-hospital bleeding. However, major bleeding was reduced in the bivalirudin arm (3.1% versus 4.6%, RR, 0.66; 95% CI, 0.49–0.90; $P = 0.008$).

Glycoprotein IIb/IIIa inhibitors/bivalrudin

The Acute Catheterization and Urgent Interventional Triage strategY (ACUITY) trial[46] compared three strategies for patients presenting with ACS, the majority of whom underwent PCI. The three anticoagulation arms included were unfractionated or low molecular weight heparin plus glycoprotein (GP) IIb/IIIa inhibitor, bivalirudin plus GP IIb/IIIa inhibitor, or bivalirudin alone. The composite primary endpoint included the usual ischemic endpoints of death, MI, and unplanned revascularization for ischemia, plus major bleeding. In the PCI group (7789 patients), the ischemic endpoint was 8% with heparin plus GP IIb/IIIa inhibitor group and 9% of the bivalirudin monotherapy. Major bleeding was reduced from 7% with heparin and GP IIb/IIIa inhibitor therapy to 4% with bivalirudin. The net clinical outcome was comparable with 13% of patients reaching the combined ischemic and bleeding endpoints with heparin plus GP IIb/IIIa inhibitor and 12% with bivalirudin monotherapy. An interesting substudy showed that patients with major bleeding episodes had higher mortality at 35 days compared with those who did not bleed.[47] This observation has led to the inclusion of ischemic events plus bleeding as the primary endpoint in some of the current trials. A similar strategy was tested in the Harmonizing Outcomes with Revascularization and Stents in acute Myocardial Infarction (HORIZONS-AMI) trial[48] that compared heparin plus GP IIb/IIIa inhibitor with bivalirudin monotherapy in patients with STEMI. The 30-day outcome showed a net benefit with bivalirudin for ischemic and bleeding endpoints (9.2% vs. 12.1%). Ischemic MACE was equivalent, but there was less bleeding with bivalirudin (4.9% vs. 8.3%). These two trials have resulted in a significant reduction in the use of GP IIb/IIIa

inhibitor therapy in both ACS and AMI in favor of bivalirudin therapy.

DUAL ANTIPLATELET THERAPY

The combination of aspirin and a $P2Y_{12}$ inhibitor is indicated for a minimum of 6 months and 1 month after DES and BMS, respectively. Clopidogrel and prasugrel are thienopyridines that require, to varying degrees, hepatic conversion to the active metabolite. While the bioactivity of clopidogrel is determined by genetic polymorphisms in the CYP2C19 *2 allele, prasugrel is minimally impacted. Ticagrelor, a nonthienopyridine agent, requires no hepatic activation and is the most potent of the three.

Although aspirin and clopidogrel resistance have been linked to increased MACE, the role of antiplatelet resistance in ST remains less certain. Part of the challenge relates to the lack of definition uniformity for platelet resistance. Additionally, accompanying confounders such as lesion complexity, stent deployment techniques, and clinical characteristics have made analyses difficult in the absence of large randomized trials. Currently, routine genetic polymorphism or platelet function assessment has not been demonstrated to impact clinical outcomes and is not recommended.

In the era of newer-generation DESs, the optimal duration for DAPT poststent implantation remains undefined. While some studies have demonstrated enhanced benefit from prolonged treatment duration (>1 year), others have reported equivalent primary endpoints but with reduced bleeding from shorter treatment durations (<1 year).[49–53] In the DAPT trial,[54] the authors observed 2% versus 1.5% all-cause mortality for longer versus shorter treatment, respectively. However, the prolonged treatment group had decreased incidences of major adverse cardiovascular and cerebrovascular events (MACCE), MI, and ST. Of note, there was no difference in cardiac mortality between groups. Until definitive evidence becomes available, DAPT duration should be individualized to the patient's specific demographics and bleeding and thrombotic risks (Table 30.5).[55]

ACCESS

In the United States, the most common PCI access site is transfemoral. The ideal puncture site is at the level of the femoral head; this can be easily identified by placing a hemostat over the area under fluoroscopic guidance. Access too far above or below this level can be associated with significant vascular complications such as arteriovenous fistulae, pseudoaneurysms, or retroperitoneal hematomas.

In many countries, however, transradial intervention (TRI) is now the default approach. Vascular access site and bleeding complications significantly increase the morbidity, mortality, and cost of PCI.[47] These issues are essentially alleviated by TRI. The radial versus femoral access for coronary intervention (RIVAL) trial,[56] randomized 7,021 ACS patients to either approach. Patients in the transradial arm

Table 30.5 Recommendations for DAPT in patients with DES (summarized from the joint scientific advisory from the American Heart Association, American College of Cardiology, Society for Cardiovascular Angiography and Interventions, American College of Surgeons, and American Dental Association, with representation from the American College of Physicians[51])

1. DES should only be implanted in patients able to comply with 12 months of DAPT, from economic and clinical considerations.
2. For patients undergoing PCI who are likely to undergo invasive or surgical procedures within the next 12 months, BMS implantation or stand-alone balloon angioplasty should be considered.
3. Healthcare providers should more thoroughly educate patients regarding the indications of DAPT as well as the risks of premature termination.
4. Patients should be advised to contact their cardiologist prior to interruption of DAPT, even if instructed to do so by another healthcare provider.
5. Healthcare providers who perform invasive or surgical procedures should be aware of potentially serious sequelae of premature DAPT interruption. They should contact the patient's cardiologist if unsure of safety of cessation of therapy.
6. Elective invasive or surgical procedures associated with significant bleeding risk should be postponed, if possible, until appropriate DAPT course is completed (12 months for DES and 1 month for BMS).
7. For DES patients undergoing invasive or surgical procedures mandating DAPT interruption, aspirin should be continued if at all feasible. The second antiplatelet agent should be re-initiated as soon as possible after procedure.
8. Healthcare industry, insurers, U.S. Congress, and pharmaceutical industry should ensure that cost issues do not cause premature DAPT discontinuation, as this can result in devastating consequences.

Source: Reprinted from Chen, J.P., et al., *JACC Cardiovasc. Interv.*, 2(7), 583–593, 2009.
Note: BMS, bare-metal stent; DAPT, dual antiplatelet therapy; DES, drug-eluting stents; PCI, percutaneous coronary intervention.

in large TRI volume centers had significantly lower rates of vascular complications. Additionally, a reduction in combined endpoint of death, MI, or stroke was observed in STEMI patients undergoing TRI in the highest tertile TRI volume centers.

Similarly, the Radial Versus Femoral Randomized Investigation in ST-Elevation Acute Coronary Syndrome (RIFLE-STEACS) Study[57] randomized 1,001 STEMI patients to TRI versus transfemoral intervention (TFI) and reported a significant cardiac mortality benefit (5.2% vs. 9.2%, $P = 0.02$). Furthermore, patients in the TRI arm experienced less bleeding (7.8% vs. 12.2%, $P = 0.026$) as well as shorter hospital stays (5 vs. 6 days, $P = 0.03$).

Decreases in vascular complications, transfusions, lengths of stay, and postprocedural nursing needs combine to provide significant cost savings for hospitals performing TRI. In one analysis, total savings, procedural savings, and postprocedural savings were estimated at $830, $130, and $705 per patient, respectively. Additionally, within each category, the observed savings varied directly with the individual patient's predicted bleeding risk.[58]

Finally, early ambulation associated with TRI allows for lower nursing needs and same-day discharge. The STRIDE study found no adverse events occurring between 6 and 24 hours after PCI, the time period during which same versus next day discharge would have impacted outcomes.[59] More recent data supporting the safety, financial benefits, and feasibility of ambulatory discharge after uncomplicated TRI have prompted the SCAI and ACC to endorse this strategy in an expert consensus document.[60] Enhanced safety, cost savings, and patient preference make TRI an attractive access strategy in today's PCI arena.

SPECIAL CLINICAL SCENARIOS

ST-segment elevation myocardial infarction

Coronary thrombosis accounts for approximately 70% of cardiovascular morbidity and mortality. Plaque rupture, or less frequently plaque erosion, is the substrate for superimposed thrombosis. Other, less common causes of MI include coronary spasm, spontaneous coronary dissection, coronary embolism, coronary vasculitis, and anomalous coronary arteries.[61] Primary PCI for STEMI remains the only clinical scenario in which survival benefit from PCI has been unequivocally demonstrated.

Pharmacology

The enhanced thrombotic milieu necessitates potent antithrombotic and antiplatelet therapy; thus, STEMI patients are at markedly elevated risk for bleeding. Significant bleeding, as well as the need for transfusion, has been found to predict 1-year mortality.[46,47] The HORIZONS-AMI trial[48] demonstrated lower combined endpoints and major bleeding for bivalirudin as compared with heparin plus a GP IIb/IIIa inhibitor. Additionally, while overall MACE was equivalent, 30-day mortality was significantly less for bivalirudin (2.1% vs. 3.1%, $P = 0.047$). Of note, the rate of acute thrombosis (<24 hours, ARC definite or probable thrombosis) was higher with bivalirudin, although the overall 30-day stent thrombosis rates were similar.

TECHNICAL CONSIDERATIONS

Multiple randomized trials have demonstrated the superiority of primary PCI over fibrinolytic therapy in STEMI.[62–64]

The door-to-balloon time should be within 90 minutes. A triage system involving immediate notification of the on-call interventionalist and catheterization laboratory staff by the emergency department facilitates this process. Nonetheless, many eligible patients still fail to receive optimal care. An analysis of 20,279 STEMI patients found that patients presenting during off-hours were less likely to receive PCI (OR, 0.93; 95% CI, 0.89–0.98), had longer door-to-balloon times (median, 110 minutes vs. 85 minutes; $P < 0.0001$), and had lower rates of under 90-minute door-to-balloon times (adjusted OR, 0.34; 95% CI, 0.29–0.39).[65]

Although previously controversial, DES implantation during STEMI appears to be safe and efficacious. Mauri and co-investigators reviewed 7,217 primary PCI cases, 4,016 with DES and 3,201 with BMS. Utilizing propensity-score matching, they found superior 2-year risk-adjusted mortality rates for patients treated with DES versus BMS (10.7% vs. 12.8%, $P = 0.02$). The DES advantage was present for STEMI (8.5% vs. 11.6%, $P = 0.008$) and non-STEMI (12.8% vs. 15.6%, $P = 0.04$). Moreover, recurrent MI rates were reduced for non-STEMI patients treated with DES; and repeat revascularization rates were superior for DES patients in all groups. The authors concluded that DES implantation resulted in superior 2-year mortality and repeat revascularization rates compared with BMS.[66]

Fragmentation of a fresh, friable thrombus can lead to distal microembolization during primary PCI. Angiographic "slow-flow" or "no-reflow" represents microembolization of fibrin and platelet into the arteriolar bed. Selection of slightly longer stent length may help "trap" some of the extruded materials.

Aspiration thrombectomy in the Thrombus Aspiration during Percutaneous coronary intervention in Acute myocardial infarction Study (TAPAS)[67] improved angiographic and 1-year clinical outcomes. However, subsequent studies have failed to reproduce these findings. Accordingly, routine aspiration thrombectomy is not recommended. However, this device may be considered in cases of large, visible thrombus.

When no-reflow is encountered, intracoronary administration of vasodilators, such as nitroprusside, adenosine, or calcium-channel blockers, through the central lumen of an over-the-wire balloon catheter into the distal vascular bed frequently provides prompt resolution. It is important to bear in mind that surgical revascularization offers no benefit in cases of refractory no-reflow. The over-the-wire system is further useful in distal visualization of a totally occluded artery. After initial guidewire lesion penetration, the balloon can be advanced distally then retracted, without inflation. The slightly higher balloon profile often results in a sufficient channel to allow visualization of the distal coronary artery. If distal flow is still not achieved at this point, the balloon is then advanced distally followed by removal of the guidewire. Contrast is subsequently injected through the central balloon lumen to opacify the distal artery, confirming intraluminal position. For predilatation, use of a smaller diameter balloon (2 or 2.5 mm), just sufficient to allow stent passage, is recommended. Additionally, a single, high-pressure stent inflation may minimize the "cheese-grating" extrusion and subsequent downstream embolization of friable plaque.

CARDIOGENIC SHOCK

The incidence of cardiogenic shock has notably declined in recent years, coincident with the increasingly widespread practice of primary PCI for STEMI. This complication occurs in 5%–8% and 2.5% of patients with STEMI and non-STEMI, respectively. In-hospital mortality is approximately 50%. Clinical risk factors for development of cardiogenic shock include anterior STEMI, left bundle-branch block, older age, multivessel CAD, and history of heart failure, diabetes, hypertension, prior MI, or angina. Although commonly diagnosed clinically by signs or symptoms of LV or biventricular failure, formal criteria for cardiogenic shock include hypotension (systolic pressure <80 mmHg or reduction of baseline mean arterial pressure by 30 mmHg) and pump failure (cardiac index <1.8 L/min × m²) in the presence of adequate filling pressures (LV end-diastolic pressure >18 mmHg).[68]

Mechanical complications comprise a minority of the causes of shock but usually have dramatic presentations. Acute mitral regurgitation results from papillary muscle ischemia or rupture, and acute ventricular septal rupture can result in large left-to-right shunt. These two entities have clinically similar presentations of marked pulmonary congestion, hypotension, and holosystolic murmurs. The harsh and turbulent flow across the interventricular septum may be associated with a palpable thrill along the sternal border, whereas most mitral regurgitant murmurs are not. Echocardiography and/or sequential blood oxygen saturations obtained from the right atrium and pulmonary artery can frequently distinguish these etiologies. Additionally, while free-wall rupture, resulting in immediate tamponade, is almost universally fatal, a contained rupture may allow time for urgent diagnosis and intervention. For all mechanical causes of cardiogenic shock, emergent surgical repair is crucial and potentially life-saving.

Most commonly, however, cardiogenic shock results from significant LV dysfunction. While Takotsubo cardiomyopathy (also known as the "broken heart" or "apical ballooning" syndrome)[69] has become an increasingly recognized etiology of STEMI and cardiogenic shock, the majority of cardiogenic shock occurs in the setting of coronary occlusion and STEMI. Of note, the degree of LV dysfunction may not be predictive of clinical presentation. In the Should We Emergently Revascularize Occluded Coronaries for Cardiogenic Shock (SHOCK)[70] trial, Hochman and associates reported a mean left ventricular ejection fraction of (LVEF) almost 30%. Nonetheless, LVEF remains a strong predictor of prognosis.[68]

Right heart catheterization can be helpful in diagnosing and monitoring these patients. Constant pulmonary arterial pressure and frequent cardiac index assessments guide titration of inotropic and pressor agents. Aside from aggressive pharmacologic and ventilatory support measures, emergent angiography and revascularization as well as mechanical circulatory devices are warranted. The intra-aortic balloon pump provides robust augmentations in diastolic coronary perfusion, cardiac index, and mean arterial blood pressure. Data from the National Registry of Myocardial Infarction suggested a survival advantage associated with intra-aortic balloon counterpulsation.[71] Intra-aortic counterpulsation is contraindicated in cases of significant aortic insufficiency and aortic dissection.

Total circulatory support may be needed in refractory cases. LV assist devices drain blood from the left heart and pump it back into the systemic arterial circulation. The TandemHeart device (Cardiac Assist, Inc, Pittsburgh, PA) is a percutaneously inserted device consisting of a transseptal left atrial inflow catheter and a femoral arterial outflow catheter. The Impella device (Abiomed, Inc, Danvers, MA) operates on a similar principle but is inserted across the aortic valve. Extracorporeal circulatory devices additionally pass the venous blood through a membrane oxygenator, thereby incorporating oxygenation with perfusion support. Although LV assist devices offer superior hemodynamic support over intra-aortic balloon counterpulsation, current data fail to demonstrate a survival difference.[72]

Urgent revascularization was shown to impart a 13% absolute increase in survival for patients in the SHOCK trial (NNT < 8).[70] The ACC/AHA guidelines assign class I and class II priorities to urgent revascularization for cardiogenic shock in patients younger and older than 75, respectively. Adherence to the STEMI 90-minute door-to-device time is less important in the setting of shock, with survival benefit demonstrated up to 48 hours after acute MI and 18 hours after shock onset. If significant delay to primary PCI is anticipated, fibrinolytic therapy can be administered, although the scope of benefit is clearly diminished. Multivessel disease can be treated with either CABG or PCI. Two-thirds of patients who underwent PCI in the SHOCK trial had multivessel disease.[70] A follow-up study of the SHOCK registry reported promising 3- and 6-year survival rates of 41.4% and 32.8%, respectively for patients receiving early PCI.[73]

Isolated or predominant right ventricular shock accounts for 5% of cardiogenic shock. The mainstay of initial therapy consists of volume resuscitation and inotropic support. Not infrequently, LV function may also be compromised by impaired filling due to leftward shift of the interventricular septum as well as decreased preload.[74]

BIFURCATION LESIONS

Despite dramatic improvements in PCI techniques and equipment, bifurcation lesions remain a serious challenge for the modern interventionalist. Turbulent flow dynamics and high shear stress likely predispose to plaque formation in such locations. These lesions comprise 15%–20% of the total number of PCI. Compared with other interventions, bifurcation PCI is associated with lower procedural success rates, higher procedural costs, longer hospitalizations, and higher clinical and angiographic restenosis rates. Some studies have reported bifurcation lesions as an independent risk factor for subacute and late stent thrombosis.[75,76] Compared with BMS, DES are associated with less TLR and main branch restenosis in this anatomic subset.[77]

LESION CLASSIFICATION

The presence of a atheromatous plaque causing >50% stenosis in both the main and side branches is considered the definition of a true bifurcation lesion. Several classification schema of varying complexity have been proposed. The Duke classification is ordered A through F according to the main-branch and side-branch locations.

Lefevre et al.[78] have proposed an alternate classification based on the side-branch to main-branch angle and lesion morphology; bifurcation lesions are classified as Y-shaped or T-shaped (side-branch to main-branch angle less than or greater than 70°, respectively). In most cases, Y-shaped lesions allow easier side-branch access but may be associated with greater plaque shift. The converse is generally true for T-shaped lesions. By this scheme, type 1 lesions are defined as true bifurcation lesions involving the main branch, proximal and distal to the bifurcation, as well as the side-branch ostium. Type 2 lesions involve only the main branch at the bifurcation, sparing the side-branch ostium. Type 3 lesions are located in the main branch proximal to the bifurcation. Type 4 lesions involve only the bifurcation, without proximal or distal disease in either branch. The latter is further divided into subtypes 4A and 4B, isolated to the main branch and side branch, respectively.

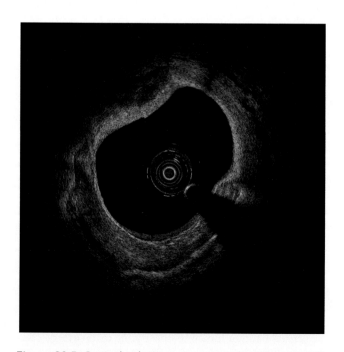

Figure 30.5 Optical coherence tomography. (Courtesy of St. Jude Medical, Inc.)

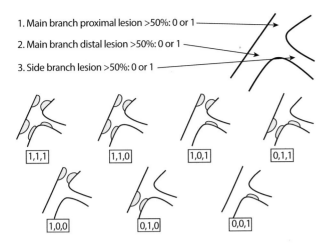

1. Main branch proximal lesion >50%: 0 or 1

2. Main branch distal lesion >50%: 0 or 1

3. Side branch lesion >50%: 0 or 1

1,1,1   1,1,0   1,0,1   0,1,1

1,0,0   0,1,0   0,0,1

Figure 30.6 The Medina Bifurcation Lesion Classification.

The Medina classification[79] is a simplified, practical system involving binary allocation of "1" or "0" based on the respective presence or absence of significant plaque burden in the proximal main branch, distal main branch, or side branch. A "1,1,0" BL, for instance, would indicate proximal and distal main-branch involvement, with sparing of the side branch (Figure 30.6). The location of the bifurcation lesion relative to the carina is a crucial determinant in the decision regarding a single- or double-stent strategy.

Techniques

DEBULKING TECHNIQUES

Plaque shift or "snow-plowing" can occur in 4.5%–26% of bifurcation PCI[79,80] and is more frequent with smaller side-branch reference diameters, side-branch origination within the main branch lesion, and ACS presentation.[80] Occlusion of the SB often results in periprocedural biomarker elevation, which may negatively impact long-term MACE, including TLR/TVR.[81] Fortunately, more than 75% of side-branch occlusions are patent at angiographic follow-up.[82]

Present debulking strategies utilizing rotational, directional, or laser atherectomy have been proposed to minimize potential plaque shift. The FLEXI-CUT[83] study evaluated directional coronary atherectomy-assisted single-vessel stenting of left main bifurcation lesions. The procedural success rate was 96.7%, with 10.3% TLR and 6.9% overall MACE rates. Karvouni and colleagues found that present directional atherectomy resulted in a lower procedural success rate (87.1% vs. 100%, $P = 0.03$), due to higher non-Q wave MI rates (12.9% vs. 0%, $P = 0.03$). However, directional atherectomy-stenting was associated with greater acute gain, as well as a trend toward reduced MACE at follow-up. The role of rotational atherectomy in present debulking of bifurcation lesions is unclear. While this strategy may improve acute side-branch patency, long-term clinical benefits have not been demonstrated.[84] In clinical practice, the relative technical complexity of these approaches limits

their applicability, and single- or double-vessel stent strategies remain preferred in the majority of cases.

STENT TECHNIQUES

While expert opinion varies regarding the preferred technique for treating bifurcation lesions, implantation of at least one DES is recommended in most cases. When the risk for compromising a large side branch is low, main-branch stenting with provisional side-branch stenting frequently offers the simplest and most practical solution. The Nordic Bifurcation Study[85] was a DES study comparing the results of two-vessel stenting versus main-branch stenting with provisional side-branch stenting. At 6 months, there were no differences in MACE; however, two-vessel stenting was associated with significantly greater procedural and fluoroscopic times, contrast volumes, and rates of postprocedural biomarkers elevations. The 5-year follow-up study likewise confirmed persistent equivalency in clinical event rates.[86]

In cases requiring double-stent implantation, several techniques have been proposed. The T-stent technique[87] involves stenting the side-branch ostium after initial stent deployment in the main branch. A second wire is initially left in the side branch and jailed by the main-branch stent. The favorable side-branch angle modification and angiographic reference offered by the jailed wire facilitates subsequent side-branch access through the deployed stent using the main-branch wire. After dilating the stent struts, a second stent is meticulously implanted at the side-branch ostium with a final kissing balloon dilation. The technique is best suited to bifurcation lesions with an angle close to or equal to 90°. Nonetheless, incomplete coverage of the side-branch ostium remains a major limitation.

In the modified T-stenting technique, the side-branch stent is advanced into position followed by the main-branch stent positioning without deployment. The former is then carefully positioned at the ostium and deployed first with only the proximal stent marker protruding into the main branch. Following removal of delivery catheter and guidewire from the side branch, the main-branch stent is then deployed across the ostium of the side branch. The side branch is then rewired for performance of a final kissing balloon dilation.

The crush technique[88] ensures complete lesion coverage at the side-branch ostium. As in the modified T-stenting technique, the side-branch stent is positioned and deployed first; however, in this case, the proximal side-branch stent marker is placed 2–3 mm proximal to the bifurcation within the main branch. After withdrawal of the side-branch wire and stent delivery catheter, the main-branch stent is subsequently inflated, crushing the proximal segment of SB stent. Three layers of stent struts are thus compressed against the ipsilateral main-branch wall. Finally, kissing balloon dilation is undertaken (through the triple layer of stent struts at the bifurcation). This last step is essential to ensure adequate carinal and side-branch ostial patency and to reduce long-term TLR of either branch.

The ability to access the side branch through a double stent layer can be challenging. Accordingly, Chen and colleagues have reported increased success rate of final kissing balloon dilation in the double-kissing crush variation of the strategy. In this technique, there is an additional main-branch balloon crush of the initially deployed side-branch stent, followed by kissing balloon inflation in both vessels. The main-branch stent is then deployed, with subsequent side-branch rewiring and a final kissing balloon dilation. The technique involves wire access through only a single stent layer.[89] In their IVUS comparison of double-kissing versus classic crush techniques, the authors reported that the former was associated with more complete side-branch stent crushing. This resulted in reduced hyperplasia, greater minimal lumen area, and lower ISR rates.[90]

The culotte (or "pant-leg") technique[91] ensures complete bifurcation carinal coverage. In its original description, after double-wire insertion, the first stent is deployed in the more sharply angulated artery (usually the side branch) at high pressure (12–14 atm). The main branch wire is thus trapped, and a third wire is introduced to recross the struts of the initial stent into the other branch. After removal of the jailed wire, balloon predilation through the stent struts facilitates passage of a second stent into the other artery. The procedure ends with a FKBI. Technical complexity and high rates of postprocedural events and restenosis in registry reports have limited the popularity of this strategy.

The simultaneous kissing stent technique is usually reserved for bifurcation lesions with similar-sized branches and large proximal vessel reference diameter. The procedure involves wiring the main and side branches and allows maintenance of access to both during the entire procedure. Both stents are positioned side by side and sequentially inflated, followed by a FKBI. A "double-barrel" configuration results, and the carina is thus extended proximally.[92] The simultaneous stent deployment minimizes plaque shift. Kim and colleagues[93] reported a procedural success rate of 100%. At 26-month follow-up, there were no deaths, MI, or stent thromboses. TLR occurred in five patients (14%), with four (13%) in the main branch and three (10%) in the SB. Of note, in 14 patients (47%), a membranous film coating the double-layered carina was noted both angiographically and by IVUS. However, no clinical sequelae were associated with this membrane.

The V-stent variant involves proximal alignment of both stents at the carina. While this strategy minimizes proximal main branch dissection, carinal coverage may not be assured. Y-stenting is performed by additional deployment of a proximal main branch stent juxtaposed against the proximal edges of both V-stents. This technique was developed to allow complete lesion coverage but is limited by its procedural complexity and the need for three stents.

The proximal optimization technique (POT) involves a final high-pressure main branch stent dilatation before the bifurcation with a short noncompliant balloon optimally sized to at least the diameter of the proximal stent segment. This strategy improves subsequent guidewire or balloon entry into the SB through a distal, rather than proximal main-branch stent cell. Distal positioning of the side-branch

opening through the main-branch stent may reduce strut malapposition. Additionally, while final kissing balloon dilation facilitates carinal and side-branch ostial optimization, the maneuver frequently results in an ovoid deformation of the proximal main-branch stent segment; the POT frequently restores a circular cross-sectional shape.[94]

Despite the myriad of bifurcation stenting techniques, however, the Keep It Simple Strategy (KISS) should be the default strategy in most cases. Angiography has been shown to be a poor and overly sensitive predictor of functional side-branch compromise, as assessed by FFR. In general, a small side branch with preserved flow after main-branch stenting is associated with favorable outcomes.[95]

LIMITATIONS OF PERCUTANEOUS CORONARY INTERVENTION

Percutaneous coronary intervention versus medical therapy

Despite widespread popularity, PCI has not been shown to decrease mortality in patients with stable CAD. Conversely, primary PCI provides a survival advantage compared with fibrinolytic therapy in STEMI.

In the Clinical Outcomes Utilizing Revascularization and Aggressive Drug Evaluation (COURAGE)[96] trial, over 35,000 patients with stable angina and angiographically documented CAD were screened for randomization to OMT with or without PCI. Inclusion criteria included >70% stenosis in a proximal major epicardial artery, Canadian Cardiovascular Society (CCS) class I to III angina, and precatheterization objective evidence of ischemia. Patients with uncontrolled angina, complicated post-MI course, ejection fraction <30%, or cardiogenic shock were excluded. Only 2,287 patients (<10%) were enrolled (1,149 OMT and 1,138 OMT with PCI). Few patients received DES in this trial. No difference was observed for the primary combined endpoint of death or MI at median of 4.6 years follow-up ($P = 0.62$). Subsequent revascularization for ischemia was required in 21% of PCI and 32.6% of medical patients.

The 314-patient nuclear stress test substudy reported significantly greater ischemic burden reductions in the PCI arm versus OMT alone (78% vs. 52%, $P = 0.007$). Additionally, those patients deriving significant ischemia improvement also demonstrated lower unadjusted mortality or MI rates ($P = 0.037$). The unadjusted primary endpoint reduction was especially pronounced in those individuals with moderate to severe baseline ischemia ($P = 0.001$). While DES use would not likely have impacted mortality results, it probably would have decreased TVR and recurrent angina rates (Table 30.6).[97] It would thus seem reasonable that patients with CAD and moderate to severe ischemia could be considered for PCI as an adjunct to OMT.

The Medicine, Angioplasty, or Surgery Study (MASS II)[98] compared medical therapy, PCI, and CABG in patients with stable multivessel CAD. At 5 years, no significant differences were observed in subsequent revascularization and

Table 30.6 Summary of DES safety and recommendations for DES use (summarized from the Statement from the Food and Drug Administration-Center for Devices and Radiological Health Expert Advisory Committee, the Circulatory System Devices Panel)

- When compared with BMS, DES are associated with a small but definite increase in risk of LAST, predominately manifesting after 1 year post-implantation.
- When used according to "on-label" indications, DES result in no overall increase in mortality or MI rates when compared with BMS. This finding is likely related to the marked decrease in repeat revascularization associated with DES.
- DES and BMS carry the same overall all-cause mortality.
- Larger and longer pre-market clinical trials are needed, with longer follow-up durations, more uniform stent thrombosis definitions, and closer attention to DAT therapy.
- At this time, when deployed according to approved indications, the risks of DES do NOT outweigh their benefits, as compared to BMS.
- When used in non-approved patient and anatomic subsets, a higher risk of DES thrombosis, MI, or death may be expected than observed in previous trials.
- Due to limited data for "off-label" DES use (accounting for at least 60% of present-day DES implantation), more studies are needed to determine the safety and efficacy of these devices in such scenarios. DES labeling should state that "off-label" use may not yield the same results as those observed in the clinical trials which led to marketing approval.
- Studies suggest that prolonged anti platelet therapy beyond product label recommendations may be beneficial.
- The optimal DAT duration is unknown, and continued DAT does not guarantee against DES thrombosis.
- Patients at low risk of bleeding are recommended to extend DAT to 12 months post-implantation.

Source: Modified from Chen, J.P., et al., *JACC Cardiovasc. Interv.*, 2(7), 583–593, 2009.
Note: BMS, bare-metal stent; DAT, dual antiplatelet therapy; DES, drug-eluting stent; LAST, late angiographic stent thrombosis; MI, myocardial infarction.

overall MACE rates between medically treated and revascularized patients.

Individuals with type 2 diabetes mellitus represent a high-risk subset of cardiovascular patients. The BARI 2D trial randomized 2,368 patients with type 2 diabetes and stable CAD in a 2×2 fashion to either OMT alone or OMT plus coronary revascularization, and to insulin-provision versus insulin-sensitization therapies. The revascularization group was further subdivided into PCI versus CABG. At 5 years, no survival differences were observed between either revascularization strategy or medical therapy or between insulin provision versus insulin sensitization. However, within the revascularization group, CABG was associated with a lower MACE rate versus medical therapy (22.4% vs. 30.5%, *P* = 0.01), while equivalent results were observed between the PCI and medical therapy groups.[99]

Left main and multivessel coronary artery disease

While CABG has traditionally been recommended for patients with triple-vessel and left main CAD, the enhanced safety and restenosis benefits of PCI due to technical and device improvements have prompted randomized trials comparing PCI and CABG. No significant mortality or MI differences have been demonstrated, although TVR was greater in PCI patients.

The SYNergy between percutaneous coronary intervention with TAXus and cardiac surgery (SYNTAX)[100] trial randomized patients with left main or triple-vessel CAD to multivessel PCI or CABG. The study protocol was reflective of modern PCI strategies using DES and optimal CABG techniques, with overall and bilateral mammary arterial

conduit rates of 97% and 27.6%, respectively. Additionally, coronary anatomy was complex with 84% bifurcation or trifurcation lesions, 22% CTOs, and 39% significant left main disease. A mean of 4.6 DES was implanted per patient with a mean total stent length of 86 mm (with one-third of patients >100 mm).

There was a higher MACCE rate for PCI (17.8% vs. 12.1% for CABG, *P* = 0.0015). Hence, the noninferiority primary endpoint for PCI was not achieved. Despite challenging anatomy, TVR with PCI was much less than that observed in previous PCI versus CABG trials. Interestingly, rates of symptomatic bypass graft occlusion and stent thrombosis were equivalent. While the SYNTAX Score is based purely on angiographic criteria, subsequent proposed risk scores, such as the NEw Risk Score (NERS), incorporate clinical, demographic, and angiographic characteristics.[101]

CONCLUSION

Despite recent advances in treating structural heart disease, PCI remains the cornerstone of interventional cardiology, and technical improvements have dramatically improved outcomes. A continuing challenge will be appropriate use of PCI. In addition, OMT must be applied to achieve optimal long-term outcomes for PCI patients.

REFERENCES

1. King SB 3rd, et al. 2007 focused update of the ACC/AHA/SCAI 2005 Guideline Update for Percutaneous Coronary Intervention: A report of the American College of Cardiology/American Heart Association Task Force on Practice Guidelines: 2007 Writing Group to Review New Evidence and Update the 2005 ACC/AHA/SCAI Guideline

Update for Percutaneous Coronary Intervention, Writing on Behalf of the 2005 Writing Committee. *Circulation* 2008;117(2):261–295.

2. Antman EM, et al. The TIMI risk score for unstable angina/non-ST elevation MI: A method for prognostication and therapeutic decision making. *JAMA* 2000;284(7):835–842.

3. Granger CB, et al. Predictors of hospital mortality in the global registry of acute coronary events. *Arch Intern Med* 2003;163(19):2345–2353.

4. Mehta SR, et al. Routine versus selective invasive strategies in patients with acute coronary syndromes: A collaborative meta-analysis of randomized trials. *JAMA* 2005;293(23):2908–2917.

5. De Winter RJ, et al. Early invasive versus selectively invasive management for acute coronary syndromes. *N Engl J Med* 2005;353(11):1095–1104.

6. Invasive compared with non-invasive treatment in unstable coronary artery disease: FRISC II prospective randomized multicenter study. FRagmin and Fast Revascularisation during Instability in Coronary artery disease Investigators. *Lancet* 1999;354(9180):708–715.

7. Cannon CP, et al. Comparison of early invasive and conservative strategies in patients with unstable coronary syndromes treated with the glycoprotein IIb/IIIa inhibitor tirofiban. *N Engl J Med* 2001;344(25):1879–1887.

8. Levine GN, et al. 2011 ACCF/AHA/SCAI Guideline for Percutaneous Coronary Intervention: Executive summary: A report of the American College of Cardiology Foundation/American Heart Association Task Force on Practice Guidelines and the Society for Cardiovascular Angiography and Interventions. *Circulation* 2011;124(23):2574–2609.

9. Patel MR, et al. ACCF/SCAI/AATS/AHA/ASE/ASNC/HFSA/HRS/SCCM/SCCT/SCMR/STS 2012 Appropriate use criteria for diagnostic catheterization. *Cathet Cardiovasc Interv* 2012;80(3):E50–E81.

10. Chen JP, et al. Appropriate use criteria for cardiac catheterization and coronary revascularization. *Chin Med J* 2014;127(6):1161–1165.

11. Ryan TJ, et al. Guidelines for percutaneous transluminal coronary angioplasty. A report of the American College of Cardiology/American Heart Association Task Force on Assessment of Diagnostic and Therapeutic Cardiovascular Procedures (Subcommittee on Percutaneous Transluminal Coronary Angioplasty). *Circulation* 1988;78(2):486–502.

12. Krone RJ, et al. Evaluation of the ACC/AHA and the SCAI lesion classification system in the current "stent" era of coronary interventions (from the ACC-national Cardiovascular Data Registry). *Am J Cardiol* 2003;92(4):389–394.

13. Fumiaki I, Yeung AC. Equipment for PCI. In King SB 3rd (ed). *Interventional Cardiology*. New York: McGraw Hill Medical, 2007:93–106.

14. Mauri L, Kinlay S. Adjunctive devices: Atherectomy, thrombectomy, embolic protection, IVUS, Doppler and pressure wires. In King SB 3rd (ed). *Interventional Cardiology*. New York: McGraw Hill Medical, 2007:93–106.

15. Margheri M, et al. Thrombus aspiration with export catheter in ST elevation myocardial infarction. *J Interv Cardiol* 2007;20(1):38–43.

16. Jolly SS, et al. Randomized trial of primary PCI with or without routine manual thrombectomy. *N Engl J Med* 2015; 372(15):1389–1398.

17. Baim DS, et al. Randomized trial of a distal embolic protection device during percutaneous intervention of saphenous vein aorto-coronary bypass grafts. *Circulation* 2002;105(11):1285–1290.

18. Stone GW, et al. Randomized comparison of distal protection with at filter-based catheter and a balloon occlusion and aspiration system during percutaneous intervention of diseased saphenous vein aorto-coronary bypass grafts. *Circulation* 2003;108(5):548–553.

19. Bittl JA. Role of adjunctive devices: Cutting balloon, thrombectomy, laser, ultrasound, and atherectomy. In Topol EJ (ed). *Textbook of Interventional Cardiology*, 5th edn. Philadelphia, PA: Saunders Elsevier, 2008:619–639.

20. Whitlow PL, et al. Results of the Study to Determine Rotablator and Transluminal Angioplasty Strategy (STRATAS). *Am J Cardiol* 2001;87(6):699–705.

21. von Dahl J, et al. Rotational atherectomy does not reduce recurrent in-stent restenosis: Results of the Angioplasty versus Rotational Atherectomy for Treatment of Diffuse In-stent Restenosis Trial (ARTIST). *Circulation* 2002;105(5):583–588.

22. Parikh KH, et al. Safety and feasibility of orbital atherectomy for the treatment of calcified coronary lesions: The ORBIT I trial. *Cathet Cardiovasc Interv* 2013;81(7):1134–1139.

23. Chambers JW, et al. Pivotal trial to evaluate the safety and efficacy of the orbital atherectomy system in treating de novo, severely calcified coronary lesions (ORBIT II). *JACC Cardiovasc Interv* 2014;7(5):510–518.

24. Stone G. *Coronary Orbital Atherectomy System Study (COAST), NCT02132611, ClinicalTrials. gov identifier.*

25. Stankovic G, et al. Comparison of directional coronary atherectomy and stenting versus stenting alone for the treatment of de novo and restenotic coronary artery narrowing. *Am J Cardiol* 2004;93(8):953–958.

26. Deckelbaum LI, et al. Effect of intracoronary saline on dissection during excimer laser coronary angioplasty: A randomized trial. *J Am Coll Cardiol* 1995;26(5):1264–1269.

27. Reifart N, et al. Randomized comparison of angioplasty of complex lesions at a single center. Excimer Laser, Rotational Atherectomy, and Balloon Angioplasty Comparison (ERBAC) study. *Circulation* 1997;96(1):91–98.

28. Appelman YEA, et al. Randomised trial of excimer laser versus balloon angioplasty for treatment of obstructive coronary artery disease. *Lancet* 1996;347(8994):79–84.

29. U.S. Food and Drug Administration CDRH. *Update to FDA Statement on Coronary Drug-Eluting Stents*. http://www.fda.gov/cdrh/news/010407.html. 2007 (accessed January 11, 2016).

30. Morice MC, et al. A randomized comparison of a sirolimus-eluting stent with a standard stent for coronary revascularization. *N Engl J Med* 2002;346(23):1773–1780.

31. Moses JW, et al. Sirolimus-eluting stents versus standard stents in patients with stenosis in a native coronary artery. *N Engl J Med* 2003;349(14):1315–1323.

32. Stone GW, et al. A polymer-based paclitaxel-eluting stent in patients with coronary artery disease. *N Engl J Med* 2004;350(3):221–231.

33. Serruys P. Arterial Revascularization Therapies Study Part II of the sirolimus-eluting stent in the treatment of patients with multivessel de novo coronary artery lesions [abstract]. [Presented at American College of Cardiology. 54th Annual Scientific Session. March 6–9, 2015; Orlando, FL] *J Am Coll Cardiol* 2005;45(suppl A):7A.

34. Cutlip De, et al. Clinical end points in coronary stent trials: A case for standardized definitions. *Circulation* 2007;115(17):2344–2351.

35. James S. *SCAAR—Long term mortality after drug eluting stents in Sweden, an additional year of follow-up. Presented at: The European Society of Cardiology Annual Congress*; September 1–5, 2007; Vienna, Austria. (Clinical Trial Update I; 1021).

36. Stettler C, et al. Outcomes associated with drug-eluting and bare-metal stents: A collaborative network meta-analysis. *Lancet* 2007;370(9591):937–948.

37. Patti G, et al. Meta-analysis comparison (nine trials) of outcomes with drug-eluting stents versus bare metal stents in patients with diabetes mellitus. *Am J Cardiol* 2008;102(10):1328–1334.

38. Park D-W, et al. Long-term mortality after percutaneous coronary intervention with drug-eluting stent implantation versus coronary artery bypass surgery for the treatment of multivessel coronary artery disease. *Circulation* 2008;117(16):2079–2086.

39. Stefanini GG, Holmes DR. Drug-eluting coronary-artery stents. *N Engl J Med* 2013;368:254–265.

40. Mauri L, et al. Stent thrombosis in randomized clinical trials drug-eluting stents. *N Engl J Med* 2007;356(10):1020–1029.

41. Ormiston JA, et al. First serial assessment at 6 months and 2 years of the second generation of absorb everolimus-eluting bioresorbable vascular scaffold: A multi-imaging modality study. *Circ Cardiovasc Interv* 2012;5(5):620–632.

42. Meredith IT, et al. Primary endpoint results of the EVOLVE trial: A randomized evaluation of a novel bioabsorbable polymer-coated, everolimus-eluting coronary stent. *J Am Coll Cardiol* 2012;59(15):1362–1370.

43. Schachinger V, et al. A randomized trial of polyteterfluoroethylene-membrane covered stents compared with conventional stents in aorto-coronary saphenous vein grafts. *J Am Coll Cardiol* 2003;42(8):1360–1369.

44. Tearney GJ, et al. Consensus standards for acquisition, measurement, and reporting of intravascular optical coherence tomography studies: A report from the International Working Group for Intravascular Optical coherence Tomography Standardization and Validation. *J Am Coll Cardiol* 2012;59(12):1058–1072.

45. Kastrati A, et al. Bivalirudin versus unfractionated heparin during percutaneous coronary intervention. *N Engl J Med* 2008;359(7):688–696.

46. Stone GW, et al. Bivalirudin in patients with acute coronary syndromes undergoing percutaneous coronary intervention: A subgroup analysis from the Acute Catheterization and Urgent Intervention Triage strategy (ACUITY) trial. *Lancet* 2007;369(9569):907–919.

47. Manoukian SV, et al. Impact of major bleeding on 30-day mortality and clinical outcomes in patients with acute coronary syndromes: An analysis from the ACUITY Trial. *J Am Coll Cardiol* 2007;49(12):1362–1368.

48. Stone GW, et al. Bivalirudin during primary PCI in acute myocardial infarction. *N Engl J Med* 2008;358(21):2218–2230.

49. Thukkani A, et al. Long-term outcomes in patients with diabetes mellitus related to prolonging clpidogrel more than 12 months after coronary stenting. *J Am Coll Cardiol* 2015;66(10):1091–1101.

50. Lee CW, et al. Optimal duration of dual antiplatelet therapy after drug-eluting stent implantation: A randomized, controlled trial. *Circulation* 204;129(3):304–312.

51. Witberg G, et al. Optimal duration of dual antiplatelet therapy after coronary stent implantation. *Am J Cardiol* 2015;116(10):1631–1636.

52. Bonaca MP, et al. Long-term use of ticagrelor in patients with prior myocardial infarction. *N Engl J Med* 2015;372(19):1791–1800.

53. Giustino G, et al. Duration of antiplatelet therapy after drug-eluting stent implantation. A systematic review and meta-analysis of randomized controlled trials. *J Am Coll Cardiol* 2015;65(13):1298–1310.

54. Mauri L, et al. Twelve or 30 months of diual antiplatelet therapy after drug-eluting stents. *N Engl J Med* 2014;371(23):2155–2166.

55. Abizaid AS, et al. Long-term follow-up after percutaneous transluminal coronary angioplasty was not performed based on intravascular ultrasound findings: Importance of lumen dimensions. *Circulation* 1999;100(3):256.

56. Jolly SS, et al. Radial versus femoral access for coronary angiography and intervention in patients with acute coronary syndromes (RIVAL): A randomised, parallel group, multicentre trial. *Lancet* 2011;377(9775):1409–1420.

57. Romagnoli E, et al. Radial versus femoral randomized investigation in ST-segment elevation acute coronary syndrome : The RIFLE-STEACS (Radial Versus Femoral Randomized Investigation in ST-Elevation Acute Coronary Syndrome) study. *J Am Coll Cardiol* 2012;60(24):2481–2489.

58. Amin AP, et al. Costs of transradial percutaneous coronary intervention. *JACC Cardiovasc Interv* 2013;6(8):827–834.

59. Jabara R, et al. Ambulatory discharge following transradial coronary intervention: Preliminary U.S. single-center experience (Same-day Trans-Radial Intervention and Discharge Evaluation, the STRIDE Study). *Am Heart J* 2008;156(6):1141–1146.

60. Chambers CE, et al. Defining the length of stay following percutaneous coronary intervention: An expert consensus document from the Society for Cardiovascular Angiography and Inerventions. Endorsed by the American College of Cardiology Foundation. *Cathet Cardiovasc Interv* 2009;73(7):847–858.

61. Virmani R, et al. Lessons from sudden coronary death: A comprehensive morphological classification scheme for atherosclerotic lesions. *Arterioscler Thromb Vasc Biol* 2000;20(5):1262–1275.

62. Keeley EC, et al. Primary angioplasty versus intravenous thrombolytic therapy for acute myocardial infarction: A quantitative review of 23 randomised trials. *Lancet* 2003;361(9351):13–20.

63. Grines C, et al. Primary coronary angioplasty compared with intravenous thrombolytic therapy for acute myocardial infarction: Six-month follow up and analysis of individual patient data from randomized trials. *Am Heart J* 2003;145(1):47–57.

64. Grzybowski M, et al. Mortality benefit of immediate revascularization of acute ST-segment elevation myocardial infartction in patients with contraindications to thrombolytic therapy: A propensity analysis. *JAMA* 2003;290(14):1891–1898.

65. Jneid H, et al. Impact of time of presentation on the care and outcomes of acute myocardial infarction. *Circulation* 2008;117(19):2502–2509.

66. Mauri L, et al. Drug-eluting or bare-metal stents for acute myocardial infarction. *N Engl J Med* 2008;359(13):1330–1342.

67. Vlaar PJ, et al. Cardiac death and reinfarction after 1 year in the Thrombus Aspiration during Percutaneous coronary intervention in Acute myocardial infarction Study (TAPAS): A 1-year follow-up study. *Lancet* 2008;371(9628):1915–1920.

68. Reynolds HR, Hochman JS. Cardiogenic shock: Current concepts and improving outcomes. *Circulation* 2008;117(5):686–697.

69. Jabara R, et al. Comparison of the clinical characteristics of apical and non-apical variants of "broken heart" (Takotsubo) syndrome in the United States. *J Invasive Cardiol* 2009;21(5):216–222.

70. Hochman JS, et al. Early revascularization in acute myocardial infarction complicated by cardiogenic shock: SHOCK Investigators: Should We Emergently Revascularize Occluded Coronaries for Cardiogenic Shock. *N Engl J Med* 1999;341(9):625–634.

71. Chen EW, et al. Relation between hospital intra-aortic balloon counterpulsation volume and mortality in acute myocardial infarction complicated by cardiogenic shock. *Circulation* 2003;108(8):951–957.

72. Burkhoff D, et al. A randomized multicenter clinical study to evaluate the safety and efficacy of the TandemHeart percutaneous ventricular assist device versus conventional therapy with intraaortic balloon pumping for treatment of cardiogenic shock. *Am Heart J* 2006;152(3):469 E1–E8.

73. Hochman JS, et al. Early revascularization and long-term survival in cardiogenic shock complicating acute myocardial infarction. *JAMA* 2006;295(21):2511–2515.

74. Jacobs AK, et al. Cardiogenic shock caused by right ventricular infarction: A report from the SHOCK registry. *J Am Coll Cardiol* 2003;41(8):1273–1279.

75. Joner M, et al. Pathology of drug-eluting stents in humans: Delayed healing and late thrombotic risk. *J Am Coll Cardiol* 2006;48(1):193–202.

76. Kuchulakanti PK, et al. Correlates and long-term outcomes of angiographically proven stent thrombosis with sirolimus- and paclitaxel-eluting stents. *Circulation* 2006;113(8):1108–1113.

77. Gordon PC, et al. In-hospital and one year outcomes with drug-eluting versus bare metal stents in large native coronary arteries: A report from the Evaluation of Drug-Eluting Stents and Ischemic Events registry. *Cathet Cardiovasc Interv* 2013;82(4):E356–E364.

78. Lefevre T, et al. Stenting of bifurcation lesions: Classification, treatments, and results. *Catheter Cardiovasc Interv* 2000;49(3):274–283.

79. Medina A, et al. A new classification of coronary bifurcation lesions. *Rev Esp Cardiol* 2006;59(2):183–184.

80. Poerner TC, et al. Natural history of small and medium-sized side branches after coronary stent implantation. *Am Heart J* 2002;143:627–635.

81. Pan M, et al. Follow-up patency of side branches covered by intracoronary Palmaz-Schatz stent. *Am Heart J* 1995;129(3):436–440.

82. Califf RM, et al. Myonecrosis after revascularization procedures. *J Am Coll Cardiol* 1998;31(2):241–251.

83. Dahm JB, et al. Directional atherectomy facilitates the interventional procedure and leads to a low rate of recurrent stenosis in left anterior descending and left circumflex artery ostium stenoses: Subgroup analysis of the FLEXI-CUT study. *Heart* 2006;92(9):1285–1289.

84. Ito H, et al. Long-term outcomes of plaque debulking with rotational atherectomy in side-branch ostial lesions to treat bifurcation coronary disease. *J Invasive Cardiol* 2009;21(11):598–601.

85. Steigen TK, et al. Randomized study on simple versus complex stenting of coronary artery bifurcation lesions: The Nordic bifurcation study. *Circulation* 2006;114(18):1955–1961.

86. Maeng M, et al. Long-term results after simple versus complex stenting of coronary artery bifurcation lesions: Nordic Bifurcation Study 5-year follow-up results. *J Am Coll Cardiol* 2013;62(1):30–34.

87. Teirstein PS. Kissing Palmaz-Schatz stents for coronary bifurcation stenoses. *Cathet Cardiovasc Diagn* 1996;37(3):307–310.

88. Colombo A, et al. Modified T-stenting technique with crushing for bifurcation lesions: Immediate results and 30-day outcome. *Catheter Cardiovasc Interv* 2003;60(2):145–151.

89. Chen SL, et al. A randomized clinical study comparing double kissing crush with provisional stenting for treatment of coronary bifurcation lesions: Results from the DKCRUSH-II (Double Kissing Crush versus Provisional Stenting Technique for Treatment of Coronary Bifurcation Lesions) trial. *J Am Coll Cardiol* 2011;57(8):914–920.

90. Chen SL, et al. Serial intravascular ultrasound analysis comparing double kissing and classical crush stenting for coronary bifurcation lesions. *Cathet Cardiovasc Interv* 2011;78(5):729–736.

91. Chevalier B, et al. Placement of coronary stents in bifurcation lesions by the "culotte" technique. *Am J Cardiol* 1998;82(8):943–949.

92. Sharma SK, et al. Simultaneous kissing stents (SKS) technique for treating bifurcation lesions in medium-to-large size coronary arteries. *Am J Cardiol* 2004;94(7):913–917.

93. Kim YH, et al. Long-term outcome of simultaneous kissing stenting technique with sirolimus-eluting stent for large bifurcation coronary lesions. *Cathet Cardiovasc Interv* 2007;70(6):840–846.

94. Lassen JF, et al. Percutaneous coronary intervention for coronary bifurcation disease: Consensus from the first 10 years of the European Bifurcation Club meetings. *Eurointervention* 2014;10(5):545–560.

95. Ahn JM, et al. Functional assessment of jailed side branches in coronary bifurcation lesions using fractional flow reserve. *JACC Cardiovasc Interv* 2012;5(2):155–161.

96. Boden WE, et al. Optimal medical therapy with or without PCI for stable coronary disease. *N Engl J Med* 2007;356(15):1503–1526.

97. Shaw LJ, et al. Optimal medical therapy with or without percutaneous coronary intervention to reduce ischemic burden: Results from the Clinical Outcomes Utilizing Revascularization and Aggressive Drug Evaluation (COURAGE) trial nuclear substudy. *Circulation* 2008;117(10):1283–1291.

98. Hueb W, et al. Five-year follow-up of the Medicine, Angioplasty, or Surgery Study (MASS II): A randomized controlled clinical trial of 3 therapeutic strategies for multivessel coronary artery disease. *Circulation* 2007;115(9):1082–1089.

99. BARI 2D Study Group, et al. A randomized trial of therapies for type 2 diabetes and coronary artery disease. *N Engl J Med* 2009;360(24):2503–2515.

100. Serruys PW, et al. Percutaneoous coronary intervention versus coronary-artery bypass grafting for severe coronary artery disease. *N Engl J Med* 2009;360(10):961–972.

101. Chen SL, et al. Comparison between the NERS (New Risk Stratification) score, and the SYNTAX (Synergy Between Percutaneous Coronary Intervention With Taxus and Cardiac Surgery) score in outcome prediction for unprotected left main stenting. *JACC Cardiovasc Interv* 2010;3(6):632–641.

31

Guiding catheters and wires

DAVID W. M. MULLER AND ROBERTO SPINA

GUIDING CATHETERS

Introduction

Selection of an appropriate guiding catheter is fundamental to the success of every coronary interventional procedure. The catheter should provide coaxial access to the coronary artery to facilitate passage of a guidewire, stability for delivery of balloons and bulky devices, and sufficient contrast flow to adequately visualize the coronary anatomy. It should have a soft atraumatic tip to minimize the risk of injury to the coronary ostium. Changes in procedural complexity over the past two decades have had important influences in guide catheter selection. Bulky inflexible devices such as the directional atherectomy catheter and early generation coronary stents required considerable support from the guide and gentle deflectable curves distally. A progressive decrease in the bulk of devices, an increase in their flexibility, and technical improvements in guiding catheter design have permitted a gradual reduction in guiding catheter caliber. Guide catheter size is defined by the outer diameter measurement, and is commonly expressed in French size (Fr). Whereas only 59% of guiding catheters were 6-Fr in 2000, the estimated distribution of catheter diameters in the United States market in 2007 was 79% 6-Fr, 14% 7-Fr, and 7% 8-Fr (Boston Scientific [BSC], Natick, MA). The approximate inner diameter of contemporary 6-Fr guiding catheters is 0.07-in, compared with 0.08-in for 7-Fr guides and 0.09-in for 8-Fr guides. Whereas catheter size is determined by the outer diameter measurement, sheath size is determined by the inner diameter measurement.

Guide construction

Guiding catheters are typically constructed with three individual layers. The outer polyurethane or polyethylene layer provides support, pushability, and curve retention with low thrombogenicity (Figure 31.1). The middle wire braid layer is a flat or round, woven stainless steel or Kevlar layer that determines the catheter's torque responsiveness and kink resistance. Tungsten may be incorporated to increase its radiopacity. The weave of the braid varies (e.g. 2×2 or 2×4) and its density is expressed as pic units. High pic values are associated with a high-torque responsiveness of the catheter. The inner layer is usually polytetrafluoroethylene (Teflon) to provide a low coefficient of friction and easy passage of devices through the catheter. Attached to the distal end is a soft radiopaque tip. Sideholes may be incorporated close to the catheter tip, particularly in large caliber catheters, to limit the hypoperfusion caused by partial occlusion of the coronary ostium. The benefit of the sideholes may, however, be offset by a reduction in visualization of the distal coronary artery, an increase in the volume of contrast used, and loss of pressure damping, an important indicator of coronary flow limitation.

Catheters are constructed in a variety of shapes to cater to differences in coronary anatomy. They all have a primary curve close to the tip and a secondary curve that varies according to the catheter size and shape. Subtle differences in construction along the length of the catheter give more support and torqueability to the catheter shaft, and greater flexibility to segments closer to the tip (Figure 31.2a and b). Variation in characteristics of these zones or segments can greatly influence catheter performance.

ACTIVE VERSUS PASSIVE GUIDE SUPPORT

Depending on the design characteristics of the catheter, a guide may be best used passively or actively. Passive guide support relies on the inherent properties of the catheter and its interaction with the walls of the aortic root. Passive support can be increased by increasing the caliber of the guide (e.g., 8-Fr vs. 6-Fr), by selecting a shape that provides greater

contact with the contralateral aortic wall, or by selecting a catheter with a stiffer shaft and power zone. A guide that is used actively is manipulated, for example, by deep seating into the proximal coronary artery (or beyond), to maximize backup support. This requires a soft atraumatic catheter tip and a flexible primary curve. Some guides, such as the Vista Brite Tip (Cordis Corporation, Miami Lakes, FL), Launcher (Medtronic, Santa Rosa, CA), and Runway (Boston Scientific, Natick, MA), are better suited to provide passive support, whereas others such as the Mach1 (BSC), Zuma2 (Medtronic), and Viking (Abbott Vascular, Redwood City, CA) catheters can be manipulated actively.

CATHETER SHAPE AND VARIATIONS IN CORONARY ANATOMY

The left main coronary and the right coronary artery (RCA) usually arise horizontally from the left and right coronary cusps, respectively. It is not uncommon, however, for their position to be anterior or posterior to the usual position and for their takeoff to be superior or inferior to the horizontal (Figure 31.3).[1] The left main coronary artery (LMCA) may be long or short, or the left anterior descending (LAD) artery and circumflex may arise from separate ostia.[1,2] The RCA often arises high and anterior to its usual position. It may arise from the left coronary cusp adjacent to the LMCA. The circumflex can take origin from the proximal RCA.[2] In this position, it can be difficult to cannulate using a guiding catheter that seats deeply in the proximal RCA. Changes in the size and shape of the aortic root and ascending aorta, and whether access is obtained from the femoral or radial artery, also have an important influence on the optimal size and shape of the guiding catheter.

To accommodate the complexity of coronary anatomy, a wide variety of catheter shapes have been developed (Figure 31.4).

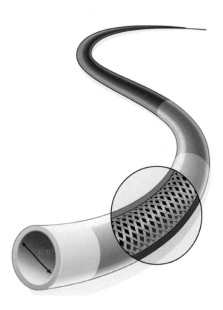

Figure 31.1 Guide catheter construction showing middle wire braid layer. (Courtesy of Boston Scientific.)

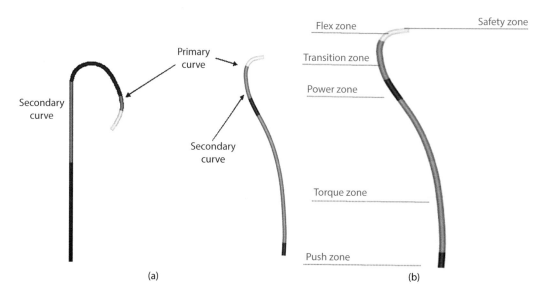

Figure 31.2 **(a)** Primary and secondary curves of Judkins left and right guiding catheters. **(b)** Functional zones of a right Judkins guiding catheter. (Courtesy of Boston Scientific.)

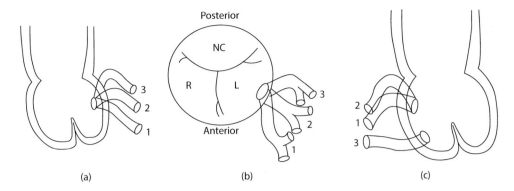

Figure 31.3 Variations in orientation of the left and right coronary artery. The orientation of the left coronary artery **(a)** may be inferior (1), orthogonal (2), or superior (3). In the anteroposterior orientation **(b)**, it may lie anteriorly (1), orthogonally (2), or posteriorly (3). The right coronary artery **(c)** may also arise orthogonally (1), superiorly (Shepherd's crook) (2), or from the inferior margin of the sinus (3). (From Casserly, I.P., and Franco, I., Guides and wires in percutaneous coronary intervention, in Ellis, S.G., and Holmes, D.R., (eds.), *Strategic Approaches in Coronary Intervention*, 3rd ed., Lippincott Williams and Wilkins, Philadelphia, PA, 2006, pp. 91–100. With permission.)

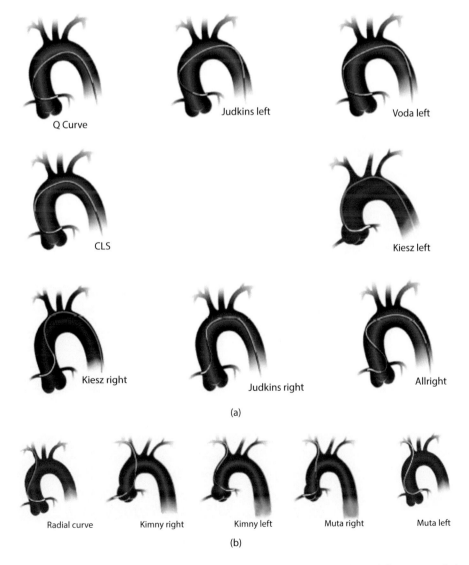

Figure 31.4 **(a)** Guide catheter shapes for transfemoral access. **(b)** Guide catheter shapes for transradial access. (Courtesy of Boston Scientific.)

Normal anatomy

Traditional curves, such as the left Judkins (JL or FL) catheter, provide adequate backup for many left coronary interventions (Figure 31.5). More supportive shapes such as the EBU, XB, Voda, and DC curves provide better support for complex interventions and, in some catheter laboratories, have become the standard choice for all left coronary procedures. These shapes have the added advantage of less angulated primary and secondary curves that facilitate the passage of bulky devices. Gentle advancement with clockwise rotation can be used to selectively engage the LAD. Counterclockwise rotation can be used to selectively engage the circumflex coronary artery. Other curves that provide excellent backup in the left coronary artery include the Amplatz curve (AL1 or AL2), the CLS (contralateral support) curve, and the Q curve (Figure 31.4a).

The RCA is most commonly cannulated using a right Judkins curve (Figure 31.5) but, unless actively deep-seated, this provides relatively little support for complex anatomy. If greater support is required, alternative curves include the Hockey stick, Amplatz (AL1), XB or Voda right, allRight, and Kiesz Right (Figure 31.4a). On occasions, the right coronary has a very superior takeoff (Shepherd's crook). If the artery is calcified or severely diseased, instrumentation of these arteries requires excellent backup using Shepherd's crook, Amplatz (AL1), or Hockey stick curves. In this, and other circumstances in which the guide is deep-seated, great care must be taken to avoid guide catheter–related dissection of the proximal artery.

Bypass grafts

Saphenous vein grafts (SVGs) to the RCA are best approached with a multipurpose catheter if the takeoff is vertical, or a right Judkins or right coronary bypass (RCB) catheter if it is more horizontal. Vein grafts to the left coronary artery can be cannulated with a right Judkins, an internal mammary artery (IMA), a left coronary bypass (LCB), or an AL1 curve though none of these provides contralateral wall support. An IMA curve is used for interventions performed through an IMA graft.

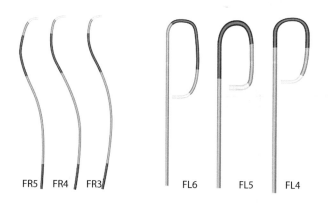

FR5 | FR4 | FR3 | FL6 | FL5 | FL4

Figure 31.5 Judkins right and left curves.

Anomalous origins

Right coronary arteries arising from the left coronary cusp can usually be cannulated with an Amplatz left catheter. Circumflex arteries arising from the proximal RCA are best approached with a short-tipped JR catheter, and AL1 or an AR1.

GUIDE CATHETERS FOR TRANSRADIAL INTERVENTION

The increasing popularity of transradial intervention (TRI) has provided the impetus for recent developments in coronary guide catheter technology. Although TRI may be performed using standard guide catheters developed for transfemoral intervention (TFI), the catheter support is generally less since the angles of approach to the coronary ostia differ markedly in transradial versus TFI. Catheters designed for TFI do not always provide coaxial engagement and optimal support in TRI. In addition, the smaller-sized radial artery limits catheter size available for TRI. Hence, both the configuration and profile of guide catheters have evolved to suit the specific requirements of the radial approach.

Extra backup catheters (e.g., EBU, XB, Voda, Q-Curve, Muta) or modified long-tip catheters (e.g., Ikari, Power Backup, Fajadet catheters) are the commonly used guide catheters for TRI (Figures 31.5, 31.6, and 31.7). These guide catheters derive extra backup support from either the sinus of Valsalva (for EBU, XB, Voda, Q-Curve) or from the contralateral aortic wall (Ikari, Muta, Kimny) (Figure 31.4b). The catheters enter the ascending aorta facing the right coronary sinus. They can be advanced and torqued toward the left coronary sinus over a 0.035-in guidewire making a large J-shaped loop in the sinus of Valsalva. The guidewire is then withdrawn and the catheter tip gently manipulated to engage the left coronary artery. An inherent drawback of these catheters is the tendency for deep intubation into LAD or left circumflex (LCX) when the LMCA is short.

Whereas extra backup catheters were originally designed for use in the femoral approach to percutaneous coronary intervention (PCI), the modified long-tip catheters (Ikari, Kimny, etc.) have been specifically developed for TRI. Their three-dimensional (3D) shape better conforms to the angle between the brachiocephalic trunk and the ascending aorta, and provide better backup support, through contact with the contralateral aortic wall. The Ikari catheter is one example of a radial PCI-specific catheter that has recently become widely adopted in some parts of the world.[3] The Ikari left-guide catheter evolved from the Judkins left through three modifications: (1) a shorter length between the third and the fourth angles, (2) longer length between the second and the first angles, and (3) a new first angle added to conform to the angle between brachiocephalic artery and ascending aorta (Figure 31.8). Engagement maneuvers are similar to those used with the Judkins left. The Ikari guide catheter may be used actively in the power position by deeply engaging the left main coronary ostium. The soft distal tip reduces

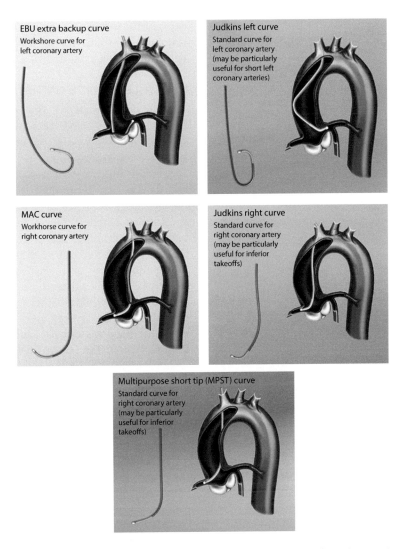

Figure 31.6 Medtronic transradial family guide catheters–basic curves. (Courtesy of Medtronic Corporation, Minneapolis, MN.)

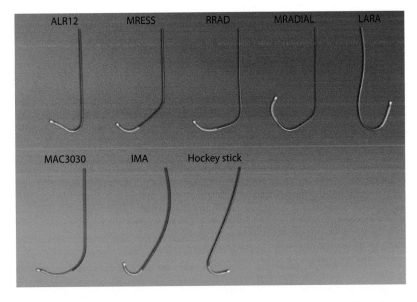

Figure 31.7 Medtronic transradial family guide catheters–additional curves. (Courtesy of Medtronic Corporation, Minneapolis, MN.)

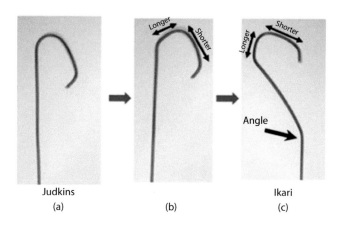

Judkins (a)   (b)   Ikari (c)

Figure 31.8 Ikari Left Guide Catheter. The Judkins left (JL) catheter **(a)** and the Ikari left catheter (**b** and **c**). Two modifications were added to the JL: (1) a shorter length between the third and the fourth angles, (2) longer length between the second and the first angles, and (3) the new first angle was added to conform to the angle between the brachiocephalic artery and the aorta.

the risk of intimal dissection when used actively. The Ikari left catheter may be used to engage the RCA as well.

For the left coronary artery, XB, EBU, and Judkins guide catheters are usually employed despite providing less support from the arm compared to the femoral approach (Figures 31.5 through 31.7). When a JL4 catheter is used from the radial approach, the point of contact with the contralateral wall shifts upward, and the resultant backup support is less than the support it provides when used transfemorally. Hence, for TRI using a Judkins catheter via the right radial artery, it is recommended either to downsize by 0.5-Fr from what is used for femoral approach (i.e., JL4 for TFI becomes JL3.5 for TRI), or to engage deeply the JL4 catheter. The Judkins catheter is suitable for noncomplex lesions or left main PCI when catheter support is not critical.

For RCA TRI, Judkins right and Amplatz right catheters are commonly used (Figures 31.5 through 31.7). Despite the lack of backup support, the Judkins right catheter in sizes similar to TFI is the first-choice catheter for noncomplex or ostial RCA lesions. Ikari right, Fajadet right, and Multi-Aortic Curves (MAC) curve are modified long-tip catheters designed for RCA TRI, providing backup support using the contralateral aortic wall (Figures 31.6 and 31.7). Care must be exercised not to dissect the aortic root or RCA ostium when manipulating these catheters.

IMA TRI is usually performed using an IMA or JR catheter via ipsilateral radial access. Cannulation of a vein graft or radial graft (with origin in the ascending aorta) is easier from the left radial approach, with standard catheters such as JR, LCB, AL, or multipurpose (Figures 31.6 and 31.7). Their cannulation can be difficult from the right radial access due to the proximity of the origin to the innominate (brachiocephalic) artery. From the right radial approach, Judkins right and Amplatz right catheters can be used to engage SVG to left coronary arteries (Figures 31.6 and 31.7). Cannulation of inferior-pointing SVG to the RCA can be performed using a multipurpose catheter (Figure 31.6).

SHEATHLESS GUIDE CATHETERS

The smaller diameter of the radial artery compared to the femoral artery, and the associated risk of radial vasospasm, often limits guide catheter size selection, and may therefore constrain options in percutaneous intervention, particularly for complex coronary lesions requiring adjunctive devices and techniques that may be delivered only through large-diameter catheters. The introduction of the sheathless Eaucath guide catheter (Asahi Intec, Nagoya, Japan), a hydrophilic-coated guide catheter (Figure 31.9) that does not require an introducer sheath, offers a potential solution to this problem. Its outer diameter is approximately 2-Fr smaller than those of the sheath required for a conventional guide catheter. For example, the outer diameter of a 7.5-Fr sheathless guide catheter (2.49 mm) is smaller than that of a 6-Fr introducer sheath (2.70 mm) (Figure 31.10a). The internal diameter of a 7.5-Fr Eaucath catheter (2.06 mm) is the same as the internal diameter of a 7-Fr standard catheter. However, the sheathless guide requires no introducer sheath and therefore its outer diameter is 2.49 mm, whereas the latter requires a 7-Fr sheath whose outer diameter is 3 mm (Figure 31.10b). The sheathless Eaucath guiding catheter possesses a hydrophilic coating layer, which enhances catheter trackability, and reduces the risk of radial artery spasm. A long dilator is provided with each catheter (Figure 31.9). This is removed once the catheter tip approaches the coronary ostium.

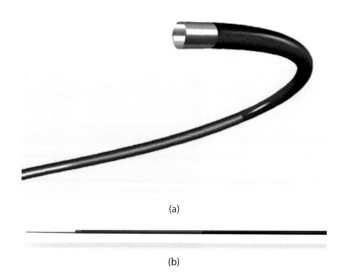

(a)

(b)

Figure 31.9 The Eaucath sheathless guiding catheter. The sheathless Eaucath guiding catheter **(a)** is designed to provide a large inner lumen size by avoiding the need for an introducer sheath. The hydrophilic coating enhances catheter trackability, and reduces the risk of radial artery spasm. A long dilator is provided with each catheter to ease introduction into the artery **(b)**.

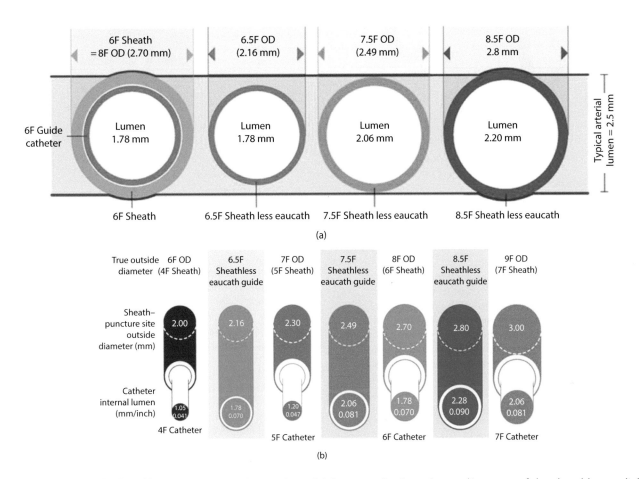

Figure 31.10 Eaucath Sheathless Comparative Dimensions. **(a)** Comparative inner/outer diameters of the sheathless radial guide catheter and standard radial sheaths. **(b)** Comparative outer and inner diameters of the sheathless radial guide catheter and standard radial sheaths. The outer diameter of a 6-Fr radial introducer sheath (2.70 mm) is aproximately the same as the outer diameter of an 8.5-Fr Eaucath sheathless catheter (2.80 mm). The internal diameter of a 7.5-Fr Eaucath catheter (2.06 mm) is the same as the internal diameter of a 7-Fr standard catheter. However, the latter requires no introducer sheath and therefore its outer diameter is 2.49 mm, whereas the former requires a 7-Fr sheath whose outer diameter is 3 mm. F, French; mm, millimeters; OD, outside diameter.

TRI performed through a sheathless guide catheter may be effective and safe in elective PCI[4,5] and in primary PCI.[6] A Italian[7] and French[8] series of 134 and 83 patients, respectively, undergoing bifurcation PCI demonstrated feasibility and safety of the sheathless catheter, with no crossover to the femoral approach and no major complications recorded. Sheathless guide catheter TRI in ST-segment elevation myocardial infarction (STEMI) proved to be safe and effective in a large Japanese series of 478 patients.[6] Procedural success was achieved in 97% of cases. 4% of the patients subsequently developed radial artery occlusion.

TECHNIQUES FOR ENHANCING GUIDE CATHETER SUPPORT

Despite the wide variety of catheter curves and sizes available, optimal support for complex percutaneous intervention may not be achievable with current guide catheters in the setting of severe vessel tortuosity, unfavorable anatomy, lesion calcification, and distal vessel lesion location. Techniques to enhance guide catheter support may prove valuable in these complex settings.

These techniques may be broadly divided into three groups: (1) techniques that rely on increased passive guide support, (2) techniques requiring active guide support, and (3) hybrid techniques.[9]

Increasing passive support involves using large (7- to 8-Fr), rigid guide catheters that sit in a more stable position in the ostium of the target coronary artery (Figure 31.11a). In addition to conferring more support compared to 5- to 6-Fr guides, these catheters allow the advancement of two over-the-wire balloons, simultaneous deployment of two stents, and the use of large intracoronary devices such as large rotational atherectomy burrs. The potential disadvantages of using 7 to 8-Fr guide catheters are that the large size may impair coronary flow, and may increase the risk of damaging the artery with catheter manipulation.

In contrast to the techniques described above, achieving greater active support involves the use of smaller (5- to 6-Fr) guide catheters, which are advanced deep into the proximal or even mid-segment of the target coronary artery (Figure 31.11b). Advancing the guide catheter into

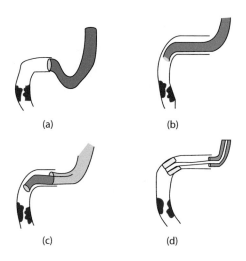

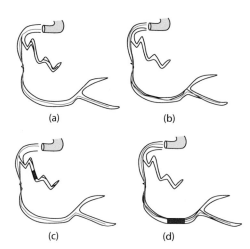

Figure 31.11 Techniques to enhance guide catheter support. Catheter support and hybrid techniques. **(a)** Passive support: a left Amplatz guide catheter engages the right coronary artery (RCA)—the catheter, deriving firm support from the coronary sinus, combines good support and a large lumen. **(b)** Active support: a 5- or 6-Fr Judkins right catheter is deeply engaged into the proximal segment of the RCA, providing excellent support. **(c)** "Mother-and-child" technique: dual coaxial guide catheter technique with a smaller inner ("child") catheter inserted into the target artery via a larger (6- to 8-Fr) "mother" guide. **(d)** Proxis: the proxis proximal occlusion balloon is inflated near the ostium of the RCA providing support as well as protection from distal embolization. (Reproduced from Di Mario, C., and Ramasami, N., *Cathet. Cardiovasc. Interv.*, 72, 505–512, 2008. With permission.)

Figure 31.12 Coronary wire and balloon anchoring techniques. Hybrid support anchoring wires and balloons. **(a)** "Anchor" wire in atrial branch of the right coronary artery (RCA) proximal to the lesion. **(b)** "Buddy" wire in the posterior descending artery (PDA) distal to the lesion. **(c)** "Anchoring balloon" in atrial branch of the RCA proximal to the lesion. **(d)** "Anchoring balloon" inflated in the distal third segment of the RCA. (Reproduced, with permission, from Di Mario et al.[9])

the artery over a coronary wire and balloon rail with gentle rotational movement minimizes the risk of arterial dissection. A balloon inflated at low pressure within the artery may also help intubate the vessel deeply. The limitations of this approach include poor visualization and high resistance to contrast injection through small-bore catheters. In addition, deep intubation may induce profound ischemia, a complication not always mitigated by the presence of sideholes. Air embolism may occur with aspiration through the Y-connector when the catheter is deeply engaged with a dampened backpressure. Finally, small guide catheter size may limit the therapeutic options available to the operator.

Hybrid techniques to enhance guide catheter support involve the use of coronary wires and balloons to stabilize the system. Additional coronary wires may be used proximal or distal to the target lesion (Figure 31.12a and b). Examples of proximal wire support are the use of right ventricular branch, sinus node, or conus branches for the RCA; the diagonal branches for the LAD coronary artery; and the obtuse marginal (OM) branches for the LCX coronary artery. Distal wire support (also known as "buddy wire technique") is achieved by advancing a second or third wire distal to the target lesion, either in the main vessel or into a distal branching vessel.[10] The additional wires provide

increased support and straighten tortuous segments of the artery.

Balloon-anchoring techniques to strengthen guide catheter support may also be categorized into distal and proximal according to the location of the anchoring balloon (Figure 31.12c and d). Proximal balloon anchoring involves inflating a balloon at low pressure into a branch proximal to the lesion to secure catheter position in the ostium of the target coronary artery. Gentle inflation of a balloon distal to the target lesion may be helpful where the use of a buddy wire has provided insufficient support to advance a stent across a tortuous or calcified proximal vessel.

In addition to the maneuvers described above to enhance guide support, adjunctive devices that increase the deliverability of intracoronary devices have emerged recently. The guide catheter extension is a prominent example of an adjunctive device available for use in complex PCI today.

GUIDE CATHETER EXTENSION SYSTEMS

Guide catheter extensions include over-the-wire devices such as the 5-Fr in 6-Fr Heartrail II and 4-Fr in 6-Fr Kiwami catheters (Terumo Corporation, Tokyo, Japan), and the rapid exchange GuideLiner catheter (Vascular Solutions, Maple Grove, MN). The "mother-and-child" principle behind guide extension postulates that by intubating the vessel deeply, the smaller, softer "child" catheter extension provides greater active support safely for the larger, more rigid "mother" guide catheter.

The GuideLiner device consists of a flexible, 20 cm long, straight, flexible, soft-tipped extension tube that is connected via a metal collar to a thin 115 cm-long

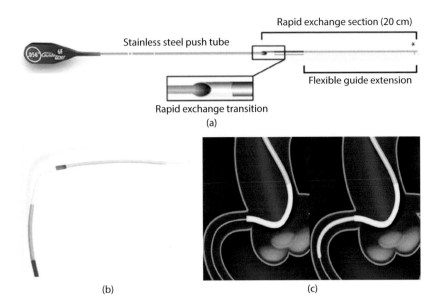

Figure 31.13 The GuideLiner guide catheter extension system. The GuideLiner is a rapid exchange guide extension system with a 20 cm long, straight, flexible tubular end with a soft tip (**a** and **b**), which can be deeply advanced into target vessels over a coronary guidewire, and through a "mother" guide catheter (**c**). See text for full procedural details. (Reproduced from De Man, F., et al., *Eurointervention*, 20, 336–344, 2012. With permission.)

stainless steel shaft (Figure 31.13). The extension tube has a silicon coating for enhanced lubricity. The procedure involves the following steps: (1) the "mother" guide catheter is positioned into the ostium of the target epicardial coronary artery, (2) the coronary guidewire is advanced across the target lesion, and (3) the GuideLiner is advanced over the guidewire through the hemostatic valve of the Y-adapter (in a similar fashion to regular balloons and stents) to intubate the target coronary artery (Figure 31.10). The GuideLiner reduces the inner diameter of the mother guide by approximately 1-Fr, but it does not lengthen the section of guide outside the patient's body. When the GuideLiner is in place, balloons and stents may be delivered over the coronary guidewire. The GuideLiner is available in sizes of 6-Fr, 7-Fr, and 8-Fr.

De Man et al. used a GuideLiner catheter extension in 65 consecutive patients with predominantly complex (B2/C) and distal lesions with a success rate of 93% and without any major complications.[11] A series of 28 cases of GuideLiner-facilitated PCI to chronic total occlusion (CTO) lesions resulted in a successful delivery of a microcatheter or small balloon across the culprit lesion in 86% cases.[12] Another series of 83 patients stated a procedural success rate of 73% without major complications.[13] Despite very deep intubation and aggressive intervention techniques, no cases of vessel dissection, perforation, or distal embolization have been reported in the literature. In summary, guide extension systems may safely provide greater backup resistive force and improved alignment for stent delivery in unfavorably tortuous coronary arteries and compex, heavily calcified and often distally located lesions, which otherwise may have been considered unsuitable for PCI.

GUIDEWIRES

Introduction

As originally conceived and developed by Gruntzig,[14] balloon dilatation catheters had a closed end attached to a short, fixed, nonsteerable, and relatively atraumatic guidewire. The inability to direct the wire to, and through, stenotic coronary lesions was a major limitation of the technique. As a consequence, the primary technical success rate reported in the National Heart, Lung, and Blood Institute (NHLBI) percutaneous transluminal coronary angioplasty (PTCA) registry in 1982 was only 59%.[15] In the same year, Simpson and colleagues reported the use of an over-the-wire system that allowed a central guidewire to be advanced independently of the dilatation catheter.[16] This adjustment improved the success and safety of the procedure by allowing the operator to exchange or reshape the wire without removing the balloon catheter, to minimize ischemia time by wiring the distal vessel before attempting to cross with the balloon catheter, and to exchange the balloon catheter without having to also remove the guidewire. Soon thereafter, technical success rates approaching 90% were reported.[17]

Technical advances in guidewire technology followed. In the mid-1980s, 0.018 and 0.016-in wires were constructed from a stainless steel core shaft that tapered distally and was covered by a flexible stainless steel coil spring (Figure 31.14a). The shaping ribbon was added to the tip to improve shaping and steerability of the wire. Visibility of the tip was enhanced by adding a platinum alloy spring coil segment, and tip flexibility and steerability were manipulated by varying the length and diameter of the central core taper. Trackability was enhanced by coating the distal coil with hydrophilic or

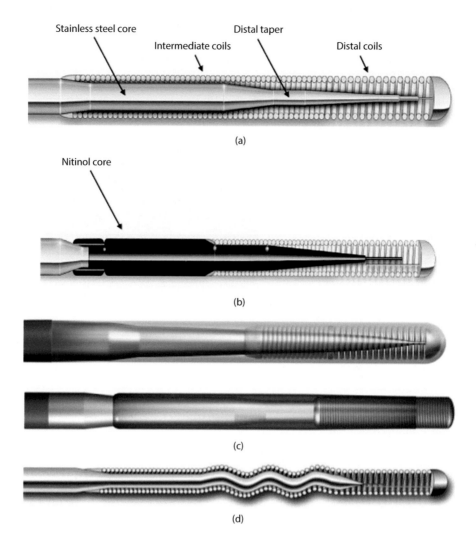

Figure 31.14 (a) Coiled tip workhorse wire with segmentally tapering stainless steel core. **(b)** Nitinol core improves durability of the wire (increases resistance to kinking). The intermediate coils have been eliminated to improve trackability. **(c)** *Upper image*. Transitionless coil-to-tip taper with a polymer sleeve and hydrophilic coating improves trackability (Whisper wire). *Lower image*. High tensile stainless steel core with polymer sleeve covering all but the distal 5 mm designed to increase tactile sense. Core-to-tip design tapering to 0.009-in to increase penetration power (Hi-Torque Progress wire). **(d)** The Wiggle wire has a series of corrugations designed to exert a tangential force in heavily calcified or previously stented arteries. (Courtesy of Abbott Vascular.)

hydrophobic materials (e.g., Teflon, silicone). This spring coil construction has remained dominant as the workhorse wire design in the two decades since then, but other refinements have been introduced to improve wire performance in specific situations. In addition, several manufacturers have developed wires with polymer coatings covering part of or the entire distal segment to facilitate passage of the wire through complex lesions and chronic total occlusions. The wire may or may not have an underlying spring coil supporting the polymer.

WIRE CHARACTERISTICS

Contemporary wires can vary considerably in a variety of important performance characteristics. The *torque response* of a wire refers to the extent of wire tip rotation in response to rotation of the wire shaft. Wires with high torque respond to very fine movements of the wire shaft and are therefore more steerable than less torqueable wires.

Wire support relates to the stiffness of the working length of the wire. Stiffer more supportive wires more readily allow passage of a balloon catheter or stent through noncompliant arteries. *Wire trackability* refers to the ease with which a wire can be advanced through a tortuous artery without buckling, kinking, or prolapsing. *Pushability* relates to the extent to which pressure applied to the shaft is transmitted to the wire tip. *Durability and shape retention* describe the impact of repeated use of the wire on the integrity of the shaft and shape of the distal tip. *Tip flexibility* refers to the ease with which a wire tip is deflected from an object. Very flexible, floppy-tipped wires are less likely to cause plaque disruption, dissection, or perforation than less flexible wires, but are also less likely to cross complex lesions and subtotal or total occlusions. *Tip malleability* refers to the ease with which the wire tip can be shaped. *Tactile sense* is the ease with which the operator can recognize changes in movement of the wire tip. *Tip load* refers to the force required to buckle the distal tip (10 mm) of a wire. This is typically measured in grams. The higher the tip load, the greater the ease with which a wire will penetrate fibrous or calcified occlusions and the greater the risk of arterial injury (dissection or perforation). *Penetration power* is derived from the tip load and the area of the tip (tip load/tip area [kg/in²]).

WORKHORSE WIRES

Coiled tip wires

The most frequently used workhorse wires are still stainless steel coiled spring wires. These wires have a 0.014-in stainless steel shaft that tapers distally to a 30–40-cm-long stainless steel core (Table 31.2). The core typically tapers segmentally and terminates before the end of the overlying coils (Figure 31.14a) with a shaping ribbon between the end of the core and the tip weld. This wire construction provides good torque control, good pushability, and light support. Examples of this include the Hi-Torque Floppy II wire (Abbott Vascular), the Asahi Light (Asahi Intec Co. Ltd., Nagoyashi, Aichi, Japan), and the Boston Scientific Forte. The performance of this type of wire can be modified by increasing the diameter of the core to increase wire support and torqueability. This may require shortening or eliminating the intermediate coils between the shaft and the floppy tip. Greater trackability and flexibility can be achieved by reducing the diameter of the core, by reducing the abruptness

of the taper (transitionless core), by increasing the length of the taper to extend to the wire tip (core-to-tip), or by changing the shape of the taper (e.g., parabolic taper).

Other modifications to this original design and construction were introduced to further enhance wire performance. Changing the core material to nitinol (e.g., Hi-Torque Balance Middleweight, IQ wire, Cougar), a highly elastic alloy of nickel and titanium, improved the durability (kink resistance) and flexibility of the wire while maintaining a moderate degree of support (Figure 31.14b). The price paid for this improvement may be a reduction in torque control of the tip. Changing the core material to a high tensile strength stainless steel (e.g., Hi-Torque Advance, Asahi Prowater/Rinato) also improved wire durability, shape retention, and torque control. Particularly good torque control is evident in the Asahi family of wires that are based on a unique method of processing the shaft and core as a single piece with a transitionless, core-to-tip taper (Tru-Torque) and eliminating the joint between the stainless steel and the platinum coil segments at the tip.

Polymer-coated wires

To maximize trackability, wires have been developed with polymer sleeves coating the distal tip (Figure 31.14c). These include wires with polymer-coated coils (e.g., Hi-Torque Whisper, Advance, Fielder, and Pilot wires), those with polymer-coated core wires (e.g., PT², PT Graphix, and ChoICE PT wires), and hybrid combinations of both (BMW Universal, Hi-Torque All Star) (Tables 31.1 through 31.4).

Table 31.1 Wires suitable for standard anatomy

Wire	Manufacturer	Core	Tip	Tipcoating	Tip stiffness	Rail support
Hi-torque floppy	Abbott	SS	Coil	Silicone	Floppy	Light
BMW	Abbott	SE Nitinol	Coil	Silicone	Floppy	Light
Light/soft	Asahi	SS	Coil	Hybrid	Floppy	Light
Choice floppy	Boston	SS	Coil	Hydrophilic	Floppy	Light
Forte	Boston	SS	Coil	Hydrophilic	Floppy	Light
Zinger	Medtronic	SS	Coil	Hydrophilic	Floppy	Light/mod

Note: SE, superelastic; SS, stainless steel.

Table 31.2 Wires suitable for tortuous arteries

Wire	Manufacturer	Core	Tip	Tip coating	Tip stiffness	Rail support
IQ	Boston	Nitinol	Coil	Silicone	Floppy	Light
Luge	Boston	SS	PCC	Hydrophilic	Floppy	Moderate
PT	Boston	Nitinol	Polymer	Hydrophilic	Intermediate	Light/mod
Prowater (Rinato)	Asahi	HTSS	Coil	Hydrophilic	Floppy	Moderate
Fielder	Asahi	SS	PCC	Hydrophilic	Floppy	Light
Whisper	Abbott	SS	PCC	Hydrophilic	Intermediate	Light/mod
Advance	Abbott	HTSS	PCC	Hydrophilic	Floppy	Light
Wizdom	Cordis	SS	PCC	Silicone	Floppy	Light
Cougar	Medtronic	Nitinol	Coil	Silicone	Floppy	Light/mod

Note: HTSS, high tensile stainless steel; PCC, polymer-coated coil; SS, stainless steel.

Table 31.3 Wires providing extra support

Wire	Manufacturer	Core	Tip	Tip coating	Tip stiffness	Rail support
Extra S'Port	Abbott	SS	Coil	Silicone	Floppy	Extra
Stabilizer Plus	Cordis	SS	Coil	Silicone	Floppy	Extra
Thunder	Medtronic	SS	Coil	Silicone	Floppy	Extra
Ironman	Boston	SS	Coil	Silicone	Floppy	Super
Mailman	Boston	SS	Coil	Hydrophilic	Floppy	Super
Grand Slam	Asahi	SS	Coil	Silicone	Floppy	Super

Note: SS, stainless steel.

Table 31.4 Commonly used wires for coronary chronic total occlusion recanalization

Use		Manufacturer	Name	Tip load	Coating	Cover	Tapered/ non-tapered tip
Antegrade Access and Microchannel Crossing	1	Asahi	Fielder XT	0.8 gr	Hydrophilic	Polymer	Tapered (0.014-in shaft, 0.009-in tip)
	2	Terumo	Runthrough NS Intermediate	3.6 gr	Hydrophilic	None	Non-tapered (0.014-in shaft)
	3	Asahi	SION blue	0.5 gr	Hydrophilic with hydrophobic tip	None	Non-tapered (0.014-in shaft)
Collateral Crossing	1	Asahi	Fielder FC	0.8 gr	Hydrophilic	Polymer	Non-tapered (0.014-in shaft)
	2	Abbott Vascular	Pilot 50	1.5 gr	Hydrophilic	Full polymer	Non-tapered (0.014-in shaft)
	3	Asahi	SION	0.7 gr	Hydrophilic	None	Non-tapered (0.014-in shaft)
	4	Asahi	SION black	0.8 gr	Hydrophilic	Polymer	Non-tapered (0.014-in shaft)
Direct Penetration	1	Asahi	Confianza Pro family	9–20 gr	Hydrophilic with hydrophobic tip	None	Tapered (0.014-in shaft, 0.009-in tip)
	2	Abbott Vascular	Progress 200T	4.1 gr	Hydrophilic, uncoated tip	Intermediate polymer	Tapered (0.014-in shaft, 0.009-in tip)
	3	Asahi	Gaia family	1.7–4.5 gr	Hydrophilic	None	Tapered (0.014-in shaft, 0.010-in–0.011-in–0.012-in tip)
	4	Abbott Vascular	Pilot 200	4.1 gr	Hydrophilic	Full polymer	Non-tapered (0.014-in shaft)
Knuckling	1	Asahi	Fielder XT	0.8 gr	Hydrophilic	Polymer	Tapered (0.014-in shaft, 0.009-in tip)
	2	Abbott Vascular	Pilot 50	1.5 gr	Hydrophilic	Full polymer	Non-tapered (0.014-in shaft)

(Continued)

Table 31.4 (Continued) Commonly used wires for coronary chronic total occlusion recanalization

Use		Manufacturer	Name	Tip load	Coating	Cover	Tapered/non-tapered tip
Lumen ReEntry	1	Asahi	Confianza Pro family	9–20 gr	Hydrophilic with hydrophobic tip	None	Tapered (0.014-in shaft, 0.009-in tip)
	2	Boston Scientific	Stingray wire	12 gr	Hydrophilic	None	Tapered (0.014-in shaft, 0.0035-in tip)
Externalization	1	Asahi	RG3	3 gr	Hydrophilic	None	Tapered (0.014-in shaft, 0.010-in tip)
	2	CSI	Viper-Wire Advance	N/A	Hydrophobic	None	Non-tapered (0.014-in shaft)

Source: Adapted from Green, P., et al., *Eurointervention*, 11, 1077–1079, 2016. With permission of Europa Digital & Publishing.

The polymer is typically impregnated with a material such as tungsten to add radiopacity to the tip. The reduced friction attributable to the polymer sleeve enhances passage of the guidewire through tortuous, severely diseased arterial segments, and through the microchannels of chronic total coronary occlusions. The major disadvantages of the coating are a loss of tactile sense and an increased risk of arterial perforation. Wires without underlying tip coils may be difficult to shape and may have a reduced torque response. Some of these limitations have been addressed with the Hi-Torque Progress family of wires (Abbott Vascular). These have a polymer sleeve coating all but the distal 5 mm of coils that are left bare to improve the tactile feel of the wire and to reduce the risk of perforation (Figure 31.14c).

SPECIFIC PURPOSE WIRES

Angulated lesions

Highly angulated lesions require wires that have exceptional torque control to allow fine movements of the tip. The tip should also be malleable with excellent shape retention. Polymer-coated wires may provide an advantage in very diseased arterial segments but only if torque control and shape retention are not compromised. Wires such as the Fielder and Fielder XT (Asahi) and the Whisper wire (Abbott Vascular) combine the benefits of excellent tip control with a polymer coating and work well in this situation.

Angled bifurcations/tortuous arteries

When the target vessel arises at a considerable angle from an adjacent artery (e.g., retroflexed circumflex, acutely angle OM branch, or stented artery side branch), many wires prolapse into the larger adjacent vessel rather than track around the acute bend. This is particularly true of wires that have an abrupt transition zone or rapidly tapering core. Wires with a transitionless core or long taper are most effective in negotiating bends without prolapse of the wire tip. Suitable wires for this situation include the Luge and IQ wires (BSC), the Advance and Whisper wires (Abbott Vascular), and the Fielder wire (Asahi) (Table 31.2). The major downside to these wires is a reduction in support for delivery of bulky devices.

Calcified tortuous arteries

When strong support is required to deliver a device to a distal lesion in an artery that is calcified or very tortuous, extra support wires are valuable. These typically have a large diameter inner core with a short taper at the tip. The PT2 Moderate Support (Boston Scientific), for example, has a core diameter of 0.097-in compared with 0.075-in in the PT2 Light Support. Other examples of support wires include the Balance Heavyweight (Abbott Vascular), the Stabilizer (Cordis), and the ChoICE PT Extra Support wire (Boston Scientific). Even greater support can be obtained using the Ironman (Boston Scientific), Grand Slam (Asahi), or Mailman (Boston Scientific) wires (Table 31.3). The downside to these very rigid, heavily supportive wires is a tendency to distort angulated segments of the artery causing pleating and potentially even transient closure of the artery. An alternative strategy, if additional support is required, is to place a second wire (buddy wire) alongside the first wire to help straighten curves in the artery and to increase the stability of the guiding catheter.

Subtotal occlusions/short or recent total occlusions

A major stimulus for the development of the plethora of wires currently available was recognition that traditional wires do not adequately address the needs of operators treating CTOs. Considerable effort has been expended in improving our understanding of the pathology of chronic occlusions. For example, the presence of microchannels and partial recanalization has implications for wire selection. For subtotal chronic occlusions, and those with visible microchannels, polymer-coated wires with excellent tip control are very effective. Occlusions due to recent myocardial infarction (MI) can usually be crossed readily with a soft or floppy tipped wire. Care does need to be taken to avoid dissection due to passage of the wire into the base of an ulcerated or aneurysmal lesion.

Chronic total occlusions

CTOs vary considerably in the duration of occlusion, in the extent of calcification, angulation, and proximal tortuosity, and in the presence of adjacent side branches. As a result, there is no single wire design that is best suited to this subset of lesions. It is commonly necessary to use an array of wires to deal with the specific characteristics of individual lesions. Most chronic occlusions that are more than 6 months old have a proximal fibrous cap that is difficult to penetrate with conventional wires.

Percutaneous methods for treating CTOs may be subdivided into two groups. The first group consists of wire escalation techniques, whereby the coronary guidewire is manipulated through the diseased segment, often with the additional help of a microcatheter or an over-the-wire balloon. Wires with different properties are used at different stages of the procedure. The approach may be either antegrade or retrograde (antegrade wire escalation [AWE] or retrograde wire escalation [RWE]).[18–20]

Wire-based strategies are usually successful in recanalizing simple CTOs, whereas with complex, calcified, or long lesions, more advanced techniques, known as dissection techniques, may be required. The latter techniques entail creating a dissection plane around the lesion, rather than penetrating directly through the lesion. Dissection techniques, similarly to wire escalation techniques, may be either antegrade or retrograde.[18–21] Dissection through or around the occlusion, whether antegrade or retrograde, may be achieved either with a coronary guidewire or with dedicated equipment (CrossBoss; Boston Scientific, Fremont, CA). In the first approach, a looped, polymer-jacket wire (termed *knuckle wire*) is advanced distally without rotation through the chronically occluded segment. The principle underlying this approach is that the knuckled wire, being blunt, will slide under the distensible adventitia layer, without causing perforation. Typically, the leading end of the knuckled wire will be the stiff-to-floppy transition point near the ribbon/coils of the guidewire. The knuckled wire is less likely to be directed into and subsequently perforate small branches. Stiff guidewires, by contrast, may penetrate the adventitia because more force is directed to the relatively small area of the tip. Another dissection-based technique involves using a dedicated catheter system, the CrossBoss catheter. The latter is a metal over-the-wire microcatheter with a rounded tip that is advanced in the subintimal space by rapid rotation by means of a fast-spin

torque device (Figure 31.15). The rounded tip reduces risk of vessel perforation. The hydrophilic coating, coupled with a multiwire coiled shaft, provides precise turn-for-turn response (Figure 31.15).

Re-entering the intravascular space distal to the lesion requires either a standard guidewire (Subintimal Tracking and Reentry [STAR] [20] or Limited Antegrade Subintimal Tracking [LAST]) or specific, dedicated equipment (Stingray balloon and Stingray guidewire; Boston Scientific). The Stingray balloon is a flat balloon with three exit ports connected to the same guidewire lumen (Figure 31.16). Hydrophilic coating on the balloon shaft ensures smooth device delivery, and two radiopaque marker bands facilitate accurate placement and positioning. The self-orienting balloon hugs the vessel once inflated at low pressure (4 atm), automatically positioning one exit port toward the true lumen. Reentry into the true lumen is subsequently achieved with the Stingray guidewire. The latter has an angled tip and distal probe (Figure 31.16). Diametrically opposed and offsetting exit ports enable selective guidewire reentry.

Retrograde and antegrade approaches may be combined.[21] Retrograde dissection reentry (RDR or reverse controlled antegrade and retrograde subintimal tracking [reverse CART]) is an example of such an approach. A microcatheter is navigated retrogradely through collateral vessels from the donor artery and into the CTO segment over a guidewire. Simultaneously, a coronary wire is advanced antegradely into the CTO segment. An angioplasty balloon is advanced over the antegrade wire and placed adjacent to the retrograde microcatheter. When antegrade and retrograde equipment are overlapping, a

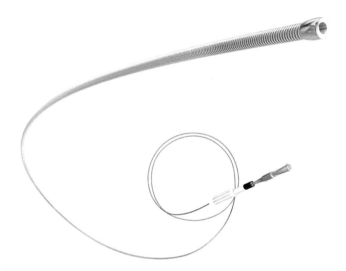

Figure 31.15 The CrossBoss coronary chronic total occlusion crossing catheter (Boston Scientific, Fremont, CA). The CrossBoss is designed to facilitate passage of coronary guidewires via either the true lumen or a subintimal pathway. The rounded tip reduces risk of perforation. A hydrophilic coated, multiwire coiled shaft provides precise turn-for-turn response. The Fast-Spin torque device allows rapid rotation of the catheter to facilitate crossing.

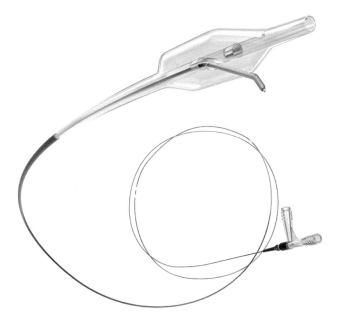

Figure 31.16 The Stingray coronary chronic occlusion reentry system (Boston Scientific, Fremont, CA). The Stingray system, consisting of a self-orienting, flat balloon and diametrically opposed and offsetting exit ports, allows the operator to accurately target and re-enter the true lumen from a subintimal position. Two radiopaque marker bands facilitate accurate placement and positioning. The hydrophilic coating on the balloon shaft ensures smooth device delivery. The balloon, when inflated, hugs the vessel, automatically positioning one exit port toward the true lumen, enabling selective guidewire reentry. The Stingray guidewire has an angled tip for easier reentry into the true lumen.

balloon is inflated, thereby connecting antegrade and retrograde spaces. Before balloon inflation, the antegrade and retrograde systems may reside in the same subadventitial space, within the CTO plaque, or in combination. Balloon angioplasty creates a connection between the two spaces. A retrograde wire can then be passed into the proximal vessel, and wire externalization or retrograde balloon angioplasty can be performed.

With the above techniques in mind, coronary guidewires utilized in the recanalization of CTOs may be classified according to their intended use in each sequence of the CTO crossing process.

For antegrade access to the proximal CTO cap, and for microchannel or soft tissue probing, hydrophilic and/or polymer-jacket 0.0014-in, low gram-force guidewires with a tapered 0.0009-in tip are most useful. The Fielder XT (Asahi Intecc, Nagoya, Japan) and the Runthrough taper wire (Terumo Corporation, Tokyo, Japan) are examples of these classes of wire. Retrograde collateral channel crossing requires nontapered, polymer-jacket hydrophilic 0.014-in coronary guidewires such as the Fielder FC (Asahi intecc), the Pilot family wires (Abbott Vascular, Santa Clara, CA), and/or the Asahi SION family of wires. For dissection techniques utilizing the wire knuckle or loop, the Fielder XT

or FC and the Pilot series wires are most suitable. Direct penetration into the CTO segment requires a moderately high-gram-force (4–6 gr), polymer-jacket, nontapered wire such as the Pilot 200 (Abbott Vascular) guidewire. This wire is also useful for long and complex lesions, knuckling and very tortuous segments with an ambiguous course. Lumen reentry following dissection plane creation often requires a high-gram-force (8–12 gr and above) 0.014-in guidewire, with a tapered 0.009-in nonjacketed tip for direct penetration, such as the Confianza Pro family (Asahi) and the Gaia family (Asahi). Such wires are also useful for cap puncture, complex lesion crossing, and various penetration techniques. The Stingray guidewire (Boston Scientific) is also specifically designed for lumen reentry, as described above. Finally, externalization of the retrograde wire is achieved by the use of a long wire through a (retrograde) microcatheter, into the antegrade guide catheter and out of the antegrade guide hub. The Viper-Wire Advance guidewire (CSI, St. Paul, MN) is 335 cm long, provides excellent support, and is the preferred wire for externalization for many operators.

Suggested recommendations of preferred wires for each CTO technique are given in Table 31.4.

OTHER SPECIALTY WIRES

Wiggle wire

This has a series of corrugations in the distal wire to promote passage of the wire and balloon catheter through heavily calcified or previously stented lesions (Figure 31.14d). The angulated segment of the wire displaces it from the wall or the stent struts allowing free movement of the wire and balloon.

ROTAWIRE

This dedicated rotational atherectomy wire has a 0.009-in shaft that tapers to 0.005-in distally. Attached to the tip is a 2.2 or 2.8 cm long, 0.014-in diameter spring coil tip. Floppy and Extra Support versions of the wire are available.

Fractional flow reserve guidewires

Coronary fractional flow reserve (FFR) measurements have traditionally been performed with a 0.014-in guidewire incorporating a piezoelectric pressure sensor in its distal end (e.g., Certus; St. Jude Medical, St. Paul, MN; Primewire Prestige; Volcano Corp, San Diego, CA). The FFR guidewire shaft is a thin-walled hollow tube separated from the tapered tip by the rigid housing unit for the piezoelectric pressure sensor (Figure 31.17). The abrupt transition around the solid rigid housing element makes the wire prone to kinking, diminishes torque control, and makes it difficult to deliver through tortuous vessels. A recent innovation in FFR delivery systems consists of the RXi system (ACIST Medical Systems, Eden Prairie, MN). With the RXi system, FFR measurements are performed, thanks to an optical pressure sensor located on the distal tip of an ultrathin

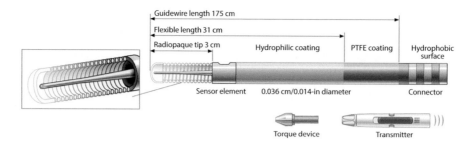

Figure 31.17 The St Jude Medical Systems coronary fractional flow reserve guidewire. St Jude FFR coronary guidewire. The FFR guidewire shaft is a thin-walled hollow tube separated from the tapered tip by the rigid housing unit for the piezoelectric pressure sensor. PTFE, polytetrafluoroethylene.

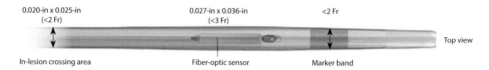

Figure 31.18 RXi fractional flow reserve microcatheter. With the RXi system, FFR measurements are performed thanks to an optical pressure sensor located on the distal tip of an ultrathin monorail microcatheter.

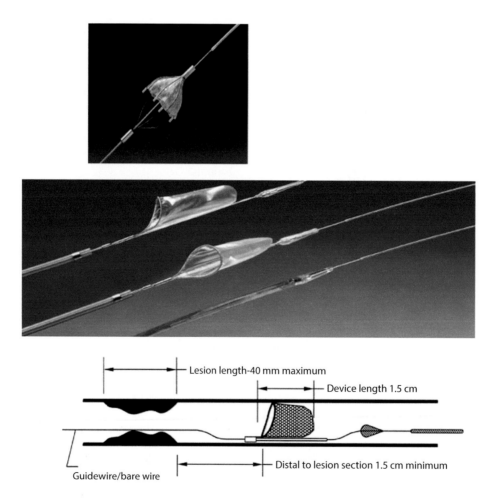

Figure 31.19 AngioGuard (upper panel) and FilterWire (lower two panels) distal protection devices. (Courtesy of Cordis Corporation and Boston Scientific, respectively.)

monorail microcatheter (Navvus; ACIST Medical Systems) (Figure 31.18). Unlike the traditional FFR guidewire systems, the ACIST system allows the operator to choose the coronary guidewire best suited to the patient's coronary anatomy. The disadvantage of the ACIST system is the larger diameter of the catheter (0.022-in diameter, compared with the 0.014-in guidewire).

DISTAL PROTECTION WIRES

Balloon dilatation and stenting of coronary or peripheral stenoses may liberate embolic material causing ischemic injury to the distal bed. Numerous guiding wires designed to collect and retrieve embolic debris are now available (Figure 31.19).[22] The shaft of the wires is usually sufficiently robust to allow stenting in most situations. If greater support is required, a buddy wire system can be used.

CONCLUSIONS

Although a vast and potentially daunting array of guiding catheter and guidewire designs are currently available, most coronary interventions can be performed with a small number of safe and reliable workhorse guides and wires. Specialty wires and guides should be used less frequently to treat the specific lesions for which they were designed.

REFERENCES

1. Casserly IP, Franco I. Guides and wires in percutaneous coronary intervention. In: Ellis SG, Holmes DR, eds. *Strategic approaches in coronary intervention.* 3rd edn. Philadelphia, PA: Lippincott Williams and Wilkins 2006;91–100.
2. Kimbiris D, et al. Anomalous aortic origin of coronary arteries. *Circulation* 1978;58:606–615.
3. Ikari Y, et al. Initial characterization of Ikari Guide catheter for transradial coronary intervention. *J Invasive Cardiol* 2004;16(2):65–68.
4. Mamas M, et al. Use of the sheathless guide catheter during routine transradial percutaneous coronary intervention: A feasibility study. *Catheter Cardiovasc Interv* 2010;75:596–602.
5. Harding SA, et al. Complex transradial percutaneous coronary intervention using a sheathless guide catheter. *Heart Lung Circ* 2013;22:188–192.
6. Miyasaka M, et al. Sheathless guide catheter in transradial percutaneous coronary intervention for ST-segment elevation myocardial infarction. *Catheter Cardiovasc Interv* 2016;7(6):1111–1117.
7. Sciahbasi A, et al. Transradial percutaneous coronary interventions using sheathless guiding catheters: A multicenter registry. *J Interv Cardiol* 2011;24:407–412.
8. Cheaito R, et al. Multicentric experience with the use of sheathless 6.5 french-size catheter in coronary angioplasty for bifurcation lesions: Feasibility and safety. *Ann Cardiol Angiol* 2012;61:405–412.
9. Di Mario C, Ramasami N. Techniques to enhance guide catheter support. *Catheter Cardiovasc Interv* 2008;72:505–512.
10. Saucedo JF, et al. Facilitated passage of the palmaz-schatz stent delivery system with the use of an adjacent 0.018″ stiff wire. *Cathet Cardiovasc Diagn* 1996;39:106–110.
11. De Man F, et al. Usefulness and safety of the guideliner catheter to enhance intubation and support of guide catheter: Insights from the Twente GuideLiner registry. *Eurointervention* 2012;20(8):336–344.
12. Kovacic J, et al. GuideLiner mother-and-child guide catheter extension: A simple adjunctive tool in PCI for balloon uncrossable chronic total occlusions. *J Interven Cardiol* 2013;26:343–350.
13. Duong T, et al. Frequency, indications, and outcomes of guide catheter extension use in percutaneous coronary interventions. *J Invasive Cardiol* 2015;27:E211–E215.
14. Gruntzig AR. Transluminal dilatation of coronary artery stenoses. *Lancet* 1978;1:263.
15. Kent KM, et al. Percutaneous transluminal coronary angioplasty: Report from the Registry of the National Heart, Lung, and Blood Institute PTCA Registry. *Am J Cardiol* 1982;49:2011–2020.
16. Simpson JB, et al. New catheter system for coronary angioplasty. *Am J Cardiol* 1982;49:1216–1222.
17. Detre K, et al. Percutaneous transluminal coronary angioplasty in 1985–1968 and 1977–1981. The NHLBI PTCA Registry. *N Engl J Med* 1988;318:265–270.
18. Green P, et al. Tools and techniques—clinical update on coronary guidewires 2016: Chronic total occlusions. *Eurointervention* 2016;11:1077–1079.
19. Brilakis E, et al. A percutaneous treatment algorithm for crossing coronary chronic total occlusions. *JACC Cardiovasc Interv* 2012;5:367–397.
20. Colombo A, et al. Treating chronic total occlusions using subintimal tracking and reentry: The STAR technique. *Catheter Cardiovsc Int* 2005;64:407–411.
21. Joyal D, et al. The retrograde technique for recanalization of chronic total occlusions. *JACC Interv* 2012;5:1–11.
22. Morís C, et al. Embolic protection in saphenous percutaneous interventions. *EuroIntervention* 2009;5:D45–D50.

32

Coronary artery stenting

RAFFAELE PICCOLO AND STEPHAN WINDECKER

INTRODUCTION

The safety and efficacy of percutaneous coronary intervention (PCI) has continuously improved since its inception nearly 40 years ago. The breathtaking growth of PCI reflects its widespread acceptance as the preferred revascularization strategy, surpassing coronary artery bypass graft surgery (CABG). Stents have remarkably improved the safety of PCI by reducing periprocedural acute closure due to coronary dissection[1] and the need for emergent CABG.[2]

The basic principles underlying short-term efficacy are common to all coronary stents and include the following:

1. Increasing the arterial lumen by scaffolding the arterial wall
2. Fixating intimal flaps between the stent surface and arterial wall
3. Sealing medial dissections

Historical perspective

The word *stent* was coined in 1916 by Jan F. Esser, a Dutch plastic surgeon, and referred to a dental impression compound developed formerly by Charles Thomas Stent. The first vascular stent was developed and implanted in 1968 by Charles Dotter in a canine popliteal artery.[3]

The first coronary stent resulted from discussions between two Swedish expatriates in Switzerland: Hans Wallsten, a paper engineer, and Ake Senning, the chief cardiac surgeon collaborating with Andreas Grüntzig during the first coronary angioplasty procedures in Zurich. The first coronary stent (Wallstent) was self-expanding and was developed by Medinvent in cooperation with Ulrich Sigwart. It was first implanted in March 1986 by Jacques Puel (Toulouse, France) in a 63-year-old male suffering from restenosis after balloon angioplasty of the left anterior descending (LAD) artery. The first bailout stenting was performed by Ulrich Sigwart during a live course (Lausanne, Switzerland) in June 1986 in a 50-year-old female suffering from occlusive dissection of the LAD artery after balloon angioplasty (Figure 32.1). Shortly after these successful procedures, an unanticipated bane of stent implantation emerged: stent thrombosis. To limit this serious complication, aggressive anticoagulant regimens were introduced.

GIANTURCO–ROUBIN STENT

The Gianturco–Roubin stent, a balloon-expandable stent, had a coil design manufactured from a single strand of stainless steel wire.[4] The stent was approved in the United States in 1993 for the treatment of coronary dissection during balloon angioplasty. Similar to the Wallstent, the Gianturco–Roubin stent had a great degree of flexibility but poor radial strength, resulting in increased rates of restenosis and stent thrombosis.

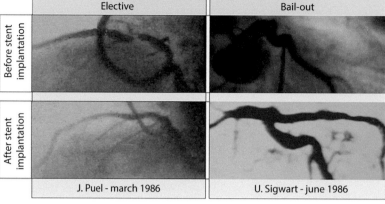

Figure 32.1 The first coronary stent implantations.

PALMAZ–SCHATZ STENT

In the late 1980s, Julio Palmaz, an Argentine radiologist, designed a vascular stent from a model taken from a piece of lathed metal. Together with Richard Schatz, a cardiologist from San Antonio, Texas, he modified the initial version of this prototype into the first tubular slotted balloon-expandable stent. In October 1987, the first peripheral Palmaz stent was implanted in Freiburg, Germany, and in December of the same year, the first Palmaz–Schatz coronary stent was implanted in São Paulo, Brazil. The stents were crimped on the coronary angioplasty balloon by the interventional cardiologists, a method that was prone to stent loss.

IMPROVEMENT OF BARE-METAL STENTS AND ANTIPLATELET REGIMEN

The widespread acceptance of coronary artery stenting resulted from the Belgian Netherlands STENT (BENESTENT)[5] and the Stent Restenosis Study (STRESS)[6] trials, which showed superiority of coronary stents compared with balloon angioplasty in reducing the risk of restenosis and the need for repeat revascularization. Since then, tremendous progress has been made in improving stent material, design, and processing, resulting in superior deliverability and procedural success. The improved results with coronary artery stenting over time were also related to expansion of the indications for stent implantation and the insight that dual antiplatelet therapy (DAPT), instead of oral anticoagulation, lowered both the incidence of stent thrombosis and hemorrhagic complications. On the basis of their efficacy, coronary artery stents have emerged as the preferred tool for PCI and are currently deployed in more than 90% of procedures.[7]

DRUG-ELUTING STENTS

Drug-eluting stents (DES) were introduced into clinical practice more than 10 years ago. DES deliver site-specific, controlled release of therapeutic agents. Heparin had been used as a stent coating in an attempt to reduce the thrombogenic potential and risk of acute/subacute stent thrombosis.[8] When used in the setting of acute myocardial infarction (AMI), one study showed a reduced rate of stent thrombosis and recurrent myocardial infarction (MI) at 30 days with a heparin-coated stent.[9] Although heparin has anti-inflammatory effects, no effect was observed on restenosis. Sirolimus-eluting stents (SES) were first implanted in 2001 and subsequently became the first DES that significantly reduced the risk of restenosis inherent with bare-metal stents (BMS). This was followed by paclitaxel-eluting stents (PES), which also consistently reduced the rate of restenosis and the need for repeat revascularization procedures compared with BMS. Both of these early generation stents are no longer used in clinical practice.

TECHNICAL CONSIDERATIONS

The key prerequisites for a modern coronary artery stent are as follows:

1. Deliverability with favorable flexibility and low profile
2. Radial strength to prevent elastic recoil (usually <4%) and limit foreshortening (usually <3%)
3. Sufficient plaque coverage (usually 10%–25%) to avoid tissue prolapse
4. Access to side branches with limited stent deformation when opening struts for stent deployment in bifurcation lesions

Bare-metal stents

The available stents may vary in their metallic composition, strut design and thickness, delivery system, and coating. These different parameters play an important role in deliverability, visibility, scaffolding performance, and procedural success.

Some of the parameters can also influence the occurrence of adverse events during the hospital stay (e.g., periprocedural myocardial necrosis, and stent thrombosis) and long-term follow-up (restenosis).[10]

The importance of stent design on acute vascular injury and the subsequent proliferative response are well-established. In animal models, changes in stent design lead to diverse degrees of vascular injury, thrombosis, and neointimal hyperplasia.[11] Furthermore, stents that allow a circular rather than angular vessel lumen lessen neointimal proliferation.[12] However, only a few randomized trials have addressed the role of stent design on clinical outcome. Compared with the Palmaz–Schatz stent, the Gianturco–Roubin II stent was shown to be inferior for the prevention of restenosis.[13] Several second-generation BMS have been directly compared with the Palmaz–Schatz stent in noncomplex lesions without showing differences in terms of stent thrombosis, restenosis, or major adverse cardiac events (MACE).[14–16]

METALLIC COMPOSITION

Stainless steel (316L) was, until recently, the most frequently used component of coronary stents due to its excellent processing characteristics, sufficient radial force, and low elastic recoil (<5%). As a stent material, stainless steel has limitations, including limited radiopacity, reduced flexibility, and a relatively high nickel content that has been linked to an increased risk of restenosis due to allergic reactions.[17] Cobalt chrome (L605 CoCr) alloys have become a more recent alternative and constitute the most frequently used stent material today. L605 CoCr is stronger, more radiopaque, and contains less nickel than 316L stainless steel. As corollary, stents manufactured from L605 CoCr have greater radiographic visibility and thinner struts (with no compromise to radial strength), thereby providing improved deliverability compared with 316L stainless steel stents. Historical data from stainless steel stents suggest that a reduction in strut thickness may be associated with lower rates of restenosis and repeat revascularization.[16,18] However, assessment of neointimal hyperplasia by late lumen loss reveals no superiority of CoCr stents. Experimental data suggest that strut thickness is positively correlated with the propensity for thrombus formation and may therefore impact the risk of stent thrombosis.[19]

More recently, platinum alloys were introduced, offering several distinct advantages over conventional stent materials. Platinum is two times denser than iron or cobalt, malleable, corrosion resistant, fracture resistant, and fully incorporated into the platinum chromium (PtCr) alloy. Consequently, the PtCr stent offers the advantage of increased radiopacity and thinner stent struts. Importantly, initial benchmark studies indicated that, despite these thinner struts, the PtCr alloy stent had better radial strength, lower acute recoil, and better vessel conformability compared to conventional stent platforms. Moreover, the nickel content is reduced when compared with 316L stainless steel, thus reducing the risk of allergic reactions. Notwithstanding, this alloy is only present in a few available platforms.

STRUT DESIGN AND THICKNESS

Basic stent characteristics—coil versus slotted tube versus modular, percent metal coverage, number of struts, strut thickness, and strut morphology—are summarized in Figure 32.2. Currently, most stents have a slotted tube design, which can be further categorized into closed-cell and open-cell design. The closed-cell design provides better coverage of the luminal surface and conveys greater radial strength. Cell size is minimally affected with

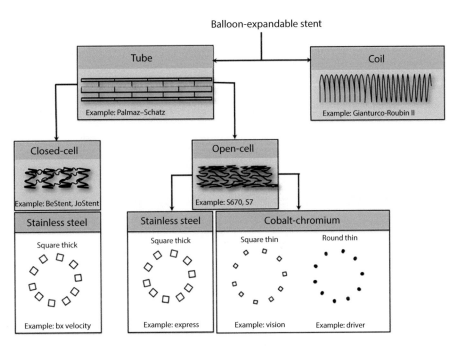

Figure 32.2 Basic stent characteristics.

a closed-cell stent design deployed in a tortuous site. However, it is less flexible and may be more difficult to deliver in tortuous and calcified arteries. In addition, side-branch access may be more challenging. The open-cell design allows for a greater flexibility of the stent and easier access to side branches. The drawbacks are a weaker radial strength, changes in cell size in tortuous anatomy, and less coverage of the lumen, particularly on the outer curvature of the artery. To further improve flexibility, the number of crowns has been increased accompanied by a decrease in strut length and strut thickness. Finally, the geometry of the cross section of the strut has been improved and most of the struts are rounded to limit edge dissections and perforation.

DELIVERY SYSTEM

Many balloon-expandable and a few self-expanding coronary stents have been developed for clinical use over the past several years. None of the self-expanding stents have found broad application in the coronary circulation.

Covered stents

The use of polytetrafluoroethylene (PTFE)-covered stents has been evaluated in saphenous vein graft (SVG) interventions. The rationale is that a covered stent may be able to entrap friable degenerated material, decrease the probability of distal embolization, and reduce neointimal hyperplasia. However, a randomized trial of 400 patients undergoing PCI of SVGs yielded disappointing results, showing no benefit in terms of restenosis or MACE over BMS.[20] In the coronary circulation, the use of covered stents is confined to the emergency treatment of coronary perforations and exclusion of coronary aneurysms.[21] Recently, the PK Papyrus covered stent (Biotronik AG, Bülach, Switzerland), which is

based on a single-layer covered design resulting in a lower crossing profile, has received the Conformité Européene (CE) mark of approval.

Drug-eluting stents

Apart from the delivery system and the platform, which are basically the same as for BMS, DES contain two additional, specific parts: the surface polymer coating and the drug.[22] A schematic representation of coronary stent technologies is summarized in Figure 32.3. With respect to drug elution, the geometric configuration of the platform is critical to accommodate the required dose of the agent on the drug-carrying units (the struts) and to allow adequate diffusion to ensure optimal tissue drug levels. Strut-based drug delivery has been shown to be highly space dependent. Accordingly, an increased strut number has been associated with higher mean arterial wall drug concentrations, and inhomogeneous strut placement has been shown to significantly affect local concentrations.[23]

POLYMERIC DRUG RELEASE

The stent coating consists of one to three layers. The most important layer is the polymer, which contains the drug and allows for drug elution into the arterial wall. Supplemental layers are found in most DES and consist of either top coatings to delay drug release (e.g., poly n-butyl methacrylate [PBMA]) or base coatings to increase polymer adhesion to the stent struts (e.g., Parylene C). While in the early development stage durable (nonbiodegradable) polymers dominated, new-generation stents preferentially use biodegradable polymer carriers. Coatings are typically spray coated or dip coated.

Polymers have been pivotal for the development of local drug delivery, and in particular DES. Polymeric materials

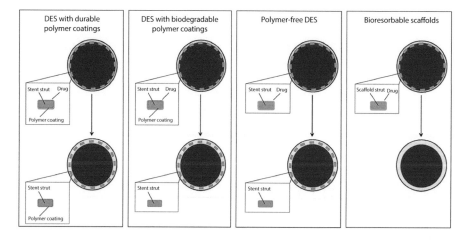

Figure 32.3 Coronary stent technologies. From left to right: Drug-eluting stents (DES) with durable polymer coatings, DES with biodegradable polymer coatings, polymer-free DES, and fully bioresorbable coronary scaffolds. The top panels summarize the features of the coronary cross sections and stent cross sections at the time of implantation, whereas the bottom panels show the same features after the completion of drug release. In the coronary cross sections, the vessel lumen is displayed in red, the intima in yellow, and the stent struts in gray. (Reproduced from Stefanini, G.G., et al., *Heart*, 100, 1051–1061, 2014. With permission.)

act as a drug reservoir and allow for controlled drug release over time. The drug may be dissolved either in a reservoir surrounded by a polymer film or within a polymeric matrix. Controlled drug release can occur by diffusion, chemical reaction, or solvent activation. Biodegradable polymers allow drug release by both drug diffusion and matrix degradation, whereas nondegradable polymers enable drug release by particle dissolution.[24] Early efforts to identify suitable polymers for stent coating were characterized by exuberant inflammatory and thrombotic responses, resulting in excessive neointimal hyperplasia and arterial occlusion.[25] These adverse effects have been attributed in part to inappropriate polymer degradation and the molecular weight of the compounds. More recently, a wide variety of biocompatible polymers, some of which trigger no or minimal inflammatory response, have been developed as carriers for DES. Furthermore, some stents have only an abluminal polymer coating (asymmetric coating) (Figure 32.4). The investigation of new drugs for local delivery therefore mandates addressing not only the drug itself but also the biocompatibility of the polymeric carrier.

NONPOLYMERIC DRUG RELEASE

Attempts to eliminate the polymer as a potential source of adverse events have provoked the development of polymer-free drug carrier systems. Nonpolymeric stents offer the potential advantages of avoiding the long-term adverse effects of a polymer, thereby improving healing and maintaining the integrity of the stent's surface, owing to the absence of a polymer cracking, webbing, and peeling off.

Several different techniques are available to enable drug elution from stents in the absence of a polymer:

- The bioactive substance can be directly attached to the stent surface using covalent bonding, or crystallization/chemical precipitation on the stent surface.
- The bioactive agent can be dissolved in a nonpolymeric biodegradable carrier on the stent surface.
- The bioactive agent in its pure form can be impregnated into the porous surface of the stent, or the stent's body.

RESERVOIR TECHNOLOGY

A third option for drug release is modification of stent design by providing laser cut reservoirs within stent struts, the so-called *reservoir technology*. Each strut may contain several reservoirs, which can be located abluminally or luminally, or feature an entire hole. The drug-filled stent (DFS, Medtronic, Santa Rosa, CA) is a novel polymer-free DES technology that features a novel trilayer wire design, which allows the inner sacrificial layer to become a lumen continuously coated with a drug. The drug (sirolimus) is contained on the inside of the stent and is released from a single continuous inner lumen through multiple laser-drilled holes on the abluminal side (outer surface) of the stent. Drug elution is controlled and sustained through passive diffusion via direct interaction with the vessel wall with an elution profile comparable to durable-polymer DES. Preliminary results of the RevElution study showed excellent strut coverage and low occurrence of malapposition among 14 patients undergoing optical coherence tomography (OCT) at 1-month follow-up.[26]

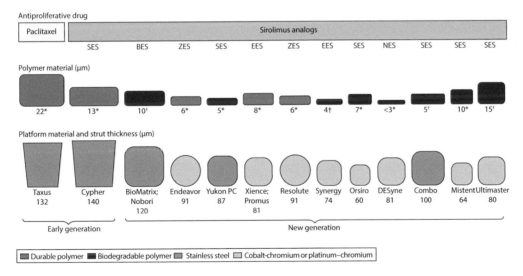

Figure 32.4 Type and composition of available metallic drug-eluting stents. Taxus and Cypher represent early generation drug-eluting stents. All other devices are regarded as new-generation drug-eluting stents, which were developed featuring thinner stent struts, more biocompatibility or biodegradable polymers, and different antiproliferative drugs than Taxus and Cypher. Boston Scientific (Marlborough, MA) makes Taxus, Promus, and Synergy. Cordis (Eastbridgewater, NJ) makes Cypher. Biosensors International Ltd. (Jalan Tukang, Singapore) makes BioMatrix. Terumo (Tokyo, Japan) makes Nobori and Ultimaster. Medtronic (Minneapolis, MN) makes Endeavor and Resolute. Translumina (Hechnigen, Germany) makes Yukon PC. Abbott Vascular (Santa Clara, CA) makes Xience. Biotronik (Berlin, Germany) makes Orsiro. Elixir Medical Corporation (Sunnyvale, CA) makes DESyne. Orbus Neich (Hong Kong, China) makes Combo. Micell Technologies (Durham NC) makes Mistent. BES, biolimus-eluting stent; EES, everolimus-eluting stent; NES; novolimus-eluting stent; SES, sirolimus-eluting stent; ZES, zotarolimus-eluting stent. *Circumferential. †Abluminal. (Reproduced from Piccolo, R., et al., *Lancet*, 386, 702–713, 2015. With permission.)

DRUG

The drug aims to limit neointimal proliferation, and the drug's ideal profile should be characterized by:

1. A wide therapeutic window
2. Low inflammatory potential
3. Selectivity for smooth muscle cell proliferation without toxicity to the medial and adventitial cell layers
4. Promotion of re-endothelialization

The efficacy of candidate drugs is not only dependent on biological activity *in vitro* but is also determined by local pharmacokinetics and physicochemical drug properties. Drug distribution is mediated by stent strut configuration and the balance between convective and diffusive forces.[23] Hydrophilic drugs, such as heparin, readily permeate into tissue but are also rapidly cleared. In contrast, lipophilic agents, such as paclitaxel or limus analogues, are water-insoluble and bind to hydrophobic sites in the arterial wall. Although both hydrophilic and hydrophobic drugs show large spatial concentration gradients in the arterial wall, lipophilic agents distribute better and more homogenously into the arterial wall than hydrophilic drugs. To date, immunosuppressive (limus family) and antiproliferative (paclitaxel) drugs are used.

Most DES use drugs that are analogs of sirolimus (limus family). The principal therapeutic agents of the limus family include sirolimus, zotarolimus, everolimus, biolimus, novolimus, and myolimus. These agents bind to the intracellular receptor FKBP-12 and inhibit a phosphoinositide 3-kinase mammalian target of rapamycin, thereby reversibly inhibiting the growth factor – and cytokine-stimulated cell proliferation in the G1 phase of the cell cycle. Vascular smooth muscle cells are usually quiescent, proliferate at low indices (<0.05%), and remain in the G0 phase of the cell cycle. However, stimulated by vascular injury or growth factors, vascular smooth muscle cells reenter the cell cycle at G1 and advance into S phase.

- *Sirolimus.* Sirolimus, a highly lipophilic drug, was the first member of the limus family to be used for prevention of restenosis following PCI. Following experimental studies showing potent suppression of vascular smooth muscle cell proliferation, local delivery of sirolimus from stents also effectively inhibited neointimal proliferation.[27]
- *Everolimus.* Everolimus is a sirolimus derivative in which the hydroxyl group at position C40 of sirolimus has been alkylated with a 2-hydroxy-ethyl group. It is slightly more lipophilic than sirolimus; therefore, it is more rapidly absorbed into the arterial wall. Although binding of everolimus to the FKBP-12 domain is threefold and immunosuppressive activity *in vitro* two- to five-fold lower than with sirolimus, oral everolimus proved at least as potent as sirolimus in models of autoimmune disease and heart transplantation.[28]
- *Zotarolimus.* Zotarolimus is another sirolimus analog in which the C40 position is modified by a tetrazole ring, resulting in a shorter circulating half-life of the drug. Although the binding affinity to the FKBP 12 domain for zotarolimus and sirolimus is similar and the antiproliferative activities of zotarolimus are also comparable to those of sirolimus, the immunosuppressive activity *in vivo* is three- to four-fold lower.

- *Biolimus-A9.* The chemical structure of Biolimus A9 consists of a 31-membered triene macrolide lactone that preserves the core sirolimus ring structure with a 2-ethoxyethyl group addition to the hydroxy group at position C(40) of the sirolimus molecule. The rationale for the ethoxyethyl group was to increase lipophilicity and, in turn, improve uptake by the coronary vessel wall and reduce risk of systemic immunosuppression and toxicity.[29] Biolimus A9 is used as a matrix together with the polylactic acid (PLA) polymer (15.6 mg each 1 mm stent length in 1:1 ratio) abluminally. Biolimus-A9 eluted from PLA has been used as therapeutic agent on several stent platforms: (1) Biomatrix (Biosensors International Pte Ltd, Singapore); (2) Biofreedom (Biosensors International Pte Ltd, Singapore); (3) Nobori (Terumo Corporation, Tokyo, Japan); (4) Axxess bifurcation stent (Biosensors International Pte Ltd, Singapore); and (5) the Xtent modular system (Xtent, Inc, Menlo Park CA) with multiple, interdigitated 6 mm CoCr stent segments. The BioMatrix biolimus-eluting stent (BES) is coated by an automated autopipette proprietary technology, whereas the Nobori BES is not coated using an automated process. Furthermore, the BioMatrix Flex BES has no parylene coating, whereas Biomatrix and Biomatrix II BES share the same parylene coating of Nobori BES.
- *Novolimus.* Novolimus is a macrocyclic lactone, which has been developed by removal of a methyl group from carbon C16. Notably, this differs from the other macrocyclic lactone agents that are used in DES, which have mainly been developed through modifications on the carbon C40 of the macrocyclic ring. Nevertheless, in a similar fashion to these other agents, novolimus inhibits the mechanistic target of rapamycin (mTOR). *In vitro* studies demonstrate it to have a potency to inhibit human smooth muscle cells comparable to that of sirolimus. Novolimus is used on two CoCr–based stents, which have a strut thickness of 81 microns, a drug load of 85 micrograms, and a maximum polymer thickness of 3 microns. The difference between the two stents relate to the polymer; while the Elixir DESyne (Elixir Medical, Sunnyvale, CA) has a durable PBMA polymer, which is similar to that found on the Cypher SES, the Elixir DESyne BD (Elixir Medical, Sunnyvale, CA) has a PLA biodegradable polymer. The polymer facilitates controlled release of novolimus, such that 80% of the drug is released over 12 weeks, with elution complete by 6 months.
- *Myolimus.* Myolimus is macrocyclic lactone that is produced by replacement of the oxygen on C32 of the macrocyclic ring, which has a comparable potency, in terms of inhibition of smooth muscle cells to sirolimus. The myolimus-eluting Elixir stent (Elixir Medical, Sunnyvale, CA) is a CoCr stent with a strut thickness of 80 micron, which is coated with a PLA polymer without any underlying primer coating.
- *Paclitaxel.* Paclitaxel stabilizes polymerized microtubules and enhances microtubule assembly, forming numerous unorganized and decentralized microtubules inside the cytoplasm. As a result, cell replication is inhibited, and this effect is seen predominantly in the G0/G1 and G2/M phases of the cell cycle. Paclitaxel was shown to effectively inhibit vascular smooth muscle cell migration and proliferation.[30] In addition, it has several favorable characteristics for stent-based local drug delivery, such as a high degree of lipophilicity and a long-lasting antiproliferative effect following a single-dose application at low concentrations. In the porcine restenosis model, implantation of stents dip-coated with paclitaxel at

increasing doses resulted in a dose-dependent inhibition of neointimal formation at 28 days. However, the beneficial effects of paclitaxel on neointimal formation were complicated by local cytotoxic effects manifested as a decrease in medial wall thickness, focal neointimal and medial wall hemorrhage, and cell necrosis.[31]

The devices that have been most commonly used for stent-based paclitaxel delivery were the TAXUS Express[2] stent (Boston Scientific, Natick, MA) and TAXUS Liberté, both made of stainless steel and manufactured with the same polymer and dose of paclitaxel. However, the Liberté stent uses a more uniform cell geometry, allowing for enhanced and uniform drug delivery, thinner struts (97 μm vs. 132 μm), a smaller profile, and separate stent designs depending on stent diameter. Paclitaxel has lost its role in newer-generation DES, but is commonly used as an antiproliferative agent released from drug-coated balloons.

DRUG-ELUTING STENT PLATFORMS

Several DES platforms are currently available for clinical use. In this section, we restrict consideration to DES with published evidence of at least one randomized clinical trial. An overview of U.S. Food and Drug Administration (FDA)-approved new-generation DES is provided in Figure 32.5 and Table 32.1. A list of CE-approved DES is reported in Table 32.2.

Early generation drug-eluting stents

SIROLIMUS-ELUTING STENTS

The first SES was the Cypher stent (developed by Cordis Corporation, Warren, NJ). It consisted of sirolimus in a concentration of 140 μg/cm² incorporated in an amalgam of two biostable polymers, with the polymer/drug matrix then applied onto the tubular 316L stainless steel BX Velocity stent. The Cypher stent was the first DES to receive

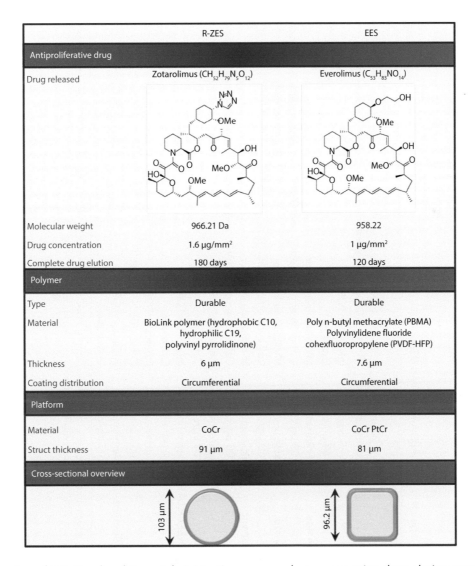

Figure 32.5 Overview of U.S. Food and Drug Administration-approved new-generation drug-eluting stents. CoCr, cobalt chromium; EES, everolimus-eluting stent; PtCr, platinum chromium; R-ZES, resolute zotarolimus-eluting stent. (Reproduced from Piccolo, R., et al., *Circ. Cardiovasc. Interv.*, 8, e002223, 2015. With permission.)

Table 32.1 Specifications of FDA-approved DES

Stent	Drug (concentration)	Drug mechanism	Polymer	Polymer thickness (μm)	Release kinetics (Days)	Metal	Geometry	Strut thickness (μm)
CYPHER	Sirolimus (140 μg/cm²)	Inhibits mTOR Cytostatic	Polyethelyne co-vinyl acetate & PBMA	12.6	80% (28)	SS	Closed-cell	140
TAXUS Express	Paclitaxel (100 μg/cm²)	Microtubule inhibitor Cell cycle arrest in G0/G1 and G2/M	Poly(styrene-b-isobutylene-b-styrene)	16	<10% (28)	SS	Open-cell	132
TAXUS Liberté	Paclitaxel (100 μg/cm²)	Microtubule inhibitor Cell cycle arrest in G0/G1 and G2/M	Poly(styrene-b-isobutylene-b-styrene)	16	<10% (28)	SS	Hybrid	97
TAXUS Element	Paclitaxel (100 μg/cm²)	Microtubule inhibitor Cell cycle arrest in G0/G1 and G2/M	Poly(styrene-b-isobutylene-b-styrene)	15	<10% (90)	PtCr	Open-cell	81
Endeavor	Zotarolimus (100 μg/cm²)	Inhibits mTOR Cytostatic	Phosphorylcholine	4.1	95% (14)	CoCr	Open-cell	91
Endeavor RESOLUTE	Zotarolimus (10 μg/mm)	Inhibits mTOR Cytostatic	Biolinx	4.1	85% (60)	CoCr	Open-cell	91
Xience V	Everolimus (100 μg/cm²)	Inhibits mTOR Cytostatic	PBMA & PVDF-HFP	7	80% (90)	CoCr	Open-cell	81
PROMUS Element	Everolimus (100 μg/cm²)	Inhibits mTOR Cytostatic	PBMA & PVDF-HFP	7	80% (90)	PtCr	Open-cell	81

Note: CoCr, cobalt chromium; DES, drug-eluting stents; FDA, Food and Drug Administration; mTOR, mechanistic target of rapamycin; PBMA, poly n-butyl methacrylate; PtCr, platinum chromium; PVDF-HFP, polyvinylidene fluoride co-hexafluoropropylene; SS, stainless steel.

Table 32.2 List of Conformité Européene (CE)-approved drug-eluting stents and bioresorbable scaffolds

Device name	Producer	Device name	Producer
Absorb	Abbott	MAGICAL	EuroCor
Acrobat SES	Svelte	MiStent	MiCell
Active	Cordynamic	Neo:DrugStar ST	MeoMedical
Amazonia PAX	Minvasys	Nevo	Cordis
Apollo	Intek	Nile PAX and Delta PAX	Minvasys
ARTAX	Aachen Resonance	NOBORI	Terumo
AXXESS	Biosensors	Omega	Globamed
BioFreedom	Biosensors	OPTIMA JET	CID
BioMatrix	Biosensors	ORSIRO	Biotronik
BioMime Aura/Morph	Meril	PARTNER	Lepu
BiOSS Expert	Balton	PAXEL	Balton
BiOSS LIM	Balton	Pico Elite PES	AMG
CARLO S	Balton	PROLIM	Balton
Combo	OrbusNeich	PROMUS	Boston Scientific
Coracto SES	Alvimedica	PROMUS Element	Boston Scientific
Coraxel	Alvimedica	ProTAXX	Vascular Concepts
Coroflex Please	B. Braun	Release-R	Relisys
Coroflex ISAR	B. Braun	Release-T	Relisys
Cre8	CID	Resolute/Resolute Integrity	Medtronic
Cypher/Cypher select	Cordis	Self-Apposing PES	Stentys
DESolve/DESolve 100	Elixir Medical	Sparrow	Biosensors
DESyne BD	Elixir Medical	Supralimus	Sahajanand
DESyne Nx	Elixir Medical	Supralimus-Core	Sahajanand
Endeavor	Medtronic	Synergy	Boston Scientific
Eucatax PES	Eucatech	TAXCOR/TAXCOR Plus	EuroCor
Firebird	Microport	TAXCOR Polymer Free	EuroCor
Genuis TAXCOR	Eurocor	TAXUS Express/Liberté/Element/ION	Boston Scientific
Indolimus	Sahajanand	Ultimaster	Terumo
Infinnium	Sahajanand	Vita Stent	Aachen Resonance
Intrepide	Clearstream	XIENCE V/PRIME/SBA/nano/Xpedition	Abbott
Itrix	AMG	XLIMUS	Cardionovum
Janus	CID	YUKON Choice PC	Translumina
Luc-Chopin2	Balton	YUKON Choice PF	Translumina
M'Sure-S	Multimedics	ZoMaxx	Abbott

CE-mark in April 2002 and was subsequently approved by the FDA in 2003. An analysis of individual data on 4,958 patients enrolled in 14 randomized trials comparing SES with BMS showed a significant 57% relative reduction in the risk of death, MI, or reintervention favoring SES.[32] This benefit was largely driven by a pronounced reduction in the need for repeat revascularization. Despite its efficacy, the use of SES was associated with a higher risk of very late stent thrombosis, particularly in more complex patient and lesion subsets.[33] The manufacturer ceased production at the end of 2011.

PACLITAXEL-ELUTING STENTS

The first TAXUS PES (Boston Scientific, Natick, MA) consisted of paclitaxel contained within a polyolefin derivative biostable polymer coated on the stainless steel near infrared (NIR) platform. The TAXUS PES gained FDA approval in 2004. A meta-analysis of TAXUS-I, TAXUS-II, TAXUS-IV, TAXUS V, and TAXUS VI trials, including 3,513 patients randomly assigned to PES or BMS, revealed that the rate of target lesion revascularization decreased from 20% with BMS to 10.1% with PES at 4 years (HR 0.46, 95% CI: 0.38–0.55, $P < 0.001$).[34] Moreover, the rate of all-cause mortality or MI was similar between patients randomized to PES or BMS (12.4% vs. 11.8%, $P = 0.78$). Similarly, there were no significant differences in the overall rate of stent thrombosis (1.3% vs. 0.9%, $P = 0.30$). However, between 1 and 4 years, the rates of stent thrombosis were significantly increased with PES (0.7% vs. 0.2%, $P = 0.028$).[34]

New-generation drug-eluting stents with durable polymer coating

Table 32.3 summarizes findings from randomized clinical trials comparing new-generation DES with the everolimus-eluting stents.

Everolimus-eluting stents

The Xience everolimus-eluting stent (EES) (Xience V or Xience Prime, Abbott Vascular, Santa Clara, CA) has a strut thickness of 81 µm, and is coated with a 7.6 µm

thick, nonerodible, copolymer of polyvinylidene fluoride co-hexafluoropropylene (PVDF-HFP) and PBMA, which facilitates elution of everolimus over 120 days. This stent was also commercially available until 2012 as the Promus (Boston Scientific, Natick, MA) stent. The Xience EES was CE-marked in 2006 and approved by the FDA in July 2008. Several lines of evidence indicate the Xience EES as the benchmark of safety and efficacy among coronary stent devices.[35] A meta-analysis of five randomized trials comparing EES versus BMS in 4,896 patients showed that EES were associated with a significant reduction of cardiac mortality (HR 0.67, 95%CI 0.49–0.91, $P = 0.01$), MI (HR 0.71,

Table 32.3 Randomized clinical trials comparing new-generation drug-eluting stents vs. everolimus-eluting stents

	N	Primary endpoint	FU (years)	Primary endpoint	TLR	Definite or probable ST
Resolute ZES						
RESOLUTE AC	2,292	Cardiac death, TV-MI, or clinically indicated TLR	5	35.3% vs. 32%, $P = 0.11$	10.2% vs. 8.9%, $P = 0.35$	2.8% vs. 1.8%, $P = 0.12$
TWENTE	1,391	Cardiac death, TV-MI, or clinically indicated TVR	3	12.1% vs. 13.4, $P = 0.50$	5.3% vs. 3.9%, $P = 0.21$	1.4% vs. 1.6%, $P = 0.82$
Platinum–chromium EES						
PLATINUM	1,530	Cardiac death, TV-MI, or clinically indicated TLR	1	2.9% vs. 3.4%, $P = 0.60$	1.9% vs. 1.9%, $P = 0.96$	0.4% vs. 0.4%, $P = 1.00$
BES						
COMPARE II	2,707	Cardiac death, MI, or TVR	3	11.9% vs. 11.1%, $P = 0.54$	5.6% vs. 5.5%, $P = 0.88$	1.3% vs. 1.4%, $P = 0.76$
NEXT	3,255	Efficacy: TLR. Safety: Cardiac death or MI	3	9.9% vs. 10.3%, $P = 0.7^*$	7.1% vs. 7.4%, $P = 0.8$	0.31% vs. 0.26, $P = 0.74^†$
BASKET-PROVE II	1,530	Cardiac death, MI, or clinically indicated TVR	2	7.6% vs. 6.8%, $P = 0.58$	5.0% vs. 4.7%, $P = 0.84^¥$	0.4% vs. 0.7%, $P = 0.48$
Yukon SES						
ISAR TEST 4	1,951	Cardiac death, TV-MI, or TLR	5	20.5% vs. 19.5%, $P = 0.71$	13.9% vs. 12.6%, $P = 0.46$	1.2% vs. 1.4%, $P = 0.67$
Orsiro SES						
BIOSCIENCE	2,119	Cardiac death, TV-MI, or clinically indicated TLR	1	6.7% vs. 6.7%, $P = 0.95$	4.0% vs. 3.1%, $P = 0.27$	1.8% vs. 2.2%, $P = 0.53$
Synergy EES						
EVOLVE II‡	1,648	Cardiac death, TV-MI, or clinically indicated TLR	1	6.2% vs. 6.7%, $P = 0.83$	2.6% vs. 1.7%, $P = 0.21$	0.4% vs. 0.6%, $P = 0.50$
Ultimaster SES						
CENTURY II	1,123	Cardiac death, TV-MI, or clinically indicated TLR	1	4.4% vs. 4.9%, $P = 0.66$	2.2% vs. 1.6, $P = 0.51$	0.9% vs. 0.9%, $P = 0.99$

Source: Only studies with a primary clinical endpoint are reported. Non-inferiority was established in all randomized trials.

Note: BES, biolimus-eluting stent; DES, drug-eluting eluting stent; EES, everolimus-eluting stent; FU, follow-up; MI, myocardial infarction; SES, sirolimus-eluting stent; ST, stent thrombosis; TLR, target lesion revascularization; TV, target vessel; TVR, target vessel revascularization; ZES, zotarolimus-eluting stent.

* Cardiac death or MI.
† Definite ST.
‡ Non-inferiority established with the platinum chromium EES.
¥ Rates of TVR are reported.

95%CI 0.55–0.92, $P = 0.01$), definite stent thrombosis (HR 0.41, 95%CI 0.22–0.76, $P = 0.005$), and target vessel revascularization (HR 0.29, 95%CI 0.20–0.41, $P < 0.001$) at a median follow-up of 2 years.[36] Consistently, other meta-analyses comparing EES with early generation SES and PES found improved safety and efficacy with EES.[37,38] Of interest, a network meta-analysis of 51 trials ($n = 52,158$) reported a reduction in the risk of mortality for EES compared with BMS (HR 0.81, 95%CI 0.64–1), PES (HR 0.81, 95%CI 0.68–1), and SES (HR 0.70, 95%CI 0.70–1).[39] Another larger network meta-analysis of 113 trials with 90,584 patients showed that EES were associated with the lowest risk of stent thrombosis compared with all stents, including biodegradable polymer BES at all times after stent implantation.[40] The use of EES among patients with ST-segment elevation myocardial infarction (STEMI) undergoing primary PCI has been tested in the EXAMINATION trial.[41] At 5-year follow-up, the trial demonstrated a significant reduction in the risk of the primary composite endpoint of all-cause death, any MI, or any revascularization favoring EES compared with BMS (HR 0.80, 95%CI 0.65–0.98, $P = 0.033$).[42] Several other trials have tested newer DES platforms against the EES, which served as control arm. The most relevant results of such studies are reported in the following paragraphs describing other new-generation DES.

ZOTAROLIMUS-ELUTING STENTS

Two stents eluting zotarolimus have been introduced. Both are based on the Driver stent platform (Medtronic, Inc., Minneapolis, MN) with a strut thickness of 91 μm made of a CoCr alloy, and have coatings with both hydrophilic and hydrophobic moieties. The FDA-approved Endeavor zotarolimus-eluting stent (ZES) (E-ZES) is absorbed into a 5-μm-thick phosphorylcholine layer with a zotarolimus concentration of approximately 1.6 μg/mm^2 stent surface area. In contrast to the sirolimus-eluting Cypher stent, which elutes approximately 80% of its drug during the first 30 days, the Endeavor stent releases the same proportion of zotarolimus within only 10 days. The Resolute ZES (R-ZES) uses the BioLinx polymer system for release of zotarolimus from the Driver stent platform. BioLinx consists of three polymers, a hydrophilic C19 polymer, water-soluble polyvinyl pyrrolidinone (PVP), and a hydrophobic C10 polymer and allows for a more delayed release of the same zotarolimus concentration as on the original Endeavor stent (1.6 μg/mm^2 stent surface area) with approximately 50% of the drug released during the first 7 days, and 85% of the drug released at 60 days after stent implantation.

Although the ENDEVOR II trial ($n = 1197$) demonstrated a greater antirestenotic efficacy of the E-ZES compared with BMS,[43] the SORT-OUT III ($n = 2332$) and the PROTECT ($n = 8800$) trials reported a higher risk of target lesion revascularization with E-ZES compared with SES during the first year of follow-up. Thereafter, the efficacy of E-ZES and SES were comparable, but the E-ZES was associated with a lower risk of very late stent thrombosis.[44,45] However, results from an adjusted indirect comparison showed that R-ZES

significantly reduced the risk of target vessel revascularization compared with E-ZES (odds ratio, OR, 0.54, 95%CI 0.37 to 0.78, $P = 0.001$).[46] The efficacy and safety of R-ZES compared with EES has been investigated in five randomized trials including a total of 9,899 patients. A pooled meta-analysis of these trials at longest available follow-up reported a similar risk of target vessel revascularization (risk ratio, RR, 1.06, 95%CI, 0.90–1.24, $P = 0.50$), definite or probable stent thrombosis (RR, 1.26, 95%CI, 0.86–1.85, $P = 0.24$), cardiac death (RR, 1.01; 95%CI, 0.79–1.30; $P = 0.91$), and target vessel MI (RR, 1.10, 95%CI, 0.89–1.36, $P = 0.39$). Moreover, R-ZES and EES had similar risks of late definite or probable very late stent thrombosis (RR, 1.06, 95%CI, 0.53–2.11, $P = 0.87$).[47] Taken together, these data support an equivalent efficacy and safety profile of the two FDA-approved, new-generation DES.

PROMUS ELEMENT EVEROLIMUS-ELUTING STENT

The PROMUS Element stent (Boston Scientific, Natick, MA) has a PtCr platform, a PBMA primer coating, a PVDF-HFP polymer, and is loaded with 1 μg/mm^2 of everolimus, 80% of which is eluted within 90 days of stent implantation. Three randomized studies proved the noninferiority of the Promus Element EES compared with the Promus Xience V EES (PLATINUM trial, $n = 1532$) and R-ZES (DUTCH PEERS, $n = 1811$; HOST-ASSURE, $n = 3755$).[48–50] Since in both DUTCH PEERS and HOST ASSURE trials there were 16 cases of longitudinal stent deformation in the EES arm, the PROMUS Premier was recently introduced. This new platform has undergone a design modification consisting of additional proximal connectors to reinforce longitudinal strength in the area where distortions most frequently occur.

NOVOLIMUS-ELUTING STENT

The performance of the novolimus-eluting stent (NES) has been assessed in a first-in-man study ($n = 15$) and in the EXCELLA II study, which randomized (2:1) a total of 210 patients to NES or E-ZES. At 9 months, the in-stent late lumen loss was significantly lower in the NES arm (0.11 ± 0.32 mm vs. 0.63 ± 0.42 mm, NES vs. E-ZES, $P < 0.0001$). However, there was no significant difference in the device-oriented endpoints (2.9% versus 5.6%, NES vs. E-ZES, $P = 0.45$).[51] At 5-year follow-up, patients in the NES group had a significantly lower incidence of the patient-oriented (HR 0.53, 95% CI: 0.32–0.87, $P = 0.013$) and device-oriented (HR 0.38, 95% CI: 0.17–0.83, $P = 0.011$) composite endpoints, mainly driven by a trend toward reduction in MI and repeat revascularization in the NES group.[52]

New-generation drug-eluting stents with biodegradable polymer coating

BIOLIMUS-ELUTING STENTS

Three large trials have evaluated the performance of the Biomatrix BES: the LEADERS, COMFORTABLE-AMI, and SORT-OUT VI trials. The LEADERS ($n = 1707$) reported at

5 years the noninferiority of BES compared with SES for the primary endpoint of cardiac death, MI, or clinically indicated target vessel revascularization (22.3% vs. 26.1%, p for noninferiority <0.001; p for superiority = 0.069). Of interest, BES was associated with a significant reduction in very late stent thrombosis between 1 and 5 years (0.7% vs. 2.5%, P = 0.003).[53] The COMFORTABLE-AMI trial (n = 1161) demonstrated the superiority of BES over BMS in patients with STEMI.[54] At year 2, the rate of major adverse events was significantly lower in the BES group (5.8% vs. 11.9%, P < 0.001), with clinical differences mainly driven by a significantly reduced risk for the composite of cardiac death or target vessel reinfarction (4.2% vs. 7.2%, P = 0.036), as well as target vessel reinfarction (BES 1.3% vs. BMS 3.4%, P = 0.0023), and ischemia-driven target lesion revascularization (3.1% vs. 8.2%, P < 0.001).[55] The SORT-OUT VI trial (n = 2999) demonstrated the noninferiority of Biomatrix BES with R-ZES at 12-month follow-up, with respect to the primary composite endpoint of cardiac death, target vessel MI, and target lesion revascularization (5% vs. 5.3%, p for noninferiority = 0.004).[56] The individual components of the primary endpoint did not differ significantly between stent types at 12 months.

The Nobori BES has been compared with SES (Nobori Japan, n = 335; SORT-OUT V, n = 2468), PES (Nobori I Phase 1, n = 120; Nobori I Phase 2, n = 243), and EES (COMPARE II, n = 2707; NEXT, n = 3235).[29] A meta-analysis of these trials comparing the Nobori BES with other DES (early and new-generation DES) found a comparable risk of target lesion revascularization (OR 0.94, 95%CI 0.66–1.34, P = 0.74), mortality (OR 1, 95%CI 0.78–1.28, P = 0.98), MI (OR 1.10, 95%CI 0.87–1.40, P = 0.42), and definite or probable stent thrombosis (OR 1.01, 95%CI 0.45–2.29, P = 0.99).[57] However, the Nobori BES significantly reduced the risk of target lesion revascularization compared with PES (OR 0.31, 95%CI 0.10–0.90, P = 0.03).[57] The 3-year follow-up of the COMPARE II trial reported a similar rate of MACE in patients randomized to BES vs. EES (11.9% vs. 11.1%, P = 0.57) with a comparable occurrence of death or MI (9.3% vs. 8.4%, P = 0.52) and target vessel revascularization (7.6% vs. 6.5%, P = 0.52).[58] Along the same line, the 3-year follow-up of the NEXT trial showed an equivalent rate of the primary endpoint of death or MI with BES compared with EES (9.9% vs. 10.3%, P = 0.70), with a similar cumulative incidence of target lesion revascularization (7.4% vs. 7.1%, P = 0.80).[59] In both studies, there was no significant difference in the risk of stent thrombosis between BES and EES.

ORSIRO SIROLIMUS-ELUTING STENT

The Orsiro SES (Biotronik AG, Bülach, Switzerland) combines a biodegradable poly-L-lactic acid (PLLA) polymer with an ultrathin strut CoCr platform (60 μm for stent diameters up to 3 mm, 80 μm for stent diameters >3 mm). Sirolimus is eluted over a period of approximately 100 days. The polymer matrix has an asymmetric design that allows for the release of a greater drug dose on the abluminal than luminal side. Three randomized studies have investigated the efficacy and safety of Orsiro SES. The BIOFLOW-II trial (n = 452) showed angiographic noninferiority of Orsiro SES compared with EES in terms of in-stent late loss at 9 months (0.10 ± 0.32 vs. 0.11 ± 0.29 mm, p for noninferiority <0.001).[60] The BIOSCIENCE trial (n = 2119) demonstrated the noninferiority of Orsiro SES compared with EES for the primary endpoint target lesion failure at 12 months (6.5% vs. 6.6%, p for noninferiority <0.004).[61] Of note, there was a significant interaction for the primary endpoint favoring the use of Orsiro SES in patients with STEMI.[62] At 2 years, the primary endpoint occurred at comparable rate in the Orsiro SES and EES groups (10.5% vs. 10.4%, P = 0.987), with a sustained benefit in the subgroup of patients with AMI.[63] The SORT OUT VII (n = 2525) showed the noninferiority of Orsiro SES compared with the Nobori BES at 12-month follow-up (3.8% vs. 4.6%, p for noninferiority <0.004), and reported a lower rate of definite stent thrombosis in patients randomized to Orsiro SES (0.4% vs. 1.2%, P = 0.03).[64]

ULTIMASTER SIROLIMUS-ELUTING STENT

The Ultimaster SES (Terumo Corporation, Tokyo, Japan) is made of a CoCr bare metal platform with thin struts (80 μm), open-cell design, and a biodegradable polymer (poly-DL-lactic acid [PDLLA] and polycaprolactone copolymer) applied to the abluminal side only. The polymer elutes the drug sirolimus (3.9 μg/mm stent length), which degrades during a period of 3–4 months. The CENTURY II trial (n = 1123) showed the noninferiority of Ultimaster SES compared with EES, with a freedom from target lesion failure, a composite of cardiac death, target vessel MI, and target lesion revascularization of 95.6% with Ultimaster SES and 95.1% with EES (p for noninferiority <.001).[65] The composite of cardiac death and MI rate was 2.9% and 3.8% (P = 0.40), respectively, and target vessel revascularization was 4.5% with Ultimaster SES and 4.2% with the permanent polymer-EES (P = 0.77). The stent thrombosis rate was 0.9% in both arms.[65]

SYNERGY EVEROLIMUS-ELUTING STENT

The SYNERGY stent (Boston Scientific Corporation, Marlborough, MA) is a thin-strut (74–81 μm), PtCr metal alloy platform with an ultrathin (4 μmol/L) biodegradable (D,L-lactide-co-glycolide) abluminal polymer, which elutes everolimus (100 μg/cm²). The EVOLVE I trial (n = 291) found SYNERGY EES to be noninferior to the Promus EES for the angiographic endpoint of in-stent late lumen loss at 6 months.[66] The EVOLVE II included 1,684 patients undergoing PCI for stable coronary artery disease or non-ST-segment elevation acute coronary syndrome randomized to SYNERGY EES or Promus Element EES.[67] At 12 months, the trial demonstrated the noninferiority of two devices (6.7% vs. 6.5%, p for noninferiority = 0.0005), with similar rates of target lesion revascularization (2.6% vs. 1.7%, P = 0.21) and definite or probable stent thrombosis (0.4% vs. 0.6%, P = 0.50).[67]

MISTENT SIROLIMUS-ELUTING STENT

The MiStent (Micell Technologies, Durham, NC) combines sirolimus, polylactide-co-glycolic acid (PLGA), and a CoCr stent platform. PLGA carries a crystalline form of sirolimus. The PLGA-sirolimus combination is eliminated from the stent within 45–60 days and PLGA is fully absorbed within 90 days. Crystalline sirolimus remains in the tissue and continues to elute the drug into the surrounding tissue for up to 9 months. The DESSOLVE II trial (2:1) showed the superiority for in-stent late lumen loss at 9 months for the MiStent compared with E-ZES (0.27 ± 0.46 mm vs. 0.58 ± 0.41 mm, $P < .001$).[68] At year 2, the rate of major adverse events was 6.7% in the MiStent group and 13.3% in the E-ZES group ($P = 0.17$).[68]

COMBO SIROLIMUS-ELUTING STENT

The Combo stent (OrbusNeich Medical, Ft. Lauderdale, FL) is a 100-μm-thick stainless steel stent covered abluminally with a biodegradable polymer matrix allowing a controlled release of sirolimus. An additional circumferential layer of anti-CD34 antibodies is applied on the stent struts on top of the polymer aiming to accelerate endothelial coverage. The Combo stent was tested in the REMEDEE trial, an angiographic noninferiority study that compared in-stent late loss at 9 months between the Combo stent and the Taxus Liberté PES in a total of 183 patients (2:1 randomization).[69] The primary endpoint was met with an in-stent late loss amounting to 0.39 ± 0.45 mm in the Combo compared with 0.44 ± 0.56 mm in the Taxus Liberté stent group (p for noninferiority $= 0.0012$).[69]

TIVOLI SIROLIMUS-ELUTING STENT

The Tivoli SES (EssenTech, Beijing, China) is a thin-strut (80 μm), CoCr metal platform with a PLGA polymer, which elutes sirolimus (8 μg/mm). Approximately 75% of the sirolimus is eluted at 28 days. The I-LOVE-IT 2 trial ($n = 2737$) reported the noninferiority for the primary endpoint target lesion failure at 12 months between the Tivoli SES and the durable polymer Firebird SES (6.3% vs. 6.1%, p for noninferiority $= 0.002$).[70]

Polymer-free, new-generation drug-eluting stents

YUKON SIROLIMUS-ELUTING STENT

The Yukon SES (Translumina, GmbH, Hechingen, Germany) presents a specifically designed surface with micropores (2 μm deep) wherein the antiproliferative agent sirolimus is deposited. The Yukon Choice 4 has a stainless steel platform, while the Yukon Chrome is made of a CoCr alloy. A pooled analysis of ISAR-TEST and LIPSIA Yukon trials ($n = 682$) comparing polymer-free Yukon SES with PES reported a similar in-stent late loss (0.53 mm vs. 0.46 mm, $P = 0.15$), with a comparable risk of target lesion revascularization (13.6% vs. 13.7%, $P = 0.93$), and death or MI (12.4% vs. 12.6%, $P = 0.71$).[71]

BIOFREEDOM BIOLIMUS-ELUTING STENT

The Biofreedom BES (Biosensors International Pte Ltd, Singapore) is made of stainless steel with a strut thickness of 112 μm and a microstructured, polymer-free surface alteration at the abluminal stent side. The investigation of drug release kinetics revealed that >90% of the drug is released within 50 hours with biolimus detectable in neointima and myocardium surrounding stent struts at 28 days. In the LEADERS FREE trial, a total of 2,466 patients at high risk for bleeding were randomized to the Biofreedom BES or BMS.[72] Elderly patients (≥75 years) and indication for oral anticoagulation after PCI were the two most common criteria to qualify for high-risk bleeding status. All patients received 1 month of DAPT. At 390 days, the rate of the primary safety endpoint—a composite of cardiac death, MI, or stent thrombosis—was significantly lower with the Biofreedom BES (9.4% vs. 12.9%, $P = 0.005$). Moreover, Biofreedom BES was associated with a lower risk of target lesion revascularization (5.1% vs. 9.8%, $P < 0.001$).[72]

AMPHILIMUS-ELUTING STENT

The amphilimus-eluting stent (AES) (Cre8, Alvimedica, Istanbul, Turkey) is made of a CoCr alloy with an 80 μm strut thickness and has an ultrathin (0.3 μm) passive carbon coating. The AES does not have polymer, and the antiproliferative drug (sirolimus, 90 μg/cm^2) is loaded into reservoirs, which are dug on the stent's abluminal surface. The sirolimus is formulated with a mixture of long-chain fatty acids (*amphilimus*) to act as a carrier and to control the drug release. Thus, 65 to 70% of the drug is released within the first 30 days, and the remainder is completely eluted by 90 days. In the NEXT trial ($n = 323$), the AES proved both noninferiority and superiority for the primary endpoint of in-stent late loss compared with PES (0.14 ± 0.36 mm vs. 0.34 ± 0.40 mm, p for noninferiority <0.0001, p for superiority <0.0001), with comparable clinical event rates at 12 months.[73] In the RESERVOIR trial, which was conducted in patients with diabetes mellitus ($n = 112$), the AES was noninferior to EES for the primary endpoint of neointimal volume obstruction assessed by OCT at 9-month follow-up ($11.97 \pm 5.94\%$ vs. $16.11 \pm 18.18\%$, p for noninferiority $= 0.0003$).[74]

INDICATIONS FOR CORONARY ARTERY STENTS

The advent of BMS resolved the issue of threatening or abrupt vessel closure following balloon angioplasty, thus eliminating the need for stand-by surgical backup. Subsequently, DES, with the release of antiproliferative drugs during the first months after implantation, successfully addressed the problem of restenosis inherent to BMS due to potent suppression of neointimal hyperplasia. A relevant shortcoming of early generation DES was a delayed healing response of the stented coronary vessel that was associated with a small but notable increase in late thrombotic events. New-generation DES were developed featuring thinner stent struts, novel durable or biodegradable polymer coatings, and different antiproliferative agents at lower dosages. These refinements resulted not only in a significant reduction in the risk of stent thrombosis compared with BMS and early generation DES during long-term follow-up, but also in improved efficacy (lower risk of repeat revascularization) and safety (lower risk of death and MI). Accordingly, new-generation DES represent the standard of care among patients undergoing PCI and are indicated in almost all patient and lesion subsets.[75] Figure 32.6 summarizes the results of a systematic review of 158 randomized trials by showing clinical outcomes at 9–12 months with BMS, early generation DES, and new-generation DES.[76]

Treatment of abrupt or threatened closure after balloon angioplasty

Coronary stents effectively scaffold coronary dissections complicating balloon angioplasty, and the availability of stents has nearly eliminated the need for emergency CABG (<1% of all PCI procedures). The initial approval of coronary stents for this "bailout" indication was based on a multicenter registry of patients with angioplasty complications who were treated with the Gianturco-Roubin II stent.[4]

Stable coronary artery disease

A recent network meta-analysis (100 trials in 93,553 patients) comparing revascularization by means of CABG and several PCI techniques compared with medical therapy found that CABG and new-generation DES (EES: 0.75, 0.59–0.96; R-ZES: 0.65, 0.42–1)—but not balloon angioplasty, BMS, or early generation DES—were associated with improved survival compared with a strategy of initial medical treatment (Figure 32.7). Similarly, the risk of MI was lower with CABG and new-generation DES, an observation confirmed by other studies.[77]

Acute coronary syndromes

Current guidelines indicate new-generation DES as the coronary devices of choice for patients with acute coronary syndrome undergoing PCI.[75,78] Several meta-analyses of randomized trials comparing early generation DES with BMS in patients undergoing primary PCI consistently showed that the benefits of early generation DES, such as a reduction in the risk of target vessel revascularization and a trend toward less definite stent thrombosis, were offset in subsequent years by an increase in the risk of very late stent thrombosis.[33,79,80] Two main trials supported the benefit of new-generation DES over BMS in patients undergoing primary PCI: the COMFORTABLE-AMI (n = 1161) and EXAMINATION (n = 1498).[41,54] A pooled analysis of

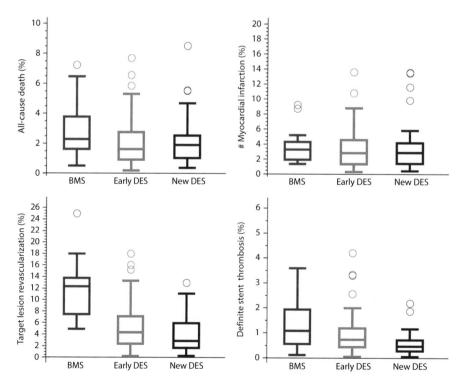

Figure 32.6 Clinical outcomes with bare-metal stents (BMS), early generation drug-eluting stents (DES), and new-generation DES. Clinical outcomes at 9–12 months. Median rates per 100 person-years. Median rates and interquartile range per 100 person-year for the clinical endpoints all-cause death, myocardial infarction, target lesion revascularization, and definite stent thrombosis. (Reproduced from Byrne, R.A., et al. *Eur. Heart J.*, 36, 2608–2620, 2015. With permission.)

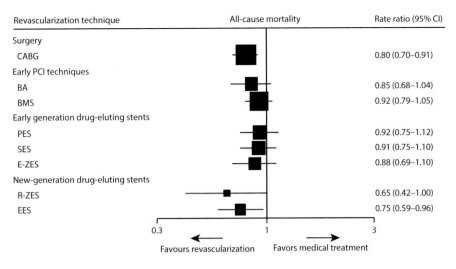

Figure 32.7 All-cause mortality for different revascularization techniques compared with medical treatment. Data are from a network meta-analysis of 100 randomized trials (95,553 patients, 262,090 patient-years follow-up). BA, balloon angioplasty; BMS, bare-metal stents; CABG, coronary artery bypass grafting; EES, everolimus-eluting stent; E-ZES, endeavor zotarolimus-eluting stent; PCI, percutaneous coronary intervention; PES, paclitaxel-eluting stent; R-ZES, resolute zotarolimus-eluting stent; SES, sirolimus-eluting stent. (Reproduced from Piccolo, R., et al., *Lancet*, 386, 702–713, 2015. With permission.)

these two trials reported a significant reduction with new-generation DES in the risk of target lesion revascularization (RR 0.33, 95%CI 0.20–0.52, $P < 0.0001$), target vessel reinfarction (RR 0.36, 95%CI 0.14–0.92, $P = 0.03$), and definite stent thrombosis (RR 0.35, 95%CI 0.16–0.75, $P = 0.006$).[81] The 5-year follow-up data of the EXAMINATION trial showed a significant reduction in the risk of patient-oriented outcomes of all-cause death, any MI, or any revascularization favoring EES compared with BMS (HR 0.80, 95%CI 0.65–0.98, $P = 0.033$).[42]

Diabetes mellitus

Diabetic patients undergoing PCI incur higher rates of restenosis and stent thrombosis following PCI. An alleged benefit of PES in diabetic patients was observed in a pooled analysis of the SPIRIT II, III, IV, and COMPARE trials with a significant interaction for the treatment effect of EES vs. PES according to diabetic status with respect to MI ($P = 0.01$), stent thrombosis ($P = 0.0006$), and target lesion revascularization ($P = 0.02$).[82] However, in a network meta-analysis of 42 randomized trials that compared various stents and included 22,844 patient-years of follow-up of patients with diabetes, EES as compared with other DES and BMS, were found to be the most effective and safe stents, and they had a high probability of being associated with the lowest rate of restenosis, MI, and stent thrombosis.[83] More recently, the TUXEDO trial randomized 1,830 diabetic patients to EES vs. PES.[84] At 1-year follow-up, EES were associated with a lower rate of the primary endpoint of target vessel failure (2.9% vs. 5.6%, $P = 0.005$), along with a significant reduction in spontaneous MI (1.2% vs. 3.2%, $P = 0.004$), stent thrombosis (0.4% vs. 2.1%, $P = 0.002$), and target vessel revascularization (1.2% vs. 3.4%, $P = 0.002$).[84] In aggregate, these

findings support the use of new-generation DES among patients with diabetes.

In-stent restenosis

Although the use of coronary stents for the treatment of in-stent restenosis invariably introduces a new stent layer, new-generation DES are highly effective in the treatment of this lesion subset. A network meta-analysis of 27 trials with 5,923 patients reported a significant reduction in the diameter stenosis at angiographic follow-up with EES compared with drug-coated balloons (–9%, 95%CI –15.8% to –2.2%).[85] The angiographic effectiveness of new-generation DES was particularly evident for the comparison of EES vs. balloon angioplasty (–24.2%, 95%CI –32.2% to –16.4%).[85]

Complex coronary lesions

The likelihood of treatment failure after PCI directly correlates with the complexity of coronary artery disease. Therefore, the treatment effect of new-generation DES may be camouflaged by the overriding effect of underlying coronary artery disease. Nonetheless, a pooled analysis of four trials ($n = 6081$) showed that the efficacy and safety of new-generation over early generation DES not only is preserved across the spectrum of disease, but is also even more evident in patients with increased SYNTAX score.[86]

LEFT MAIN DISEASE

Relevant unprotected left main disease is observed in 5%–7% of patients undergoing coronary angiography. Although no direct randomized trials have compared new-generation vs. early generation DES in this setting, the use of DES is recommended over BMS. A meta-analysis including early generation DES vs. CABG reported no significant difference between the two techniques for the risk of death and MI, but a higher risk of target vessel revascularization with DES and a lower risk of stroke among patients treated with PCI.[87] In the ISAR-LEFT-MAIN 2 trial, patients with left main disease were randomized to R-ZES (n = 324) or EES (n = 326). At 1 year, the composite of death, MI, or target vessel revascularization was not significantly different between R-ZES and EES (17.5% vs. 14.3%, P = 0.25).[88]

CHRONIC TOTAL OCCLUSION

The percutaneous treatment of chronic total occlusion (CTO) is challenged by failure to cross the lesion and restenosis. A meta-analysis of five randomized trials (n = 1077) comparing new-generation vs. early generation DES in patients undergoing PCI of CTO lesions found a lower risk of death (OR 0.37, 95%CI 0.15–0.91, P = 0.03) and target vessel revascularization (OR 0.59, 95%CI 0.40–0.87, P = 0.007) associated with newer devices.[89]

SAPHENOUS VEIN GRAFTS

SVG stenosis after CABG may ensue in up to 50% of patients at year 5. PCI of vein graft stenoses accounts for about 6% of total PCI volume. The ISAR-CABG trial (n = 610) showed a significant reduction in the risk of the primary endpoint of death, MI, or target lesion revascularization at 1 year with DES compared with BMS (15% vs. 22%, P = 0.02), mainly driven by a lower rate of target lesion revascularization (7% vs. 13%, P = 0.01).[90] A retrospective analysis including 2,471 patients undergoing PCI of SVGs reported a similar rate of procedural complications with DES and BMS, but a lower risk of long-term mortality with DES (HR 0.72, 95%CI 0.57–0.89).[91]

BIORESORBABLE VASCULAR SCAFFOLDS

The introduction of bioresorbable vascular scaffolds (BVS/BRS), which provide transient vessel support with drug delivery capability, has represented a further iteration in the field of coronary devices with the potential to overcome the limitations of permanent metallic stents.[92] The concept of BRS is not entirely novel to the field of interventional cardiology since a first clinical description of a fully biodegradable device—the Igaki-Tamai stent (Kyoto Medical Planning Co., Ltd., Kyoto, Japan)—traces back to the early years of the 21st century.[93] There are two main potential advantages of BRS: (1) the reduction of late complications related to permanent implants (i.e., very late stent thrombosis, neoatherosclerosis, late catch-up phenomenon, aneurysm formation); and (2) the restoration of anatomical and physiological properties in the coronary vessel (permanent side-branch occlusion, vessel vasomotion, adaptive shear stress, late luminal enlargement, and late positive remodeling).

Scaffold composition

Current BRS are made of either a polymer or bioresorbable metal alloy. The scaffold composition is of great importance as it entails different chemical compositions, mechanical properties, and subsequent resorption times. The two most frequently used materials in the current generation of BRS are PLLA and magnesium.

POLY-L-LACTIC ACID

PLLA is the most commonly used polymer for BRS and strut thickness generally amounts to 150 μm in PLLA-based BRS. PLLA are degraded through hydrolysis, with the final conversion of lactates into CO_2 and O_2 in the Krebs cycle. However, PLLA degradation is a complex process, which requires months to years.[94] The degradation of PLLA-BRS can be modulated by altering the ratio between semicrystalline and amorphous polymer status.[95]

MAGNESIUM

Magnesium is mixed with rare earth metals to increase radial strength and control the degradation process. Magnesium degradation requires up to 12 months according to its composition, and magnesium-based BRS are finally converted into soft amorphous hydroxyapatite. Of note, magnesium is more electronegative than other materials, and antithrombotic properties related to electronegative charges have been described.

OTHER MATERIALS

Other materials for BRS include tyrosine polycarbonate which require 2–3 years for resorption; it is used in the REVA BRS and REVA ReZolve (Reva Medical, San Diego, CA). Poly-lactic anhydride, which takes approximately 15 months for resorption, is used in the Idea BioStent (Xenogenics Corp, Canton, MA).[96]

Conformité Européene-approved bioresorbable vascular scaffolds

So far, two BRS have received the CE-mark of approval for coronary use: the Absorb vascular scaffold (BVS 1.1, Abbott Vascular, Santa Clara, CA) and the DESolve scaffold (Elixir Medical Corporation, Sunnyvale, CA). However, most clinical data are available for the BVS 1.1, which currently represents the only BRS to have been investigated in randomized trials.

ABSORB BIORESORBABLE VASCULAR SCAFFOLD

The BVS is an everolimus-eluting, balloon-expandable BRS consisting of a PLLA matrix (150 μm) coated with a 1:1 mixture of poly-D,L-lactide and everolimus (8.2 μg/mm). Preclinical and imaging-based studies have shown favorable healing characteristics, with restoration of vasomotor function of the treated segment and a positive vessel remodeling after resorption.[97] Currently, six randomized trials have compared BVS 1.1 with new-generation DES, mainly Xience EES: ABSORB China (n = 480), ABSORB II (n = 501), ABSORB III (n = 2008), ABSORB Japan (n = 400), EVERBIO II (n = 158), and TROFI II (n = 191). A study-level meta-analysis of these trials (n = 3738) showed that

BVS compared with EES had a similar 12-month risk of target lesion failure (OR 1.20, 95%CI 0.90–1.60, $P = 0.21$), target lesion revascularization (OR 0.97, 95%CI 0.66–1.43, $P = 0.87$), MI (OR 1.36, 95%CI 0.98–1.89, $P = 0.06$), and death (OR 0.95, 95%CI 0.45–2, $P = 0.89$).[98] However, patients treated with BVS had a higher risk of definite or probable stent thrombosis than those treated with metallic stents (OR 1.99, 95%CI 1–3.98, $P = 0.05$), with the highest risk observed between 1 and 30 days after implantation (OR 3.11, 95%CI 1.24–7.82, $P = 0.02$).[98] In a patient-level meta-analysis of ABOSORB II, ABSORB Japan, ABOSORB China, and ABSORB III, BVS compared with EES has a similar 1-year risk of patient-oriented (RR 1.09, 95%CI 0.89–1.34, $P = 0.38$) and device-oriented clinical endpoints (RR 1.22, 95%CI 0.91–1.64, $P = 0.17$). However, treatment with BVS was associated with a significantly higher risk of target vessel MI (RR 1.45, 95%CI 1.02–2.07, $P = 0.04$) due in part to a numerically higher rate of periprocedural MI and stent thrombosis (RR 2.09, 95%CI 0.92–4.75, $P = 0.08$).[99] When addressing angiographic efficacy by using the primary endpoint of in-segment late lumen loss, BVS was found to be associated with somewhat greater late lumen loss than metallic DES (0.05 mm; 95%CI 0.01–0.09—data from four studies [$n = 1131$]).[100] Therefore, it seems reasonable to improve procedural techniques for BVS implantation, such as more aggressive plaque modification before BRS deployment, routine use of high-pressure, noncompliant balloon postdilatation to ensure sufficient scaffold expansion, and more frequent use of intravascular imaging.[101]

DESOLVE SCAFFOLD

The DESolve BRS is made of PLLA and elutes a mixture of novolimus and PLLA. The strut thickness is 150 µm (more recently 100 µm) and >95% of the device is resorbed after approximately 1 year. The first-in-man study ($n = 15$) reported a late lumen loss at 6-month angiographic follow-up amounting to 0.19 ± 0.19 mm.[102]

CONCLUSIONS

Coronary artery stents constitute the most important advance in the field of PCI since the introduction of balloon angioplasty. Stents are used in more than 90% of coronary procedures today and have enabled the technique to become one of the most frequently performed therapeutic interventions in medicine. The most important benefit of coronary artery stents has been the effective treatment of abrupt or threatened vessel closure, eliminating the need of emergency bypass surgery required in 5%–8% of patients in the balloon angioplasty era. In addition, the technique of coronary artery stenting has reproducible results and allows for short, minutes-long procedures in uncomplicated cases. Moreover, the ease and predictable outcome in the context of excellent periprocedural safety, as well as cost considerations, contribute to the justification for ad hoc procedures as the preferred approach for patient care. Controlled release

of antiproliferative drugs from polymer coatings immobilized on the stent surface was realized in the form of DES. These devices effectively reduce restenosis and lower the need for repeat revascularization of the target lesion to below 5%. Of note, new-generation DES seem to have overcome the only limitation of first-generation DES—the problem of very late stent thrombosis—thus combining improved safety while maintaining an excellent efficacy profile.

REFERENCES

1. Sigwart U, et al. Intravascular stents to prevent occlusion and restenosis after transluminal angioplasty. *N Engl J Med* 1987;316(12):701–706.
2. Lindsay J, et al. Effects of endoluminal coronary stents on the frequency of coronary artery bypass grafting after unsuccessful percutaneous transluminal coronary vascularization. *Am J Cardiol* 1996;77(8):647–649.
3. Dotter CT. Transluminally-placed coilspring endarterial tube grafts. Long-term patency in canine popliteal artery. *Invest Radiol* 1969;4(5):329–332.
4. Roubin GS, et al. Intracoronary stenting for acute and threatened closure complicating percutaneous transluminal coronary angioplasty. *Circulation* 1992;85(3):916–927.
5. Serruys PW, et al. A comparison of balloon-expandable-stent implantation with balloon angioplasty in patients with coronary artery disease. *New Engl J Med* 1994;331(8):489–495.
6. Fischman DL, et al. A randomized comparison of coronary-stent placement and balloon angioplasty in the treatment of coronary artery disease. *N Engl J Med* 1994;331(8):496–501.
7. Praz L, et al. Percutaneous coronary interventions in Europe in 2005. *Eurointervention* 2007;3(4):442–446.
8. Serruys PW, et al. Randomised comparison of implantation of heparin-coated stents with balloon angioplasty in selected patients with coronary artery disease (Benestent II). *Lancet* 1998;352(9129):673–681.
9. Lev EI, et al. Comparison of outcomes up to six months of Heparin-Coated with noncoated stents after percutaneous coronary intervention for acute myocardial infarction. *Am J Cardiol* 2004;93(6):741–743.
10. Kastrati A, et al. Increased risk of restenosis after placement of gold-coated stents: Results of a randomized trial comparing gold-coated with uncoated steel stents in patients with coronary artery disease. *Circulation* 2000;101(21):2478–2483.
11. Rogers C, Edelman ER. Endovascular stent design dictates experimental restenosis and thrombosis. *Circulation* 1995;91(12):2995–3001.
12. Garasic JM, et al. Stent and artery geometry determine intimal thickening independent of arterial injury. *Circulation* 2000;101(7):812–818.
13. Lansky AJ, et al. Randomized comparison of GR-II stent and Palmaz-Schatz stent for elective treatment of coronary stenoses. *Circulation* 2000;102(12):1364–1368.
14. Baim DS, et al. Final results of a randomized trial comparing the MULTI-LINK stent with the Palmaz-Schatz stent for narrowings in native coronary arteries. *Am J Cardiol* 2001;87(2):157–162.

15. Baim DS, et al. Final results of a randomized trial comparing the NIR stent to the Palmaz-Schatz stent for narrowings in native coronary arteries. *Am J Cardiol* 2001;87(2):152–156.

16. Kastrati A, et al. Intracoronary stenting and angiographic results: Strut thickness effect on restenosis outcome (ISAR-STEREO) trial. *Circulation* 2001;103(23):2816–2821.

17. Koster R, et al. Nickel and molybdenum contact allergies in patients with coronary in-stent restenosis. *Lancet* 2000;356(9245):1895–1897.

18. Pache J, et al. Intracoronary stenting and angiographic results: Strut thickness effect on restenosis outcome (ISAR-STEREO-2) trial. *J Am Coll Cardiol* 2003;41(8):1283–1288.

19. Kolandaivelu K, et al. Stent thrombogenicity early in high-risk interventional settings is driven by stent design and deployment and protected by polymer-drug coatings. *Circulation* 2011;123(13):1400–1409.

20. Turco MA, et al. Pivotal, randomized U.S. study of the Symbiot covered stent system in patients with saphenous vein graft disease: Eight-month angiographic and clinical results from the Symbiot III trial. *Catheter Cardiovasc Interv* 2006;68(3):379–388.

21. Eshtehardi P, et al. Giant coronary artery aneurysm: Imaging findings before and after treatment with a polytetrafluoroethylene-covered stent. *Circ Cardiovasc Interv* 2008;1:85–86.

22. Stefanini GG, et al. Coronary stents: Novel developments. *Heart* 2014;100:1051–1061.

23. Hwang CW, et al. Physiological transport forces govern drug distribution for stent-based delivery. *Circulation* 2001;104(5):600–605.

24. Langer R. New methods of drug delivery. *Science* 1990;249(4976):1527–1533.

25. van der Giessen WJ, et al. Marked inflammatory sequelae to implantation of biodegradable and nonbiodegradable polymers in porcine coronary arteries. *Circulation* 1996;94(7):1690–1697.

26. Worthley S, et al. Stent strut coverage and apposition at 1 and 3 months after implantation of a novel drug-filled coronary stent: First report from the RevElution Study. *J Am Coll Cardiol* 2016;67(13_S):422.

27. Poon M, et al. Overcoming restenosis with sirolimus: From alphabet soup to clinical reality. *Lancet* 2002;359(9306):619–622.

28. Joner M, et al. Endothelial cell recovery between comparator polymer-based drug-eluting stents. *J Am Coll Cardiol* 2008;52(5):333–342.

29. Piccolo R, et al. The Nobori biolimus-eluting stent: Update of available evidence. *Expert Rev Med Devices* 2014;11(3):275–282.

30. Axel DI, et al. Paclitaxel inhibits arterial smooth muscle cell proliferation and migration in vitro and in vivo using local drug delivery. *Circulation* 1997;96(2):636–645.

31. Heldman AW, et al. Paclitaxel stent coating inhibits neointimal hyperplasia at 4 weeks in a porcine model of coronary restenosis. *Circulation* 2001;103(18):2289–2295.

32. Kastrati A, et al. Analysis of 14 trials comparing sirolimus-eluting stents with bare-metal stents. *N Engl J Med* 2007;356:1030–1039.

33. Piccolo R, et al. Long-term clinical outcomes following sirolimus-eluting stent implantation in patients with acute myocardial infarction. A meta-analysis of randomized trials. *Clin Res Cardiol* 2012;101(11):885–893.

34. Stone GW, et al. Safety and efficacy of sirolimus- and paclitaxel-eluting coronary stents. *N Engl J Med* 2007;356(10):998–1008.

35. Palmerini T, et al. Stent thrombosis with drug-eluting and bare-metal stents: Evidence from a comprehensive network meta-analysis. *Lancet* 2012;379(9824):1393–1402.

36. Valgimigli M, et al. Effects of cobalt-chromium everolimus eluting stents or bare metal stent on fatal and non-fatal cardiovascular events: Patient level meta-analysis. *BMJ* 2014;349:g6427.

37. Cassese S, et al. Twelve-month clinical outcomes of everolimus-eluting stent as compared to paclitaxel- and sirolimus-eluting stent in patients undergoing percutaneous coronary interventions. A meta-analysis of randomized clinical trials. *Int J Cardiol* 2011;150(1):84–89.

38. Park KW, et al. Safety and efficacy of everolimus- vs. sirolimus-eluting stents: A systematic review and meta-analysis of 11 randomized trials. *Am Heart J* 2013;165(2):241–250.e4.

39. Palmerini T, et al. Long-term safety of drug-eluting and bare-metal stents: Evidence from a comprehensive network meta-analysis. *J Am Coll Cardiol* 2015;65(23):2496–2507.

40. Kang SH, et al. Biodegradable-polymer drug-eluting stents vs. bare metal stents vs. durable-polymer drug-eluting stents: a systematic review and Bayesian approach network meta-analysis. *Eur Heart J* 2014;35(17):1147–1158.

41. Sabate M, et al. Everolimus-eluting stent vs. bare-metal stent in ST-segment elevation myocardial infarction (EXAMINATION): 1 year results of a randomised controlled trial. *Lancet* 2012;380(9852):1482–1490.

42. Sabate M, et al. Clinical outcomes in patients with ST-segment elevation myocardial infarction treated with everolimus-eluting stents vs. bare-metal stents (EXAMINATION): 5-year results of a randomised trial. *Lancet* 2016;387(10016):357–366.

43. Fajadet J, et al. Randomized, double-blind, multi-center study of the Endeavor zotarolimus-eluting phosphorylcholine-encapsulated stent for treatment of native coronary artery lesions: Clinical and angiographic results of the ENDEAVOR II trial. *Circulation* 2006;114(8):798–806.

44. Maeng M, et al. Differential clinical outcomes after 1 year vs. 5 years in a randomised comparison of zotarolimus-eluting and sirolimus-eluting coronary stents (the SORT OUT III study): A multicentre, open-label, randomised superiority trial. *Lancet* 2014;383(9934):2047–2056.

45. Wijns W, et al. Endeavour zotarolimus-eluting stent reduces stent thrombosis and improves clinical outcomes compared with cypher sirolimus-eluting stent: 4-year results of the PROTECT randomized trial. *Eur Heart J* 2014;35(40):2812–2820.

46. Cassese S, et al. Two zotarolimus-eluting stent generations: A meta-analysis of 12 randomised trials vs. other limus-eluting stents and an adjusted indirect comparison. *Heart* 2012;98(22):1632–1640.

47. Piccolo R, et al. Safety and efficacy of resolute zotarolimus-eluting stents compared with everolimus-eluting stents: A meta-analysis. *Circ Cardiovasc Interv* 2015;8:e002223.

48. Park KW, et al. A randomized comparison of platinum chromium-based everolimus-eluting stents vs. cobalt chromium-based Zotarolimus-Eluting stents in all-comers receiving percutaneous coronary intervention: HOST-ASSURE (harmonizing optimal strategy for treatment of coronary artery stenosis-safety & effectiveness of drug-eluting stents & anti-platelet regimen), a randomized, controlled, noninferiority trial. *J Am Coll Cardiol* 2014;63(25 Pt A):2805–2816.

49. Stone GW, et al. A prospective, randomized evaluation of a novel everolimus-eluting coronary stent: The PLATINUM (a Prospective, Randomized, Multicenter Trial to Assess an Everolimus-Eluting Coronary Stent System [PROMUS Element] for the Treatment of Up to Two de Novo Coronary Artery Lesions) trial. *J Am Coll Cardiol* 2011;57(16):1700–1708.

50. von Birgelen C, et al. Third-generation zotarolimus-eluting and everolimus-eluting stents in all-comer patients requiring a percutaneous coronary intervention (DUTCH PEERS): A randomised, single-blind, multicentre, non-inferiority trial. *Lancet* 2014;383(9915):413–423.

51. Serruys PW, et al. A randomised comparison of novolimus-eluting and zotarolimus-eluting coronary stents: 9-month follow-up results of the EXCELLA II study. *Eurointervention* 2010;6(2):195–205.

52. Iqbal J, et al. DESyne novolimus-eluting coronary stent is superior to Endeavor zotarolimus-eluting coronary stent at five-year follow-up: Final results of the multicentre EXCELLA II randomised controlled trial. *EuroIntervention* 2016;12(11):e1336–e1342.

53. Serruys PW, et al. Improved safety and reduction in stent thrombosis associated with biodegradable polymer-cased biolimus-eluting stents vs. durable polymer-based sirolimus-eluting stents in patients with coronary artery disease: Final 5-year report of the LEADERS (Limus Eluted From A Durable Vs. ERodable Stent Coating) randomized, noninferiority rrial. *JACC Cardiovasc Interv* 2013;6(8):777–789.

54. Raber L, et al. Effect of biolimus-eluting stents with biodegradable polymer vs bare-metal stents on cardiovascular events among patients with acute myocardial infarction: The COMFORTABLE AMI randomized trial. *JAMA* 2012;308(8):777–787.

55. Raber L, et al. Biolimus-eluting stents with biodegradable polymer vs. bare-metal stents in acute myocardial infarction: Two-year clinical results of the COMFORTABLE AMI trial. *Circ Cardiovasc Interv* 2014;7:355–364.

56. Raungaard B, et al. Zotarolimus-eluting durable-polymer-coated stent vs. a biolimus-eluting biodegradable-polymer-coated stent in unselected patients undergoing percutaneous coronary intervention (SORT OUT VI): A randomised non-inferiority trial. *Lancet* 2015;385(9977):1527–1535.

57. Danzi GB, et al. Nobori biolimus-eluting stent vs. permanent polymer drug-eluting stents in patients undergoing percutaneous coronary intervention. *Circ J* 2014;78(8):1858–1866.

58. Vlachojannis GJ, et al. Long-term clinical outcomes of biodegradable polymer biolimus-eluting stents vs. durable polymer everolimus-eluting stents in patients with coronary artery disease: Three-year follow-up of the COMPARE II (Abluminal biodegradable polymer biolimus-eluting stent vs. durable polymer everolimus-eluting stent) trial. *EuroIntervention* 2015;11(3):272–279.

59. Natsuaki M, et al. Final 3-year outcome of a randomized trial comparing second-generation drug-eluting stents using either biodegradable polymer or durable polymer: NOBORI biolimus-eluting vs. XIENCE/PROMUS everolimus-eluting stent trial. *Circ Cardiovasc Interv* 2015;8(10):e002817.

60. Windecker S, et al. Comparison of a novel biodegradable polymer sirolimus-eluting stent with a durable polymer everolimus-eluting stent: Results of the randomized BIOFLOW-II trial. *Circ Cardiovasc Interv* 2015;8(2):e001441.

61. Pilgrim T, et al. Ultrathin strut biodegradable polymer sirolimus-eluting stent vs. durable polymer everolimus-eluting stent for percutaneous coronary revascularisation (BIOSCIENCE): A randomised, single-blind, non-inferiority trial. *Lancet* 2014;384(9960):2111–2122.

62. Pilgrim T, et al. Biodegradable polymer sirolimus-eluting stents vs. durable polymer everolimus-eluting stents for primary percutaneous coronary revascularisation of acute myocardial infarction. *EuroIntervention* 2016;12(11):e1343–e1354.

63. Zbinden R, et al. Ultrathin strut biodegradable polymer sirolimus-eluting stent vs. durable polymer everolimus-eluting stent for percutaneous coronary revascularization: Two year results of the BIOSCIENCE trial. *J Am Heart Assoc* 2016;5:e003255.

64. Jensen LO. Randomised comparison of a sirolimus-eluting stent with a biolimus-eluting stent in patients treated with PCI: The SORT OUT VII trial. *Am Heart J* 2015;170(2):210–215.

65. Saito S, et al. A randomized, prospective, intercontinental evaluation of a bioresorbable polymer sirolimus-eluting coronary stent system: The CENTURY II (Clinical Evaluation of New Terumo Drug-Eluting Coronary Stent System in the Treatment of Patients with Coronary Artery Disease) trial. *Eur Heart J* 2014;35(30):2021–2031.

66. Meredith IT, et al. Primary endpoint results of the EVOLVE trial: A randomized evaluation of a novel bioabsorbable polymer-coated, everolimus-eluting coronary stent. *J Am Coll Cardiol* 2012;59(15):1362–1370.

67. Kereiakes DJ, et al. Efficacy and safety of a novel bioabsorbable polymer-coated, everolimus-eluting coronary stent: The EVOLVE II randomized trial. *Circ Cardiovasc Interv* 2015;8(4):e002372.

68. Wijns W, et al. Evaluation of a crystalline sirolimus-eluting coronary stent with a bioabsorbable polymer designed for rapid dissolution: Two-year outcomes from the DESSOLVE I and II trials. *EuroIntervention* 2016;12(3):352–355.

69. Haude M, et al. The REMEDEE trial: A randomized comparison of a combination sirolimus-eluting endothelial progenitor cell capture stent with a paclitaxel-eluting stent. *JACC Cardiovasc Interv* 2013;6(4):334–343.

70. Han Y, et al. A randomized comparison of novel biodegradable polymer- and durable polymer-coated cobalt-chromium sirolimus-eluting stents. *JACC Cardiovasc Interv* 2014;7(12):1352–1360.

71. Cassese S, et al. Polymer-free sirolimus-eluting vs. polymer-based paclitaxel-eluting stents: An individual patient data analysis of randomized trials. *Rev Esp Cardiol (Engl Ed)* 2013;66:435–442.

72. Urban P, et al. Polymer-free drug-coated coronary stents in patients at high bleeding risk. *N Engl J Med* 2015;373(21):2038–2047.

73. Carrie D, et al. A multicenter randomized trial comparing amphilimus- with paclitaxel-eluting stents in de novo native coronary artery lesions. *J Am Coll Cardiol* 2012;59(15):1371–1376.

74. Romaguera R, et al. A randomized comparison of reservoir-based polymer-free amphilimus-eluting stents vs. everolimus-eluting stents with durable polymer in patients with diabetes mellitus: The RESERVOIR clinical trial. *JACC Cardiovasc Interv* 2016;9(1):42–50.

75. Windecker S, et al. 2014 ESC/EACTS Guidelines on myocardial revascularization: The Task Force on Myocardial Revascularization of the European Society of Cardiology (ESC) and the European Association for Cardio-Thoracic Surgery (EACTS)Developed with the special contribution of the European Association of Percutaneous Cardiovascular Interventions (EAPCI). *Eur Heart J* 2014;35(37):2541–2619.

76. Byrne RA, et al. Report of a European Society of Cardiology-European Association of Percutaneous Cardiovascular Interventions task force on the evaluation of coronary stents in Europe: Executive summary. *Eur Heart J* 2015;36(38):2608–2620.

77. Windecker S, et al. Revascularisation vs. medical treatment in patients with stable coronary artery disease: Network meta-analysis. *BMJ* 2014;348:g3859.

78. Roffi M, et al. 2015 ESC Guidelines for the management of acute coronary syndromes in patients presenting without persistent ST-segment elevation: Task Force for the Management of Acute Coronary Syndromes in Patients Presenting without Persistent ST-Segment Elevation of the European Society of Cardiology (ESC). *Eur Heart J* 2016;37(3):267–315.

79. Kalesan B, et al. Comparison of drug-eluting stents with bare metal stents in patients with ST-segment elevation myocardial infarction. *Eur Heart J* 2012;33(8):977–987.

80. Piccolo R, et al. Long-term safety and efficacy of drug-eluting stents in patients with acute myocardial infarction: A meta-analysis of randomized trials. *Atherosclerosis* 2011;217(1):149–157.

81. Sabate M, et al. Comparison of newer-generation drug-eluting with bare-metal stents in patients with acute ST-segment elevation myocardial infarction: A pooled analysis of the EXAMINATION (clinical Evaluation of the Xience-V stent in Acute Myocardial INfArcTION) and COMFORTABLE-AMI (Comparison of Biolimus Eluted From an Erodible Stent Coating With Bare Metal Stents in Acute ST-Elevation Myocardial Infarction) trials. *JACC Cardiovasc Interv* 2014;7(1):55–63.

82. Stone GW, et al. Differential clinical responses to everolimus-eluting and Paclitaxel-eluting coronary stents in patients with and without diabetes mellitus. *Circulation* 2011;124(8):893–900.

83. Bangalore S, et al. Outcomes with various drug eluting or bare metal stents in patients with diabetes mellitus: Mixed treatment comparison analysis of 22,844 patient years of follow-up from randomised trials. *BMJ* 2012;345:e5170.

84. Kaul U, et al. Paclitaxel-eluting vs. everolimus-eluting coronary stents in diabetes. *N Engl J Med* 2015;373(18):1709–1719.

85. Siontis GC, et al. Percutaneous coronary interventional strategies for treatment of in-stent restenosis: A network meta-analysis. *Lancet* 2015;386(9994):655–664.

86. Piccolo R, et al. Comparative effectiveness and safety of new-generation vs. early-generation drug-eluting stents according to complexity of coronary artery disease: A patient-level pooled analysis of 6,081 patients. *JACC Cardiovasc Interv* 2015;8(13):1657–1666.

87. Athappan G, et al. Left main coronary artery stenosis: A meta-analysis of drug-eluting stents vs. coronary artery bypass grafting. *JACC Cardiovasc Interv* 2013;6(12):1219–1230.

88. Mehilli J, et al. Zotarolimus- vs. everolimus-eluting stents for unprotected left main coronary artery disease. *J Am Coll Cardiol* 2013;62(22):2075–2082.

89. Lanka V, et al. Outcomes with first-vs. second-generation drug-eluting stents in coronary chronic total occlusions (CTOs): A systematic review and meta-analysis. *J Invasive Cardiol* 2014;26(7):304–310.

90. Mehilli J, et al. Drug-eluting vs. bare-metal stents in saphenous vein graft lesions (ISAR-CABG): A randomised controlled superiority trial. *Lancet* 2011;378(9796):1071–1078.

91. Aggarwal V, et al. Safety and effectiveness of drug-eluting vs. bare-metal stents in saphenous vein bypass graft percutaneous coronary interventions: Insights from the Veterans Affairs CART program. *J Am Coll Cardiol* 2014;64(17):1825–1836.

92. Piccolo R, et al. Stable coronary artery disease: Revascularisation and invasive strategies. *Lancet* 2015;386(9994):702–713.

93. Tamai H, et al. Initial and 6-month results of biodegradable poly-l-lactic acid coronary stents in humans. *Circulation* 2000;102(4):399–404.

94. Raber L, et al. Very late scaffold thrombosis: Intracoronary imaging and histopathological and spectroscopic findings. *J Am Coll Cardiol* 2015;66(17):1901–1914.

95. Onuma Y, Serruys PW. Bioresorbable scaffold: The advent of a new era in percutaneous coronary and peripheral revascularization? *Circulation* 2011;123(7):779–797.

96. Wiebe J, et al. Current status of bioresorbable scaffolds in the treatment of coronary artery disease. *J Am Coll Cardiol* 2014;64(23):2541–2551.

97. Iqbal J, et al. Bioresorbable scaffolds: Rationale, current status, challenges, and future. *Eur Heart J* 2014;35(12):765–776.

98. Cassese S, et al. Everolimus-eluting bioresorbable vascular scaffolds vs. everolimus-eluting metallic stents: A meta-analysis of randomised controlled trials. *Lancet* 2016;387(10018):537–544.

99. Stone GW, et al. 1-year outcomes with the Absorb bioresorbable scaffold in patients with coronary artery disease: A patient-level, pooled meta-analysis. *Lancet* 2016;387(10025):1277–1289.

100. Windecker S, et al. Bioresorbable scaffolds vs. metallic drug-eluting stents: Are we getting any closer to a paradigm shift? *J Am Coll Cardiol* 2015;66(21):2310–2314.

101. Tamburino C, et al. Contemporary practice and technical aspects in coronary intervention with bioresorbable scaffolds: A European perspective. *EuroIntervention* 2015;11(1):45–52.

102. Verheye S, et al. A next-generation bioresorbable coronary scaffold system: From bench to first clinical evaluation: 6- and 12-month clinical and multimodality imaging results. *JACC Cardiovasc Interv* 2014;7(1):89–99.

33

Primary PCI in ST-elevation myocardial infarction

MOTAZ MOUSSA AND JAMES E. TCHENG

INTRODUCTION

ST-elevation myocardial infarction (STEMI) is the most urgent of presentations among the acute coronary syndromes (ACSs). Ideally, the patient presenting with STEMI mobilizes the numerous health care resources needed to rapidly restore coronary artery perfusion, maximize myocardial salvage, and improve patient survival. A comprehensive knowledge of STEMI and percutaneous coronary intervention (PCI) guidelines, as well as an understanding of the reperfusion strategies, adjunctive treatments, and the local health care system competencies and constraints is required to optimally manage these potentially complex patients. This chapter specifically focuses on the role of the cardiac catheterization laboratory in STEMI.

GOALS OF REPERFUSION THERAPY

In patients with STEMI, reperfusion choices include primary PCI, fibrinolytic therapy, and (rarely) acute surgical revascularization. The emphasis should be on the appropriate and timely use of the form of reperfusion therapy most appropriate to the local health care system. It is well established that the benefits of reperfusion are time-dependent. The greater the delay to reperfusion, the less the potential to salvage myocardium and improve outcomes. To facilitate rapid coronary reperfusion, the primary approach (pharmacologic or interventional) should be decided on quickly. Major factors impacting the selection of approach include the local resources (catheterization laboratory availability, clinician and team expertise, time-to-treatment) and patient characteristics (comorbidities, hemodynamic stability, duration of symptoms) balanced against the risks of the reperfusion strategy.

TRIAGE AND TRANSFER DECISIONS FOR ST-ELEVATION MYOCARDIAL INFARCTION PATIENTS

Compared with fibrinolytic therapy, primary PCI produces higher rates of reperfusion and lower rates of reinfarction, recurrent ischemia, and intracranial hemorrhage.[1] A 25% relative risk reduction in 1-year mortality can be expected. Guidelines recommend that a STEMI system of care achieve a time of 90 minutes or less from first medical contact (FMC) to first device activation.[2] A number of factors can influence the total time from onset to reperfusion, including prehospital factors (symptom onset to FMC, transport time, prehospital emergency medical system [EMS] activation, EMS-administered medications) and in-hospital factors (cath lab staff availability, procedural time, patient variables). Critically, hospital "door-to-balloon" (D2B) time is significantly correlated with mortality, with faster reperfusion times associated with reductions in mortality. Data from the National Cardiovascular Data Registry (NCDR) demonstrate a continuous relationship between in-hospital mortality and DTB time, suggesting that any delay is associated with a concomitant increase in mortality even when D2B time is <90 minutes.[3] Only in rare conditions, namely, where the delay from FMC to D2B is anticipated to be longer than 120 minutes, should a fibrinolytic strategy be considered the primary approach. Current guidelines regarding triage, transfer, and treatment of STEMI patients are summarized in Figure 33.1 and Table 33.1.

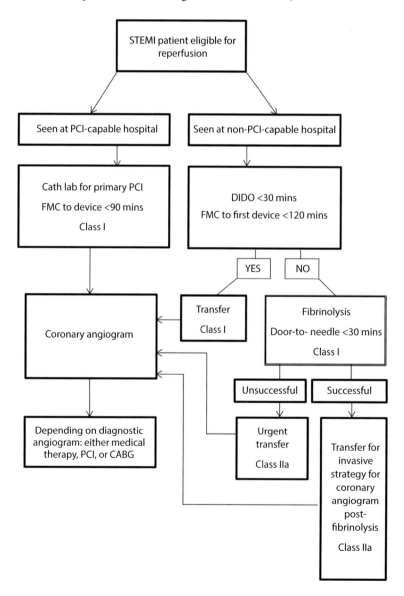

Figure 33.1 Current guidelines regarding triage, transfer, and treatment of STEMI patients. CABG, coronary artery bypass graft; DIDO, door-in-door-out; FMC, first medical contact; LOE, level of evidence; MI, myocardial infarction; PCI, percutaneous coronary intervention; STEMI, ST-elevation myocardial infarction.

Table 33.1 Current guidelines regarding triage, transfer, and treatment of STEMI patients

Class I

1. A systematic approach to regional STEMI care should be implemented and maintained across all communities.
2. In patients with symptoms consistent with acute ischemic heart disease, an ECG should be obtained as quickly as possible by EMS personnel.
3. In patients with STEMI symptoms of less than 12 hours duration, primary treatment should be directed at reperfusion strategies.
4. The recommended triage strategy for patients with STEMI is transport directly to a PCI-capable hospital, with an FMC-to-PCI device activation time goal of 90 minutes or less.
5. In patients presenting to a hospital without emergency PCI capabilities, immediate transfer to a PCI-capable hospital is the recommended triage strategy, with an FMC-to-PCI device activation time goal of 120 minutes or less.
6. In patients presenting to a hospital without emergency PCI capabilities where the anticipated FMC-to-PCI device activation time exceeds 120 minutes, fibrinolytic therapy should be administered (in the absence of contraindications), with a door-to-needle time goal of 30 minutes or less.

Class IIa

1. In patients with STEMI symptoms of 12–24 hours duration and ongoing clinical and/or ECG evidence of ischemia, pursuing a reperfusion strategy is reasonable, with primary PCI preferred over thrombolytic therapy.

Source: Adapted from 2013 ACCF/AHA Guideline for the Management of ST-Elevation Myocardial Infarction.
Note: ECG, electrocardiogram; EMS, emergency medical services; FMC, first medical contact; PCI, percutaneous coronary intervention; STEMI, ST-elevation myocardial infarction.

HOSPITALS WITHOUT PERCUTANEOUS CORONARY INTERVENTION-CAPABILITY

For patients presenting to a hospital without PCI capability, a key decision is whether to transfer the patient immediately to a hospital with PCI capability or to administer fibrinolytic therapy. A rapid, directed assessment including symptom duration, risk of bleeding, hemodynamic stability, presence of cardiogenic shock, and the time required for transfer to a hospital with PCI capability should be quickly performed. These critical factors inform the primary reperfusion therapy decision. Every hospital without PCI capability should establish a standard protocol for STEMI.

Immediate transfer to a hospital with PCI capability is the preferred strategy. The DANAMI (Danish Multicenter Randomized Study on Thrombolytic Therapy Versus Acute Coronary Angioplasty in Acute Myocardial Infarction)-2 study evaluated the immediate transfer strategy for 1,572 patients with STEMI randomized to either primary PCI or intravenous alteplase.[4] The composite of death, reinfarction, or stroke at 3 years was reduced in the cohort transferred for primary PCI compared with on-site fibrinolytic therapy (19.7% vs. 25%, P = .006). Outcomes were driven primarily by a reduction in reinfarction rates. In a propensity-matched study of 19,012 STEMI patients treated with primary PCI and fibrinolysis enrolled in the National Registry of Myocardial Infarction (NRMI), there was no survival advantage with primary PCI when transfer times exceeded 120 minutes from FMC.[5] Based on these data, interhospital transfer to a hospital with PCI capability is the recommended strategy if PCI can be performed within 120 minutes of FMC.

To accomplish this, minimizing the time spent at the hospital without PCI capability is paramount. Minimizing door-in–door-out (DIDO) time, defined as the time from arrival to discharge at the referral hospital, is key. A retrospective cohort of 14,871 patients with STEMI in the ACTION Registry-Get With the Guidelines demonstrated that patients with a DIDO time within 30 minutes were more likely to achieve a D2B time within 90 minutes compared with patients with a DIDO time greater than 30 minutes (60%; 95% CI, 57%–62% vs. 13%; 95% CI 12%–13%, P = 0.001).[6] In-hospital mortality rates were higher in the group with a DIDO time of 30 minutes or greater compared to within 30 minutes (5.9% vs.2.7%). Of note, the median DIDO time was 68 minutes and a DIDO time within 30 minutes was achieved in only 11% of patients.

When a 120-minute time goal cannot be met, in the absence of contraindications, fibrinolytic therapy should be administered within 30 minutes of patient presentation. The benefits of fibrinolytic therapy are well established, with a time-dependent reduction in both mortality and morbidity rates during the initial 12 hours after symptom onset.[7-13] Even when interhospital transport times are short, there may be benefits with the immediate administration of fibrinolytic therapy in patients who present within the first 1–2 hours of symptom onset, particularly when there are delays to primary PCI. A benefit of fibrinolytic therapy in patients who present >12 hours after symptom onset has not been established, although there remains consensus that fibrinolytic therapy should be considered in symptomatic patients presenting >12 hours after symptom onset who have a large area of myocardium at risk, or if hemodynamic instability is present and primary PCI is unavailable.

The guidelines for fibrinolytic therapy are summarized in Table 33.2. A summary of the characteristics and contraindications of fibrinolytic agents is presented in Tables 33.3 and 33.4.

Table 33.2 Indications for fibrinolytic therapy in STEMI patients

Class I

In patients with STEMI symptoms of less than 12 hours duration where the anticipated FMC-to-PCI device activation time exceeds 120 minutes, fibrinolytic therapy should be administered (in the absence of contraindications).

Class IIa

In patients with STEMI symptoms of 12–24 hours duration and ongoing clinical and/or ECG evidence of ischemia, and with either a large area of myocardium at risk or hemodynamic instability, fibrinolytic therapy is reasonable to administer.

Class III

In patients with symptoms consistent with acute ischemic heart disease and ST depression on the ECG, fibrinolytic therapy should not be given unless the primary diagnosis is posterior (inferobasal) acute STEMI.

Source: Adapted from 2013 ACCF/AHA Guideline for the Management of ST-Elevation Myocardial Infarction.
Note: ECG, electrocardiogram; EMS, emergency medical services; FMC, first medical contact; PCI, percutaneous coronary intervention; STEMI, ST-elevation myocardial infarction.

Table 33.3 Summary of characteristics of fibrinolytic agents

Fibrinolytic agent	Dose	Fibrin specificity	90-minute TIMI 2 or 3 flow
Tenecteplase	Single IV dose, weight specific (30–50 mg IV bolus)	+++	~85%
Reteplase	Two 10 unit IV boluses 30 minutes apart	++	~85%
Alteplase	15 mg IV bolus, 0.75 mg/kg (max 50 mg) infusion over 30 minutes, followed by 0.5 mg/kg (max 30 mg) over 60 minutes	++	~75–85%

Note: IV, intravenous; TIMI, thrombolysis in myocardial infarction.

Table 33.4 Contraindications to the administration of fibrinolytic therapy

Absolute contraindications
History of/current intracranial hemorrhage
History of/current structural cerebrovascular lesion (e.g., arteriovenous malformation)
History of/current malignant intracranial neoplasm (primary or metastatic)
History of/current bleeding diathesis (excluding menses)
Recent/current ischemic stroke (within 3 months, except acute ischemic stroke within 4.5 hours)
Recent/current significant closed-head or facial trauma (within 3 months)
Recent/current intracranial or intraspinal surgery (within 2 months)
Current suspected aortic dissection
Current ongoing bleeding
Current uncontrolled hypertension, unresponsive to therapy

Relative contraindications
History of poorly controlled severe hypertension
History of ischemic stroke (>3 months)
History of dementia
History of/current intracranial pathology not included in absolute contraindications
Recent major surgery (<3 weeks)
Recent internal bleeding (<4 weeks)
Current pregnancy
Current peptic ulcer
Current non-compressible vascular puncture
Severe hypertension (SBP > 180 mmHg or DBP > 110 mmHg) at presentation
Prolonged (>10 min) or traumatic CPR at presentation

Source: Adapted from 2013 ACCF/AHA Guideline for the Management of ST-Elevation Myocardial Infarction.
Note: CPR, cardiopulmonary resuscitation; DBP, diastolic blood pressure; SBP, systolic blood pressure.

INDICATIONS FOR PERCUTANEOUS CORONARY INTERVENTION AFTER FIBRINOLYTIC THERAPY

Rescue percutaneous coronary intervention

Even with modern fibrinolytic agents, failure to achieve normal coronary flow at 60–90 minutes occurs in nearly half of patients.[14] Rescue PCI is the immediate, emergency referral of a patient to the cardiac catheterization laboratory for PCI-based management of presumed reperfusion failure. A number of variables have been evaluated and found to be reasonably predictive of successful coronary reperfusion with fibrinolytic therapy, including the reduction and/or relief of chest pain, resolution of ST-segment elevation, and the presence of reperfusion arrhythmias. Conversely, >50% residual ST-segment elevation, ongoing chest discomfort, and the absence of reperfusion arrhythmias 60–90 minutes after treatment is indicative of reperfusion failure. Concern for reperfusion failure should prompt strong consideration to proceed with immediate coronary angiography and "rescue" PCI.

The REACT study was a multicenter trial involving 427 patients with STEMI who failed fibrinolytic therapy.[15] Patients were randomized to repeated fibrinolytic therapy, conservative management, or rescue PCI within 90 minutes after fibrinolytic therapy. The primary endpoint was a composite of death, reinfarction, stroke, and heart failure at 6 months. The rate of event-free survival was highest with rescue PCI (84.6%) compared with 70.1% in the conservative group, and was lowest, 68.7%, in the repeat fibrinolytic group ($P < 0.004$). Of note, the benefit was driven primarily by a reduction in reinfarction; there was no survival benefit or difference in major bleeding among the three groups. The rescue PCI approach should be balanced against the higher rates of periprocedural bleeding and stroke reported with this strategy than in patients treated conservatively.[16] The benefits of transferring a patient for rescue PCI are likely heightened when cardiogenic shock, significant hypotension, severe heart failure, or ECG evidence of an extensive area of myocardial jeopardy are present. On the other hand, conservative treatment might be reasonable in the patient with stable hemodynamics, improving symptoms, and a limited inferior infarction even in the presence of persistent ST-elevation.

Cardiogenic shock

Patients with STEMI complicated by cardiogenic shock are a subgroup benefiting from preferential referral for emergency primary PCI. The SHOCK (Should We Emergently Revascularize Occluded Coronaries for Cardiogenic Shock) trial randomized 302 patients presenting with cardiogenic shock to emergency revascularization (with either PCI or CABG) or immediate medical stabilization and delayed revascularization.[17] Of note, 56% of patients received fibrinolytic therapy. One-year survival was 46.7% in the revascularization group compared with 33.6% in the medically managed group (relative risk [RR] for death 0.72; 95% CI, 0.54–0.95). Importantly, the benefit of the emergency invasive strategy was similar in patients transferred versus those admitted directly to a PCI-capable hospital. For patients with cardiogenic shock, the benefit of emergency revascularization was apparent across a very wide time window, extending up to 54 hours after MI and 18 hours after shock onset. The time window for benefit in cardiogenic shock thus appears to be prolonged, arguing for a lower threshold for referral for cardiac catheterization-based management in this situation.

Routine transfer for immediate percutaneous coronary intervention after fibrinolytic therapy

One common question faced by hospitals without PCI capability is whether to immediately transfer the patient following administration of a fibrinolytic agent to a hospital with PCI capability (so-called "drip and ship"), or to delay transfer for 60–90 minutes and determine whether transfer for rescue PCI is indicated. Most trials have demonstrated improvement in clinical outcomes in patients transferred for early catheterization, particularly in higher-risk patients.[18] In the GRACIA (Grupo de Analisis de la Cardiopatia Isquemica Aguda) study, 500 stable patients were randomized to either early catheterization within 6–24 hours of successful fibrinolysis or an ischemia-guided approach.[19] The primary endpoint was the combined rate of death, reinfarction, or revascularization at 12 months. Patients in the invasive group had a lower frequency of the primary endpoint (9% vs. 21%, $P = 0.0008$).

The TRANSFER-AMI (Trial of Routine Angioplasty and Stenting after Fibrinolysis to Enhance Reperfusion in Acute Myocardial Infarction) study was the largest randomized trial evaluating immediate transfer for coronary angiography and revascularization.[20] In this study, 1,059 patients were randomized to immediate transfer for PCI after fibrinolytic therapy or standard treatment (including rescue PCI if indicated). This trial demonstrated a significant reduction in the combined primary endpoint of death, recurrent MI, recurrent ischemia, new or worsening heart failure, or shock at 30 days (11% in the immediate transfer group compared with 17.2% in the standard treatment group, RR with early PCI, 0.64; 95% CI, 0.47–0.87; $P = 0.004$) and no difference in rates of major bleeding between groups, thus favoring the early transfer and revascularization strategy.

The NORDISTEMI (Norwegian Study on District Treatment of ST-Elevation Myocardial Infarction) investigators[21] randomized 226 STEMI patients who lived in rural areas (more than 90 minute transfer time to a PCI-capable hospital) to immediate routine transfer for catheterization after fibrinolytic therapy versus a conservative strategy with either ischemia-guided treatment in the hospital without PCI capability or transfer for rescue PCI. The primary composite endpoint of death, recurrent MI, stroke, or recurrent ischemia at 12 months occurred in 28 patients (21%) in the immediate transfer group compared with 36 patients (27%) in the conservative group (HR:0.72,95% CI: 0.44–1.18, $P = 0.19$). In the immediate transfer group, the incidence of the composite of death, recurrent MI, or stroke at 1 year was significantly lower in the invasive group compared with the conservative group (8 patients [6%] vs. 21 patients [16%], HR: 0.36, 95% CI: 0.16–0.81, $P = 0.01$). A meta-analysis published in 2010 evaluated the seven randomized clinical trials of immediate routine transfer for catheterization following fibrinolytic therapy. The study revealed the invasive strategy to be associated with a statistically significant reduction in the incidence of death or MI at 30 days and at 1 year, without an increase in the risk of major bleeding.[22] The meta-analysis identified an advantage of immediate transfer even in patients without high-risk features.

In stable patients who exhibit clinical evidence of reperfusion and are not transferred immediately, early cardiac catheterization should still be considered routine. However, because of the associated increased bleeding risk of anticoagulation coupled with mild fibrinogen depletion, cardiac catheterization may be deferred for at least several hours after administration of fibrinolytic therapy. Conversely, emergency cardiac catheterization should be reserved for patients with evidence of failed fibrinolysis and significant myocardial jeopardy in whom rescue PCI would be appropriate. Indications for transfer for angiography after fibrinolytic therapy are summarized in Table 33.5.

Other approaches to the administration of fibrinolytic therapy

Administration of fibrinolytic therapy by EMS in the prehospital phase is not uncommon in some regions of Europe, and facilitates a reduction in the time from symptom onset to treatment. The logistics of administration typically involve a trained EMS unit either with a physician on board or a hospital-based physician in contact with the EMS team. A meta-analysis of six randomized trials ($n = 6,434$) that compared prehospital fibrinolytic therapy with in-hospital fibrinolytic therapy demonstrated a significant decrease in all-cause mortality with prehospital fibrinolytic therapy (OR, 0.83; 95% CI 0.70–0.98) and a significant decrease in time from establishing the diagnosis of STEMI to the administration of fibrinolytic therapy (104 minutes for prehospital compared with 162 minutes for in-hospital fibrinolytic therapy [$P = 0.007$]).[23]

THE OCCLUDED ARTERY AT ELECTIVE (DELAYED) CATHETERIZATION

In patients found to have an occluded infarct artery more than 24 hours after symptom onset (at the time of a delayed elective cardiac catheterization), PCI should only be considered for patients with cardiogenic shock, acute severe heart failure, postinfarction angina, or a large area of residual ischemia by provocative testing. Delayed PCI of a totally occluded infarct artery should not be performed in the otherwise stable patient. In the OAT (Occluded Artery Trial), 2,166 patients with an occluded infarct artery 1–28 days following acute myocardial infarction were randomized to PCI or medical therapy.[24] There was no difference in the composite endpoint of death, reinfarction, or class IV heart failure at a median follow-up of 5.8 years between patients randomized to PCI and those treated medically. Furthermore, infarction rates tended to be higher in the PCI group.

FACILITATED PERCUTANEOUS CORONARY INTERVENTION

With a facilitated PCI strategy, STEMI patients are administered a fibrinolytic agent as an intentional adjunctive treatment to emergency primary PCI. This approach has fallen into disfavor because of the negative results of the ASSENT-4 PCI (Assessment of the Safety and Efficacy of a New Treatment Strategy with Percutaneous Coronary Intervention) and FINESSE (Facilitated Intervention with Enhanced Reperfusion Speed to Stop Events) trials.[25,26] In the ASSENT 4 trial, 1,667 STEMI patients were randomized to full-dose tenecteplase and primary PCI or primary PCI alone.[25] Early termination of the trial was recommended

Table 33.5 Indications for transfer for angiography after fibrinolytic therapy

Class I

1. In patients with STEMI who develop cardiogenic shock or severe heart failure, immediate transfer to a PCI-capable hospital is the recommended.

Class IIa

1. In patients treated with fibrinolytic therapy for acute STEMI where there is evidence of reperfusion failure or reinfarction, urgent transfer to a PCI-capable hospital for cardiac catheterization is reasonable.
2. In patients treated with fibrinolytic therapy for acute STEMI who are hemodynamically stable and have clinical evidence of reperfusion, transfer to a PCI-capable hospital for cardiac catheterization is reasonable; PCI should be performed 3–24 hours following administration of the fibrinolytic agent.

Source: Adapted from 2013 ACCF/AHA Guideline for the Management of ST-Elevation Myocardial Infarction.
Note: PCI, percutaneous coronary intervention; STEMI, ST-elevation myocardial infarction.

by the data safety monitoring board as the group receiving fibrinolytic therapy had an increased incidence of the composite endpoint of death, cardiogenic shock, or congestive heart failure (19% [151 of 810] patients in the facilitated PCI group vs. 13% [110 of 819] in the primary PCI group [RR 1.39, 95% CI 1.11–1.74; $P = 0.004$]) In the FINESSE trial, 2,452 STEMI patients were randomized to one of three approaches: abciximab followed by PCI, abciximab and half-dose reteplase followed by PCI, or primary PCI with abciximab given in the catheterization lab.[26] The primary efficacy outcome did not differ among the groups, but there was a significant increase in major and minor bleeding in patients who received fibrinolytic therapy. Given these results, fibrinolytic therapy-facilitated PCI is no longer recommended.

REPERFUSION AT A HOSPITAL WITH PERCUTANEOUS CORONARY INTERVENTION-CAPABILITY

As mentioned previously, primary PCI of the infarct artery is the preferred strategy when D2B delays are short and the patient presents to a PCI-capable hospital. Multiple studies have demonstrated that primary PCI results in higher rates of coronary patency and TIMI 3 flow in the infarct artery, along with lower rates of recurrent ischemia, repeat revascularization, intracranial hemorrhage, and death.[1] Early successful PCI also decreases the rate of complications that result from longer ischemic times (ventricular septal defect, ventricular rupture, cardiogenic shock), allowing earlier hospital discharge. Furthermore, the greatest survival benefit for primary PCI is in the highest-risk patients.

Primary PCI is now routinely performed in hospitals without on-site surgical backup with excellent outcomes.[27] In hospitals without surgical backup, however, primary PCI should not be performed unless there is a proven plan for rapid transport to a cardiac surgery hospital accompanied by appropriate hemodynamic support.

For hospitals to be classified as PCI-capable, the total volume of PCI procedures should exceed 400 per year, ideally with more than 36 being primary PCIs, though, volumes of 200 PCI procedures per year are acceptable.[28] In terms of operator experience, it is recommended that individual operator volumes of PCI exceed 75 PCIs per year with at least 11 cases being primary PCIs, although 50 PCIs per year are acceptable. Guidelines for primary PCI are summarized in Table 33.6.

Serious complications with primary PCI can be expected to occur in 10%–20% of patients and include events attributable to MI, vascular access site complications, adverse reactions to contrast media, technical and other procedural complications, and reperfusion events. Of these, the "no-reflow phenomenon" is one of the most serious of the reperfusion complications. This term refers to suboptimal myocardial perfusion despite restoration of epicardial artery flow in the infarct artery. No-reflow is attributed to multiple processes, including the inflammatory response, endothelial injury, atheroembolization, vasospasm, and reperfusion injury at the myocyte level. Treatment strategies include the use of GP IIb/IIIa antagonists and vasodilators (intracoronary nitroprusside, calcium channel blockers, and/or adenosine). However, none of the strategies have been proven to be consistently effective.[29]

BALLOON ANGIOPLASTY ALONE VERSUS PLANNED STENT IMPLANTATION IN PRIMARY PERCUTANEOUS CORONARY INTERVENTION

In the current era, balloon angioplasty alone is no longer the treatment of choice. Studies comparing balloon angioplasty and primary stenting demonstrate balloon angioplasty to be associated with a higher risk of reinfarction and repeat target-vessel revascularization (TVR). In meta-analyses, stent PCI significantly reduced the incidence of overall major adverse cardiac events (MACE) (OR: 0.49 [0.40–0.59]), primarily driven by a reduction in TVR (OR 0.44 [0.36–0.54]), with a nonsignificant trend toward a decrease in reinfarction.[30,31] These studies document that reocclusion rates following balloon angioplasty are approximately 15% versus 5% with stent implantation.

Table 33.6 Guidelines for primary PCI

Class I

1. In patients with STEMI symptoms of less than 12 hours duration, primary PCI should be performed, with a FMC-to-PCI device activation time goal of less than 90 minutes.
2. In patients with STEMI symptoms of less than 12 hours duration who have contraindications to fibrinolytic therapy, primary PCI should be performed irrespective of the amount of time anticipated to PCI device activation.

Class IIa

1. In patients with STEMI symptoms of 12–24 hours duration and ongoing clinical and/or ECG evidence of ischemia, primary PCI is reasonable.

Source: Adapted from 2013 ACCF/AHA Guideline for the Management of ST-Elevation.
Note: ECG, electrocardiogram; EMS, emergency medical services; FMC, first medical contact; PCI, percutaneous coronary intervention; STEMI, ST-elevation myocardial infarction.

TYPE OF STENT IN PRIMARY PERCUTANEOUS CORONARY INTERVENTION

During primary PCI, implantation of a drug-eluting stent (DES) is preferred over a bare-metal stent (BMS), given the lower rates of restenosis and target lesion revascularization (TLR) associated with DES. The only real consideration is whether the patient is a reasonable candidate for prolonged treatment with a $P2Y_{12}$ inhibitor. Potential barriers that might limit compliance with prolonged treatment include financial or social barriers, anticipated invasive surgery in the subsequent year, a high bleeding risk or indication for long-term anticoagulation, or comorbidities with a poor prognosis. In these patients, BMS implantation may be the preferred strategy. The safety of DES in STEMI has been studied extensively with the conclusion that while DES implantation is not associated with a significant reduction in mortality, there is a marked reduction in rates of restenosis, TLR, and TVR.

Several studies have specifically addressed the question of DES versus BMS in primary PCI. In the GRACE registry, an analysis of 5,093 STEMI patients showed mortality to be similar between DES and BMS at 6-months follow-up, although the mortality rate was higher in the DES group at 1–2-year follow-up.[32] The HORIZONS AMI study randomized 3,006 STEMI patients to receive paclitaxel DES or BMS. Results showed a reduction in the 1-year rate of ischemia-driven TLR in the paclitaxel DES cohort (4.5% vs. 7.5%; HR 0.59; 95% CI; 0.43–0.83; $P = 0.002$) and TVR (5.8% vs. 8.7%; HR 0.65; 95% CI: 0.48–0.89; $P = 0.006$), with no significant difference in the composite safety endpoint (stent thrombosis, reinfarction, stroke, and death).[33] Rates of death and stent thrombosis at 12 months were similar between groups, while restenosis at 13 months was significantly decreased in the DES group (10% vs. 22.9%; HR 0.44; 95% CI 0.33–0.57; $P < 0.001$). Results at 3 years showed that the group randomized to paclitaxel DES experienced a reduction in the 3-year rate of ischemia-driven TLR compared with those receiving a BMS, from 15.1% to 9.4% (40% relative risk reduction). The study also showed that higher-risk patient subgroups (patients with insulin-dependent diabetes, vessel size <3 mm and lesion length >30 mm) benefited from DES compared with BMS.

In summary, the benefit of DES compared with BMS in STEMI patients is mainly in reducing restenosis and the need for repeat revascularization, while not affecting rates of recurrent MI or death. Critically, stent thrombosis does not appear to be increased with DES compared with BMS in trials, although it does remain a concern in the real-world setting. Guidelines for stent implantation are summarized in Table 33.7.

ANTIPLATELET THERAPY IN THE ACUTE ST-ELEVATION MYOCARDIAL INFARCTION PATIENT

A dose of 325 mg of aspirin should be administered once the diagnosis of STEMI is suspected. Based on the results of the CURRENT-OASIS (Clopidogrel Optimal Loading Dose Usage to Reduce Recurrent Events-Organization to Assess Strategies in Ischemic Syndromes)-7 trial, there is no difference in the efficacy of a maintenance dose of 81 mg versus 325 mg of aspirin, while the higher dose is associated with an increased risk of bleeding.[34] Given these results, current guidelines recommend a maintenance dose of 81 mg aspirin indefinitely in patients presenting with STEMI.

A loading dose of a $P2Y_{12}$ inhibitor should be administrated as soon as primary PCI is decided upon, with the intent to continue a maintenance dose for 1 year (in the absence of complications). Choices include clopidogrel, prasugrel, and ticagrelor. In terms of the loading dose of clopidogrel, results of the CURRENT-OASIS 7 subgroup analysis demonstrated a 600 mg loading dose of clopidogrel to have more rapid and extensive platelet inhibition[35]; this loading dose is generally preferred in primary PCI. Prasugrel is a thienopyridine that achieves a greater degree of platelet inhibition than clopidogrel. In the TRITON-TIMI (The Trial to Assess Improvement in Therapeutic Outcomes by Optimizing Platelet Inhibition with Prasugrel-Thrombolysis in Myocardial Infarction)-38 trial, 13,608 patients with ACS undergoing PCI were randomized to either prasugrel (60 mg loading dose and 10 mg maintenance dose) or clopidogrel (300 mg loading dose and 75 mg maintenance dose).[36] Median follow-up was 14.5 months. Results showed that the primary efficacy endpoint (death from cardiovascular causes, nonfatal MI, or nonfatal stroke) and the individual components occurred less frequently in the prasugrel cohort (primary endpoint 9.9% vs. 12.1%. HR 0.81; 95% CI 0.73–0.90; $P < 0.001$; TVR 3.7% vs. 2.5%, $P < 0.001$; and stent thrombosis 2.4% vs. 1.1%, $P < .001$). Offsetting the advantages in efficacy were increases in major bleeding (2.4% vs. 1.8%, HR 1.32; 95% CI 1.03–1.68, $P = 0.03$) and

Table 33.7 Use of stents in primary PCI for STEMI

Class I

1. In patients treated with PCI for STEMI, implantation of a bare-metal or drug-eluting stent is preferred over balloon angioplasty alone.
2. In patients at high risk of bleeding who will have difficulty with prolonged compliance with dual antiplatelet therapy or who have surgery planned within 1 year, bare-metal stent implantation is preferred over drug-eluting stent placement.

Source: Adapted from 2013 ACCF/AHA Guideline for the Management of ST-Elevation Myocardial Infarction.
Note: PCI, percutaneous coronary intervention; STEMI, ST-elevation myocardial infarction.

fatal bleeding (0.4% vs. 0.1%, $P = 0.002$). It should be noted that clopidogrel was not routinely administered prior to primary PCI, and the loading dose of clopidogrel was limited to 300 mg, which may have contributed to differences in efficacy between the two groups.[37] In addition, the prasugrel package insert includes a black box warning about administration to patients with a history of stroke or transient ischemic attack, those who are older than 75 years, and those who weigh less than 60 kg.[38] If a patient has a high risk of bleeding, lower maintenance doses of 5 mg daily may be considered.

Ticagrelor is a reversible $P2Y_{12}$ receptor antagonist that does not require metabolic conversion to active metabolite for the antiplatelet effects. The PLATO (Platelet Inhibiton and Patient Outcomes) trial compared ticagrelor (180 mg loading dose, 90 mg twice daily maintenance dose) with clopidogrel (300 or 600 mg loading dose, 75 mg daily maintenance dose) in 18,624 patients presenting with ACS, of whom 7,544 patients presented with STEMI.[39] During a median follow-up of 10 months, the primary endpoint (composite of death from vascular causes, MI, or stroke) occurred in 7.9% of patients randomized to ticagrelor versus 8.6% in the clopidogrel group (HR 0.91, 95% CI 0.75–1.12, $P = 0.38$). Ticagrelor reduced the risk of stent thrombosis (HR 0.58, 95 %CI 0.37–0.89, $P = .013$), with major bleeding as defined in the protocol occurring at similar rates (6.7% vs. 6.8%; HR 0.97, 95% CI 0.77–1.22; $P = 0.79$).[40] Noteworthy, a subgroup analysis of the PLATO trial showed the opposite effect of ticagrelor in North America compared with other regions of the world.[41] Given the observation of both lower efficacy and a higher risk of bleeding in patients in the PLATO trial receiving 325 mg per day of aspirin, it is recommended that the dose of aspirin not exceed 100 mg when given with ticagrelor.

PLATELET GLYCOPROTEIN IIB/IIIA INHIBITORS

The benefits of platelet glycoprotein (GP) IIb/IIIa inhibition during PCI (before the availability of prasugrel and ticagrelor) are well-documented. A meta-analysis that included three trials demonstrated a reduction in the endpoint of death and reinfarction with the use of abciximab in patients with STEMI (12.9% vs. 19% at 3 years of follow-up, RR 0.633, 95%CI 0.452–0.887, $P = 0.008$).[42] Major bleeding was 2.5% in the abciximab group versus 2% in the placebo group. The CADILLAC (Controlled Abciximab and Device Investigation to Lower Late Angioplasty Complications) trial[43] was the largest trial that compared the use of abciximab with placebo. In this trial of 1,036 patients presenting with STEMI, there was a significant reduction in the 30-day composite endpoint of death, recurrent MI, and TVR in the abciximab cohort (6.8% vs. 4.6%, $P = 0.01$).

In the current era of potent oral dual antiplatelet therapy, the efficacy of these agents is less certain. Based on recent guidelines, treatment with abciximab, eptifibatide, or tirofiban remains a class IIa recommendation in selected patients presenting with STEMI; they are most commonly used in

patients with a large thrombus burden and in patients not adequately loaded with $P2Y_{12}$ receptor antagonists.[2] The routine use of these agents prior to catheterization lab arrival is a class III recommendation.

ANTICOAGULANT THERAPY TO SUPPORT PRIMARY PERCUTANEOUS CORONARY INTERVENTION

The use of intravenous unfractionated heparin (UFH) for adjunctive anticoagulation in primary PCI during STEMI is currently the most common approach. Enoxaparin and fondaparinux have also been studied in this setting. The ATOLL (Acute STEMI Treated with Primary PCI and IV Enoxaparin or UFH to Lower Ischemic and Bleeding Events at Short- and Long-term Follow-up) trial compared intravenous enoxaparin 0.5 mg/kg with UFH titrated to ACT levels during primary PCI.[44] The trial was statistically underpowered and the primary endpoint of mortality, MI, procedure failure, or major bleeding was negative. Although the trial showed decreased mortality with enoxaparin, it did not reduce infarct size or bleeding risk, or improve TIMI flow. In the absence of a clear explanation for decreased mortality, it is likely that results were due to chance. Fondaparinux has been associated with catheter thrombosis and should not be relied on as the sole anticoagulant during primary PCI.[45]

The primary alternative to heparin is bivalirudin, a short-acting direct thrombin inhibitor. In combination with oral dual antiplatelet therapy, it is considered a reasonable anticoagulant alternative for primary PCI, especially in patients at higher risk of bleeding. The HORIZONS-AMI (Harmonizing Outcomes with Revascularization and Stents in Acute Myocardial Infarction) trial randomized 3,602 patients undergoing primary PCI to treatment with heparin plus a GP IIb/IIIa inhibitor or bivalirudin alone.[46] Bivalirudin resulted in a reduced 30-day rate of net adverse clinical events (9.2% vs. 12.1%; RR 0.76; 95% CI 0.63–0.92; $P = 0.005$), lower rates of major bleeding (4.9% vs. 8.3%), and a lower 30-day all-cause mortality (2.1% vs. 3.1%). However, within the first 24 hours, stent thrombosis occurred in 17 more patients in the bivalirudin group than in the group receiving heparin plus a GP IIb/IIIa inhibitor (1.3% vs. 0.3%, $P < 0.001$).

Table 33.8 summarizes loading dose and maintenance dose recommendations for antiplatelet and anticoagulant agents, along with corresponding guidelines, class of recommendation, and level of evidence.

PERCUTANEOUS CORONARY INTERVENTION OF A NONINFARCT ARTERY BEFORE HOSPITAL DISCHARGE

Multivessel primary PCI in hemodynamically stable patients presenting with STEMI, either at the time of primary PCI or as a staged procedure, has been upgraded from a class III (possible harm) to a class IIb recommendation in the 2015 Guidelines update.[47] Physicians should determine the

Table 33.8 Loading dose and maintenance dose recommendations for antiplatelet and anticoagulant agents

	Loading dose	Maintenance dose	COR	LOE
Antiplatelet				
Aspirin	324 mg once	81 mg po daily for life	I	B
Clopidogrel	600 mg once	75 mg po daily for 1 year	I	B
Prasugrel	60 mg once	10 mg po daily for 1 year	I	B
Ticagrelor	180 mg once	90 mg po twice daily for 1 year	I	B
GP IIb/IIIa Inhibitors				
Abciximab	0.25 mg/kg IV bolus, then 0.125 mcg/kg/min infusion		IIa	A
Eptifibatide	2 boluses, 180 mcg/kg, 10 minutes apart, then 2 mcg/kg/min infusion; reduce infusion dose by 50% if CrCl < 50 ml/min		IIa	B
Tirofiban	25 mg/kg IV bolus, then 0.15 mcg/kg/min infusion; reduce infusion dose by 50% if CrCl < 30 ml/min		IIa	B
Anticoagulant Therapy				
UFH	70-100 U/kg bolus if a GP IIb/IIIa inhibitor is not given 50–70 U/kg if a GP IIb/IIIa inhibitor is given		I	C
Bivalirudin	0.75 mg/kg IV bolus, then 1.75 mg/kg/h infusion. If CrCl < 30, infusion should be adjusted to 1 mg/kg/h		I	B

Note: COR, class of recommendation; CrCL, creatinine clearance; GPIIb/IIIa, glycoprotein IIb/IIIa; IV, intravenous; LOE, level of evidence; PO, oral; UFH, unfractionated heparin.

optimal time for noninfarct artery PCI depending on factors including patient comorbidities, lesion complexity, risk of contrast nephropathy, and radiation dose limits. The prior class III recommendation, mainly based on multiple observational trials, was changed as a result of three randomized trials. In the PRAMI (Preventive Angioplasty in Acute Myocardial Infarction) trial, 465 patients presenting with STEMI and multivessel disease were randomized to either complete revascularization or culprit vessel–only primary PCI.[48] The composite primary outcome of cardiac death, nonfatal MI, or refractory angina occurred in 21 patients (9%) in the multivessel PCI group versus 53 patients (22%) in the culprit vessel–only PCI group (HR: 0.35; 95% CI: 0.21–0.58; $P < 0.001$). The CvLPRIT (Complete Versus Culprit-Lesion-Only Primary PCI) trial randomized 296 patients to culprit vessel–only PCI or multivessel PCI during the index hospitalization.[49] The multivessel PCI group experienced lower rates of the composite primary outcome of death, reinfarction, revascularization, and heart failure (15 patients [10%] vs. 31 patients [21%]; HR 0.49; 95% CI 0.24–0.84; $P = 0.008$). Similarly, the DANAMI 3 PRIMULTI (Third Danish Study of Optimal Acute Treatment of Patients with ST-segment Elevation Myocardial Infarction) trial randomized 627 patients to multivessel PCI or culprit vessel–only PCI, guided by fractional flow reserve assessment of the noninfarct artery.[50] Lower rates of the composite primary endpoint of all-cause death, MI, and revascularization were found in the multivessel PCI group (13% vs. 22%; HR: 0.56; 95% CI 0.38–0.83; $P = 0.004$).

At this time, there is still insufficient data to unequivocally argue the optimal timing of nonculprit artery PCI (i.e., whether it should be performed at the time of the primary PCI or at a later point in time). Both patient and lesion characteristics must also be considered in the timing decision.

ASPIRATION THROMBECTOMY

The prior class IIa recommendation for aspiration thrombectomy has been downgraded in the 2015 Guidelines update.[47] Routine aspiration thrombectomy is not currently considered beneficial (class III) based on several large trials. The previous class IIa recommendation for performing aspiration thrombectomy during primary PCI was based primarily on the results of the TAPAS (Thrombus Aspiration During Primary Percutaneous Coronary Intervention in Acute Myocardial Infarction) trial, a single-center trial that randomized 1,071 patients presenting with STEMI to aspiration thrombectomy prior to primary PCI or primary PCI without thrombectomy.[51,52] Results showed benefit with aspiration thrombectomy, measured as myocardial blush (myocardial blush grade 0 or 1 occurred in 17.1% in the thrombectomy group vs. 26.3% in the primary PCI group, $P < 0.001$). At 1 year, cardiac death was 3.6% in the thrombectomy group versus 6.7% in the conventional PCI group (hazard ratio [HR] 1.93; 95% CI 1.11–3.37; $P = 0.020$). Following TAPAS, multiple trials of routine aspiration thrombectomy have failed to replicate those results. In the INFUSE-AMI (Intracoronary Abciximab and Aspiration Thrombectomy in Patients with Large Anterior Myocardial Infarction) trial, 452 patients were randomized in an open-label, 2 × 2 factorial design to bolus intracoronary abciximab versus no abciximab and to routine aspiration thrombectomy versus no thrombectomy.[53] The findings included a significant reduction in 30-day infarct size in patients randomized to intracoronary abciximab (median, 15.1%; IQR 6.8%–22.7% vs. 17.9%; IQR 10.3%–25.4%, $P = 0.03$), but no benefit in patients randomized to aspiration thrombectomy (median, 17% IQR 9%–22.8% vs. 17.3% IQR 7.1%–25.5%, $P = 0.51$). In the TASTE (Thrombus Aspiration During ST-Segment Elevation Myocardial Infarction) trial, 7,244 patients presenting with STEMI were randomized to aspiration thrombectomy versus primary PCI without routine thrombectomy.[54,55] The primary endpoint of all-cause mortality at 30 days was similar between both groups (2.8% vs. 3% HR 0.94; 95% CI 0.72–1.22; $P = 0.63$), and no significant differences were observed at 1 year or across any of the subgroups. Finally, the TOTAL (Trial of Routine Aspiration Thrombectomy with PCI versus PCI Alone in Patients with STEMI) trial randomized 10,732 patients with STEMI to aspiration thrombectomy prior to PCI or to primary PCI alone.[56] The endpoint of death, recurrent MI, and heart failure was similar between both groups, with consistent findings across subgroups, including patients with large thrombus burden (6.9% vs. 7%, HR 0.99; 95% CI 0.85–1.15). Of note, there was a small but statistically significant increase in the rate of stroke in the aspiration thrombectomy group. There are insufficient data to assess the potential benefit of "bailout aspiration thrombectomy" when used during PCI because of unsatisfactory initial results. The current recommendation is that aspiration thrombectomy should be evaluated on a case-by-case basis, rather than being considered as a universally applicable strategy.

CORONARY ARTERY BYPASS GRAFT SURGERY IN ST-ELEVATION MYOCARDIAL INFARCTION

Coronary bypass graft surgery has a limited role in the acute phase of STEMI. It may be considered in failed PCI, for coronary anatomy not amenable to PCI, or if a mechanical defect, such as ventricular septal, papillary muscle, or ventricular free-wall rupture occurs. In patients presenting with three-vessel disease but with an occluded culprit artery with ongoing ischemia, it is not unreasonable to consider balloon-only infarct-related artery in preparation for bypass surgery and thus avoid the need for a thienopyridine or ticagrelor during the perioperative period.

In patients on dual antiplatelet therapy who require urgent coronary bypass surgery, it is recommended that aspirin be continued through the perioperative period. The P2Y$_{12}$ antagonist should be discontinued for at least 24–48 hours prior to surgery unless benefits of revascularization outweigh the risks of bleeding.

Of note, recent guidelines consider emergency PCI of the left main artery an appropriate option in patients presenting with STEMI, even when the left main is unprotected and particularly if it is the culprit lesion. Only PCI can be performed more rapidly and safely than emergency coronary bypass surgery. This approach has a class IIa recommendation.[57]

KEY POINTS

- The greatest emphasis should be placed on the delivery of reperfusion therapy as rapidly as possible to the patient.
- PCI achieves higher rates of infarct artery TIMI grade 3 flow and superior outcomes compared with fibrinolytic therapy.
- Current guidelines recommend a systems goal of 90 minutes or less from first medical contact to first interventional device activation for hospitals with PCI capability.
- Current guidelines recommend transfer of high-risk patients who receive fibrinolytic therapy to a hospital with PCI capability as soon as possible.
- Patients presenting to a non-PCI-capable facility with acute STEMI should be transferred to a PCI-capable hospital if transfer can be achieved within 120 minutes of first medical contact.
- Facilitated PCI is not beneficial and should be avoided.
- New guidelines consider PCI of significant noninfarct artery lesions to be reasonable, either at time of initial presentation or during index hospitalization.
- Compared with BMS implantation, DES reduces restenosis and repeat revascularization rates but does not reduce the incidence of death or recurrent MI.
- Recent guidelines classify routine aspiration thrombectomy as a class III recommendation in patients undergoing primary PCI. Selective aspiration thrombectomy is considered a class IIb strategy and should be applied only on a case-by-case basis.

REFERENCES

1. Keeley EC, et al. Primary angioplasty vs. intravenous thrombolytic therapy for acute myocardial infarction, a quantitative review of 23 randomized trials. *Lancet* 2003;361(9351):13–20.
2. O'Gara PT, et al. 2013 ACCF/AHA guideline for the management of ST-elevation myocardial infarction: A report of the American College of Cardiology Foundation/ American Heart Association Task Force on practice guidelines. *J Am Coll Cardiol* 2013;61(4):e78–e140.
3. Rathore SS, et al. Association of door-to-balloon time and mortality in patients admitted to hospital with ST elevation myocardial infarction national cohort study. *BMJ* 2009;338:b1807.

4. Andersen HR, et al. Danish multicenter randomized study on fibrinolytic therapy versus acute coronary angioplasty in acute myocardial infarction: Rationale and design of the DANish trial in Acute Myocardial Infarction-2 (DANAMI-2). *Am Heart J* 2003;146(2):234–241.

5. Armstrong PW, Boden WE. Reperfusion paradox in ST-segment elevation myocardial infarction. *Ann Intern Med* 2011;155(6):389–391.

6. Wang TY, et al. Association of door-in to door-out time with reperfusion delays and outcomes among patients transferred for primary percutaneous coronary intervention. *JAMA* 2011;305(24):2540–2547.

7. Bode C, et al. Randomized comparison of coronary thrombolysis achieved with double-bolus reteplase (recombinant plasminogen activator) and front loaded, accelerated alteplase (recombinant tissue plasminogen activator) in patients with acute myocardial infarction. *Circulation* 1996;94(5):891–898.

8. ISIS-3 (Third International Study of Infarct Survival) Collaborative Group. ISIS-3: A randomised comparison of streptokinase vs tissue plasminogen activator vs anistreplase and of aspirin plus heparin vs aspirin alone among 41,299 cases of suspected acute myocardial infarction. *Lancet* 1992;339(8796):753–770.

9. Llevadot J, et al. Bolus fibrinolytic therapy in acute myocardial infarction. *JAMA* 2001;286(4):442–449.

10. The Global Use of Strategies to Open Occluded Coronary Arteries (GUSTO III) Investigators. A comparison of reteplase with alteplase foracute myocardial infarction. *N Engl J Med* 1997;337:1118–1123.

11. The GUSTO Investigators. An international randomized trial comparing four thrombolytic strategies for acute myocardial infarction. *N Engl J Med* 1993;329(10):673–682.

12. Van De Werf F, et al. Single-bolus tenecteplase compared with front-loaded alteplase in acute myocardial infarction: TheASSENT-2 double-blind randomised trial. *Lancet* 1999;354(9180):716–722.

13. Wilcox RG, et al. Trial of tissue plasminogen activator for mortality reduction in acute myocardial infarction: Anglo-Scandinavian Study of Early Thrombolysis (ASSET). *Lancet* 1988;2(8610):525–530.

14. Lincoff AM, Topol EJ. Illusion of reperfusion. Does anyone achieve optimal reperfusion during acute myocardial infarction? *Circulation* 1993;88(3):1361–1374.

15. Gershlick AH, et al. Rescue angioplasty after failed thrombolytic therapy for acute myocardial infarction. *N Engl J Med* 2005;353(26):2758–2768.

16. Wijeysundera HC, et al. Rescue angioplasty or repeat fibrinolysis after failed fibrinolytic therapy for ST-segment myocardial infarction: A meta-analysis of randomized trials. *J Am Coll Cardiol* 2007;49(4):422–430.

17. Hochman JS, et al. One-year survival following early revascularization for cardiogenic shock. *JAMA* 2001;285(2):190–192.

18. Tcheng JE, Kinney KJ. After fibrinolysis: Is cardiac catheterization the answer? *J Am Coll Cardiol* 2006;48(7):1336–1338.

19. Fernandez-Avilés F, et al. Routine invasive strategy within 24 hours of thrombolysis versus ischaemia-guided conservative approach for acute myocardial infarction with ST-segment elevation (GRACIA-1): A randomised controlled trial. *Lancet* 2004;364(9439):1045–1053.

20. Cantor WJ, et al. Routine early angioplasty after fibrinolysis for acute myocardial infarction. *N Engl J Med* 2009;360(26):2705–2718.

21. Bøhmer E, et al. Efficacy and safety of immediate angioplasty versus ischemia-guided management after thrombolysis in acute myocardial infarction in areas with very long transfer distances results of the NORDISTEMI (NORwegian study on DIstrict treatment of ST-elevation myocardial infarction). *J Am Coll Cardiol* 2010;55(2):102–110.

22. Borgia F, et al. Early routine percutaneous coronary intervention after fibrinolysis vs. standard therapy in ST segment elevation myocardial infarction: A meta-analysis. *Eur Heart J* 2010;31(17):2156–2169.

23. Morrison LJ, et al. Mortality and prehospital thrombolysis for acute myocardial infarction: A meta-analysis. *JAMA* 2000;283(20):2686–2692.

24. Hochman JS, et al. Long-term effects of percutaneous coronary intervention of the totally occluded infarct related artery in the subacute phase after myocardial infarction. *Circulation* 2011;124(21):2320–2328.

25. ASSENT-4 PCI Investigators. Primary PCI versus tenecteplase-faciliatated percutaneous coronary intervention in patients with ST-segment elevation acute myocardial infarction (ASSENT-4 PCI): Randomized trial. *Lancet* 2006;367(9510):569–578.

26. Ellis SG, et al. Facilitated PCI in patients with ST-elevation myocardial infarction. *N Engl J Med* 2008;358(21):2205–2217.

27. Aversano T, et al. Thrombolytic therapy vs primary percutaneous coronary intervention for myocardial infarction in patients presenting to hospitals without on-site cardiac surgery: A randomized controlled trial. *JAMA* 2002;287(15):1943–1951.

28. Kushner FG, et al. 2009 focused updates: ACC/AHA guidelines for the management of pateints with ST-elevation myocardial infarction and ACC/AHA/ SCAI guidelines on percutaneous coronary intervention: A report of the American College of Cardiology Foundation/ American Heart Association Task Force on Practice Guidelines. *Circulation* 2009;120(22):2271–2306.

29. Wong DT, et al. Myocardial "no-reflow"—diagnosis, pathophysiology and treatment. *Int J Cardiol* 2013;167(5):1798–1806.

30. Nordmann AJ, et al. Clinical outcomes of primary stenting versus balloon angioplasty in patients with myocardial infarction: A meta-analysis of randomized clinical trials. *Am J Med* 2004;116(4):253–262.

31. Zhu MM, et al. Primary stent implantation compared with primary balloon angioplasty for acute myocardial infarction: A meta-analysis of randomized trials. *Am J Cardiol* 2001;88(3):297–301.

32. Steg PG, et al. Mortality following placement of drug-eluting and bare-metal stents for ST-segment elevation acute myocardial infarction in the global registry of acute coronary events. *Eur Heart J* 2009;30(3):321–329.

33. Stone GW, et al. Paclitaxel-eluting stents versus bare-metal in acute myocardial infarction. *N Engl J Med* 2009;360(19):1946–1959.

34. Mehta SR, et al. Dose comparisons of clopidogrel and aspirin in acute coronary syndromes. *N Engl J Med* 2010;363(10):930–942.

35. Mehta SR, et al. Double-dose versus standard-dose clopidogrel and high-dose versus low-dose aspirin in individuals undergoing percutaneous coronary intervention for acute coronary syndromes (CURRENT-OASIS 7): A randomised factorial trial. *Lancet* 2010;376(9748):1233–1243.

36. Wiviott SD, et al. Prasugrel versus clopidogrel in patients with acute coronary syndromes. *N Engl J Med* 2007;357(20):2001–2015.

37. Montalescot G, et al. Prasugrel compared with clopidogrel in patients undergoing percutaneous coronary intervention for ST-elevation myocardial infarction (TRITON-TIMI 38): Double-blind, randomised controlled trial. *Lancet* 2009;373(9665):723–731.

38. AstraZeneca. *Brilinta REMS Document*. Available at: www.fda.gov/downloads /Drugs/DrugSafety/PostmarketDrugSafetyInformationforPatientsandProviders/UCM264004.pdf. Accessed July 26, 2012.

39. Wallentin L, et al. Ticagrelor versus clopidogrel in patients with acute coronary syndromes. *N Engl J Med* 2009;361:(11)1045–1057.

40. Steg PG, et al. Ticagrelor versus clopidogrel in patients with ST-elevation acute coronary syndromes intended for reperfusion with primary percutaneous coronary intervention: A Platelet Inhibition and Patient Outcomes (PLATO) trial subgroup analysis. *Circulation* 2010;122(21):2131–2141.

41. Mahaffey KW, et al. Ticagrelor compared with clopidogrel by geographic region in the Platelet Inhibition and Patient Outcomes (PLATO) trial. *Circulation* 2011;124(5):544–554.

42. Montalescot G, et al. Abciximab in primary coronary stenting of ST-elevation infarction: A European meta-analysis on individual patients' data with long-term follow-up. *Eur Heart J* 2007;28(4):443–449.

43. Stone GW, et al. A comparison of angioplasty with stenting, with or without abciximab, in acute myocardial infarction. *N Engl J Med* 2002;346(13):957–966.

44. Montalescot G, et al. Intravenous enoxaparin or unfractionated heparin in primary percutaneous coronary intervention for ST-elevation myocardial infarction: The international randomized open-label ATOLL trial. *Lancet* 2011;378(9792):693–703.

45. Yusuf S, et al. Effects of fondaparinux on mortality and reinfarction in patients with acute ST-segment elevation myocardial infarction: The OASIS-6 randomized trial. *JAMA* 2006;295(13):1519–1530.

46. Stone GW, et al. Bivalirudin during primary PCI in acute myocardial infarction. *N Engl J Med* 2008;358(21):2218–2230.

47. Levine GN, et al. 2015 ACC/AHA/SCAI focused update on primary percutaneous coronary intervention for patients with ST-elevation myocardial infarction: An update of the 2011 ACCF/AHA/SCAI guideline for percutaneous coronary intervention and the 2013 ACCF/AHA guideline for the management of ST-elevation myocardial infarction. *J Am Coll Cardiol* 2016;67(10):1235–1250.

48. Wald DS, et al. Randomized trial of preventive angioplasty in myocardial infarction. *N Engl J Med* 2013;369(12):1115–1123.

49. Gershlick AH, et al. Randomized trial of complete versus lesion-only revascularization in patients undergoing primary percutaneous coronary intervention for STEMI and multivessel disease: The CvLPRIT trial. *J Am Coll Cardiol* 2015;65(10):963–972.

50. Engstrøm T, et al. Complete revascularisation versus treatment of the culprit lesion only in patients with ST-segment elevation myocardial infarction and multivessel disease (DANAMI 3-PRIMULTI): An open-label, randomised controlled trial. *Lancet* 2015;386(9994):665–671.

51. Vlaar PJ, et al. Cardiac death and reinfarction after 1 year in the Thrombus Aspiration during Percutaneous coronary intervention in Acute myocardial infarction Study (TAPAS): A 1-year follow-up study. *Lancet* 2008;371(9628):1915–1920.

52. Svilaas T, et al. Thrombus aspiration during primary percutaneous coronary intervention. *N Engl J Med* 2008;358(6):557–567.

53. Stone GW, et al. Intracoronary abciximab and aspiration thrombectomy in patients with large anterior myocardial infarction: The INFUSE-AMI randomized trial. *JAMA* 2012;307(17):1817–1826.

54. Fröbert O, et al. Thrombus aspiration during ST-segment elevation myocardial infarction. *N Engl J Med* 2013;369(17):1587–1597.

55. Lagerqvist B, et al. Outcomes 1 year after thrombus aspiration for myocardial infarction. *N Engl J Med* 2014;371(12):1111–1120.

56. Jolly SS, et al. Randomized trial of primary PCI with or without routine manual thrombectomy. *N Engl J Med* 2015;372(15):1389–1398.

57. Levine GN, et al. 2011 ACCF/AHA/SCAI guideline for percutaneous coronary intervention: A report of the American College of Cardiology Foundation/American Heart Association task force on practice guidelines and the Society for Cardiovascular Angiography and Interventions. *Circulation* 2011;124(23):e574–e651.

34

Cardiogenic shock

ARIF JIVAN AND MARK J. RICCIARDI

INTRODUCTION

Circulatory shock is characterized by inadequate systemic tissue perfusion due to altered physiology and reduced blood supply. Tissue perfusion, a function of systemic vascular resistance (SVR) and cardiac output (CO), is significantly reduced when SVR is low and CO is elevated (vasodilatory shock), or where SVR is elevated and CO is reduced. When the latter is accompanied by inadequate intravascular volume, hypovolemic shock is present. Depressed CO with elevated SVR in the presence of adequate intravascular volume indicates cardiogenic shock (CS).[1] Specifically, the National Cardiovascular Data Registry (NCDR) defines CS as sustained (>30 min) hemodynamic compromise with systolic blood pressure (SBP) <90 mmHg and/or cardiac index <2.2 L/min/m² determined to be secondary to cardiac dysfunction and/or the need for inotropic or vasopressor agents or mechanical circulatory support (e.g. intra-aortic balloon pump [IABP], extracorporeal circulation, or ventricular assist devices) to maintain blood pressure and cardiac index above those specified levels. Transient episodes of hypotension that are easily reversed with intravenous (IV) fluid or atropine do not fall under the definition of CS. Furthermore, the *International Classification of Diseases, Tenth Revision* (*ICD-10*) diagnosis coding of CS requires a state of end-organ hypoperfusion due to cardiac failure with persistent hypotension defined as above (also including a mean arterial pressure 30 mmHg lower than baseline), as well as a reduction in cardiac index <1.8 L/min/m² without, and <2.2 L/min/m² with, inotropic support and adequate filling pressures. Moreover, left ventricular end-diastolic pressure (LVEDP) must be >18 mmHg and/or right ventricular end-diastolic pressure >10 mmHg. Table 34.1 summarizes the clinical and hemodynamic findings in CS.

FUNDAMENTALS OF CARDIOGENIC SHOCK

The pathophysiology of CS due to pump failure usually begins with profound depression of myocardial contractility and/or other mechanisms that reduce CO and forward flow. This, in turn, leads to hypotension, insufficient coronary blood flow, myocardial ischemia, further reduction in contractility, and compensatory systemic vasoconstriction. Without intervention, continued decline in tissue perfusion, pathologic vasodilatation, organ failure, and death may rapidly ensue. Acute myocardial infarction (AMI) with resultant ventricular dysfunction accounts for approximately 80% of cases of CS.[1] Left ventricular (LV) pump failure is often due to large ST-segment elevation myocardial infarction (STEMI) that results in extensive LV infarction, but can also be caused by smaller infarction in the presence of preexisting LV dysfunction, right ventricular (RV) involvement, or mechanical complications (papillary muscle rupture, ventricular septal rupture [VSR], or free wall rupture [FWR] with ensuing tamponade).

In clinical practice, two related phenomena are often encountered: *pre-shock* and *mixed shock*. Patients may develop a state of *pre-shock* where hypoperfusion is present but compensatory increases in heart rate and peripheral vasoconstriction allow for the maintenance of CO and systemic blood pressure. *Pre-shock* can be present at the time of hospital admission for AMI. Indeed, most patients with CS complicating AMI develop shock after initial presentation to the hospital.[2] In the Global Utilization of Streptokinase and Tissue Plasminogen Activator for Occluded Coronary Arteries (GUSTO-I) trial, five times the number of patients developed shock after admission than had it on presentation.[3] In CS complicating non-STEMI, the delay may be even more pronounced.[4,5] The *pre-shock* state may provide a

Table 34.1 Hemodynamic criteria for cardiogenic shock

Clinical
SBP < 90 mmHg for > 30 min or MAP 30 mmHg below baseline
Signs of end-organ hypoperfusion: cool extremities, urine output < 30 mL/h, heart rate > 60 bpm
Hemodynamic
Cardiac index < 1.8 mL/min/m² without inotropic support OR CI < 2.2 mL/min/m² with inotropic support
LV end-diastolic pressure > 18 mmHg
RV end-diastolic pressure > 10 mmHg

Note: BPM, beats per minute; CI, cardiac index; LV, left ventricular; MAP, mean arterial pressure; RV, right ventricular; SBP, systolic blood pressure.

window of opportunity for aggressive reperfusion and supportive strategies. In the case of *mixed shock*, evidence for vasodilatation or underfilling confuses the classic paradigm of CS. In fact, the average SVR in the Should We Emergently Revascularize Occluded Coronaries for Cardiogenic Shock (SHOCK) trial was not elevated with wide variability between patients.[2] Normal SVR, therefore, even in the presence of vasopressor therapy, does not preclude the presence of CS. Together, these two frequently encountered clinical scenarios of *pre-shock* and *mixed shock* raise the possibility of alternate mechanisms of hypotension in CS (such as systemic inflammation and vasodilatation) and iatrogenic contributions to the disorder (vasodilation with angiotensin-converting enzyme inhibitors, excessive diuresis and preload reduction, and IV beta-blocker therapy).

ETIOLOGIES

The focus of the remainder of this chapter will be CS complicating AMI. Over 90% of cases fit into one of five etiologic categories with approximately 80% of these due to pump failure (left or right ventricular) and the remainder due to mechanical complications.[1] Non-AMI-related etiologies of CS, including decompensated severe valvular heart disease, acute myocarditis, and arrhythmogenic causes, are beyond the scope of this chapter (Figure 34.1).[7]

Left ventricular pump failure

LV pump failure is the dominant category of CS.[1,5–9] The vast majority of CS resulting from LV pump failure is due to large, often anterior, infarction; a minority is due to smaller infarctions in patients with preexisting LV dysfunction resulting in cumulative loss of >40% of LV mass.[8,9] Multivessel or left main disease is present in up to 80%[9] and CS may be present despite only moderate degrees of LV systolic dysfunction.[1] Data from the National Registry of Myocardial Infarction (NRMI) database and the recent CathPCI registry suggest that the incidence of CS due to LV failure after AMI ranges from 5% to 15%.[4–6,10] CS remains the leading cause of death

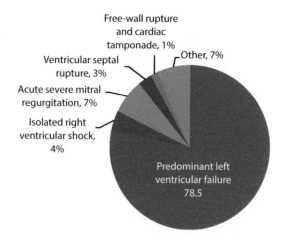

Figure 34.1 Etiologies of cardiogenic shock. (Modified from Hochman, J.S., et al., *J. Am. Coll. Cardiol.*, 36, 1063–1070, 2000.)

in AMI with reported mortality rates of 40%–60%. Data from contemporary registries show an increase in adjusted in-hospital mortality in AMI complicated by CS from 27.6% in 2005–2006 versus 30.6% in 2011–2013. Moreover, Goldberg et al. reported 30-year trends in one regional area of the United States and noted that patients who developed CS had a significantly greater risk of dying during their index hospitalization (65.4% vs. 10.6%, *P* < 0.001). Whether this is due to sicker patients, changes in anticoagulation and antiplatelet medical therapy, or varying considerations underlying revascularization and/or use of mechanical circulatory support, remains to be further investigated.[10] Also, whether the incidence of CS has decreased over the past few decades is contentious; some observational studies suggest that the downward trend reported is explained by earlier hospital presentation, not a decrease in incidence.[5–7]

CLINICAL MANIFESTATIONS

CS due to LV pump failure is characterized by certain physical, laboratory, and hemodynamic parameters. Physical examination is highly variable. A typical patient, however, may manifest ashen skin, cool extremities, altered sensorium, oliguria, tachycardia to maintain CO, narrow pulse pressure, low pulse volume, distant heart sounds, and an audible and palpable left S_3 gallop. Distended neck veins may or may not be present; pulmonary congestion is often present.[1] A 12-lead electrocardiogram (ECG) usually shows STEMI or evidence for prior infarction with new ST-segment depression, or left bundle branch block. Tachy- and bradyarrhythmias are common. Laboratory findings are consistent with rising creatinine, transaminase, and lactate values. Bedside, hemodynamic monitoring typically shows persistent (>30 minutes) hypotension with systolic blood pressure <90 mmHg or vasopressors required to achieve a systolic blood pressure ≥90 mmHg, cardiac index <2.2 L/m²/min, and a pulmonary capillary wedge pressure >18 mmHg. Furthermore, patients in CS typically have an elevated SVR.[1]

MANAGEMENT

Addressing metabolic perturbations, respiratory insufficiency, arrhythmias, and supportive care take on special urgency with CS. If initial assessment suggests hypovolemia as a possible etiology (i.e., no obvious pulmonary congestion), small boluses of normal saline (100 cc at a time) may be used with careful assessment of its effects on systemic blood pressure, heart rate, and urine output. When CS (or *pre-shock*) is suspected, quickly establishing the diagnosis and ruling out mechanical complications with immediate echocardiographic, hemodynamic, and angiographic evaluations is necessary. Because LV failure CS is directly related to the degree of myocardial tissue loss, strategies that limit infarct size are paramount. The benefits of early revascularization for CS due to LV failure complicating MI have been well described in the SHOCK trial.[11,12] Comparing early revascularization—either percutaneous coronary intervention (PCI) or coronary artery bypass grafting (CABG)—with initial medical stabilization with fibrinolysis, inotropes, and vasopressor support when indicated, this landmark study demonstrated a numerical, albeit not a statistically significant, difference in survival at 30 days with early revascularization[11,12] that ultimately became statistically significant by 6 months and persisted at the 6-year follow-up.[12,13] The number needed to treat with early revascularization compared with initial medical stabilization was less than eight. Intra-aortic balloon pump (IABP) counterpulsation was used in 86% of patients. Those randomized within 6 hours of MI onset and those younger than 75 years had particular benefit with early revascularization. Equally beneficial effects were seen with PCI (64%) and CABG (36%). While unselected patients age >75 years in the SHOCK trial appeared to have worse outcomes with early revascularization,[12] nonrandomized data from the SHOCK Registry[13] and a subsequent study in 2009[14] suggest that patients >75 years of age who are otherwise good candidates for early revascularization may also benefit and should be considered for revascularization.[15] As a result, the 2013 American College of Cardiology/American Heart Association (ACC/AHA) guidelines provide a class IIb recommendation for emergent/early revascularization with either PCI or CABG in suitable patients with CS secondary to LV pump failure after acute STEMI irrespective of the time of symptom onset.[16]

As is usually performed with CABG, complete revascularization with PCI should be the goal in the setting of AMI with shock.[17-19] Several observational studies have shown that mortality in CS patients treated with guideline-recommended early revascularization has decreased to 30%–40% compared with 70%–80% when treated without revascularization.[20,21] Assessment of LV myocardial viability can be considered at a later time if staged revascularization is the goal, as myocardial tissue may be ischemic, stunned, hibernating, or completely infarcted without reversible improvement. The 2014 European Society of Cardiology (ESC) and the European Association of Cardio-Thoracic Surgery (EACTS) guidelines on myocardial revascularization give a class IIa recommendation for multivessel PCI in CS.[18,19,22,23]

The need for hemodynamic support with inotropic therapy, IABP counterpulsation, and/or mechanical circulatory support (MCS) should be assessed on the basis of individual need, as the data for morbidity and mortality benefit are conflicting and somewhat limited. However, the risk–benefit ratio often favors the early use of MCS (IABP for pre-shock and more supportive therapies for true CS). Indeed, there are data suggesting that MCS device use prior to revascularization may improve outcomes.[24,25] The early use of such devices can help protect ischemic myocardium before irrevocable injury occurs.

While early use of MCS is often the key measure to protecting end-organ perfusion, inotropic and vasopressor medications are often needed as well. The agents to be considered include IV dopamine (5–15 mcg/kg/min), dobutamine (2–20 mcg/kg/min), and norepinephrine (0.5–30 mcg/min)[26]—the latter when a significant vasodilatory component is present.[26,27] Pure α-adrenergic agents, such as phenylephrine, should be reserved for the rare cases when vasodilation predominates. The use of IV beta-blockers at the time of presentation for patients with acute coronary syndromes (ACS) and STEMI should be avoided. As noted above, many patients initially present with *pre-shock* and can easily deteriorate to CS by limiting both stroke volume and heart rate with acute beta-blockade.

Dopamine, a precursor to norepinephrine, acts on dopaminergic and adrenergic receptors to promote a variety of dose-dependent effects. At low doses (0.5–3 mcg/kg/min), stimulation of dopaminergic D_1 and D_2 receptors concentrated in the coronary, renal, mesenteric, cerebral, and vascular beds promote vasodilatation and increased perfusion to these tissues. At intermediate doses (3–10 mcg/kg/min), dopamine binds to beta 1-adrenergic receptors promoting inotropy and results in a mild increase in SVR. At higher doses (10–20 mcg/kg/min), dopamine preferentially binds α_1-adrenergic receptors, causing peripheral vasoconstriction. Dobutamine has a strong affinity for both beta 1- and beta 2-adrenergic receptors causing an increase in cardiac contractility and a mild increase in chronotropy. Dobutamine, however, significantly increases myocardial oxygen consumption, which can adversely affect ischemic myocardium. Norepinephrine with α_1-adrenergic receptor agonist and modest β-agonist activity is particularly useful in patients who are hypotensive and where vasodilatation predominates (SVR <1,800 dynes/s/cm⁵). Norepinephrine (in doses ranging 2–10 mg/min) can increase contractility as well as diastolic arterial pressure, which in turn maintain coronary perfusion. Data from the Sepsis Occurrence in Acutely Ill Patients (SOAP) II trial showed that CS patients who were randomized to treatment with dopamine (versus norepinephrine) had an increased rate of the predetermined primary endpoint of death at 28 days (RR = 0.75, 95% CI 0.55–0.93, P = 0.03).[27] Additionally, in the total cohort, dopamine was associated with more arrhythmic events compared with norepinephrine (24.1% vs. 12.4%, P < 0.001).

Vasodilators may be used to decrease afterload and LVEDP, thus improving Frank–Starling mechanics in an effort to increase CO. This often comes at a cost, as lowering the already reduced coronary perfusion pressure can further compromise myocardial perfusion, thus worsening the burden of ischemia.

Despite being relatively ineffective as a stand-alone therapy, IABP counterpulsation may be useful for patients with STEMI complicated by CS who present to hospitals without primary angioplasty and without advanced interventional capabilities. In this scenario, STEMI treatment with fibrinolytic therapy plus IABP counterpulsation, followed by immediate transfer for PCI or CABG, has been shown to be effective.[28] With inflation of the IABP during diastole and active deflation during systole, higher diastolic pressures improve perfusion pressure in the coronary arteries and reduce LV afterload, LV wall stress, and myocardial oxygen demand during systole. IABP counterpulsation can increase CO by 15%–30%, with the largest increases observed in patients with significantly reduced CO. In the largest randomized control trial to date, the Intraaortic Balloon Pump in CS II (IABP-SHOCK II) trial, in which patients undergoing early revascularization and optimum medical therapy were randomized to IABP support or control, IABP support did not reduce 30-day or 1-year all-cause mortality.[29] As such, the current ACC/AHA guidelines downgrade the use of IABP from a previous class I recommendation to class IIa for patients with CS who do not quickly stabilize with pharmacologic therapy.[16]

Given the high mortality associated with AMI complicated by CS and the rising incidence of resultant heart failure, nondurable MCS devices have been increasingly used for CS.[30] Along these lines, Kapur et al. showed that mechanical unloading of the LV to reduce LV wall stress prior to coronary reperfusion decreases the extent of myocardial injury during AMI in an animal model.[31]

Currently available ventricular assist devices include the percutaneously placed Impella CP, the surgically placed Impella 5 (Abiomed), and the percutaneously placed TandemHeart (Cardiac Assist, Inc.).[32] In addition, the Impella RP was recently approved for right heart support (see below). Veno-arterial extracorporeal membrane oxygenation (VA-ECMO) has been available for decades and may be used in cases of shock and severe respiratory failure requiring membrane oxygenation.[33] A percutaneously placed "portable ECMO" is also available (CARDIOHELP, Maquet Medical Systems). These devices will be discussed elsewhere in the text.

There are only limited prospective randomized studies that provide evidence-based guidance on the use of these devices in CS. While they can be associated with complications such as limb ischemia, embolization of atherosclerotic plaque and/or thrombus, stroke, infection, access site bleeding, and hemolysis, LV assist devices provide better hemodynamic support than IABP but with no data showing survival benefit.[28–30,34,35] The 2013 ACC/AHA guidelines for

management of STEMI assign a class IIb indication (with level of evidence C) to LV assist devices in refractory CS.[16]

Controversy exists regarding the use of invasive hemodynamic monitoring in the critical care setting,[36–38] with several shock (albeit primarily septic) and decompensated heart failure studies showing that the use of a pulmonary artery catheter provided no mortality benefit.[37] However, in expert hands, the use of pulmonary artery catheterization for CS can be very helpful, particularly in the setting of biventricular or RV failure. The 2007 ACC/AHA guideline update for the management of STEMI suggests that pulmonary artery catheterization should be performed, or is considered useful, in the majority of cases of CS or suspected shock; however, this is not addressed in the most recent guidelines.[16]

Right ventricular pump failure

Although some degree of RV infarction is seen in up to 50% of inferior wall MI,[39] resultant severe RV dysfunction leading to CS is less common. Isolated RV infarction and shock is rare.[2,39,40]

CLINICAL MANIFESTATIONS

The classic presentation of RV shock is that of CS without pulmonary congestion, but with elevated right-sided filling pressures (manifest by elevated jugular venous distention, Kussmaul's sign, pulsus paradoxus, and pressure waveforms with steep right atrial y-decent and RV dip and plateau), ST-segment elevation in the right precordial ECG leads, and RV chamber enlargement and dysfunction. Marked CO depression is present. On occasion, elevated right-sided filling pressures can lead to right-to-left shunting through a patent foramen ovale (PFO) and manifest as unexpected degrees of hypoxemia. The clinical presentation of RV shock can include components of LV dysfunction depending on the relative involvement of the inferior LV. Patients with predominant RV shock are more likely to have single- or double-vessel disease and less likely to have triple-vessel disease than patients with LV shock, and as expected, RV shock is rare with acute left anterior descending artery occlusion.[40] RV shock need not only occur due to occlusion of the proximal right coronary artery (RCA) leading to cessation of blood flow to the RV marginal artery. It can also be seen in conjunction with posterior LV infarction and distal RCA or distal dominant circumflex occlusion.[41,42]

MANAGEMENT

Immediate reperfusion therapy, either with fibrinolysis or PCI, is the goal of therapy for RV shock. Avoidance of medications that decrease preload (nitroglycerin or morphine) or depress CO (beta-blockers) is important. Maintaining or augmenting RV preload with volume expansion constitutes initial therapy for predominant RV shock. If hypotension is not reversed after 1–2 L of fluid, CO augmentation with dobutamine may be necessary, especially if there is a delay to reperfusion therapy or while awaiting recovery of RV function after reperfusion. The loss of atrioventricular (AV) synchrony can result in marked reduction in RV filling and systemic hypotension. Atrial or AV pacing, or cardioversion may provide benefit in such circumstances.[43] Typically, however, when patients are promptly diagnosed, adequately supported, and treated with immediate reperfusion therapy, return of sinus rhythm and improved RV filling often are forthcoming and pacing unnecessary. Finally, if RV failure persists despite optimal medical therapy or for extreme forms of RV shock, mechanical assistance should be considered. Emerging and early data from the RECOVER RIGHT study suggest that the use of a percutaneous right ventricular assist device, the Impella RP, is safe and efficacious. The Impella RP is a 22-Fr catheter-based percutaneous microaxial pump that is positioned across the tricuspid and pulmonary valves with the inflow port in the inferior vena cava (IVC) and outflow in the pulmonary artery. RECOVER RIGHT was a prospective trial consisting of 30 patients, five with post-MI RV-CS. The authors showed a significant improvement in hemodynamics after initiation of Impella RP support with an increase in cardiac index from 1.82 ± 0.04 to 3.3 ± 0.23 L/min/m^2 and decrease in central venous pressure from 19.2 ± 0.7 to 12.6 ± 1 mmHg.[44]

PROGNOSIS

Surprisingly, predominant RV and LV shock resulted in similar mortality in the SHOCK registry, despite younger age, less LV wall injury, and less multivessel disease in RV shock patients.[40] Anecdotal experience and single-center studies of patients undergoing primary PCI for predominant RV shock, however, suggest they do better than their LV shock counterparts,[45] often recover quickly, and represent a particularly gratifying subgroup of shock patients to treat. In patients who

do survive, return of RV function to normal is common.[45,46] Figure 34.2 summarizes MCS strategies for pump failure CS.[24]

Myocardial rupture

The three categories of myocardial rupture following MI have unique presentations and usually require surgery for survival. The time course of these complications post-MI has a bimodal distribution with an occurrence that typically happens within 3–5 days but can occur up to 2 weeks postinfarction (Table 34.2).

PAPILLARY MUSCLE RUPTURE

Acute mitral regurgitation (MR) due to papillary muscle rupture and dysfunction was responsible for 7% of CS in the SHOCK Registry of CS complicating AMI; however, more contemporary data suggest the incidence of papillary muscle rupture is approximately 1%.[1,2]

CLINICAL MANIFESTATIONS

The posteromedial papillary muscle is supplied by a single vascular source—the right or left circumflex coronary artery. Inferior MI due to thrombosis of either of these arteries can therefore lead to posteromedial papillary necrosis and rupture. Because the dually supplied anterolateral papillary muscle is relatively protected from necrosis after thrombotic coronary occlusion, anterior wall MI less commonly leads to acute MR. Acute MR shock typically presents with profound hypotension and pulmonary edema. The lack of an audible murmur is not uncommon and does not rule out acute MR due to papillary rupture. Immediate echocardiography for suspected

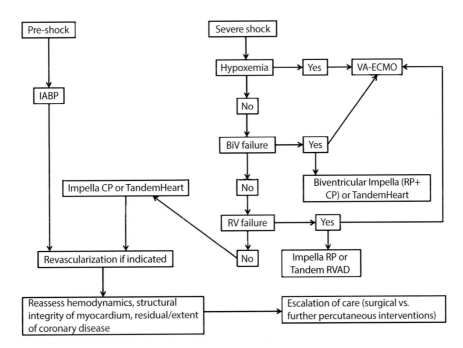

Figure 34.2 Management of cardiogenic shock. (Modified from Atkinson, T.M., et al., *JACC Cardiovasc. Interv.*, 9, 871–883, 2016.) BiV, biventricular; IABP, intraortic balloon pump; RV, right ventricular; RVAD, right ventricular assist device; VA-ECMO, veno-arterial extracorporeal membrane oxygenation.

Table 34.2 Cardiogenic shock due to myocardial rupture

	PMR	VSR	FWR
Location	3/4 inferior	2/3 anterior	1/2 anterior
Exam	Murmur in 50%	Murmur in 90%	JVD, PEA
Thrill	Rare	Common	No
Echocardiography	Regurgitant jet	Shunt	Effusion
PA catheterization	C-V wave in wedge tracing	O2 step-up	Diastolic equalization

Note: FWR, free-wall rupture; JVD, jugular venous distension; PA, pulmonary artery; PEA, pulsus electrical activity; PMR, papillary muscle rupture; VSR, ventricular septal rupture.

acute MR is diagnostic. Dislocation of the tip of the papillary muscle or choral rupture is often seen. As expected, LV ejection fraction may be better preserved than those with CS due to LV failure. The pulmonary capillary wedge tracing may show tall V waves.

MANAGEMENT

Immediate mitral valve surgery (repair or replacement) with revascularization is the only currently established treatment. All other efforts should be aimed at stabilizing the patient prior to surgery. MCS should be used and, if the augmented systemic blood pressure allows, afterload reduction with IV sodium nitroprusside should be started. Patients with papillary muscle necrosis and rupture (and not simply ischemia) would not be expected to benefit from revascularization alone, and primary PCI does not appear to reduce MR in the setting of severe acute papillary rupture complicating STEMI.[47]

PROGNOSIS

Like all cases of myocardial rupture complicating MI, survival with or without aggressive surgical intervention is poor. In the nonrandomized SHOCK registry, patients undergoing mitral valve surgery for acute MR fared poorly, albeit significantly better than those managed medically.[48]

Ventricular septal rupture

VSR complicating MI was responsible for 3% of CS in the SHOCK Registry and represents a particularly challenging group because of the difficulties of operative management and very poor prognosis.[2]

CLINICAL MANIFESTATIONS

Patients with VSR complicating MI often fit the classic rupture dictum "first MI in an older hypertensive patient presenting late."[49–51] In the SHOCK registry, VSR patients were less likely to have had prior MI compared to those with LV failure CS, and the average age was 72 years.[51]

Other risk factors included female gender, advanced age, and an absence of collateral flow to the affected myocardial territory. It is postulated that VSR complicates a first MI because there is a lack of ischemic preconditioning from prior ischemic events or routine ischemic insults that protect against transmural myocardial necrosis and resultant rupture. Unlike acute MR, VSR is almost always accompanied by a murmur (harsh holosystolic) and thrill. Color Doppler echocardiography visualizes the left-to-right shunt, and oxygen saturation step-up in the RV is present. Both anterior and inferior infarction can lead to VSR.

MANAGEMENT

CS due to VSR is nearly uniformly fatal and requires immediate surgery or repair. Delaying surgery in patients who do not have overt CS is appealing in concept as it may allow for healing of the defect margins. Unfortunately, waiting risks the development of shock, which is unpredictable and significantly worsens surgical survival. Because of the high mortality of immediate surgical repair, treatment with less-invasive acute percutaneous VSR closure using septal occlusion devices may be considered. This less-invasive approach to treating acute VSR does not appear to offer an advantage over surgery, especially when CS is present.[39,52]

PROGNOSIS

VSR with CS carries one of the worst survival rates of all cardiac conditions.[2] In a small retrospective analysis by Poulsen et al., 30-day mortality after VSR was 62%.[49] Despite high operative mortality, surgical repair offers an improved chance of survival.[51] Although not all surgical series agree,[53] VSR complicating inferior MI can be particularly challenging for two reasons. First, RV involvement is more likely with inferior infarction. Second, proximal RCA occlusion leading to basal septal VSR is more difficult to repair than the apical defects often seen with anterior MI.[54] In deciding whether to proceed to surgery in patients with multiple comorbidities and advanced age, the location of the VSD may help determine the usefulness or futility of going forward with surgery.

Free-wall rupture and hemorrhagic tamponade

The most devastating complication of MI, FWR, was responsible for 1% of CS in the SHOCK Registry, with an incidence of 0.3%–6.2% in contemporary literature.[2]

CLINICAL MANIFESTATIONS

Like other forms of myocardial rupture complicating MI, FWR often presents with a first MI and may be more common in hypertensive women.[50,55,56] Typically, the infarct is large and anterior.[56,57] Because acute FWR and hemopericardium can lead to abrupt hemodynamic collapse, electromechanical dissociation, and near instant death, many of the clinical manifestations of FWR reported in the literature may represent a subacute variety of FWR in which the rupture is contained within the pericardial space. FWR exists on a spectrum—catastrophic to subacute—with initial clinical presentation varying from pericardial chest pain to hypotension or immediate death. Whether fibrinolytic therapy increases the likelihood of rupture is in dispute and was not found to be the case in the SHOCK trial registry.[57] Furthermore, percutaneous transluminal coronary angioplasty (PTCA), but not fibrinolytic therapy, improved risk. The lack of pulmonary edema is more likely in FWR than LV pump failure CS (17% vs. 55%) and may provide a diagnostic clue.[57] Echocardiography has obvious utility in diagnosis and is specific for FWR when the pericardial effusion is large.[58] Because small effusions and tamponade physiology may be missed, up to 25% of patients with FWR may not have a visibly identifiable pericardial effusion by echocardiography.[58,59]

MANAGEMENT

Early recognition and swift operative repair are imperative. Contained ruptures may allow for the institution of temporizing supportive measures like IABP counterpulsation, vasopressor therapy, and pericardiocentesis in preparation for definitive management. Long-term survival without surgery has been reported (using pericardiocentesis, bed rest, and blood pressure control with beta-blocker therapy) for patients surviving initial FWR and tamponade;[59] however, prompt surgical repair is recommended.

PROGNOSIS

Many patients die almost instantly with rapid and irreversible electromechanical dissociation. Patients presenting with subacute FWR and hemopericardium appear to have survival rates similar to CS due to LV pump failure.[56,57] Survival requires prompt recognition of tamponade, aggressive stabilization, and prompt surgery.

CONCLUSIONS

The high mortality of CS in conjunction with the importance of establishing the correct etiology makes the management of CS challenging and fascinating. Despite advances in therapy and a potential decrease in the incidence of CS, CS fatality remains high. Pump failure CS complicating AMI is best treated with urgent (usually percutaneous) revascularization and stabilizing medical therapies. The early use of MCS with newer devices that provide more hemodynamic support than IABP is intuitively attractive, but survival data are limited. All CS therapies are most beneficial when instituted early. The early diagnosis of CS is therefore paramount.

REFERENCES

1. Mann DL, et al. *Braunwald's Heart Disease: A Textbook of Cardiovascular Medicine* Volume 2. Elsevier Saunders: Philadelphia, PA. 2015.
2. Webb JG, et al. Implications of the timing of onset of cardiogenic shock after acute myocardial infarction: A report from the SHOCK Trial Registry. Should we emergently revascularize Occluded Coronaries for cardiogenic shocK? *J Am Coll Cardiol* 2000;36(3 Suppl A):1084–1090.
3. Holmes DR Jr., et al. Contemporary reperfusion therapy for cardiogenic shock: The GUSTO-I trial experience. The GUSTO-I Investigators. Global Utilization of Streptokinase and Tissue Plasminogen Activator for Occluded Coronary Arteries. *J Am Coll Cardiol* 1995;26(3):668–674.
4. Babaev A, et al. Trends in management and outcomes of patients with acute myocardial infarction complicated by cardiogenic shock. *JAMA* 2005;294(4):448–454.
5. Goldberg RJ, et al. Thirty-year trends (1975 to 2005) in the magnitude of, management of, and hospital death rates associated with cardiogenic shock in patients with acute myocardial infarction: A population-based perspective. *Circulation* 2009;119(9):1211–1219.
6. Jeger RV, et al. Ten-year incidence and treatment of cardiogenic shock. *Ann Intern Med* 2008;149(9):618–626.
7. Hochman JS, et al. Cardiogenic shock complicating acute myocardial infarction—etiologies, management and outcome: A report from the SHOCK Trial Registry. SHould we emergently revascularize Occluded Coronaries for cardiogenic shocK? *J Am Coll Cardiol* 2000;36(3 Suppl A):1063–1070.
8. Holmes DR Jr, et al. Cardiogenic shock in patients with acute ischemic syndromes with and without ST-segment elevation. *Circulation* 1999;100(20):2067–2073.
9. Holmes DR Jr. Cardiogenic shock: A lethal complication of acute myocardial infarction. *Rev Cardiovasc Med* 2003;4(3):131–135.
10. Wayangankar S, Bangalore S, McCoy LA, et al. Temporal trends and outcomes of patients undergoing percutaneous coronary interventions for cardiogenic shock in the setting of acute myocardial infarction. *JACC Cardiovasc Interv* 2016;9(4):341–351.
11. Hochman JS, et al. Early revascularization and long-term survival in cardiogenic shock complicating acute myocardial infarction. *JAMA* 2006;295(21):2511–2515.
12. Hochman JS, et al. Early revascularization in acute myocardial infarction complicated by cardiogenic shock. SHOCK Investigators. Should We Emergently Revascularize Occluded Coronaries for Cardiogenic Shock. *N Engl J Med* 1999;341(9):625–634.

13. Dzavik V, et al. Early revascularization is associated with improved survival in elderly patients with acute myocardial infarction complicated by cardiogenic shock: A report from the SHOCK Trial Registry. *Eur Heart J* 2003;24(9):828–837.

14. Lim HS, et al. Survival of elderly patients undergoing percutaneous coronary intervention for acute myocardial infarction complicated by cardiogenic shock. *JACC Cardiovasc Interv* 2009;2(2):146–152.

15. Hochman JS, Skolnick AH. Contemporary management of cardiogenic shock: Age is opportunity. *JACC Cardiovasc Interv* 2009;2(2):153–155.

16. O'Gara PT, et al. 2013 ACCF/AHA guideline for the management of ST-elevation myocardial infarction: Executive summary: A report of the American College of Cardiology Foundation/American Heart Association Task Force on Practice Guidelines. *Circulation* 2013;127(4):529–555.

17. Kornowski R, et al. Prognostic impact of staged vs. "one-time" multivessel percutaneous intervention in acute myocardial infarction: Analysis from the HORIZONS-AMI (harmonizing outcomes with revascularization and stents in acute myocardial infarction) trial. *J Am Coll Cardiol* 2011;58(7):704–711.

18. Hannan EL, et al. Culprit vessel percutaneous coronary intervention vs. multivessel and staged percutaneous coronary intervention for ST-segment elevation myocardial infarction patients with multivessel disease. *JACC Cardiovasc Interv* 2010;3(1):22–31.

19. Vlaar PJ, et al. Culprit vessel only vs. multivessel and staged percutaneous coronary intervention for multivessel disease in patients presenting with ST-segment elevation myocardial infarction: A pairwise and network meta-analysis. *J Am Coll Cardiol* 2011;58(7):692–703.

20. Goldberg RJ, et al. Recent magnitude of and temporal trends (1994–1997) in the incidence and hospital death rates of cardiogenic shock complicating acute myocardial infarction: The second national registry of myocardial infarction. *Am Heart J* 2001;141(1):65–72.

21. Kolte D, et al. Trends in incidence, management, and outcomes of cardiogenic shock complicating ST-elevation myocardial infarction in the United States. *J Am Heart Assoc* 2014;3(1):e000590.

22. Toma M, et al. Non-culprit coronary artery percutaneous coronary intervention during acute ST-segment elevation myocardial infarction: Insights from the APEX-AMI trial. *Eur Heart J* 2010;31(14):1701–1707.

23. Windecker S, et al. 2014 ESC/EACTS Guidelines on myocardial revascularization: The Task Force on Myocardial Revascularization of the European Society of Cardiology (ESC) and the European Association for Cardio-Thoracic Surgery (EACTS) Developed with the special contribution of the European Association of Percutaneous Cardiovascular Interventions (EAPCI). *Eur Heart J* 2014;35(37):1–100.

24. Atkinson TA, et al. A practical approach to mechanical circulatory support in patients undergoing percutaneous coronary intervention. *JACC Cardiovasc Interv* 2016;9(9):871–883.

25. Rab T. Disappointing results, but we must carry on. *JACC Cardiovasc Interv* 2016;9(4):352–354.

26. Overgaard CB, Dzavik V. Inotropes and vasopressors. *Circulation* 2008;118(10):1047–1056.

27. De Backer D, et al. Comparison of dopamine and norepinephrine in the treatment of shock. *N Engl J Med* 2010;362(9):779–789.

28. Sanborn TA, et al. Impact of thrombolysis, intra-aortic balloon pump counterpulsation, and their combination in cardiogenic shock complicating acute myocardial infarction: A report from the SHOCK Trial Registry. SHould we emergently revascularize Occluded Coronaries for cardiogenic shocK? *J Am Coll Cardiol* 2000;36(3 Suppl A):1123–1129.

29. Thiele H, et al. Intra-aortic balloon counterpulsation in acute myocardial infarction complicated by cardiogenic shock (IABP-SHOCK II): Final 12 month results of a randomized, open-label trial. *Lancet* 2013;382(9905):1638–1645.

30. Morine KJ, Kapur NK. Percutaneous mechanical circulatory support for cardiogenic shock. *Curr Treat Options Cardiovasc Med* 2016;18(6):1–14.

31. Kapur NK, et al. Mechanical unloading the left ventricle before coronary reperfusion reduces left ventricular wall stress and myocardial infarct size. *Circulation* 2013;128(4):328–336.

32. Burkhoff D, et al. TandemHeart Investigators Group. A randomized multicenter clinical study to evaluate the safety and efficacy of the TandemHeart percutaneous ventricular assist device vs. conventional therapy with intraaortic balloon pumping for treatment of cardiogenic shock. *Am Heart J* 2006;152(3):469.e1–469.e8.

33. Sheu JJ, et al. Early extracorporeal membrane oxygenator-assisted primary percutaneous coronary intervention improved 30-day clinical outcomes in patients with ST-segment elevation myocardial infarction complicated with pro- found cardiogenic shock. *Crit Care Med* 2010;38(9):1810–1817.

34. Thiele H, et al. Randomized comparison of intra-aortic balloon support with a percutaneous left ventricular assist device in patients with revascularized acute myocardial infarction complicated by cardiogenic shock. *Eur Heart J* 2005;26(13):1276–1283.

35. Seyfarth M, et al. A randomized clinical trial to evaluate the safety and efficacy of a percutaneous left ventricular assist device vs. intra-aortic balloon pumping for treatment of cardiogenic shock caused by myocardial infarction. *J Am Coll Cardiol* 2008;52(19):1584–1588.

36. Connors AF Jr., et al. The effectiveness of right heart catheterization in the initial care of critically ill patients. SUPPORT Investigators. *JAMA* 1996;276(11):889–897.

37. Harvey S, et al. Pulmonary artery catheters for adult patients in intensive care. *Cochrane Database Syst Rev* 2006;3:CD003408.

38. Binanay C, et al. Evaluation study of congestive heart failure and pulmonary artery catheterization effectiveness: The ESCAPE trial. *JAMA* 2005;294(13):1625–1633.

39. Kinch JW, Ryan TJ. Right ventricular infarction. *N Engl J Med* 1994;330(17):1211–1217.

40. Jacobs AK, et al. Cardiogenic shock caused by right ventricular infarction: A report from the SHOCK registry. *J Am Coll Cardiol* 2003;41(8):1273–1279.

41. Andersen HR, et al. Right ventricular infarction: Frequency, size and topography in coronary heart disease: A prospective study comprising 107 consecutive autopsies from a coronary care unit. *J Am Coll Cardiol* 1987;10(6):1223–1232.

42. Isner JM, Roberts WC. Right ventricular infarction complicating left ventricular infarction secondary to coronary heart disease. Frequency, location, associated findings and significance from analysis of 236 necropsy patients with acute or healed myocardial infarction. *Am J Cardiol* 1978;42(6):885–894.

43. Topol EJ, et al. Hemodynamic benefit of atrial pacing in right ventricular myocardial infarction. *Ann Intern Med* 1982;96(5):594–597.

44. Anderson MB, et al. Benefits of a novel percutaneous ventricular assist device for right heart failure: The prospective RECOVER RIGHT study of Impella RP device. *J Heart Lung Transplant* 2015;34(12):1549–1560.

45. Brodie BR, et al. Comparison of late survival in patients with cardiogenic shock due to right ventricular infarction versus left ventricular pump failure following primary percutaneous coronary intervention for ST-elevation acute myocardial infarction. *Am J Cardiol* 2007;99(4):431–435.

46. Dell'Italia LJ, et al. Hemodynamically important right ventricular infarction: Follow-up evaluation of right ventricular systolic function at rest and during exercise with radionuclide ventriculography and respiratory gas exchange. *Circulation* 1987;75(5):996–1003.

47. Tcheng JE, et al. Outcome of patients sustaining acute ischemic mitral regurgitation during myocardial infarction. *Ann Intern Med* 1992;117(1):18–24.

48. Thompson CR, et al. Cardiogenic shock due to acute severe mitral regurgitation complicating acute myocardial infarction: A report from the SHOCK Trial Registry. SHould we use emergently revascularize Occluded Coronaries in cardiogenic shocK? *J Am Coll Cardiol* 2000;36(3 Suppl A):1104–1109.

49. Poulsen SH, et al. Ventricular septal rupture complicating acute myocardial infarction: Clinical characteristics and contemporary outcome. *Ann Thorac Surg* 2008;85(5):1591–1596.

50. Figueras J, et al. Relevance of delayed hospital admission on development of cardiac rupture during acute myocardial infarction: Study in 225 patients with free wall, septal or papillary muscle rupture. *J Am Coll Cardiol* 1998;32(1):135–139.

51. Menon V, et al. Outcome and profile of ventricular septal rupture with cardiogenic shock after myocardial infarction: A report from the SHOCK Trial Registry. SHould we emergently revascularize Occluded Coronaries in cardiogenic shocK? *J Am Coll Cardiol* 2000;36(3 Suppl A):1110–1116.

52. Thiele H, et al. Immediate primary transcatheter closure of postinfarction ventricular septal defects. *Eur Heart J* 2009;30(1):81–88.

53. Deja MA, et al. Post infarction ventricular septal defect—can we do better? *Eur J Cardiothorac Surg* 2000;18(2):194–201.

54. Moore CA, et al. Postinfarction ventricular septal rupture: The importance of location of infarction and right ventricular function in determining survival. *Circulation* 1986;74(1):45–55.

55. Shapira I, et al. Cardiac rupture in patients with acute myocardial infarction. *Chest* 1987;92(2):219–223.

56. Honan MB, et al. Cardiac rupture, mortality and the timing of thrombolytic therapy: A meta-analysis. *J Am Coll Cardiol* 1990;16(2):359–367.

57. Slater J, et al. Cardiogenic shock due to cardiac free-wall rupture or tamponade after acute myocardial infarction: A report from the SHOCK Trial Registry. Should we emergently revascularize occluded coronaries for cardiogenic shock? *J Am Coll Cardiol* 2000;36(3 Suppl A):1117–1122.

58. Lopez-Sendon J, et al. Diagnosis of subacute ventricular wall rupture after acute myocardial infarction: Sensitivity and specificity of clinical, hemodynamic and echocardiographic criteria. *J Am Coll Cardiol* 1992;19(6):1145–1153.

59. Figueras J, et al. Medical management of selected patients with left ventricular free wall rupture during acute myocardial infarction. *J Am Coll Cardiol* 1997;29(3):512–518.

35

A clinical approach and comprehensive review of percutaneous revascularization of coronary chronic total occlusion

SUBRATA KAR, DEBABRATA MUKHERJEE, AND DAVID E. KANDZARI

INTRODUCTION

Chronically occluded coronary arteries remain a formidable challenge in the evolving field of interventional cardiology. Total coronary occlusion is identified in approximately one-third of diagnostic cardiac catheterizations; however, attempted revascularization accounts for less than 8% of all percutaneous coronary interventions (PCIs).[1] In the Emory Angioplasty versus Surgery Trial (EAST), the presence of a chronic total occlusion (CTO) was the most common reason for physician referral to coronary artery bypass graft (CABG) surgery.[2] Such a disparity between their frequency and treatment underscores not only the technical and procedural frustrations associated with these complex lesions, but also the clinical uncertainties regarding which patients may benefit from CTO revascularization. CTOs remain the single most important reason not to attempt PCI in favor of CABG or medical treatment. In the multivessel PCI versus CABG Synergy between PCI with TAXUS and Cardiac Surgery (SYNTAX) study, the prevalence of CTO in the randomized arm was 27% compared with 59% in the CABG registry cohort.[3]

Unlike PCI of nonocclusive coronary disease, CTOs have fewer studies describing the procedural and clinical outcomes among patients undergoing attempted revascularization. Moreover, they are limited by their retrospective, observational design, variability in operator skills, and inconsistencies regarding the definition of CTO and patient selection. Since the duration of an occluded artery is an independent predictor of procedural outcome,[4,5] an inability to date these lesions, in addition to their heterogeneous composition, has restricted the evaluation of novel revascularization technologies. Until recently, many of the technologies promoted for the treatment of CTOs were modeled after devices applied to nonocclusive disease, even though the pathophysiology between these lesion subsets are not similar.

ANATOMIC CONSIDERATIONS

The definition of a coronary CTO is reflective of the degree of lumen stenosis, the amount of antegrade blood flow, and the age of the occlusion. The degree of stenosis can range from complete occlusion (Thrombolysis in Myocardial Infarction [TIMI] grade 0 flow), frequently called a "true" CTO, to 99% occlusion with minimal contrast penetration through the lesion (TIMI grade 1 flow), referred to as a "functional" total occlusion. Without serial angiograms, the duration of coronary occlusion is difficult to determine with any certainty and must be estimated from available clinical information, such as the timing of the event that caused the occlusion, clinical history of myocardial infarction (MI), or sudden change in angina pattern with electrocardiographic changes consistent with the location of the occlusion. In most patients, the age of the CTO cannot be precisely defined. Furthermore, the temporal criterion used to define a CTO has varied among registries, trials, and databases, ranging from >2 weeks[6–8] to >3 months,[9] which in part explains interstudy differences in lesion characteristics and procedural success. In general, a total occlusion duration of >3 months may be considered "chronic."

Chronic total occlusion histopathology

CTOs most often arise from thrombotic occlusion followed by thrombus organization and tissue aging.[10,11] On histopathological examination, approximately half of all CTOs are <99% stenotic, despite the angiographic appearance of total occlusion with TIMI grade 0 antegrade flow. Moreover, minimal to no relationship exists between the severity of the histopathological lumen stenosis and either plaque composition or lesion age.

The typical atherosclerotic plaque of a CTO consists of intracellular and extracellular lipids, smooth muscle cells, extracellular matrix, and calcium. Collagens are the major structural components of the extracellular matrix,[8,12] with predominance of types I and III (and minor amounts of IV, V, and VI) in the fibrous stroma of atherosclerotic plaques.[13] The concentration of collagen-rich fibrous tissue is particularly dense at the proximal and distal ends of the lesion,

contributing to a column-like lesion of calcified, resistant, fibrous tissue surrounding a softer core of organized thrombus and lipids.

Key histopathological attributes of CTOs are calcification extent, inflammation, and neovascularization. The typical CTO may be classified as "soft," "hard," or a mixture of both (Figures 35.1 and 35.2). Soft plaque consists of cholesterol-laden cells and foam cells with loose fibrous tissue and neovascular channels, which is more frequent in younger occlusions (<1 year old). Soft plaque is more likely to allow guidewire passage either directly through tissue planes or via neovascular channels into the distal lumen. Conversely, hard plaques are characterized by dense fibrous tissue and often contain large fibrocalcific regions without neovascular channels. During PCI, such occlusions are more likely to deflect coronary guidewires into the subintimal area, creating dissection planes. Hard plaques are more prevalent with increasing CTO age (>1 year old). However, areas of calcification frequently occur even in CTOs of <3 months of age, although the extent and severity of calcification increase with occlusion duration. This age-related increase in calcium and collagen content of CTOs partially explains the progressive difficulty during PCI in crossing older occlusions.

Inflammatory cell infiltrates in CTOs consist of macrophages, foam cells, and lymphocytes. Inflammation may exist in the intima, media, and adventitia, although it is most predominant in the intima. As fibrotic CTO lesions age, the vessels typically undergo negative remodeling with decreasing dimension of the external elastic membrane, a phenomenon due to adventitial vascular responses. Occasionally, plaque hemorrhage and inflammation may

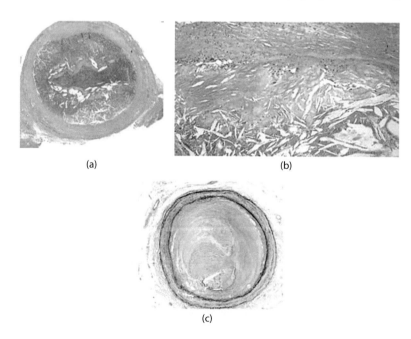

(a)   (b)

(c)

Figure 35.1 **(a)** CTO, soft plaque (hematoxylin–eosin stain; magnification 1×). **(b)** Magnified view of **(a)** showing cholesterol clefts and loose fibrous tissue (hematoxylin–eosin stain; magnification 10×). **(c)** CTO, hard plaque, dense fibrous tissue, and calcium (elastic van Gieson stain; magnification 1×). CTO, chronic total occlusion. (From Stone, G.W., et al., *Circulation*, 112, 2364–2372, 2005. With permission.)

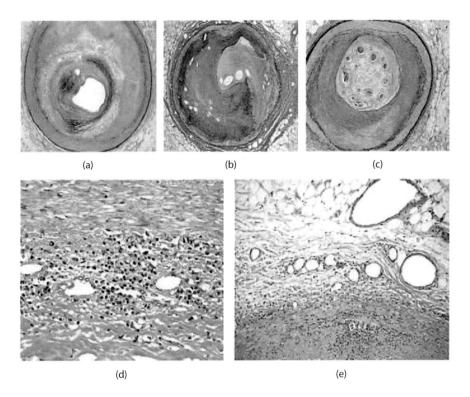

(a)   (b)   (c)

(d)   (e)

Figure 35.2 **(a)** A single large channel is seen in this CTO (elastic van Gieson stain; magnification 1×). **(b)** Traversing capillaries connect with the small recanalization channels in the center of this CTO (elastic van Gieson stain; magnification 1×). **(c)** Small recanalization vascular channels are seen in the center of this CTO (elastic van Gieson stain; magnification 1×). **(d)** Inflammation is found adjacent to vascular channels of the adventitia in this vessel (hematoxylin–eosin stain; magnification 25×). **(e)** Adventitial capillaries have grown to large size in this CTO (hematoxylin–eosin stain; magnification 40×). CTO, chronic total occlusion. (From Stone, G.W., et al., *Circulation*, 112, 2364–2372, 2005. With permission.)

result in positive remodeling.[14] Another hallmark of CTOs is extensive neovascularization, which occurs throughout the extent of the vessel wall. Capillary density and angiogenesis increase with advancing occlusion age. In CTOs <1 year old, new capillary formation is greatest in the adventitia. In CTOs >1 year old, the number and size of capillaries in the intima have increased to a similar or greater extent than those present in the adventitia. Relatively large (>250 mm) capillaries are frequently (47%–67%) present throughout the CTO vessel wall, even in young occlusions, suggesting that angiogenesis within the CTO is an early event. Frequent co-localization of inflammation and neovascularization within the intimal plaque and adventitia suggest that these findings are closely related, although it is unclear whether inflammation is a cause or an effect of neovascularization in CTOs. Lymphocytes and monocytes/macrophages may play an active role in both angiogenesis and atherosclerotic lesion progression by producing a variety of mitogenic and angiogenic factors.[15]

A rich neovasculature network often traverses the CTO vessel wall, arising from the adventitial vasa vasorum across the media and into the lesion intima, suggesting that vessel ingrowth proceeds from the adventitia in younger lesions. An autopsy study of subtotal atherosclerotic lesions demonstrated that new intimal vessels originate in the adventitial vasa vasorum of lesions with >70% stenosis, but rarely

from the coronary lumen.[16] Such microchannels, which can recanalize the distal lumen, may result from thrombus-derived angiogenic stimuli[17] and are suggested on an angiogram of an old CTO without a well-defined proximal cap or stump. The distinction should be made between ipsilateral epicardial angiographic "bridging" collateral vessels and true microvascular collaterals. Neochannels may also develop with the organization of thrombus, connecting the proximal and distal lumens; this is suggested by a tapered CTO proximal cap on an angiogram. Such channels may serve as a route for a guidewire to reach the distal vessel for therapeutic intervention.

Collaterals and chronic total occlusions

Collaterals preserve myocardial function and prevent cell death in the distribution of the occluded artery. A CTO that is well collateralized is functionally equivalent to a 90% stenosis (Figure 35.3).[18] The myocardium remains viable but produces ischemia during periods of increased oxygen demand. Thus, patients with these lesions are likely to have exertional angina. The risk of unstable angina or acute coronary syndrome due to the lesion is unlikely as it is totally occluded. The myocardium supplied by the CTO can result in acute coronary syndrome if the arteries supplying the collaterals become compromised.

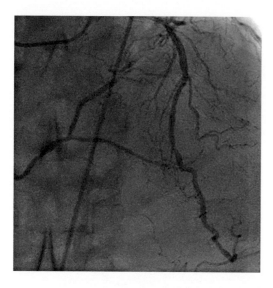

Figure 35.3 Angiogram with the injection of contrast into the left coronary artery showing the extensive collaterals supplying the right coronary artery.

Recovery of impaired left ventricular function after revascularization of a CTO is not directly related to the quality of collateral function, as collateral development does not appear to require the presence of viable myocardium.

Clinical impact relative to target vessel

Scant data exist regarding the differential benefit of CTO recanalization on particular target vessels; for example, the left anterior descending (LAD), left circumflex (LCX), or right coronary artery (RCA). A large, single-center registry suggests that PCI for CTO of the LAD, but not LCX or RCA, is associated with improved long-term survival.[19] The study included 2,608 patients and the LAD was the target vessel in 936 (36%), the LCX in 682 (26%), and the RCA in 990 (38%) patients. Angiographic success rates were 77%, 76%, and 72%, respectively. Procedural success compared with failure was associated with improved 5-year survival in the LAD cohort (88.9% vs. 80.2%, $P < 0.001$), but not in the LCX (86.1% versus 82.1%, $P = .21$) and RCA groups (87.7% vs. 84.9%, $P = 0.23$). In multivariable analysis, CTO PCI success in the LAD group remained associated with decreased mortality risk (Hazard ration [HR] 0.61; 95% CI, 0.42–0.89).

INDICATIONS FOR REVASCULARIZATION

In general, when the CTO represents the only significant lesion in the coronary tree, PCI is warranted when the following conditions are all present:[8]

1. The occluded artery is responsible for the patient's symptoms of chest pain or heart failure despite maximal medical therapy. PCI may also be considered in selected cases of silent ischemia if a large myocardial territory is in jeopardy.
2. If the CTO territory is associated with significant left ventricular dysfunction, viability is demonstrated within the myocardial territory supplied by the occluded artery.

3. The likelihood of success is moderate to high (>60%), with an anticipated major complication rate of death of <1% and MI of <5%.
4. The goal is to achieve complete revascularization.[20]

If the PCI attempt is unsuccessful, further management will depend on the symptomatic status and the extent of jeopardized ischemic myocardium. Repeated PCI following initial failure (typically with an allowance of several weeks for vessel healing in the case of dissection) or CABG may be warranted if a large myocardial territory is ischemic or the patient is very symptomatic. Alternatively, conservative therapy may be appropriate if repeated PCI is unlikely to be successful and the patient's symptoms can be managed with antianginal medications.

In patients with multivessel disease and one or more CTOs, the relative risks and benefits of CABG compared with PCI should be considered. The presence of any of the following may favor CABG[8]:

1. Left main artery disease
2. Complex triple-vessel disease (e.g., SYNTAX score >32), especially in the patient with insulin-dependent diabetes, severe left ventricular dysfunction, or chronic kidney disease (CKD)
3. An occluded proximal LAD (supplying a viable anterior wall), which is not favorable for PCI
4. Multiple CTOs with a relatively low anticipated success rate

Other patients with multivessel disease, including a CTO, may be appropriately managed by PCI, with the goal of complete revascularization whenever possible. In the All-Comers Synergy Between Percutaneous Coronary Intervention with Taxus and Cardiac Surgery (SYNTAX) trial,[20] incomplete revascularization was associated with significantly higher 4-year mortality, all-cause revascularization, major adverse cardiac and cerebrovascular events, and stent thrombosis.

George et al.[21] analyzed 13,443 patients and showed that successful CTO revascularization (10,199 cases, 70.6%) was associated with improved long-term survival (HR of 0.72, 95% CI of 0.62–0.83; $P < 0.001$). Furthermore, complete revascularization (regardless of the diseased vessel) was associated with greater survival benefit compared with incomplete (HR 0.70, CI 0.56–0.87, $P = 0.002$) or failed revascularization (HR 0.61, CI 0.50–0.74, $P < 0.001$). The multivariable predictors of death for CTO PCI included heart failure, advanced age, smoking, renal disease, and insulin-dependent diabetes.

Typically, in patients presenting with acute coronary syndrome or with stable angina in whom the nonoccluded vessels can be reliably stented with a low rate of complication, angioplasty of the CTO should be performed after PCI of nonoccluded lesions. The one exception to this rule would be in patients in whom failed PCI of the CTO would result in referral for CABG, in which case, the CTO should be approached first unless conditions dictate otherwise.

Patients with medically refractory angina or a moderate to large ischemic burden deserve consideration for PCI, particularly if the symptoms or jeopardized myocardial territory is enough to warrant CABG as an option. In several large databases, only 11%–15% of patients undergoing PCI for CTO were asymptomatic.[19,22] Conversely, the proportion of patients presenting with unstable angina due to a CTO is also fairly low (9%–18%).[8,23] Thus, the majority of patients undergoing PCI for CTO have stable or progressive angina, whereas many asymptomatic patients with CTO are managed medically. A history of prior MI has been reported in 42%–68% of patients with an angiographically demonstrated CTO.

Stress-induced ischemia can typically be elicited in patients with CTOs, especially in the absence of a history of prior MI. One study identified reversible perfusion defects using stress myocardial single-photon emission computed tomography (SPECT) in 83% of 71 patients without history of prior MI and with single-vessel disease involving a CTO.[24] Similarly, another study documented severe and extensive stress perfusion defects in 56 patients with no prior MI and single-vessel CTO with the presence of collaterals.[25] Adenosine SPECT imaging may be even more sensitive than exercise-induced stress imaging to detect perfusion defects in patients with CTO.

Temporal changes in contractility and hyperemic and resting myocardial blood flow (MBF) in CTO-dependent and remote myocardium after PCI of CTOs were investigated using cardiovascular magnetic resonance (CMR) imaging.[26] Three groups were prospectively studied: 17 patients scheduled for CTO PCI, 17 scheduled for PCI of a nonocclusive coronary artery stenosis (non-CTO), and 6 patients with CTO who were not scheduled for revascularization. Contractility in treated segments was improved at 24 hours and 6 months after CTO PCI, but only at 6 months after non-CTO PCI. In both PCI groups, successfully revascularized segments demonstrated normalized MBF or contractility similar to remote segments. In patients with untreated CTO segments, however, MBF and wall thickening did not improve at follow-up.

Debate and conflicting data exist regarding the optimal timing for revascularization of a total coronary occlusion resulting from a recent infarction. In the Occluded Artery Trial (OAT),[27] PCI of infarct arteries 3–28 days after MI did not reduce death, recurrent MI, or congestive heart failure over 4 years. Notably, exclusion criteria included multivessel coronary disease, rest angina, or demonstration of at least moderate ischemia by noninvasive stress testing. The Total Occlusion Study of Canada (TOSCA-2) substudy[28] of this trial also reported no improvement in left ventricular function with revascularization at 1 year. Consequently, it may be best to allow recovery from acute MI for patients similar to those included in this trial who present within this time period. Conversely, a meta-analysis of randomized control trials demonstrated that PCI of the infarct artery performed late (12 hours to 60 days) after MI is associated with significant improvements in cardiac function and survival.[29] Angiographic documentation of total occlusion was an inclusion criterion in 5 of the 10 studies, and 3 additional studies required either a total occlusion or significant stenosis. The analysis included 3,560 patients with median time from MI to randomization of 12 days (range 1–26 days) and follow-up of 2.8 years (42 days to 10 years). Randomization allocated 1,779 subjects to PCI and 1,781 to medical treatment. There were 112 (6.3%) PCI and 149 (8.4%) medical therapy deaths, yielding significantly improved survival in the PCI group (odds ratio [OR] 0.49; 95% CI, 0.26–0.94; $P = 0.030$). In the PCI group, such benefits were associated with favorable effects on cardiac remodeling, including improved left ventricular ejection fraction (LVEF) (+4.4% change; 95% CI, 1.1–7.6; $P = 0.009$). Successful CTO PCI is associated with increased patient survival, improved ejection fraction and exercise tolerance, attenuation of angina, decreased need for CABG, and enhanced tolerance of future acute coronary syndromes.[30]

PROCEDURAL FUNDAMENTALS

The technical and procedural success rates of PCI in CTOs have significantly increased over the last 10 years because of greater operator experience and improvements in equipment and procedural techniques.[31] However, CTOs remain the lesion subtype in which PCI is most likely to fail. In recent contemporary series, procedural success rates have ranged from 55% to greater than 90%, with the variability reflecting differences in operator technique and experience, availability of advanced guidewires, CTO definition, and case selection. The most common PCI failure mode for CTOs is inability to successfully pass a guidewire across the lesion into the true lumen of the distal vessel.

Most studies have consistently reported that increasing age of the occlusion, greater lesion length, presence of a nontapered stump, origin of a side branch at the occlusion site, excessive vessel and lesion tortuosity, calcification, ostial occlusion, and lack of visibility of the distal vessel course negatively affect the ability to successfully cross a CTO.[31] In the past, the presence of bridging collaterals was also consistently identified as a determinant of failed CTO PCI, but in more recent experiences, success rates may no longer be inversely correlated with the presence of bridging collaterals and other angiographic characteristics. Bridging collaterals may reflect the chronicity of the lesion and signify the requirement for stiffer and/or tapered tip wires to penetrate the occlusion. The availability of enhanced force wires with greater torque response, tapered tip guidewires, and adoption of retrograde and antegrade dissection reentry techniques have clearly increased the success rates with bridging collaterals and similar angiographic complexities such that CTOs should no longer be avoided for solely these reasons.

A multicenter CTO registry identified predictors of unsuccessful recanalization.[32] This study documented experiences with 1,362 patients at three centers from 2000 to 2007. Both angiographic and clinical outcomes were measured over long-term follow-up (3 years for the majority of patients). Recanalization was successful in 65.5% of native vessels and 76.6% of in-stent restenosis cases. In the overall cohort, a longer lesion, blunt appearance of the proximal occlusion, vessel calcification, and prior CABG were all associated with procedural failure.

CLINICAL AND PROCEDURAL CONSIDERATIONS FOR CHRONIC TOTAL OCCLUSION REVASCULARIZATION

In CTO interventions, characterization of the plaque (e.g. extent of calcification and CTO origin) and visualization of the distal vessel must be optimized. In most instances, invasive angiography with contralateral injection of contrast into the artery supplying collaterals to the distal vessel (Figure 35.4) may provide the necessary information. If there is any doubt regarding the location of the true lumen or the anatomical course of the occluded vessel segment, a coronary computed tomography (CT) angiogram with three-dimensional (3D) reconstruction may be particularly useful (Figure 35.5). Furthermore, in selected cases, coronary CT angiography may improve patient selection for CTO recanalization, decrease the time and contrast media

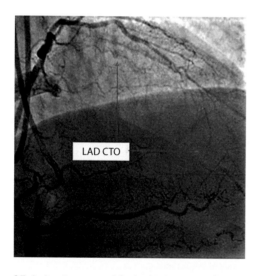

Figure 35.4 Angiogram with dual injections showing a chronic total occlusion (CTO) of the left anterior descending artery (LAD).

needed for the procedure, decrease complications, and ultimately, improve procedural outcome.[32]

To increase the likelihood of success, larger caliber guiding catheters (e.g. 7- or 8-Fr diameter) are recommended, although favorable procedural success has also been reported using transradial vascular access.[33] Extended-length sheaths will provide additional support. Larger guide catheters provide excellent support for guidewire penetration but may also be associated with increased contrast utilization. Larger-diameter guiding catheters also enable delivery of covered stent grafts in uncommon instances of coronary perforation after successful recanalization. If a second angiographic catheter is used for contralateral injection, a 5- or 6-Fr catheter may be inserted into the contralateral femoral artery or either the brachial or radial artery. For RCA CTOs, an Amplatz guide will provide maximal support, while any supportive catheter with extra backup can be used for the left coronary system. One exception is the retrograde approach (described below), in which a short guide (<90 cm) is required in the "donor" artery that supplies the collateral flow.

Intravascular ultrasound (IVUS) can be very useful in the evaluation and treatment of CTOs. Using an antegrade approach to the lesion, IVUS can be used to:

1. Identify the proximal cap location using the IVUS catheter in the side branch.
2. Confirm the wire penetration into the proximal cap.
3. Redirect the wire into the true lumen after penetrating the subintimal space.
4. Optimize stent placement, expansion, and apposition.

When performing a retrograde approach, IVUS can be used to help guide the retrograde wire into the proximal lumen of the CTO (Figure 35.6).

Antithrombotic therapy

Unfractionated heparin (UFH) is the preferred antithrombin therapy during percutaneous CTO revascularization. In cases of coronary perforation, UFH can be rapidly reversed with administration of protamine (10 mg reverses 1,000 U of UFH to maximum dose 50 mg), unlike presently available

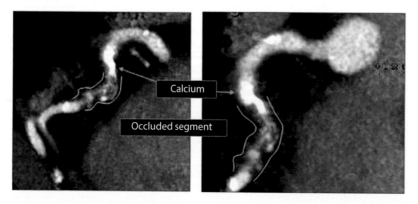

Figure 35.5 Computed tomography angiogram of a known chronic total occlusion (CTO) of the right coronary artery (RCA) demonstrating heavy calcification at the site of occlusion and a significant bend in the RCA within the occluded segment.

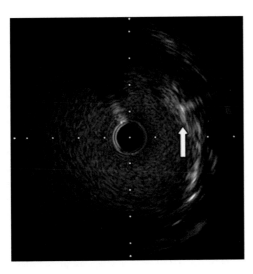

Figure 35.6 Intravascular ultrasound of the ostial left main coronary artery showing a retrograde guidewire penetrating from the subintimal space into the aorta (*white arrow*).

direct thrombin inhibitors. In most cases, an initial bolus dose of UFH is administered to achieve an activated clotting time (ACT) of approximately 250–300 seconds for antegrade CTO procedures, and greater than 300 seconds for retrograde procedures. Bivalirudin and glycoprotein (GP) IIb/IIIa inhibitors are usually avoided at the start of the procedure because of the increased procedural risk of bleeding complications (e.g. tamponade) in instances of coronary perforation. If indicated, GP IIb/IIIa inhibitors may be administered once the guidewire has successfully crossed the lesion and is confirmed to be intraluminal. Pretreatment with clopidogrel has anecdotally not been associated with increased risk of CTO procedural complications but has not been well studied. Similar to other PCI procedures, if the patient is naive to thienopyridine therapy, a loading dose may be administered before, during, or immediately at the end of the procedure.

Guidewire technology and selection

Crossing the CTO with a guidewire is the most important and challenging step of the procedure. This is the most frequent cause for failed CTO intervention. There are three separate steps to crossing a CTO: penetrating the proximal fibrous cap, traversing the body of the CTO to reach the distal fibrous cap, and penetrating the distal fibrous cap to enter the true lumen. Wires designed for treating CTOs can be broadly divided into two major groups: polymer-jacketed and/or hydrophilic guidewires, and stiffer, nonpolymer (nonhydrophilic or hydrophilic) guidewires. Both wire categories may be available in standard (0.014-in diameter) or tapered (0.009–0.010-in diameter) tip configurations. The stiffer, nonhydrophilic guidewires are typically more controllable, provide improved tactile sensation, and are less likely to cause vessel dissection. It is generally recommended to initially attempt CTO penetration with a less stiff guidewire and progress to graduated tip-load wires if resistance to penetration is encountered.

Hydrophilic wires advance with minimal resistance and tactile sensation, even down minute branches and false channels, contributing to an increased risk of coronary perforation. These guidewires offer maneuverability in tortuous vessels and may be steered more easily in a true lumen immediately after sharp bends. However, they are more likely than noncoated wires to penetrate beneath plaque and cause subintimal dissections. Furthermore, they may, less commonly, maintain their tip shape compared with nonpolymer coated wires and do not offer precise tip control. A hydrophilic wire may be passed for long distances in a false channel without resistance. The course of hydrophilic wires must be assessed in at least two orthogonal views to confirm the wire is in the true lumen. The most commonly used polymer-coated wires are the Asahi Fielder (Regular, FC, and XT), and the Abbott Pilot (ranging in support from 50 to 200) guidewire series. Additionally, commonly used tapered tip hydrophilic wires include the Asahi Gaia series. Once a CTO-specific guidewire has crossed the occlusion and passed into the distal lumen, the wire should be exchanged with a soft, floppy-tipped wire to minimize the risk of distal wire perforation or dissection.

A microcatheter or an over-the-wire (OTW) 1.5 mm balloon catheter can be used for support as well as access for ease of exchanging wires. The most commonly used support catheter in both antegrade and retrograde CTO methods is the Corsair catheter (Asahi, Inc.). In addition, current 1.2 and 1.25 mm compliant balloons are very low profile and are able to cross lesions in a majority of cases. Although less navigable than the Corsair catheter, a balloon catheter also offers the option of treatment with dilation of the vessel as well as added support by using it as an anchoring device within the vessel for enhanced guidewire support.

Inability to cross a CTO with a balloon catheter despite successful guidewire recanalization is infrequent. Assuming adequate guiding catheter support, one method is to use a second angioplasty balloon in a side-branch vessel proximal to the CTO ("anchoring balloon" technique). In some instances, incremental inflations with a small diameter (1.5 mm) balloon within the proximal segment of a CTO may facilitate eventual crossing. Other options include laser atherectomy using a 0.9 mm laser catheter, rotational atherectomy (which requires passage of specialized rotablator guidewire), or the Tornus (Asahi Intec, Aichi, Japan) support catheter. The Tornus catheter is a braided stainless steel support catheter that is advanced in a counterclockwise fashion over the guidewire to create a passage in highly stenosed lesions and facilitate subsequent balloon catheter delivery.

Guidewire techniques: Antegrade, retrograde, controlled dissection and hybrid approach

The antegrade approach is the most common initial strategy for attempted recanalization of a CTO.[34] Starting equipment may vary depending on lesion characteristics and anatomy.

A support catheter (OTW balloon or microcatheter) with either a stiff nonhydrophilic guidewire (e.g., Miracle Bros 3 g, Asahi Intec/Abbott Vascular, Redwood City, CA) or a tapered hydrophilic wire (e.g., Fielder XT, Abbott Vascular) is used to initially probe the lesion. If the proximal cap cannot be penetrated or the wire is unable to be advanced within the lesion, progressively stiffer wires may be substituted. For some experienced CTO interventionalists, high-penetrating force wires (e.g., 9–12 g tip load), specialized polymer-jacketed guidewires (e.g., Pilot 200), or selected tapered tip hydrophilic guidewires (e.g., Gaia series) are often selected as the initial guidewire. With the use of the stiffer (and hydrophilic) guidewires, however, the operator must be aware of the increased risk of complications (e.g. coronary perforation or major dissection). Wire shaping for the antegrade approach of CTOs is markedly different than for nonocclusive disease. In general, the initial wire should have a bend with an angle <30° approximately 1 mm from the tip. If more angulated bends are required to access the CTO, this should be done with a soft, floppy wire and then exchanged for a dedicated CTO wire.

The parallel wire technique is a common method to approach CTO PCI (Figure 35.7). Occasionally, a guidewire may exit the true lumen of the occluded vessel and enter a subintimal dissection plane. In this scenario, the wire is left in place as a visual landmark to avoid further vessel trauma and to obstruct entry into the false lumen. A second wire (stiff or hydrophilic, depending on the lesion characteristics) is advanced to the point of the first wire's exit and then redirected toward the true lumen. A twin-pass dual-access exchange catheter (Vascular Solutions, Inc., Minneapolis, MN) can be very useful when introducing the second wire. An alternative method is the subintimal tracking and reentry (STAR) technique (Figure 35.8).[35] This is a method of

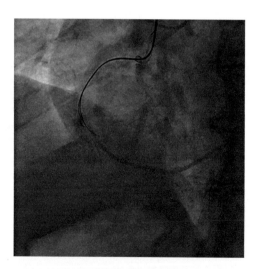

Figure 35.7 Angiogram of a CTO of the right coronary artery using a parallel wire technique. The first guidewire entered the subintimal space and was left in place. A second guidewire was passed adjacent to the first one and directed toward the true lumen. CTO, chronic total occlusion.

intentional subintimal dissection using a hydrophilic wire typically shaped with a prolapsed tip. The wire is advanced beyond the occlusion adjacent to the distal lumen and may spontaneously reenter the true lumen in the main vessel, or more commonly at the confluence of bifurcating side branches. Ultimately, an extensive dissection is created, which typically requires treatment with several stents. This technique may not only be associated with a higher risk of coronary perforation but also can result in shearing and occlusion of side branches and should be reserved as a bail-out technique for highly symptomatic patients refractory to medical therapy.

More complex techniques for difficult CTOs include the retrograde approach, as well as the controlled antegrade and retrograde subintimal tracking (CART) and reverse CART methods (Figure 35.9).[36,37] These advanced techniques are generally reserved for passing wires in a retrograde course through septal or occasionally epicardial collaterals, although manipulations in epicardial collaterals are higher risk for perforation. Since the collaterals often originate from the contralateral coronary artery, dual arterial catheter access is required, and shortened guiding catheters (85–90 cm) are essential (at least for the retrograde donor catheter) to enable appropriate working length. Dedicated angiography focusing on the collaterals is essential to define the location, size, and tortuosity of the vessels. Once localized, the collateral can be crossed with a hydrophilic wire such as a Fielder FC or more commonly Sion guidewire (Asahi) and microcatheter. A specialized guidewire is then used to penetrate the proximal cap via a retrograde approach followed by balloon dilatation and then antegrade crossing. Alternatively, in cases of successful retrograde, the retrograde wire (325 cm in length) may be externalized through the antegrade guiding catheter and then exchanged and followed by antegrade PCI. IVUS from the proximal portion of the CTO may also assist in guiding the wire into the true lumen.

In cases of primary retrograde crossing failure, variations on the retrograde approach include controlled dissection techniques termed *CART* and *reverse CART*. With CART, a balloon is inflated in the distal portion of the CTO over the retrograde wire that is located in the false lumen. A second antegrade wire is introduced distal to the proximal cap and into the subintimal space. When the retrograde balloon is inflated, expanding the subintimal space, the antegrade wire is then directed toward the retrograde balloon as it is deflated. Once the antegrade wire enters the space occupied by the balloon, it may then be advanced distally into the true lumen parallel to the path taken by the retrograde wire and balloon. The more commonly applied reverse CART is the same concept, although the roles are reversed; a balloon is inflated in the proximal portion of the CTO on the antegrade wire, and the retrograde wire is advanced into the subintimal space. These techniques are highly specialized so they require dedicated equipment and unique skills acquired from extensive training.

Since CTO interventions are time-consuming and usually require a high contrast load, the hybrid approach utilizes

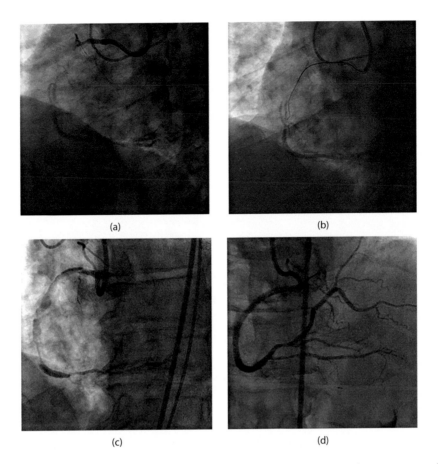

(a)

(b)

(c)

(d)

Figure 35.8 Angiogram showing the subintimal tracking and reentry (STAR) technique for treatment of a right coronary artery chronic total occlusion (a). This is a method of intentional subintimal dissection using a hydrophilic wire with a prolapsed tip. The wire is advanced beyond the occlusion adjacent to the distal lumen (b). It may spontaneously reenter the true lumen in the main vessel, or more commonly in side branches. Ultimately, an extensive dissection is created, which needs to be treated with several stents (c,d).

a combination of all the aforementioned techniques to achieve success in the safest, most efficient, and most effective manner, while using the least amount of radiation and contrast. Wire escalation is a key component of the hybrid strategy, using anterograde and retrograde approaches as necessary to maximize time efficiency.[38] A general time frame of 5–10 minutes should not be exceeded for a specific technique if progress is not being achieved.[38] Next, a change in the wire, microcatheter, or alternative lesion crossing approaches (i.e., anterograde to retrograde) should be implemented.[35] The hybrid approach can also increase the chance of successful CTO PCI even in non-CTO operators based on the experience of a tertiary care hospital.[39] The hybrid algorithm[40] with dual injection includes four criteria to determine whether the antegrade or retrograde approach should be used:

1. Ambiguous proximal cap
2. Poor distal target
3. Good interventional collaterals
4. Major side branch at distal cap

If the lesion length is less than 20 mm, antegrade wire escalation may be initially attempted followed by antegrade

dissection reentry if unsuccessful. Subsequent attempts may progress to retrograde wire escalation followed by eventual retrograde dissection reentry.[41] Conversely, if the lesion length is greater than 20 mm, the initial approach may include antegrade dissection reentry followed by retrograde dissection reentry if unsuccessful.[40] This hybrid algorithm is described by Wilson et al.[40] who showed that 1,156 patients who underwent CTO PCI by experienced hybrid CTO operators can achieve success rates of 90% in real-world practice (first attempt success rates of 79%, 90% overall; 30-day MACE of 1.6%). Patients with lower five-point Multicenter CTO registry of Japan (J-CTO) scores had higher first attempt success (J-CTO ≤ 1, 92% vs. J-CTO ≥ 2, 74%; $P < 0.001$). The J-CTO score is defined as 0 = easy, 1 = intermediate, 2 = difficult, ≥3 = very difficult.

Innovative technologies include true lumen crossing and intraluminal reentry devices. The most commonly applied method for successful recanalization when an antegrade guidewire passes into a subintimal dissection plane is the antegrade dissection reentry method (ADR). Using the facilitated antegrade steering technique (FAST), both the CrossBoss CTO catheter and the Stingray CTO reentry system (Bridgepoint Technologies, Minneapolis, MN) may

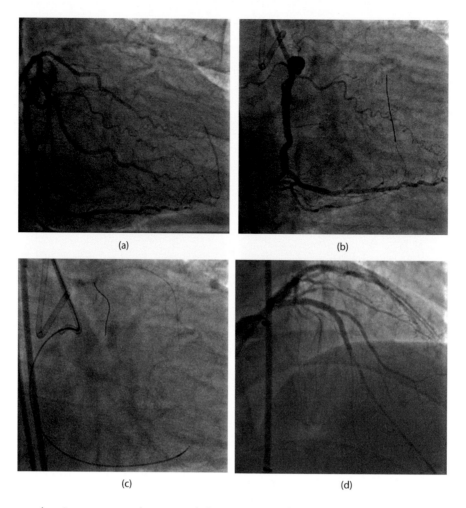

(a)

(b)

(c)

(d)

Figure 35.9 Angiogram showing a retrograde approach for treatment of a chronic total occlusion of the left anterior descending artery (a). After selecting a septal collateral, a polymer-coated wire is advanced to the distal edge of the occlusion (b). The proximal lumen is accessed and treated with angioplasty. Next, guidewires are introduced from an antegrade approach (c), and the vessel is treated definitively (d).

provide increased success rates and safety compared with guidewires alone. The Boston Scientific Coronary CTO Crossing System (BridgePoint Medical System) consists of the CrossBoss CTO catheter, and the Stingray balloon and guidewire.[42] The CrossBoss CTO catheter tracks over a wire via a FAST spin technique to create a longitudinal dissection plane that is parallel to the occluded segment.[42] Specifically, the catheter has a highly torqueable coiled-wire shaft, and the spin technique reduces the amount of forward force required to cross the CTO. The Stingray system is a balloon catheter with a flat shape and opposing exit ports for selective guidewire reentry when positioned within a dissection plane adjacent to the true vessel lumen. The Stingray guidewire is designed specifically for reentry into the distal true lumen. The Facilitated Antegrade Steering Technique in Chronic Total Occlusions (FAST-CTOs) trial[43] evaluated this novel device, the CrossBoss catheter, and Stingray re entry system (BridgePoint Medical System, BridgePoint Medical, Plymouth, MN) for the treatment of refractory CTOs. A total of 147 patients with 150 CTOs were enrolled in a prospective, multicenter, single-arm trial. In the first 75 treated

CTOs, 67% were successful, which increased to 87% in the remaining 75 CTOs (77% overall success rate). Coronary perforation occurred in 14 patients (9.3%) and the 30-day major adverse cardiac event (MACE) rate was 4.8% (similar to historical controls, P = .40). The study concluded that the new antegrade crossing and re entry system resulted in high success rates without a significant increase in complication for patients who failed standard CTO crossing techniques (Table 35.1). Therefore, the CrossBoss and Stingray system with the appropriate training and experience safely allows successful CTO recanalization with relatively short crossing times, limited contrast use, and radiation utilization.

Danek et al.[41] evaluated ADR outcomes in 1,313 CTO PCIs performed in 11 centers in the United States, which showed that ADR had lower technical success rates (86.9% vs. 91.8%, P = 0.005) and procedural success (85% vs. 90.7%, P = 0.002), compared with non-ADR cases, with similar MACE risk (2.9% vs. 2.2%, P = 0.42). ADR was also associated with longer procedure time, longer fluoroscopy time, and greater contrast volume (P < 0.001). However, if retrograde cases were excluded, ADR and antegrade wire escalation

Table 35.1 Drug-eluting stent clinical trials, multicenter registries, and meta-analysis in chronic total occlusions

Trial	n; Stent type	Follow-up	Results	Conclusions
Clinical Trials				
PRISON III trial (89)	304; SES vs ZES (Endeavor or Resolute ZES)	3 years	TLR:12.2 vs. 19.6% ($P = 0.49$) (Phase 1) TLR:10 vs. 5.9% ($P = 0.42$) (Phase 2)	No significant difference in TLR and TVF. Similar incidence of definite or probable stent thrombosis.
EXPERT CTO trial (96)	250; EES	1 year	TLR: 6.3%	EES: significantly lower composite adverse events intent-to-treat (18.5%, $P = 0.025$) and per protocol populations (8.2%, $P < 0.0001$).
FAST-CTO trial (43)	147; DES; BridgePoint Medical System- CrossBoss and Stingray Balloon catheters	30 days	MACE 30 days 4.8% ($P = 0.40$)	Overall success rate 77% (antegrade and retrograde crossing). 30 day mortality ($n = 2$). Coronary perforations (14, 9.3%).
Multicenter Clinical Registries				
Michael et al. (72) (U.S. Registry-3 centers)	1,361; unspecified PCI	retro-spective	Technical and procedural success rates (85.5%, 84.2%), antegrade (66%) and retrograde.	Multivariate analysis-independent predictors of success: female gender, no initiation of CTO PCI at each center. Major complications (24, 1.8%; antegrade 0.9%, retrograde 3.4%, $P < 0.001$).
ERCTO (97) (European Registry-44 centers)	1,395; DES (85.4%), BMS (2.4%), both (9.7%), PTCA only (2.2%)	24.7 ±15.0 months	Procedural and clinical success rates (75.3%, 71.2%). Successful CTO PCI: cardiac death (0.6% vs. 4.3%, $P < 0.001$), major adverse cardiac and cerebrovascular events (8.7% vs 23.9%, $P < 0.001$). Retrograde primary strategy (1193, 76.2%). Retrograde, after failed antegrade (202, 23.8%)	Retrograde CTO PCI: high success, low complications, good long-term outcomes. Independent predictors of major cardiac and cerebrovascular events: female sex, prior PCI, low EF, J-CTO score ≥3, and procedural failure. Retrograde > complications (coronary perforation and tamponade).
Meta-Analysis				
Khan et al. (91)	16,490 (25 studies); PTCA, BMS, DES	none; in-hospital: outcomes	Failed CTO PCI: higher in-hospital mortality (1.44% vs. 0.5%, $P < 0.001$), MACE (8.88% vs. 3.75%, $P = 0.001$), MI (3.17% vs. 2.4%, $P = 0.03$), increased risk for urgent CABG (4.0% vs. 5.0%, $P < 0.001$)	Failed CTO PCI = higher risk of adverse in-hospital outcomes. Higher rates of coronary perforations and cardiac tamponade ($P < 0.001$).
Pancholy et al. (92)	3,932 (13 studies); Mainly DES. Remainder, BMS, and PTCA. Stents >70% of patients.	≥1 year	Successful CTO PCI: short-term mortality reduction (OR: 0.218, CI: 0.095–0.498, $P < 0.001$). Long-term mortality reduction (OR: 0.391, CI: 0.311–0.493, $P = 0.001$.	Successful CTO PCI = significant reduction in short- and long-term mortality. Coronary perforation association = unsuccessful CTO PCI (OR: 0.168, CI: 0.104–0.271, $P < 0.001$).

(Continued)

Table 35.1 (Continued) Drug-eluting stent clinical trials, multicenter registries, and meta-analysis in chronic total occlusions

Trial	n; Stent type	Follow-up	Results	Conclusions
Christakopoulos et al (93)	28,486 (25 studies); DES, BMS, or PTCA.	3.11 years	Successful CTO PCI: lower mortality (OR 0.52, CI: 0.43–0.63), less residual angina (OR 0.38, CI: 0.24–0.6), lower stroke risk (OR 0.72, CI 0.60–0.88), less need for later CABG (OR 0.18, CI: 0.14 0.22), and lower MACE (OR 0.59, CI: 0.44–0.79). No difference in TVR or MI.	Overall CTO PCI success 71% (51–87%). Successful CTO PCI = lower risk of death, stroke, CABG, and recurrent angina. No outcome differences: DES, BMS, or PTCA.
Yang et al. (94)	9,140 (29 studies); DES (4132) vs. BMS -5008	60 months	DES vs. BMS CTO PCI: DES in-stent thrombosis > BMS (36 months, $P < 0.05$); DES MACE-free survival improved (60 months); DES all-cause death > BMS at 6 months; lower 12 months . DES less MI at 12 months.	DES CTO PCI: less MACE, restenosis, reocclusion, improved MACE-free survival in long-term follow-up. DES > in-stent thrombosis at 36 months.

Note: BMS, bare-metal stent; CABG, coronary artery bypass graft; CI, confidence interval; CTO, chronic total occlusion; DES, drug-eluting stent; EES, everolimus-eluting stent; EF, ejection fraction; MACE, major adverse cardiovascular event; MI, myocardial infarction; OR, odds ratio; PCI, percutaneous coronary intervention; PTCA, percutaneous transluminal coronary angioplasty; SES, sirolimus-eluting stent; TLR, target-lesion revascularization; TVF, target-vessel failure; TVR, target-vessel revascularization; ZES, zotarolimus-eluting stent.

had similar technical success (92.7% vs. 94.2%, $P = 0.43$), procedural success (91.8% vs. 94.1%, $P = 0.23$), and MACE (2.1% vs. 0.6%, $P = 0.12$), with ADR cases being more difficult (greater lesion length, $P < 0.001$, and J-CTO score, $P = 0.004$), thus showing the benefits of ADR. Furthermore, in a multi-center U.S. Registry of 1,363 patients, Michael et al.[44] performed a retrospective analysis that showed that operator experience and a greater number of years performing CTO PCI were associated with increased technical success (85.5%, odds ratio [OR] = 1.52, 95% CI = 1.52–1.70, $P < 0.001$), and lower fluoroscopy times (OR = 0.84, 95% CI = 0.75–0.95, $P = 0.005$), and contrast use (OR = 0.84, 95% CI = 0.62–0.79, $P < 0.001$). Also, the retrograde approach (OR = 3.36, 95% CI = 2.42–4.69, $P < 0.001$) and failed CTO PCI (OR =1.97, 95% CI = 1.37–2.80, $P < 0.001$) were associated with greater fluoroscopy times and contrast use.

CORONARY STENT OUTCOMES IN CHRONIC TOTAL OCCLUSION REVASCULARIZATION

Six randomized trials of bare-metal stent (BMS) placement compared with balloon angioplasty alone have been reported (Table 35.2). Collectively, these trials have shown that BMS implantation achieves statistically significant and clinically meaningful reductions in angiographic restenosis and reocclusion rates. Compared with angioplasty alone, BMS also confer a long-term benefit with fewer repeat revascularization procedures.[45,46] Despite these results, outcomes with BMS in CTOs are more similar to outcomes with balloon angioplasty in less complex, nonocclusive disease.[47–49] In the TOSCA trial,[50] rates of restenosis and reocclusion in complex lesions exceeded 50% and 10%, respectively. At 3-year follow-up, the occurrence of reocclusion was associated with a trend toward higher mortality and significant increase in the need for repeat revascularization.[51]

Although these trials have varied considerably regarding enrollment criteria, antithrombotic regimen, and trial design, their results are remarkably concordant, demonstrating significant reductions in restenosis and reocclusion associated with BMS. Additional studies have demonstrated statistically significant, yet modest improvement in left ventricular function and regional wall motion with CTO revascularization.[52–57] Importantly, an increase in left ventricular function may be conditional on vessel patency at follow-up and revascularization of total occlusions of shorter duration (<6 weeks).[59]

Two observations suggest the necessity for systematic evaluation of drug-eluting stents (DES) in CTO revascularization: (1) advances in CTO technical and procedural success have been disproportionate to the increasing number of PCI procedures that involve nonacute occlusions and (2) outcomes with stenting in CTOs with BMS are more similar to balloon angioplasty than to stenting in nonocclusive lesions.

Drug-eluting stents

SIROLIMUS-ELUTING STENTS

Against the background of several nonrandomized observational studies demonstrating improved angiographic and clinical outcomes with DES for CTOs, only one randomized trial comparing DES with BMS for CTOs has been performed. In the Primary Stenting of Occluded Native Coronary Arteries (PRISON) II trial, 200 CTO patients were randomized in a single-blinded fashion at two centers in the Netherlands to treatment with either sirolimus-eluting stents (SES; Cypher, Cordis Corporation, Bridgewater, NJ); or the bare-metal BX Velocity stent (Cordis Corporation).[60] Patients enrolled in this study

Table 35.2 Randomized clinical trials of angioplasty versus stenting for chronic total coronary occlusions

Trial	N	Reocclusion			Restenosis			TVR		
		PTCA (%)	Stent (%)	P	PTCA (%)	Stent (%)	P	PTCA (%)	Stent (%)	P
Stenting in chronic coronary occlusion (SICCO) (47)	114	26	16	0.058	74	32	<0.001	42	22	0.025
Gruppo Italiano di Studi sulla Stent nelle Occlusioni coronariche (GISSOC) (45)	110	34	8	0.004	68	32	0.0008	22	5	0.04
Mori et al. (49)	96	11	7	0.04	57	28	0.005	49	28	<0.05
Stent vs. percutaneous angioplasty in chronic Total occlusion (SPACTO) (58)	85	24	3	0.01	64	32	0.01	40	25	NS
Total occlusion Study of Canada (TOSCA) (50)	410	20	11	0.02	70	55	<0.01	15	8	0.03
Stents in total occlusion for restenosis prevention (STOP) (46)	96	17	8	NS	71	42	0.032	42	25	NS

Note: NS, not significant; PTCA, percutaneous transluminal coronary angioplasty; TVR, target vessel revascularization.

underwent 6-month angiographic follow-up to assess the primary endpoint of in-segment binary restenosis (50% reduction in minimal lumen diameter). At 6 months, treatment with SES was associated with statistically significant reductions in both in-stent (7% vs. 36%; $P < 0.0001$) and in-segment (11% vs. 41%; $P < 0.001$) angiographic restenosis (Figure 35.10). Reocclusion was also significantly reduced with SES (4% vs. 13%; $P < 0.04$), despite treatment in both groups with aspirin and clopidogrel for a minimum duration of 6 months. The clinical benefit with SES paralleled the relative benefit observed with angiographic measures. Specifically, target lesion revascularization (TLR) at 12 months occurred in 21% and 5% of BMS and SES patients, respectively ($P = 0.001$).

Several observational studies examining clinical outcomes among patients treated with DES in CTO revascularization

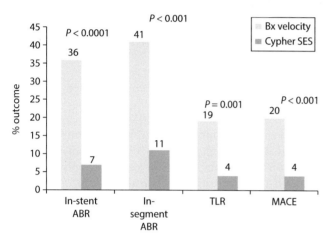

Figure 35.10 Six-month angiographic results from the PRISON II Trial. ABR, angiographic binary restenosis. MACE, major adverse cardiac events; SES, sirolimus-eluting stents; TLR, target lesion revascularization. (Adapted from Lotan, C., et al., *Eur. Heart J.*, 21, 1960–1966, 2000.)

have supported the notion that DES may achieve reductions in target vessel revascularization (TVR) (Table 35.3).[61-73] In a retrospective study of 122 patients with CTOs treated with SES ($n = 144$ lesions), clinical and angiographic outcomes were compared with a historical control of 259 patients treated with BMS ($n = 286$ lesions).[63] At 6 months, overall MACE were significantly lower with SES (16.4% vs. 35.1%; $P < 0.001$), principally due to a significantly lower rate of TLR (7.4% vs. 26.3%; $P < 0.001$). Restenosis was identified in 9.2% of patients in the SES group and 33.3% in the BMS group ($P < 0.001$).

In the Rapamycin-Eluting Stent Evaluated at Rotterdam Cardiology Hospital (RESEARCH) registry, among 56 patients treated with SES following CTO revascularization, the 1-year occurrence of TVR was 3.6%, compared with 17.9% among a historical control group of BMS patients.[65] Among 180 patients undergoing SES implantation for CTO revascularization in Asia, the 6-month occurrences of angiographic binary restenosis and TVR were 1.5% and 2.3%, respectively.[73]

As part of a multicenter Asian registry evaluating DES, clinical, and angiographic outcomes among 60 patients who underwent SES implantation during CTO revascularization were compared with a matched control of 120 CTO patients treated with BMS.[74] At 6-month angiographic follow-up, treatment with SES was associated with significant reductions in in-stent late loss, restenosis, and reocclusion. TLR was significantly lower at 6 months (2% vs. 23%; $P = 0.001$), and the LVEF also significantly improved among the SES patients (51.8% baseline vs. 57% at 6 months; $P < 0.01$). This latter finding implies that maintenance of vessel patency with DES may be an important predictor of improvement in left ventricular function. In a related study of 226 patients undergoing CTO revascularization (SES 106, BMS 120), treatment with SES was associated with a sustained, significant reduction in MACE through 4-year follow-up (7.5% vs. 33.8%; $P < 0.001$).[66]

Table 35.3 Clinical trials evaluating drug-eluting stents in total coronary occlusions

Trial	N	6 month			1 year	
		Angiographic restenosis (%)	TVR (%)	MACE (%)	TVR (%)	MACE (%)
SICCO (52)	25	0	8.0	12.0	12.0	12.0
e-Cypher Registry (62)	360		1.4[a]	3.1	–	–
RESEARCH Registry (63)	56	9.1	3.6	3.6	–	–
Werner et al. (64)	48	8.3	–	–	6.3	12.5
Nakamura et al. (65)	60	2.0	3.0	–	3.0	
Ge et al. (66)	122	9.2	9.0	16.4	–	–
WISDOM Registry (67)	65	–	–	–	6.7	1.7
TRUE Registry (68)	183	17.0	16.9	17.1	–	–
Buellesfeld et al. (69)	45	13.2	13.2	15.6	–	–
ACROSS/TOSCA-4 (70)	200	7.5	6.0	6.5	–	–

Note: MACE, major adverse cardiac events; TVR, target-vessel revascularization.

[a] Denotes target-lesion revascularization.

The Approaches to Chronic Occlusions with Sirolimus-Eluting Stents/Total Occlusion Study of Coronary Arteries-4 (ACROSS)/TOSCA-4 trial prospectively enrolled 200 patients undergoing CTO revascularization with SES using contemporary techniques and crossing technologies (Figure 35.11).[70] In this nonrandomized study, clinical and 6-month angiographic outcomes were compared with a historical control of patients receiving BMS in the prior TOSCA-1 trial. Compared with the BMS group, patients treated with SES were significantly older, had more CTOs (i.e., >6 weeks), smaller caliber vessels, a higher proportion of diabetes, and longer lesion and stent lengths. However, despite higher complexity in the SES cohort, treatment with SES was associated with an unadjusted 66% relative reduction in the primary endpoint of angiographic binary restenosis within the treated segment (19% vs. 55%; $P < 0.001$), defined as the length of contiguous target segment exposed to balloon dilation prior to stent placement. Following adjustment for baseline characteristics predictive of restenosis, the treatment effect increased to an 84% relative reduction in treated segment restenosis. Rates of in-segment and in-stent restenosis were 11.5% and 6.5%, respectively. At 6-month clinical follow-up, rates of MI and TLR were 1% and 6%, respectively, contributing to a 6% occurrence of the composite endpoint of target vessel failure (cardiovascular death, MI, or TVR).

In a multicenter U.S. registry of 1,361 CTO patients, Michael et al.[72] retrospectively evaluated the immediate and in-hospital CTO PCI outcomes by experienced operators, which revealed that CTO PCI can be safely performed with 85.5% technical and 84.2% procedural success (34% retrograde approach) and minimal major complications (24, 1.8%). In a multivariate analysis, the independent predictors of CTO PCI success included female gender, no history of prior CABG, and number of years since the initiation of performing CTO PCI at each hospital.

PACLITAXEL-ELUTING STENTS

Limited evidence exists for using paclitaxel-eluting stents (PES) in CTO revascularization. One study examined treatment with PES (Taxus, Boston Scientific Corporation, Natick, MA) in 48 patients undergoing CTO PCI and compared them with a historical control group of similar clinical and angiographic characteristics.[64] At 6 months, both restenosis (8.3% vs. 51.1%; $P < 0.001$) and reocclusion (2.1% vs. 23.4%; $P < 0.005$) were significantly reduced among patients treated with PES. One year following the index revascularization, repeat revascularization occurred in 3 patients in the PES group and 21 patients in the BMS group (6.3% vs. 43.8%; $P < 0.001$).

In the European TRUE Registry of 183 patients with CTOs who were treated with PES, 7-month rates of restenosis and TVR were 17% and 16.9%, respectively.[68] Among 65 patients with CTOs in the international WISDOM registry, treatment with PES resulted in freedom from MACE and TVR at 1 year in 93.3% and 98.3%, respectively.[69]

A subgroup analyses of CTO patients included in the SYNTAX trial[62] was conducted at 62 European sites and 23 sites in the United States. The SYNTAX trial randomized 1,800 patients to either CABG ($N = 897$) or PCI ($N = 903$) with PES to examine a primary endpoint of 12-month MACE and cerebrovascular events (MACCE). Overall, less than 50% of the CTOs were successfully treated with PCI; if CTO PCI was attempted, the success rate was 78%. Safety outcomes (all-cause death, stroke, MI) for patients with CTOs were similar between PCI and CABG patients, although CTO lesions treated with PCI had a higher rate of repeat revascularization compared with CABG.

Comparative bare-metal and drug-eluting stent trials in chronic total occlusion revascularization

Examination of the similarities of safety, clinical efficacy, and angiographic outcomes between differing DES has only recently been determined.[64,65] Despite more predictable variance in measures of neointimal hyperplasia by angiography and IVUS, demonstration of differences in clinical outcome across individual trials has been less consistent.[75–85] However, whether disparities in angiographic and clinical outcome emerge in more complex lesion morphologies is an issue of ongoing study and is particularly relevant to CTOs.

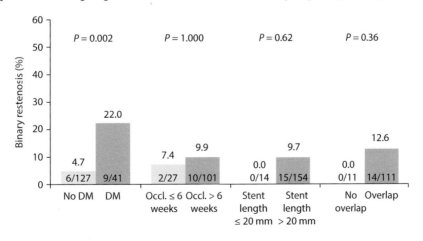

Figure 35.11 Rates of 6-month angiographic in-stent binary restenosis for selected patient subgroups. DM, diabetes mellitus. (Adapted from Kandzari, D.E., et al., *JACC Cardiovasc. Interv.*, 2, 97–106, 2009.)

Four comparative trials of SES and PES have been performed (Table 35.4). In general, these studies have been limited by their small study populations that limit statistical comparisons, variability in trial design, and limited clinical and angiographic follow-up. In the single-center Rotterdam registry (RESEARCH and T-SEARCH) comparing clinical outcomes among CTO patients treated with BMS ($N = 26$), SES ($N = 76$) and PES ($N = 57$), 1-year freedom from repeat TVR was significantly greater with DES compared with BMS (97.4% with SES; 96.4% with PES; 80.8% with BMS; $P = 0.01$ for comparison), despite significantly greater stent number and length per patient with DES.[83] Similarly, the open-label, multicenter Asian CTO registry reported no significant differences in 1-year TVR rates of 3.6% and 6.7% for SES ($N = 396$) and PES ($N = 526$).[85] In a subgroup of patients with 3-year follow-up, MACE was significantly lower in the SES group (10.9% SES vs. 16.3% PES; $P = 0.03$), although rates of TLR were statistically similar (7.7% SES vs. 9.5% PES).[86] These same investigators reported results from a prospective registry of 1,149 CTO patients treated with SES ($N = 365$), PES ($N = 482$), zotarolimus-eluting stents (ZES) ($N = 154$), tacrolimus-eluting stents (TES) ($N = 109$), or endothelial progenitor cell (EPC) capture stents ($N = 39$).[85] At 9 months, TLR was significantly lower with SES compared with ZES, TES, and EPC stents, but did not statistically differ from PES. In another nonrandomized comparison of CTO patients treated with SES ($N = 107$) and PES ($N = 29$), statistically significant differences were observed regarding angiographic restenosis (9.4% with SES vs. 28.6% with PES; $P < 0.05$), although rates of TVR did not statistically vary (3.7% with SES vs. 6.9% with PES).[88] Finally, a modest-sized randomized trial comparing SES ($N = 60$) and PES ($N = 58$) in CTO PCI also demonstrated no significant difference in the 8-month TVR rates of 3.3% and 7% in the SES and PES cohorts, respectively.[87–88]

The recent PRISON III trial[89] evaluated the safety and efficacy of SES versus ZES-Endeavor (Medtronic, Minneapolis,

MN) and Resolute ZES (Medtronic, Minneapolis, MN) for CTO interventions in two study phases (304 patients). In the first phase, 51 patients were randomized to receive SES and 46 to receive Endeavor ZES. In the second phase, 103 patients were randomized to SES while 104 were randomized to Resolute ZES. In the 3-year clinical follow-up of the first phase study, no significant differences were noted in rates of target lesion revascularization (12.2 vs. 19.6%, $P = 0.49$) or target vessel failure (14.3 vs. 19.6%, $P = 0.68$). Also, rates of definite or probable stent thrombosis (4.1% vs. 2.2%) were similar between SES and Endeavor ZES. In the second phase, no significant differences were noted in the rates of target lesion revascularization (10% vs. 5.9%, $P = 0.42$) or target vessel failure (10% vs. 7.9%, $P = 0.79$). Moreover, rates of definite or probable stent thrombosis (1% vs. 0%) were also similar between SES and Resolute ZES. However, the study was not powered for clinical endpoints. A study with longer term follow-up reported that successfully revascularized CTO confers a significant 10-year survival advantage compared with failed revascularization.[90]

In a recent meta-analysis of 25 studies (16,490 patients), Khan et al.[91] evaluated successful vs. failed CTO PCI. Failed CTO PCI was associated with a greater in-hospital mortality (1.44% vs. 0.5%, $P < 0.001$), higher risk of in-hospital MACE (8.88% vs. 3.75%, $P < 0.001$), higher risk of in-hospital MI (3.17% vs. 2.4%, $P = 0.03$), increased need for urgent CABG (4% vs. 0.5%, $P < 0.001$), higher rates of coronary perforations (relative risk of 5, CI 3.93–6.59, $P < 0.001$), and higher rates of cardiac tamponade (relative risk of 5, CI 1.97–12.69, $P < 0.001$). The most common cause of failed intervention was inability to cross or dilate the lesion. The overall CTO PCI success rate was 75%.

Another meta-analysis of 13 studies performed by Pancholy et al.[92] evaluated the effects on mortality between successful and failed CTO PCI. Successful CTO PCI was associated with a reduction in short- and long-term mortality (respectively, odds ratio [OR] 0.218, 95% CI 0.095–0.498,

Table 35.4 Comparative drug-eluting stent trials in total coronary occlusions

Trial	N (SES:PES)	Angiographic restenosis (%)		TVR (%)		MACE (%)	
		SES	PES	SES	PES	SES	PES
RESEARCH/T-SEARCH Registry (Ref below)[a] Nakamura et al.	76:57	–	–	2.6	3.6	–	–
Asian Registry (85)[a]	396:526	4.0	6.7	3.6	6.7	3.6	6.7
de Lezo et al. (86)[b,c]	60:58	7.4	19.0	3.3	7.0	3.0	7.0
Jang et al. (87)	107:29	9.4	28.6[d]	3.7	6.9	4.2	14.2[d]

Note: MACE, major adverse cardiac events; PES, paclitaxel-eluting stents; SES, sirolimus-eluting stents; TVR, target-vessel revascularization.

  P, not significant for all comparisons unless otherwise noted.

[a] One-year outcomes. Wholey MH. Recanalization of peripheral total occlusions. Endovascular Today 2003;2:1–4.

[b] Eight-month outcomes.

[c] Angiographic follow-up in only 48% of patients.

[d] $P < 0.05$.

$P < 0.001$; OR 0.391, 95% CI 0.311–0.493, $P < 0.001$)]. Also, coronary perforations were associated with unsuccessful PCI (OR 0.168, 95% CI 0.014–0.271, $P < 0.001$).

Furthermore, a recent meta-analysis by Christakopoulos et al.[93] of 25 studies (1990–2014; 28,486 patients; 29,315 CTO PCIs) evaluated the long-term outcomes (weighted mean follow-up of 3.11 years) of successful vs. failed CTO PCI. The results showed that successful CTO PCI compared with failed CTO PCI was associated with lower mortality (OR 0.52, 95% CI 0.43–0.63), less residual angina (OR 0.38, 95% CI 0.24–0.60), lower risk of stroke (OR 0.72, 95% CI 0.60–0.88), less need for subsequent CABG (OR 0.18, 95% CI 0.14–0.22), and lower risk for MACE (OR 0.59, 95% CI 0.44–0.79). No differences in outcomes were noted with balloon angioplasty only vs. bare-metal or drug-eluting stents, or in the incidence of target vessel revascularization (OR 0.66, 95% CI 0.36–1.23) or MI (OR 0.73, 95% CI 0.52–1.03).

In another meta-analysis, Yang et al.[94] compared the safety and efficacy of DES vs. BMS CTO PCI of 29 studies (9,140 patients: 4,132 DES, 5,008 BMS) at various follow-up durations. The risk of all-cause death using DES was higher at 6 months but lower at 12 months. No significant differences were noted at 24, 36, and 60 months. DES had lower risk of MI at 12 months, but there was no difference compared with BMS at 6, 24, 36, and 60 months. The DES MACE-free survival was significantly better compared with BMS at 6, 12, 24, 36, and 60 months (respectively, 73%, 68%, 49%, 40%, and 37%). DES did show a greater risk of in-stent thrombosis at 36 months.

The Canadian Multicenter CTO registry[95] of 14,439 patients who underwent nonemergent coronary angiography showed that 2,630 patients (18.2%) with CAD had at least one coronary CTO. In 44%, the CTOs were treated medically, 26% were referred for CABG (88% were actually bypassed), and 30% were referred for PCI (only 10% attempted with 70% success). Overall, 64% of CTOs were managed medically. CTO patients compared with non-CTO patients were more likely to be older and sicker with a greater likelihood of heart failure and peripheral and cerebrovascular disease. However, these patients were less likely to present with acute coronary syndrome.

The recent Evaluation of the XIENCE Coronary Stent, Performance, and Technique in Chronic Total Occlusions (EXPERT CTO) trial[96] evaluated the safety and efficacy of everolimus-eluting stents (EES) (XIENCE V and XIENCE PRIME, Abbott Vascular, Santa Clara, CA) for elective CTO PCI in a prospective, nonrandomized, multicenter trial of 20 centers in the United States using contemporary techniques. In 250 consecutive patients, the procedural in-hospital comes 1-year primary endpoint of death, MI, and target lesion revascularization (MACE) were analyzed with overall procedural success rate of 96.4% (antegrade-only methods, 97.9%; retrograde/combined methods, 86.2%). EES was associated with significantly lower composite adverse events for both the intent-to-treat (18.5%, one-sided upper CI: 23.4%, $P = 0.025$) and per-protocol populations (8.2%, one-sided upper CI: 12.3%, $P < 0.0001$). At 1 year, EES revealed a

significant reduction in adverse events with 1-year mortality of 1.9%, target lesion revascularization of 6.3%, subacute definite stent thrombosis in two patients (0.9%), and late probable stent thrombosis in one patient (0.5%).

Furthermore, the multicenter European Registry of CTOs (ERCTO)[97] evaluated CTO PCI using mainly the retrograde approach. They evaluated 1,395 patients; the retrograde approach was initially used in 76.2% or after failed antegrade approach in 23.8% of patients. Procedural and clinical success rates were 75.3% and 71.2%. Patients who had successful retrograde CTO PCI had lower rates of cardiac death (0.6% vs. 4.3%, $P < 0.001$), MI (2.3% vs. 5.4%, $P = 0.001$), further revascularization (8.6% vs. 23.6%, $P < 0.001$), and MACE (8.7% vs. 23.9%, $P < 0.001$). The independent predictors of MACCE at long-term follow-up (mean follow-up of 24 ± 15 months) included female sex (HR: 2.06; 95% CI: 1.33–3.18; $P = 0.001$), prior PCI (HR: 1.73; 95% CI: 1.16–2.60; $P = 0.011$), low ejection fraction (HR: 2.43; 95% CI: 1.22–4.83; $P = 0.011$), J-CTO (Multicenter CTO Registry in Japan) score ≥ 3 (HR: 2.08; 95% CI: 1.32–3.27; $P = 0.002$), and procedural failure (HR: 2.48; 95% CI: 1.72–3.57; $P < 0.001$). Also, CTO PCI success decreased with advanced age, diabetes, and history of stroke. Furthermore, operator experience directly correlated to procedural success for the retrograde approach. Therefore, several different approaches and newer devices currently exist that can improve CTO PCI success to improve patient outcomes.

CHRONIC TOTAL OCCLUSION COMPLICATIONS

CTO PCI has traditionally been considered benign because of the assumption that the artery is already occluded with collateral circulation; therefore, damage cannot be done. However, observational studies demonstrate that CTO PCI carries similar risk as conventional PCI.[90] Coronary perforation is the most feared complication of CTO intervention. Perforation may not occur at the occluded segment or be related to the guidewire itself; rather, adjunctive devices including balloon inflation, stent implantation, or atherectomy may be responsible. Coronary perforation may also occur in epicardial or septal collateral branches related to catheter delivery during retrograde procedures. Perforation is not always manifest during the procedure. In one case series, 45% of 31 tamponade events were diagnosed after the patient had left the catheterization laboratory.[98] Although infrequent, coronary perforation and cardiac tamponade may have severe clinical consequences. Among patients developing cardiac tamponade, rates of death, emergency surgery, MI, and transfusion occurred in 42%, 39%, 29%, and 65% of patients, respectively.[98] Aside from early recognition, management of coronary perforation requires simultaneous action on behalf of multiple catheterization laboratory personnel, including (1) prolonged inflation across the perforation with an occluding balloon or perfusion balloon catheter; (2) reversal of anticoagulation; (3) covered stent placement, emergency surgery, or embolization; and/or

(4) pericardiocentesis. In the absence of clinically evident perforation, an operator should be vigilant if a perforation is suspected. Angiography of the contralateral vessel must be performed to exclude the possibility of extravasation via the collaterals. Close monitoring with a pulmonary artery catheter and serial echocardiograms may also be necessary. Finally, aside from coronary perforation, additional procedural-related complications that may result in MI include thrombus formation, coronary dissection, and side-branch or collateral occlusion. CTO complications are more likely in the elderly, female patients, patients with depressed ejection fraction, and the presence of triple vessel disease.[99] Thus, such patients may be predisposed to higher risk from CTO interventions so operators may weigh these factors and consider extra vigilance and preparation for such cases. Furthermore, CTO PCI is associated with increased fluoroscopy and procedure times which may induce radiation dermal injury along with contrast-induced nephropathy.[100] Given the higher risk of complications from CTO PCI, operators experienced in such interventions or specialized CTO centers should be considered for optimal success and excellent patient outcomes.

FUTURE DIRECTIONS

Although the angiographic results of intended revascularization are unmistakable (i.e., either failed or successful epicardial recanalization), the effects of total occlusion and reperfusion at the level of the myocardium are less apparent. To identify which patients might benefit from revascularization, delayed-enhancement contrast magnetic resonance imaging (MRI) may be useful for the identification of viable and ischemic myocardium subtended by a CTO. Clinical experience has been useful in identifying viable myocardial tissue in spite of matched, regional wall motion abnormalities by other imaging methods.[101] Among 44 patients with 58 CTO segments, 37 patients (64%) had 50% transmural infarction with 12 patients (21%) having no evidence of infarction. Further, the presence of collateral flow did not predict either myocardial viability or improvement following revascularization. Territories without extensive infarction at baseline demonstrated significant regional wall motion improvement following revascularization, and more recent evaluations with adenosine stress MRI following percutaneous revascularization have demonstrated resolution of ischemia. Thus, application of noninvasive imaging with coronary CT angiography and MRI may inform patient selection by assisting in prediction of both procedural success (coronary CT angiography) and clinical improvement (MRI).

CONCLUSIONS

The implications of improving early procedural and long-term clinical outcomes with CTOs are considerable. Currently, no technology is available to reliably predict procedural success in those undergoing CTO revascularization.

Even following successful guidewire crossing compared with revascularization in nonocclusive lesions, the unfavorable results with coronary stenting reflect the complexity of CTOs with regard to lesion length, plaque burden, negative vascular remodeling, thrombus, and calcification.

Our evolving understanding of the benefits of CTO revascularization has resulted in an increased interest in CTOs, thus generating an increasing number of CTO procedures, development of novel technologies, and the design of trials dedicated to CTO revascularization. Over the last decade, a number of alternative technologies to guidewires have advanced, including mechanical techniques, ablation, microdissection, and transvascular reentry. Further clinical trials with DES and drug-eluting balloons are also underway. Recent evaluations with MRI in patients with CTOs provide further support toward improvement in left ventricular function, which may translate into favorable clinical outcomes for successful CTO revascularization. CTOs reflect the current insufficiencies in PCI techniques for achieving initial procedural success and sustaining vessel patency after success. However, CTOs also represent a unique opportunity to flourish in one of the most common and complex lesion subsets in the dynamic field of interventional cardiology.

REFERENCES

1. Srinivas VS, et al. Contemporary percutaneous coronary intervention versus balloon angioplasty for multi-vessel coronary artery disease: A comparison of the National Heart, Lung and Blood Institute Dynamic Registry and the Bypass Angioplasty Revascularization Investigation (BARI) study. *Circulation* 2002;106(13):1627–1633.
2. King SB 3rd, et al. A randomized trial comparing coronary angioplasty with coronary bypass surgery. Emory Angioplasty versus Surgery Trial (EAST). *N Engl J Med* 1994;331(16):1044–1150.
3. Serruys PW, van Geuns RJ. Arguments for recanalization of chronic total occlusions. *JACC Cardiovasc Interv* 2008;1(1):54–55.
4. Bell MR, et al. Initial and long-term outcome of 354 patients after coronary balloon angioplasty of total coronary artery occlusions. *Circulation* 1992;85(3):1003–1011.
5. Noguchi T, et al. Percutaneous transluminal coronary angioplasty of chronic total occlusions. Determinants of primary success and long-term clinical outcome. *Catheter Cardiovasc Interv* 2000;49(3):258–264.
6. Werner GS, et al. Regression of collateral function after recanalization of chronic total coronary occlusions: A serial assessment by intracoronary pressure and Doppler recordings. *Circulation* 2003;108:2877–2882.
7. Tamai H, et al. Frequency and time course of reocclusion and restenosis in coronary artery occlusions after balloon angioplasty versus Wiktor stent implantation: Results from the Mayo-Japan Investigation for Chronic Total Occlusion (MAJIC) trial. *Am Heart J* 2004;147(3):E9.
8. Stone GW, et al. Percutaneous recanalization of chronically occluded coronary arteries: A consensus document: Part I. *Circulation* 2005;112(11):2364–2372.

9. Zidar FJ, et al. Prospective, randomized trial of prolonged intracoronary urokinase infusion for chronic total occlusions in native coronary arteries. *J Am Coll Cardiol* 1996;27(6):1406–1412.

10. Katsuragawa M, et al. Histologic studies in percutaneous transluminal coronary angioplasty for chronic total occlusion: Comparison of tapering and abrupt types of occlusion and short and long occluded segments. *J Am Coll Cardiol* 1993;21(3):604–611.

11. Srivatsa SS, et al. Histologic correlates of angiographic chronic total coronary artery occlusions: Influence of occlusion duration on neovascular channel patterns and intimal plaque composition. *J Am Coll Cardiol* 1997;29(5):955–963.

12. Hosoda Y, et al. Age-dependent changes of collagen and elastin content in human aorta and pulmonary artery. *Angiology* 1984;35(10):615–621.

13. Katsuda S, et al. Collagens in human atherosclerosis. Immunohistochemical analysis using collagen type-specific antibodies. *Arterioscler Thromb* 1992;12(4):494–502.

14. Burke AP, et al. Morphological predictors of arterial remodeling in coronary atherosclerosis. *Circulation* 2002;105(3):297–303.

15. Sueishi K, et al. Atherosclerosis and angiogenesis. Its pathophysiological significance in humans as well as in an animal model induced by the gene transfer of vascular endothelial growth factor. *Ann NY Acad Sci* 1997;811(Atherosclerosis IV):311–324.

16. Kumamoto M, et al. Intimal neovascularization in human coronary atherosclerosis: Its origin and pathophysiological significance. *Hum Pathol* 1995;26(4):450–456.

17. Sakuda H, et al. Media conditioned by smooth muscle cells cultured in a variety of hypoxic environments stimulates in vitro angiogenesis. A relationship to transforming growth factor-beta 1. *Am J Pathol* 1992;141(6):1507–1516.

18. Puma JA, et al. Support for the open-artery hypothesis in survivors of acute myocardial infarction: Analysis of 11,228 patients treated with thrombolytic therapy. *Am J Cardiol* 1999;83(4):482–487.

19. Safley DM, et al. Improvement in survival following successful percutaneous coronary intervention of coronary chronic total occlusions: Variability by target vessel. *JACC Cardiovasc Interv* 2008;1(3):295–302.

20. Farooq V, et al. The negative impact of incomplete angiographic revascularization on clinical outcomes and its association with total occlusions: The SYNTAX (Synergy Between Percutaneous Coronary Intervention with Taxus and Cardiac Surgery) trial. *J Am Coll Cardiol* 2013;61(3):282–294.

21. George S, et al. Long-term follow-up of elective chronic total coronary occlusion angioplasty: Analysis from the U.K. Central Cardiac Audit Database. *J Am Coll Cardiol* 2014;64(3):235–243.

22. Olivari Z, et al. Immediate results and one-year clinical outcome after percutaneous coronary interventions in chronic total occlusions: Data from a multicenter, prospective, observational study (TOAST-GISE). *J Am Coll Cardiol* 2003;41(10):1672–1678.

23. Serruys PW, et al. Total occlusion trial with angioplasty by using laser guidewire. The TOTAL trial. *Eur Heart J* 2000;21(21):1797–1805.

24. He ZX, et al. Myocardial perfusion in patients with total occlusion of a single coronary artery with and without collateral circulation. *J Nucl Cardiol* 2001;8(4):452–457.

25. Aboul-Enein F, et al. Influence of angiographic collateral circulation on myocardial perfusion in patients with chronic total occlusion of a single coronary artery and no prior myocardial infarction. *J Nucl Med* 2004;45(6):950–955.

26. Cheng AS, et al. Percutaneous treatment of chronic total coronary occlusions improves regional hyperemic myocardial blood flow and contractility: Insights from quantitative cardiovascular magnetic resonance imaging. *JACC Cardiovasc Interv* 2008;1(1):44–53.

27. Hochman JS, et al. Coronary intervention for persistent occlusion after myocardial infarction. *N Engl J Med* 2006;355(23):2395–2407.

28. Dzavik V, et al. Randomized trial of percutaneous coronary intervention for subacute infarct-related coronary artery occlusion to achieve long-term patency and improve ventricular function: The Total Occlusion Study of Canada (TOSCA)-2 trial. *Circulation* 2006;114:2449–2457.

29. Abbate A, et al. Survival and cardiac remodeling benefits in patients undergoing late percutaneous coronary intervention of the infarct-related artery: Evidence from a meta-analysis of randomized controlled trials. *J Am Coll Cardiol* 2008;51(9):956–964.

30. Sianos G, et al. Theory and practical based approach to chronic total occlusions. *BMC Cardiovasc Disord* 2016;16:33.

31. Stone GW, et al. Percutaneous recanalization of chronically occluded coronary arteries: A consensus document: Part II. *Circulation* 2005;112(16):2530–2537.

32. Mehran R. *Analysis of the Columbia-Milan CTO Registry.* Presented at: The Sixth International Chronic Total Occlusion Summit, New York, 2009.

33. Rinfret S, et al. Retrograde recanalization of chronic total occlusions from the transradial approach; early Canadian experience. *Catheter Cardiovasc Interv* 2011;78(3):366–374.

34. Wilson W, Spratt JC. Advances in procedural techniques—antegrade. *Curr Cardiol Rev* 2014;10(2):127–144.

35. Colombo A, et al. Treating chronic total occlusions using subintimal tracking and reentry: The STAR technique. *Catheter Cardiovasc Interv* 2005;64(4):407–411; discussion 412.

36. Surmely JF, et al. Coronary septal collaterals as an access for the retrograde approach in the percutaneous treatment of coronary chronic total occlusions. *Catheter Cardiovasc Interv* 2007;69(6):826–832.

37. Surmely JF, et al. New concept for CTO recanalization using controlled antegrade and retrograde subintimal tracking: The CART technique. *J Invasive Cardiol* 2006;18(7):334–338.

38. Brilakis ES, et al. A percutaneous treatment algorithm for crossing coronary chronic total occlusions. *JACC Cardiovasc Interv* 2012;5(4):367–379.

39. Shammas NW, et al. The learning curve in treating coronary chronic total occlusion early in the experience of an operator at a tertiary medical center: The role of the hybrid approach. *Cardiovasc Revasc Med* 2016;17(1):15–18.

40. Wilson WM, et al. Hybrid approach improves success of chronic total occlusion angioplasty. *Heart* 2016;102(18):1486–1493.

41. Danek BA, et al. Use of antegrade dissection re-entry in coronary chronic total occlusion percutaneous coronary intervention in a contemporary multicenter registry. *Int J Cardiol* 2016;214:428–437.

42. Drozd J, et al. Percutaneous recanalisation of chronically occluded coronary arteries with the CrossBoss/Stingray system: First experience (report of three cases). *Kardiol Pol* 2015;73(9):711–721.

43. Whitlow PL, et al. Use of a novel crossing and re-entry system in coronary chronic total occlusions that have failed standard crossing techniques: Results of the FAST-CTOs (Facilitated Antegrade Steering Technique in Chronic Total Occlusions) trial. *JACC Cardiovasc Interv* 2012;5(4):393–401.

44. Michael TT, et al. Temporal trends of fluoroscopy time and contrast utilization in coronary chronic total occlusion revascularization: Insights from a multicenter United States registry. *Catheter Cardiovasc Interv* 2015;85(3):393–399.

45. Rubartelli P, et al. Coronary stent implantation is superior to balloon angioplasty for chronic coronary occlusions: Six-year clinical follow-up of the GISSOC trial. *J Am Coll Cardiol* 2003;41(9):1488–1492.

46. Lotan C, et al. Stents in total occlusion for restenosis prevention. The multicentre randomized STOP study. The Israeli Working Group for Interventional Cardiology. *Eur Heart J* 2000;21(23):1960–1966.

47. Sirnes PA, et al. Stenting in Chronic Coronary Occlusion (SICCO): A randomized, controlled trial of adding stent implantation after successful angioplasty. *J Am Coll Cardiol* 1996;28:1444–1451.

48. Engelstein E, et al. Improved global and regional left ventricular function after angioplasty for chronic coronary occlusion. *Clin Investig* 1994;72:442–447.

49. Mori M, et al. Comparison of results of intracoronary implantation of the Plamaz-Schatz stent with conventional balloon angioplasty in chronic total coronary arterial occlusion. *Am J Cardiol* 1996;78:985–989.

50. Buller CE, et al. Primary stenting versus balloon angioplasty in occluded coronary arteries: The Total Occlusion Study of Canada (TOSCA). *Circulation* 1999;100(3):236–242.

51. Buller CE, et al. Three year clinical outcomes from the Total Occlusion Study of Canada (TOSCA). *Circulation* 2000;102:II-1885.

52. Sirnes PA, et al. Sustained benefit of stenting chronic coronary occlusion: Long-term clinical follow-up of the Stenting in Chronic Coronary Occlusion (SICCO) study. *J Am Coll Cardiol* 1998;32(2):305–310.

53. Serruys PW, et al. A comparison of balloon-expandable-stent implantation with balloon angioplasty in patients with coronary artery disease. Benestent Study Group. *N Engl J Med* 1994;331(8):489–495.

54. Serruys PW, et al. Randomised comparison of implantation of heparin-coated stents with balloon angioplasty in selected patients with coronary artery disease (Benestent II). *Lancet* 1998;352(9138):673–681.

55. Dzavik V, et al. Predictors of improvement in left ventricular function after percutaneous revascularization of occluded coronary arteries: A report from the Total Occlusion Study of Canada (TOSCA). *Am Heart J* 2001;142(2):301–308.

56. Melchior JP, et al. Improvement of left ventricular contraction and relaxation synchronism after recanalization of chronic total coronary occlusion by angioplasty. *J Am Coll Cardiol* 1987;9(4):763–768.

57. Sallam M, et al. Predictors of re-occlusion after successful recanalization of chronic total occlusion. *J Invasive Cardiol* 2001;13(7):511–515.

58. Hoher M, et al. A randomized trial of elective stenting after balloon recanalization of chronic total occlusions. *J Am Coll Cardiol* 1999;34(3):722–729.

59. Sirnes PA, et al. Improvement in left ventricular ejection fraction and wall motion after successful recanalization of chronic coronary occlusions. *Eur Heart J* 1998;19(2):273–281.

60. Suttorp MJ, et al. Primary Stenting of Totally Occluded Native Coronary Arteries II (PRISON II): A randomized comparison of bare metal stent implantation with sirolimus-eluting stent implantation for the treatment of total coronary occlusions. *Circulation* 2006;114(9):921–928.

61. Serruys P. *Syntax Trial: Chronic total occlusion subsets, 1 year results from the SYNTAX Trial.* Presented at: Cardiovascular Research Technologies, Washington, D.C., 2009.

62. Holmes D. *Complex lesions in the e-Cypher Registry.* Presented at: Transcatheter Cardiovascular Therapeutics, Washington, D.C., 2004.

63. Hoye A, et al. Significant reduction in restenosis after the use of sirolimus-eluting stents in the treatment of chronic total occlusions. *J Am Coll Cardiol* 2004;43(11):1954–1958.

64. Werner GS, et al. Prevention of lesion recurrence in chronic total coronary occlusions by paclitaxel-eluting stents. *J Am Coll Cardiol* 2004;44(12):2301–2306.

65. Nakamura S, et al. Impact of sirolimus-eluting stent on the outcome of patients with chronic total occlusions. *Am J Cardiol* 2005;95:161–166.

66. Ge L, et al. Immediate and mid-term outcomes of sirolimus-eluting stent implantation for chronic total occlusions. *Eur Heart J* 2005;26:1056–1062.

67. Abizaid A, et al. Twelve-month outcomes with a paclitaxel-eluting stent transitioning from controlled trials to clinical practice (the WISDOM Registry). *Am J Cardiol* 2006;98(8):1028–1032.

68. Grube E, et al. Assessing the safety and effectiveness of TAXUS in 183 patients with chronic total occlusions: Insights from the TRUE study. *Am J Cardiol* 2005;96:37H.

69. Buellesfeld L, et al. Polymer-based paclitaxel-eluting stent for treatment of chronic total occlusions of native coronaries: Results of a Taxus CTO registry. *Catheter Cardiovasc Interv* 2005;66:173–177.

70. Kandzari DE, et al. Clinical and angiographic outcomes with sirolimus-eluting stents in total coronary occlusions: The ACROSS/TOSCA-4 (Approaches to Chronic Occlusions With Sirolimus-Eluting Stents/Total Occlusion Study of Coronary Arteries-4) trial. *JACC Cardiovasc Interv* 2009;2(2):97–106.

71. Nakamura S, et al. Impact of sirolimus-eluting stents on the outcome of patients with chronic total occlusions: Multicenter registry in Asia. *J Am Coll Cardiol* 2003;43:35A.

72. Michael TT, et al. Procedural outcomes of revascularization of chronic total occlusion of native coronary arteries (from a multicenter United States registry). *Am J Cardiol* 2013;112(4):488–492.

73. Schomig A, et al. A meta-analysis of 16 randomized trials of sirolimus-eluting stents versus paclitaxel-eluting stents in patients with coronary artery disease. *J Am Coll Cardiol* 2007;50(14):1373–1380.

74. Nakamura S, et al. Four-year durability of sirolimus-eluting stents in patients with chronic total occlusions compared with bare metal stents: Multicenter registry in Asia. *Am J Cardiol* 2007;100:93L.

75. Dibra A, et al. Paclitaxel-eluting or sirolimus-eluting stents to prevent restenosis in diabetic patients. *N Engl J Med* 2005;353:663–670.

76. Goy JJ, et al. A prospective randomized comparison between paclitaxel and sirolimus stents in the real world of interventional cardiology: The TAXi trial. *J Am Coll Cardiol* 2005;45(2):308–311.

77. Kastrati A, et al. Sirolimus-eluting stents vs paclitaxel-eluting stents in patients with coronary artery disease: Meta-analysis of randomized trials. *JAMA* 2005;294(7):819–825.

78. Kastrati A, et al. Sirolimus-eluting stent or paclitaxel-eluting stent vs balloon angioplasty for prevention of recurrences in patients with coronary in-stent restenosis: A randomized controlled trial. *JAMA* 2005;293(2):165–171.

79. Morice MC, et al. Sirolimus- vs paclitaxel- eluting stents in de novo coronary artery lesions: The REALITY trial: A randomized controlled trial. *JAMA* 2006;295(8):895–904.

80. Stettler C, et al. Outcomes associated with drug-eluting and bare-metal stents: A collaborative network meta-analysis. *Lancet* 2007;370(9591):937–948.

81. Windecker S, et al. Sirolimus-eluting and paclitaxel-eluting stents for coronary revascularization. *N Engl J Med* 2005;353(7):653–662.

82. de Lezo JS, et al. Drug-eluting stents for complex lesions: Latest angiographic data from the randomized rapamycin versus paclitaxel CORPAL study. *J Am Coll Cardiol* 2005;45:75A.

83. Hoye A, et al. Drug-eluting stent implantation for chronic total occlusions: Comparison between the sirolimus- and paclitaxel-eluting stent. *EuroIntervention* 2005;1(2):193–197.

84. Nakamura S, et al. Comparison of efficacy and safety between sirolimus-eluting stent and paclitaxel-eluting stent on the outcome of patients with chronic total occlusions: Multicenter registry in Asia. *Am J Cardiol* 2005;96:38H.

85. Nakamura S, et al. Drug-eluting stents for the treatment of chronic total occlusion: A comparison of sirolimus, paclitaxel, zotarolimus, tacrolimus-eluting and EPC capture stents: Multicenter registry in Asia. *Am J Cardiol* 2007;100:16L.

86. de Lezo JS, et al. Drug-eluting stents for the treatment of chronic total occlusions: A randomized comparison of rapamycin- versus paclitaxel-eluting stents. *Circulation* 2005;112:II477.

87. Jang JS, et al. Comparison between sirolimus- and paclitaxel-eluting stents for the treatment of chronic total occlusions. *J Invasive Cardiol* 2006;18:205–208.

88. Nakamura S, et al. Comparison of efficacy and durability of sirolimus-eluting stents and paclitaxel-eluting stents in patients with chronic total occlusions: Multicenter registry. *Am J Cardiol* 2007;100:93L.

89. Teeuwen K, et al. Three-year clinical outcome in the Primary Stenting of Totally Occluded Native Coronary Arteries III (PRISON III) trial: A randomised comparison between sirolimus-eluting stent implantation and zotarolimus-eluting stent implantation for the treatment of total coronary occlusions. *EuroIntervention* 2015;10(11):1272–1275.

90. Suero JA, et al. Procedural outcomes and long-term survival among patients undergoing percutaneous coronary intervention of a chronic total occlusion in native coronary arteries: A 20-year experience. *J Am Coll Cardiol* 2001;38(2):409–414.

91. Khan MF, et al. Comparison of procedural complications and in-hospital clinical outcomes between patients with successful and failed percutaneous intervention of coronary chronic total occlusions: A meta-analysis of observational studies. *Catheter Cardiovasc Interv* 2015;85(5):781–794.

92. Pancholy SB, et al. Meta-analysis of effect on mortality of percutaneous recanalization of coronary chronic total occlusions using a stent-based strategy. *Am J Cardiol* 2013;111(4):521–525.

93. Christakopoulos GE, et al. Meta-analysis of clinical outcomes of patients who underwent percutaneous coronary interventions for chronic total occlusions. *Am J Cardiol* 2015;115(10):1367–1375.

94. Yang SS, et al. Efficacy of drug-eluting stent for chronic total coronary occlusions at different follow-up duration: A systematic review and meta-analysis. *Eur Rev Med Pharmacol Sci* 2015;19(6):1101–1116.

95. Fefer P, et al. Current perspectives on coronary chronic total occlusions: The Canadian Multicenter Chronic Total Occlusions Registry. *J Am Coll Cardiol* 2012;59(11):991–997.

96. Kandzari DE, et al. Safety and effectiveness of everolimus-eluting stents in chronic total coronary occlusion revascularization: Results from the EXPERT CTO Multicenter Trial (Evaluation of the XIENCE Coronary Stent, Performance, and Technique in Chronic Total Occlusions). *JACC Cardiovasc Interv* 2015;8(6):761–769.

97. Galassi AR, et al. Retrograde recanalization of chronic total occlusions in Europe: Procedural, in-hospital, and long-term outcomes from the multicenter ERCTO Registry. *J Am Coll Cardiol* 2015;65(22):2388–2400.

98. Fejka M, et al. Diagnosis, management, and clinical outcome of cardiac tamponade complicating percutaneous coronary intervention. *Am J Cardiol* 2002;90(11):1183–1186.

99. Stone GW, et al. Procedural outcome of angioplasty for total coronary artery occlusion: An analysis of 971 lesions in 905 patients. *J Am Coll Cardiol* 1990;15(4):849–856.

100. Shah PB. Management of coronary chronic total occlusion. *Circulation* 2011;123(16):1780–1784.

101. Kim HW, et al. Assessment of viability in patients with chronic total occlusions. *Circulation* 2003;108:IV–698.

36

Saphenous vein grafts

CLAUDIA P. HOCHBERG, ION BOTNARU, AND JOSEPH P. CARROZZA

INTRODUCTION

In 1969, René G. Favaloro described the first use of coronary artery bypass graft surgery (CABG) for the treatment of myocardial ischemia due to coronary artery disease.[1] Subsequent advances in myocardial preservation and surgical techniques led to improvements in outcomes and the widespread use of CABG. Whereas CABG improves long-term prognosis in high-risk subsets, such as in patients with significant left main and three-vessel disease with decreased left ventricular function, for most patients CABG is a palliative, rather than a curative procedure. The use of the internal mammary artery (IMA) and other arterial conduits revolutionized CABG because of the relative resistance of arterial conduits to accelerated atherosclerosis compared with saphenous vein bypass grafts (SVGs).[2,3] Recurrent ischemic events occur in a time-dependent manner and may result from progression of disease in the native coronary arteries. However, the most common cause of adverse cardiac events in the post-CABG patient is atherosclerosis and attrition of SVGs.[4]

ANATOMIC CONSIDERATIONS

SVG patency and predictors of SVG failure

Ischemia in myocardial territories supplied by a SVG is often highly dependent on the time from implantation. Historically, the perioperative SVG occlusion rate was 10% and the 10-year occlusion rate was 50%.[5] A more recent assessment reported improved 10-year SVG patency rates but lower IMA patency rates than had previously been described.[6] At 7–10 days, 95% of SVGs were patent by angiography. One-week patency was associated with a 76% 6-year patency rate and a 68% 10-year patency rate (Figure 36.1). The overall 10-year SVG patency rate was 61%. IMA patency at 1 week was 99% and was associated with 90% 6-year and 88% 10-year patency rates. The overall 10-year IMA patency rate was 85%.[6]

Early SVG failure may result from any process that contributes to flow reduction and thrombosis, such as prothrombotic states, surgical misadventure (e.g., constrictive sutures) (Figure 36.2), nonlaminar flow patterns secondary to SVG-coronary artery size mismatch, compromised outflow from

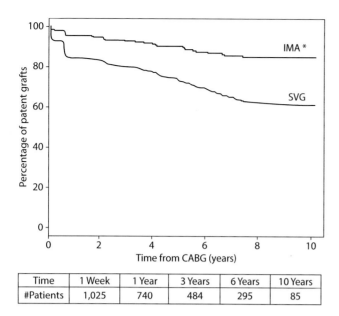

Time	1 Week	1 Year	3 Years	6 Years	10 Years
#Patients	1,025	740	484	295	85

Figure 36.1 Plot of time-related graft patency (or freedom from graft occlusion) for SVG and IMA grafts. *P* < 0.001 (IMA versus SVG) (*). CABG, coronary artery bypass grafting; IMA, internal mammary artery; SVG, saphenous vein graft. (From Goldman, S., et al., *J. Am. Coll. Cardiol.*, 44, 2149–2156, 2004. With permission.)

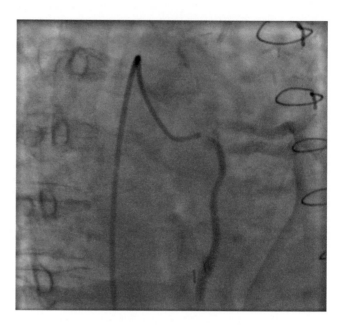

Figure 36.2 A 50-year-old man underwent coronary artery bypass surgery. Three days later he developed recurrent chest pain and ST-segment elevation. Angiography revealed a subtotal occlusion at the aorto-ostial anastomosis of the vein graft to the posterior descending artery.

distal coronary artery disease, and venous varicosities. Predictors of SVG patency include the location of the SVG, with left anterior descending artery SVGs having a 69% 10-year patency rate compared with 56% for right coronary artery SVGs, and 58% for left circumflex artery SVGs. The diameter of the recipient artery by angiography was also highly predictive. Grafting of arteries >2 mm in diameter had an 88% 10-year patency rate compared with arteries <2 mm that had a 55% 10-year patency rate (*P* < 0.001).[6] Clinical presentations of early SVG failure can be protean and include exertional chest pain, acute coronary syndromes, ventricular arrhythmias, hemodynamic compromise, or may be clinically silent, especially if the grafted artery subtends a minimal amount of viable myocardium.

Pathology of SVG failure

Within 1 year following CABG, most SVGs have developed some degree of concentric intimal proliferation similar to the smooth muscle cell proliferative response observed after vascular injury induced by percutaneous coronary intervention (PCI). The development of intimal hyperplasia in "arterialized" veins is a ubiquitous process commencing approximately 4 weeks after implantation. While this proliferative response often results in mild luminal narrowing throughout the SVG, it may be of sufficient magnitude to obstruct blood flow. The etiology of this pathologic response probably involves endothelial cell damage or denudation occurring during harvesting, vascular ischemia when vasa vasorum are severed, and barotrauma resulting from exposure of the vein to arterial pressure. This proliferative response is often most exuberant

at anastomotic sites, suggesting greater injury at these loci (Figure 36.3). Even if intimal hyperplasia does not result in ischemia within the first year following CABG, its presence may provide the substrate for accelerated SVG atherosclerosis.[5] Canos et al. compared the clinical, angiographic, and intravascular ultrasound (IVUS) characteristics of early (mean SVG age 6 months) and late (mean SVG age 105 months) SVG failure. Early SVG failures were more likely to be ostial (37.5% vs. 17.5%, *P* < 0.001) and had smaller pretreatment reference diameters (2.47 ± 0.86 vs. 3.26 ± 0.83, *P* < 0.001), smaller minimum lumen diameters (MLD) (0.80 ± 0.64 vs. 1.08 ± 0.64, *P* < 0.001), and greater pretreatment diameter stenosis (71.6 ± 19% vs. 66.7 ± 17.7%, *P* < 0.017). Additionally, early SVG failure was associated with lower thrombolysis in myocardial infarction (TIMI) flow rates and SVGs that failed late were more likely to have degenerated, diffuse atheroma. IVUS analysis suggested that SVGs that fail early are diffusely diseased conduits without positive remodeling, resulting in smaller lumen size.[7] While it is controversial whether SVGs undergo positive remodeling, the lack of positive remodeling may contribute to early SVG failure.

Premature atherosclerosis is the major factor contributing to SVG attrition and accounts for the majority of acute ischemic syndromes in the post-CABG patient. While the pathophysiology of atherosclerosis in SVGs generally resembles that of native coronary arteries, there are important differences. Compared with native arteries, SVG atherosclerosis is often rapidly progressive, more diffuse, associated with greater numbers of foam and inflammatory cells, lacks a fibrous cap, and is generally more friable (Figure 36.4). Furthermore, since SVGs lack side

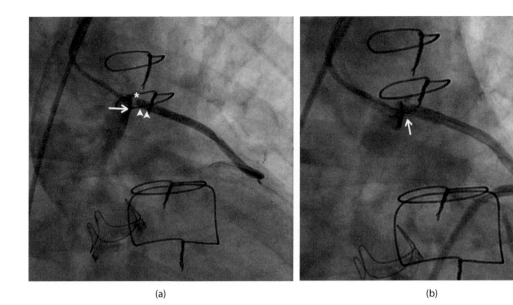

(a)　　　　　　　　　　　　　　(b)

Figure 36.3 **(a)** A high-grade aorto-ostial stenosis is present in a 5-month-old venous graft. The patient presented with acute coronary syndrome. The inner lumen of the ascending aorta is marked with an arrow. The origin of the saphenous vein graft (two arrowheads) is free of significant disease. The radiolucent segment represents hyperplastic in-growth within the wall of the aorta (asterisk). **(b)** Following stent placement, the lesion is significantly improved, but some narrowing is still present at the site of the original lesion (arrow).

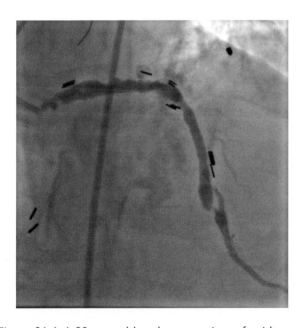

Figure 36.4 A 20-year-old saphenous vein graft with diffuse atheromatous degeneration.

branches, any process resulting in decreased flow may precipitate secondary thrombosis. Arterial bypass conduits are relatively resistant to atherosclerosis, thus offering a greater likelihood of long-term freedom from ischemic events.[8] However, focal stenoses may develop within the first year, especially at anastomotic sites. Repeat CABG is technically more challenging than the first operation and is associated with increased procedural morbidity and mortality.[9]

FUNDAMENTALS

Percutaneous SVG intervention: The "pre-stent era"

Compared with the treatment of native coronary arteries, balloon angioplasty of SVG stenoses is associated with poorer acute outcomes as the friable nature of SVG atheroma and greater plaque burden make balloon dilatation less predictable.[8] Angioplasty of SVGs that are older, degenerated, diffusely diseased, or totally occluded, is associated with a markedly higher incidence of procedural complications, including a high frequency of creatine kinase-MB (CK-MB) elevations.[9] In addition, the long-term clinical and angiographic results of balloon angioplasty are limited by an incidence of angiographic and clinical restenosis that may exceed 50% for lesions located at the ostium or within the body of the SVG.[10] One large series reported a 5-year, event-free survival rate of only 26% for patients treated with balloon angioplasty for SVG stenoses.[11] The use of debulking techniques has also been associated with suboptimal outcomes. Directional or extraction atherectomy has been limited by a high incidence of distal embolization, and excimer laser angioplasty has been associated with high residual stenoses with rates of restenosis exceeding 50%.[12–14]

SVG stenting: Early experience

The favorable angiographic and clinical outcomes observed after stenting native coronary arteries provided a rationale for investigating the use of stents for the treatment of SVG disease. Several single and multicenter observational studies reported on the use of the Palmaz–Schatz coronary stent.[15-17] The multicenter Palmaz–Schatz Stent Registry enrolled 589 patients with 624 focal SVG stenoses. Procedural success was high (>98%), and major adverse cardiac events such as myocardial infarction (MI), urgent CABG, and death occurred in only 2.9%. Stent thrombosis within the first month was diagnosed in only 1.4% of patients. However, there was a high incidence of hemorrhagic complications (14.3%) secondary to the mandated use of aspirin, heparin, dextran, dipyridamole, and warfarin. Quantitative angiographic analysis of a subset of patients in the registry revealed an overall restenosis rate of 34%,[15] with significantly higher rates of restenosis observed for previously treated (51% vs. 22%) and aorto-ostial (61% vs. 28%) stenoses. Debulking of ostial SVG stenoses before stent implantation did not appear to confer improved long-term outcomes compared with stenting alone.[18] This relatively high incidence of restenosis may have been due, in part, to the absence of stents designed to optimally treat vessels larger than 4 mm in diameter.

The first multicenter, prospective randomized trial of SVG stenting was the Saphenous Vein in De Novo (SAVED) trial, in which 220 patients were randomized to Palmaz–Schatz stenting or balloon angioplasty for the treatment of relatively focal de novo stenoses in 3–5 mm SVGs.[19] The primary endpoint of the trial was angiographic restenosis at 6 months. Procedural success (defined as a reduction in diameter stenosis of <50%, in the absence of major cardiac complications) was significantly higher with stenting compared with balloon angioplasty (92% vs. 69%), although the incidence of major hemorrhagic complications was also higher in the stent cohort. The post-treatment minimal luminal diameter was significantly larger in the stent group (2.81 mm vs. 2.16 mm), and at 6 months despite a greater late loss (1.06 mm vs. 0.66 mm), stenting conferred both a significantly greater net gain (0.85 mm vs. 0.54 mm) and larger minimal luminal diameter (1.73 mm vs. 1.49 mm). Whereas the angiographic restenosis rates were not statistically different (37% vs. 46%, P = 0.11), because of inadequate sample size, freedom from major adverse cardiac events (MACE), defined as freedom from death, MI, repeat CABG, or target lesion revascularization (TLR), was significantly improved in the stent group (73% vs. 58%, P = 0.03) (Figure 36.5). Although the SAVED trial did not *conclusively* demonstrate a reduction in angiographic restenosis with stenting, the favorable *clinical* results from the trial, as well as the limitations of other devices, has established stenting as the predominant percutaneous treatment modality for SVG disease. While stand-alone balloon angioplasty can be performed with similar safety and efficacy as stenting at the distal anastomosis of SVG, adjunctive stenting improves long-term outcome by reducing the need for repeat revascularization.[20]

SVG stenting: Contemporary experience

On the basis of the findings of the SAVED trial and the more recent BENESTENT trial, the implantation of stents

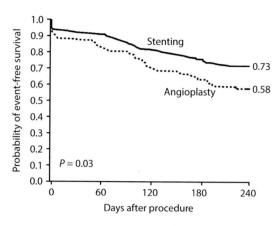

Figure 36.5 Saphenous Vein in De Novo (SAVED) trial. Kaplan–Meier survival curves for freedom from major cardiac events. Event-free survival was significantly higher among patients assigned to stenting than among those assigned to angioplasty. The relative risk of a major cardiac event after stenting was 0.82 (95% confidence interval, 0.68–0.98); after adjustment for diabetes, the relative risk was 0.82 (95% confidence interval, 0.68–0.99). (From Savage, M.P., et al., *N. Engl. J. Med.*, 337, 740–747, 1997. With permission.)

in diseased SVGs has become the standard of care for the endovascular treatment of SVG stenoses.[21] Despite improved angiographic results and clinical outcomes after bare metal stent (BMS) implantation, the rate of BMS restenosis in SVGs is higher than in native coronary arteries, with restenosis rates over 30%.[19] The introduction of drug-eluting stents (DES) has conclusively decreased the rates of angiographic and clinical restenosis, as well as target vessel revascularization (TVR) in native coronary arteries compared with BMS. It is unknown whether there is comparable benefit to DES implantation in SVGs. Several registries and one small randomized trial evaluating both short- and long-term outcomes of DES and BMS in the treatment of SVG disease have been completed.[22-30] The Reduction of Restenosis in Saphenous Vein Grafts with Sirolimus-Eluting Stents (RRISC) trial randomized 75 patients with SVG stenoses (distal graft anastomotic stenoses were excluded) to receive BMS or sirolimus DES.[22] In-stent late loss was significantly lower with DES (0.38 ± 0.51 vs. 0.79 ± 0.66 mm) compared with BMS, and both binary in-stent and in-segment restenosis were reduced (11.3% vs. 30.6% and 13.6% vs. 32.6%, respectively). Additionally, both TLR and TVR were significantly reduced with DES compared with BMS, but there were no significant differences in rates of death or MI between the two groups. However, intermediate-term follow-up (median 32 months) reported an excess mortality in the cohort randomized to DES with 11 deaths in the DES group compared with 0 deaths in the BMS group (P < 0.001) (Figure 36.6a). A post hoc analysis of the RRISC trial suggests that the reduction in repeat revascularization in the DES group seen at 6 months was lost at later follow-up (Figure 36.6b).[31]

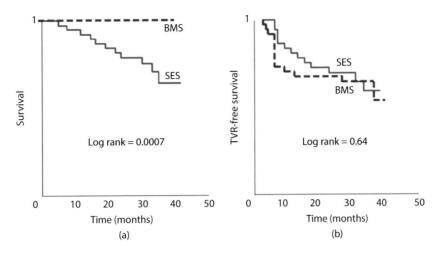

Figure 36.6 (a) Kaplan–Meier estimates for survival by type of randomized stent. **(b)** Kaplan–Meier estimates for target vessel revascularization (TVR)-free survival by type of randomized stent. BMS, bare metal stent; SES, sirolimus-eluting stent. (From Vermeersch, P., et al., *J. Am. Coll. Cardiol.*, 50, 261–267, 2007. With permission.)

One possible mechanism for DES failure in SVGs is the potential for stent-SVG size mismatch. Many SVGs are >4 mm in diameter and DES are not currently manufactured larger than 4 mm. This potential size mismatch may lead to stent undersizing and increased rates of restenosis. Another possibility is that although DES implantation in SVGs is associated with a lower early risk of restenosis, there may be a significant "catch-up phenomenon" (similar to that seen with brachytherapy) resulting in later events.

Results from the Registro Regionale Angiolastiche (REAL) Emilia-Romagna Registry from Italy also suggested similar long-term clinical outcomes for DES compared with BMS in the treatment of SVG disease.[29] The registry contained 288 BMS patients and 72 DES patients. The incidence of MACE at 12 months was similar in the two groups (17.8% with DES and 20.3% with BMS, $P = 0.46$). Nor was there a difference in the individual components of the primary endpoint. Additionally, the TLR was not significantly different between the two groups, although there was a twofold increase in TLR in the BMS group compared with the DES group (8.1% vs. 4.3%).[29] In contrast, a single-center study with 61 DES and 89 BMS showed cumulative MACE rates at 6 months to be 11.5% in the DES group compared with 28.1% in the BMS group ($P = 0.02$) and TLR rates of 3.3% versus 19.8%, respectively.[23] Similarly, Lee et al. looked at 139 patients undergoing SVG PCI and found that DES was associated with a lower incidence of MI (4.3% vs. 20%, $P = 0.04$), and TVR (1.01% vs. 36.9%, $P = 0.035$) at a mean follow-up of 9.1 months.[24] In a recent analysis of nearly 50,000 patients who had undergone SVG stenting from the NCDR registry, Brennan et al. concluded that DES use was not linked to increased rates of death, MI, or urgent revascularization.[32]

Bioresorbable stents

Bioresorbable stents, or bioresorbable vascular scaffolds (BVS), are relatively novel devices that were intended to serve the same purpose as the traditional metal stents, while overcoming some of their long-term limitations. Their role in our armamentarium is still being defined and today there have been limited data on BVS use in SVGs. A small case series of six patients from the OCTOPUS registry[25] evaluated the use of ABSORB (Abbott Laboratories) BVS in patients with SVGs and reported that the healing of BVS in SVGs is not impaired. However, serious clinical trials are needed to properly assess the role of BVS implantation in SVGs.

PREVENTION OF SVG FAILURE

Several interventions aimed at extending SVG patency have been evaluated. Prevention of SVG disease progression via early stenting of nonobstructive stenoses was evaluated in the VELETI trial.[26] This promising study demonstrated a significant decrease in MACE at 1-year follow-up (3% vs. 19%, $P = 0.09$).

The VEST trial examined the use of an external stent (VGS FLUENT, RAD BioMed) to prevent SVG dilatation. Thirty patients undergoing CABG had one of their SVGs stented, and another SVG served as the control. At 1-year follow-up, SVG patency did not differ significantly but external stenting seemed to have reduced intimal hyperplasia and ectasia.[27] Another trial looking at using an eSVS external nitinol mesh (Kips Bay Medical) revealed a decrease in 1-year patency rates (76% vs. 100%).[28] Given such discouraging signals, we do not expect external support devices to gain much acceptance in the near future.

It is worth mentioning that the type of technique utilized in the harvesting the venous conduit seems to also play a role in long-term SVG patency. The "no-touch" technique, which refers to vein removal with minimal trauma, appears to produce SVG patency rates comparable to the venerable left internal mammary artery (LIMA).

COMPLICATIONS OF SVG STENTING

Distal embolization and no-reflow

The major limitation of SVG stenting is the occurrence of acute ischemic events secondary to distal embolization and no-reflow. When serial cardiac biomarkers are measured routinely following SVG stenting, the incidence of periprocedural CK-MB elevation may be as high as 50% with an incidence of large (>5 times normal) CK-MB release of 15%.[33] The pathophysiology of distal embolization following SVG stenting is multifactorial. Compared with native coronary arteries, diseased SVGs are on average 0.3 mm larger in diameter and more diffusely diseased, thus containing a greater plaque burden.[34] Furthermore, the friable nature of SVG atheroma, with its abundance of cholesterol-laden foam cells and thin fibrous caps, renders it prone to embolization following high-pressure dilation commonly employed to optimize stent expansion. Aspirates from stented SVGs are enriched with atheromatous elements including foam cells, inflammatory cells, fibrous caps, and necrotic cores.[35] Older, degenerated SVGs often contain abundant fresh and organized thrombus, which develop in SVGs with reduced or nonlaminar flow resulting from vascular ectasia, flow-limiting atheroma, poor distal outflow, and systemic prothrombotic states associated with comorbidities, such as diabetes mellitus.[36] Disruption of fresh thrombus may lead to no-reflow from the embolization of platelet aggregates or intense microvascular constriction following the release of soluble mediators of vasoconstriction such as serotonin or thromboxane A2.[37] Risk factors for distal embolization include angiographically visible thrombus, intervention for acute coronary syndromes, plaque ulceration, and SVG degeneration.[38]

The inability to restore TIMI 3 flow is associated with a 32% incidence of Q-wave, or large (CK-MB > 50 IU/L) non–Q wave MI, and an 8% in-hospital mortality, underscoring the link between reduced postintervention TIMI flow and clinical outcome.[39] Rates of periprocedural MI in one study were 41.7% with postprocedure TIMI 1 or 2 flow, and only 5.6% with TIMI 3 flow.[30] However, it is important to remember that even in the absence of angiographic complications or impaired flow, patients who undergo successful SVG stenting are at risk for periprocedural myonecrosis. The incidence and consequences of distal embolization following SVG stenting are best illustrated by a retrospective analysis of 1,056 patients by Hong et al.[33] Seventy percent of the patients did not experience an angiographic complication; however, post-treatment CK-MB elevation was still an important determinant of mortality at 12 months, indicating that angiography is inadequate to completely evaluate downstream microperfusion. Postprocedure enzyme elevation and diabetes mellitus were the strongest independent predictors of long-term mortality. This strong association between periprocedural myonecrosis and poor prognosis in post-CABG patients (compared with patients undergoing stenting of native arteries) is best explained by the observation that this population is older, and has a greater incidence of comorbidities such as congestive heart failure, diabetes mellitus, and reduced ejection fraction.[34] A recent registry analysis notes a higher risk of MI, TLR, and stent thrombosis in patients with SVG PCI compared with CABG patients who underwent PCI of native coronaries.[40] A more recent pooled analysis of five randomized control trials and one registry study conducted by Coolong et al. evaluated embolic protection devices (EPDs) in SVG PCI. The univariate predictors of increased risk were current smoking, history of MI, glycoprotein (GP) IIb/IIIa inhibitor use, the angiographic presence of thrombus and two novel angiographic determinants: the SVG degeneration score, and the estimated plaque volume.[41] The SVG degeneration score is determined by estimating the degree of luminal irregularities or ectasia making up >20% of the reference normal segment. Multivariate analysis found that the strongest independent predictors of MACE were the SVG degeneration score ($P < 0.0001$) and the estimated plaque volume ($P < 0.001$). However, the presence of thrombus, increasing patient age, the use of a GP IIb/IIIa inhibitor, and current smoking still carried lesser independent risk. The use of GP IIb/IIIa inhibitors was not randomized in these studies; therefore, a detrimental effect could not be determined. The finding that GP IIb/IIIa inhibitor use was associated with a higher risk of MACE, independent of the angiographic predictors, may reflect that these medications are chosen for use in patients with a perceived higher preprocedural risk.[41] Likewise, in a post hoc analysis of the PRIDE study, Kirtane found that lesion length was an independent predictor of both CK-MB release and adverse events in patients undergoing SVG PCI with EPDs.[42] These studies underscore the unequivocal link between SVG atheroma, procedural events, and clinical outcome. The use of an EPD offers a 25%–40% reduction in 30-day MACE; however, the lack of other effective treatments or strategies to prevent distal embolization is the impetus for a large body of research focusing on adjunctive pharmacologic and mechanical treatments to render SVG stenting safer and more predictable.

There is some evidence that direct stenting of the SVG (i.e., without pre-dilation) may be associated with a reduction in the volume of atheroembolic debris.[35] Another strategy to reduce distal embolization during SVG stenting is to deploy a self-expanding stent such as the Wallstent without pre-dilation. It was hypothesized that primary stenting with these self-expanding endovascular prostheses might reduce the likelihood of distal embolization by trapping friable atheroma before high-pressure balloon dilatation. However, this strategy has not been validated in a prospective clinical trial.

ADJUNCTIVE THERAPY AND EQUIPMENT

Pretreatment with vasodilators

An important mediator of no-reflow is downstream microvascular vasoconstriction. The intragraft administration of a variety of microvascular vasodilators, such as verapamil, diltiazem, adenosine, nicardipine, and nitroprusside, have been shown to improve flow in no-reflow events.[43-45] Prophylactic treatment of SVGs before the intervention with verapamil and nicardipine has been shown to decrease no-reflow rates. One study reported no cases of no-reflow in the verapamil-treated population compared with 33.3% in the placebo group.[45] Among patients pretreated with intragraft nicardipine, only 4.4% had a CK-MB >3 times normal and the total MACE at 30 days was 4.4%, with no deaths, MI, or repeat TVR from hospital discharge to 30 days.[45] Prophylactic use of intragraft nitroprusside was associated with lower frequency and magnitude of CK-MB elevation (CK-MB >5 times, 1.6% vs. 10.9%, $P = 0.02$).[46]

Prophylactic intragraft administration of a vasodilator can decrease the rates of no-reflow and periprocedural elevations of CK-MB in patients treated without EPDs; however, the role of medical pretreatment in conjunction with EPDs has not been studied. Combined mechanical and medical therapy may offer an additive benefit for reducing MACE and long-term mortality after SVG PCI. Clearly, adjunctive therapies, in addition to EPD, are needed to further reduce the high MACE rates after SVG PCI.

Antithrombotic and fibrinolytic therapy

Many operators still routinely administer a GP IIb/IIIa receptor antagonist before SVG PCI, although administration of these agents in randomized trials failed to demonstrate a decrease in periprocedural complications, such as distal embolization, with a significant increase in hemorrhagic events.[41] Moreover, a meta-analysis of five randomized trials of intravenous GP IIb/IIIa receptor antagonists also failed to demonstrate improved outcomes in 627 patients undergoing SVG PCI.[47] At 30 days, death, MI, or TVR occurred in 16.5% of patients treated with GP IIb/IIIa receptor antagonists, versus 12.6% in the placebo group. One small series demonstrated that *local* delivery of abciximab significantly reduced the lesion percent diameter stenosis and TIMI thrombus grade.[48] Use of GP IIb/IIIa inhibitors during SVG PCI currently carries a class III indication in the 2011 ACCF/AHA/SCAI PCI guidelines.

Fibrinolytic agents, such as urokinase, are moderately effective in recanalizing occluded SVGs, but are associated with a high incidence (>10%) of hemorrhagic complications.[49] Intragraft administration of fibrinolytics to treat nonocclusive thrombus burden in SVGs has not been studied. One approach to reducing the thrombus burden before SVG stenting, without exposing the patient to the risk of systemic fibrinolysis, is mechanical thrombectomy. The Angiojet (Possis Medical, Inc., Minneapolis, MN) utilizes the Venturi principle to create a low-pressure vortex around the catheter tip, macerating fresh thrombus before aspiration (Figure 36.7). In the VEGAS trial, 351 patients with thrombotic lesions, the majority of which were SVGs, were randomized to prolonged urokinase infusion or thrombectomy with the Angiojet.[50] Randomization to

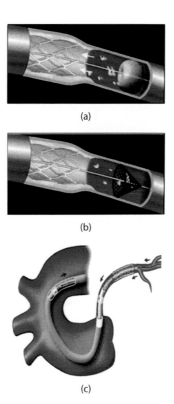

Figure 36.7 Mechanism of action of the embolic retrieval devices. Distal occlusion **(a)**, distal filtration **(b)**, and proximal occlusion **(c)**. (From Mauri, L., et al., *Circulation*, 113, 2651–2656, 2006. With permission.)

Angiojet treatment was associated with greater procedural success, reduced incidence of MACE, shorter length of hospitalization, and a reduction in in-hospital cost. However, despite a significant reduction in angiographic thrombus, 11% of patients still had periprocedural MI, affirming the growing understanding that factors beyond thrombosis, for example, atheroembolism and soluble mediators, are major contributors to adverse events after SVG stenting. Thrombus aspiration using hollow-lumen catheters, such as the Export catheter (Medtronic, Inc., Santa Rosa, CA), have also been used to remove thrombus in SVGs prior to stenting.

Bivalirudin, a direct thrombin inhibitor, is increasingly administered instead of unfractionated heparin as an anticoagulant during PCI of native coronary arteries. It has been associated with lower rates of bleeding without increased ischemic complications. Bivalirudin has been compared with heparin in SVG PCI with adjunctive EPDs. The use of bivalirudin was safe and associated with a trend toward fewer in-hospital non–Q wave MI, TVR, and vascular complications, and had a significantly lower rate of periprocedural CK-MB increases >5 times normal.[51]

Debulking prior to SVG stenting

Mechanical approaches to plaque removal before stenting include directional atherectomy, excimer laser angioplasty, and extraction atherectomy.[12,14,52] The CAVEAT II trial randomized patients with SVG stenoses to treatment with directional atherectomy versus PTCA. Directional atherectomy was associated with an increased incidence of distal embolization (13.4% vs. 5.1%) and non–Q wave MI (10.1% vs. 5.8%).[12] These disappointing results dampened any enthusiasm for the use of directional atherectomy in the treatment of SVG disease. The transluminal extraction catheter combines both atherectomy and thrombectomy features and has been used in diffusely diseased, thrombus-laden SVGs with the aim off minimizing distal embolization. Safian analyzed the results of extraction atherectomy in 146 patients with SVG disease and reported a 21% incidence of acute angiographic complication, including distal embolization (11.3%), no-reflow (4.4%), and abrupt closure (5%).[13] Results from the X-SIZER (EV3, Inc., Plymouth, MN) for Treatment of Thrombus and Atherosclerosis in Coronary Interventions Trial (X-TRACT) comparing short-term outcomes in patients with SVG disease randomized to stenting alone or pretreatment with the X-SIZER device (EndiCOR Medical, Inc., San Clemente, CA) showed a benefit of this atherothrombectomy device.[53] Thirty-day events included one death (2%), Q- or non–Q wave MI in 4.1%, TVR in 6%, and any MACE in 6%. Pretreatment with the X-Sizer was associated with a lower incidence of large MI and the need for bailout GP IIb/IIIa receptor blockade.

Adjunctive excimer laser before balloon angioplasty of SVGs has been evaluated in retrospective studies; however, its use has been plagued by a high rate of restenosis and total occlusion.[14,53] Ahmed compared debulking with excimer laser prior to stand-alone stenting for treatment of aorto-ostial SVG stenoses and found no difference in procedural safety or efficacy.[18]

The ATLAS study randomized patients with acute coronary syndromes undergoing SVG PCI to acolysis (ultrasound thrombolysis) or abciximab. The acolysis probe delivers a therapeutic level of ultrasound, which leads to a cavitation effect, resulting in a vortex that pulls thrombus toward the catheter tip. The study was terminated prematurely because of a significantly higher number of adverse clinical outcomes in the acolysis arm, with a 25% 30-day incidence of MACE with acolysis compared to 12% with abciximab ($P = 0.036$).[54] Debulking methods have mostly been abandoned.

Embolic protection

Considerable research has focused on the prevention of embolization of thrombotic and atheromatous material by EPDs. These devices are grouped into three classes: distal occlusion balloons, distal filters, and proximal occlusion balloons. The prototypic balloon occlusion distal EPD is the Guardwire (Medtronic, Inc., Santa Rosa, CA) (Figure 36.8). A nitinol hypotube inside a 0.014-in guidewire functions as an inflation lumen for a compliant balloon located near the distal end of the wire. After the balloon is inflated in the distal SVG, balloon angioplasty or stenting is performed over the Guardwire, which serves as the interventional guidewire throughout the procedure (Figure 36.8). A hollow-lumen catheter attached to a large syringe is passed over the wire, allowing aspiration of material dislodged from the SVG lumen. Webb reported favorable outcomes in the first 23 procedures performed with the PercuSurge Guardwire, with an incidence of periprocedural MI of only 3.7%.[35]

The pivotal Saphenous Vein Graft Angioplasty Free of Emboli Randomized (SAFER) trial randomized 801 patients

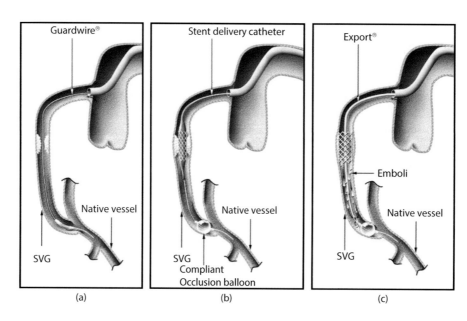

Figure 36.8 The PercuSurge embolic protection system. The GuardWire (Medtronic, Inc., Santa Rosa, CA) is positioned in the distal SVG (a). With the distal protection balloon inflated, a stent is deployed across the stenosis (b). Embolic debris liberated during balloon expansion is aspirated with the Export (Medtronic, Inc., Santa Rosa, CA) catheter (c). SVG, saphenous vein graft.

who underwent SVG stenting to conventional therapy or distal protection using the PercuSurge Guardwire system.[55] The primary composite endpoint of death, emergency CABG, MI, or TLR at 30 days was reduced by 42% in patients assigned to the PercuSurge EPD (Figure 36.9). This reduction in adverse events was driven primarily by a lower incidence of no-reflow and MI. These findings were independent of GP IIb/IIIa inhibitor use. Use of distal EPDs was associated with a trend toward reduced mortality (1% vs. 2.3%). Interestingly, in a subset analysis of the SAFER trial, embolic protection was associated with significantly lower rates of MACE, even in patients who were directly stented (14.1% in the nonprotected group vs. 5.5% in the protected group, $P < 0.001$). The SAFER trial served as an important "proof of concept," establishing EPD technology as the first adjunctive therapy to dramatically improve the safety of SVG stenting. Embolic protection with the Guardwire was also found to be highly cost effective.[56]

An example of a different approach toward embolic protection is the Proxis (St. Jude Medical, St. Paul, MN) device, which occludes inflow proximal to the target lesion. Inflation of the balloon interrupts antegrade flow in the SVG during the PCI. The stagnated column of blood can be aspirated throughout the procedure to remove debris particles and must be done before restoring flow. Advantages to the Proxis system include choice of guidewires, the establishment of protection before a wire or bulky device crosses the lesion, and the ability to protect arteries with multiple side branches or distal lesions that prohibit the use other distal EPDs.[57] The Proximal Protection During Saphenous Vein Graft Intervention Using the Proxis Embolic Protection System (PROXIMAL) trial was a multicenter, prospective randomized trial comparing proximal protection with distal protection using either a balloon occlusion or a filter wire. The primary composite endpoint of death, MI, or TVR at 30 days by intention-to-treat analysis occurred in 10% of the distal protection group and in 9.2% of the proximal protection group (p for noninferiority = 0.006). Secondary analyses suggested that among patients whose lesions were

amenable to either method of protection, proximal protection was associated with a numerically lower, although not statistically significant, 30-day MACE rate. This study established noninferiority of the Proxis device in preventing 30-day MACE and suggested a possible benefit of protecting the SVG prior to crossing the lesion with a wire or device.[58] However, this device is no longer marketed.

A second class of distal EPDs includes embolic protection filters that trap debris in semiporous membranes while allowing antegrade perfusion (Figure 36.8). Filter wires offer several theoretic benefits over balloon occlusion devices. Since flow is maintained during stent deployment, angiographic landmarks can guide accurate stent placement. In addition, maintenance of flow reduces the occurrence of prolonged no-flow ischemia, which may result in hemodynamic compromise if the treated SVG subtends a large amount of myocardium or if left ventricular function is significantly compromised. Potential limitations include flow compromise from filter sludging, failure to block soluble mediators of no-reflow, embolization of particles during filter recovery, and the embolization of small (<100 mm) particles. The randomized FIRE trial compared the filter-based FilterWire EX (Boston Scientific, Natick, MA) to distal protection with the Guardwire.[59] The 30-day outcomes of SVG PCI using the FilterWire EX system were noninferior to those with the Guardwire balloon occlusion system. The postprocedural measures of epicardial blood flow and angiographic complications were similar between the two groups, although there was a slightly higher rate of GP IIb/IIIa inhibitor use for bailout therapy in the GuardWire group. The 6-month outcomes from the FIRE trial revealed a 3.5% all-cause mortality in the entire study population, MI in 12% of patients at 6 months, and TVR in 9%. Although the outcomes between the two groups were similar at 6 months, the rates of MACE in both groups were not insignificant.[60]

The favorable results of the SAFER and FIRE trials affirm the causal link between distal embolization and clinical events following SVG stenting and establish the practice

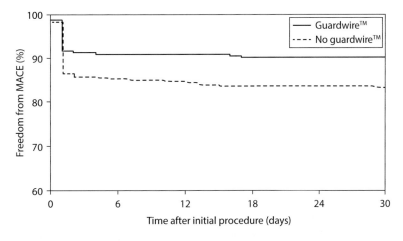

Figure 36.9 Survival free from MACE (at 30 days): event-free survival ±1.5 SEM in all patients. MACE, major adverse cardiac event; SEM, standard error of the mean. (From Baim, D.S., et al., *Circulation*, 105(11):1285–1290. With permission.)

standard for prevention of these complications. However, the 6-month outcomes from the FIRE trial reinforce the fact that long-term outcomes after SVG PCI remain poor. The FIRE trial showed parity between balloon occlusion and filter wires but did not analyze the particulate matter retrieved after intervention. Rogers et al. characterized the size and volume of debris retrieved from either a balloon occlusion device or a filter wire during SVG stenting and demonstrated that with both methods of protection, most particles were <100 mm in the longest dimension. Additionally, both types of EPDs had a similar total embolic load per lesion supporting the findings of equivalency from the FIRE trial, assuming that soluble mediators are not major contributors to MACE post-stenting.[61]

Newer filter protection systems, such as the Spider (EV3, Inc., Plymouth, MN), allow the operator to cross the stenosis with any 0.014 inch guidewire and deliver the filter system over that wire. Despite these technological improvements, major adverse events still occur in 5%–10% of patients, and half of SVG PCIs are performed without EPDs.[57]

Covered stents

Another approach to the prevention of distal embolization following SVG stenting is the use of covered stents. Stents covered with a variety of organic and synthetic compounds have been deployed to exclude aneurysms and seal perforations. The GraftMaster (Abbott Vascular, Abbott Park, IL) polytetrafluoroethylene (PTFE)-covered stent was approved by the U.S. Food and Drug Administration under a Humanitarian Device Exemption for treatment of coronary perforation (Figure 36.10). It was anticipated that covered stents might also exclude friable atheroma, thereby reducing atheroembolic complications and no-reflow states during SVG stenting. In a multicenter series of 109 consecutive patients, Baldus reported successful deployment of the JoMed PTFE stent in all but one of 109 patients, with an incidence of periprocedural MI of only 1%.[62] In a small series of patients treated with either a PTFE-covered stent or a BMS, those treated with a PTFE-covered stent had a lower incidence of non–Q wave MI.[63] However, tempering this initial enthusiasm for the use of PTFE-covered stents in SVGs was a report from the Randomized Evaluation of Covered Stent in Saphenous Vein Graft (RECOVERS) trial in which 201 patients with SVG disease were randomized to treatment with either the Jostent Flex BMS or the PTFE-covered JoMed stent. The incidence of no-reflow (5.8% vs. 2.1%) and 30-day major adverse events (15.3% vs. 12.4%) were higher in patients randomized to the PTFE-covered stent.[64] A more recent trial, SYMBIOT, which randomized patients to either the Symbiot (Boston Scientific, Natick, MA) covered stent or BMS showed no benefit of the covered stents in the treatment of degenerated SVGs. The rates of binary restenosis in the stented segment were similar (29.1% Symbiot vs. 21.9% BMS, P = 0.17); however, more patients in the Symbiot group had binary restenosis at the proximal edge (9% Symbiot vs. 1.8% BMS, P = 0.0211). There was no

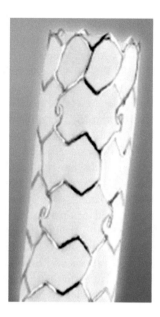

Figure 36.10 The GraftMaster polytetrafluoroethylene-covered stent.

difference in MACE between the groups (30.6% Symbiot vs. 26.6% BMS, P = 0.43).[65] The hypothesis that covered stents may reduce periprocedural complications by potentially preventing distal embolization and serving as a possible barrier to cell migration, thereby reducing restenosis, appears to have been invalidated.

CLINICAL OUTCOMES AND SPECIAL CONSIDERATIONS

Restenosis, recurrent events, and long-term outcome following SVG stenting

Although the SAVED trial demonstrated improvement in the long-term outcome of stenting compared with balloon angioplasty, and newer technologies such as EPDs have improved procedural safety, the long-term outcomes after SVG PCI are still suboptimal. Recurrent ischemic events are quite common (>50% by 18 months) in patients who have undergone successful SVG stenting.[16,66–69] There is controversy as to whether the incidence, time course, and biology of restenosis differs in SVGs compared with native coronary arteries following stenting. More clinical events occur beyond 6–12 months in stented SVGs compared with native coronary arteries, suggesting that the restenotic hazard in SVGs has a prolonged time course. Whereas the incidence of TVR and non-TVR is higher in patients with SVGs, the rate of revascularization driven by failure of the target lesion is similar to that of native coronary arteries.[67] Thus, the incidence of clinical events approaches 50% by 5 years because of the progression of disease at nontarget sites within the treated SVG, the attrition of other SVGs, and the progression of native coronary artery disease.[70] Depre and colleagues examined the histology of previously stented SVGs and reported "long-term restenosis" occurs in at least 30% of cases and results from a combination of cellular hyperplasia, thrombosis, and progressive atherosclerosis.[71] Another histologic study found abnormal adherence of inflammatory cells and platelets as late as 10 months after implantation, suggesting a propensity toward late thrombosis.[72] While this may partly explain the observation that late reocclusion often accompanies in-stent restenosis, it is important to remember that other factors, such as the absence of side branches and the rapid progression of atherosclerosis at other loci within the SVG, may also predispose the patient to thrombotic occlusion. The presence of diabetes mellitus, nonobstructive stenosis in other SVG segments, restenosis, placement of multiple stents, SVG degeneration, peripheral vascular disease, and congestive heart failure were all predictors of MACE following SVG stenting.[8,73–75] Although female gender was associated with periprocedural and 30-day MACE, clinical outcome at 12 months was independent of gender.[76]

Predictors of *angiographic* restenosis following SVG stenting include previously dilated lesions, smaller reference diameter, diabetes mellitus, and smaller post-treatment diameter stenosis.[17] SVG in-stent restenosis has been treated by a variety of approaches, including repeat balloon dilation, excimer laser angioplasty; and directional, rotational, and extraction atherectomy.[68,77,78] Repeat PCI does not appear to entail the high risk of distal embolization associated with the treatment of de novo lesions. In a series of 54 patients who underwent treatment of in-stent restenosis, distal embolization resulting in MACE was not observed.[79] Despite excellent acute angiographic and clinical outcome, the incidence of recurrent restenosis approaches 50%.

Contemporary approaches to the technique of SVG stenting

First-generation coronary devices, such as the Gianturco-Roubin and Palmaz–Schatz stents, were designed to treat focal lesions in native coronary arteries. SVG are larger and contain more diffuse, friable atheroma than native coronary arteries.[8] Consequently, multiple stents were commonly required and plaque prolapse was frequently observed when stents designed to treat vessels 3–4 mm in diameter were overexpanded to treat larger SVGs. In an effort to provide better scaffolding by increasing the metal-to-surface area ratio, hand-crimped larger biliary stents were used to treat diseased SVGs.[80] However, these stents were difficult to deliver because of their high profile, rigidity, and suboptimal anchoring of the stent to the delivery balloon. This necessitated the use of 8-Fr or 9-Fr guiding catheters, lesion predilation, and relatively stiff guidewires for delivery. This prompted several vendors to develop modified balloon-expandable stents to treat larger vessels. These balloon-expandable delivery systems are the platforms for both BMS and DES. These large vessel stents are compatible with 6-Fr guiding catheters, have relatively low crimped profiles and greater flexibility, and increased surface area coverage to minimize plaque prolapse. Additionally, with

the development of DES and the decreased rates of restenosis seen in native coronary arteries, the use of DES in SVG PCI has rapidly increased. Guiding catheter selection is an important component of successful SVG stenting. Ideally, the operator should choose a guiding catheter whose shape allows selective, coaxial intubation of the SVG. For an SVG anastomosed to branches of the left coronary artery, a right Judkins catheter will generally engage the SVG and is usually adequate for diagnostic angiography. However, the right Judkins guiding catheter often provides minimal backup support and frequently disengages from the ostium during balloon or stent delivery. A Hockey stick or Amplatz left guiding catheter will allow deeper intubation of the SVG, especially if the SVG has a vertical take-off or if maximum support is needed to facilitate delivery of longer stents or through tortuous segments. Care must be taken when manipulating such aggressive catheters, as the post-CABG patient often has friable atheroma in the ascending aorta that can dislodge when traumatized. Occasionally, when grafting the left circumflex artery, the surgeon will place the aortic anastomosis on the posterior surface of the aorta. These SVGs can be successfully cannulated with either a multipurpose or right Judkins guiding catheter. SVGs to the right coronary artery typically are sutured to the posterior surface of the aorta and usually have a downward orientation. The multipurpose or AR-1 guiding catheters generally provide adequate visualization and support.

Given the dramatic reduction in no-reflow and its clinical sequelae observed in both the SAFER and FIRE trials, the use of an EPD is recommended. Exceptions to this recommendation include SVGs less than a year old or treatment of in-stent restenosis. Stenting of SVGs with large amounts of angiographic thrombus can be especially challenging. Subgroup analysis from the SAFER trial identified angiographic thrombus as an important predictor of MACE. While the use of GP IIb/IIIa receptor antagonists has not been associated with the same benefit during SVG stenting compared with treatment of native coronary arteries, their use should be considered if a large thrombus burden is angiographically apparent or suspected clinically, for example, when intervention is performed for an acute coronary syndrome or the graft is freshly occluded. Intragraft administration of abciximab may reduce thrombus burden. Alternatively, the use of a thrombus aspiration catheter, such as the Export catheter with an EPD, may be helpful.

Generally, with the propensity of SVG atheroma to embolize, a "less is better" approach to stenting may be warranted even when the EPD is employed. Primary stenting (i.e., without predilatation) should be strongly considered. Webb has shown that primary stenting is associated with a reduced volume of embolized debris.[35] Contemporary stents are mounted on balloons that can be inflated to high pressure. Thus, if the operator chooses the correct stent size, post-dilatation can be avoided in most cases. However, occasionally one encounters a noncompliant lesion resulting from significant adventitial fibrosis that requires high-pressure post-dilation with a noncompliant balloon. It is important that all subsequent inflations be performed with an EPD as embolism and slow flow can occur even with post-dilation. Occasionally, balloon rupture or severe barotrauma may lead to perforation of the SVG. Usually, small perforations do not lead to hemodynamic compromise as they rarely cause pericardial tamponade and extensive fibrosis often seals the perforation. When the perforation is large, or associated with hemodynamic instability, the perforation can be reliably sealed with a PTFE-covered stent.[81] Before the advent of EPDs, moderate stenoses were often left untreated to avoid additional plaque manipulation. However, since these nonflow-limiting plaques may be associated with rapid disease progression and future ischemic events,[67,69] the availability of reliable, easy-to-use EPDs allows the operator to take a more proactive, aggressive approach to these lesions. When patients with SVG stents develop recurrent symptoms, angiography should be performed since progressive flow impairment may result in thrombotic occlusion of the SVG. Unless clinically contraindicated because of hypotension, we routinely pretreat with vasodilators to decrease rates of no-reflow. One series has reported a low rate of adverse events with vasodilator pretreatment.[45]

TREATMENT OF EARLY (<1 MONTH) SVG FAILURE

Early ischemic events may manifest as recurrent chest pain, MI, hemodynamic instability, or heart failure and are usually precipitated by SVG thrombosis resulting from a combination of a prothrombotic milieu and technical misadventure. Treatment of thrombosed SVG usually involves a combination of platelet inhibition with a $P2Y_{12}$ receptor inhibitor and thrombectomy, followed by balloon dilatation and or stent placement, usually at the aorto-ostial or distal anastomosis.[82] Since the flow-limiting lesion is usually located at a freshly sutured site, excessive pressure needed to expand the stent may disrupt the sutures, resulting in severe hemorrhage or tamponade. This risk may be highest for stents placed at the distal anastomosis when sutures are placed through the back wall of the native coronary artery.

TREATMENT OF CHRONIC SVG TOTAL OCCLUSIONS

Chronic total occlusions (CTOs) of venous grafts are very different from native artery CTOs. They are usually very challenging to treat with relatively low success rates and a high incidence of adverse events. PCI of SVG CTOs has been assigned a class III indication by the 2011 ACCF/AHA/SCAI guidelines.

CONCLUSIONS

SVG disease after CABG is common. One year after surgery, up to 15% of SVGs are occluded and only 61% of SVGs are patent at 10 years. Of the patent SVGs, many are diffusely diseased and repeat CABG is associated with increased morbidity and mortality. Therefore, PCI is the preferred revascularization strategy for SVG disease. However, it is limited by a substantial risk of MACE caused mainly by periprocedural MI as a result of no-reflow and distal embolization. Treatment of SVG disease is associated with a high rate of restenosis, ranging from 20% to 37%, and high rates of TVR. Recent advances in SVG PCI have included the development of EPDs that have reduced the rates of 30-day MACE by 42%. Nonetheless, SVG PCI is still associated with worse long-term outcomes than native coronary artery PCI and research is needed to develop pharmacological as well as mechanical devices to improve the outcomes of SVG PCI.

REFERENCES

1. Favaloro RG. Saphenous vein autograft replacement of severe segmental coronary artery occlusion: Operative technique. *Ann Thorac Surg* 1968;5(4):334–339.
2. Shelton ME, et al. A comparison of morphologic and angiographic findings in long-term internal mammary artery and saphenous vein bypass grafts. *J Am Coll Cardiol* 1988;11(2):297–307.
3. Cameron A, et al. Clinical implications of internal mammary artery bypass grafts: The Coronary Artery Surgery Study experience. *Circulation* 1988;77(4):815–819.
4. Chen L, et al. Angiographic features of vein grafts versus ungrafted coronary arteries in patients with unstable angina and previous bypass surgery. *J Am Coll Cardiol* 1996;28(6):1493–1499.
5. Morrison DA, et al. Percutaneous coronary intervention versus repeat bypass surgery for patients with medically refractory myocardial ischemia: AWESOME randomized trial and registry experience with post-CABG patients. *J Am Coll Cardiol* 2002;40(11):1951–1954.
6. Goldman S, et al. Long-term patency of saphenous vein and left internal mammary artery grafts after coronary artery bypass surgery: Results from a Department of Veterans Affairs Cooperative Study. *J Am Coll Cardiol* 2004;44(11):2149–2156.
7. Canos DA, et al. Clinical, angiographic, and intravascular ultrasound characteristics of early saphenous vein graft failure. *J Am Coll Cardiol* 2004;44(1):53–56.
8. de Feyter PJ, et al. Balloon angioplasty for the treatment of lesions in saphenous vein bypass grafts. *J Am Coll Cardiol* 1993;21(7):1539–1549.
9. Platko WP, et al. Percutaneous trans-luminal angioplasty of saphenous vein graft stenosis: Long-term follow-up. *J Am Coll Cardiol* 1989;14(7):1645–1650.
10. Reeves F, et al. Long-term angiographic follow-up after angioplasty of venous coronary bypass grafts. *Am Heart J* 1991;122(3 Pt 1):620–627.
11. Plokker HW, et al. The Dutch experience in percutaneous transluminal angioplasty of narrowed saphenous veins used for aortocoronary arterial bypass. *Am J Cardiol* 1991;67(5):361–366.
12. Holmes DR Jr., et al. A multicenter, randomized trial of coronary angioplasty versus directional atherectomy for patients with saphenous vein bypass graft lesions. CAVEAT-II Investigators. *Circulation* 1995;91(7):1966–1974.
13. Safian RD, et al. Clinical and angiographic results of trans-luminal extraction coronary atherectomy in saphenous vein bypass grafts. *Circulation* 1994;89(1):302–312.

14. Strauss BH, et al. Early and late quantitative angiographic results of vein graft lesions treated by excimer laser with adjunctive balloon angioplasty. *Circulation* 1995; 92(3):348–356.

15. Fenton SH, et al. Long-term angiographic and clinical outcome after implantation of balloon expandable stents in aortocoronary saphenous vein grafts. *Am J Cardiol* 1994;74(12):1187–1191.

16. Piana RN, et al. Palmaz-Schatz stenting for treatment of focal vein graft stenosis: Immediate results and long-term outcome. *J Am Coll Cardiol* 1994;23(6):1296–1304.

17. Wong SC, et al. Immediate results and late outcomes after stent implantation in saphenous vein graft lesions: The multicenter U.S. Palmaz-Schatz stent experience. The Palmaz-Schatz Stent Study Group. *J Am Coll Cardiol* 1995;26(3):704–712.

18. Ahmed JM, et al. Comparison of debulking followed by stenting versus stenting alone for saphenous vein graft aortoostial lesions: Immediate and one-year clinical outcomes. *J Am Coll Cardiol* 2000;35(6):1560–1568.

19. Savage MP, et al. Stent placement compared with balloon angioplasty for obstructed coronary bypass grafts. Saphenous Vein De Novo Trial Investigators. *N Engl J Med* 1997;337(11):740–747.

20. Gruberg L, et al. In-hospital and long-term results of stent deployment compared with balloon angioplasty for treatment of narrowing at the saphenous vein graft distal anastomosis site. *Am J Cardiol* 1999;84(12):1381–1384.

21. Hanekamp CE, et al. Randomized study to compare balloon angioplasty and elective stent implantation in venous bypass grafts: The Venestent study. *Catheter Cardiovasc Interv* 2003;60(4):452–457.

22. Vermeersch P, et al. Randomized double-blind comparison of sirolimus-eluting stent versus bare-metal stent implantation in diseased saphenous vein grafts: Six-month angiographic, intravascular ultrasound, and clinical follow-up of the RRISC Trial. *J Am Coll Cardiol* 2006;48(12):2423–2431.

23. Ge L, et al. Treatment of saphenous vein graft lesions with drug-eluting stents: Immediate and midterm outcome. *J Am Coll Cardiol* 2005;45(7):989–994.

24. Lee MS, et al. Drug-eluting stenting is superior to bare metal stenting in saphenous vein grafts. *Catheter Cardiovasc Interv* 2005;66(4):507–511.

25. Roleder T, et al. Bioresorbable vascular scaffolds in saphenous vein grafts (data from OCTOPUS registry). *Postepy Kardiol Interwencyjnej* 2015;11(4):323–326.

26. Rodes-Cabau J, et al. Comparison of plaque sealing with paclitaxel-eluting stents versus medical therapy for the treatment of moderate nonsignificant saphenous vein graft lesions: The moderate vein graft lesion stenting with the Taxus stent and intravascular ultrasound (VELETI) pilot trial. *Circulation* 2009;120:1978–1986.

27. Taggart DP, et al. A randomized trial of external stenting for saphenous vein grafts in coronary bypass grafting. *Ann Thorac Surg* 2015;99(6):2039–2045.

28. Inderbitzin DT, et al. One-year patency control and risk analysis of eSVS-mesh-supported coronary saphenous vein grafts. *J Cardiothorac Surg* 2015;10:108.

29. Vignali L, et al. Long-term outcomes with drug-eluting stents versus bare metal stents in the treatment of saphenous vein graft disease (results from the Registro Regionale AngioPLastiche Emilia-Romagna registry). *Am J Cardiol* 2008;101(7):947–952.

30. Pucelikova T, et al. Short- and long-term outcomes after stent-assisted percutaneous treatment of saphenous vein grafts in the drug-eluting stent era. *Am J Cardiol* 2008;101(1):63–68.

31. Vermeersch P, et al. Increased late mortality after sirolimus-eluting stents versus bare-metal stents in diseased saphenous vein grafts: Results from the randomized DELAYED RRISC Trial. *J Am Coll Cardiol* 2007;50(3):261–267.

32. Brennan JM, et al. Safety and clinical effectiveness of drug-eluting stents for saphenous vein graft intervention in older individuals: Results from the medicare-linked National Cardiovascular Data Registry® CathPCI Registry® (2005–2009). *Catheter Cardiovasc Interv* 2016;87(1):43–49.

33. Hong MK, et al. Creatine kinase-MB enzyme elevation following successful saphenous vein graft intervention is associated with late mortality. *Circulation* 1999;100(24):2400–2405.

34. Carrozza JP Jr., et al. Acute and long-term outcome after Palmaz-Schatz stenting: Analysis from the New Approaches to Coronary Intervention (NACI) registry. *Am J Cardiol* 1997;80(10A):78K–88K.

35. Webb JG, et al. Retrieval and analysis of particulate debris after saphenous vein graft intervention. *J Am Coll Cardiol* 1999;34(2):468–475.

36. Motwani JG, Topol EJ. Aortocoronary saphenous vein graft disease: Pathogenesis, predisposition, and prevention. *Circulation* 1998;97(9):916–931.

37. Golino P, et al. Local effect of serotonin released during coronary angioplasty. *N Engl J Med* 1994;330(8):523–528.

38. Sdringola S, et al. Risk assessment of slow or no-reflow phenomenon in aortocoronary vein graft percutaneous intervention. *Catheter Cardiovasc Interv* 2001;54(3):318–324.

39. Piana RN, et al. Incidence and treatment of "no-reflow" after percutaneous coronary intervention. *Circulation* 1994;89(6):2514–2518.

40. Yamaji K, et al. Percutaneous coronary intervention in patients with previous coronary artery bypass grafting (from the j-Cypher Registry). *Am J Cardiol* 2013;112(8):1110–1119.

41. Coolong A, et al. Saphenous vein graft stenting and major adverse cardiac events: A predictive model derived from a pooled analysis of 3958 patients. *Circulation* 2008;117(6):790–797.

42. Kirtane AJ, et al. Correlates of adverse events during saphenous vein graft intervention with distal embolic protection: A PRIDE substudy. *JACC Cardiovasc Interv* 2008;1(2):186–191.

43. Kaplan BM, et al. Treatment of no-reflow in degenerated saphenous vein graft interventions: Comparison of intracoronary verapamil and nitroglycerin. *Cathet Cardiovasc Diagn* 1996;39(2):113–118.

44. Weyrens FJ, et al. Intracoronary diltiazem for microvascular spasm after interventional therapy. *Am J Cardiol* 1995;75(12):849–850.

45. Fischell TA, et al. "Pharmacologic" distal protection using prophylactic, intragraft nicardipine to prevent no-reflow and non-Q-wave myocardial infarction during elective saphenous vein graft intervention. *J Invasive Cardiol* 2007;19(2):58–62.

46. Rha SW, et al. Bivalirudin versus heparin as an antithrombotic agent in patients who undergo percutaneous saphenous vein graft intervention with a distal protection device. *Am J Cardiol* 2005;96(1):67–70.

47. Roffi M, et al. Lack of benefit from intravenous platelet glycoprotein IIb/IIIa receptor inhibition as adjunctive treatment for percutaneous interventions of aortocoronary bypass grafts: A pooled analysis of five randomized clinical trials. *Circulation* 2002;106(24):3063–3067.

48. Barsness GW, et al. Reduced thrombus burden with abciximab delivered locally before percutaneous intervention in saphenous vein grafts. *Am Heart J* 2000;139(5):824–829.

49. Teirstein PS, et al. Low- versus high- dose recombinant urokinase for the treatment of chronic saphenous vein graft occlusion. *Am J Cardiol* 1999;83(12):1623–1628.

50. Kuntz RE, et al. A trial comparing rheolytic thrombectomy with intracoronary urokinase for coronary and vein graft thrombus [the Vein Graft AngioJet Study (VeGAS 2)]. *Am J Cardiol* 2002;89(3):326–330.

51. Zoghbi GJ, et al. Pretreatment with nitroprusside for microcirculatory protection isaphenous vein graft interventions. See comment in PubMed Commons below. *J Invasive Cardiol* 2009;21(2):34–39.

52. Braden GA, et al. Transluminal extraction catheter atherectomy followed by immediate stenting in treatment of saphenous vein grafts. *J Am Coll Cardiol* 1997;30(3):657–663.

53. Bittl JA, et al. Predictors of outcome of percutaneous excimer laser coronary angioplasty of saphenous vein bypass graft lesions. The Percutaneous Excimer Laser Coronary Angioplasty Registry. *Am J Cardiol* 1994;74(2):144–148.

54. Singh M, et al. Treatment of saphenous vein bypass grafts with ultrasound thrombolysis: A randomized study (ATLAS). *Circulation* 2003;107(18):2331–2336.

55. Baim DS, et al. Randomized trial of a distal embolic protection device during percutaneous intervention of saphenous vein aorto-coronary bypass grafts. *Circulation* 2002;105(11):1285–1290.

56. Cohen DJ, et al. Cost-effectiveness of distal embolic protection for patients undergoing percutaneous intervention of saphenous vein bypass grafts: Results from the SAFER trial. *J Am Coll Cardiol* 2004;44(9):1801–1808.

57. Cragun DT, Heuser RR. Embolic protection devices in saphenous vein graft interventions. *J Interv Cardiol* 2006;19(6):525–529.

58. Mauri L, et al. The PROXIMAL trial: proximal protection during saphenous vein graft intervention using the Proxis Embolic Protection System: A randomized, prospective, multicenter clinical trial. *J Am Coll Cardiol* 2007;50(15):1442–1449.

59. Stone GW, et al. Randomized comparison of distal protection with a filter-based catheter and a balloon occlusion and aspiration system during percutaneous intervention of diseased saphenous vein aorto-coronary bypass grafts. *Circulation* 2003;108(5):548–553.

60. Halkin A, et al. Six-month outcomes after percutaneous intervention for lesions in aortocoronary saphenous vein grafts using distal protection devices: Results from the FIRE trial. *Am Heart J* 2006;151(4):915.e1–e7.

61. Rogers C, et al. Embolic protection with filtering or occlusion balloons during saphenous vein graft stenting retrieves identical volumes and sizes of particulate debris. *Circulation* 2004;109(14):1735–1740.

62. Baldus S, et al. Treatment of aortocoronary vein graft lesions with membrane-covered stents: A multicenter surveillance trial. *Circulation* 2000;102(17):2024–2027.

63. Briguori C, et al. Polytetrafluoroethylene-covered stent for the treatment of narrowings in aorticocoronary saphenous vein grafts. *Am J Cardiol* 2000;86(3):343–346.

64. Stankovic G, et al. Randomized evaluation of polytetrafluoroethylene-covered stent in saphenous vein grafts: The Randomized Evaluation of polytetrafluoroethylene COVERed stent in Saphenous vein grafts (RECOVERS) Trial. *Circulation* 2003;108(1):37–42.

65. Turco MA, et al. Pivotal, randomized U.S. study of the Symbiottrade mark covered stent system in patients with saphenous vein graft disease: Eight-month angiographic and clinical results from the Symbiot III trial. *Catheter Cardiovasc Interv* 2006;68(3):379–388.

66. Frimerman A, et al. Long-term follow-up of a high risk cohort after stent implantation in saphenous vein grafts. *J Am Coll Cardiol* 1997;30(5):1277–1283.

67. Laham RJ, et al. Long-term (4- to 6-year) outcome of Palmaz-Schatz stenting: paucity of late clinical stent-related problems. *J Am Coll Cardiol* 1996;28(4):820–826.

68. Le May MR, et al. Predictors of long-term outcome after stent implantation in a saphenous vein graft. *Am J Cardiol* 1999;83:681–686.

69. de Jaegere PP, et al. Long-term clinical outcome after stent implantation in saphenous vein grafts. *J Am Coll Cardiol* 1996;28(1):89–96.

70. Mauri L, et al. Devices for distal protection during percutaneous coronary revascularization. *Circulation* 2006;113(22):2651–2656.

71. Depre C, et al. Pathology of restenosis in saphenous bypass grafts after long-term stent implantation. *Am J Clin Pathol* 1998;110(3):378–384.

72. van Beusekom HM, et al. Histology after stenting of human saphenous vein bypass grafts: Observations from surgically excised grafts 3 to 320 days after stent implantation. *J Am Coll Cardiol* 1993;21(1):45–54.

73. Keeley EC, et al. Long-term clinical outcome and predictors of major adverse cardiac events after percutaneous interventions on saphenous vein grafts. *J Am Coll Cardiol* 2001;38(3):659–665.

74. Ahmed JM, et al. Influence of diabetes mellitus on early and late clinical outcomes in saphenous vein graft stenting. *J Am Coll Cardiol* 2000;36(4):1186–1193.

75. Ellis SG, et al. Late myocardial ischemic events after saphenous vein graft intervention–importance of initially "nonsignificant" vein graft lesions. *Am J Cardiol* 1997;79(11):1460–1464.

76. Ahmed JM, et al. Influence of gender on early and one-year clinical outcomes after saphenous vein graft stenting. *Am J Cardiol* 2001;87(4):401–405.

77. Virk SJ, et al. Transluminal extraction atherectomy for stent restenosis in a saphenous vein bypass graft. *Eur Heart J* 1997;18(2):350–351.

78. Dangas G, et al. Acute and long-term results of treatment of diffuse in-stent restenosis in aortocoronary saphenous vein grafts. *Am J Cardiol* 2000;86(7):777–779, A6.

79. Ashby DT, et al. Effect of percutaneous coronary interventions for in-stent restenosis in degenerated saphenous vein grafts without distal embolic protection. *J Am Coll Cardiol* 2003;41(5):749–752.

80. Friedrich SP, et al. Investigational use of the Palmaz-Schatz biliary stent in large saphenous vein grafts. *Am J Cardiol* 1993;71(5):439–441.

81. Hernandez-Antolin RA, et al. Successful sealing of an angioplasty-related saphenous vein graft rupture with a PTFE-covered stent. *J Invasive Cardiol* 2000;12(11):589–593.

82. Hanratty CG, et al. Angioplasty and stenting of the distal coronary anastomosis for graft failure immediately after coronary artery bypass grafting. *Am J Cardiol* 2002;90(9):1009–1011.

37

Emboli protection devices, atherectomy, and thrombus aspiration devices

FERNANDO CURA AND JOSE ANDRÉS NAVARRO

INTRODUCTION

There is a large armamentarium of medical devices available for the percutaneous treatment of a variety of coronary atherosclerosis lesions. This chapter describes several aspects related to the biological components of the atherosclerotic plaque and the rationale, clinical evidence, and indications for different interventional devices. The scope of this chapter will range from devices that prepare very hard atherosclerotic plaques prior to stenting, for example, rotational atherectomy, to devices that are either used to remove very soft, friable, or thrombotic lesions, such as thrombectomy, or those preventing distal embolization during intervention by temporary vessel occlusion or filter placement.

PLAQUE COMPOSITION AND SELECTION OF INTERVENTIONAL STRATEGY

Normal human coronary arteries have three thin layers: the intima, media, and adventitia. The intima interfaces with the arterial lumen and is composed of endothelial cells. The media is composed of smooth muscle cells, collagen, fibroblast, and intercellular matrix molecules, and it regulates vascular contraction. The media is separated from the intima and adventitia by the internal and external elastic membranes, respectively. Coronary atherosclerosis is a complex inflammatory-infiltrative disorder affecting the three vessel layers.[1] During life, the presence of acquired and inherent coronary artery disease (CAD) risk factors triggers a series of events that leads to atherosclerosis. Prior results from animal studies have suggested that the first step

in atherosclerosis is endothelial cell dysfunction and lipoprotein particle accumulation at the intima level.[2] At this stage, lipid oxidation, local release of interleukins, cytokines, reactive oxygen species, and pro-oxidative enzymes generate white blood cell chemotaxis and adhesion to the endothelial surface.[3-5] Then, leukocytes and monocytes penetrate endothelial cells into the arterial wall, engulfing lipid particles constituting foam cells.[6,7] Foam cells progress to fatty streaks and ultimately to raised atheromatous plaques.[1] Several other factors are also involved in the development of atherosclerosis. Laminar flow elicits atheroprotective properties.[8] On the contrary, turbulent flow, especially at branch points, leads to the atheromas plaque formation. In fact, during plaque growth, lumen reduction increases blood flow velocity, thus elevating shear stress. There is a large amount of evidence that indicates high levels of shear stress stimulate outward vascular remodeling of the arterial wall, probably in an attempt to preserve endoluminal dimensions.[9,10] At still an unpredictable point in the atherosclerosis process, outward remodeling may fail or just simply stop due to an excess of plaque burden or inherent poor vascular ability to produce outward remodeling, and significant arterial luminal stenosis ensues. Despite the previous belief that the presence of high shear stress and continuous outward remodeling were only protective factors, their presence, in conjunction with high plaque burden and a thin fibrous cap, represent the classic scenario leading to a ruptured and/or eroded plaque.[11] This metabolically active, unstable plaque expresses several prothrombotic cytokines leading to thrombus formation and vasoconstriction. This is the most common underlying coronary lesion among patients with acute coronary syndromes (ACS). In particular, patients with ST-segment elevation acute myocardial infarction (STEMI) have highly thrombotic lesions. In addition, these patients have different levels of myocardial damage with microvascular embolization, interstitial edema, and vasoconstriction.[12]

Coronary stenosis due primarily to negative remodeling is associated with relatively low plaque burden and thick fibrous cap, usually present in stable coronary syndromes.[13] Some of these patients have dense fibrocalcific coronary plaques, which are sometimes difficult to be adequately addressed with balloon angioplasty or stenting alone. These types of lesions have been the target of numerous devices, chiefly designed to remove or alter the plaque as an adjunctive measure prior to stenting. Devices such as directional coronary atherectomy, rotational atherectomy, excimer laser and cutting-balloon, among others, have been tested.[14,15] The two most commonly used devices for severely fibro-calcified stable coronary lesions in current practice are rotational atherectomy and cutting balloon angioplasty.

Atherectomy devices

The year 2016 marks the 29th year since rotational atherectomy[16] (RA) was first introduced in the market for the treatment of chronic endovascular lesions.[17] It is commercially available as the Rotablator System (Boston Scientific, Scimed) (Figure 37.1) and consists of a nickel-plated, diamond chip–coated brass burr rotating at 140,000–190,000 rotations per minute (rpm). Eight burr sizes are available, ranging from 1.25 to 2.5 mm. Rotational atherectomy works by the physical principle of differential cutting.[18] This principle enables destruction of only inelastic material, such as atherosclerotic, calcified, and fibrotic plaques while preventing normal elastic tissue from becoming damaged. Debris dislodged after rotational atherectomy are less than 12 μm, and with careful technique, should not create a significant impact on the epicardial and myocardial blood flow. However, creatine kinase myocardial b fraction (CK-MB) release (myocardial infarction [MI]) rates after rotational atherectomy are significantly higher than after conventional angioplasty.[19–21] Selection of burr size should not exceed a burr/artery diameter ratio of 0.7. In fact, for undilatable lesions, the use of very small burrs is less aggressive and usually sufficient to physically alter the plaque surface, allowing balloon dilatation and stenting. During the bare-metal stent (BMS) era, substantial evidence indicated that despite achieving greater acute gain with the use of rotational atherectomy, restenosis remained unchanged and increased the risk of the procedure due to distal embolization or slow flow.[21] Increased operator experience using shorter runs (less than 20 seconds) with <5,000 rpm decrements, the use of smaller burr size, along with device improvements, have reduced periprocedural complications. Prophylactic use of intracoronary "Rota Flush Cocktail" with different concentrations of nitroglycerin, verapramil, and heparin has improved the epicardial flow after rotational atherectomy.[22] However, ventricular arrhythmias, coronary dissection, and vessel perforation are still a concern, especially among patients with severe vessel tortuosity or angulated lesions.[23] Thus, the popularity of rotational atherectomy has decreased in the past decade, and in recent series, rotational atherectomy use has fallen to 3%–5% in select high-volume centers and <1% in others.[24] It is predominantly utilized for undilatable lesions or delivery failure. Unfortunately, the complexity of this device requires proper operator training and experience to be comfortable to use this unique tool. In systematic research done in 2013, the authors established the fundamental "steps" of optimal technique: single burr with burr-to-artery ratio of 0.5–0.6, rotational speed of 140,000–150,000 rpm, gradual burr advancement using a pecking motion, short ablation runs of 15s–20s, avoidance of decelerations >5,000 rpm, and final polishing run.[25] This should increase the success of rotational atherectomy and more importantly, decrease the incidence of complications.

Although intravascular ultrasound (IVUS) studies have demonstrated that suboptimal deployment, incomplete apposition, and failure to achieve adequate stent dimensions may lead to stent thrombosis[26–28] and repeat target vessel revascularization, the available anecdotal data comparing rotational atherectomy use prior to drug-eluting stent (DES) deployment versus DES alone do not support its systematic use.[29] The first randomized trial to directly test the impact of rotational atherectomy on long-term outcomes of DES placement, called ROTAXUS (Rotational Atherectomy Prior to

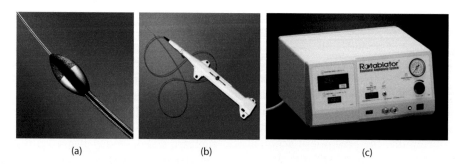

(a)   (b)   (c)

Figure 37.1 The Rotablator system: **(a)** burr, **(b)** advancer, and **(c)** control console. (Courtesy of Boston Scientific, SCIMED, Maple Grove, MN.)

Taxus Stent Treatment for Complex Native Coronary Artery Disease), did not show long-term benefit.[30] However, several case series have reported intermediate and long-term outcomes with adjunctive rotational atherectomy, with rates of target lesion revascularization <10% within 1–2 years,[25,31–33] and with better outcomes with lower major adverse cardiac events (MACE), compared to BMS.[34–36] However, vigorous manipulation of DES through calcified lesions could potentially damage polymer coating integrity and lower DES efficiency. Although there are still some concerns regarding local delivery of drugs through a calcified lesion, clinical trials with the paclitaxel-eluting stent did not reveal differences in in-stent restenosis or thrombosis rates between calcified and noncalcified lesions.[37]

In under-expanded stents, high-pressure balloons, drug-coated balloons, or sometimes cutting balloon dilation are preferred.[38] On the other hand, when the lesion cannot be crossed by a balloon, when multiple jail side branches exist, or when metallic stent struts contribute directly to luminal obstruction,[39] rotational atherectomy has been utilized; however, this maneuver may only be used in select cases with experienced operators since the chance of burr entrapment may be increased.

The percutaneous and endovascular system—Diamondback 360° Coronary Orbital Atherectomy System (OAS) (Cardiovascular Systems, Inc., St. Paul, MN)—is a peripheral device adapted for use in calcified coronary arteries. It is a control handled, eccentrically mounted, diamond-coated crown that orbits over an atherectomy wire at high speeds to incorporate the use of centrifugal force and differential sanding to modify calcified lesions. The orbital atherectomy procedure removes the calcified stenotic lesion material to increase vessel compliance prior to balloon angioplasty and stent placement, which may lead to reduced acute vascular injury.[40] The pivotal ORBIT II Trial, a single-arm trial, enrolled 443 subjects at 49 U.S. sites with severely calcified lesions that are usually excluded from randomized trials. The orbital atherectomy system was utilized for plaque modification before stent implantation, where 88.2% were DES. The 1-year follow-up (with a median of 16.7 months) showed a MACE rate of 16.4%. The target lesion revascularization rate was 4.7%, and stent thrombosis occurred in one patient (0.2%). These findings are promising as 1-year adverse ischemic events were low compared with historical controls, giving us an option for the treatment of calcified lesions.[41]

Cutting balloon angioplasty represents another alternative to overcome fibro-calcified plaques.[42,43] It consists of a balloon catheter with three or four atherotomes or microsurgical blades, which are three to five times sharper than conventional surgical blades.[43] Atherotomes are placed longitudinally on the outer surface of a noncomplaint balloon. The radial expansion of the cutting balloon produces longitudinal incisions in the plaque and vessel, reducing tensile vessel stress[44] and elastic recoil.[45] Balloon sizes are 2–3.2 mm and its unique design protects the vessel from the edges of the atherotomes when the balloon is deflated. The latter is vital in order to diminish the risk of vessel trauma during device delivery to the lesion or balloon retrieval from the vessel. Usually, lower balloon inflation pressures (4–8 atmospheres) are required. Currently, cutting balloon use is limited to undilatable coronary artery stenosis, preferable with a reference vessel diameter ranging from 2 to 4 mm in diameter, without extreme vessel tortuosity.[46] Highly tortuous and angulated lesions are technically difficult to access due to the presence of the longitudinal atherotomes in the cutting balloon. Shorter cutting balloons (10 mm) are usually more deliverable than the longer (15 mm) ones in passing a moderately tortuous vessel. Cutting balloons can also be used in aorto-ostial lesions.[47] It is used to prepare patients with heavily calcified coronary lesions (HCCLs) who are undergoing percutaneous intervention with DES, and has similar outcomes as rotational atherectomy and plain old balloon angioplasty (POBA).[48] Its anecdotal popularity for patients with in-stent restenosis has been replaced with the overwhelming data supporting the use of DES.[49,50]

Thrombus removal and prevention of distal embolization

Unstable coronary syndromes are associated with soft, friable, thrombotic, and metabolically active atherosclerotic lesions.[51] At sites of plaque formation there is substantial inflammation with proliferation of vasa vasorum from the adventitia into the endoluminal surface of the plaque,[52,53] clustered with macrophages, which release proteolytic enzymes such as matrix metalloproteinases that are responsible for thinning elastic internal and external membranes as well as fibrous cap, ultimately leading to plaque erosion or rupture and thrombus formation.[54] Besides atherothrombotic debris, unstable plaques contain a milieu of humoral factors that, if released downstream during PCI, have the potential for damaging the distal microcirculation. During STEMI, primary PCI of the thrombotic lesion requires particular care to reduce distal atherothrombotic embolization and its complications. The angiographic observance of distal embolization is rather common (~15%) during primary PCI, and translates into poor left ventricular recovery and clinical outcome.[55] Even in the absence of this complication and despite successful epicardial recanalization, inadequate myocardial reperfusion at the tissue level, reflected by incomplete ST-segment resolution, is frequently observed immediately following the procedure (~40%).[56,57] Suboptimal myocardial reperfusion at the end of the intervention is associated with reduced myocardial salvage and worse long-term outcome than patients achieving adequate reperfusion.[58,59] Lack of myocardial reperfusion or no-reflow is due to mechanical obstruction of the microcirculation, partly explained by the complex interplay of distal atherothromboic embolization, postischemic arteriolar damage, myocardial edema, reperfusion injury, and the downstream release of vasoconstrictors and prothrombotic mediators.[60] Although distal embolization is a common phenomenon, the amount and composition of distal debris vary largely. Consequently, a variety of techniques have been designed to either reduce or prevent the amount of debris that migrates distally during the procedure. These devices are divided into nonocclusive (distal embolic filter protection) and occlusive devices (proximal or distal vessel occlusion).

Distal embolic protection with filter devices

These devices provide the ability to maintain distal perfusion, while protecting against macroembolization. Thus, they enable antegrade flow and allow the operator to inject contrast during the procedure. Nevertheless, several potential disadvantages should be mentioned. Depending on the filter design, small debris (<80–100 μm) and humoral mediators can go through the filter pores. Moreover, there is a potential risk of embolization while crossing the lesion with the device, especially if predilatation is required in order to advance the filter distally. Unlike proximal protection, distal filters do not protect side branches proximal to the device. In the setting of STEMI, it can be challenging to perform blinded distal filter placement in patients with baseline epicardial thrombolysis in myocardial infarction (TIMI) flow 0–1.

Several studies have shown the benefit of distal protection in carotid stenting[61,62] and saphenous veins graft (SVG) intervention.[63,64] These positive results encouraged their use in the native coronary circulation among patients with ACS. Initial anecdotal data reported an improvement in myocardial reperfusion parameters using different surrogates, such as myocardial blush grade or ST-segment resolution.[65]

However, the PROMISE (Protection Devices in PCI-Treatment of Myocardial Infarction for Salvage of Endangered Myocardium) trial[66] utilized the FilterWire EZ Embolic Protection System (Boston Scientific, CA) and randomized 200 patients undergoing PCI for STEMI and non-STEMI. Surrogate markers, such as maximal adenosine-induced flow velocity, infarct size, and incidence of distal embolization, as well as 30-day mortality, did not differ between the two groups. The inclusion of non-STEMI patients in this trial may have blunted any differences between the two treatment groups.

The PREMIAR (Protection of Distal Embolization in High-Risk Patients with Acute ST-Segment Elevation Myocardial Infarction) trial[56] was a prospective, randomized, controlled study that tested a low-profile distal protection filter device (SpideRX, ev3, Inc, MN; Figure 37.2), during PCI

in STEMI patients at high risk for embolic events. Thus, by protocol, only patients with TIMI grade flow between 0 and 2 were included. The study randomized 150 patients, and visible macroscopic atherothrombotic debris was noted by visual assessment in the filters in 48% of cases. Histopathologic analysis was performed in a subgroup of patients demonstrating that particles were recovered in all analyzed filters. The number of particles ranged from 8 to 48 per filter. Particles size ranged from 101 to 1,299 μm in maximum diameter and from 212 to 1,487 μm² in area. Most particles were composed of platelet clumps, red cells, and fibrin, which led to the diagnosis of fresh thrombus. All patients underwent 24-hour ST-segment monitoring in order to measure the extent of ST-segment recovery. In this trial, the adjunctive use of a distal filter device did not improve myocardial reperfusion either by ST-segment resolution or quantitative angiographic markers (TIMI blush grade, TIMI flow, and TIMI frame count). Furthermore, left ventricular function and 6-month clinical outcome did not differ between groups. There were no specific subgroups discerned that derived benefit from adjunctive distal protection.

In a published meta-analysis (*n* = 1,467) including eight randomized clinical trials, the role of distal protection with either filter or balloon occlusion during primary PCI did not show improvement in extent of reperfusion or 30-day mortality when compared to PCI alone. In summary, due to the lack of positive results and potential disadvantages, the routine use of distal filter protection during primary PCI in native coronary arteries cannot be recommended. Nonetheless, these studies have demonstrated the use of distal filters to be feasible and safe.

Although it is not a filter device, the stent system MGuard (InspireMD, Tel Aviv, Israel; Figure 37.3)[67] is a reasonable alternative during intervention of thrombotic or friable plaques. In addition to its low profile, it has an ultrathin polyethylene terephthalate microfiber sleeve that

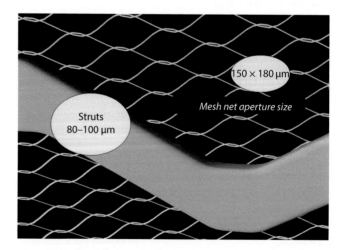

Figure 37.3 The MGuard Coronary Stent System. Note its mesh sleeve covering the stent, which allows a less traumatic stent dilation and adequate entrapment of plaque debris behind the stent. (Courtesy of InspireMD, Ltd., Tel Aviv, Israel.)

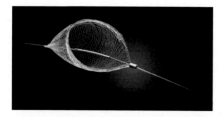

Figure 37.2 The SpideRX Distal Filter. (Courtesy of SpideRX, ev3, Inc., MN.)

wraps the stent, which traps plaque material behind the stent and reduces vessel trauma during stent deployment. Nowadays, there are two types: the MGuard stent and the MGuard Prime, mostly differing in the L605 cobalt chromium alloy platform (strut thickness 80 μm), while the MGuard has a 316L stainless steel frame with strut thickness of 100 μm.[68] Two randomized trials have compared the use of MGuard stent to conventional PCI in STEMI patients. In the MASTER I trial, 433 STEMI patients were randomized in a 1:1 fashion to the MGuard stent versus BMS or DES. The MGuard stent was associated with better reperfusion indices with higher ST-segment resolution (57.8% vs. 44.7%; $P = 0.008$), and TIMI 3 flow (91.7% vs. 82.9%, $P = 0.006$), with a trend toward lower mortality at 30 days (0% vs. 1.9%, $P = 0.06$) and 1 year (1% vs. 3.3%, P = 0.09). The more profound impact that favored the MGuard stent was seen among subgroups with the presence of large thrombus[69] or long delay time.[70] However, there was a higher incidence of repeat revascularization (8.6% vs. 0.9%, $P = 0.0003$).[71] The MASTER II enrolled 1,114 patients to demonstrate superiority of the MGuard stent versus conventional PCI on the reduction of clinical events, such as death or MI. However, due to stent dislodgement, the study was voluntarily suspended in April 2014 after enrollment of 310 patients (155 patients per group). Analysis of the enrolled cohort showed no benefit of the MGuard stent in any of the analyzed endpoints (ST-segment resolution was 56.9% vs. 59.3% in the control group, $P = 0.68$; mortality was 0.6% vs. 1.9% in the control group, $P = 0.62$). Similarly, a pooled analysis of the MASTER I and II trials ($n = 743$) failed to show better myocardial reperfusion (ST-segment resolution 57.5% for the MGuard vs. 50.7% for the control group, $P = 0.07$), although mortality at 30 days was significantly lower (0.3% vs. 1.9%, $P = 0.03$).[72]

Thus, data from randomized trials suggest that the use of the MGuard stent may reduce distal embolization and may improve survival at 30 days compared with other commercially available coronary stents, although further randomized studies are warranted to confirm this hypothesis. Also, further research is needed to understand if the restenosis rate is only related to the lack of drug elution or, by contrast, if there is also an antigenic stimulus caused by the polyethylene terephthalate mesh.[73,74]

Distal embolic protection with occlusive devices

This system is based on transient distal balloon occlusion coupled with an aspiration catheter to prevent plaque debris embolization. Similar to distal filters, this system requires passage through the lesion and does not provide protection to proximal side branches. In addition, it may not have an adequately visible landing zone in the presence of baseline TIMI 0. Unlike distal filters, balloon occlusion provokes myocardial ischemia due to blood flow stagnation, and hence, its duration should remain as short as possible. Examples of distal occluding devices include PercuSurge

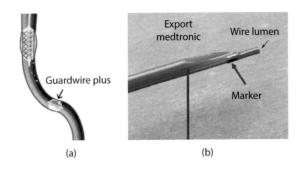

Figure 37.4 **(a)** PercuSurge GuardWire Distal Protection Device (PercuSurge, Minneapolis, MN). Note the distal balloon occluding the coronary vessel. **(b)** Export thromboaspiration catheter. (Courtesy of Medtronic, Minneapolis, MN.)

GuardWire Distal Protection Device[75] (Medtronic, PA; Figure 37.4a) and TriActive System (Kensey, PA).

The PercuSurge Guardwire Protection Device occludes distally with a balloon while the Export catheter (Medtronic, PA; Figure 37.4b) is used to aspirate the stagnated debris-containing blood. Thromboaspiration is performed after balloon dilation and stent deployment. This device has been used with success in a large multicenter randomized trial— The SVG Angioplasty Free of Emboli Randomized (SAFER) trial. A total of 801 patients were randomized to SVG intervention with and without the PercuSurge Guardwire Protection Device System.[55] The primary endpoint of the study, MACE rate at 30 days, was defined as the composite of death, MI, emergent bypass surgery or target vessel revascularization within 30 days of the index procedure. There was a 6.9% absolute reduction (42% relative reduction) in 30-day MACE (9.6% for GuardWire vs. 16.5% for controls, $P = 0.001$). This reduction in MACE was driven primarily by MI (8.6% vs. 14.7%, $P = 0.008$) and no-reflow (3% vs. 9%, $P = 0.02$). The same protection system was evaluated in the EMERALD trial in the setting of STEMI. The Enhanced Myocardial Efficacy and Recovery by Aspiration of Liberalized Debris (EMERALD) trial randomized 501 patients who presented within 6 hours from symptom onset for primary (81%) or rescue PCI (19%) to receive PCI with the GuardWire Plus (*Medtronic*) distal balloon occlusion system compared to angioplasty without distal protection.[42] Although visible debris were retrieved from 73% of patients randomized to the device, this did not result in improved microvascular flow, reperfusion success, reduced infarct size, or enhanced event-free survival.

Embolic protection with proximal occlusion

Proximal occlusion devices cause blood flow stagnation by occluding the target coronary artery "upstream" from the lesion. With flow temporarily interrupted, thromboaspiration is performed and the stent or balloon is delivered to the lesion. Then, thromboaspiration is performed again and the proximal balloon is deflated, which restores blood flow. Advantages of proximal occlusion devices over distal occlusion or filters are several. First, proximal occlusions do not need to cross the lesion, thereby avoiding device-induced embolization. Second, device delivery is not affected as much by tortuous vessels. Third, the landing zone is always seen at the beginning of the procedure. Fourth, side branches are protected and humoral mediators theoretically do not reach the microcirculation. However, proximal occlusion devices may not have an adequate landing zone in ostial or proximal lesions.

The most studied proximal protection device is the Proxis Proximal Protection System Device (St. Jude Medical, MN; Figure 37.5). A single-center STEMI registry[76] (N = 177) has shown encouraging results, with 96% final TIMI 3 and 80% complete ST-segment resolution at 60 minutes with a 30-day MACE rate of 4%. The PREPARE (Prospective Randomized Trial of Proximal Microcirculatory Protection in Patients with Acute Myocardial Infarction Undergoing Primary PCI) trial enrolled 284 primary PCI patients with the adjunctive use of the Proxis device versus PCI alone. In this study, immediate percentage ST-segment resolution was higher in the device group; however, similar ST-segment resolution was seen at 30, 60, and 90 minutes

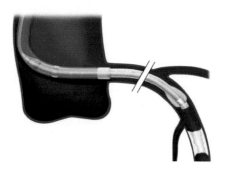

Figure 37.5 The Proxis Proximal Protection System for proximal balloon occlusion and thromboaspiration. (Courtesy of St. Jude Medical, Inc., MN.)

after the procedure. There was also no difference in 30-day clinical outcome. According to the investigators (personal communication), there was a correlation between early ST-segment resolution and myocardial salvage and long-term outcomes. Based on these findings, a larger randomized trial is planned with this device.

Thrombectomy devices

Thromboaspiration devices are used to remove thrombus from the coronary lesions during primary PCI in order to reduce distal embolization. There are, however, other potential advantages for thrombus removal prior to stent implantation, possibly more so in the DES era. Following primary PCI, an IVUS study has detected high rates of late stent malapposition. This finding might partially explain the increased risk of stent thrombosis in this population when compared to more elective procedures. Stent implantation may compress thrombotic material behind the stent struts, which eventually dissolves in the long term, rendering the stent malapposed. In a primary PCI study,[77] thrombus burden was graded from 0 to 4 according to thrombus length. The highest grade (grade 4) was defined as the presence of thrombus length ≥2 times vessel diameter. Patients with the highest thrombus grade had significantly higher late stent thrombosis than patients with lower thrombus grades (Figure 37.6). In this retrospective study, the adjunctive use of mechanical thrombectomy was independently associated with a reduction in the development of late stent thrombosis. Further retrospective analysis performed by these investigators only in patients with large thrombus burden (n = 266) showed that adjunctive thromboaspiration (72/266, 28.2%) was associated with an improvement in myocardial perfusion and a 2-year survival benefit (92% vs. 83%, P = 0.051)[78] when compared to primary PCI alone. Thus, thrombus removal appears to confer short- and long-term benefits, possibly avoiding the development of stent

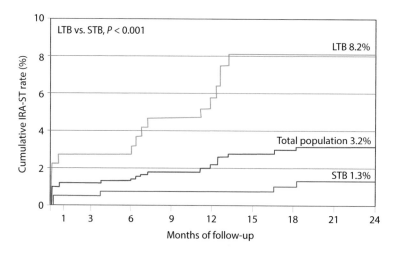

Figure 37.6 Two-year cumulative infarct-related artery (IRA) drug-eluting stent thrombosis (ST) rate for the overall population and patients with large thrombus burden (LTB or grade 4) and small thrombus burden (STB). (Reproduced from Sianos, G., et al., *J. Am. Coll. Cardiol.*, 50, 573–583, 2007. With permission.)

malapposition and, hence, reducing stent thrombosis rates. Again, however, prospective randomized clinical trials are needed to confirm this hypothesis.

Numerous thrombectomy devices have been tested during primary PCI. Although there is an ample heterogeneity in designs, aspiration capacity, and operational principles, thrombectomy devices can be further divided into manual and mechanical.

MANUAL THROMBECTOMY DEVICES

Manual thrombectomy devices are user friendly; they have a minimal learning curve and do not impact overall procedural time. The most studied and widely used devices include the Export Catheter (Medtronic, MN; see Figure 37.4b), Diver CE (Invatec, Roncadelle, Italy; Figure 37.7), the Rescue catheter (Boston Scientific), the Pronto catheter (Vascular Solutions, Inc., Minneapolis, MN), and the QuickCat (Kensey, PA).

The use of routine aspiration thrombectomy, plus primary PCI versus PCI alone in patients presenting with STEMI has been a subject of debate.

In the TAPAS (Thrombus Aspiration during Percutaneous coronary intervention in Acute myocardial infarction Study) trial,[79] a single-center randomized clinical trial ($n = 1071$) evaluated the adjunctive use of Export catheter in an unselected STEMI population undergoing primary PCI. Manual thromboaspiration resulted in great improvement in myocardial perfusion, as assessed by the percentage of complete ST-segment resolution (Figure 37.8), TIMI blush grade, and TIMI 3 flow, which translated into a significant reduction in 12-month cardiac death (3.6 vs. 6.7%; OR 1.93; 95% CI 1.11–3.37; $P = .020$) and reinfarction (2.2 vs. 4.3%; $P = .05$).[80] In fact, this landmark randomized trial is the first to report a significant benefit in clinical hard endpoints with the use of an adjunctive distal protection tool during primary PCI.

A meta-analysis of nine randomized trials, including 2,417 STEMI patients undergoing primary PCI with or without adjunctive manual thrombectomy, was previously published[81] demonstrating that the use of manual thromboaspiration significantly improved myocardial reperfusion and 30-day mortality. These results suggested that manual thromboaspiration offers a significant clinical benefit prior to stenting during primary PCI, and its use should be encouraged, in particular, among patients with large thrombus, and large and proximal vessels.

However, particular attention has to be paid to the technical management of the aspiration and guiding catheter to avoid thrombus dislodgement during retrieval, which may explain the incremental stroke risk.

In contrast, the TOTAL (Trial of Routine Aspiration Thrombectomy With PCI versus PCI Alone in Patients With STEMI) trial,[82] the largest clinical trial on this topic, did not observe a benefit in clinical outcomes. This study randomized a total of 11,063 patients to either aspiration thrombectomy followed by PCI ($n = 5,033$) or conventional PCI alone ($n = 5,030$) to compare outcomes after routine adjunctive aspiration thrombectomy versus conventional PCI in patients with STEMI undergoing primary PCI. The results of this trial evidenced that routine thrombus aspiration during primary PCI is associated with no improvement on clinical outcomes at 1 year compared with conventional PCI alone (with use of bailout thrombectomy as needed). Moreover, 30-day stroke risk was higher with aspiration thrombectomy.[82]

Therefore, although the TAPAS trial demonstrated a reduction in cardiovascular death, INFUSE-AMI,[83] TASTE,[84,85] and TOTAL, the largest clinical trial on this topic, did not observe a benefit in clinical outcomes with aspiration thrombectomy compared to conventional PCI.

MECHANICAL THROMBECTOMY DEVICES

The Angiojet Rheolytic Thrombectomy System[86] (Possis Medical, Inc., MN) creates an extremely high negative pressure zone (–600 mmHg) at its distal tip by high-velocity saline jets that are directed back within the catheter, resulting in removal of thrombus by suction through the outflow lumen using the Ventouri and Bernoulli effects (Figure 37.9). Compared to mechanical, manual thromboaspiration achieves a much lower negative suction pressure (–10 mmHg). Furthermore, more powerful suction due to the outflow pressure also generates clot fragmentation while entering into the catheter. Moreover,

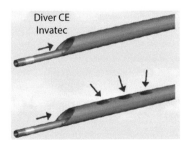

Figure 37.7 Diver catheter. (Courtesy of Invatec, Roncadelle, Italy.)

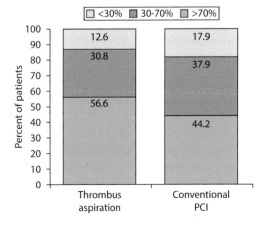

Figure 37.8 TAPAS trial: the percentages of patients are shown according to the degree of resolution of ST-segment elevation. PCI, percutaneous coronary intervention.

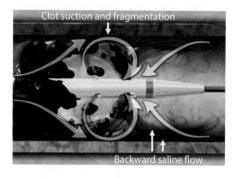

Figure 37.9 The Angiojet Rheolytic Thrombectomy System. (Courtesy of Possis Medical, Inc., MN.)

manual aspiration may face catheter occlusion during clot aspiration. In experimental models, clot mass removal is significantly higher using mechanical compared to manual thromboaspiration.

The multicenter AiMI (AngioJet Rheolytic Thrombectomy in Patients Undergoing Primary Angioplasty for Acute MI) trial[87] included 480 STEMI patients evaluating the adjunctive use of the Angiojet device during primary PCI versus primary PCI alone. In this study, myocardial reperfusion and myocardial salvage were worse in the thrombectomy group when compared to PCI alone. These results further translated into more 30-day adverse events in the thrombectomy group (6.7% vs. 1.7%; P = 0.01). To be fair, the control group experienced a surprisingly low mortality rate (0.8% vs. 4.6%; P = 0.02), much lower than normally observed in STEMI trials. The data safety monitoring committee of the AiMI trial felt the deaths in the thrombectomy arm were not specifically caused by the device. However, ventricular arrhythmias, hemolysis, and coronary perforation are potential complications associated with this device. This trial included a high percentage of patients without angiographically visible thrombus. The use of this device may derive greater benefit in patients with large thrombus burden.[78] Thus, the JETSTENT multicenter trial is enrolling STEMI patients with high thrombus grade to PCI with the adjunctive Angiojet thromboaspiration or PCI alone. Technical aspects related to the use of Angiojet have also been modified to take the greatest advantage of this device and to diminish procedural risk. Until these study results are available, no clearly foreseeable recommendation for its use can be given.

CONCLUSION

The majority of these devices require that each case be carefully considered, balancing risk and benefit of the chosen device. Such evaluation depends on patient demographics, clinical presentation, and coronary anatomy. The profound knowledge of the underlying coronary pathophysiology is crucial in order to determine the feasibility, safety, and benefit of using any adjunctive interventional device. At this juncture, emboli protection devices are warranted in particular cases of carotid and vein graft interventions. However, the totality of evidence does not support the routine use of manual aspiration thrombectomy in primary PCI.

REFERENCES

1. Libby P, Theroux P. Pathophysiology of coronary artery disease. *Circulation* 2005;111(25):3481–3888.
2. Kruth HS. Sequestration of aggregated low-density lipoproteins by macrophages. *Curr Opin Lipidol* 2002;13(5):483–488.
3. Kruth HS, et al. Macrophage foam cell formation with native low density lipoprotein. *J Biol Chem* 2002;277(37):34573–34580.
4. Libby P. Inflammation in atherosclerosis. *Nature* 2002;420(6917):868–874.
5. Swirski FK, et al. Ly-6Chi monocytes dominate hypercholesterolemia-associated monocytosis and give rise to macrophages in atheromata. *J Clin Invest* 2007;117(1):195–205.
6. Yano T, et al. Atherosclerotic plaques composed of a large core of foam cells covered with thin fibrous caps in twice-injured carotid arterial specimens obtained from high cholesterol diet-fed rabbits. *J Atheroscler Thromb* 2000;7(2):83–90.
7. Cybulsky MI, et al. Leukocyte recruitment to atherosclerotic lesions. *Can J Cardiol* 2004;20 Suppl B:24B–28B.
8. Yamawaki H, et al. Fluid shear stress inhibits vascular inflammation by decreasing thioredoxin-interacting protein in endothelial cells. *J Clin Invest* 2005;115(3):733–738.
9. Pasterkamp G, et al. Expansive arterial remodeling: Location, location, location. *Arterioscler Thromb Vasc Biol* 2004;24(4):650–657.
10. Krams R, et al. Shear stress in atherosclerosis, and vascular remodelling. *Semin Interv Cardiol* 1998;3(1):39–44.
11. Slager CJ, et al. The role of shear stress in the destabilization of vulnerable plaques and related therapeutic implications. *Nat Clin Pract Cardiovasc Med* 2005;2(9):456–464.
12. Alfayoumi F, et al. The no-reflow phenomenon: Epidemiology, pathophysiology, and therapeutic approach. *Rev Cardiovasc Med* 2005;6(2):72–83.
13. Nakamura M, et al. Impact of coronary artery remodeling on clinical presentation of coronary artery disease: An intravascular ultrasound study. *J Am Coll Cardiol* 2001;37(1):63–69.
14. Holmes DR, Jr., et al. Coronary angioplasty versus excisional atherectomy trial: CAVEAT. *Int J Cardiol* 1992;35(2):143–146.
15. Lefkovits J, et al. Predictors and sequelae of distal embolization during saphenous vein graft intervention from the CAVEAT-II trial. Coronary Angioplasty Versus Excisional Atherectomy Trial. *Circulation* 1995;92(4):734–740.
16. Moussa I, et al. Coronary stenting after rotational atherectomy in calcified and complex lesions. Angiographic and clinical follow-up results. *Circulation* 1997;96(1):128–136.
17. Ritchie JL, et al. Rotational approaches to atherectomy and thrombectomy. *Z Kardiol* 1987;76 Suppl 6:59–65.
18. Meany TB, et al. Coronary rotational atherectomy: Clinical application. *J Invasive Cardiol* 1991;3(1):19–24.
19. Suguta M, et al. Increase in serum troponin-I following rotational atherectomy reliably predicts the occurrence of reversible wall motion abnormalities. *Int J Cardiol* 2006;107(1):78–84.
20. Kini A, et al. Reduction in periprocedural enzyme elevation by abciximab after rotational atherectomy of type B2 lesions: Results of the Rota ReoPro randomized trial. *Am Heart J* 2001;142(6):965–969.

21. MacIsaac AI, et al. High speed rotational atherectomy: Outcome in calcified and noncalcified coronary artery lesions. *J Am Coll Cardiol* 1995;26(3):731–736.

22. Fischell TA, et al. Nicardipine and adenosine "flush cocktail" to prevent no-reflow during rotational atherectomy. *Cardiovasc Revasc Med* 2008;9(4):224–228.

23. Villanueva EV, et al. Percutaneous transluminal rotational atherectomy for coronary artery disease. *Cochrane Database Syst Rev* 2003;(4):CD003334.

24. Mota P SR, et al. Facts on rotational atherectomy for coronary artery disease: Multicentric registry (abstr). Paris, France. Paper presented at: EuroPCR; 2013 May 21.

25. Tomey MI, et al. Current status of rotational atherectomy. *JACC Cardiovasc Interv* 2014;7(4):345–353.

26. Hong MK, et al. Late stent malapposition after drug-eluting stent implantation: An intravascular ultrasound analysis with long-term follow-up. *Circulation* 2006;113(3):414–419.

27. Siqueira DA, et al. Late incomplete apposition after drug-eluting stent implantation: Incidence and potential for adverse clinical outcomes. *Eur Heart J* 2007;28(11):1304–1309.

28. Cook S, et al. Incomplete stent apposition and very late stent thrombosis after drug-eluting stent implantation. *Circulation* 2007;115(18):2426–2434.

29. Tran T, et al. An evidence-based approach to the use of rotational and directional coronary atherectomy in the era of drug-eluting stents: When does it make sense? *Catheter Cardiovasc Interv* 2008;72(5):650–662.

30. Abdel-Wahab M, et al. High-speed rotational atherectomy before paclitaxel-eluting stent implantation in complex calcified coronary lesions: The randomized ROTAXUS (Rotational Atherectomy Prior to Taxus Stent Treatment for Complex Native Coronary Artery Disease) trial. *JACC Cardiovasc Interv* 2013;6(1):10–19.

31. Abdel-Wahab M, et al. Long-term clinical outcome of rotational atherectomy followed by drug-eluting stent implantation in complex calcified coronary lesions. *Catheter Cardiovasc Interv* 2013;81(2):285–291.

32. Naito R, et al. Comparison of long-term clinical outcomes between sirolimus-eluting stents and paclitaxel-eluting stents following rotational atherectomy. *Int Heart J* 2012;53(3):149–153.

33. Benezet J, et al. Drug-eluting stents following rotational atherectomy for heavily calcified coronary lesions: Long-term clinical outcomes. *J Invasive Cardiol* 2011;23(1):28–32.

34. Rathore S, et al. Rotational atherectomy for fibro-calcific coronary artery disease in drug eluting stent era: Procedural outcomes and angiographic follow-up results. *Catheter Cardiovasc Interv* 2010;75(6):919–927.

35. Mangiacapra F, et al. Comparison of drug-eluting versus bare-metal stents after rotational atherectomy for the treatment of calcified coronary lesions. *Int J Cardiol* 2012;154(3):373–376.

36. Tamekiyo H, et al. Clinical outcomes of sirolimus-eluting stenting after rotational atherectomy. *Circ J* 2009;73(11):2042–2049.

37. Moussa I, et al. Impact of coronary culprit lesion calcium in patients undergoing paclitaxel-eluting stent implantation (a TAXUS-IV sub study). *Am J Cardiol* 2005;96(9):1242–1247.

38. Dangas GD, et al. In-stent restenosis in the drug-eluting stent era. *J Am Coll Cardiol* 2010;56(23):1897–1907.

39. Lee S, et al. Stentablation of an underexpanded stent in a heavily calcified lesion using rotational atherectomy. *J Cardiovasc Med (Hagerstown)* 2012;13(4):284–288.

40. Bhatt P, et al. Orbital atherectomy system in treating calcified coronary lesions: 3-Year follow-up in first human use study (ORBIT I trial). *Cardiovasc Revasc Med* 2014;15(4):204–208.

41. Genereux P, et al. Orbital atherectomy for treating de novo severely calcified coronary narrowing (1-year results from the pivotal ORBIT II trial). *Am J Cardiol* 2015;115(12):1685–1690.

42. Dahm JB, et al. Laser-facilitated thrombectomy: A new therapeutic option for treatment of thrombus-laden coronary lesions. *Catheter Cardiovasc Interv* 2002;56(3):365–372.

43. Barath P, et al. Cutting balloon: A novel approach to percutaneous angioplasty. *Am J Cardiol* 1991;68(11):1249–1252.

44. Liao CK, et al. Arterial response during cutting balloon angioplasty: A volumetric intravascular ultrasound study. *J Formos Med Assoc* 2002;101(11):756–761.

45. Kawaguchi K, et al. Reduction of early elastic recoil by cutting balloon angioplasty as compared to conventional balloon angioplasty. *J Invasive Cardiol* 2002;14(9):515–519.

46. Bertrand OF, et al. Management of resistant coronary lesions by the cutting balloon catheter: Initial experience. *Cathet Cardiovasc Diagn* 1997;41(2):179–184.

47. Dahm JB, et al. Cutting-balloon angioplasty effectively facilitates the interventional procedure and leads to a low rate of recurrent stenosis in ostial bifurcation coronary lesions: A subgroup analysis of the NICECUT multicenter registry. *Int J Cardiol* 2008;124(3):345–350.

48. Tian W, et al. Comparison of rotational atherectomy, plain old balloon angioplasty, and cutting-balloon angioplasty prior to drug-eluting stent implantation for the treatment of heavily calcified coronary lesions. *J Invasive Cardiol* 2015;27(9):387–391.

49. Stone GW, et al. Paclitaxel-eluting stents vs vascular brachytherapy for in-stent restenosis within bare-metal stents: The TAXUS V ISR randomized trial. *JAMA* 2006;295(11):1253–1263.

50. Holmes DR, Jr., et al. Sirolimus-eluting stents vs vascular brachytherapy for in-stent restenosis within bare-metal stents: The SISR randomized trial. *JAMA* 2006;295(11):1264–1273.

51. Schoenhagen P, et al. Coronary plaque morphology and frequency of ulceration distant from culprit lesions in patients with unstable and stable presentation. *Arterioscler Thromb Vasc Biol* 2003;23(10):1895–1900.

52. Fuster V, et al. Atherothrombosis and high-risk plaque: Part I: Evolving concepts. *J Am Coll Cardiol* 2005;46(6):937–954.

53. Virmani R, et al. Pathology of the vulnerable plaque. *J Am Coll Cardiol* 2006;47(8 Suppl):C13–C18.

54. Fukuda D, et al. Comparison of levels of serum matrix metalloproteinase-9 in patients with acute myocardial infarction versus unstable angina pectoris versus stable angina pectoris. *Am J Cardiol* 2006;97(2):175–180.

55. Henriques JP, et al. Incidence and clinical significance of distal embolization during primary angioplasty for acute myocardial infarction. *Eur Heart J* 2002;23(14):1112–1117.

56. Cura FA, et al. Protection of Distal Embolization in High-Risk Patients with Acute ST-Segment Elevation Myocardial Infarction (PREMIAR). *Am J Cardiol* 2007;99(3):357–363.

57. Stone GW, et al. Distal microcirculatory protection during percutaneous coronary intervention in acute ST-segment elevation myocardial infarction: A randomized controlled trial. *JAMA* 2005;293(9):1063–1072.

58. De Luca G, et al. Combination of electrocardiographic and angiographic markers of reperfusion in the prediction of infarct size in patients with ST-segment elevation myocardial infarction undergoing successful primary angioplasty. *Int J Cardiol* 2007;117(2):232–237.

59. Prasad A, et al. Impact of ST-segment resolution after primary angioplasty on outcomes after myocardial infarction in elderly patients: An analysis from the CADILLAC trial. *Am Heart J* 2004;147(4):669–675.

60. Ito H, et al. Clinical implications of the "no reflow" phenomenon. A predictor of complications and left ventricular remodeling in reperfused anterior wall myocardial infarction. *Circulation* 1996;93(2):223–228.

61. Cremonesi A. The SPIDER embolic protection device performance evaluation in the carotid artery during percutaneous transluminal angioplasty and or stenting. *J Invasive Cardiol* 2005;17(9):463–467.

62. Zahn R, et al. Embolic protection devices for carotid artery stenting: Is there a difference between filter and distal occlusive devices? *J Am Coll Cardiol* 2005;45(11):1769–1774.

63. von Korn H, et al. Safety and efficacy of a new filter-based protection system for aorto-coronary bypass graft interventions: The ev3 Spider device. *J Invasive Cardiol* 2005;17(7):352–355.

64. Stone GW, et al. Distal filter protection during saphenous vein graft stenting: Technical and clinical correlates of efficacy. *J Am Coll Cardiol* 2002;40(1):1882–1888.

65. Limbruno U, et al. Thrombectomy for thrombus removal, filters for whatever else. *J Cardiovasc Med (Hagerstown)* 2008;9(4):408–409.

66. Guetta V, et al. Safety and efficacy of the FilterWire EZ in acute ST-segment elevation myocardial infarction. *Am J Cardiol* 2007;99(7):911–915.

67. Kaluski E, et al. Coronary stenting with MGuard: First-in-man trial. *J Invasive Cardiol* 2008;20(10):511–515.

68. Gracida M, et al. The MGuard coronary stent: Safety, efficacy, and clinical utility. *Vasc Health Risk Manag* 2015;11:533–539.

69. Costa RA, et al. Impact of thrombus burden on outcomes after standard versus mesh-covered stents in acute myocardial infarction (from the MGuard for acute ST elevation reperfusion trial). *Am J Cardiol* 2015;115(2):161–166.

70. Dudek D, et al. Efficacy of an embolic protection stent as a function of delay to reperfusion in ST-segment elevation myocardial infarction (from the MASTER Trial). *Am J Cardiol* 2014;114(1):1485–1489.

71. Dudek D, et al. Mesh-covered embolic protection stent implantation in ST-segment-elevation myocardial infarction: Final 1-year clinical and angiographic results from the MGUARD for acute ST elevation reperfusion trial. *Circ Cardiovasc Interv* 2015;8(2):e001484.

72. Stone GW. *The MASTER II trial. Comparison of the MGuard embolic protection stent with standard stent in acute myocardial infarction.* The International Conference for Innovations Meeting. Tel Aviv, Israel; 2014.

73. Lung HL, et al. Allergic contact dermatitis to polyethylene terephthalate mesh. *J Investig Allergol Clin Immunol* 2009;19(2):161–162.

74. Stone GW, et al. Prospective, randomized, multicenter evaluation of a polyethylene terephthalate micronet mesh-covered stent (MGuard) in ST-segment elevation myocardial infarction: The MASTER Trial. *J Am Coll Cardiol* 2012;60(19):1975–1984.

75. Stone GW, et al. Randomized comparison of distal protection with a filter-based catheter and a balloon occlusion and aspiration system during percutaneous intervention of diseased saphenous vein aorto-coronary bypass grafts. *Circulation* 2003;108(5):548–553.

76. Koch KT, et al. Proximal embolic protection with aspiration in percutaneous coronary intervention using the Proxis device. *Rev Cardiovasc Med* 2007;8(3):160–166.

77. Sianos G, et al. Angiographic stent thrombosis after routine use of drug-eluting stents in ST-segment elevation myocardial infarction: The importance of thrombus burden. *J Am Coll Cardiol* 2007;50(7):573–583.

78. Sianos G, et al. Rheolytic thrombectomy in patients with ST-elevation myocardial infarction and large thrombus burden: The Thoraxcenter experience. *J Invasive Cardiol* 2006;18 Suppl C:3C–7C.

79. Svilaas T, et al. Thrombus aspiration during percutaneous coronary intervention in Acute myocardial infarction Study (TAPAS)—study design. *Am Heart J* 2006;151(3):597. e1–e7.

80. Vlaar PJ, et al. Cardiac death and reinfarction after 1 year in the thrombus aspiration during percutaneous coronary intervention in acute myocardial infarction Study (TAPAS): A 1-year follow-up study. *Lancet* 2008;371(9628):1915–1920.

81. De Luca G, et al. Adjunctive manual thrombectomy improves myocardial perfusion and mortality in patients undergoing primary percutaneous coronary intervention for ST-elevation myocardial infarction: A meta-analysis of randomized trials. *Eur Heart J* 2008;29(24):3002–3010.

82. Jolly SS, et al. Outcomes after thrombus aspiration for ST elevation myocardial infarction: 1-year follow-up of the prospective randomised TOTAL trial. *Lancet* 2016;387(10014):127–135.

83. Stone GW, et al. Intracoronary abciximab and aspiration thrombectomy in patients with large anterior myocardial infarction: The INFUSE-AMI randomized trial. *JAMA* 2012;307(17):1817–1826.

84. Frobert O, et al. Thrombus aspiration in ST-elevation myocardial infarction in Scandinavia (TASTE trial). A multicenter, prospective, randomized, controlled clinical registry trial based on the Swedish angiography and angioplasty registry (SCAAR) platform. Study design and rationale. *Am Heart J* 2010;160(6):1042–1048.

85. Frobert O, et al. ST-elevation myocardial infarction, thrombus aspiration, and different invasive strategies. A TASTE trial substudy. *J Am Heart Assoc* 2015;4(6):e001755.

86. Antoniucci D. Rheolytic thrombectmy in acute myocardial infarction: The Florence experience and objectives of the multicenter randomized JETSTENT trial. *J Invasive Cardiol* 2006;18 Suppl C:32C–34C.

87. Ali A, et al. Rheolytic thrombectomy with percutaneous coronary intervention for infarct size reduction in acute myocardial infarction: 30-day results from a multicenter randomized study. *J Am Coll Cardiol* 2006;48(2):244–252.

38

Complications of PCI: Stent loss, coronary perforation, and aortic dissection

AMIR-ALI FASSA AND MARCO ROFFI

Various complications may occur during percutaneous coronary interventions (PCIs) (Table 38.1). These may be related to the devices used during the procedure (e.g., coronary perforation, stent loss, or thrombosis) or to the intervention itself (e.g., abrupt vessel closure, distal embolization, or side-branch occlusion). The vascular system may also be affected in cases of aortic dissection, peripheral vascular complications, or atheroembolic events. In addition, access site complications may occur. Finally, PCIs may be complicated by systemic events in relation to adjunctive therapies and other aspects of the procedure (e.g., contrast nephropathy, non-access-site-related bleeding events, or allergic reactions). These complications may result in adverse events, such as myocardial infarction (MI), renal failure, stroke, bleeding, or death.

Despite the increasing procedural complexity and higher-risk profile of patients treated with PCI over the years, there has been a marked reduction of related in-hospital MI and mortality rates, as well as for the need of emergency coronary artery bypass graft (CABG) surgery.[1,2] This trend is likely the result of technological and pharmacological advancements, as well as of the increasing experience of operators in the management of high-risk situations and prevention and treatment of procedural complications.

The present chapter focuses on three major complications of PCI, including stent loss, coronary perforations, and aortic dissection. Access site complications are described in Chapter 8.

STENT LOSS

Introduction

Stents are currently used in 93%–96% of PCIs.[3,4] Failure to deliver a stent to the target site occurs in 3.9%–8.3% of the procedures, mostly due to excessive tortuosity, and/or calcification of the target lesion and/or of the proximal vessel segments.[5-7] As a consequence, the undeployed stent needs to be retrieved from the guiding catheter. This may lead to stent dislodgement from the delivery balloon catheter and subsequent stent embolization/loss. According to early studies, stent loss occurred in 0.9%–3.4% of the procedures, but the incidence has decreased to 0.2%–0.5% in the most recent studies.[6-18] This progress is likely due, in part, to the fact that manually crimped stents are no longer on the market; further factors may include the major improvements in stent profile, flexibility, and stent adhesion to the balloon catheter; finally, operators have gained experience with stent utilization.[11] Importantly, this favorable trend has been observed despite the increasing complexity of coronary lesions treated by endovascular means.[1,2]

Factors associated with stent loss include vessel anatomy, operator technique, and equipment characteristics. The most common situation associated with stent loss is the retraction of an undeployed stent into the guiding catheter without having a coaxial alignment between the guiding catheter and the stent. Most of the time, the need for stent retrieval follows an attempt to cross a calcified

Table 38.1 Complications of percutaneous coronary intervention

Coronary Complications
    Coronary perforation
    Stent loss
    Coronary dissection
    Abrupt vessel closure
    Distal embolization
    Side branch occlusion
    Stent thrombosis
Vascular Complications
    Access site
        Bleeding
        Pseudoaneurysm
        Arteriovenous fistula
        Arterial thrombosis
        Venous thrombosis
        Infection
    Retroperitoneal hematoma
    Dissection or perforation of peripheral vessels
    Iatrogenic aortic dissection
    Atheroembolism
Other
    Contrast nephropathy
    Gastrointestinal bleeding
    Radiation exposure
    Allergic reactions
    Ventricular arrhythmia, conduction disturbances

Table 38.2 Conditions associated with coronary stent loss

Moderate to severe vessel calcification
Proximal tortuosity/angulation
Incomplete lesion preparation
Insufficient guiding catheter and/or guidewire support
Advancing or retrieving a stent through a previously placed stent
Retraction of undeployed stent into small-French guiding catheter
Guiding catheter not co-axial with wire during retrieval
Use of longer stents
Use of manually crimped stents

and/or tortuous lesion that has not been sufficiently prepared with balloon predilatation or rotational atherectomy. Other mechanisms and factors associated with stent loss are listed in Table 38.2. Key points in preventing stent loss include adequate lesion preparation, sufficient guiding catheter and guidewire support, verification of proper alignment between the guiding catheter and the ostial portion of the vessel while retrieving an undelivered stent, use of short and low-profile stents, and stenting of distal segments first, if multiple stents are required. Facilitation of stent delivery

with the use of guiding catheter extensions, such as the Guideliner (Vascular Solutions, Inc., Minneapolis, MN) or the Heartrail (Terumo Corp., Tokyo, Japan), is particularly indicated for avoidance of this complication during complex procedures.[19] Importantly, once a stent is retrieved, it should be carefully checked for integrity (i.e., no protruding stent struts) before further attempting to place the stent.

Outcomes

Stent loss is associated with a high rate of adverse events. In a meta-analysis of 919 procedures by Alomar et al., stent loss was associated with a mortality of 4% and a major adverse event rate of 19% (which included death, nonfatal MI, CABG, bleeding requiring transfusion, vascular access complications, and cerebrovascular accident).[18] The rate of adverse events depends on the location of the embolized stent and on the management of the complication. In a series of 387 procedures complicated by stent loss (from a total of 25,558 procedures), Bolte et al. showed that the major in-hospital adverse events rate was as high as 89% among patients with an undeployed stent left in the coronary tree ($n = 47$).[8] Conversely, less unfavorable outcomes were observed with successful stent retrieval ($n = 111$, adverse event rate of 9%), peripheral stent embolization ($n = 157$, event rate of 15%), and successful intracoronary exclusion (crushing) or deployment of the lost stent ($n = 72$, event rate of 31%). In a series of 20 patients by Eggbrecht et al., three patients died following urgent CABG after stent embolization.[10] Similarly, Brilakis et al. reported increased rates of hospital mortality (3%) and emergency CABG (5%) following stent embolization.[11]

These outcomes may or may not be directly related to stent embolization. For instance, maneuvers to retrieve a lost stent may result in coronary or peripheral artery injury. Likewise, an undeployed stent left in the coronary tree may also result in vessel thrombosis and MI. Moreover, if stenting is applied to treat a dissection, failure to deliver the stent at the target lesion may lead to abrupt vessel closure. Finally, stent loss likely identifies a population of patients with complex coronary anatomy and advanced disease who are at increased risk of adverse clinical events in addition to any consequence of the stent loss. As a general rule, peripheral stent embolization is associated with a more favorable clinical course than stent embolization in the coronary tree, the former rarely resulting in limb ischemia or stroke.[9–11] On the basis of the potentially catastrophic complications of stent embolization, appropriate management is of paramount importance.

Management

Percutaneous treatments of lost coronary stents include retrieval, exclusion from circulation (crushing), or deployment at the embolization site. To that purpose, several tools and techniques have been described, such as the use of small-diameter balloon catheters, guidewires, vascular loop snares, vascular baskets, vascular forceps/bioptomes, and dedicated fragment retrieval devices. In a meta-analysis by Alomar et al., of 1,048 lost stents, 66% could be retrieved from the coronary circulation, of which 55% could be removed from the body, and 45% were embolized into the peripheral circulation.[18]

SMALL-DIAMETER BALLOON CATHETER TECHNIQUE

The use of a small-diameter balloon catheter is probably the simplest way to attempt stent retrieval. This technique may be used if the stent gets stripped off the balloon, as long as the stent remains on the guidewire. A small-caliber balloon catheter (typically with a diameter of 1–1.5 mm) is passed through the undeployed stent and is inflated distally. Subsequently, the balloon catheter, the guidewire, the guiding catheter, and the stent are all removed as a unit (Figures 38.1 and 38.2).[11] To prevent possible embolization to the cerebral circulation, the whole system should always be pulled down into the descending aorta (in case of femoral access) or the axillary artery (in case of radial approach) before attempting to pull the stent-loaded balloon catheter into the guiding catheter.[9] Alternatively, some authors have also described use of small-diameter balloon catheters to attempt the advancement of the stent and the deployment at the target lesion site.[10]

DOUBLE-WIRE TECHNIQUE

The double-wire method is also a relatively straightforward technique that can be used if the stent remains on the guidewire. A second guidewire is advanced distal to the stent, following which the two guidewires are twisted to intermingle their distal ends, therefore allowing entrapment of the stent, which can then be retrieved by pulling both wires back to the tip of the guide catheter.

LOOP SNARE

If the stent is not on the guidewire, a loop snare can be used to retrieve the stent. Loop snares are commercially available (e.g., Microvena Amplatz Goose Neck Snare, Microvena Corp., Plymouth, MN) or can be prepared *de novo* in the catheterization laboratory using an exchange-length 0.014-in guidewire and a diagnostic multipurpose catheter.

SPECIFIC VASCULAR RETRIEVAL DEVICES

The biliary or vascular forceps consists of a curved, finger-like projection that can be expanded/extended or contracted/retracted, allowing for the entrapment of lost stents. The Cook retained fragment retriever (Cook Medical, Bloomington, IN) has an articulating arm operable from the proximal hub, which allows for grasping and retrieving fragments. The basket retrieval device (Cook Medical) consists of several helically arranged loops that can be expanded or collapsed, allowing entrapment of the embolized stent, in particular, if it has been deformed. These devices may not be available in all cardiac catheterization laboratories, and usage should be limited to experienced operators who are

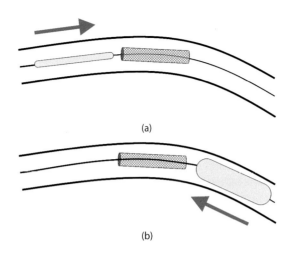

Figure 38.1 Small-diameter balloon catheter technique for lost stent retrieval. A small-diameter balloon catheter is advanced on the guidewire toward the lost stent **(a)**. The catheter is advanced beyond the stent and inflated. Then, the balloon catheter is pulled back, allowing retrieval of the lost stent **(b)**.

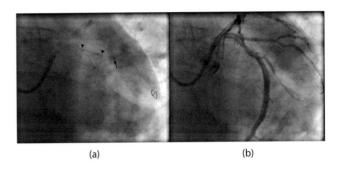

(a)   (b)

Figure 38.2 A stent was lost in the first obtuse marginal branch of the circumflex artery (*arrowheads*, a, left anterior oblique-caudal view). A small balloon catheter was advanced through the stent (*arrow*, **a**), allowing successful retrieval of the lost stent in the absence of complications, as documented in the final angiogram (**b**, left anterior oblique-caudal view).

familiar with them. Importantly, because of their size, these devices cannot be used in the coronary vasculature but are typically used to treat stents embolized into large vessels, such as the aorta, the iliac, and the femoral arteries.[11]

The appropriate strategy for managing stent loss depends on whether the stent has embolized in a coronary artery or into the peripheral circulation, and whether the stent is still on the guidewire (Figure 38.3). If the stent has stripped off the delivery balloon catheter in the coronary artery but remains on the guidewire, recovery with a small-profile balloon catheter or the double-wire technique should be attempted. Use of a loop snare should be considered if the stent is no longer on the guidewire. Alternative options include deployment of the stent at the embolization site (using initially a small-caliber balloon and then increasing the balloon size) or exclusion from the coronary circulation by crushing the undeployed stent with an additional one. However, the two latter strategies should be avoided if the stent is located in the left main trunk or at other critical locations.[11] In fact, both an undersized stent and an undeployed stent crushed against the vessel wall put the patient at risk of subacute or late stent thrombosis. If none of these retrieval or exclusion options is possible, efforts should be made to move the stent into the aortic root, as peripheral embolization usually has a more benign prognosis than coronary embolization.[8] Management options of peripheral stent embolization include retrieval with the small-diameter balloon catheter or double-wire techniques or using the dedicated tools mentioned above (i.e., snare, basket, forceps, or Cook retrieval set) (Figure 38.4). While deployment of a coronary stent at a peripheral arterial site is rarely possible due to the mismatch between the stent and the vessel size, crushing the embolized device with a peripheral stent is an option. Because of the larger vessel size, this maneuver is far less likely to be associated with vessel thrombosis than in the coronary tree. Overall, leaving an undeployed stent in the peripheral circulation should be considered, as the technical difficulties and risk related to retrieval maneuvers may outweigh the risk of local complications related to the embolized device (Figure 38.5).[11] In addition, the location

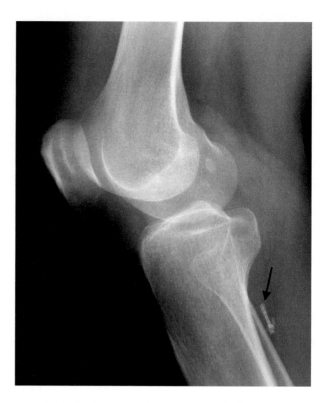

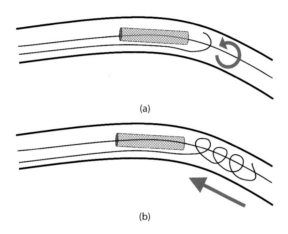

Figure 38.3 Double-wire technique for lost stent retrieval: A second guidewire is advanced distal to the lost stent **(a)**. The two guidewires are twisted to intermingle their distal ends, allowing entrapment of the stent, which can then be retrieved by pulling both wires **(b)**.

Figure 38.5 Radiograph showing an embolized stent in infrapopliteal circulation (*arrow*). No retrieval maneuver was attempted following stent embolization. The patient remained asymptomatic during follow-up.

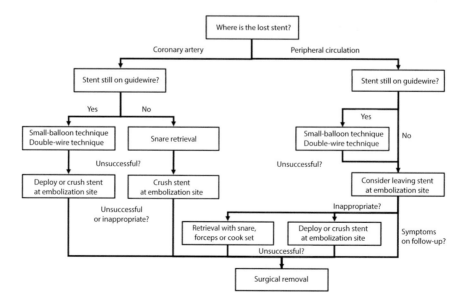

Figure 38.4 Suggested algorithm for management of stent loss.

of the stent embolized in the peripheral circulation often remains unknown.

If percutaneous efforts to treat the lost stent in the coronary tree fail, surgical retrieval should be considered—along with CABG if the target lesion is left untreated—because of the intrinsic risk of vessel thrombosis. Conversely, surgical retrieval of a stent that has embolized in the peripheral circulation should be performed only in the presence of symptoms resulting from device embolization.

Conclusion

Stent loss is a rare complication of PCI, which is associated with a high rate of adverse outcomes if the stent is lost in the coronary tree. Stent embolization may be prevented by proper patient selection, equipment, and technique. Percutaneous treatment of an embolized or undeployed stent, including retrieval, deployment at embolization site, and exclusion are effective. Operators should be familiar with these techniques to properly manage this potentially serious complication. In case of failure to retrieve or exclude undeployed stents in the coronary vasculature, cardiac surgery should be considered. Stent embolization into the peripheral vasculature has a more benign prognosis and usually does not require treatment.

CORONARY PERFORATIONS

Introduction

Coronary perforation is a rare but potentially life-threatening complication that occurs in 0.2%–0.9% of PCIs.[20–40] With atheroablative techniques such as directional or rotational atherectomy and excimer laser angioplasty, the risk is somewhat higher (0.3%–3.3%).[23–25,41–43] The overall incidence of coronary perforation during PCI has remained unchanged over the last 20 years. This is likely explained by a balance between the expected decrease due to improvements in equipment and technique—such as the more selective use of atheroablative techniques and the abandonment of high-pressure angioplasty with oversized or compliant balloon catheters—and the likely increase due to the greater number of high-risk interventions (e.g., chronic total occlusions) and the use of stiff and hydrophilic guidewires.[24,25,44]

The diagnosis of coronary perforation is usually made immediately by visualization of contrast extravasation on coronary angiogram.[44,45] However, in case of wire perforation, the diagnosis may be missed initially and made only later in the presence of hemodynamic compromise and pericardial effusion on echocardiography.[20,21] Patients with frank perforation may complain of severe chest pain, dizziness, nausea, and vomiting—out of proportion to what is typically observed during balloon inflation. Heart rate usually increases and blood pressure falls, with a rise in central venous pressure when tamponade develops. At times, vagal-mediated bradycardia may occur. ST-segment elevation or

Table 38.3 Classification of coronary perforations

Type I	Extraluminal crater without contrast extravasation
Type II	Pericardial or myocardial blush without contrast jet extravasation
Type III	Extravasation through frank (≥1 mm) perforation
Cavity spilling	Perforation into an anatomic cavity (i.e., ventricle, coronary sinus)

Source: From Ellis, S.G., et al., *Circulation*, 90(6), 2725–2730, 1994. With permission.

depression may ensue due to vessel occlusion at the level of the perforation or distally.[44]

Ellis et al. proposed a classification of coronary perforation based on angiographic appearance (Table 38.3).[20] Type I perforations are characterized by a focal extraluminal crater limited to the media or adventitia in the absence of contrast extravasation; these cannot be differentiated angiographically from the previously described National Heart, Lung, and Blood Institute (NHLBI) type C dissection, suggesting a continuum between dissection and perforation.[46,47] Type II perforations include pericardial or myocardial blush without contrast jet extravasation (Figure 38.6), while type III perforations involve persistent extravasation with streaming or a jet of contrast through a frank (≥1 mm) perforation (Figure 38.7). If the jet is directed into an anatomic cavity (e.g., ventricle or coronary sinus), the perforation is classified as cavity spilling (CS), type IV, or alternatively, type IIIB, as opposed to type IIIA where the jet is directed toward the pericardium. The most frequent type of perforation is type II (37%–61%), while type I and III occur less often (18%–44% and 19%–36%, respectively), and type CS is rarely encountered (2%–5%).[24,27,31] Most type I and II perforations are caused by guidewires, while type III are more frequently associated with the use of stents or atheroablative techniques.[22,24,30] Muller et al. proposed a modification of the Ellis classification, adding a type V perforation to describe distal coronary perforations by guidewires.[48]

Based on a series of 1,762 coronary perforations recorded from 527,121 PCI procedures in the British Cardiovascular Intervention Society database, Kinnaird et al. determined the predictive factors of coronary perforation by multivariate analysis. These included age, female gender, history of CABG, left main or chronic total occlusion interventions, and use of rotational atherectomy.[40] In other smaller series, congestive heart failure, heavy calcification, extreme vessel tortuosity, small vessel diameter, balloon catheter or stent oversizing, and the use of intravascular ultrasound (IVUS)–guided lumen optimization have also been associated with an increased incidence of coronary perforation[22,24,25,49] (Table 38.4). The latter is probably explained by the more frequent use of IVUS during the treatment of complex lesions or procedures with unexpanded stents in resistant lesions.[36,45] Moreover, although distal perforation caused by guidewires has been largely reported as a common

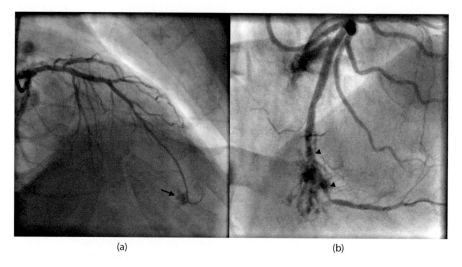

Figure 38.6 **(a)** Left anterior oblique view of a distal type II perforation of the left anterior descending coronary artery induced by a hydrophilic guidewire with pericardial extravasation (*arrow*). **(b)** Right anterior oblique cranial view of a type II perforation in the left circumflex coronary artery with myocardial staining following implantation of an oversized stent (*arrowheads*).

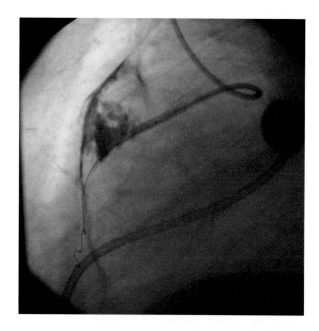

Figure 38.7 Left lateral view of a type III perforation of the mid-left anterior descending artery following post-dilatation of an implanted stent with direct staining of the pericardial space.

cause, the data on whether the incidence of this complication is specifically increased with the use of hydrophilic or stiff guidewires remain conflicting.[20–34,36,50,51] In addition, a large registry based on cutting balloon angioplasty has shown that the use of this device was associated with a higher risk of coronary perforation than plain balloon angioplasty or stenting.[52] However, results from the more recent and larger British Cardiovascular Intervention Society registry suggested that the use of cutting balloons was associated with a reduced occurrence of perforations.[40]

Following the widespread use of glycoprotein (GP) IIb/IIIa inhibitors, concern of a potential increase in the occurrence of coronary perforation during administration of these potent drugs was raised. Nevertheless, several series have shown that GP IIb/IIIa inhibitors are not associated with a higher incidence of coronary perforations. Yet, coronary perforations occurring in patients under GP IIb/IIIa inhibitors are associated with a higher rate of adverse events, suggesting that these antiplatelet drugs may increase the harmful consequences but not necessarily the occurrence of coronary perforation. In this respect, the association of GP IIb/IIIa inhibitors and hydrophilic wires appears somewhat risky.[21,22,24,27,40]

Table 38.4 Predictive factors of coronary perforations

Clinical	Anatomical	Procedural
Female gender	Complex lesions[a]	Atheroablative techniques
Chronic renal failure	Chronic total occlusion	Use of intravascular ultrasound
Prior CABG	Heavy calcification	Balloon catheter or stent oversizing
Elderly	Extreme tortuosity	Stiff or hydrophilic guidewires
Congestive heart failure	Small vessel diameter	
Unstable angina/NSTEMI	Graft anastomosis	

Source: From Marco Roffi and Amir Fassa.
Note: CABG, coronary artery bypass surgery; NSTEMI, non-ST segment elevation myocardial infarction.
[a] ACC/AHA type B2/C.

The mainstay of perforation prevention is the cautious use of atheroablative techniques and of hydrophilic guidewires in complex anatomy, especially if there is concomitant administration of potent antithrombotic therapy. Of paramount importance is the stable position of the guidewire (especially if it is hydrophilic) during advancement and retrieval of balloon catheters or stents, as distal perforation is frequently the result of an unnoticed distal wire movement. Finally, provided that the anatomy is suitable, debulking with rotational atherectomy should be favored for preparation of severely calcified lesions resistant to conventional angioplasty over the use of oversized balloons inflated at high pressures.

Outcomes

Coronary perforation is clearly associated with an increased rate of in-hospital and long-term adverse events, which include MI, bleeding, stroke, emergency CABG, and death.[25,33,40] In the British Cardiovascular Intervention Society registry, coronary perforation was associated with a 4-fold increase of in-hospital stroke, a 20-fold increase of in-hospital bleeding, and a 5-fold increase of 30-day mortality.[40] These adverse events are mostly the consequence of hemodynamic compromise, resulting from pericardial effusion and tamponade, or of ischemia due to failure to treat the target lesion or vessel occlusion. According to the literature, tamponade may complicate 12%–55% of coronary perforations.[24,26] However, the true incidence is likely lower because of underreporting of "benign" perforations. Tamponade usually appears immediately after coronary perforation, although a late occurrence has been reported in 21%–52% of patients, appearing as late as 3 days after PCI.[21,26,50,53–55] Tamponade rarely develops in patients with prior CABG due to obliteration of the pericardial space by adhesions between the epicardium and pericardium, as well as the persistence of partial pericardiotomy following surgery.[56]

Emergency surgery, usually consisting of pericardial drainage with or without CABG or repair or ligation of the perforated artery, was reported in ~20%–40% of perforations in earlier studies.[20,42] More recent reports show a much lower frequency (2%–3%).[32,40] This reduction is likely related to improved early detection of coronary perforations, a decreased use of atheroablative devices, a higher proportion of guidewire-induced distal coronary perforations that can be managed conservatively or percutaneously, the availability of covered stents and coils, and the increasing experience of operators.[44]

MI, which can be due to vessel occlusion, either as a direct consequence or as an intended treatment of coronary perforation, may occur in 5%–37% of cases.[27,28]

The mortality rate associated with coronary perforations ranges from 0 to 17% (11% at 30 days in the British Cardiovascular Intervention Society registry).[26,30,40] Predictors of mortality include age, diabetes, prior myocardial MI, renal disease, requirement for ventilator and/

or circulatory support, GP IIb/IIIa inhibitor use, and coronary flow other than TIMI 3 at the end of the procedure.[40] Furthermore, type III perforations are clearly associated with far worse outcomes than types I, II, and CS (mortality of 19%–22% for type III and <6% for types I, II, and CS).[24,29]

Fasseas et al. reported that patients receiving GP IIb/IIIa inhibitors at the time of coronary perforation more frequently required the placement of a covered stent or emergency surgery in comparison to patients not treated with these agents.[24] A retrospective analysis has shown that guidewire-induced coronary perforation was associated with a significantly lower incidence of major adverse cardiac events when bivalirudin was used as an adjunctive therapy compared with unfractionated heparin.[32] In addition, a pooled analysis from three randomized controlled trials showed that outcomes following coronary perforation with bivalirudin as an adjunctive therapy were not inferior in comparison with unfractionated heparin (UFH).[33] These results suggest that bivalirudin may be as safe as UFH in the presence of a coronary perforation. This is possibly explained by the short half-life of the drug, although in the presence of frank perforation, the antithrombotic effect of bivalirudin cannot be immediately reversed, while in patients treated with UFH, protamine can be administered. However, as described below, the value of reversing anticoagulation with protamine remains controversial.

Subepicardial (or intramyocardial) hematoma has been reported as an extremely rare consequence of coronary perforation but is likely underreported as the diagnosis can hardly be made by angiography. This dreadful complication is characterized by a bleed that can progress in a relentless fashion, dissecting the epicardium and the epicardial vessels from the underlying myocardium and avulsing perforator vessels, which in turn bleed further, establishing a self-propagating process that may continue even though the initial perforation site may have been successfully sealed.[57–60] It is believed that subepicardial hematoma is more frequent in patients with prior CABG because of adhesions between the epicardium and the pericardium that can prevent blood from accumulating in the pericardial space. However, cases of subepicardial hematoma in patients without prior CABG have also been reported. Finally, it is worth mentioning that bypass graft perforation may result in tamponade, mediastinal hemorrhage, hemoptysis, and subepicardial hematoma.[27,56,58,59,61]

Management

The first step in the treatment of coronary perforation is prompt detection and classification of the type of perforation, as this will dictate the immediate management strategy (Figure 38.8).[20] Type I perforations can generally be managed either conservatively or by the implantation of a conventional stent, based on the size and prognostic importance of the vessel.[44,46] Similarly, type CS perforations may also be treated conservatively, with the vascular communication often closing spontaneously later on. Type

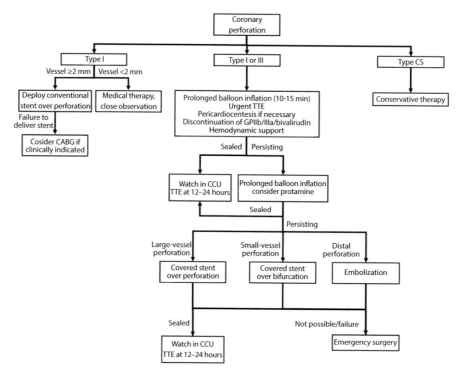

Figure 38.8 Suggested algorithm for management of coronary perforation. CABG, coronary artery bypass grafting; CCU, coronary care unit; CS, cavity spilling; TTE, transthoracic echocardiogram.

II perforation management depends on the extent of the extravasation, as limited pericardial and myocardial staining can usually be observed and treated conservatively with the discontinuation of anticoagulants and/or GP IIb/IIIa inhibitors. Larger type II perforations should be treated aggressively, with prolonged balloon inflation, reversal of anticoagulation and platelet transfusion if indicated, and echocardiographic assessment of pericardial effusion. Finally, type III perforations require immediate action with prolonged balloon inflation, discontinuation and reversal of antiplatelet and antithrombotic therapy (if possible), hemodynamic supportive therapy, echocardiographic assessment of pericardial effusion and, if needed, pericardiocentesis, and percutaneous (e.g., placement of a covered stent) or surgical treatment of perforation. In this respect, the balance between the ongoing ischemia (caused by the management of the perforation) and the hemodynamic instability (caused by the perforation or by the ongoing ischemia) is key.[62] Following successful treatment of coronary perforation, surveillance in a coronary care unit for at least 24 hours is indicated, as delayed tamponade may occur.

PROLONGED BALLOON INFLATION

In large type II and all type III perforations, the first maneuver, even before starting cardiopulmonary resuscitation, pericardiocentesis, or reversal of anticoagulation, should be the placement of a balloon catheter (with balloon-to-artery diameter ratio of 0.9–1) at the site of perforation or upstream in case of distal perforation, inflated at a low pressure (2–6 atm). Serial angiographic assessments of the perforation should be performed after one or more 10–15 minute inflation periods. In the case of incomplete perforation sealing, the use of a perfusion balloon has been suggested to reduce myocardial ischemia and the risk of proximal thrombosis, but the availability of these devices in catheterization laboratories has markedly decreased.[22,45,48,63]

CESSATION AND REVERSAL OF ADJUNCTIVE THERAPY

If the patient is receiving GP IIb/IIIa inhibitors or bivalirudin, the drugs should be immediately discontinued in type II and III perforations.

In large, persisting perforations despite prolonged balloon inflation and/or sealing attempt, reversal of UFH with protamine sulfate should be considered. However, due to the possibly increased risk of thrombosis, heparin reversal should be performed cautiously in the setting of ongoing prolonged balloon inflation or implantation of a conventional or covered stent during the procedure, and partial reversal can be performed (i.e., half protamine dosage). Reversal of anticoagulation cannot be quickly achieved in patients receiving low-molecular-weight heparin (LMWH), fondaparinux, or bivalirudin, though protamine does partially reverse the effect of LMWH.

If the patient was receiving abciximab, the platelet inhibitory function of this potent drug can be reversed by platelet transfusions, as abciximab binds platelets with high affinity and has low, free plasma levels. Conversely, small molecules like tirofiban and eptifibatide maintain high plasma concentration, and their antiplatelet properties therefore remain unaffected by platelet transfusions. However, in the presence of normal renal function, small molecules are cleared from plasma within a few hours.

HEMODYNAMIC SUPPORT THERAPY

Intravenous fluids should be administered immediately. Vasopressor and inotropic therapy, as well as cardiopulmonary resuscitation, may become rapidly necessary following coronary perforation.[22] Placement of percutaneous ventricular assist devices or extracorporeal membrane oxygenation may also be required in the presence of depressed left ventricular function or large-territory ongoing ischemia.[64]

PERICARDIOCENTESIS

The details of pericardiocentesis are described in Chapter 14. If a sizable coronary perforation is observed, an echocardiogram should be performed emergently to assess the presence of pericardial effusion. In case of tamponade, pericardiocentesis is a life-saving maneuver.[65] If there is an ongoing hemodynamically significant effusion despite implementation of adequate measures (such as prolonged balloon-inflation and perforation sealing), direct autotransfusion of the blood recovered from the pericardium to the femoral vein can be performed.[66] However, due to the risk of thrombosis or disseminated intravascular coagulopathy, the use of a cell-salvage system may be preferable in this setting.[67]

Following pericardiocentesis, the catheter should be maintained until the next day. In the absence of recurrent effusion on the echocardiogram, the catheter can then be removed. Observation for an additional day in a regular unit with a subsequent echocardiogram is warranted before discharge.[22]

PERFORATION SEALING

Coronary perforations with persistent extravasation despite prolonged balloon inflation can successfully be treated with implantation of a covered stent.[68-75] Two devices have been approved by the U.S. Food and Drug Administration (FDA).

The Graftmaster RX device (Abbott Vascular Devices, Abbott Park, IL) consists of an ultrathin, biocompatible, and expandable polytetrafluoroethylene layer sandwiched between two coaxial balloon-expandable stents. A major limitation of this device is its high profile and low flexibility that may prevent delivery in small, calcified or tortuous vessels (which are typical anatomical characteristics of arteries at risk for perforation).[75] Reported successful deployment rates range from 81% to 96%.[71,73] The Aneugraft (previously known as the Over and Under) device (ITGI Medical, Or Akiva, Israel) is a highly flexible, laser-cut stent covered by a single layer of equine pericardium. Its low profile appears to result in better deliverability than the Graftmaster.[72,74,75]

The Papyrus PK (Biotronik, Berlin, Germany) device received the CE mark at the end of 2013, though has not been approved by the FDA. It consists of a 90 μm thick polyurethane membrane electrospinned around a single metallic stent with thin struts (60–120 μm). It also achieves greater flexibility and a smaller crossing profile in comparison to the Graftmaster.[76,77] Occasional use of autologous venous-covered stents has been described. The preparation is cumbersome and unsuitable for emergency situations, although time intervals from vein harvest to stent deployment of 20–45 minutes have been reported.[78,79]

Complete sealing rates of coronary perforation after successful deployment of one or several covered stents vary from 85% to 100%.[36,68-72] Moreover, the use of covered stents appears to have reduced the need for emergency surgery.[70] Covered stents should be placed either at the level of the perforation or at a bifurcation upstream from the perforation site to seal the vessel. In order to reduce the delay between the deflation of the balloon sealing the perforation and the implantation of the covered stent, the use of a second guiding catheter using an additional arterial access to deliver the covered stent may be useful.[80] Furthermore, delivery of a covered stent may be facilitated with the use of guiding catheter extensions, such as the Guideliner or the Heartrail.[19,81,82] Importantly, implantation of a covered stent to exclude a branch with a perforation should be considered only if the branch is minor and not collateralized, otherwise bleeding would persist.

Dual antiplatelet therapy (DAPT) with aspirin and clopidogrel should also be continued at least 6 months following covered stent implantation because of delayed endothelialization and the increased risk of stent thrombosis. Indeed, the reported risk of stent thrombosis varies from 0 to 33% at 3–6 months, with the lowest rates reported in series using IVUS-guided deployment and prolonged DAPT (3–6 months).[71-73,75] The off-label use of more potent P2Y$_{12}$ inhibitors (i.e., prasugrel or ticagrelor) and/or extension of the dual antiplatelet treatment to 12 months should be considered.[72] Furthermore, reported rates of in-stent restenosis for covered stents range from 7% to 50% at 3–6 months.[71-73,75] If the patient survives coronary perforation treated by covered stents, the short-term outcomes are quite favorable, with mortality rate of 0–6% at 3–6 months.[71,75]

In case of guidewire-induced distal coronary perforation or perforation of a branch that can be "sacrificed," coil embolization has proved to be effective (Figure 38.9).[51,83,84] Coils are made of steel or platinum. Use of detachable coils, which allow for confirmation of the position before release and retrieval, is preferable over pushable coils, which cannot be retrieved. Most coils (such as the Azur Hydrocoil, Terumo Corp) must be delivered through a large microcatheter (≥2.3-Fr), although some (such as the Cook microcoils, Cook Medical) can be delivered through smaller microcatheters like the Finecross (Terumo Corp).[84]

Other reported percutaneous strategies include embolization of Gelfoam, polyvinyl alcohol, thrombin, collagen, glue, autologous blood clot, or subcutaneous fat.[84-91]

EMERGENCY SURGERY

In the presence of persistent coronary perforation with hemodynamic compromise or large ischemic territory

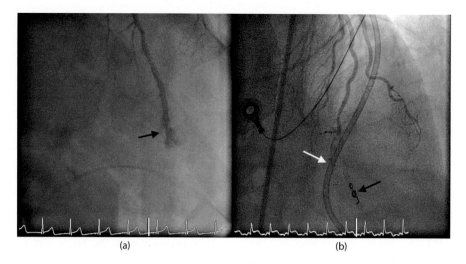

(a)   (b)

Figure 38.9 Cranial view showing a guidewire-induced perforation of the distal left anterior descending artery (*arrow*, **a**). Successful coil embolization was performed (*black arrow*, **b**) following pericardiocentesis (*white arrow*, b, showing the pigtail in the pericardium).

despite optimal nonoperative measures, surgical management should be considered. Emergency surgery can involve pericardial drainage—if percutaneous drainage failed or is insufficient—perforation repair or vessel ligation, and bypass grafting to vessels with significant stenoses. Before transferring the patient to the operating room, a balloon catheter should be kept inflated at low pressure at the perforation site, as previously described, and then removed during surgery.

Conclusion

Coronary perforation is a life-threatening complication of PCI, which usually occurs in high-risk anatomical settings or with the use of atheroablative devices or hydrophilic wires. Prompt recognition of this complication may be life saving, allowing for effective percutaneous, or rarely, surgical treatment of the perforation as well as its hemodynamic consequences.

AORTIC DISSECTION

Introduction

Iatrogenic aortic dissection (IAD) is an extremely rare complication of cardiac catheterization. Reported incidence ranges from 2 to 6 cases per 10,000 cardiac catheterizations. The incidence is higher during PCI (3–15 cases per 10,000 procedures) than during diagnostic coronary angiography (4–10 cases per 100,000 catheterizations). This complication is more frequently observed in the setting of acute MI (19 cases per 10,000 procedures).[92-95] IAD are usually caused by catheter manipulation during cannulation of coronary ostia. Two types of IAD have been reported: an antegrade form (61% of cases), usually with an entry point inside a coronary artery that extends into the aortic root, and a retrograde form (39%) without the involvement of the coronary arteries.[95]

Table 38.5 Classification of iatrogenic coronary dissections with retrograde extension into the aortic root

Class I	Aortic dissection involving only the ipsilateral cusp
Class II	Aortic dissection involving cusp and extending up the aorta <40 mm
Class III	Aortic dissection involving cusp and extending up the aorta >40 mm

Source: From Dunning, D.W., et al., *Catheter Cardiovasc. Interv.*, 51(4), 387–393, 2000. With permission.

The diagnosis of IAD is usually straightforward on angiography, characterized by contrast medium stagnating at the level of the aortic root or even extending to the ascending aorta. The spectrum of associated symptoms ranges from none to excruciating chest or back pain. Hypotension, hemodynamic compromise, and shock may ensue.[96] On the basis of the extent of the aortic dissection, a classification of IAD was proposed by Dunning et al.[92] Class I is defined as a focal dissection, limited to the ipsilateral cusp of the dissected coronary artery. Classes II and III include dissections that extend up the aorta <40 mm and >40 mm, respectively (Table 38.5; Figures 38.10 and 38.11).

IAD originate most frequently from the ostium of the right coronary artery. In a review of 67 cases published, Carstensen et al. reported that the dissection spread from the right coronary ostium, left coronary ostium, and ostium of a saphenous vein graft in 87%, 12%, and 1% of the cases, respectively.[97] IAD occurs more often when deep intubation of the guiding catheter in the coronary artery is required (e.g., in the treatment of chronic total occlusions). The use of left Amplatz guiding catheters also may be associated with a higher risk of IAD.[92,93] As previously mentioned, IAD appears to occur more frequently during PCI for acute MI. This is most likely due to the urgency of the situation and operator haste in attempting to rapidly achieve myocardial reperfusion; however, an increased vulnerability of vessel walls in relation with the ongoing inflammatory process cannot be excluded.[92,94] Finally, although underlying conditions may cause spontaneous aortic dissection, such as Marfan syndrome or bicuspid aortic valve, no apparent increase in incidence of IAD has been reported in such settings. Likewise, although cases of IAD in patients with cystic medial necrosis have been described, it is believed that it does not represent a risk factor for IAD, as low grades of degeneration are nonspecific and associated with advanced age.[92]

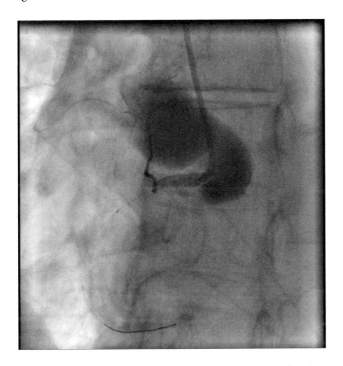

Figure 38.10 Class II iatrogenic aortic dissection following retrograde extension of a right coronary artery dissection.

Outcomes

IAD can lead to extensive dissection involving the ascending aorta, the aortic arch, the supra-aortic vessels, and even the descending aorta. Furthermore, extension of the intimal flap toward the aortic valve may cause significant acute aortic regurgitation as well as hemopericardium and tamponade. In earlier studies, emergency surgery (which usually associates repair or replacement of the ascending aorta with the treatment of the aortic valve, and CABG or pericardial drainage, if required) was performed in 6%–33% of cases following IAD.[92–94,97] A more recent study on 74 patients with IAD reported by Núñez-Gil et al. showed that surgery was necessary in only a minority of patients (4%).[95] In-hospital mortality rates after IAD range between 0 and 25%.[92–95,97]

Management

When a coronary artery is involved, the accepted management strategy is immediate stent implantation at the ostium of the coronary artery from where the intimal flap has spread. Earlier studies have supported that following sealing of the coronary dissection, a conservative approach of watchful waiting was warranted for class I and II IAD, while class III dissections should undergo immediate surgical treatment.[92–94,97] However, a larger and more recent publication from Núñez-Gil et al. suggests that surgery is only rarely necessary, even in type III dissections, and that stenting of the coronary ostium is sufficient.[95] This strategy appears reasonable if the patient is in a relatively stable hemodynamic condition and if stent implantation successfully seals the dissection. Concerning retrograde IAD (without coronary involvement), a conservative approach usually leads to an uneventful outcome.[95]

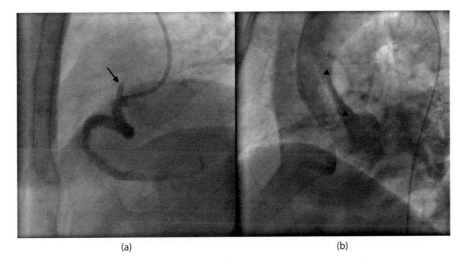

(a)   (b)

Figure 38.11 Left lateral view of an aortic dissection following retrograde extension of a right coronary artery ostial dissection (*arrow*, **a**), rapidly progressing to a class III dissection involving the entire aorta (arrowheads indicating dissection flap on aortography, **b**). Note also the filling of the left ventricle as a sign of associated aortic regurgitation (*arrow*, **b**).

Immediate assessment of the extension of the IAD can be achieved with aortography. Additional diagnostic techniques for the acute phase include transthoracic and transesophageal echocardiography. In asymptomatic patients with class II or III aortic dissection initially treated conservatively, it is reasonable to perform electrocardiogram-gated computed tomography angiography immediately after coronary angiography and after 12–24 hours in order to exclude progression of the dissection.

Conclusion

IAD is a rare complication of cardiac catheterization, which occurs more frequently in the setting of PCI for acute MI. When a coronary artery is involved with its dissection as an entry point, it should be sealed with a stent.

REFERENCES

1. Venkitachalam L, et al. Twenty-year evolution of percutaneous coronary intervention and its impact on clinical outcomes: A report from the National Heart, Lung, and Blood Institute-sponsored, multicenter 1985–1986 PTCA and 1997–2006 Dynamic Registries. *Circ Cardiovasc Interv* 2009;2(1):6–13.
2. Singh M, et al. Twenty-five-year trends in in-hospital and long-term outcome after percutaneous coronary intervention: A single-institution experience. *Circulation* 2007;115(22): 2835–2841.
3. Williams DO, et al. Outcomes of 6906 patients undergoing percutaneous coronary intervention in the era of drug-eluting stents: Report of the DEScover Registry. *Circulation* 2006;114(20):2154–2162.
4. Fokkema ML, et al. Population trends in percutaneous coronary intervention: 20-year results from the SCAAR (Swedish Coronary Angiography and Angioplasty Registry). *J Am Coll Cardiol* 2013;61(12):1222–1230.
5. Lohavanichbutr K, et al. Mechanisms, management, and outcome of failure of delivery of coronary stents. *Am J Cardiol* 1999;83(5):779–781, A9.
6. Nikolsky E, et al. Stent deployment failure: Reasons, implications, and short- and long-term outcomes. *Catheter Cardiovasc Interv* 2003;59(3):324–328.
7. Cantor WJ, et al. Failed coronary stent deployment. *Am Heart J* 1998;136(6):1088–1095.
8. Bolte J, et al. Incidence, management, and outcome of stent loss during intracoronary stenting. *Am J Cardiol* 2001;88(5):565–567.
9. Alfonso F, et al. Stent embolization during intracoronary stenting. *Am J Cardiol* 1996;78(7):833–835.
10. Eggebrecht H, et al. Nonsurgical retrieval of embolized coronary stents. *Catheter Cardiovasc Interv* 2000;51(4):432–440.
11. Brilakis ES, et al. Incidence, retrieval methods, and outcomes of stent loss during percutaneous coronary intervention: A large single-center experience. *Catheter Cardiovasc Interv* 2005;66(3):333–340.
12. Dunning DW, et al. The long-term consequences of lost intracoronary stents. *J Interv Cardiol* 2002;15(5):345–348.
13. Kozman H, et al. Long-term outcome following coronary stent embolization or misdeployment. *Am J Cardiol* 2001;88(6):630–634.
14. Kammler J, et al. Long-term follow-up in patients with lost coronary stents during interventional procedures. *Am J Cardiol* 2006;98(3):367–369.
15. Colkesen AY, et al. Coronary and systemic stent embolization during percutaneous coronary interventions: A single center experience. *Int Heart J* 2007;48(2):129–136.
16. Roffi M, et al. Failure to retrieve undeployed paclitaxel-eluting coronary stents. *Am J Cardiol* 2006;97(4):502–505.
17. Iturbe JM, et al. Frequency, treatment, and consequences of device loss and entrapment in contemporary percutaneous coronary interventions. *J Invasive Cardiol* 2012;24(5):215–221.
18. Alomar ME, et al. Stent loss and retrieval during percutaneous coronary interventions: A systematic review and meta-analysis. *J Invasive Cardiol* 2013;25(12):637–641.
19. Chan PH, et al. Extended use of the GuideLiner in complex coronary interventions. *EuroIntervention* 2015;11(3):325–335.
20. Ellis SG, et al. Increased coronary perforation in the new device era. Incidence, classification, management, and outcome. *Circulation* 1994;90(6):2725–2730.
21. Gunning MG, et al. Coronary artery perforation during percutaneous intervention: Incidence and outcome. *Heart* 2002;88(5):495–498.
22. Dippel EJ, et al. Coronary perforation during percutaneous coronary intervention in the era of abciximab platelet glycoprotein IIb/IIIa blockade: An algorithm for percutaneous management. *Catheter Cardiovasc Interv* 2001;52(3):279–286.
23. Gruberg L, et al. Incidence, management, and outcome of coronary artery perforation during percutaneous coronary intervention. *Am J Cardiol* 2000;86(6):680–682, A8.
24. Fasseas P, et al. Incidence, correlates, management, and clinical outcome of coronary perforation: Analysis of 16,298 procedures. *Am Heart J* 2004;147(1):140–145.
25. Stankovic G, et al. Incidence, predictors, in-hospital, and late outcomes of coronary artery perforations. *Am J Cardiol* 2004;93(2):213–216.
26. Fukutomi T, et al. Early and late clinical outcomes following coronary perforation in patients undergoing percutaneous coronary intervention. *Circ J* 2002;66(4):349–356.
27. Witzke CF, et al. The changing pattern of coronary perforation during percutaneous coronary intervention in the new device era. *J Invasive Cardiol* 2004;16(6):257–301.
28. Eggebrecht H, et al. Acute and long-term outcome after coronary artery perforation during percutaneous coronary interventions. *Z Kardiol* 2004;93(10): 791–798.
29. Ramana RK, et al. Coronary artery perforation during percutaneous coronary intervention: Incidence and outcomes in the new interventional era. *J Invasive Cardiol* 2005;17(11):603–605.
30. Javaid A, et al. Management and outcomes of coronary artery perforation during percutaneous coronary intervention. *Am J Cardiol* 2006;98(7):911–914.
31. Kiernan TJ, et al. Coronary artery perforations in the contemporary interventional era. *J Interv Cardiol* 2009;22(4):350–353.
32. Kini AS, et al. Changing outcomes and treatment strategies for wire induced coronary perforations in the era of bivalirudin use. *Catheter Cardiovasc Interv* 2009;74(5):700–707.

33. Doll JA, et al. Outcomes of patients with coronary artery perforation complicating percutaneous coronary intervention and correlations with the type of adjunctive antithrombotic therapy: Pooled analysis from REPLACE-2, ACUITY, and HORIZONS-AMI trials. *J Interv Cardiol* 2009;22(5):453–459.

34. Shimony A, et al. Incidence, risk factors, management and outcomes of coronary artery perforation during percutaneous coronary intervention. *Am J Cardiol* 2009;104(12):1674–1677.

35. Romaguera R, et al. Outcomes of coronary arterial perforations during percutaneous coronary intervention with bivalirudin anticoagulation. *Am J Cardiol* 2011;108(7):932–935.

36. Al-Lamee R, et al. Incidence, predictors, management, immediate and long-term outcomes following grade III coronary perforation. *JACC Cardiovasc Interv* 2011;4(1):87–95.

37. Shimony A, et al. Coronary artery perforation during percutaneous coronary intervention: A systematic review and meta-analysis. *Can J Cardiol* 2011;27(6):843–850.

38. Hendry C, et al. Coronary perforation in the drug-eluting stent era: incidence, risk factors, management and outcome: The UK experience. *EuroIntervention* 2012;8(1):79–86.

39. Bauer T, et al. Fate of patients with coronary perforation complicating percutaneous coronary intervention (from the Euro Heart Survey Percutaneous Coronary Intervention Registry). *Am J Cardiol* 2015;116(9):1363–1367.

40. Kinnaird T, et al. Incidence, determinants, and outcomes of coronary perforation during percutaneous coronary intervention in the United Kingdom between 2006 and 2013: An analysis of 527 121 cases from the British Cardiovascular Intervention Society Database. *Circ Cardiovasc Interv* 2016;9(8). pii:e003449.

41. Bittl JA, et al. Coronary artery perforation during excimer laser coronary angioplasty. The percutaneous Excimer Laser Coronary Angioplasty Registry. *J Am Coll Cardiol* 1993;21(5):1158–1165.

42. Holmes DR, Jr., et al. Coronary perforation after excimer laser coronary angioplasty: The Excimer Laser Coronary Angioplasty Registry experience. *J Am Coll Cardiol* 1994;23(2):330–335.

43. Cohen BM, et al. Coronary perforation complicating rotational ablation: The U.S. multicenter experience. *Cathet Cardiovasc Diagn* 1996;Suppl 3:55–59.

44. Klein LW. Coronary artery perforation during interventional procedures. *Catheter Cardiovasc Interv* 2006;68(5):713–717.

45. Nair P, Roguin A. Coronary perforations. *EuroIntervention* 2006;2(3):363–370.

46. Rogers JH, Lasala JM. Coronary artery dissection and perforation complicating percutaneous coronary intervention. *J Invasive Cardiol* 2004;16(9):493–499.

47. Coronary artery angiographic changes after PTCA. In: *Manual of Operations. NHLBI PTCA Registry*. Bethesda, MD: National Heart, Lung, and Blood Institute, 1985:6–9.

48. Muller O, et al. Management of two major complications in the cardiac catheterisation laboratory: The no-reflow phenomenon and coronary perforations. *EuroIntervention* 2008;4(2):181–183.

49. Smith SC Jr., et al. ACC/AHA guidelines for percutaneous coronary intervention (revision of the 1993 PTCA guidelines)-executive summary: A report of the American College of Cardiology/American Heart Association task force on practice guidelines (Committee to revise the 1993 guidelines for percutaneous transluminal coronary angioplasty) endorsed by the Society for Cardiac Angiography and Interventions. *Circulation* 2001;103(24):3019–3041.

50. Teis A, et al. Coronary artery perforation by intracoronary guide wires: Risk factors and clinical outcomes. *Rev Esp Cardiol* 2010;63(6):730–734.

51. Stathopoulos I, et al. Guidewire-induced coronary artery perforation and tamponade during PCI: In-hospital outcomes and impact on long-term survival. *J Invasive Cardiol* 2014;26(8):371–376.

52. Mauri L, et al. Cutting balloon angioplasty for the prevention of restenosis: Results of the Cutting Balloon Global Randomized Trial. *Am J Cardiol* 2002;90(10):1079–1083.

53. Von Sohsten R, et al. Cardiac tamponade in the "new device" era: Evaluation of 6999 consecutive percutaneous coronary interventions. *Am Heart J* 2000;140(2):279–283.

54. Fejka M, et al. Diagnosis, management, and clinical outcome of cardiac tamponade complicating percutaneous coronary intervention. *Am J Cardiol* 2002;90(11):1183–1186.

55. Ajluni SC, et al. Perforations after percutaneous coronary interventions: Clinical, angiographic, and therapeutic observations. *Cathet Cardiovasc Diagn* 1994;32(3):206–212.

56. Lowe R, et al. Prior CABG does not prevent pericardial tamponade following saphenous vein graft perforation associated with angioplasty. *Heart* 2005;91(8):1052.

57. Rahman N, et al. Intramyocardial hematoma after coronary perforation during percutaneous coronary intervention—Anticipated and treated. *J Invasive Cardiol* 2008;20(7):E224–E228.

58. Quan VH, et al. Coronary artery perforation by cutting balloon resulting in dissecting subepicardial hematoma and avulsion of the vasculature. *Catheter Cardiovasc Interv* 2005;64(2):163–168.

59. Shekar PS, et al. Dissecting sub-epicardial hematoma—challenges to surgical management. *Eur J Cardiothorac Surg* 2004;26(4):850–853.

60. Inoue Y, et al. Teflon felt wrapping repair for coronary perforation after failed angioplasty. *Ann Thorac Surg* 2006;82(6):2312–2314.

61. Shammas NW, et al. Perforation of saphenous vein graft during coronary stenting: A case report. *Cathet Cardiovasc Diagn* 1996;38(3):274–276.

62. Satler LF. A revised algorithm for coronary perforation. *Catheter Cardiovasc Interv* 2002; 57(2):215–216.

63. Harries I, et al. Tools & Techniques—Clinical: Management of coronary perforation. *EuroIntervention* 2014;10(5):646–647.

64. Myat A, et al. Percutaneous circulatory assist devices for high-risk coronary intervention. *JACC Cardiovasc Interv* 2015;8(2):229–244.

65. Holmes DR, Jr., et al. Iatrogenic pericardial effusion and tamponade in the percutaneous intracardiac intervention era. *JACC Cardiovasc Interv* 2009;2(8):705–717.

66. Morton AC, Gunn J. A case of autotransfusion from pericardium to femoral vein. *Heart* 2006;92(12):1727.

67. Venkatachalam KL, et al. Use of an autologous blood recovery system during emergency pericardiocentesis in the electrophysiology laboratory. *J Cardiovasc Electrophysiol* 2009;20(3):280–283.

68. Lansky AJ, et al. Treatment of coronary artery perforations complicating percutaneous coronary intervention with a polytetrafluoroethylene-covered stent graft. *Am J Cardiol* 2006;98(3):370–374.

69. Ly H, et al. Angiographic and clinical outcomes of polytetrafluoroethylene-covered stent use in significant coronary perforations. *Am J Cardiol* 2005;95(2):244–246.

70. Briguori C, et al. Emergency polytetrafluoroethylene-covered stent implantation to treat coronary ruptures. *Circulation* 2000;102(25):3028–3031.

71. Kawamoto H, et al. Short-term and long-term outcomes after polytetrafluoroethylene-covered stent implantation for the treatment of coronary perforation. *Am J Cardiol* 2015;116(12):1822–1826.

72. Secco GG, et al. Indications and immediate and long-term results of a novel pericardium covered stent graft: Consecutive 5 year single center experience. *Catheter Cardiovasc Interv* 2016;87(4):712–719.

73. Copeland KA, et al. Long-term follow-up of polytetrafluoroethylene-covered stents implanted during percutaneous coronary intervention for management of acute coronary perforation. *Catheter Cardiovasc Interv* 2012;80(1):53–57.

74. Colombo A, et al. The pericardium covered stent (PCS). *EuroIntervention* 2009;5(3):394–399.

75. Romaguera R, Waksman R. Covered stents for coronary perforations: Is there enough evidence? *Catheter Cardiovasc Interv* 2011;78(2):246–253.

76. Di Mario C, et al. Exclusion of a giant aneurysm post-Kawasaki disease with novel polyurethane covered stents. *Int J Cardiol* 2015;184:664–666.

77. Lattuca B, et al. New polyurethane covered stent with low profile for treatment of a large aneurysm after left anterior descending artery stenting: First experience. *Int J Cardiol* 2015;201:208–209.

78. Caputo RP, et al. Successful treatment of a saphenous vein graft perforation with an autologous vein-covered stent. *Catheter Cardiovasc Interv* 1999;48(4):382–386.

79. Colombo A, et al. Successful closure of a coronary vessel rupture with a vein graft stent: Case report. *Cathet Cardiovasc Diagn* 1996;38(2):172–174.

80. Ben-Gal Y, et al. Dual catheter technique for the treatment of severe coronary artery perforations. *Catheter Cardiovasc Interv* 2010;75(5):708–712.

81. Fujimoto Y, et al. Successful delivery of polytetrafluoroethylene-covered stent through 5 French guiding catheter. *J Invasive Cardiol* 2012;24(9):E199–E201.

82. Fujimoto Y, et al. Successful delivery of polytetrafluoroethylene-covered stent using rapid exchange guide extension catheter. *Cardiovasc Interv Ther* 2017;32(2):142-145.

83. Assali AR, et al. Successful treatment of coronary artery perforation in an abciximab-treated patient by microcoil embolization. *Catheter Cardiovasc Interv* 2000;51(4):487–489.

84. Shemisa K, et al. Management of guidewire-induced distal coronary perforation using autologous fat particles versus coil embolization. *Catheter Cardiovasc Interv* 2017;89(2):253–258 . doi:10.1002/ccd.26542.

85. Cordero H, et al. Intracoronary autologous blood to seal a coronary perforation. *Herz* 2001;26(2):157–160.

86. Storger H, Ruef J. Closure of guide wire-induced coronary artery perforation with a two-component fibrin glue. *Catheter Cardiovasc Interv* 2007;70(2):237–240.

87. Yoo BS, et al. Guidewire-induced coronary artery perforation treated with transcatheter injection of polyvinyl alcohol form. *Catheter Cardiovasc Interv* 2001;52(2):231–234.

88. Fischell TA, et al. Successful treatment of distal coronary guidewire-induced perforation with balloon catheter delivery of intracoronary thrombin. *Catheter Cardiovasc Interv* 2003;58(3):370–374.

89. Dixon SR, et al. Gelfoam embolization of a distal coronary artery guidewire perforation. *Catheter Cardiovasc Interv* 2000;49(2):214–217.

90. George S, et al. Guidewire-induced coronary perforation successfully treated with subcutaneous fat embolisation: A simple technique available to all. *Catheter Cardiovasc Interv* 2015;86(7):1186–1188.

91. Aleong G, et al. Collagen embolization for the successful treatment of a distal coronary artery perforation. *Catheter Cardiovasc Interv* 2009;73(3):332–335.

92. Dunning DW, et al. Iatrogenic coronary artery dissections extending into and involving the aortic root. *Catheter Cardiovasc Interv* 2000;51(4):387–393.

93. Gomez-Moreno S, et al. Iatrogenic dissection of the ascending aorta following heart catheterisation: Incidence, management and outcome. *EuroIntervention* 2006;2(2):197–202.

94. Yip HK, et al. Unusual complication of retrograde dissection to the coronary sinus of valsalva during percutaneous revascularization. *Chest* 2001;119(2):493–501.

95. Nunez-Gil IJ, et al. Incidence, management, and immediate and long-term outcomes after iatrogenic aortic dissection during diagnostic or interventional coronary procedures. *Circulation* 2015;131(24):2114–2119.

96. Januzzi JL, et al. Iatrogenic aortic dissection. *Am J Cardiol* 2002;89(5):623–626.

97. Carstensen S, Ward MR. Iatrogenic aortocoronary dissection: The case for immediate aortoostial stenting. *Heart Lung Circ* 2008;17(4):325–329.

Intra-aortic balloon pump counterpulsation and percutaneous left ventricular support

AMIRREZA SOLHPOUR AND RICHARD W. SMALLING

INTRODUCTION

Over the past few years it has been shown that short-term mechanical cardiac assistance may be appropriate in a few well-defined circumstances.[1-4] The 2013 American Heart Association (AHA)/American College of Cardiology (ACC) Guidelines for the Management of ST-Elevation Myocardial Infarction (STEMI) assigns a level IIb/c indication for left ventricular assist devices (LVADs) in refractory cardiogenic shock.[5] This includes centrifugal pump systems, such as the TandemHeart and extracorporeal membrane oxygenation (ECMO). In the setting of acute myocardial infarction (MI) with severely compromised ventricular function, temporary mechanical support unloads the left ventricle (LV) and augments cardiac output. Improving cardiac output mitigates end-organ damage, potentially limiting the systemic inflammatory response. In the case of chronic heart failure, temporary LV support reverses the acute metabolic derangements associated with decompensation. If the ventricle is able to recover sufficiently, medical management may be resumed. If ventricular function remains inadequate, temporary support may serve as a bridge to more definitive therapy. Finally, during high-risk percutaneous coronary intervention (PCI), temporary support provides circulatory protection in the event of acute vessel closure or catastrophic LV compromise.

Cardiogenic shock occurs in approximately 7% of patients hospitalized for acute STEMI and is the leading cause of death in post-MI patients.[6] Despite maximal medical management, including early thrombolysis and intra-aortic balloon counterpulsation (IABC), 30-day mortality from cardiogenic shock following acute MI remains unacceptably high, roughly 50%.[7] A strategy of early, aggressive PCI appears to have a positive, sustained influence at 1-year and on late survival.[8,9] However, even with successful mechanical reperfusion, viable myocardium may be stunned and noncontractile for up to a week.[10] Without adequate LV support during this period of myocardial recovery, the cycle of shock and further ischemic damage goes unchecked, leading to more profound pump failure, propagation of the systemic inflammatory response syndrome, and eventually death.[11]

The safety and durability of PCI have improved dramatically in the past 10 years due to better antiplatelet agents and improved stent technology. Attendant reductions in periprocedural complications, a decreased need for target lesion revascularization, and mortality comparable to conventional bypass grafting have led to greater acceptance of more aggressive PCI strategies.[12,13] Despite noteworthy procedural success, early attempts at percutaneous coronary transluminal angioplasty (PTCA) in high-risk individuals demonstrated unacceptable in-hospital mortality and required frequent target lesion revascularization. The studies with supported PTCA demonstrated a role for temporary LV assistance during high-risk procedures.[14,15]

ANATOMIC CONSIDERATIONS

The primary anatomic considerations limiting percutaneous LV support are access site disease, aortic valve dysfunction, and integrity of the thoracic and abdominal aorta.

All of the devices detailed in this chapter require relatively large arterial access conduits. With the exception of sheathless intra-aortic balloon pump (IABP) insertion, all forms of percutaneous LV support described require a minimum of 7.5-Fr arterial access. Furthermore, there is a significant trade-off between the degree of LV support provided and the size of arterial cannula required. The IABP offers minimal augmentation of cardiac output (0.5 L/min), but sheathed insertion is nominal at 7.5-Fr. The TandemHeart offers excellent cardiac assistance, 4 L/min, but requires 21-Fr venous access and unilateral 15- to 17-Fr or bilateral 12- to 15-Fr arterial access. The Impella LP2.5 is intermediate and the Impella CP provides better support, requiring a single 13- to 14-Fr (14-Fr for CP) arterial cannula and offering up to 2.5 L/min with LP2.5 (and slightly greater with CP). Due to the prevalence of significant peripheral vascular disease in our patients, if vessel anatomy is unknown at the time of intervention, angiography of the aorta with runoff is generally performed prior to device insertion.

Device selection is also limited by aortic valve disorders and diseases of the aorta. Moderate to severe aortic regurgitation is a contraindication to Impella and IABP support. All of these devices can potentially worsen the severity of aortic regurgitation, negating the benefits of LV assistance. In addition, due to its transvalvular design, the Impella cannot be used in patients with moderate to severe aortic stenosis or in individuals with mechanical aortic valves. Last, severe atherosclerotic disease or significant aneurysm of the thoracoabdominal aorta is a relative contraindication to IABP, ECMO, and Impella support. Repeated balloon inflations and the associated mechanical stress may lead to dislodgement and embolization of atherosclerotic debris with the IABP. The same repetitive forces combined with systemic anticoagulation may lead to devastating rupture of aortic aneurysms. Patients with severe disease of the aorta have generally been excluded from previous Impella trials; therefore, safety of the Impella in this population is uncertain.

FUNDAMENTALS

Two basic concepts provide the rationale for LV assistance during acute MI, cardiogenic shock, and high-risk PCI. First, augmentation of cardiac output enhances systemic hemodynamics and improves end-organ perfusion. Second, left ventricular unloading modestly improves coronary artery blood flow while reducing myocardial oxygen demand, thus limiting adverse remodeling. Animal experiments and human trials have demonstrated superior hemodynamics and improved left ventricular unloading with mechanical LV support. An early trial with the Hemopump (Medtronic Inc, Minneapolis, MN) elegantly demonstrated enhanced systemic hemodynamics in patients suffering from cardiogenic shock.[16] Fifty-three patients meeting criteria for cardiogenic shock (CI < 2 L/min*m², PCWP > 18 mmHg, SBP < 90 mmHg) were assigned to Hemopump insertion. In the 41 patients with successful placement, cardiac index (CI) increased from 1.6 to 2.2 L/min*m², pulmonary capillary wedge pressure (PCWP) decreased from 27 to 17 mmHg, and mean arterial pressure (MAP) increased from 56 to 67 mmHg. Later, in a sheep model of anterior MI, Meyns et al. demonstrated that the Impella 5.0 improved cardiac output and increased MAP while decreasing myocardial oxygen consumption.[17] In this trial, fully supported animals demonstrated lower left ventricular end-diastolic pressure (LVEDP) during ischemia and reperfusion compared to the unsupported group. Furthermore, despite increased MAP, device-supported animals demonstrated a lower dP/dt max and reduced myocardial volume oxygen (MVO2) consumption. Improved systemic hemodynamics, including increased CI and cardic output (CO), decreased PCWP and increased MAP, as well as reduced cardiac work have also been demonstrated with the Impella LP2.5[18] and in trials with the TandemHeart.[19,20]

In addition to improving systemic hemodynamics, mechanical left ventricular support has a positive effect on coronary blood flow while reducing myocardial oxygen demand, therefore reducing infarct size. In 1992, our lab demonstrated a modest improvement in regional myocardial blood flow and concomitant reduced myocardial oxygen demand in a canine model of anterior MI with LV assistance. When infarction was expressed as a percentage of the myocardium at risk, Hemopump and IABP-supported animals suffered infarcts of 22% and 27%, respectively, compared to unsupported controls with infarcts of 63%. This difference in infarct size was not significant comparing IABP and Hemopump supported animals; however, there was a striking contrast between infarct size in supported versus unsupported animals.[21] In the Meyns' sheep model of anterior MI, as detailed earlier, investigators also demonstrated a significant decrease in the size of infarct in Impella-supported animals. Furthermore, they showed that infarct size was related to both timing and the degree of mechanical support. Animals supported throughout the infarct and recovery period developed infarctions roughly one-quarter the size of unsupported animals, and approximately half the size of animals receiving support only during the reperfusion period.[17] It had been shown that as Impella support increased, hyperemic coronary flow velocity increased as well. An inverse relationship between Impella support and coronary microvascular resistance was also noted.[22] This combination of improved systemic hemodynamics, along with superior myocardial oxygen supply and decreased metabolic demand, suggests a compelling argument for mechanical left ventricular support during acute MI.

INDICATIONS

Clinical applications of the IABP, TandemHeart, and ECMO are fairly well-established and generally similar. As a much newer device, indications for the Impella LP2.5 and CP are evolving. Based on data from the Benchmark Registry, the most common applications of IABC are hemodynamic support during cardiac catheterization procedures (21%), cardiogenic shock (19%), weaning from bypass

Table 39.1 Indications for temporary cardiac support

Cardiogenic Shock
  Myocardial infarction
  Mechanical complications of acute myocardial infarction
  Papillary muscle rupture
  Ventricular septal defect
Acute Myocarditis
Cardiac Arrest
Incessant Ventricular Arrhythmias
Cath Lab Procedures
  High-risk percutaneous coronary intervention
  Low ejection fraction with
  Left main disease
    Three-vessel disease
    Last remaining patent conduit
High-Risk Valvular Procedures
Heart Failure
  Acutely decompensated chronic heart failure
    Reinitiation of medical therapy
    Bridge to transplant
    Bridge to bridge
    Bridge to destination
Post-Operative Allograft Dysfunction
Surgical
  Peri-operative support of high-risk patients
  Failure to wean from bypass
  Postcardiotomy syndrome

(16%), perioperative support in high-risk patients (13%), and refractory unstable angina (12%).[23] Common indications for TandemHeart, Impella, and ECMO, and in general for temporary cardiac support, are summarized in Table 39.1.

EQUIPMENT

Over the past several years, a great deal has been learned from previous generations of cardiac assist devices. The ideal temporary left ventricular support system could be quickly and easily inserted in the catheterization laboratory, would offer near complete cardiac support with LV unloading, and could remain in place for days to weeks. Traditional ventricular assist devices (VADs), such as the HeartMate II (St. Jude Medical) and HVAD (HeartWare), are safe, durable, and capable of complete cardiac assistance, but these devices are not well-suited for short-term or emergent use.[24] A technology that initially showed promise was percutaneous cardiopulmonary bypass (pCPB).

Cardiopulmonary bypass was introduced to the surgical theater in the early 1950s and the first report of pCPB was published in 1983.[25] In its simplest form, CPB consists of a venous intake cannula, oxygenator, blood pump, and an arterial return cannula. In 1990, two independent groups, Shawl and colleagues and Vogel et al., reported separate experiences of pCPB supported coronary angioplasty. Each registry reported a high degree of procedural success; however, they also encountered significant vascular

and hematologic complications. Access site complications ranged from 26% to 46% and the need for transfusion was between 30% and 43%.[26,27] The frequencies of access site complications and bleeding were likely related to the size of cannulae used, 18-Fr arterial and 20-Fr venous, as well as the high level of anticoagulation needed during pump initiation with an activated clotting time (ACT) >400 seconds. Another limitation of pCAB is the inability to adequately vent the LV. Although pCAB supports systemic circulation, percutaneous bypass actually increases LV wall stress. In the presence of ongoing myocardial ischemia, this increased wall stress leads to further myocardial damage. In contrast, devices such as the TandemHeart and Impella actively decompress the LV, leading to a reduction in wall stress, which is beneficial.

Percutaneous CPB-supported PTCA has largely been abandoned, but the recent publication of the first-in-human trials with a new pCPB device, the Lifebridge B2T (LifebridgeMedizintechnik GmbH, Ampfing, Germany), offers tempered optimism. The Lifebridge B2T is described as a modular "plug-and-play" device. Weighing about 20 kg and easily transported, the device employs 15-Fr arterial and 17-Fr venous access to circulate up to 4 L of oxygenated blood. Initially demonstrated in a swine model, in-human support for three-vessel disease and left-main PCI has been promising.[28-30] The new device does not overcome many of the pitfalls of previous bypass machines, including suboptimal LV decompression, the large blood–foreign body interface, and limited runtime, but the intake and outflow cannula are considerably smaller than predecessors and the modular construction is well-suited for emergent use. Further testing is necessary to define a role for the Lifebridge in the modern catheterization laboratory.

Surgical VADs are impractical in the acute setting, and pCPB is currently unproven. Veno-arterial ECMO (VA ECMO) is a device similar to the LifeBridge Device, which can be inserted quickly, even at bedside, and can have substantial hemodynamic support for heart, lung, or both until definitive therapy can be achieved. The TandemHeart offers excellent LV support, but even in skilled hands, it may take up to 30 minutes to insert and activate. By virtue of its left atrial cannulation, it effectively unloads the LV and does not require an oxygenator in the circuit. The balloon pump can be rapidly inserted; however, an IABP may not adequately support a failing ventricle, particularly in the setting of arrhythmia or extreme tachycardia. The device poised to fill the gap is the catheter-based axial flow pump.

The first percutaneous axial flow blood pump was developed and tested by Wampler and colleagues. In its initial forms, the Hemopump (Medtronic Inc., Minneapolis, MN), a 21-Fr femoral and a 24-Fr sternal pump, required surgical access. These devices were capable of flows from 3.5 to 5 L/min depending on loading conditions.[31]

Later, a 14-Fr device intended for percutaneous femoral insertion and capable of 2.5 L/min was introduced.

Initial testing with Hemopump was promising. In an animal model, the Hemopump demonstrated modestly improved regional myocardial blood flow, better LV unloading, and reduced infarct size when compared to the IABP.[21] Initial in-human trials also demonstrated improved systemic hemodynamics and suggested a survival benefit in select patients.[16,32] Despite these early successes, further testing demonstrated an unacceptable incidence of access site complications, hemolysis, and bleeding.[33] The Hemopump did not receive FDA approval, but these early experiences laid the groundwork for the next generation of transvalvular axial blood pumps.

Intra-aortic balloon pump

With a lack of easy access to VA ECMO and the fact that the other support devices are not easily and quickly implanted for cardiac support, the IABP has been essential in the management of high-risk patients. The IABP was conceived by two separate groups, Dr. Dwight Harken and Drs. Adrian and Arthur Kantrovitz.

Early models demonstrated decreased LVEDP, a reduction in left ventricular work index, and increased peak diastolic pressure.[34] Subsequent developments have resulted in devices that no longer require surgical insertion or large arteriotomies, and the current generation of IABP can be placed quickly and easily by experienced cardiologists.

When is hemodynamic support needed for PCI, and what defines "high-risk" PCI? Califf et al. devised the jeopardy score, a scoring system based on coronary anatomy and the presence of coronary disease as a prognostic indicator for major cardiovascular outcomes. In 462 nonsurgically treated patients, investigators demonstrated that patients with a score of 2 had a 5-year survival of 97%, and those with a score of 12 had a 5-year survival of 56%.[35] Further analysis indicated that left ventricular ejection fraction had a similar correlation with prognosis. Adding the degree of stenosis to each vessel, in particular the left anterior descending artery, further increased the prognostic value of the jeopardy score. The jeopardy score has been validated and is a good prognostic indicator in patients undergoing coronary artery bypass surgery and PCI.

Briguori et al., examined the use of prophylactic IABP placement in 133 high-risk patients undergoing elective PCI with left ventricular dysfunction (EF <30%) and a jeopardy score of greater than 6. Sixty-one patients had elective preprocedural IABP placement and 72 individuals had conventional PCI. Patients with an IABP suffered fewer intraprocedural complications (0% vs. 15%; $P = 0.001$).[36] Using stepwise regression analysis, high-risk predictors of intraprocedural complications were provisional versus prophylactic insertion of an IABP, female sex, and jeopardy score. Based on data from the National Registry of Supported Angioplasty, older patients (>70 years old) and those with left main stenosis are also at increased risk of intraprocedural complications, and may merit consideration of prophylactic IABP support.[27]

The question of when to place an IABP during an acute MI has been studied in several trials. PAMI II investigators looked at the use of prophylactic IABP placement in high-risk, hemodynamically stable patients with acute MI undergoing PTCA. The primary combined endpoint (reduction in death, reinfarction, infarct artery reocclusion, stroke, new-onset heart failure, or sustained hypotension) showed no significant difference between treatment groups (28.9% vs. 29.2%, $P = 0.95$). Unfortunately, in this study, the IABP was placed after reperfusion, which has been shown to not improve outcomes in ischemia/reperfusion.[21] Routine post-PCI IABP placement was beneficial in terms of reducing recurrent ischemia and limiting repeat unscheduled catheterizations; however, use of an IABP was also associated with a higher incidence of stroke (2.4% vs. 0%, $P = 0.03$).[37] In another study, Brodie et al. examined prophylactic IABC in high-risk acute MI. In this series, Brodie compared placement of an IABP prior to PTCA, after PTCA, and PTCA without IABP support. This study of 1,490 acute MI patients found a reduction in catheterization lab events—defined as ventricular fibrillation, cardiopulmonary arrest, or prolonged hypotension—in the group receiving IAPB support prior to PTCA (15% vs. 35%, $P = 0.009$). IABP support also demonstrated benefit in patients with an ejection fraction <30%.[38] The results of the SHOCK trial showed a marked reduction in 6-month mortality (50% vs. 63%, $P = 0.027$) in patients with cardiogenic shock who underwent emergency revascularization. In a subgroup analysis, patients who received IABP support had lower in-hospital mortality than those who did not receive an IABP (50% vs. 72%, $P = 0.0001$).[9] Additionally, patients who received revascularization and placement of an IABP had the lowest in-hospital mortality of all groups analyzed.

In the Intra-aortic Balloon Pump in Cardiogenic Shock (IABP-SHOCK) trial, 45 patients were randomized, and there was no significant difference in Acute Physiology and Chronic Health Evaluation II (APACHE II) scores in those patients assigned to IABP compared with the control group. IABP was associated with a significant reduction in serial brain natriuretic peptide levels.[39]

The same investigators, in the larger Intra-aortic Balloon Pump in Cardiogenic Shock 2 trial (IABP-SHOCK II), randomized 600 patients with cardiogenic shock complicating acute MI for whom an early revascularization strategy was planned. Once again, the IABP was not inserted prior to reperfusion, and in most, it was initiated too late in the patient's course to salvage myocardium. The IABP did not significantly reduce mortality at 30 days or at 12 months (IABP 52% and control 51%).[40,41] There were no significant differences in secondary endpoints or in process-of-care measures. Subgroup analysis in IABP-SHOCK II showed a hazard ratio in favor of IABP in those without a history of hypertension and those under 50 years. IABP-SHOCK II did not demonstrate an increased rate of major bleeding, stroke, peripheral ischemic complications, or sepsis among the IABP-treated patients, supporting that this technique is safe in primary PCI.

There are also some limitations for the IABP-SHOCKII Trial: inclusion criteria were based on readily available clinical assessments, such as systolic blood pressure of less than 90 mmHg for greater than 30 minutes, signs of end-organ hypoperfusion, and pulmonary congestion. It may be argued that a metabolic parameter, such as a serum lactate level of greater than 2 mmol/L, might have been useful to confirm the diagnosis and severity of cardiogenic shock; however, the high 30-day mortality rate of 39.7%–41.3% is consistent with previous randomized studies in cardiogenic shock MI (CSMI).[42] Between 20.4% and 23.7% of the patients had a previous MI, which may have negatively impacted their potential to benefit from circulatory support.

As mentioned previously, the timing of IABP insertion in shock MI patients (before or after PCI) may impact outcome. On one hand, placement of IABP before PCI could delay reperfusion, thereby increasing infarct size and adverse outcomes. A recent retrospective review of 173 shock MI patients[43] demonstrated greater elevations in creatine kinase when IABP was inserted prior to, rather than following, PCI. There was, however, no associated increase in mortality after a 5-year follow-up. On the other hand, IABP insertion prior to PCI will provide support during PCI when it is most needed and possibly limit the requirement for inotropic support. IABP was inserted following PCI in 84% of IABP-SHOCK II patients, and it left open the possibility that early IABP insertion might have been beneficial. It should be noted that patients with cardiogenic shock are a very difficult group to study, and it is possible that selection bias may have limited recruitment of severely shocked patients who might have benefited from IABP.

Unfortunately, in most of the early trials of IABC in the setting of acute STEMI, investigators waited until after infarct artery revascularization to initiate support. However, as early as 1986, Allen and Buckberg demonstrated the beneficial effects of LV decompression on myocardial salvage prior to reperfusion.[44] Similarly, in animal models, we have demonstrated a significant improvement in infarct salvage when LVAD or IABP support was initiated prior to reperfusion compared to support initiated after reperfusion.[45,46]

However, more recent studies, including CRISP-AMI, have not demonstrated reduced infarct size with IABP as adjunctive therapy compared with standard treatment alone in high-risk STEMI patients treated with primary PCI.[47,48] The AMI trial randomized 337 patients with anterior STEMI without cardiogenic shock to IABP inserted prior to PCI and continued for at least 12 hours, versus PCI alone, and found that counterpulsation reduces infarct size pre-PCI. There was no difference in the primary outcome measure of infarct size on cardiac magnetic resonance imaging (MRI) 3–5 days after PCI. Although the study was not powered for mortality, the 6-month mortality was 1.9% in the IABP-treated patients and 5.2% in those with PCI alone ($P = 0.12$).[47] Pre-PCI unloading occurred more than 2 hours after symptom onset in the majority of patients, which precluded the possibility of favorable impact on infarct salvage.[49,50] However, IABP unloaded patients had a much lower risk of late death, congestive heart failure, or shock, compared to control patients at 6 months, suggesting that the unloading may have reduced delayed cell death, possibly by inhibiting apoptosis.[45,46] Recent meta-analyses have demonstrated an increase in the incidence of major bleeding and stroke with IABP use in high-risk STEMI patients.[51–53]

At this stage, based on recent studies, there is no evidence to support the routine use of IABP in MI without cardiogenic shock. The ACC, the AHA, and the European Society of Cardiology (ESC) guidelines have downgraded their recommendation for IABP use in cardiogenic shock from class I to IIa and IIb, respectively.[54,55] Further trials powered to clinical endpoints should be considered, particularly in high-risk subgroups.

In brief, published meta-analyses, one small and one large RCT, show the absence of benefit of routine IABP insertion on morbidity and mortality in patients with CSMI. Given the easy insertion and widespread familiarity with the IABP, and the fact that TandemHeart, ECMO, and Impella are usually available only at tertiary-care hospitals with cardiac and vascular surgery expertise, the IABP will continue to be used in CSMI. This is because of belief in a certain understanding of pathophysiology and anecdotal experience of improved clinical status that has not, however, been confirmed by clinical benefit in randomized trials.

In patients with severely depressed left ventricular function and hemodynamic compromise who are currently awaiting cardiac transplantation, an IABP is often placed as a temporizing measure until a donor heart becomes available. There is no clinical or statistically significant difference in transplant outcomes between patients who receive IABP support before surgery compared to those who do not receive an IABP.[56] If placed before cardiac transplantation, the IABP should remain for at least 24 hours postoperatively in the event of allograft dysfunction. Potential complications with this method of treatment are increased rates of local and systemic infection and prolonged immobilization of the patient while the IABP is in place. Left axillary IABP placement may improve patient mobility prior to surgery. This method has been studied retrospectively in small number of patients. In one small series, all patients with axillary IABP insertion were successfully transplanted and discharged home.[57] The longest the ambulatory IABP was in place was for 70 days.

IABP insertion technique is well known to most cardiologists and is only reviewed briefly. Access is obtained via the femoral artery by a modified Seldinger's technique, and then a long J-tipped wire is advanced to the distal ascending aorta. A small incision is made in the skin and bluntly dilated with small curved forceps. Once dilatation has been performed, the sheath and dilator combination are inserted, and the dilator is removed. The sheath remains in place. The balloon is then advanced to the proximal descending thoracic aorta, distal to the take-off of the left subclavian artery

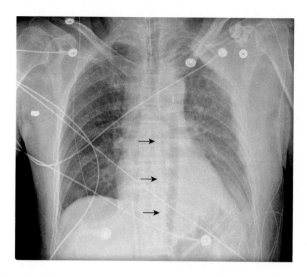

Figure 39.1 Intra-aortic balloon pump *in situ.* Appropriate positioning minimizes intra-aortic balloon pump complications. The distal balloon tip should be between the second and third intercostal spaces and 1–2 cm distal to the left subclavian artery. Note the balloon marker just distal to the calcified aortic arch. In this film, the balloon is seen fully inflated in the descending aorta. (Courtesy of RW Smalling. McGovern Medical School. The University of Texas Health Science Center at Houston. Houston, Texas.)

(Figure 39.1). Placement at this level ensures there is no obstruction of the renal arteries. Negative suction is applied in the central lumen of the balloon to remove any trapped air and debris. After flushing the central lumen, the balloon is connected to the pressure tubing and gas line. Once proper placement has been confirmed, counterpulsation can begin.

TandemHeart

Conceptually, the TandemHeart (Cardiac Assist, Inc., Pittsburgh, PA) device is similar to percutaneous cardiopulmonary bypass as described earlier; however, key modifications offer substantial benefits in the setting of acute MI and high-risk PCI. Similar to pCPB, placement of the TandemHeart requires femoral artery and vein access. Additionally, both devices employ an external pump to augment systemic circulation. However, the TandemHeart uses a unique transseptal inflow cannula that more effectively unloads the LV during pump operation. The TandemHeart also takes advantage of the individual's own pulmonary circuit for oxygenation, eliminating the external oxygenator and limiting contact between blood elements and foreign material. Theoretically, this modification minimizes the inflammatory reaction and allows longer run times.

Dennis et al. were the first to demonstrate the feasibility of percutaneous left atrial-to-femoral artery bypass. Their initial design employed a right internal jugular approach and used a stiff metallic transseptal cannula.[58] After refinements in materials and methods, the femoral approach was shown in a small study of animals and critically ill humans.[59] Further modifications led to the first modern demonstration

atrial-femoral bypass in a cohort of high-risk PCI patients.[60] But it was not until 2001 that Thiele et al. described the initial in-human trial with the TandemHeart.[60] A year after Thiele's pioneering work with the TandemHeart for support during cardiogenic shock, feasibility of TandemHeart-assisted high-risk elective PCI was described.[61,62]

Since these initial accounts, multiple papers have documented successful support of patients with cardiogenic shock and in patients undergoing high-risk procedures. Most of these accounts are small, descriptive case series indicating excellent procedural success and relatively limited complication rates.[63–66] Although the aforementioned trials are noteworthy, two small randomized trials of the IABP versus the TandemHeart merit further consideration.[60,64]

In the first of these trials, Thiele et al. randomized 41 patients suffering from cardiogenic shock following an acute MI to either IABC or TandemHeart support. All patients underwent revascularization within 24 hours of the onset of cardiogenic shock. During therapy (mean duration of support 3.5 days for the IABP and 4 days for the TandemHeart), investigators closely monitored key hemodynamic parameters and adverse events. The primary outcome measure, cardiac power index, was improved more effectively in the TandemHeart group. Similarly, other common hemodynamic parameters and metabolic indicators of perfusion demonstrated greater improvement in TandemHeart patients. Despite the impressive hemodynamic differences, investigators were unable to show a survival benefit. It is likely that the hemodynamic benefits were offset by an increase in device-related complications, including bleeding, need for transfusion, and limb ischemia. Investigators also noted higher rates of systemic inflammatory response syndrome and disseminated intravascular coagulation in the TandemHeart group.[60] In a similar study, Burkhoff and colleagues randomized 19 patients with cardiogenic shock to TandemHeart support and 14 to IABC. They also observed improved hemodynamics (decreased PCWP, increased MAP, and improved CI) with the TandemHeart as compared to the IABP, but failed to find a survival advantage. The incidence of many prespecified adverse events was similar between groups—hemolysis, thrombocytopenia, renal dysfunction, and infection. But, higher rates of arrhythmia, bleeding, and access site complications were noted in the TandemHeart group.[64] Due to slow enrollment, the trial was ended early. Thirty-day survival was 53% (10/19) in the TandemHeart group compared to 64% (9/14) in the IABP group.

The TandemHeart has been associated with significant complications. In the registry of 117 patients, one patient died after postoperative revision of a wire-related perforation of the LA following transseptal puncture; other complications included sepsis/systemic inflammatory response syndrome (SIRS) (29.9%), bleeding around the cannula site (29.1%), groin hematomas (5.1%), device-related limb ischemia (3.4%), gastrointestinal bleeding (19.7%), coagulopathy (11%), stroke (6.8%), right common femoral artery dissection (0.85%), as well as blood transfusions (71%).[67] Furthermore, the complexity of the insertion procedure limits the use of the device to centers experienced in transseptal puncture.

In its current design, the TandemHeart device consists of four major components: (1) a 21-Fr transseptal inflow cannula; (2) an extracorporeal, continuous-flow centrifugal pump; (3) a 15- to 17-Fr venous return cannula; and (4) an electronic pump control module. The inflow cannula has a unique design with a large endhole and multiple sideholes permitting high flow rates with limited resistance (Figure 39.2). The inflow cannula can be placed via a standard transseptal approach. We have modified this slightly by employing a soft-tipped stiff-core 0.014-in wire (Sparta Core, Abbot Vascular, Santa Clara, CA) inserted through the transseptal needle and directed into the left upper pulmonary vein (LUPV). Holding the needle and wire fixed, the dilator and transseptal sheath are advanced across the septum and into the LUPV. The wire, needle, and dilator are then removed, and the sheath is aspirated multiple times to eliminate air and debris. After placement is confirmed fluoroscopically, the patient is systemically heparinized through the transseptal sheath. A stiff 0.035-in exchange wire (Amplatz Super Stiff, Boston Scientific, Natick, MA) is advanced to the LUPV, which serves as the working wire. The interatrial septum is then serially dilated and the aspiration cannula is secured in place. During transseptal puncture, the Spartacore wire protects internal cardiac structures from inadvertent laceration with the transseptal needle. Thus far, this technique has proven safe and effective. The external pump unit has a dual-chamber design. The upper chamber houses a low-speed centrifugal impeller that is in direct contact with blood elements. The lower chamber is the drive unit consisting of an electromagnetic pump and liquid bearing. The liquid bearing is a heparinized solution that functions as local anticoagulation, pump lubrication, and heat sink. Systemic anticoagulation is typically withheld until successful transseptal puncture; however, during pump assembly and priming, we use a target ACT of 300 seconds. During pump operation, an ACT of 200–250 seconds is generally sufficient to limit most thrombotic complications. The control module has a simple operational design with a fully redundant battery back-up system (Figures 39.2 through 39.4). Pump flow is measured with a

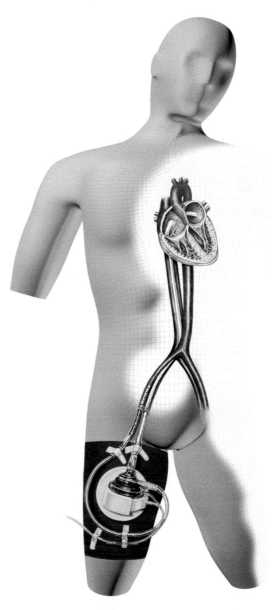

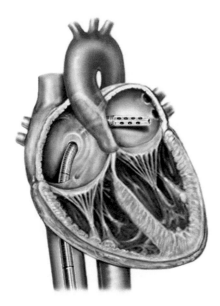

Figure 39.2 TandemHeart transseptal inflow cannula. Multiple sideholes and a large endhole permit easy aspiration of oxygenated blood from the left atrium. The 21-Fr inflow catheter traverses the interatrial septum at the level of the fossa ovalis. The catheter then descends the inferior vena cava. (Courtesy of Cardiac Assist, Inc., Pittsburgh, Pennsylvania.)

Figure 39.3 TandemHeart with thigh mounting bracket. Note same transseptal cannulation as in Figure 39.2. Also, the inflow cannula exits via the right femoral vein. Blood enters the TandemHeart pump via the central port and is propelled centrifugally out of the side port. Blood returns to the systemic circulation at the level of the right iliac via the right femoral artery. (Courtesy of Cardiac Assist, Inc., Pittsburgh, Pennsylvania.)

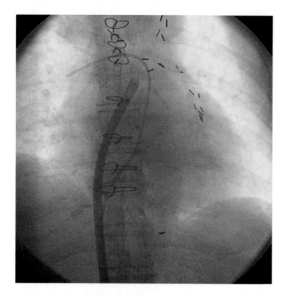

Figure 39.4 Transseptal cannulation with the TandemHeart device. The TandemHeart inflow cannula has been correctly placed via the transseptal approach in a patient with prior coronary artery bypass. Note the Swan–Ganz catheter in wedge position and surgical clips from the prior bypass. Severe calcification of the native vessels and previous stents can also be appreciated. (Courtesy of RW Smalling. McGovern Medical School. The University of Texas Health Science Center at Houston. Houston, Texas.)

trans-sonic flow probe placed on the arterial return line. Total cardiac output can be measured using a thermodilution or continuous monitoring pulmonary artery (PA) catheter. Hemodynamic parameters such as systemic vascular resistance (SVR) and pulmonary vascular resistance (PVR) should be calculated using the total CO measured from the PA catheter. Figure 39.3 shows the TandemHeart fully connected and secured to the thigh mounting bracket.

Since introduction of the TandemHeart percutaneous ventricular assist device (pVAD) in 2001, the device has been successfully performed in a multitude of settings. According to company resources, nearly 1,500 procedures were performed worldwide as of November 2008. In the past 7 years, the TandemHeart has been used for support of cardiogenic shock following acute MI and for mechanical complications of acute MI. In the setting of chronic heart failure, the TandemHeart has been used as temporary support, as a bridge to transplant, and as a bridge-to-bridge. In the surgical arena, the TandemHeart is effective support for postcardiotomy syndrome. More recently case reports have demonstrated benefit in the setting of critical aortic stenosis for support during high-risk mitral valvuloplasty and as effective right ventricular assist device (RVAD).[68] Versatility of the TandemHeart has also been demonstrated with alternative anticoagulants, including argatroban and bivalirudin. In short, the TandemHeart shows promise as a truly percutaneous, fully supportive VAD. Although a mortality benefit has not been demonstrated, increasing patient comorbidities and the escalating demand for innovative percutaneous therapies will likely necessitate a greater role for TandemHeart in coming years.

Impella

Not all patients presenting with LV compromise or undergoing high-risk PCI will require the near complete support of the TandemHeart; however, IABC may not be sufficient without some essential level of CO. Bridging this gap are relatively new devices, the Impella LP2.5 and CPX. The Impella family of devices has their basis in the early clinical experiences of the Hemopump.[69] Like the Hemopump, the Impella LP2.5 and CPX is a catheter-based transvalvular axial flow pump. The LP2.5 is the smallest of four devices developed by Abiomed Inc. for temporary cardiac support. The larger devices in the series are the CP, LD, RD, and the LP5.0 (Table 39.2). These devices are capable of higher flow rates, up to 4 L/min. The LP2.5 and CP are inserted percutaneously and the rest require either surgical access or arterial cutdown for placement. In a randomized trial of 199 coronary artery bypass grafting (CABG) patients, the combination of RD and LD support compared favorably with normothermic cardiopulmonary bypass in terms of mortality, peri-operative MI, and length of stay.[70] These devices have also demonstrated utility in the setting of shock following acute MI, acute myocarditis, postcardiotomy syndrome, and as a bridge to transplant.[71–74]

As shown in Figures 39.5 through 39.8, the Impella LP2.5 has a 12-Fr maximum outer diameter and is recommended for placement via a 13-Fr to 14-Fr sheath. The drive line is 9-Fr, and the assembly is mounted on a 6-Fr pigtail catheter. The device is advanced across the aortic valve over a stiff soft-tipped 0.018-in coronary guidewire (Platinum Plus, Boston Scientific, Natick, MA). The Impella LP2.5 is angled to approximate the couture of the aortic outflow tract. The motor unit and impeller are located at the proximal end of the device. The intake cannula sits across the aortic valve with the inflow port near the cardiac apex. The drive-line and infusate port connect to a control module and purge pump, respectively. The control module has a simple operational design. Infusate is maintained under constant pressure, with a minimum recommendation of 300 pounds per square inch (PSI), creating a liquid seal for the motor unit. Flow and aortic pressure are continuously displayed on the control module. Flow reflects an estimated flow rate based on impeller speed and transvalvular loading conditions (Figures 39.5 through 39.8).

Although the Impella LP2.5 and CP lack the power of their larger siblings, the LD and LP5.0, speed and ease of placement make it an attractive option during elective high-risk procedures and in the setting of acute MI. Valgimigli and colleagues published the first in-human use of the Impella LP2.5. The patient, a 56-year-old man with a history of multiple MIs and reduced ejection fraction (EF) (27%), underwent PCI of a dominant left circumflex artery. Swan–Ganz monitoring during the case demonstrated a marked reduction in PCWP—18–11 mmHg—during pump

Table 39.2 Impella family devices—characteristics

	Impella LP 2.5	Impella CP	Impella 5.0/LD	Impella RP
Access	Percutaneous/ femoral artery	Percutaneous/ femoral artery	Surgical (Axillary, fem or ascend aorta)	Percutaneous/ femoral vein
Output (max) L/min	Up to 2.5	Up to 3.5	5.0	4.6
Introducer size	13 F peel away	14 F peel away	Dacron graft 10 mm recommended	23 F peel away
Motor size	12 F	14 F	21 F	22 F
Guiding catheter size	9 F	9 F	9 F	11 F
RPM (max)	51,000	46,000	33,000	33,000

F, french; RPM, rotation per minute.

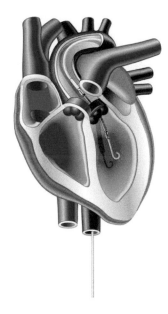

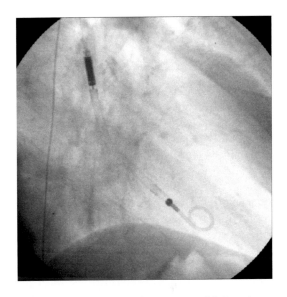

Figure 39.5 Impella LP2.5 heart schematic. The drive-line ascends the abdominal aorta. The motor unit, outflow port, and orifice of the pressure lumen are positioned appropriately in the proximal aorta. The flow cannula traverses the aortic valve. The inflow port and pigtail catheter are at the mid-cavity level and near the left ventricular apex, respectively. (Courtesy of Abiomed Inc., Danvers, Massachusetts.)

Figure 39.7 Fluoroscopic right anterior oblique view-Impella LP2.5. (*Upper left*) The opaque drive unit is superior to the aortic valve. (*Center*) The transvalvular cannula traverses the aortic valve with the pre-formed angle reflecting the normal contour of the left ventricle outflow tract. (*Lower right*) The inflow port and pigtail catheter are in the left ventricle appex. (Courtesy of Abiomed Inc., Danvers, Massachusetts.)

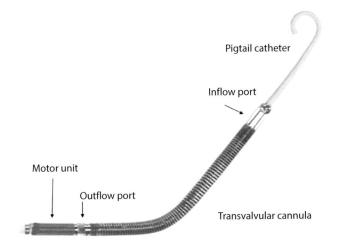

Figure 39.6 Impella LP2.5.

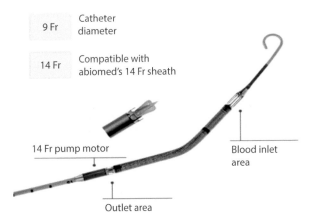

Figure 39.8 Impella CP.

operation and a similar increase in cardiac output, 6 L/min compared to 7.4 L/min, as measured by thermodilution.[18] Shortly after this initial account, safety and feasibility of Impella LP2.5 support were further demonstrated in 19 elective, high-risk PCI patients. All patients had EF's <40%, and many were older (>60 years old), diabetic (53%), and had a history of MI (74%). The Impella LP2.5 was successfully placed in all 19 patients, and no device-related deaths were recorded. Two in-hospital mortalities were noted: one following prolonged cardiac surgery and another secondary to multiorgan failure. One patient developed a large access site hematoma, and two patients required postprocedural blood transfusion.[75] At ACC 2007, Jose Henriques, MD, presented a large series of Impella LP2.5 assisted PCI cases on 109 patients. In this series, he found a relatively low rate of in-hospital MACE, 13% (14/109), and excellent tolerability, 100% device placement (109/109).[76] Several studies have shown that the Impella device is safe and hemodynamically effective in STEMI and high-risk PCI patients.[77] The unloading of the LV is associated with reduced end diastolic wall stress and an immediate decrease in PCWP.[77] Clinical trials with the Impella Recover LPw2.5 applied in a STEMI population with pre-shock (IMPRESS trial), as well as in hemodynamically unstable STEMI population (RECOVER II trial), had to be terminated due to insufficient patient enrollment.[77] With respect to the role of the Impella pump in cardiogenic shock and especially in cardiogenic shock MI, an initial report of the experience in six patients[74] was followed by two relevant studies. The multicenter Impella EUROSHOCK-Registry[2] included 120 patients with cardiogenic shock MI receiving temporary circulatory support with the Impella-2.5-pLVAD. Thirty-day mortality was 64.2%. After Impella-2.5-pLVAD implantation, lactate levels were not significantly improved. The ISAR-SHOCK randomized trial compared the Impella 2.5 with the IABP in cardiogenic shock patients.[78] CI and MAP increased more in the Impella group; furthermore, serum lactate levels were lower in the Impella group than in the IABP group. There were no differences in mortality, major bleeding, arrhythmias, infections, and distal limb ischemia.

Other studies have suggested that in severe cardiogenic shock, the Impella 5.0 device may provide superior hemodynamic support.[77,79] A lower mortality rate has been reported for Impella 5.0 in patients with post-cardiotomy low-output syndrome with a residual CO of 1 L/min[81] versus IABP.[80,81]

Currently, there is neither meta-analysis nor a randomized clinical trial available for the Impella pump family alone with mortality as an endpoint. The most important meta-analysis included three controlled trials involving a relatively small total of 100 patients with cardiogenic shock mainly due to MI; it compared the effects of LVADs—two trials with TandemHeart and one trial with the Impella PL2.5—with the effects of IABP with respect to hemodynamics and 30-day survival.[82] In total, LVAD patients had higher CI (+0.35 L min/m²), higher MAP (+12.8 mmHg), and lower PCWP (25.3 mmHg) compared with IABP patients. The 30-day mortality rate was similar between the two circulatory support groups (RR 1.06 for LVAD patients versus IABP patients, CI 0.68–1.66). There was no significant difference in the incidence of leg ischemia (RR 2.59, CI 0.75–8.97) and fever or sepsis (RR 1.11, CI 0.43–2.90) for LVAD patients versus IABP patients; however, bleeding was significantly more frequent (RR 2.35, CI 1.40–3.93) in LVAD patients versus IABP. The frequency of adverse events (i.e., leg ischemia, bleeding) was higher in the TandemHeart trials than in the Impella trial.

A subgroup evaluation—including the same LVAD trials—of a Cochrane analysis further supports that Tandem Heart and Impella 2.5LP pump support improve hemodynamics, with no improvement in survival in comparison with IABP support in small trials of patients with cardiogenic shock MI.[83]

The use of Impella support in high-risk interventions has been studied in PROTECT II, a prematurely discontinued randomized controlled trial[3,84] in which at the primary endpoint of 30-day MACE, no major difference was observed, but at 90 days, the Impella group showed a significant reduction in MACE.

It has been shown that hemodynamic parameters like cardiac power and stroke work index are powerful short-term prognostic data.[85] Nevertheless, there has been a decrease in PA catheter (Swan–Ganz) use, likely due to the controversy sparked by a prospective observational study that suggested that PA catheters were associated with poor outcomes. We feel that Swan–Ganz catheterization should be considered to evaluate the severity of cardiogenic shock, especially when mechanical cardiac assistance devices are selected.

Extracorporeal Membrane Oxygenation

Kloff and Berk in 1944 noted that blood became oxygenated as it passed through the cell-phase chambers of their artificial kidney. This concept was applied in 1953 by Gibbon who used artificial oxygenation and perfusion support for the first successful open heart operation.[86,87] In 1970, Baffes et al. reported the successful use of ECMO as support in infants with congenital heart defects undergoing cardiac surgery.[88]

ECMO has remarkably progressed over recent years; the indications are extended to more prolonged use in the intensive care unit, such as bridge to transplant for both cardiac and lung transplant, and support for lung resections in unstable patients.[89,90]

The major advantage of ECMO over other modern PVADs is the lack of need for transseptal puncture or transfer to a cardiac catheterization laboratory, that it can be placed quickly at bedside without the need for fluoroscopy, and can provide biventricular support as well as oxygenation to aid with pulmonary dysfunction. In patients with imminent circulatory collapse, ECMO is usually the best choice for cardiopulmonary support, as it provides complete biventricular and oxygenation support while being convenient enough to be quickly placed at bedside if necessary.

However, ECMO does not reduce afterload; therefore, myocardial protection and oxygen demand are not addressed by ECMO. Furthermore, it can have some complications, such as infection, limb ischemia, hemolysis, thrombocytopenia, and access site bleeding. Daily management of a patient on an ECMO circuit involves ensuring adequate flow of the device by optimizing pump speed and afterload, achieving adequate anticoagulation targets, and monitoring for ECMO complications, such as vascular compromise, thrombocytopenia, and bleeding. Although ECMO has been approved for up to 32 days of extracorporeal support, clinically, our experience has been that it is usually only used for a few days. The use of ECMO has been increasing in the institution where it is available. According to the Extracorporeal Life Support Organization (ESLO) registry, ECMO was used in over 5,000 cases in 2014.[41]

In terms of outcomes, although there is no available randomized trial, Sheu et al. compared 219 patients with cardiogenic shock as a complication of acute STEMI treated with primary PCI and adjunctive ECMO, versus a historical cohort of 115 patients treated with primary PCI without adjunctive ECMO.[91] In this retrospective study, the 30-day mortality for the non-ECMO group was significantly higher than that for the ECMO group (41.7% vs. 30.1%, $P = 0.034$). Unfortunately, the historical cohort (1993–2002) was mostly treated in the prior decade as compared to the ECMO group (2002–2009).

ECMO has also been used with or without IABP for short-term cardiopulmonary support in patients with postcardiotomy cardiogenic shock;[92] it has been used as a bridge-to-recovery device in patients with fulminant myocarditis.[93]

Similarly, an FDA-approved handheld mini-ECMO system, the CARDIOHELP system (Marquette AG, Hirrlingen, Germany), was implanted successfully and safely as a bridge-to-recovery device in out-of-hospital patients presenting with severe refractory cardiogenic shock (SRCS).[46] Finally, the LIFEBRIDGE-B2T (Medizintechnik AG, Ampfing, Germany) is a portable cardiopulmonary bypass unit that can be implanted via the femoral vessels within 15 minutes and is capable of 3–4 L/min of circulatory support (Figure 39.9). It is FDA approved for support up to 6 hours. It has been used successfully to support high-risk PCI in a patient with cardiogenic shock and to support pulmonary embolectomy in a patient with cardiovascular collapse secondary to a massive pulmonary embolism.[29]

Table 39.3 summarizes the characteristics of the currently available percutaneous LVADs.[94]

TECHNIQUE FOR ECMO PLACEMENT

During VA ECMO, blood will bypass both the heart and the lungs. Blood is extracted from the right atrium (RA) or vena cava (for drainage), and returned to the arterial system. This is done either through peripheral cannulation via femoral, axillary, or carotid arteries (for infusion) or into the ascending aorta if central cannulation is used, especially in cases of postcardiotomy ECMO, where the cannulas

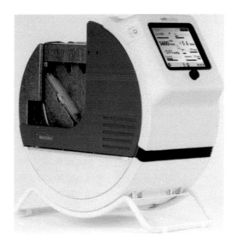

Figure 39.9 The ultracompact, lightweight, and fully self-contained Lifebridge B2T Portable Extracorporeal Life Support System.

employed for cardiopulmonary bypass can be transferred from the heart-lung machine to the ECMO circuit. Blood is drained from the RA and reinfused into the ascending aorta (Figures 39.10 and 39.11). In a special configuration when an RVAD is used as ECMO, the oxygenated blood is delivered to the PA so the blood bypasses only the right heart. Femoral access is preferred for VA ECMO in cases of emergency or cardiogenic shock because insertion is relatively less invasive and faster to institute the ECMO. The probability of ischemia of the ipsilateral lower extremity can be decreased by inserting an additional arterial cannula distal to the femoral artery cannula to perfuse the distal extremity at the time of ECMO insertion. In our institution, we use an antegrade access and place a 7-Fr arrow flex sheath using a modified Seldinger technique, and it is connected to the side port of the arterial cannula of the ECMO using a three-way stopcock. Occasionally, the femoral vessels are unsuitable for cannulation for VA ECMO (e.g., patients with severe occlusive peripheral artery disease or prior femoral arterial reconstruction). In such circumstances, the right common carotid artery (CCA) should be considered as an alternative insertion site; however, this technique is associated with an increased risk of a large watershed cerebral infarction of 5%–10%.

CONTRAINDICATIONS

As detailed earlier in anatomical considerations, many of the contraindications to temporary left ventricular support are common to the IABP, the TandemHeart and the Impella LP2.5, and CP and ECMO. For review, shared contraindications include severe peripheral vascular disease, moderate to severe aortic valve regurgitation, and uncontrolled bleeding diathesis. In the case of peripheral arterial disease, vessel diameter is the limiting factor. If the operator is skilled in peripheral interventions, these limitations may be partially overcome. We have had excellent success with balloon

Table 39.3 Currently available percutaneous left ventricular assist devices

Device	Company	Pump mechanism	Flow	Direct cardiac chamber support	Disposable costs per use
IABP	Multiple	Counterpulsation	Up to 1 L/min	LV	US $1,000
Tandem Heart	Cardiac Assist	Centrifugal flow	LV support, 4.0 L/min at 15 Fr FA cannulae, 5.0 L/min at 17 Fr FA cannulae	LV, RV, or Bi-V	US $26,000–28,000
Impella 2.5	Abiomed	Axial flow	2.5 L/min	LV	US $20,000
Impella CP	Abiomed	Axial flow	3.33 L/min	LV	US $25,000
Impella 5.0	Abiomed	Axial flow	5.0 L/min	LV	US $28,000
Impella RP	Abiomed	Axial flow	4.0 L/min	RV	TBD
ECMO	Multiple	Centrifugal flow	>4.5 L/min	Bi-V	US $3,000

Source: Modified from Abnousi, F., et al., *Curr. Cardiol. Rep.*, 17(6), 40, 2015.
Note: Bi-V, biventricular; ECMO, extracorporeal membrane oxygenation; FA, femoral artery; Fr, French size; IABP, intra-aortic balloon pump; LV, left ventricle; RV, right ventricle; TBD, to be determined.

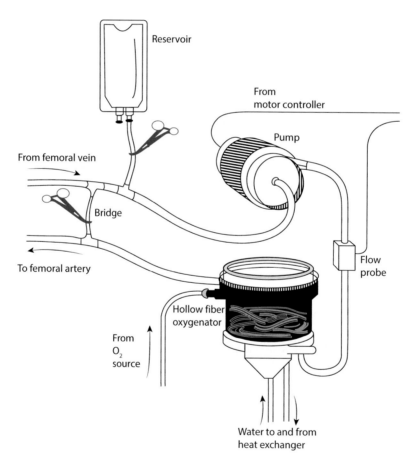

Figure 39.10 The ECMO circuit.

dilation and occasional stenting of the target artery prior to device insertion. Next, all of these devices can exacerbate aortic insufficiency; therefore, moderate to severe aortic valve regurgitation is another shared limitation. Finally, due to the inherent thrombogenicity of foreign material and the need for adequate anticoagulation during device insertion and operation, uncontrolled bleeding diathesis and conditions incompatible with normal life if the person recovers

are the shared limitations of these temporary LV support devices.

A couple of noteworthy limitations are specific to the Impella 2.5 or CP and the IABP. Because the Impella is a transvalvular blood pump, passage of the device across an already stenotic aortic valve may increase the transvalvular gradient, leading to further clinical decompensation. Therefore, insertion in patients with moderate to severe

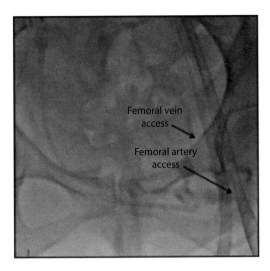

Figure 39.11 Venous-arterial extracorporeal membrane oxygenation placement of both the inflow and outflow cannulas.

Table 39.4 Contraindications to temporary mechanical support

Severe peripheral vascular disease
Moderate to severe aortic regurgitation (except for tandem heart)
Uncontrolled bleeding diathesis
Severe atherosclerosis of the thoracic or abdominal aorta[a]
Significant thoracic or abdominal aortic aneurysm[a]
Mechanical aortic valves[b]
Moderate to severe aortic valve stenosis[b]
Mural thrombus[b]

[a] Applies to intra-aortic balloon pump and Impella.
[b] Applies to Impella only.

aortic stenosis is not recommended. Similarly, passing the Impella through a mechanical prosthetic valve is likely to disrupt valve function. Therefore, the Impella should not be used in patients with prior valve replacement. In addition to these limitations, the inflow cannula of the Impella sits at the left ventricular apex; therefore, due to the risk of embolic phenomena, LV mural thrombus is another strict contraindication to Impella support. As detailed earlier in this chapter, significant disease of the thoracic or abdominal aorta—atherosclerosis or aneurysm—is a shared relative contraindication of the Impella and the IABP. Finally, although not a contraindication, the IABP works best when there is ventricle-pump synchrony. Although programming modifications and control features have largely addressed this issue, rapid or chaotic rhythms decrease the efficacy of IABP support. Table 39.4 summarizes the major contraindications to temporary mechanical LV support.

CLINICAL ASPECTS

Once a decision has been made that temporary mechanical support is required, the interventionalist must select the most appropriate device. In some hospitals, the choice may be limited by device availability. Alternatively, the interventionalist must carefully assess the urgency and degree of support required along with access limitations. Finally, issues of closure technique, cost considerations, and physician preference play a role. Not all of the devices described in this chapter will be available at every hospital.

Next, the urgency of the patient's hemodynamic requirements, the relative degree of cardiac support needed, and the duration of therapy play a role in device selection. As stated earlier, the TandemHeart offers up to 4 L/min of cardiac support; however, in a critically unstable patient, rapid device insertion and early initiation of support may be a greater concern. In such cases, VA ECMO may be the best option because it can be inserted quickly and provides

biventricular support. Alternatively, in a patient with unstable angina and severe LV dysfunction scheduled to undergo PCI of an unprotected left main, the time necessary to place the TandemHeart is likely well spent. Finally, the duration of support must be considered. The TandemHeart is FDA approved for 6 hours of extracorporeal support; however, case reports of support for up to 30 days exist. Similarly, the Impella LP2.5 and CP are intended for short-term use, but if weaning becomes difficult, prolonged support, up to 7 days, has been reported. Finally, IABP support in our institution is generally limited to the 24–48 hours following an acute MI. However, the duration of balloon pump support at our transplant centers is frequently on the order of weeks, and prolonged support in excess of 3 months is not without precedent.

As discussed earlier in this chapter, there is a significant trade-off between the size of arterial cannula required for a given device and the maximum achievable flow rate. The TandemHeart generally requires large-bore (17-Fr) arterial access; however, bilateral 12-Fr access is possible at the cost of decreasing maximum pump flow rate from 4 to 3 L/min. In a large, adult male with isolated coronary artery disease, device options are unlimited; however, in the context of a petite, elderly female with peripheral vascular disease, arterial cannulation may be impossible without prior peripheral intervention.

Finally, closure of vascular access sites, relative cost, and physician preferences play a role in device selection. Simple manual pressure is often sufficient to ensure safe and durable hemostasis following IABP removal; however, for larger arteriotomies, we prefer a pre-close technique. Our technique requires deployment of two preloaded vascular sutures prior to final dilation of the arteriotomy site. During device support, the suture ends are left untied, tagged with small hemostats, and then set aside. Following the procedure, while the large vascular conduits are being removed, gentle pressure is applied superior to the access site as the previously deployed sutures are tied and advanced.

Certainly, cost and reimbursement must be considered. The unit cost of each device is shown in Table 39.3; however, reimbursement often varies by diagnosis-related group (DRG). Based on DRG payment for the same device, the same procedure may vary by over $20,000. In general, DRGs for the Impella, TandemHeart, and ECMO will have higher payouts to cover the cost of equipment and the additional technical support required. Last, there is a very real element of physician preference and appropriate training. Even when these more advanced devices are available at any institution, only experienced operators should consider them as an option.

CONCLUSION

Percutaneous left ventricular support has finally come into the mainstream as a viable option for interventional cardiologists. The TandemHeart left ventricular support device is the only device currently available that essentially provides full support of circulation, decompression of the left ventricle, and circulation at a level commensurate with survival, which is independent of an organized heart rhythm or left ventricular ejection. Unfortunately, it requires advanced interventional skills, including transseptal puncture and manipulation of a very large cannula into the LA via the right femoral vein. Additionally, the arterial return cannula, while possible to insert percutaneously, requires either the pre-close technique for temporary use or formal femoral artery repair for removal after a more chronic implant. The Impella 2.5 device is potentially capable of pumping at a level of 2.5 liters per minute, but it is dependent on optimal loading conditions to achieve this level of support. Obviously, the Impella by itself is not capable of supporting the entire circulation except for very brief periods of time. It does, however, provide active left ventricular decompression and is not dependent on synchronization with the cardiac cycle.

The IABP is simple to insert but provides indirect support of diastolic blood flow and a modest level of left ventricular unloading. Nonetheless, animal models and observational studies in humans suggest that the level of support provided by the balloon pump is sufficient to provide meaningful left ventricular assistance and is associated with reduction in infarct size when implanted prior to reperfusion in the setting of STEMIs.

VA ECMO can have biventricular support by substantial hemodynamic improvement and decreasing the LV preload. It also increases LV after load, thereby increasing the oxygen demand and impeding myocardial protection.

Right-sided support is also feasible with the TandemHeart device utilizing two atrial cannulas, one inserted into the superior vena cava and one inserted via antegrade access from the RA through the right ventricle to the PA. Left ventricular assist in the setting of right-sided cardiogenic shock has not been beneficial; however, now that percutaneous right-sided cardiac support is available, further evaluation of this technique is warranted. It is not infrequent after implantation of a PVAD, such as the TandemHeart or Impella, for it to be necessary to wean from the LVAD to IABP support prior to complete cessation of left ventricular support.

It is indeed an exciting time in this area. We anticipate that new percutaneous devices will become available in the near future, which will significantly improve our armamentarium for treating circulatory failure without the necessity of requiring major cardiac surgery. As new devices become available, it will be imperative to compare them to the existing devices and to delineate the relative merits of each device in given clinical situations.

REFERENCES

1. Kantrowitz A, et al. Initial clinical experience with intraaortic balloon pumping in cardiogenic shock. *JAMA* 1968;203(2):113–118.
2. Lauten A, et al. Percutaneous left-ventricular support with the Impella-2.5-assist device in acute cardiogenic shock: Results of the Impella-EUROSHOCK-registry. *Circ Heart Fail* 2013;6(1):23–30.
3. O'Neill WW, et al. A prospective, randomized clinical trial of hemodynamic support with Impella 2.5 versus intra-aortic balloon pump in patients undergoing high-risk percutaneous coronary intervention: The PROTECT II study. *Circulation* 2012;126(14):1717–1727.
4. Friedman PA, et al. Percutaneous endocardial and epicardial ablation of hypotensive ventricular tachycardia with percutaneous left ventricular assist in the electrophysiology laboratory. *J Cardiovasc Electrophysiol* 2007;18(1):106–109.
5. American College of Emergency Physicians, et al. 2013 ACCF/AHA guideline for the management of ST-elevation myocardial infarction: A report of the American College of Cardiology Foundation/American Heart Association Task Force on Practice Guidelines. *J Am Coll Cardiol* 2013;61(4):e78–e140.
6. Goldberg RJ, et al. Temporal trends in cardiogenic shock complicating acute myocardial infarction. *N Engl J Med* 1999;340(15):1162–1168.
7. Hochman JS, et al. Early revascularization in acute myocardial infarction complicated by cardiogenic shock. SHOCK Investigators. Should We Emergently Revascularize Occluded Coronaries for Cardiogenic Shock. *N Engl J Med* 1999;341(9):625–634.
8. Hochman JS, et al. Early revascularization and long-term survival in cardiogenic shock complicating acute myocardial infarction. *JAMA* 2006;295(21):2511–2515.
9. Hochman JS, et al. One-year survival following early revascularization for cardiogenic shock. *JAMA* 2001;285(2):190–192.
10. McFalls EO, et al. Temporal changes in function and regional glucose uptake within stunned porcine myocardium. *J Nucl Med* 1996;37(12):2006–2010.
11. Hochman JS. Cardiogenic shock complicating acute myocardial infarction: Expanding the paradigm. *Circulation* 2003;107(24):2998–3002.
12. Hannan EL, et al. Drug-eluting stents vs. coronary-artery bypass grafting in multivessel coronary disease. *N Engl J Med* 2008;358(4):331–341.
13. Seung KB, et al. Stents coronary-artery bypass grafting for left main coronary artery disease. *N Engl J Med* 2008;358(17):1781–1792.
14. Hartzler GO, et al. "High-risk" percutaneous transluminal coronary angioplasty. *Am J Cardiol* 1988;61(14):33G–37G.

15. Ellis SG, et al. In-hospital cardiac mortality after acute closure after coronary angioplasty: Analysis of risk factors from 8,207 procedures. *J Am Coll Cardiol* 1988;11(2):211–216.

16. Wampler RK, et al. Treatment of cardiogenic shock with the Hemopump left ventricular assist device. *Ann Thorac Surg* 1991;52(3):506–513.

17. Meyns B, et al. Left ventricular support by catheter-mounted axial flow pump reduces infarct size. *J Am Coll Cardiol* 2003;41(7):1087–1095.

18. Valgimigli M, et al. Left ventricular unloading and concomitant total cardiac output increase by the use of percutaneous Impella Recover LP 2.5 assist device during highrisk coronary intervention. *Catheter Cardiovasc Interv* 2005;65(2):263–267.

19. Burkhoff D, et al. Feasibility study of the use of the TandemHeart percutaneous ventricular assist device for treatment of cardiogenic shock. *Catheter Cardiovasc Interv* 2006;68:211–217.

20. Thiele H, et al. Reversal of cardiogenic shock by percutaneous left atrial-to-femoral arterial bypass assistance. *Circulation* 2001;104(24):2917–2922.

21. Smalling RW, et al. Improved regional myocardial blood flow, left ventricular unloading, and infarct salvage using an axial-flow, transvalvular left ventricular assist device. A comparison with intra-aortic balloon counterpulsation and reperfusion alone in a canine infarction model. *Circulation* 1992;85:1152–1159.

22. Remmelink M, et al. Effects of left ventricular unloading by Impella recover LP2.5 on coronary hemodynamics. *Catheter Cardiovasc Interv* 2007;70(4):532–537.

23. Ferguson JJ 3rd, et al. The current practice of intra-aortic balloon counterpulsation: Results from the Benchmark Registry. *J Am Coll Cardiol* 2001;38(5):1456–1462.

24. Song X, et al. Axial flow blood pumps. *ASAIO J* 2003;49(4):355–364.

25. Phillips SJ, et al. Percutaneous initiation of cardiopulmonary bypass. *Ann Thorac Surg* 1983;36(2):223–225.

26. Shawl FA, et al. Percutaneous cardiopulmonary bypass support in the catheterization laboratory: Technique and complications. *Am Heart J* 1990;120(1):195–203.

27. Vogel RA, et al. Initial report of the National Registry of Elective Cardiopulmonary Bypass Supported Coronary Angioplasty. *J Am Coll Cardiol* 1990;15(1):23–29.

28. Ferrari M, et al. First use of a novel plug and-play percutaneous circulatory assist device for high-risk coronary angioplasty. *Acute Card Care* 2008;10(2):111–115.

29. Jung C, et al. Providing macro- and microcirculatory support with the Lifebridge System during high-risk PCI in cardiogenic shock. *Heart Lung Circ* 2008;18(4):296–298.

30. Mehlhorn U, et al. LIFEBRIDGE: A portable, modular, rapidly available "plug-and-play" mechanical circulatory support system. *Ann Thorac Surg* 2005;80(5):1887–1892.

31. Wampler RK, et al. Circulatory support of cardiac interventional procedures with the Hemopump cardiac assist system. *Cardiology* 1994;84(3):194–201.

32. Smalling RW, et al. Transvalvular left ventricular assistance in cardiogenic shock secondary to acute myocardial infarction. Evidence for recovery from near fatal myocardial stunning. *J Am Coll Cardiol* 1994;23(3):637–644.

33. Scholz KH, et al. Clinical experience with the percutaneous hemopump during high-risk coronary angioplasty. *Am J Cardiol* 1998; 82(9):1107–1110, A6.

34. Bolooki H. *Clinical Application of the Intra-Aortic Balloon Pump*. 3rd edn. Armonk, NY: Futura Publishing Company, Inc., 1998.

35. Califf RM, et al. Prognostic value of a coronary artery jeopardy score. *J Am Coll Cardiol* 1985;5(5):1055–1063.

36. Briguori C, et al. Elective versus provisional intra-aortic balloon pumping in high-risk percutaneous transluminal coronary angioplasty. *Am Heart J* 2003;145:700–707.

37. Stone GW, et al. A prospective, randomized evaluation of prophylactic intraaortic balloon counterpulsation in high-risk patients with acute myocardial infarction treated with primary angioplasty. Second Primary Angioplasty in Myocardial Infarction (PAMI-II) Trial Investigators. *J Am Coll Cardiol* 1997;29(7):1459–1467.

38. Brodie BR, et al. Intra-aortic balloon counterpulsation before primary percutaneous transluminal coronary angioplasty reduces catheterization laboratory events in high-risk patients with acute myocardial infarction. *Am J Cardiol* 1999;84(1):18–23.

39. Prondzinsky R, et al. Intra-aortic balloon counterpulsation in patients with acute myocardial infarction complicated by cardiogenic shock: The prospective, randomized IABP SHOCK Trial for attenuation of multiorgan dysfunction syndrome. *Crit Care Med* 2010;38(1):152–160.

40. Thiele H, et al. Intraaortic balloon support for myocardial infarction with cardiogenic shock. *N Engl J Med* 2012;367(4):1287–1296.

41. Thiele H, et al. Intra-aortic balloon counterpulsation in acute myocardial infarction complicated by cardiogenic shock (IABP-SHOCK II): Final 12 month results of a randomised, open-label trial. *Lancet* 2013;382(9905):1638–1645.

42. TRIUMPH Investigators, et al. Effect of tilarginine acetate in patients with acute myocardial infarction and cardiogenic shock: The TRIUMPH randomized controlled trial. *JAMA* 2007;297(15):1657–1666.

43. Cheng JM, et al. Impact of intra-aortic balloon pump support initiated before versus after primary percutaneous coronary intervention in patients with cardiogenic shock from acute myocardial infarction. *Int J Cardiol* 2013;168(4):3758–3763.

44. Okamoto F, et al. Reperfusion conditions: Critical importance of total ventricular decompression during regional reperfusion. *J Thorac Cardiovasc Surg* 1986;92(3 Pt 2):613–620.

45. Achour H, et al. Mechanical left ventricular unloading prior to reperfusion reduces infarct size in a canine infarction model. *Catheter Cardiovasc Interv* 2005;64(2):182–192.

46. LeDoux JF, et al. Left ventricular unloading with intra-aortic counter pulsation prior to reperfusion reduces myocardial release of endothelin-1 and decreases infarction size in a porcine ischemia-reperfusion model. *Catheter Cardiovasc Interv* 2008;72(4):513–521.

47. Patel MR, et al. Intra-aortic balloon counterpulsation and infarct size in patients with acute anterior myocardial infarction without shock: The CRISP AMI randomized trial. *JAMA* 2011;306(12):1329–1337.

48. Vijayalakshmi K, et al. Intra-aortic counterpulsation does not improve coronary flow early after PCI in a high-risk group of patients: Observations from a randomized trial to explore its mode of action. *J Invasive Cardiol* 2007;19(8):339–346.

49. Francone M, et al. Impact of primary coronary angioplasty delay on myocardial salvage, infarct size, and microvascular damage in patients with ST-segment elevation myocardial infarction: Insight from cardiovascular magnetic resonance. *J Am Coll Cardiol* 2009;54(23):2145–2153.

50. Eitel I, et al. Prognostic significance and determinants of myocardial salvage assessed by cardiovascular magnetic resonance in acute reperfused myocardial infarction. *J Am Coll Cardiol* 2010;55(22):2470–2479.

51. Cassese S, et al. Intra-aortic balloon counterpulsation in patients with acute myocardial infarction without cardiogenic shock. A meta-analysis of randomized trials. *Am Heart J* 2012;164(1):58–65.

52. Bahekar A, et al. Cardiovascular outcomes using intraaortic balloon pump in high-risk acute myocardial infarction with or without cardiogenic shock: A meta-analysis. *J Cardiovasc Pharmacol Ther* 2012;17(1):44–56.

53. Sjauw KD, et al. A systematic review and metaanalysis of intra-aortic balloon pump therapy in ST-elevation myocardial infarction: Should we change the guidelines? *Eur Heart J* 2009;30(4):459–468.

54. O'Gara PT, et al. 2013 ACCF/AHA guideline for the management of ST-elevation myocardial infarction: A report of the American College of Foundation/American Heart Association Task Force on Practice Guidelines. *Circulation* 2013;127(4):e362–e425.

55. Steg PG, et al. ESC guidelines for the management of acute myocardial infarction in patients presenting with ST-segment elevation. *Eur Heart J* 2012;33(20):2569–2619.

56. Christenson JT, et al. Optimal timing of preoperative intraaortic balloon pump support in high-risk coronary patients. *Ann Thorac Surg* 1999;68(3):934–939.

57. Cochran RP, et al. Ambulatory intraaortic balloon pump use as bridge to heart transplant. *Ann Thorac Surg* 2002;74(3):746–751; discussion 51–52.

58. Dennis C, et al. Left atrial cannulation without thoracotomy for total left heart bypass. *Acta Chir Scand* 1962;123:267–279.

59. Glassman E, et al. A method of closed-chest cannulation of the left atrium for left atrial-femoral artery bypass. *J Thorac Cardiovasc Surg* 1975;69(2):283–290.

60. Thiele H, et al. Randomized comparison of intra-aortic balloon support with a percutaneous left ventricular assist device in patients with revascularized acute myocardial infarction complicated by cardiogenic shock. *Eur Heart J* 2005;26(13):1276–1283.

61. Lemos PA, et al. Usefulness of percutaneous left ventricular assistance to support high-risk percutaneous coronary interventions. *Am J Cardiol* 2003;91(4):479–481.

62. Vranckx P, et al. Clinical introduction of the Tandemheart, a percutaneous left ventricular assist device, for circulatory support during high-risk percutaneous coronary intervention. *Int J Cardiovasc Intervent* 2003;5(1):35–39.

63. Aragon J, et al. Percutaneous left ventricular assist device: "TandemHeart" for high-risk coronary intervention. *Catheter Cardiovasc Interv* 2005;65(3):346–352.

64. Burkhoff D, et al. A randomized multicenter clinical study to evaluate the safety and efficacy of the TandemHeart percutaneous ventricular assist device versus conventional therapy with intraaortic balloon pumping for treatment of cardiogenic shock. *Am Heart J* 2006;152(3):469.e1–e8.

65. Giombolini C, et al. Percutaneous left ventricular assist device, TandemHeart, for high-risk percutaneous coronary revascularization. A single centre experience. *Acute Card Care* 2006;8(2):35–40.

66. Kar B, et al. Clinical experience with the TandemHeart percutaneous ventricular assist device. *Tex Heart Inst J* 2006;33(2):111–115.

67. Kar B, et al. The percutaneous ventricular assist device in severe refractory cardiogenic shock. *J Am Coll Cardiol* 2011;57(6): 688–696.

68. Giesler GM, et al. Initial report of percutaneous right ventricular assist for right ventricular shock secondary to right ventricular infarction. *Catheter Cardiovasc Interv* 2006;68(2):263–266.

69. Siess T, et al. From a lab type to a product: A retrospective view on Impella's assist technology. *Artif Organs* 2001;25(5):414–421.

70. Meyns B, et al. Coronary artery bypass grafting supported with intracardiac microaxial pumps versus normothermic cardiopulmonary bypass: A prospective randomized trial. *Eur J Cardiothorac Surg* 2002;22(1):112–117.

71. Garatti A, et al. Impella recover 100 microaxial left ventricular assist device: The Niguarda experience. *Transplant Proc* 2004;36(3):623–626.

72. Garatti A, et al. Different applications for left ventricular mechanical support with the Impella Recover 100 microaxial blood pump. *J Heart Lung Transplant* 2005;24:481–485.

73. Garatti A, et al. Left ventricular mechanical support with the Impella Recover left direct microaxial blood pump: A single-center experience. *Artif Organs* 2006;30(7):523–528.

74. Meyns B, et al. Initial experiences with the Impella device in patients with cardiogenic shock—Impella support for cardiogenic shock. *Thorac Cardiovasc Surg* 2003;51(6):312–317.

75. Henriques JP, et al. Safety and feasibility of elective high-risk percutaneous coronary intervention procedures with left ventricular support of the Impella Recover LP 2.5. *Am J Cardiol* 2006;97(7):990–992.

76. Henriques J. Impella 2.5 Safe to Use in High-Risk PCI: 109 Patient Study. *ACC*, 2007.

77. Ouweneel DM, Henriques JPS. Percutaneous cardiac support devices for cardiogenic shock: Current indications and recommendations. *Heart* 2012;98:1246–1254.

78. Seyfarth M, et al. A randomized clinical trial to evaluate the safety and efficacy of a percutaneous left ventricular assist device vs. intra-aortic balloon pumping for treatment of cardiogenic shock caused by myocardial infarction. *J Am Coll Cardiol* 2008;52(19):1584–1588.

79. Engstrom AE, et al. The Impella 2.5 and 5.0 devices for ST-elevation myocardial infarction patients presenting with severe and profound cardiogenic shock: The Academic Medical Center intensive care unit experience. *Crit Care Med* 2011;39(9):2072–2079.

80. Siegenthaler MP, et al. The Impella recover microaxial left ventricular assist device reduces mortality for postcardiotomy failure: A three-center experience. *J Thorac Cardiovasc Surg* 2004;127(3):812–822.

81. Jurmann MJ, et al. Initial experience with miniature axial flow ventricular assist devices for postcardiotomy heart failure. *Ann Thorac Surg* 2004;77(5):1642–1647.

82. Cheng JM, et al. Percutaneous left ventricular assist devices vs. intra-aortic balloon pump counterpulsation for treatment of cardiogenic shock: A meta-analysis of controlled trials. *Eur Heart J* 2009;30(17):2102–2108.

83. Unverzagt S, et al. Intra-aortic balloon pump counterpulsation (IABP) for myocardial infarction complicated by cardiogenic shock. *Cochrane Database Syst Rev* 2011;7:CD007398.

84. Dangas GD, et al. Impact of hemodynamic support with Impella 2.5 versus intra-aortic balloon pump on prognostically important clinical outcomes in patients undergoing high risk percutaneous coronary intervention (from the PROTECT II randomized trial). *Am J Cardiol* 2014;113(2):222–228.

85. Fincke R, et al. Cardiac power is the strongest hemodynamic correlate of mortality in cardiogenic shock: A report from the SHOCK trial registry. *J Am Coll Cardiol* 2004;44(1)340–348.

86. Kolff WJ, et al. The artificial kidney: A dialyser with a great area. 1944. *J Am Soc Nephrol* 1997;8(12):1959–1965.

87. Gibbon JH Jr. Application of a mechanical heart and lung apparatus to cardiac surgery. *Minn Med* 1954;37(3):171–185.

88. Baffes TG, et al. Extracorporeal circulation for support of palliative cardiac surgery in infants. *Ann Thorac Surg* 1970;10(4):354–363.

89. Acker MA. Mechanical circulatory support for patients with acute-fulminant myocarditis. *Ann Thorac Surg* 2001;71(3 Suppl):S73–S76; discussion S82–S85.

90. Clark JB, et al. Mechanical circulatory support for end-stage heart failure in repaired and palliated congenital heart disease. *Curr Cardiol Rev* 2011;7(2):102–109.

91. Sheu JJ, et al. Early extracorporeal membrane oxygenator-assisted primary percutaneous coronary intervention improved 30-day clinical outcomes in patients with ST-segment elevation myocardial infarction complicated with profound cardiogenic shock. *Crit Care Med* 2010;38(9):1810–1817.

92. Doll N, et al. Five- ear results of 219 consecutive patients treated with extracorporeal membrane oxygenation for refractory postoperative cardiogenic shock. *Ann Thorac Surg* 2004;77(1):151–157, discussion 157.

93. Asaumi Y, et al. Favourable clinical outcome in patients with cardiogenic shock due to fulminant myocarditis supported by percutaneous extracorporeal membrane oxygenation. *Eur Heart J* 2005;26:2185–2192.

94. Abnousi F, et al. The evolution of temporary percutaneous mechanical circulatory support devices: A review of the options and evidence in cardiogenic shock. *Curr Cardiol Rep* 2015;17(6):40.

PART 8

Structural Heart Procedures

40

Intracardiac echocardiography

LAURENS F. TOPS, VICTORIA DELGADO, DENNIS W. DEN UIJL, AND JEROEN J. BAX

INTRODUCTION

In the past years, intracardiac echocardiography (ICE) has emerged as a valuable imaging tool for interventional and electrophysiological procedures. ICE allows real-time visualization of important anatomical structures that cannot be visualized on fluoroscopy and is not associated with radiation exposure to the patient and operator. This imaging modality is used to guide and monitor interventional procedures and for early detection of complications. Importantly, as an alternative to transesophageal echocardiography (TEE), ICE can be performed without general anesthesia. Among other indications, ICE has recently been introduced for guidance of transcatheter valve procedures.

In this chapter, the basic principles and clinical applications of ICE are discussed, as well as new technologies and indications.

ANATOMIC CONSIDERATIONS

ICE is generally performed by placing the probe within the right atrium (RA) or the right ventricle (RV). The images acquired with ICE should therefore be interpreted from that perspective. Depending on the position and direction of the ultrasound catheter, all large cardiac structures, including the atria, ventricles, atrioventricular and semilunar valves, coronary sinus, and pericardium, can be visualized. Awareness of the orientation of the scanning plane and a good understanding of the three-dimensional (3D) cardiac anatomy are essential for a correct interpretation.

EQUIPMENT

Currently, two different ICE technologies are available. The first approach utilizes a mechanical ultrasound-tipped catheter, which can also be used for endovascular echocardiography. The second uses an electronic ultrasound catheter that is equipped with a phased array transducer at its tip. Both are introduced using a femoral venous approach after the application of local anesthesia.

The mechanical or rotational system uses a 9-Fr catheter equipped with a 9-MHz single-element transducer incorporated at its tip (Ultra ICE, Boston Scientific, San Jose, CA). A piezoelectric crystal inside the transducer is rotated at 1,800 revolutions per minute (RPM) in the radial dimension and provides a two-dimensional (2D) 360° scanning plane, oriented perpendicular to the catheter shaft. To adjust the imaging plane, the catheter can be withdrawn or advanced inside the heart. To prepare the catheter for use, the system has to be filled with 3–5 mL of sterile water and connected to a dedicated ultrasound machine (iLab System, Boston Scientific).

The electronic system uses an 8-, 9-, or 10-Fr ultrasound catheter equipped with a 64-element phased array transducer located at its tip (ACUSON Acunav, Siemens Medical Solutions, Mountain View, CA; and ViewFlex, St. Jude Medical, West Berlin, NJ) that generates a 90° wedge-shaped, 2D scanning plane oriented parallel to the catheter shaft. The high-resolution transducer can be used at multiple frequencies (5–10 MHz), thereby allowing depth control and enhancement of tissue penetration to a maximum of 15 cm.

The flexible catheter can be rotated around its axis, and the tip of the catheter can be deflected by manipulating the steering mechanism at the handle of the catheter. The flexibility and maneuverability of the catheter enable the operator to position it inside the RV or coronary sinus. In this way, additional views can be obtained that cannot be acquired from the RA. The phased array catheter is connected to a dedicated ultrasound machine (Sequoia, Cypress, CV70, Siemens Medical Solutions; and ViewMate1, St. Jude Medical).

Several important differences between the two ICE technologies exist. The phased-array catheter allows adjustment of the ultrasound frequency, thereby enabling depth control. Furthermore, the phased array catheter has Doppler capabilities, allowing measurement of hemodynamic and physiological variables, and has superior flexibility compared with the rotational catheter. The advantages of rotational ICE include a 360° scanning plane instead of 90° and considerably lower costs.

Recently, 3D ICE has been introduced. At present, the AcuNav V (Siemens Medical Solutions, Mountain View, CA) is the only commercially available system. It is a phased array technology incorporated in a 10-Fr catheter, providing 22 × 90° real-time volume images. These real-time 3D images may be of particular value for spatial alignment of catheters/devices and cardiac structures (e.g., interatrial septum). However, the relatively small 3D rendered volume is currently the major limitation of this technique. To date, there is only limited clinical experience to guide interventional procedures with this new technology.[1]

In daily clinical practice, phased array ICE is the most commonly used technology in the cardiac catheterization laboratory. The focus of this chapter is on phased array ICE; mechanical intravascular ultrasound is reviewed in Chapter 28.

FUNDAMENTALS

ICE can be used to visualize nearly all cardiac structures.[2] However, unlike transthoracic echocardiography (TTE) and TEE, there are no widely accepted standard views for ICE. In the following paragraphs, a clinically-oriented guide for catheter manipulation and visualization of the various cardiac structures is provided.

ICE is generally performed under conscious sedation. Using local anesthesia and a femoral vein approach, the ultrasound catheter is inserted through the inferior vena cava (IVC) into the right atrium (RA). While standing at the right side of the patient, the operator can change the orientation of the ultrasound beam by advancing or withdrawing the catheter and by rotating it around its axis. In this chapter, rotation of the ultrasound catheter away from the operator is called clockwise rotation, whereas rotation toward the operator is referred to as counterclockwise rotation. The orientation of the ultrasound beam can also be altered by deflecting the tip of the ultrasound catheter in two orthogonal planes (anterior–posterior, left–right) through manipulation of the two steering knobs at the handle of the catheter.

Even though images acquired with ICE are quite similar to TEE, the large freedom of ultrasound beam orientation can easily cause a sense of disorientation to the inexperienced operator. To gain or regain orientation, a "home view" position is defined and can be used as the starting point for all catheter manipulations. In this chapter, home view position is used as the starting point from which all catheter manipulations are described. To reach this position, the ultrasound catheter is positioned in the mid-RA with the control knobs in a neutral position. The resulting image shows the RA, tricuspid valve, and RV (Figure 40.1a). The operator can use these and other anatomical landmarks to maintain orientation during catheter manipulation. To further improve the operator's orientation, a marker is present on the ultrasound screen corresponding to the inferior portion of the ultrasound beam.

Right-sided structures

Starting from the home view position and slightly withdrawing the catheter into the inferior RA, the Eustachian ridge can be visualized (Figure 40.1b). The tissue between the Eustachian ridge and the tricuspid valve is known as the cavotricuspid isthmus and is targeted during catheter ablation for atrial flutter. By advancing the catheter back into the home view position and rotating it counterclockwise, the crista terminalis and right atrial appendage (RAA) are visualized. Clockwise rotation will first bring back the home view and will then reveal the right ventricular outflow tract, the pulmonary artery (PA), and the ascending aorta.

Left-sided structures

Clockwise rotation of the ultrasound catheter from the home view position, past the RV and right ventricular outflow tract, provides a view on the left atrium (LA), mitral valve (MV), the interatrial septum, and the coronary sinus (Figure 40.1c). By gently deflecting the catheter tip in the left direction, the left atrial appendage (LAA) can be seen (Figure 40.2a). From this view, clockwise rotation will reveal the left-sided pulmonary veins (Figure 40.2b). The left inferior pulmonary vein is visualized at the inferior portion of the ultrasound beam and the left superior pulmonary vein at the superior portion. In case of difficulty distinguishing between the left superior pulmonary vein and the LAA, Doppler flow measurements can be used to differentiate between the two structures. When further rotating clockwise, the posterior left atrial wall and the esophagus can be visualized (Figure 40.2c). Eventually, continued clockwise rotation will provide a cross-sectional view of the right-sided pulmonary veins and the right PA (Figure 40.2d). Similar to the left pulmonary veins, the right inferior pulmonary vein is visualized at the inferior portion of the ultrasound beam and the right superior pulmonary vein at the superior portion.

To acquire a long axis view of the left ventricle (LV) and MV from the home view, the catheter is withdrawn slightly

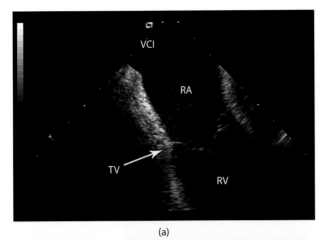

(a)

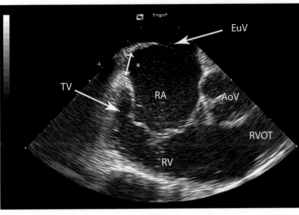

(b)

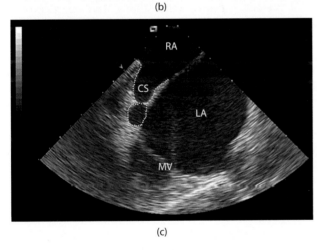

(c)

Figure 40.1 **(a)** Home view position: RA, RV, TV, and VCI; **(b)** AoV, cavotricuspid isthmus (*). EuV, and RVOT; **(c)** interatrial septum, LA, CS, and MV. AoV, aortic valve; CS, coronary sinus; EuV, Eustachian ridge/valve; LA, left atrium; MV, mitral valve; RA, right atrium; RV, right ventricle; RVOT, right ventricular outflow tract; TV, tricuspid valve; VCI, vena cava inferior.

into the inferior RA and the tip of the catheter is deflected in the anterior direction. By advancing the catheter through the tricuspid valve into the RV and rotating the catheter clockwise, the interventricular septum and LV appear (Figure 40.3a). This long axis view can be very useful to

detect pericardial effusion during interventional procedures (Figure 40.4). From the long axis view, a short axis view of the LV can be acquired by deflecting the tip of the catheter in the left or right direction (Figure 40.3b). Advancing or withdrawing the catheter will result in more apical or basal short axis views (Figure 40.3c).

INDICATIONS AND CLINICAL APPLICATIONS

ICE can be used in a wide variety of interventional procedures. These procedures are summarized in Table 40.1 and are reviewed in the following paragraphs.

Detection of intracardiac thrombus

Patients undergoing a left-sided interventional procedure are at high risk for systemic embolism.[3,4] ICE can facilitate a safe left-sided procedure by excluding intracardiac thrombus inside the LAA, LA, and LV.[5] Furthermore, ICE can be used to assess the presence of spontaneous contrast, thereby identifying patients at high risk for thrombus formation.[6] During left-sided procedures, ICE can help to detect the formation of thrombi at an early phase and allow for treatment (e.g., by increasing the dose of anticoagulant) prior to the occurrence of embolic events.[7,8]

The efficacy of TEE to detect intracardiac thrombus has been established by the Assessment of Cardioversion Using Transesophageal Echocardiography (ACUTE) trial.[9] Even though ICE provides high-quality images comparable to TEE, only a few studies have compared the sensitivity of the two imaging modalities for the detection of intracardiac thrombus. The Intracardiac Echocardiography-Guided Cardioversion to Help Interventional Procedures (ICE-CHIP) study was designed to address this issue.[10] In 95 patients with atrial fibrillation (AF) undergoing an invasive catheterization procedure (electrophysiological study, right or LAA), the interatrial septum, LA, and LAA were visualized with ICE and TEE. Primary endpoints included assessment of the presence of thrombus or spontaneous echo contrast in the LA or LAA and the presence of a patent foramen ovale (PFO), atrial septal defect (ASD), and septal aneurysm with both techniques. Although the LA could be visualized well with both techniques in 96% of the patients, there was concordance of complete imaging of the LAA with both TEE and ICE in only 85% of the patients. Spontaneous contrast of the LA was seen in 50% of the patients on ICE and in 56% on TEE, whereas spontaneous contrast of the LAA was seen in 24% on ICE and in 36% on TEE. A thrombus in the LAA was more frequently detected with TEE as compared with ICE, with concordance of both imaging techniques in only 92% of the patients.[11]

The sensitivity of ICE to detect thrombus in the LAA improves when imaging is performed from a different

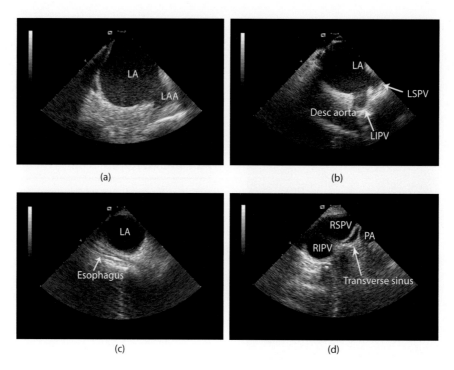

Figure 40.2 **(a)** LA and LAA; **(b)** descending aorta (Desc Aorta), LA, LSPV, and LIPV; **(c)** esophagus and posterior LA wall; and **(d)** PA, RIPV, RSPV, and transverse sinus. LA, left atrium; LAA, left atrial appendage; LIPV, left inferior pulmonary vein; LSPV, left superior pulmonary vein; PA, pulmonary artery; RIPV, right inferior pulmonary vein; RSPV, right superior pulmonary vein.

position than the RA. In 74 patients undergoing catheter ablation for AF, the LAA could be well visualized with ICE from the PA in 88% of the patients. The best agreement between ICE and TEE for the detection of LAA thrombus was noted when ICE imaging was performed from the PA.[12]

Transseptal puncture

A transseptal puncture provides antegrade access to the LA and LV during left-sided interventional procedures as an alternative to a retrograde approach through the aortic valve and MV. However, a transseptal puncture can result in serious complications, such as aortic perforation, pericardial tamponade, and perforation of the IVC.[13] The fossa ovalis is considered to be the safest site to perform a transseptal puncture to avoid these complications, although procedures such as percutaneous treatment of the MV may require an alternative puncture site within the septum. ICE allows excellent visualization of the fossa ovalis and can be used to detect a PFO or monitor the transseptal puncture.[14] A recent study demonstrated the feasibility of transseptal puncture in patients with previously repaired or scarred interatrial septum (e.g., after multiple transseptal punctures). ICE was used to guide the transseptal puncture successfully in 251 patients undergoing catheter ablation for AF. In particular, ICE allows the identification of the thinnest part of the interatrial septum (target region) and/or the relation of the puncture needle with occlusion device.[15]

At present, no prospective studies have addressed the question of whether ICE may improve the safety of transseptal punctures. To visualize the interatrial septum, the catheter is gently rotated clockwise from the home view position. The interatrial septum consists of a thicker part (limbus) and a thinner part (fossa ovalis) (Figure 40.5a). To detect a PFO, saline/contrast is injected through the femoral vein inside the RA, and the patient is instructed to perform the Valsalva maneuver (Figure 40.6a). In the presence of a patent foramen, the contrast will cross the interatrial septum into the LA (Figure 40.6b). In the absence of a PFO, a transseptal sheath with a concealed Brockenbrough transseptal needle is inserted through the femoral vein inside the RA. Using fluoroscopy and ICE, the transseptal sheath is positioned against the fossa ovalis. In case of a stable position of the sheath against the fossa ovalis, a "tenting" phenomenon can be seen on ICE (Figure 40.5b). The transseptal puncture can then be performed by pushing the needle out from the sheath through the fossa ovalis. Successful transseptal puncture can be confirmed on ICE by injecting saline/contrast through the needle inside the LA.

Closure of atrial septal defect

Percutaneous transcatheter device closure of ASD and PFO has proven to be a safe and effective alternative to open heart surgery, as detailed in Chapter 46.[16,17] While percutaneous closure of PFO may be performed under fluoroscopy guidance only, closing procedures

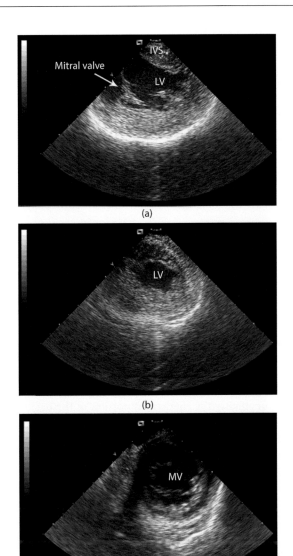

(a)

(b)

(c)

Figure 40.3 **(a)** Long axis view of the LV, IVS, and MV; **(b)** short axis view at the apical level; and **(c)** short axis view at the basal level. IVS, interventricular septum; LV, left ventricle; MV, mitral valve.

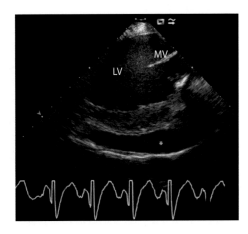

Figure 40.4 Pericardial effusion. The long-axis view of the LV shows the presence of significant pericardial effusion (*) along the posterior wall. Abbreviations: LV, left ventricle; MV, mitral valve.

Table 40.1 Applications of intracardiac echocardiography during interventional and electrophysiological procedures

- Detection of intracardiac thrombus
- Closure of patent foramen ovale or atrial septal defect
- Transseptal puncture
- Electrophysiological procedures
  - Atrial fibrillation ablation
  - Complex atrial flutter ablation
  - Ventricular tachycardia ablation
  - Left ventricular lead placement in cardiac resynchronization therapy
- Other interventional procedures
  - Biopsy of an intracardiac tumor
  - Left atrial appendage closure
  - Closure of ventricular septal defect
  - Alcohol septum ablation in hypertrophic obstructive cardiomyopathy
  - Mitral valve balloon valvuloplasty
  - Percutaneous valve procedures

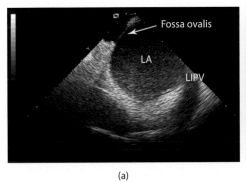

(a)

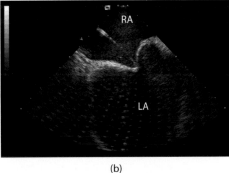

(b)

Figure 40.5 **(a)** Fossa ovalis, LA, and LIPV; and **(b)** tenting of the transseptal sheath against the fossa ovalis. LA, left atrium; LIPV, left inferior pulmonary vein; RA, right atrium.

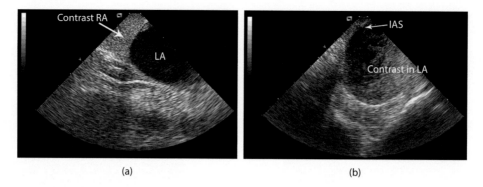

Figure 40.6 **(a)** Contrast inside the RA during Valsalva in a patient with a closed foramen ovale. **(b)** Contrast crosses the IAS from the RA to the LA during Valsalva in a patient with a patent foramen ovale. IAS, interatrial septum; LA, left atrium; RA, right atrium.

of ASDs are typically guided by TEE and fluoroscopy. However, ICE does not require general anesthesia and may provide similar images as TEE.[18,19] It has been shown that the use of ICE during transcatheter device closure may result in a reduction of fluoroscopy time (from 9.5 ± 1.6 vs. 6 ± 1.7 min, $P < 0.0001$) and procedure length (37.8 ± 5.6 vs. 33.4 ± 4.7 min, $P < 0.01$) compared with TEE-guided interventions.[18] Importantly, the high cost of an ICE catheter may be balanced by the need for general anesthesia during TEE-guided procedures.[20]

To guide the placement of a transcatheter closure device, the ultrasound catheter is positioned in the home view position and is rotated clockwise to visualize the interatrial septum and fossa ovalis (Figures 40.7a through c).

By using Doppler capacities, the flow between the LA and RA can be visualized and quantified (Figure 40.7d). A guiding wire is then placed through the ASD and inside the LA. Subsequently, the catheter that contains the closure device is advanced through the ASD and the left-sided portion of the occluder is deployed. After this step, the position of the device against the interatrial septum is carefully evaluated before deploying the right-sided portion of the occluder to avoid malposition and the associated risk of migration of the device (Figure 40.8a). Once the operator is convinced that the position is correct, the right-sided portion of the occluder is deployed (Figure 40.8b). Once again the position and the stability of the device are checked and then the occluder is released.

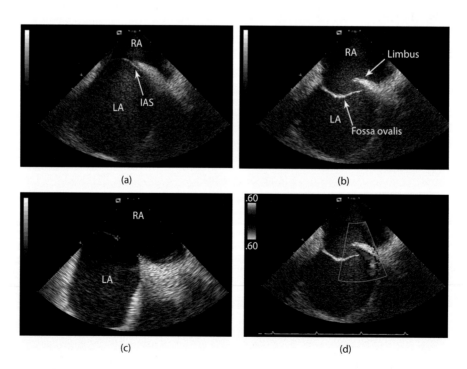

Figure 40.7 **(a)** IAS, LA, and RA. **(b)** During a Valsalva maneuver, the PFO is revealed. **(c)** A large type II atrial septal defect (*two markers*). **(d)** Doppler flow delineates the flow across PFO during a Valsalva maneuver. IAS, interatrial septum; LA, left atrium; PFO, patent foramen ovale; RA, right atrium.

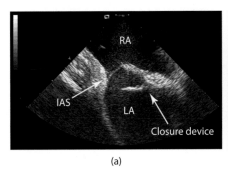 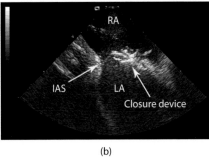

(a)   (b)

Figure 40.8 **(a)** A closure device is inserted across the IAS inside LA. Subsequently, the left-sided occluder is deployed. **(b)** After confirmation of the position of the device, the right-sided occluder is also deployed. IAS, interatrial septum; LA, left atrium; RA, right atrium.

Electrophysiological procedures

ICE has become an important imaging tool during electrophysiological procedures. In addition to thrombus detection and guidance of a transseptal puncture, ICE can be used to identify key anatomical structures to facilitate complex procedures like AF ablation and atrial flutter ablation.[21-23] ICE can visualize the exact location of the mapping catheter and confirm stable contact of the catheter against the myocardium. Moreover, ICE can be used to visualize morphological changes in the myocardium, such as increased echo density, wall thickening, and crater formation as a sign of effective lesion formation[24] and the development of microbubbles as a sign of radiofrequency energy delivered.[25] In the following paragraphs, the specific role of ICE in various electrophysiological procedures is reviewed.

ATRIAL FIBRILLATION ABLATION

Radiofrequency catheter ablation targeting the pulmonary veins is a potential curative treatment option for patients with drug-refractory AF.[26] However, it is associated with long procedure times and a small risk for severe complications, including pulmonary vein stenosis, systemic embolism, cardiac tamponade, and esophagus injury.[3] ICE can facilitate these complex procedures by visualization of the pulmonary veins and monitoring of the location of the ablation catheter and may help in avoiding complications by visualization of the esophagus and other important surrounding structures.[23,25,27] A recent study in 11,525 patients demonstrated that the use of ICE during the ablation procedure was associated with lower repeat ablation rates at 6 months (5.7% vs. 8.5%, adjusted HR 0.68 (95% CI 0.57–0.82), $P < 0.001$), but also with a higher risk of severe bleeding (1.1% vs. 0.7%, adjusted HR 1.78 [95% CI 1.11–2.83], $P = 0.02$).[28]

Several studies have shown that pulmonary vein anatomy is highly variable.[29,30] Application of radiofrequency current inside a pulmonary vein ostium may cause pulmonary vein stenosis and pulmonary hypertension.[31] Accurate visualization of the pulmonary vein region is therefore of utmost importance to safely and effectively perform catheter ablation. A head-to-head comparison between ICE

and multislice computed tomography (MSCT) demonstrated that ICE enables accurate assessment of pulmonary vein anatomy and mean ostial diameters (ICE 1.51 ± 0.22 vs. MSCT 1.45 ± 0.29 mm, P = NS). However, fewer additional pulmonary veins were detected using ICE, as compared with MSCT (ICE 2 = 8% vs. MSCT 5 = 21%).[32] This was confirmed by Jongbloed et al. who detected fewer additional pulmonary veins with ICE, as compared with MSCT (ICE 7 = 17% vs. MSCT 13 = 32%).[29] In addition, an underestimation of the ostial diameter on ICE compared with the ostial diameter in superior–inferior direction on MSCT was noted (14.9 ± 4 vs. 18.4 ± 3.4 mm, $P < 0.01$).[29] This finding suggests the need for 3D imaging to accurately visualize the shape and dimensions of the pulmonary vein ostia. Nevertheless, in a group of 259 patients, Marrouche et al. demonstrated that anatomical guidance of radiofrequency catheter ablation with ICE is both safe and effective.[25] Importantly, the use of ICE in addition to a circular catheter resulted in an improved outcome compared with a circular catheter alone.[25]

The esophagus and left atrial posterior wall are very closely related. With the use of ICE, Ren and colleagues demonstrated that the mean distance between the left atrial posterior wall and the esophagus was 5.8 ± 1.2 mm (range 3.2–10.1 mm) and that the left atrial posterior wall and the esophagus were contiguous over a mean length of 36 ± 7.7 mm (range 18–59 mm).[27] As a consequence, the temperature inside the esophagus may increase significantly during left atrial ablation.[33] Heating of the esophagus can result in esophageal injury varying from transient erythematous changes to tissue necrosis and the development of an atrioesophageal fistula.[27,34,35] While monitoring the relation between the esophagus and the ablation catheter with ICE, the ablation power and duration can be adjusted to reduce esophageal damage.[27] Monitoring lesion development and the occurrence of microbubbles as an indication of an increased esophageal temperature allows the operator to perform additional energy titration, thereby further minimizing the risk of esophageal damage.[27,33] As an alternative to anatomical guidance with ICE, image integration with MSCT or magnetic resonance imaging (MRI) is commonly used to guide radiofrequency catheter ablation for AF.[36] A 3D image of the LA can be integrated with an electroanatomical map by performing a semiautomatic registration process. However, the validity of this technique is largely dependent on the quality of the registration.[37] An inaccurate registration process can result in a large shift of landmark points of up to 5–10 mm, thereby compromising the safety and efficiency of lesion placement. Adjunctive real-time imaging with ICE can be used to confirm the accuracy of the registration process to ensure an accurate delivery of radiofrequency energy.[37]

An electroanatomical mapping system (CARTO-SOUND, Biosense Webster, Diamond Bar, CA) allows integration of ICE and electroanatomical mapping.[38] By integrating ICE and electroanatomical mapping, an accurate 3D anatomical shell of the LA and pulmonary veins can be acquired without performing a registration process.[39] A modified phased array ultrasound catheter with an embedded navigation sensor at its tip (Soundstar, Biosense Webster) is positioned inside the RA. The mapping system can detect the position and direction of the ICE catheter, thereby enabling the projection of the scanning plane inside its 3D environment. By gently rotating the ultrasound catheter, electrocardiographic (ECG)–gated images of the LA and pulmonary veins are acquired. On each image, the endocardial borders (contours) are traced manually and are thereafter assigned to a designated map (Figure 40.9a). Separate maps are created for the left atrial body and each of the pulmonary veins. All contours within a map are used to create a 3D shell of the structure (Figure 40.9b). By combining all maps, the 3D geometry of the whole LA and pulmonary veins is visualized and can be merged with a MSCT image to facilitate the ablation procedure (Figure 40.9c). Recently, it has been demonstrated that the use of image integration with ICE and MSCT results in a reduction of total X-ray time (65 ± 18 vs. 51 ± 12 min; $P = 0.001$), via a reduction in both mapping time and remaining procedure X-ray time when compared with the use of electroanatomical mapping alone.[40]

COMPLEX ATRIAL FLUTTER ABLATION

A common atrial flutter is an organized tachycardia with a reentry circuit inside the RA and a protected isthmus between the tricuspid valve and the IVC (cavo-tricuspid isthmus).[22] Ablation of a common flutter is performed by creating a linear line of block across the cavotricuspid isthmus. Even though it is considered unnecessary to use special imaging or mapping during a standard procedure, during complex cases ICE may be used to facilitate the procedure.[21] ICE can identify the cavotricuspid isthmus and other anatomical structures that can act as electrical barriers during atrial flutter, like the crista terminalis and Eustachian ridge.[22] Ablation of an atrial flutter can be complicated by complex anatomy, for example, in patients with previous surgery for congenital heart disease. Particularly in these patients, ICE can facilitate the ablation procedure by visualizing important anatomical structures and guiding catheter placement.[41]

VENTRICULAR TACHYCARDIA ABLATION

Ablation of ventricular tachycardia is usually limited to inducible and tolerated arrhythmias.[42,43] Techniques to identify the arrhythmogenic substrate without inducing the tachycardia are being developed to treat patients who do not meet these criteria. ICE allows identification of akinetic and dyskinetic (aneurysmatic) myocardial segments in patients with ischemic ventricular tachycardia, thereby visualizing the exact location and extent of the substrate in relation to the ablation catheter during the procedure.[44,45] Furthermore, ICE can be used to visualize small aneurysms of the RV in patients with suspected arrhythmogenic right ventricular dysplasia, thereby detecting the arrhythmogenic substrate in these patients.[44]

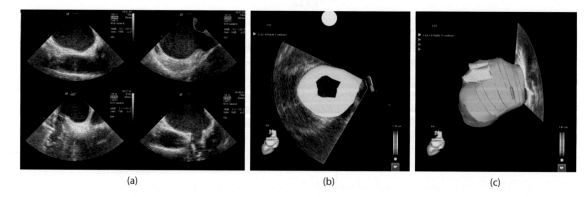

(a)   (b)   (c)

Figure 40.9 **(a)** After acquisition of an electrocardiogram-gated ultrasound image, the endocardial contours (*green*) of the LA and pulmonary veins are manually traced and are thereafter assigned to a corresponding map. **(b)** By systematically collecting images of the whole LA and marking the endocardial borders, a registered 3D reconstruction of the LA anatomy is created. **(c)** The acquired 3D geometry can be used to guide radiofrequency catheter ablation for atrial fibrillation. LA, left atrium.

Recently, the feasibility of the integration of ICE and electroanatomical mapping to guide ischemic ventricular tachycardia ablation was demonstrated.[46] By creating a 3D geometry of the LV and marking the akinetic and dyskinetic segments as seen on ICE, the ischemic substrate could be mapped and the ablation procedure could be performed successfully.

LEFT VENTRICULAR LEAD PLACEMENT IN CARDIAC RESYNCHRONIZATION THERAPY

Cardiac resynchronization therapy (CRT) has a beneficial effect on clinical symptoms, exercise capacity, and left ventricular systolic function in selected patients with drug-refractory heart failure.[47] Moreover, CRT is associated with increased survival and a reduction in the number of rehospitalizations for heart failure, as compared with optimal medical treatment.[48] However, implantation of a CRT device—usually performed under fluoroscopic and angiographic guidance—can be challenging because of venous anatomy, resulting in a failure to place the left ventricular pacing lead in up to 8% of patients.[47,48] A number of case studies report on the use of ICE to visualize the coronary sinus to guide left ventricular lead placement.[49,50] In addition, ICE may be useful to identify optimal left ventricular lead position (optimal resynchronization) during the procedure with the use of vector velocity imaging.[51]

Other interventional procedures

BIOPSY OF INTRACARDIAC MASSES

ICE can be used to visualize the origin and extent of an intracardiac mass (Figure 40.10a). Therefore, ICE may be used to guide biopsies (Figure 40.10b) and to monitor associated complications, such as perforation or bleeding, as suggested by few preliminary reports.[52–54]

LEFT ATRIAL APPENDAGE CLOSURE

Implantation of a LAA occlusion device has been advocated as strategy to reduce the risk for systemic embolism in patients with atrial fibrillation and contraindications for anticoagulation, and the procedure is typically guided by TEE. In a small group of patients, the feasibility of ICE guidance as an alternative to TEE was reported.[55] ICE provided similar visualization of the LAA and similar assessment of the LAA orifice diameter compared with TEE (ICE 22.6 ± 3.4 vs. TEE 19.5 ± 1.5 mm, P = NS). Importantly, the degree of accuracy with respect to exclusion of a thrombus inside the LAA, the exact positioning of the delivery sheath, and verification of the location and stability of the occlusion device using ICE were comparable to TEE. A more recent study in 121 patients confirmed the ability of ICE to accurately guide the implantation of the Amplatzer device, and demonstrated agreement of ICE, TEE, and angiography for assessment of LAA diameters.[56] ICE, like TEE, allows for detection of LAA thrombus (which would contraindicate closure) as well as early recognition of procedure-related complications, notably pericardial effusion.

PERCUTANEOUS VALVE PROCEDURES

In recent years, percutaneous valve procedures have become an alternative for conventional surgery in high-risk patients with selected symptomatic valvular heart conditions. In general, these procedures are guided by fluoroscopy and/or TEE. However, the need for general anesthesia and the interference of the TEE probe with fluoroscopic views may be important limitations of TEE during the procedure. ICE may provide the essential anatomical and functional information needed to guide percutaneous valve procedures.[57] This imaging modality can be used to determine the appropriate size (annular sizing) and site of deployment of the percutaneous valve as well as to monitor the anatomical and functional result of the procedure.[58]

For transcatheter aortic valve implantation, a number of recent studies have demonstrated the feasibility of ICE to guide the implantation procedure.[59–62] An example of a transcatheter aortic valve implantation guided by ICE is shown in Figure 40.11. Bartel et al. randomized 50 patients undergoing transcatheter aortic valve implantation to either ICE or TEE guidance of the procedure.[59] It was demonstrated that ICE provided comparable images

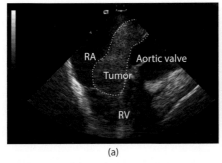
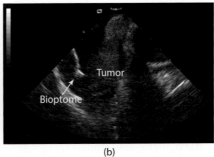

(a)   (b)

Figure 40.10 **(a)** An intracardiac mass originating from the superior vena cava is extending into the RA and tricuspid valve. **(b)** Intracardiac echocardiography is used to monitor and guide the biopsy by visualizing both tumor and bioptome. RA, right atrium; RV, right ventricle.

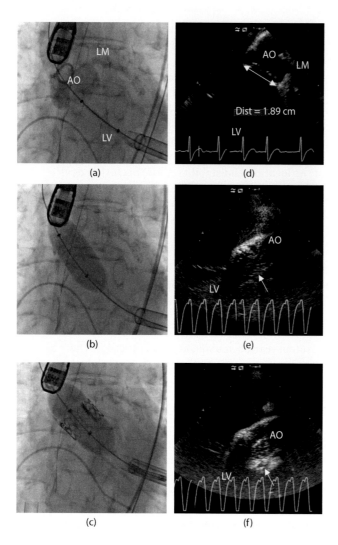

Figure 40.11 Transcatheter aortic valve implantation. Example of transapical aortic valve implantation guided by fluoroscopy (**a** through **c**) and intracardiac echocardiography (**d** through **f**). **(a)** The angiography of the aortic root and the left main coronary artery. The ICE view on **(d)** mimics the angiographic view. The aortic annulus is measured in this view (*double arrowhead*). **(b** and **e)** The ballooning of the aortic valve (*arrow*) under rapid right ventricular pacing. **(c** and **f)** The deployment of the balloon expandable bioprosthesis (*arrow*). Ao, aorta; LM, left main coronary artery; LV, left ventricle.

of the ascending aorta and coronary ostia, with less need for repositioning of the probe, as compared with TEE. Importantly, it has been demonstrated that the use of ICE during transcatheter aortic valve implantation may reduce the amount of contrast agent that is used during the procedure.[60] Recently, the feasibility of 3D ICE to guide transcatheter aortic valve implantation has been demonstrated.[61] For assessment of valve positioning and (para) valvular regurgitation, 3D ICE provided similar images as compared with 2D and 3D TEE. However, the use of ICE during these procedures is limited by higher cost, possible interference of the probe with the temporary pacemaker lead needed for rapid pacing, and the need for a second

venous sheath. Therefore, more studies are needed to define the role of ICE during percutaneous aortic valve implantation procedures.

Percutaneous balloon valvuloplasty is an accepted alternative to surgical commissurotomy in selected patients with symptomatic mitral stenosis. In this setting, ICE can be used to exclude thrombus formation at the level of the LA, assess the morphology and function of the MV, guide the transseptal puncture, monitor the positioning of the balloon, and assess any residual valvular gradient or postprocedural mitral regurgitation.[63] In addition, it may allow an early detection of complications, such as cardiac tamponade. An example of mitral balloon valvuloplasty guided by ICE is shown in Figure 40.12a through f. A recent study reported the feasibility of ICE to guide percutaneous mitral commissurotomy in 20 consecutive patients.[64] ICE enabled exclusion of LAA thrombus and guidance of the procedure without the need for general anesthesia or a separate TEE procedure.

In selected patients with severe symptomatic mitral regurgitation, percutaneous edge-to-edge repair using the MitraClip system may be an alternative to conventional MV repair.[65] Recently, the use of 2D ICE to guide percutaneous MitraClip implantation has been reported.[66] Although of potential interest, the exact value of ICE to guide MitraClip procedures needs to be elucidated in future studies.

ALCOHOL ABLATION IN HYPERTROPHIC OBSTRUCTIVE CARDIOMYOPATHY

Alcohol septal ablation is an effective treatment to reduce the intraventricular gradient in patients with hypertrophic obstructive cardiomyopathy.[67] However, the efficacy and safety of the procedure is dependent on the identification of the correct septal artery. To identify this branch, echo contrast is commonly injected into a septal artery at the time of coronary angiography, and TTE is used to detect the extent and localization of the corresponding myocardial territory. ICE allows high-quality visualization of the entire interventricular septum and may be a useful tool to guide alcohol septal ablation.[68] Recently, it has been demonstrated that the use of image integration of ICE and electroanatomical mapping may facilitate a radiofrequency ablation procedure of the interventricular septum to treat hypertrophic obstructive cardiomyopathy.[69] However, more studies are needed to define the role of ICE in alcohol septal ablation or radiofrequency ablation in patients with hypertrophic obstructive cardiomyopathy.

VENTRICULAR SEPTAL DEFECT CLOSURE

ICE can be used to guide transcatheter closure of a perimembranous ventricular septal defect (VSD).[70] This imaging modality allows identification and visualization of the defect, monitoring of the placement of a guiding wire through the defect, and the deployment of the left-sided occluder. Subsequently, ICE is used to confirm the correct

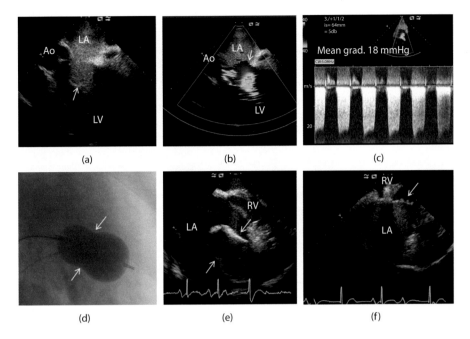

Figure 40.12 Percutaneous mitral valve balloon valvuloplasty guided with intracardiac echocardiography. Example of a 30-year-old patient with rheumatic valve disease and severe mitral stenosis. **(a)** Note the enlarged LA with spontaneous contrast due to severe stenosis of the mitral valve, which shows pliable leaflets (*arrow*). **(b)** Using color Doppler, the turbulent flow through the valve can be observed (*arrow*) and with the continuous wave Doppler recording, the mean gradient can be measured **(c)**. After transseptal puncture, the Inoue catheter is introduced in the LA and advanced through the mitral valve. **(d)** Under fluoroscopy, the balloon is inflated. The arrows show the constriction by the mitral valve. **(e)** The intracardiac echocardiographic view of the balloon valvuloplasty similar to the fluoroscopic view. **(f)** The final result with improved opening of the mitral valve (*arrow*). Ao, aorta; LA, left atrium; LV, left ventricle; RV, right ventricle.

position of the left-sided occluder against the interventricular septum before the deployment of the right-sided occluder. After deployment of the second occluder, ICE can be used to assess any residual shunt and valvular regurgitation that may have resulted from the procedure. In 12 patients, Cao et al. documented that ICE may be used as a safe and effective alternative for TEE to guide closure of a VSD.[70]

INTRAPERICARDIAL USE OF ICE

Positioning the ICE catheter inside the pericardium has the potential to provide valuable information during complex ablation procedures. The safety and feasibility of this approach were suggested in both experimental and clinical settings.[71,72] In 10 patients, endocardial structures could be visualized in great detail from various angles.[71] The ability to visualize cardiac anatomy from different angles could benefit catheter navigation. However, this invasive approach is limited to patients undergoing epicardial access for catheter ablation.

LIMITATIONS

Although phased array ICE enables adjustment of the ultrasound frequency, tissue penetration remains a limiting factor in visualizing cardiac anatomy. Use of a lower ultrasound frequency would result in a higher degree of tissue penetration allowing visualization of structures

further away from the transducer, but at the cost of lower image resolution. In addition, the costs of phased array ICE are relatively high as compared with TEE, and these expensive catheters are for single-use only. However, the cost of ICE is somewhat balanced by the need for general anesthesia and an echocardiographist during TEE. Moreover, ICE provides 2D monoplane images. This limitation can be partially overcome by the flexibility of the catheter, enabling visualization of the same structure from another angle. Nevertheless, operators who are used to multiplane TEE may still have difficulty obtaining the same views. Finally, there are no widely accepted standard views for ICE, in contrast to TEE and TTE. This may be difficult, in particular for the inexperienced operator. Standard manipulation of the ultrasound catheter starting from home view position, as well as recognition of landmark structures, may be helpful.

SPECIAL ISSUES

ICE is an invasive imaging modality, and its use is usually confined to patients undergoing a percutaneous interventional procedure. In general, the contraindications for ICE are similar to other right-sided cardiac catheterization procedures using a transfemoral access. In pediatric patients, the use of ICE is limited by the respective diameters of the femoral vein and the ultrasound catheter.

CONCLUSIONS

ICE is a valuable imaging tool for a wide variety of interventional and electrophysiological procedures. This imaging modality allows real-time visualization of anatomical structures, catheters, and devices, thereby enabling the monitoring and guidance of complex procedures like catheter ablation for AF and placement of a transcatheter closure device for ASDs or VSDs, and more recently, transcatheter heart valve replacement or repair. Since it provides images of quality comparable to TEE, ICE may be used—in the hands of an experienced operator—as an alternative to TEE to guide and monitor these procedures.

REFERENCES

1. Fontes-Carvalho R, et al. Three-dimensional intracardiac echocardiography: A new promising imaging modality to potentially guide cardiovascular interventions. *Eur Heart J Cardiovasc Imaging* 2013;14(10):1028.
2. Packer DL, et al. Intracardiac phased-array imaging: Methods and initial clinical experience with high resolution, under blood visualization: Initial experience with intracardiac phased-array ultrasound. *J Am Coll Cardiol* 2002;39(3):509–516.
3. Cappato R, et al. Updated worldwide survey on the methods, efficacy, and safety of catheter ablation for human atrial fibrillation. *Circ Arrhythm Electrophysiol* 2010;3(1):32–38.
4. Thakur RK, et al. Embolic complications after radiofrequency catheter ablation. *Am J Cardiol* 1994;74(3):278–279.
5. Jongbloed MR, et al. Thrombus in the left atrial appendage detected by intracardiac echocardiography. *Int J Cardiovasc Imaging* 2004;20(2):113–116.
6. Ren JF, et al. Increased intensity of anticoagulation may reduce risk of thrombus during atrial fibrillation ablation procedures in patients with spontaneous echo contrast. *J Cardiovasc Electrophysiol* 2005;16(5):474–477.
7. Keane D, et al. Detection by intracardiac echocardiography of early formation of left atrial thrombus during pulmonary vein isolation. *Europace* 2004;6(2):109–110.
8. Ren JF, et al. Left atrial thrombus associated with ablation for atrial fibrillation: Identification with intracardiac echocardiography. *J Am Coll Cardiol* 2004;43(10):1861–1867.
9. Klein AL, et al. Use of transesophageal echocardiography to guide cardioversion in patients with atrial fibrillation. *N Engl J Med* 2001;344(19):1411–1420.
10. Rao HB, et al. Intra-cardiac echocardiography guided cardioversion to help interventional procedures (ICE-CHIP) study: Study design and methods. *J Interv Card Electrophysiol* 2005;13 Suppl 1:31–36.
11. Saksena S, et al. A prospective comparison of cardiac imaging using intracardiac echocardiography with transesophageal echocardiography in patients with atrial fibrillation: The intracardiac echocardiography guided cardioversion helps interventional procedures study. *Circ Arrhythm Electrophysiol* 2010;3(6):571–577.
12. Baran J, et al. Intracardiac echocardiography for detection of thrombus in the left atrial appendage: Comparison with transesophageal echocardiography in patients undergoing ablation for atrial fibrillation: The Action-Ice I Study. *Circ Arrhythm Electrophysiol* 2013;6(6):1074–1081.
13. B-Lundqvist C, et al. Transseptal left heart catheterization: A review of 278 studies. *Clin Cardiol* 1986;9(1):21–26.
14. Epstein LM, et al. Nonfluoroscopic transseptal catheterization: Safety and efficacy of intracardiac echocardiographic guidance. *J Cardiovasc Electrophysiol* 1998;9(6):625–630.
15. Arkles J, et al. Feasibility of transseptal access in patients with previously scarred or repaired interatrial septum. *J Cardiovasc Electrophysiol* 2015;26(9):963–968.
16. Du ZD, et al. Comparison between transcatheter and surgical closure of secundum atrial septal defect in children and adults: Results of a multicenter nonrandomized trial. *J Am Coll Cardiol* 2002;39(11):1836–1844.
17. Javois AJ, et al. Results of the U.S. Food and Drug Administration continued access clinical trial of the GORE HELEX septal occluder for secundum atrial septal defect. *JACC Cardiovasc Interv* 2014;7(8):905–912.
18. Bartel T, et al. Intracardiac echocardiography is superior to conventional monitoring for guiding device closure of interatrial communications. *Circulation* 2003;107(6):795–797.
19. Mullen MJ, et al. Intracardiac echocardiography guided device closure of atrial septal defects. *J Am Coll Cardiol* 2003;41(2):285–292.
20. Alboliras ET, Hijazi ZM. Comparison of costs of intracardiac echocardiography and transesophageal echocardiography in monitoring percutaneous device closure of atrial septal defect in children and adults. *Am J Cardiol* 2004;94(5):690–692.
21. Morton JB, et al. Phased-array intracardiac echocardiography for defining cavotricuspid isthmus anatomy during radiofrequency ablation of typical atrial flutter. *J Cardiovasc Electrophysiol* 2003;14(6):591–597.
22. Olgin JE, et al. Role of right atrial endocardial structures as barriers to conduction during human type I atrial flutter. Activation and entrainment mapping guided by intracardiac echocardiography. *Circulation* 1995;92(7):1839–1848.
23. Verma A, et al. Pulmonary vein antrum isolation: Intracardiac echocardiography-guided technique. *J Cardiovasc Electrophysiol* 2004;15(11):1335–1340.
24. Ren JF, Marchlinski FE. Utility of intracardiac echocardiography in left heart ablation for tachyarrhythmias. *Echocardiography* 2007;24(5):533–540.
25. Marrouche NF, et al. Phased-array intracardiac echocardiography monitoring during pulmonary vein isolation in patients with atrial fibrillation: Impact on outcome and complications. *Circulation* 2003;107(21):2710–2716.
26. Haissaguerre M, et al. Spontaneous initiation of atrial fibrillation by ectopic beats originating in the pulmonary veins. *N Engl J Med* 1998;339(10):659–666.
27. Ren JF, et al. Esophageal imaging and strategies for avoiding injury during left atrial ablation for atrial fibrillation. *Heart Rhythm* 2006;3(10):1156–1161.
28. Steinberg BA, et al. Periprocedural imaging and outcomes after catheter ablation of atrial fibrillation. *Heart* 2014;100(23):1871–1877.

29. Jongbloed MR, et al. Multislice computed tomography versus intracardiac echocardiography to evaluate the pulmonary veins before radiofrequency catheter ablation of atrial fibrillation: A head-to-head comparison. *J Am Coll Cardiol* 2005;45(3):343–350.

30. Marom EM, et al. Variations in pulmonary venous drainage to the left atrium: Implications for radiofrequency ablation. *Radiology* 2004;230(3):824–829.

31. Robbins IM, et al. Pulmonary vein stenosis after catheter ablation of atrial fibrillation. *Circulation* 1998;98(17):1769–1775.

32. Wood MA, et al. A comparison of pulmonary vein ostial anatomy by computerized tomography, echocardiography, and venography in patients with atrial fibrillation having radiofrequency catheter ablation. *Am J Cardiol* 2004;93(1):49–53.

33. Cummings JE, et al. Assessment of temperature, proximity, and course of the esophagus during radiofrequency ablation within the left atrium. *Circulation* 2005;112(4):459–464.

34. Marrouche NF, et al. Randomized comparison between open irrigation technology and intracardiac-echo-guided energy delivery for pulmonary vein antrum isolation: Procedural parameters, outcomes, and the effect on esophageal injury. *J Cardiovasc Electrophysiol* 2007;18(6):583–588.

35. Pappone C, et al. Atrio-esophageal fistula as a complication of percutaneous transcatheter ablation of atrial fibrillation. *Circulation* 2004;109(22):2724–2726.

36. Tops LF, et al. Fusion of multislice computed tomography imaging with three-dimensional electroanatomic mapping to guide radiofrequency catheter ablation procedures. *Heart Rhythm* 2005;2(10):1076–1081.

37. Daccarett M, et al. Blinded correlation study of three-dimensional electro-anatomical image integration and phased array intra-cardiac echocardiography for left atrial mapping. *Europace* 2007;9(10):923–926.

38. den Uijl DW, et al. Real-time integration of intracardiac echocardiography and multislice computed tomography to guide radiofrequency catheter ablation for atrial fibrillation. *Heart Rhythm* 2008;5(10):1403–1410.

39. Kimura M, et al. Validation of accuracy of three-dimensional left atrial CartoSound and CT image integration: Influence of respiratory phase and cardiac cycle. *J Cardiovasc Electrophysiol* 2013;24(9):1002–1007.

40. Brooks AG, et al. Accuracy and clinical outcomes of CT image integration with Carto-Sound compared to electro-anatomical mapping for atrial fibrillation ablation: A randomized controlled study. *Int J Cardiol* 2013;168(3):2774–2782.

41. Forleo GB, et al. Real-time integration of intracardiac echocardiography and 3D electroanatomical mapping to guide catheter ablation of isthmus-dependent atrial flutter in a patient with complete situs inversus and interruption of the inferior vena cava with azygos continuation. *J Interv Card Electrophysiol* 2011;30(3):273–277.

42. Callans DJ, et al. Efficacy of radiofrequency catheter ablation for ventricular tachycardia in healed myocardial infarction. *Am J Cardiol* 1998;82(4):429–432.

43. Morady F, et al. Radiofrequency catheter ablation of ventricular tachycardia in patients with coronary artery disease. *Circulation* 1993;87(2):363–372.

44. Jongbloed MR, et al. Radiofrequency catheter ablation of ventricular tachycardia guided by intracardiac echocardiography. *Eur J Echocardiogr* 2004;5(1):34–40.

45. Bunch TJ, et al. Image integration using intracardiac ultrasound and 3D reconstruction for scar mapping and ablation of ventricular tachycardia. *J Cardiovasc Electrophysiol* 2010;21(6):678–684.

46. Khaykin Y, et al. Real-time integration of 2D intracardiac echocardiography and 3D electroanatomical mapping to guide ventricular tachycardia ablation. *Heart Rhythm* 2008;5(10):1396–1402.

47. Abraham WT, et al. Cardiac resynchronization in chronic heart failure. *N Engl J Med* 2002;346(24):1845–1853.

48. Cleland JG, et al. The effect of cardiac resynchronization on morbidity and mortality in heart failure. *N Engl J Med* 2005;352(15):1539–1549.

49. Scholten MF, et al. Visualization of a coronary sinus valve using intracardiac echocardiography. *Eur J Echocardiogr* 2004;5(1):93–96.

50. Shalaby AA. Utilization of intracardiac echocardiography to access the coronary sinus for left ventricular lead placement. *Pacing Clin Electrophysiol* 2005;28(6):493–497.

51. Bai R, et al. Positioning of left ventricular pacing lead guided by intracardiac echocardiography with vector velocity imaging during cardiac resynchronization therapy procedure. *J Cardiovasc Electrophysiol* 2011;22(9):1034–1041.

52. Mitchell AR, et al. Intracardiac echocardiography to guide myocardial biopsy of a primary cardiac tumour. *Eur J Echocardiogr* 2007;8(6):505–506.

53. Poommipanit P, Tobis J. Intracardiac echocardiography (ICE)—Guided biopsy of a right atrial mass. *J Invasive Cardiol* 2011;23(5):E99–E101.

54. Azzalini L, et al. Right atrial mass in a patient with breast cancer: Percutaneous transcatheter biopsy under intracardiac echocardiography guidance. *BMJ Case Rep* 2016; 2016:10.

55. Ho IC, et al. Use of intracardiac echocardiography to guide implantation of a left atrial appendage occlusion device (PLAATO). *Heart Rhythm* 2007;4(5):567–571.

56. Berti S, et al. Periprocedural intracardiac echocardiography for left atrial appendage closure: A dual-center experience. *JACC Cardiovasc Interv* 2014;7(9):1036–1044.

57. Bartel T, et al. Intracardiac echocardiography for guidance of transcatheter aortic valve implantation under monitored sedation: A solution to a dilemma? *Eur Heart J Cardiovasc Imaging* 2016;17(1):1–8.

58. Chessa M, et al. Intracardiac echocardiography during percutaneous pulmonary valve replacement. *Eur Heart J* 2008;29(23):2908.

59. Bartel T, et al. Intracardiac echocardiography: A new guiding tool for transcatheter aortic valve replacement. *J Am Soc Echocardiogr* 2011;24(9):966–975.

60. Bartel T, et al. Intracardiac echo and reduced radiocontrast requirements during TAVR. *JACC Cardiovasc Imaging* 2014;7(3):319–320.

61. Kadakia MB, et al. Intracardiac echocardiography-guided transcatheter aortic valve replacement. *Catheter Cardiovasc Interv* 2015;85(3):497–501.

62. Muller S, et al. Intracardiac Doppler echocardiography for monitoring of pulmonary artery pressures in high-risk patients undergoing transcatheter aortic valve replacement. *J Am Soc Echocardiogr* 2016;29(1):83–91.

63. Green NE, et al. Initial clinical experience with intracardiac echocardiography in guiding balloon mitral valvuloplasty: Technique, safety, utility, and limitations. *Catheter Cardiovasc Interv* 2004;63(3):385–394.

64. Saji M, et al. Use of intracardiac echocardiography to guide percutaneous transluminal mitral commissurotomy: A 20-patient case series. *Catheter Cardiovasc Interv* 2016;87(2):E69–E74.

65. Feldman T, et al. Percutaneous repair or surgery for mitral regurgitation. *N Engl J Med* 2011;364(15):1395–406.

66. Patzelt J, et al. Percutaneous mitral valve edge-to-edge repair with simultaneous biatrial intracardiac echocardiography: First-in-human experience. *Circulation* 2016;133(15):1517–1519.

67. Sorajja P, et al. Outcome of alcohol septal ablation for obstructive hypertrophic cardiomyopathy. *Circulation* 2008;118(2):131–139.

68. Alfonso F, et al. Intracardiac echocardiography guidance for alcohol septal ablation in hypertrophic obstructive cardiomyopathy. *J Invasive Cardiol* 2007;19(5):E134–E136.

69. Cooper RM, et al. Radiofrequency ablation of the interventricular septum to treat outflow tract gradients in hypertrophic obstructive cardiomyopathy: A novel use of CARTOSound(R) technology to guide ablation. *Europace* 2016;18(1):113–120.

70. Cao QL, et al. Initial clinical experience with intracardiac echocardiography in guiding transcatheter closure of perimembranous ventricular septal defects: Feasibility and comparison with transesophageal echocardiography. *Catheter Cardiovasc Interv* 2005;66(2):258–267.

71. Horowitz BN, et al. Percutaneous intrapericardial echocardiography during catheter ablation: A feasibility study. *Heart Rhythm* 2006;3(11):1275–1282.

72. Rodrigues AC, et al. Intrapericardial echocardiography: A novel catheter-based approach to cardiac imaging. *J Am Soc Echocardiogr* 2004;17(3):269–274.

41

TEE to guide interventional cardiac procedures in the catheterization laboratory

MATTHIAS GREUTMANN, CHRISTIANE GRUNER, MELLITA MEZODY, AND ERIC HORLICK

INTRODUCTION

Since its development for clinical use more than three decades ago,[1,2] transesophageal echocardiography (TEE) has seen widespread use for diagnostic purposes and has been used to guide many new interventional cardiac procedures. More recently, intracardiac echocardiography (ICE) has emerged as an alternative to TEE for some indications, as detailed in Chapter 40. The wide availability of TEE, its low cost, the long-standing clinical experience with this technique, and its well-documented safety profile, however, have preserved its role as an important tool for many interventional procedures.[3,4]

In this chapter, we discuss the role of TEE for guiding cardiac interventions with a special focus on the most commonly performed procedures and on newer developments, such as three-dimensional (3D) and real-time 3D echocardiography.

General aspects

Periprocedural echocardiographic guidance is most useful for device closure of interatrial or interventricular communications, and TEE guidance is mandatory for interventional repair of the mitral valve.[5]

When used for peri-interventional guidance, echocardiography has four fundamental roles for every single procedure:

1. Confirm the indication and exclude contraindications.
2. Guide the procedure to improve its safety and increase its success rate.
3. Confirm early procedural efficacy.
4. Identify immediate or imminent complications.

The role of TEE before, during, and after various noncoronary cardiac interventions is outlined in Table 41.1. There is a large degree of variability in its use among institutions and individual interventionalists.

Table 41.1   Role of TEE for commonly performed non-coronary cardiac interventions

Procedure	Pre-procedure	During the procedure	Immediate post-procedure	Comments
ASD	+++	+++	+++	3D promising
Baffle leak closure	+++	+	+	
PFO closure	+++	+[a]	+[a]	Not mandatory
VSD closure	+++	++	+	3D potentially helpful
Balloon aortic valve dilatation	++	+	+	Limited use, not mandatory
Aortic valve replacement	+	(+)	++	Often performed without general anesthesia in Europe, many procedures now performed without TEE
Interventional mitral valve repair, e.g. Mitra-Clip	+++	+++	+++	TEE is critical for success
Balloon mitral valvuloplasty	++	+	++	Not mandatory
'Aortic root' interventions (i.e. ruptured Sinus valsalva aneurysms)	+++	+++	+++	
Pulmonary valve interventions	-	-	-	
Transseptal puncture	+	++	+	Enhances safety
Paravalvular leak closure	+++	+++	++	3D echocardiography should be considered mandatory
PDA closure	-	-	-	
Coarctation stenting	-	-	-	

Note: 3D, three dimensional; ASD, atrial septal defect; PDA, patent ductus arteriosus; PFO, patent foramen ovale; TEE, transesophageal echocardiography; VSD, ventricular septal defect.

-, not recommended for routine use, may be helpful in individual cases; +, may be helpful in some instances; ++, very helpful but not mandatory; +++, mandatory / very helpful.

[a] Use of TEE for PFO-closure varies depending on institution.

Transesophageal echocardiography versus intracardiac echocardiography

A detailed discussion of ICE for cardiac interventions is given in Chapter 40. Compared to ICE, which costs many thousands of dollars per procedure, TEE is significantly less expensive. An important advantage of TEE above ICE is the fact that using TEE allows merging of knowledge of the echocardiographer and the interventional cardiologist, which is particularly helpful when starting a structural interventional program. ICE has been shown to lower procedure times and to be equivalent to TEE in terms of procedural success and safety for closure of atrial septal defects (ASDs).[6,7] Its main advantage is improved patient comfort and freedom from general anesthesia. In practical terms, a major advantage of ICE is freedom from additional personnel required to perform a procedure (i.e., a sonographer and an anesthetist), which add substantially to procedural costs. In many centers, the scarcity of anesthetists remains a challenge to schedule TEE-assisted procedures. For this reason, and for patient comfort, in many laboratories ICE has begun to replace TEE for guiding septal closure procedures. In pediatric structural catheterization laboratories, where general anesthesia is the rule, there is little role for ICE and TEE is the preferred modality.

The current generation of ICE probes allows for two-dimensional (2D) and 3D imaging, including color and spectral Doppler techniques, while all modern TEE systems allow multiplane imaging with rapidly evolving technology for 3D imaging. Although ICE allows for high-quality visualization of most cardiac structures, it remains mostly a tool for interventions on the atrial septum, the pulmonary valve, and the aortic root. Interventionalists have also used ICE to close the left atrial appendage (LAA). To date, there is little experience with interventions in other locations within the heart and standardized protocols for its use are lacking. For example, no literature is available about how to quantify valvar regurgitation or stenosis of left-sided valve lesions with ICE.

3D echocardiography and fusion imaging

Experience with 3D and real-time 3D TEE for various procedures has rapidly increased. Software applications and postprocessing of full-volume image acquisitions have markedly improved, allowing for simple and rapid postprocessing. 3D TEE has become the standard for the assessment of the mitral valve and for guiding interventional mitral valve repair.[8-10] 3D imaging improves the interventionalist's perception of the location of the lesion to be treated, which is often lost with omniplane 2D images. The interventionalist can gain an improved appreciation of where wires and catheters are in the 3D space related to the target. By virtue of this improved spatial resolution, 3D imaging has the potential to facilitate procedures in patients with complex cardiac anatomy or complex lesion geometry. Procedural guidance by 3D TEE remains a domain of real-time image acquisition. New generations of ICE probes capable of 3D imaging are also presently commercially available. Hybrid imaging with real-time fusion of different imaging technologies may further improve guidance for complex procedures in the future. To date, only the technology for fusion of echocardiographic images from 3D TEE with images gained from fluoroscopy allows adequate real-time image quality capable of facilitating structural heart interventions. Hybrid or fusion imaging has the potential to improve and facilitate communication between the imager and the interventionalist, reduce procedure time, and has the potential to improve procedural success. Further experience and research are needed, however, to define the role of this novel and promising technique in day-to-day life.[11]

Teamwork and communication

When handling the ICE probe, the interventionalist can immediately adjust views to his or her needs, but maintaining those views when their hands leave the probe is another matter. In contrast, when TEE is used to guide a procedure, clear communication between the echocardiographer and interventionalist is crucial. The echocardiographer should be familiar with the procedure, know the critical steps, and understand what information is relevant to the interventionalist. The echocardiographer should also be familiar with potential complications and should know what to expect and when to look for it. Using TEE for guiding interventions therefore requires optimal teamwork. As interventionalists and echocardiographers often speak in different terms, clear communication is important. In our experience, it is of great advantage to have dedicated interventionalists and echocardiographers who work together frequently. Teams who work well together use both verbal and nonverbal communication to improve procedural efficacy.

In the following sections, the role of TEE for various interventions is outlined, including detailed descriptions of selected critical steps and a summary of key points in the form of a table format checklist for some of the most important and most common interventions.

TRANSESOPHAGEAL ECHOCARDIOGRAPHY FOR DEVICE CLOSURE OF INTERATRIAL COMMUNICATIONS

General aspects

Device closure of interatrial communications is among the most frequently performed noncoronary interventions in the cardiac catheterization laboratory. TEE has evolved as a reliable method for guiding percutaneous closure of ASDs with contemporary devices. Its usefulness for planning and guiding the procedure has been demonstrated in numerous studies.[12,13,14–19] Most procedures are guided by both fluoroscopy and TEE, but even guidance with TEE alone has been shown to be feasible.[20]

The role of 3D echocardiography

Although real-time transthoracic 3D echocardiography has shown to be of increasing value for the characterization of secundum-type ASD,[21] TEE has remained the gold standard. The accuracy of transthoracic studies remains crucially dependent on image quality, being more often than not suboptimal in the adult population. There has been a rapid evolution of 3D TEE technology since the late 1990s. It has been shown to allow visualization of the changing geometry of ASDs throughout the cardiac cycle (Figure 41.1) and allows for better definition of their borders, as well as their relationship to atrioventricular (AV) valves and venous inflows.[22–26] The evolution of real-time 3D-TEE has enhanced its utility to guide procedures in the cardiac catheterization laboratory.[8] The definition of size and quality of tissue rims around the entire circumference of the ASD remains the most important aspect that determines the success and safety of ASD device closure. As tissue rims are often very thin, floppy, and mobile, 2D TEE with its high temporal and spatial resolution remains the gold standard to define tissue rims and is superior to 3D TEE in this regard. 3D TEE may facilitate the assessment of ASDs with complex geometry or multiple defects.

Transesophageal echocardiography for guidance of secundum-type atrial septal defect closure

The technical details of closure of secundum-type ASDs are outlined in Chapter 46. This section covers the role of TEE during these procedures. Due to their ease of use, high procedural success, and low complication rates, double-disc septal devices (e.g., Amplatzer and Occlutech) are currently the most frequently used septal closure devices on the market. The Gore septal occluder is favored by many because of its safety profile. Soon, a Gore device is expected to become available that will allow the closure of much larger defects. Other innovative device designs are available as well. The general principles of device implantation for ASDs are similar for all device designs. In this section we focus on the implantation of double-disc devices.

An overview of the role of TEE for these interventions is given in Table 41.2, followed by a detailed description of critical steps.

PREPROCEDURAL ASSESSMENT

Only defects confined to the oval fossa, secundum, or "true" ASD, without anomalous drainage of pulmonary veins (PVs) have classically been considered amenable to device closure.

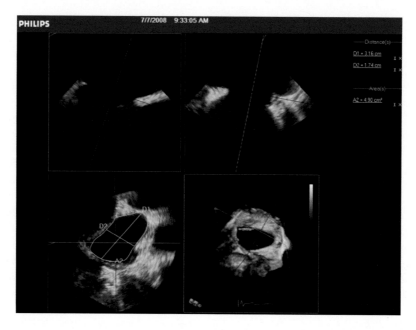

Figure 41.1 Reconstruction of the "true" size and geometry of a secundum atrial septal defect derived from postprocessing of a 3D TEE acquisition (*bottom right*). 3D, three-dimensional; TEE, Transesophageal echocardiography.

Table 41.2   TEE checklist for ASD closure

Preprocedural

✓   Rule out intracardiac thrombus in patients with atrial fibrillation
✓   Assess left ventricular diastolic function and estimate left atrial pressure
✓   Define size, anatomy and location of the defect
✓   Rule out sinus venosus, coronary sinus and primum atrial septal defects
✓   Rule out anomalous pulmonary venous drainage
✓   Assess severity of tricuspid regurgitation and estimate right ventricular systolic pressure
✓   Rule out other congenital or acquired cardiac lesions
✓   Ensure adequate tissue rims towards atrioventricular valves, caval veins and pulmonary veins (at least 5 mm with most Amplatzer® devices)
✓   Assess whether rims appear floppy or firm
✓   Rule out or define multiple defects
✓   Define presence of an atrial septal aneurysm

During the procedure

✓   Confirm position of guidewire and delivery sheath
✓   Confirm position of the sizing balloon and cessation of shunting on color Doppler when the sizing balloon is inflated.
✓   Measurement of balloon 'stop flow' size
✓   Confirm proper alignment of left atrial disc to interatrial septum
✓   Confirm proper grasping of tissue rims between discs of the device (particularly in its infero-posterior aspect)
✓   Ensure permanent pacemaker wires are not entrapped
✓   Confirm absence of entangling in Chiari network
✓   Confirm absence of prolapse of left atrial disc at aortic margin

Postprocedural

✓   Confirm proper position and alignment of the device, rule out device prolapse
✓   Confirm absence of 'rubbing' of the device against the aortic root
✓   Confirm normal function of atrioventricular valves and absence of aortic regurgitation
✓   Confirm unobstructed inflow of caval veins, right pulmonary veins and coronary sinus
✓   Confirm absence of pericardial effusion and signs of tamponade

Note: ASD, atrial septal defect; TEE, transesophageal echocardiography

However, not all patients with anomalous PV drainage are candidates for surgical redirection, and in selected patients, ASD closure, leaving the anomalous PV drainage unrepaired, may still be beneficial in such patients. The determination of the extent of the defect, the demonstration of normal drainage of the four PVs, as well as the exclusion of contraindications to percutaneous closure such as sinus venosus defect, primum ASD, and coronary sinus defect are usually performed during an outpatient preinterventional study; some programs carry out this evaluation during the index procedure. In case of incomplete assessment on those preinterventional studies, a thorough examination at the time of the planned closure procedure is mandatory (Figure 41.2).

The Amplatzer septal occluder is currently available in sizes up to 40 mm, and hence, defects larger than 38–39 mm by balloon sizing are generally not amenable to device closure. Secundum defects can extend in any direction, toward the orifices of the superior or inferior vena cava (IVC) and the coronary sinus, anterosuperior toward the aortic root, and toward the AV valves. Given the design of the double-disc devices, a tissue rim of at least 5 mm toward most of these structures is mandatory for stable device positioning. A partially deficient rim is the rule rather than the exception, and its characterization is important for procedure planning.[27] The vast majority of defects larger than 20 mm in size have an absent aortic rim. Figure 41.3 and Table 41.3 give an overview of the most valuable TEE views to define tissue rims surrounding a defect.[28]

The best angle to identify drainage of PV is highly variable and differs from patient to patient. We usually start by identifying the left upper PV at an angle of 60°–110°. It drains just above the LAA. By gently turning the probe counterclockwise and slightly increasing the angle, the left lower PV is identified. The right upper PV drains into the left atrium (LA) just posterior to the superior vena cava (SVC) and is easy to identify by turning the probe slightly clockwise from a bicaval view. When keeping the right upper PV in view, slowly decrease the plane angle toward about 30°–60° with slight clockwise rotation of the probe until the right lower PV is identified. As an alternative approach, PV can be identified from a 0° angle by gently advancing and withdrawing the probe from a midesophageal view while turning the probe either clockwise or counterclockwise. Fortunately, in the presence of a significant left-to-right shunt across the interatrial septum, PV flow is markedly increased, which helps with identifying these vessels. Finding only one PV entering the LA on one side is not an abnormal finding as PVs are often confluent before entering the LA. About 7% of patients have some abnormality of the PV. However, a high suspicion for the detection of abnormal pulmonary venous drainage needs to be maintained, especially if the dilatation of the right-sided heart chambers is out of proportion to the size of the ASD.

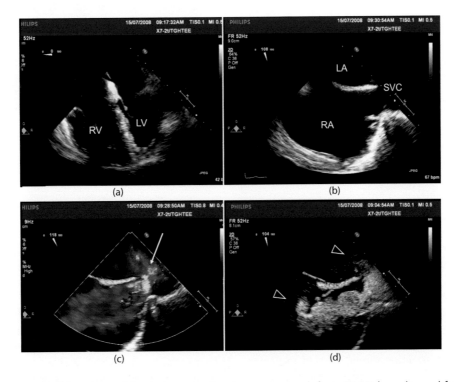

Figure 41.2 Sixty-one-year-old patient with a large superior sinus venosus defect. (a) Midesophageal four-chamber view showing enlarged right-sided heart chambers. (b) Standard bicaval view of interatrial septum does not demonstrate superior sinus venosus defect. (c) Only further withdrawing and slight clockwise rotation of the echo probe shows the large superior sinus venosus defect (*white arrow*). (d) After injection of agitated saline into left antecubital vein, immediate opacification of both atrial chambers from the SVC (*arrowheads*). LA, left atrium; LV, left ventricle; RA, right atrium; RV, right ventricle; SVC, superior vena cava.

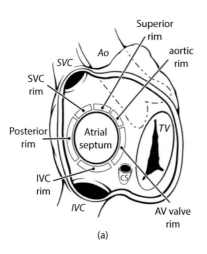
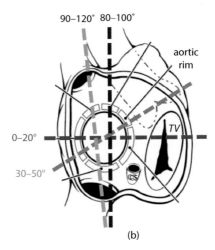

(a)　　　　　　　(b)

Figure 41.3 Classifications of atrial septal rims. **(a)** Classification and nomenclature of atrial septal rims. **(b)** Cross section of the atrial septum with standard TEE angles at midesophageal level. Ao, aorta; AV; atrioventricular; CS, coronary sinus; IVC, inferior vena cava; SVC, superior vena cava; TEE, transesophageal echocardiography; TV, tricuspid valve. (Modified from Amin, Z., *Catheter. Cardiovasc. Interv.*, 68, 778–787, 2006. With permission.)

Table 41.3 Most useful TEE views for visualization of an ASD and its surrounding structures

Structure to visualize	TEE view (may vary in individual patients)
Inferoposterior and supero-posterior (vena cava) rims	80°–120° 'bicaval view'
Posterior rim	Midesophageal 0°–20°
Anterosuperior (aortic) rim	Midesophageal 30°–50°
Rim to AV-valves	0°–40° midesophageal 4-chamber view
Rim to coronary sinus	0° view at esophago-gastric junction

Note: ASD, atrial septal defect; AV, atrioventricular; TEE, transesophageal echocardiography.

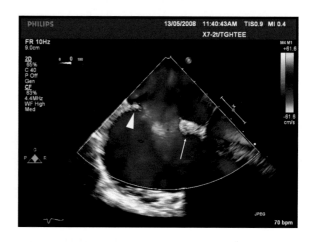

Figure 41.4 Large atrial septal defect II with small posterior tissue rim (arrowhead) and good rim towards the atrioventricular-valve level (arrow).

PROCEDURAL ASPECTS

For device stability, the size of tissue rims is important but also whether they are characterized as firm or pliable. A sufficient inferoposterior rim (Figures 41.3 and 41.4) is crucial for a stable position of the device. In case of insufficient inferoposterior rims, surgical closure may be more appropriate. In the case of an isolated absence of the anterosuperior or aortic rim (Figure 41.5),[29] device closure with stable device position is almost universally possible. As most cases of device erosion occur in patients with deficient anterosuperior rims, particular attention should be paid to device position toward the aortic root in these patients. Given that absent aortic rims are common and device erosion even in these cases is an extremely rare event, the isolated absence of the aortic rim is not regarded as a contraindication for ASD device closure. While there is agreement that impingement/protrusion of either of the discs into the aorta or other adjacent cardiac structures, as well as motion of the device relative to the heart, are detrimental (Figure 41.6), some controversy exists about straddling of the discs around the aortic root.[29,30] In these cases, one should still size to the "stop flow" point, the balloon size at which flow across the septum ceases, and not just to the point where a waist appears on the balloon. The previous strategy, which involved oversizing devices, should be avoided as it may predispose erosion of the roof of the atria and the aorta.[31,32]

There is a trend to avoid balloon sizing of ASDs before device implantation. Defect size is measured on TEE, and device size is then arbitrarily selected 4–5 mm larger. There is little evidence to suggest that this practice is safer than balloon sizing. The compliance of the septum and difficulty in predicting the true size of these defects make this technique unpalatable to many operators who prefer the traditional balloon approach.

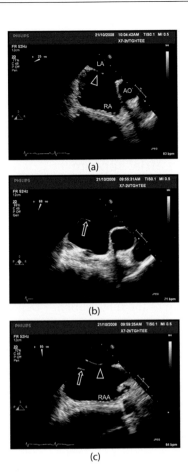

(a)

(b)

(c)

Figure 41.5 (**a** through **c**) Midesophageal TEE views of an anterosuperior-located secundum type ASD with an absent aortic rim at different degree of angulation. The large Eustachian valve (arrow) must not be mistaken for an infero-posterior tissue rim (arrowhead). (**c**) A bicaval view showing the true, in this case large, inferior rim. Ao, aorta; LA, left atrium; RA, right atrium; RAA, right atrial appendage.

To rule out multiple defects, it is crucial to probe the interatrial septum with color Doppler while the sizing balloon is inflated. If residual flow is noted with the balloon inflated, we would advocate for entry of the contralateral femoral vein to balloon size any substantial secondary defect.

The most important task of the echocardiographer during device closure of ASDs is assessment of the deployed device and the detection of imminent complications after implantation, but ideally before release of the device. We spend adequate time verifying tissue margins in multiple views, assessing residual shunting with color Doppler, and confirming the absence of impingement on surrounding structures. It is prudent to be certain of device stability before its release and to reposition or even change to another device size if uncertain. As outlined above, apart from device embolization, the most feared complication is erosion of the roof of the atrium or aorta. One should always have a high level of awareness of a developing pericardial effusion. It is also important to exclude entrapment of a pacemaker wire during device manipulation and the final deployment of a device. Some pacemaker leads may be placed in such a way that it is impossible to avoid wire entrapment, especially with large devices. This is not an absolute contraindication for device placement and may be performed under special circumstances after careful consideration of alternatives—usually it is possible to free an entrapped wire.

Deployment of the left atrial disc in the LAA or against the left atrial wall may result in damage to these structures and should be avoided. Deploying the left atrial disc after rotation has occurred in the delivery system may lead to a deformation of the device, the "cobra head" malformation, which is easily detectable on TEE. Although it is thought that only complete withdrawal of

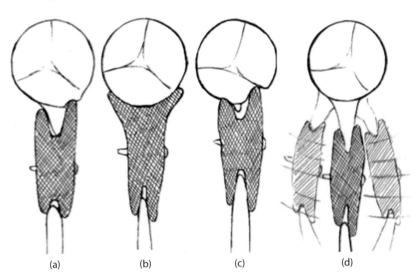

(a)   (b)   (c)   (d)

Figure 41.6 Potential risk factors for device erosion with double-disc devices. (**a**) Intermittent contact of the edges of the disc with the aortic root. (**b**) Splaying of the discs around the aortic root. (**c**) Protrusion of one of the discs into the aortic root or adjacent cardiac structures. (**d**) Mobility of the device, independent of cardiac movement. While there is general agreement that device positions, as outlined in (**a**), (**c**), and (**d**), predispose to device erosion, most experts would recommend device position as in (**b**) for patients with deficient aortic rims. (From Moore, J.W., et al. *JACC Cardiovasc Interv.*, 7, 1430–1436, 2014. With permission.)

the device and manual reshaping outside the body could resolve cobra head malformation,[33] in our experience simply advancing the left atrial disc further into the LA and opening the entire device in that location usually restores normal device configuration.

With large defects, the left atrial disc can become perpendicular to the defect itself, leading to prolapse at the aortic valve margin and preventing proper delivery of the device. This problem is less evident on fluoroscopy but can be easily recognized on TEE. We have found that a second maneuver to resolve aortic disc prolapse includes rotating the delivery system clockwise to the right side of the LA followed by usual deployment, which is often successful. In these cases, the use of a Hausdorf sheath is advocated; however, we have never required one so far in over 1,600 cases. Opening the left atrial disc in the left upper PV and rapidly exposing the right atrial disc works well for devices of more than 34 mm in size. After such a maneuver, confirming good alignment of the device toward the interatrial septum and exclusion of prolapse of the device are important to minimize the risk of subsequent device embolization.

The Gore septal occluder and Helex device have been widely used for the closure of small ASDs, usually less than 18 mm. These devices are easily seen by echo but have a different appearance than the more solid Nitinol mesh devices. Given their flexible and soft nature, they may be particularly useful in defects with partially absent rims when device protrusion into adjacent structures may be a concern. As these devices are not self-centering, careful guiding of optimal and stable device position by echocardiography is of great importance.

There are reports of entanglement of an ASD-closure device in a Chiari network, a complication that should be easily detected on TEE.[34] In our experience, however, this is a rare situation, and avoiding entanglement of pacemaker or implantable cardioverter defibrillator (ICD) leads during insertion of the sheaths and finally, when deploying the device, is of greater clinical importance.

ASSESSMENT POST DEVICE DEPLOYMENT

After deployment of the device, its position, any degree of residual shunting, functional integrity of AV and aortic valves, as well as unhindered systemic and PV inflow, must be documented. Thrombus formation on the left or right atrial disc has become rare with modern devices, proper use of full-dose heparinization, and restriction of the use of protamine. Its frequency of occurrence with older generation devices, such as the Starflex, was up to 7% in early follow-up with TEE.[35,36] After implantation, it is very important to carefully probe each margin for stability. Immediately after the procedure, it is not uncommon to note leaking through the device with color Doppler, which will cease with device thrombosis. If color Doppler flow is noted at the SVC or the aortic rim, consideration should be given to upsizing by 2 mm for devices larger than 20 mm and by 1–2 mm for devices smaller than 20 mm. In large defects, it is common to

find minimal residual leaks with color Doppler at the inferior caval vein margin. When the septum is thin, this residual color Doppler flow may be caused by small fenestrations or Thebesian veins. If the inferior septum, however, is seen within the "jaws" of the device, one is further reassured about device stability.

Closure of multiple atrial septal defects or fenestrated atrial septum

Although multiple defects are no longer considered to be a contraindication for device closure, their recognition and detailed delineation are of paramount importance for planning and executing a successful intervention. Particularly in the presence of multiple defects, 3D imaging has proven to be helpful in understanding the spatial relationship of those defects (Figure 41.7) and hence planning of the intervention.[26] Depending on the strategy chosen, it is important to ensure on TEE that the guidewire passes through either one of the central defects or the largest defect. However, it is often difficult to be certain of this in a large and aneurysmal septum. In those circumstances, we advocate crossing a defect with a wire and inflating a sizing balloon within this defect before trying to cross with another guidewire and catheter through an adjacent defect. This technique avoids the misleading possibility of crossing a single defect with multiple wires.

Device closure of patent foramen ovale

Echocardiographic guidance for device closure of patent foramen ovale (PFO) is not mandatory.[37,38] However, this issue is still contentious, and there is an ongoing debate about the safest way of closing a patent foramen ovale (PFO).[34,38,39] From a practical point of view, we use echocardiographic guidance in addition to fluoroscopy only for those patients in whom complex anatomy is anticipated. This includes large atrial septal aneurysms, severe scoliosis, cardiac malposition due to pericardial rupture or pneumonectomy, for patients with platypnea orthodeoxia, or if new devices are used, especially those that cannot be easily retrieved once deployed.[40] If TEE or ICE is not used for PFO closure, the use of angiography postimplantation, in addition to fluoroscopy, is mandatory.

Device closure of baffle leaks after atrial switch and Fontan-type operations

Baffle leaks after atrial switch operations are common. They behave functionally as ASDs. There is either predominant left-to-right shunt and associated volume load of the subpulmonic left ventricle (LV), or right-to-left shunt, typically in the presence of a concomitant distal baffle obstruction. The latter leaves the patient cyanotic and at risk for paradoxical embolism. This is especially true in the company of a transvenous pacemaker lead.

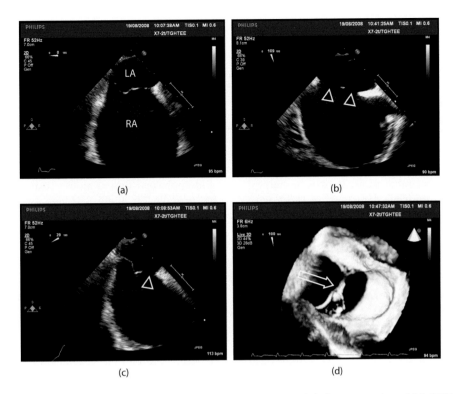

Figure 41.7 (**a** through **c**) TEE images of a large secundum type atrial septal defect at angles of 0°, 109°, and 29°. From 2D images, the impression arises that there are two defects, but only the 3D reconstruction (view from left atrium) shows the true extent of the defect being a common atrium with a narrow tissue bridge (*arrow* in [**d**]) across the atrium, rather than two separate defects (*arrowheads*). LA, left atrium; RA, right atrium; TEE, transesophageal echocardiography.

As the anatomy in these patients is often complex and distorted, a detailed understanding of the anatomy is crucial to succeed.[41] Full visualization of atrial baffles after atrial switch procedures can be difficult on TEE. To visualize the systemic venous baffles, one practical approach is to find the mitral valve (at 0–40°) and then to follow the inferior and superior cava baffles by slowly withdrawing and advancing the probe, respectively, while simultaneously rotating the probe gently to follow the baffles. A different way to assess systemic venous baffles is the modified bicaval view. The PV baffle is posterior to the systemic baffle. PV baffle obstructions are much less frequent. Visualization of PV drainage is comparable to visualization of PV in the normal heart. Bubble contrast echocardiography is the most sensitive way to detect even small right-to-left shunts. The role of TEE to guide the closure of baffle leaks is limited but should always be considered as these interventions remain increasingly rare, and additional imaging may be helpful for defining the optimal treatment strategy (e.g., treatment with a covered stent, endograft, or a closure device).[42–45]

In contrast to baffle leaks after atrial switch operations, residual fenestrations in the systemic venous limb of the Fontan circulation are often deliberately created at the time of surgery to reduce immediate postoperative complications. This occurs at the price of persistent right-to-left shunting. Many fenestrations do not close spontaneously. Elective device closure of these residual right-to-left shunts is therefore often performed when significant cyanosis persists. We rarely use TEE guidance for these procedures, but some cases have been reported where it has been useful.[46,47]

TRANSESOPHAGEAL ECHOCARDIOGRAPHY FOR DEVICE CLOSURE OF VENTRICULAR SEPTAL DEFECTS

General aspects

Device closure of congenital muscular ventricular septal defects (VSDs) or residual VSDs after open heart surgery is a well-established procedure with a low complication risk and high rate of procedural success. In contrast, device closure of perimembranous VSDs is associated with a risk of complete heart block of up to 5% in a mostly pediatric population. Device closure is therefore more contentious in patients at low risk for elective surgical repair and especially in children. Finally, post-myocardial infarction (MI) VSDs are associated with a high mortality rate both when left untreated and when treated successfully with device closure in the acute setting. Device closure of postoperative or subacute post-MI VSDs are usually associated with acceptable outcomes.

In many series, VSD device closure was performed under fluoroscopic and TEE guidance. Fluoroscopic guidance alone or guidance by fluoroscopy and transthoracic echocardiography was used in others, especially for single muscular VSDs.[48,49] In patients with complex anatomy, for example, residual postoperative shunts after complex repair of congenital heart disease, TEE usually shares the same obstacles and difficulties as angiography, namely atypical imaging planes. Shadowing artifacts created by calcified VSD patches from previous surgical repair or prosthetic valves can hamper image quality significantly. The utility of TEE can only be assessed on a case-by-case basis (Table 41.4). It may be helpful in those patients with multiple defects or in those with defects in proximity to other cardiac structures, such as AV and aortic valves. A peri-interventional diagnostic study often clarifies this. Sizing of VSDs is performed by angiography and TEE at end diastole or with a compliant sizing balloon. We universally use TEE guidance and general anesthesia for VSD closure.

Practical aspects

Detailed preprocedural echocardiography is important not only for defining defect size, location, and relationship to the surrounding structures, but also for planning the technical details of a procedure. If the defect is located anterior or toward the outlet septum, a transfemoral

Table 41.4 TEE checklist for VSD device closure

Preprocedural
- ✓ Define size, anatomy, exact location, and number of defects (multiple views)
- ✓ Rule out aortic valve cusp prolapse and malalignment VSD
- ✓ Rule out additional congenital cardiac defects
- ✓ Define relation and distance to AV-valves and aortic valve

During the procedure
- ✓ Confirm position of guidewire and delivery sheath
- ✓ Rule out pericardial effusion
- ✓ Rule out injury to tricuspid valve during deployment
- ✓ Confirm position and device stability before release (multiple views)
- ✓ Assess residual shunting before device release

Postprocedural
- ✓ Confirm proper position and alignment of the device
- ✓ Document any degree of residual shunting[a]
- ✓ Exclude significant aortic regurgitation / distortion of aortic root[b]

Note: AV, atrioventricular; TEE, transesophageal echocardiography; VSD, ventricular septal defect.
[a] Color Doppler tends to underestimate the degree of a residual shunt and one needs to be cautious not to overestimate the success of a given procedure! Even small residual shunts may predispose to hemolysis.
[b] Most important for device closure of perimembranous VSDs

approach is preferred, while in the past, for most other defect localizations, a transjugular access was chosen. In the adult heart, it is easy to form a loop in the right atrium (RA), especially with the availability of braided sheaths that mimic a jugular orientation of guidewire and delivery sheath. This allows the performance of most VSD closures from a femoral approach. If a muscular Amplatzer septal occluder is used, the distance to AV and aortic valves must be at least 4 mm.

The best views on TEE to define a muscular VSD are the midesophageal four-chamber (usually 0–20°), two-chamber (usually 70°–100°), and long-axis views (100°–135°), as well as transgastric short-axis views and deep transgastric four-chamber views (both at 0°). It is important to visualize a defect in several planes to appreciate its size and geometry. For perimembranous VSDs, in addition, a short-axis view through the base of the heart (20°–60°) is helpful. As apically located VSDs may be hard to visualize on TEE, complementary transthoracic imaging might be more helpful in these cases. As for other indications, 3D-echocardiography is particularly useful for delineation of spatial relationship between multiple defects and hence, might help planning of optimal interventional or surgical strategies.[50]

Postinfarction ventricular septal defects

VSDs after MI differ in many ways from congenital VSDs. Interventionalists can be involved in the care of these patients when they present either as acute postinfarction VSDs or when patients have residual defects after surgical closure of a postinfarction VSD. The outlook for the former is bleak when left untreated, and every intervention, either surgical or interventional, remains at very high risk. Those who survive initial conservative management and are treated in the subacute phase often have a much improved outlook. However, many patients will deteriorate and die in the acute phase. It is difficult to predict in which patients VSD closure may be postponed. Even in patients initially stable, VSD expansion may occur and lead to hemodynamic compromise with pulmonary overcirculation, heart failure, systemic hypoperfusion, and organ dysfunction. We advocate for early surgery for all post-MI VSDs. In those patients who are not candidates, we consider waiting a number of weeks to allow for scar maturation, as experience with acute closure of these defects has an exceedingly high mortality similar to medical therapy. Some patients who are poor candidates for open repair will remain stable on medical therapy long enough to undergo a semi-elective procedure later in their course when the defect rims have had time to mature.

Rather than being well-defined defects, postinfarction VSDs are often jagged-edged, irregular, and serpiginous ruptures of the interventricular septum with poorly defined borders. They often have multiple exit points toward the right ventricle (RV). To allow proper planning of interventional closure, it is therefore crucial to define defect size, location, borders, and inflow and outflows.

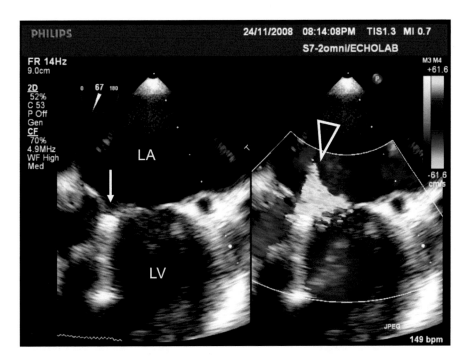

Figure 41.8 Eighty-four-year-old patient in cardiogenic shock due to subacute postmyocardial infarction VSD. The arrow points to the left ventricular disc of an Amplatzer VSD occluder (*white arrow*), entangling the subvalvular mitral valve apparatus, leading to severe mitral regurgitation (*arrowhead*). LA, left atrium; LV, left ventricle; VSD, ventricular septal defect.

As the largest dedicated double-disc device size at present is 24 mm (St Jude Post Infarct VSD Occluder), proper sizing of the defect is critical. Apart from defining defect location and morphology, echocardiography defines left ventricular function, integrity of the valvular apparatus, and defect location (Figure 41.8). It is important to detect pericardial effusion, as this may herald free wall or contained rupture. The location of the defect with respect to the rims is quite critical, as one tries to avoid putting stress on a structurally weakened septum to free wall junction, which might result in free wall rupture. As there is often more than one defect, it is also crucial to assure that at the time of intervention, the guidewire is crossing the largest defect.[51–53] We have generally seen TEE as complementary for assessing these patients. Our present practice is to obtain a gated cardiac computed tomography (CT) scan for planning, followed by the creation of a 3D printed model, or evaluation with a True 3D Echopixel workstation (Mountainview, CA). The True 3D system is approved by the U.S. Food and Drug Administration (FDA) and allows for a 3D appreciation of echo, CT, or magnetic resonance imaging (MRI) using a dedicated workstation and glasses that allow an appreciation of depth.

TRANSESOPHAGEAL ECHOCARDIOGRAPHY FOR INTERATRIAL TRANSSEPTAL PUNCTURE

Access to the LA from a systemic venous path is a prerequisite for many cardiac interventions. This includes percutaneous mitral valve repair, mitral balloon valvuloplasty, device closure of LAA, device closure of paravalvular leaks, and many electrophysiological procedures.[54] Although echocardiographic guidance is not mandatory, it provides additional safety and helps to localize the optimal site of puncture for a specific intervention (Table 41.5). Different procedures require puncture at different sites in the interatrial septum, for example, a high posterior puncture when a mitral valve clip repair is planned or a low puncture when a mitral valvuloplasty is planned (see also below).[55,56] New-generation interventionalists are increasingly dependent on TEE guidance, as transseptal puncture has become a rare procedure for most interventional practices. Proper position of the transseptal needle is confirmed by "tenting" of the interatrial septum with the needle withdrawn into the tip of the Mullins sheath. The puncture of the septum can be confirmed by injection of contrast through the transseptal needle.[57,58] Transseptal puncture across patches, baffles, or conduits in patients with repaired congenital heart disease is particularly challenging and optimal delineation of an individual's cardiac anatomy is important to enhance safety of a procedure involving this step.[59] Real-time 3D imaging has recently been shown to be helpful for some interventions. Due to its unique ability to delineate spatial relationship, it might prove useful for guiding transseptal puncture in certain patients with high-risk anatomy. This includes patients with congenital heart disease, pulmonary artery hypertension, left-to-right bowing of the septum in the presence of mitral stenosis, or cases of a thickened lipomatous septum.[60]

Table 41.5   TEE checklist for interatrial transseptal puncture

Preprocedural
✓ Define optimal site of puncture (usually in the region of the oval fossa)
✓ Define anatomical distortion due to congenital heart disease, mitral valve disease, or pulmonary hypertension
✓ Define localization of the aortic root
✓ Rule out clot in left atrium or left atrial appendage
✓ Define presence and extent of lipomatous interatrial septum

During the procedure
✓ Confirm position of transseptal needle on the interatrial septum (tenting)
✓ Confirm intra-atrial location of needle tip after puncture (saline contrast)

Postprocedural
✓ Rule out pericardial effusion or tamponade
✓ Define size of residual atrial septal defect

TRANSESOPHAGEAL ECHOCARDIOGRAPHY FOR LEFT-SIDED HEART VALVE PROCEDURES

Balloon aortic valvuloplasty

The role of TEE in guiding aortic valve balloon dilatation is limited. When used, its purpose is accurate sizing of the aortic annulus to choose the appropriate balloon size and to detect immediate complications after each dilatation. Increasing aortic regurgitation is prohibitive for further dilatations, and in the hypotensive patient after dilatation, TEE provides an excellent tool to immediately detect new wall motion abnormalities suggestive of coronary emboli or pericardial effusion, which may be related to ventricular perforation or aortic annulus rupture. In patients with significant renal dysfunction, TEE can prove very helpful to assess regurgitation between (multiple) valvuloplasties and can spare iodinated contrast.

Catheter-based aortic valve replacement

As catheter-based aortic valve replacement emerged, it was usually performed under general anesthesia with TEE guidance. This has changed over the last few years and most procedures are now performed in the awake patient, except in cases where additional procedures (e.g., concomitant transcatheter mitral valve repair or LAA occlusion) are planned. Accurate sizing of the aortic annulus is important to choose the appropriate type and size of the prosthetic valve. TEE has been shown to be more accurate than transthoracic echocardiogram (TTE) in sizing the annulus, especially in patients with heavily calcified valves.[61,62] Currently, aortic annulus measurements by CT are often used alone or in

adjunction to measurements on TEE, especially in cases of severe renal dysfunction.

The main roles for TEE include the optimal centering of the valved stent relative to the native aortic annulus, the early detection of complications, and the assessment of aortic insufficiency, which may require further intervention (Figure 41.9 and Table 41.6). With the transfemoral approach using the Edwards SAPIEN valve, the aim is for a ventricular-to-aortic ratio of the stent of 60:40 (i.e., the larger part of the stent before implantation sits in the left ventricular outflow tract [LVOT]) as a slight "travel" of the stent during deployment is expected. With the transapical approach, less aortic travel is observed, and therefore, the aim for centering is 50:50. Communication between the interventionalist and the echocardiographer during the procedure is the key to success. We have used the terms *ventricular* and *aortic* to describe the position of the valve instead of "in and out" to avoid any ambiguity during this critical step.[63] When we started using the transapical approach, TEE was even more important, as fluoroscopy in many operating rooms at the time was provided by a portable C-arm with less optimal image quality. As programs have matured, most centers now use high-quality and modern hybrid operating rooms, and increasingly use conscious sedation for transfemoral procedures, while the increasingly infrequent transapical procedures continue to be performed with general anesthesia. In those patients in whom a transapical approach is chosen, entanglement of the delivery system in the mitral valve apparatus can be life-threatening and must be immediately detected by TEE. After deployment of the stent, TEE should confirm stable stent position and define the amount of paravalvular leakage. In cases of severe paravalvular regurgitation, postdilatation with a slightly larger balloon volume might be efficacious. If the prosthesis is placed too low or high, a second valve may need to be deployed.

SINUS VALSALVA ANEURYSM AND OTHER AORTIC TO ATRIAL COMMUNICATIONS

Congenital or acquired communications between the aorta and various cardiac structures (i.e., ruptured sinus Valsalva aneurysms) are often amenable to device closure. In an individual patient, it always has to be decided whether or not device closure is expected to be equivalent to surgery, taking into account the patient's estimated perioperative risk. Figure 41.10 depicts the successful closure of a postoperative aortic to left atrial fistula after bioprosthetic aortic valve replacement, and Figure 41.11 describes an attempted device closure of a ruptured sinus Valsalva aneurysm. TEE is very helpful in exact delineation of a patient's lesion anatomy, and the most useful views are generally midesophageal short-axis view through the aortic root and long-axis views at 110°–140°. Sometimes, however, off-axis views may be required, especially for facilitating guidewire and sheath placement across a defect. Special note should be made of multiple perforations of these aneurysms, which may compromise the result.

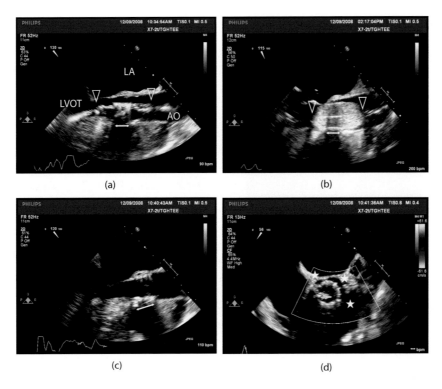

(a) (b)

(c) (d)

Figure 41.9 Catheter-based aortic valve implantation. (**a** through **d**) Long-axis views. (**a**) Placement of the valved stent (arrowheads mark edges of stent balloon; double-headed arrows mark the actual length of the valved stent). (**b**) Valve implantation, balloon inflated. (**c**) Immediate postvalve deployment with thin prosthetic valve cusps visible. (**d**) Short-axis view through base of the heart, depicting mild valvular and three small paravalvular jets (white stars) of aortic regurgitation. AO, aorta; LA, left atrium; LVOT, left ventricular outflow tract.

Table 41.6   TEE checklist for catheter-based aortic valve replacement

Preprocedural

✓   Rule out mobile clot or active endocarditis

✓   Rule out plaques, grade IV, or mobile clots in the thoracic aorta

✓   Accurate measurement of aortic annulus (between hinge-points of the valve)

During the procedure

✓   Avoid entanglement of delivery system in mitral valve apparatus in case of transapical approach

✓   Confirm optimal position of valved stent before deployment

Postprocedural

✓   Confirm stable position of the valved stent

✓   Confirm normal prosthetic valve function

✓   Assess severity and localization of paravalvular leaks

✓   Assess immediate complications (new wall motion abnormalities may help localizing the site of coronary obstruction)

Balloon valvuloplasty of the mitral valve

The most important role of TEE in balloon valvuloplasty of the mitral valve is the assessment of valve characteristics predicting the success of the procedure (thickening,

calcification, mobility of valve, and subvalvar apparatus). The procedure is discussed in detail in Chapter 43. The absence of left atrial thrombus is a prerequisite for a safe procedure and must be confirmed by TEE even in patients with therapeutic anticoagulation.[64]

During the procedure, TEE guidance is not mandatory but may ease transseptal puncture. It allows assessment of the severity of mitral regurgitation and other complications immediately after the procedure, such as pericardial effusion.[65] In addition, compared to fluoroscopy alone, it might improve placement of the dilatation balloon and decrease procedure and fluoroscopy time.[66] It is uncommon to use TEE for mitral valvuloplasty in the present era.

Percutaneous mitral valve repair

GENERAL ASPECTS

Catheter-based mitral valve repair plays an increasing role in patients with symptomatic, severe mitral regurgitation who are not surgical candidates for various reasons (advanced age, comorbidities, etc.). The device most frequently used, which is Conformité Européene (CE) marked and also FDA approved, is the MitraClip system (Abbott Vascular, IL). Initially, it was mostly used for degenerative mitral regurgitation in the A2/P2 (anatomical segment 2 of the anterior/posterior mitral valve leaflets) segment, but it is now increasingly used in patients with functional mitral

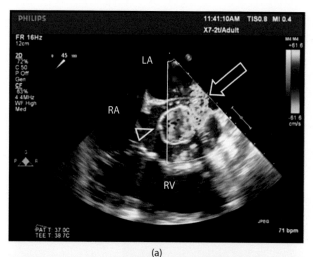

(a)

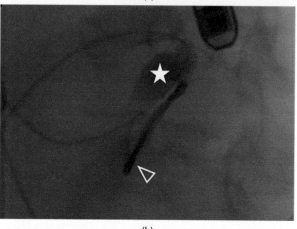

(b)

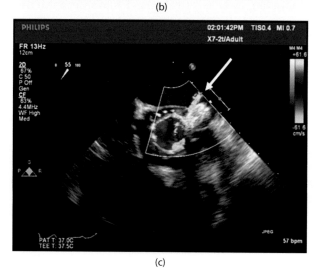

(c)

Figure 41.10 Device closure of fistula from aorta to left atrium after bioprosthetic aortic valve replacement. **(a)** Midesophageal short-axis view through aortic root. The arrowhead points to the aortic valve prosthesis; the large arrow to the shunt. **(b)** Angiographic view of sizing balloon (*white star*) measuring defect size. **(c)** Small residual left shunt after deployment of an Amplatzer duct occluder (*arrow*). LA, left atrium; RA, right atrium; RV, right ventricle.

regurgitation.[67] As other investigational devices are not yet established in clinical routine or are still in the experimental stage, we focus on the MitraClip system in this chapter. For success of mitral valve repair with the MitraClip system, TEE is key. First, it is used to evaluate detailed mitral valve anatomy prior to the intervention to determine whether or not a MitraClip insertion is even possible at all. Second, the entire procedure is guided by TEE, starting with the transseptal puncture, followed by positioning of the clip, successful grasping of the leaflets, and assessment of the result after the clip deployment.

PRACTICAL ASPECTS

MitraClip insertion is critically dependent on TEE guidance.[73] Once the interdisciplinary heart team has decided that the insertion of a MitraClip is feasible and indicated, the intervention will be performed under general anesthesia, mainly because of the need for TEE. The various steps necessary for the procedure are summarized in Table 41.7 and Figure 41.12. The actual procedure starts with the transseptal puncture, which is key for a successful intervention. For MitraClip, the puncture site should be 4–4.5 cm above the coaptation zone–meaning for degenerative mitral regurgitation, the puncture site should be higher–and for functional mitral regurgitation, it should be lower in order to provide sufficient degrees of freedom for the guiding catheter and the clip delivery system. As always, the puncture site needs to be cross checked in the aortic valve short-axis view (distance to the aortic root) and in the bicaval view. Once the guiding catheter is in place and the MitraClip delivery system is advanced through the guiding catheter into the LA, the echocardiographer needs to make sure that the interventionalist brings the clip toward the mitral valve safely without damaging the LA. The next key step is the orientation of the clip. Therefore, the interventionalist opens the clip above the valve, and it needs to be confirmed in the 3D surgeon's view that the clip is oriented perpendicular to the leaflet coaptation zone and in the area of the lesion causing the regurgitation. Then, the clip can be advanced through the valve carefully without getting entangled in the subvalvular apparatus. For leaflet grasping and leaflet insertion, ideally, the biplane mode is used, showing the commissural view and the long-axis view side by side. Enough leaflet material (at least 5 mm) should be inserted into the clip. In case the image quality from the transesophageal view is insufficient, a transgastric short-axis view can be used in order to assess leaflet insertion. After clip deployment, again careful valve interrogation is mandatory, including measurement of transvalvular diastolic gradients to assess the potential for mitral valve stenosis. A mean diastolic gradient <5 mmHg is acceptable.[68] The degree of residual mitral regurgitation needs to be assessed in color Doppler imaging in various views. In the case of insufficient results after the first clip, up to three additional clips may be inserted under careful surveillance of transvalvular diastolic gradients. After the

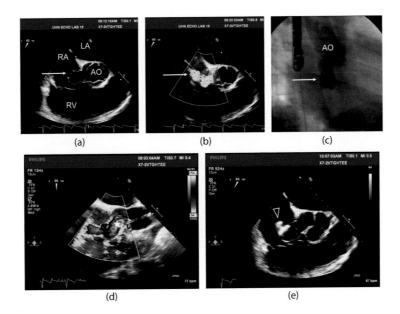

Figure 41.11 Attempted device closure of ruptured sinus valsalva aneurysm. (**a** and **b**) Midesophageal short-axis view through aortic root without and with color Doppler. The arrow points to the perforation of the sinus valsalva aneurysm toward the right atrium. (**c**) Angiographic view of the sinus valsalva aneurysm. (**d**) Balloon sizing of the defect (*white star*). (**e**) Amplatzer duct occluder sealing the perforation of the sinus valsalva aneurysm (not released). The device seals only one of three communications between the aorta and the right ventricle, leaving a large residual shunt. The device was therefore retrieved and the patient was referred for surgical repair. AO, aorta; LA, left atrium; RA, right atrium; RV, right ventricle.

Table 41.7 TEE checklist for MitraClip insertion

Preprocedural

✓ Define mitral valve lesion responsible for regurgitation: functional versus degenerative

✓ Localize lesion (ideally A2/P2) and assess coaptation length, coaptation depth, flail gap, flail width, and calcification of the anulus/leaflets

✓ Measure gradient in order to assess likelihood for mitral stenosis after clip insertion

✓ Rule out clot in left atrium or left atrial appendage

During the procedure

✓ Assess presence of pericardial effusion prior to transseptal puncture (important for comparison before and after)

✓ Define puncture site (usually 4–4.5 cm above coaptation zone in the 4 chamber view); see also separate section for transseptal puncture

✓ After puncture, confirm that guidewire is in the left upper pulmonary vein while advancing the guiding catheter

✓ Confirm that guiding catheter protrudes ca. 1 cm into the left atrium; help guiding the clip towards the valve without touching the atrial wall

✓ Confirm correct alignment of the clip in 3D surgical view

✓ Avoid entanglement of the clip and the delivery system in the subvalvular apparatus

✓ Guide grasping in biplane mode (commissural and long axis view)

✓ Check leaflet insertion in long axis view, alternative transgastric short axis view

✓ Check diastolic gradient after each clip (goal: <5 mmHg in order to avoid mitral stenosis)

✓ Check success by assessing residual mitral regurgitation in multiple views by color Doppler echocardiography

After the procedure

✓ Assess result by defining residual degree of mitral regurgitation

✓ Assess leaflet insertion, measure gradient

✓ Define size of iatrogenic atrial septal defect

✓ Rule out pericardial effusion or tamponade

Note: A2/P2, segments 2 of anterior and posterior mitral valve leaflets.

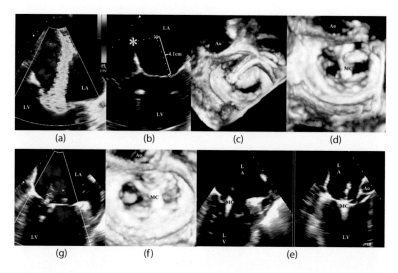

Figure 41.12 Procedural steps in MitraClip insertion. **(a)** Situation prior to clipping shows severe functional mitral regurgitation. **(b)** Necessary measurement in order to puncture the septum in the correct height, which usually should be 4–4.5 cm above the level of coaptation of the leaflets in the four-chamber view; * indicates puncture site. However, it is of great importance to double-check at a 40° angle to make sure that there is enough distance in between puncture site and the aortic root. **(c)** The guiding catheter coming across the interatrial septum into the left atrium above the mitral valve. **(d)** 3D surgeon's view of the mitral valve with the open MitraClip. This view in 3D is used in order to make sure that the clip is well-oriented. It should be perpendicular to the coaptation zone of the mitral valve leaflets and usually in the A2/P2 segment. **(e)** Commissural view (*left*) along with the long axis view (*right*), which is used to guide positioning of the clip. The commissural view is used to guide the position along the coaptation zone lateral-medial. The long-axis view is used for the leaflet grasping and evaluation of leaflet insertion. **(f)** What the result looks like on 3D surgeon's view with a double-orifice mitral valve. **(g)** The successful reduction of the severity of mitral regurgitation after MitraClip insertion in color Doppler imaging. AO, aorta; LA, left atrium; LV, left ventricle; MC, MitraClip.

procedure, the guiding catheter is pulled back under TEE control, and the iatrogenic ASD can be assessed in terms of hemodynamic impact. However, this is only very rarely necessary. At the end of the procedure, careful attention should be paid to development of new pericardial effusion, since pericardial tamponade may complicate several of the steps during MitraClip procedures.

DEVICE CLOSURE OF PARAVALVULAR LEAKS AFTER PROSTHETIC HEART VALVE SURGERY

Paravalvular leaks after surgical prosthetic heart valve replacement can cause significant morbidity due to residual regurgitation or hemolysis. To avoid the significant risk of a reoperation, device closure has become an attractive alternative to conventional surgery in poor surgical candidates.

For these technically demanding procedures, TEE plays an important role for both planning and executing these interventions (Table 41.8).[69] A detailed description of the defect localization, size, and relationship to adjacent structures is of paramount importance.[69–72] Again of great importance is clear communication between the echocardiographer and the interventionalist, as localization on echocardiography may not be easily translated into a biplane radiographic view. Due to its unique ability to delineate spatial relationships within the heart and its ability to visualize the true geometry of a defect, real-time 3D TEE is the modality of choice for guidance of these procedures (Figure 41.13).[69] During the procedure, TEE provides invaluable assistance to help target the defect with a guidewire and delivery sheaths in 3D space. In the future,

Table 41.8   TEE checklist for device closure of paravalvular leaks

Preprocedural

✓   Define localization, size and geometry of the defect

✓   Define relationship to adjacent structures (heart valves, coronary arteries)

✓   Rule out intracardiac clot and malfunction of the prosthetic valve

✓   Rule out 'rocking' of the valve and confirm stability of the prosthesis

During the procedure

✓   Guide transseptal puncture for optimal position of the delivery sheath

✓   Ease proper guidewire position (to AVOID entangling in mechanical valves)

✓   Rule out prosthesis malfunction caused by the closure device – BEFORE release

Postprocedural

✓   Confirm normal prosthetic heart valve function

✓   Detect immediate complications

✓   Define the amount of residual paravalvular leakage and assess whether a second device is necessary

✓   Define the size of the residual atrial septal defect

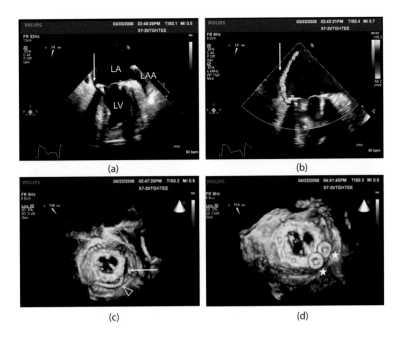

Figure 41.13 Device closure of paravalvular mitral leak (bioprosthesis). (**a** and **b**) 74° midesophageal TEE views demonstrating paravalvular mitral regurgitation (*arrow*). (**c**) Live 3D image of the mitral valve prosthesis seen from the left atrium demonstrating a large inferomedial paravalvular leak (*arrow*). The arrowhead points to the delivery sheath crossing the leak. (**d**) Live 3D image after device closure of paravalvular leak with two Amplatzer duct occluder (*white stars*). AO, aorta; LA, left atrium; LVOT, Left ventricular outflow tract; TEE, transesophageal echocardiography.

multimodality imaging, including fusion images with reconstructed images from CT, may further enhance procedural success.[11,69]

RIGHT-SIDED VALVE LESIONS

The role of TEE for guiding right-sided heart valve procedures is limited. Balloon dilatation of native pulmonary valve stenoses and implantation of percutaneous pulmonary valves are usually performed under fluoroscopy alone, and the additional yield of echocardiography is small. For optimal positioning of the stent valve in the case of percutaneous treatment of a stenosed or regurgitant conduit, calcifications within the wall of the conduit are the most important landmarks for placement of the device. The almost inevitably present heavy calcification of these conduits hampers image quality on TEE significantly because of shadowing artifacts. ICE imaging after valve implantation may inform whether regurgitation is valvular or perivalvular and guide further intervention. Interventional procedures on the tricuspid valve are rarely performed, and the role of TEE is yet to be defined.

MISCELLANEOUS INTERVENTIONS

Whether or not TEE or echocardiography is at all helpful for a particular intervention is determined by several factors. First, not surprisingly, if TEE were unable to visualize the structure of interest in high quality, we would not expect any yield in adding this modality. This is true for

any structures remote from the esophagus, as for example patent ductus arteriosus, aortopulmonary collaterals, or peripheral pulmonary artery stenoses. Some clinical scenarios preclude the use of TEE. This includes patients with esophageal disease (strictures, varices, etc.) and those in whom it is safer to perform a procedure without general anesthesia. The latter may be the case in hemodynamically unstable patients or patients with severe respiratory compromise. In those cases, we avoid the use of TEE, as we feel discouraged about the safety of TEE with topical anesthesia and sedation only. However, TEE without general anesthesia is a widely practiced technique in many European centers. ICE might be more helpful in cases of this nature.

Some lesions, such as pulmonary artery stenoses and coarctation of the aorta, are easily and fully visualized by angiography; therefore, echocardiography is not routinely used for guiding these procedures. Its role remains limited to immediate assessment of acute catastrophic complications, such as aortic dissection and tamponade.

SUMMARY AND CONCLUSIONS

The introduction of TEE into clinical practice has not only supported the development of many innovative cardiac interventions, but also become an essential tool for guiding many of them. For some interventions, ICE will likely replace TEE in the future, but with the advent of real-time 3D TEE, the role of TEE for enhancing success rates and safety for many procedures is increasing.

REFERENCES

1. Hisanaga K, et al. Transesophageal cross-sectional echocardiography. *Am Heart J* 1980;100(5):605–609.

2. Schluter M, et al. Transoesophageal cross-sectional echocardiography with a phased array transducer system. Technique and initial clinical results. *Br Heart J* 1982;48(1):67–72.

3. Daniel WG, et al. Safety of transesophageal echocardiography. A multicenter survey of 10,419 examinations. *Circulation* 1991;83(3):817–821.

4. Min JK, et al. Clinical features of complications from transesophageal echocardiography: A single-center case series of 10,000 consecutive examinations. *J Am Soc Echocardiogr* 2005;18(9):925–929.

5. Cheung YF, et al. An evolving role of transesophageal echocardiography for the monitoring of interventional catheterization in children. *Clin Cardiol* 1999;22(12):804–810.

6. Mullen MJ, et al. Intracardiac echocardiography guided device closure of atrial septal defects. *J Am Coll Cardiol* 2003;41(2):285–292.

7. Boccalandro F, et al. Comparison of intracardiac echocardiography versus transesophageal echocardiography guidance for percutaneous transcatheter closure of atrial septal defect. *Am J Cardiol* 2004;93(4):437–440.

8. Balzer J, et al. Real-time three-dimensional transoesophageal echocardiography for guidance of atrial septal defect closures. *Eur Heart J* 2008;29(18):2226.

9. Balzer J, et al. Real-time transesophageal three-dimensional echocardiography for guidance of percutaneous cardiac interventions: First experience. *Clin Res Cardiol* 2008;97(9):565–574.

10. Biaggi P, et al. Quantification of mitral valve anatomy by three-dimensional transesophageal echocardiography in mitral valve prolapse predicts surgical anatomy and the complexity of mitral valve repair. *J Am Soc Echocardiogr* 2012;25(7):758–765.

11. Biaggi P, et al. Hybrid imaging during transcatheter structural heart interventions. *Curr Cardiovasc Imaging Rep* 2015;8(9):33.

12. Hellenbrand WE, et al. Transesophageal echocardiographic guidance of transcatheter closure of atrial septal defect. *Am J Cardiol* 1990;66(2):207–213.

13. Ferreira SM, et al. Morphological study of defects of the atrial septum within the oval fossa: Implications for transcatheter closure of left-to-right shunt. *Br Heart J* 1992;67(4):316–320.

14. Chan KC, Godman MJ. Morphological variations of fossa ovalis atrial septal defects (secundum): Feasibility for transcutaneous closure with the clam-shell device. *Br Heart J* 1993;69(1):52–55.

15. Carminati M, et al. A European multicentric experience using the CardioSEal and Starflex double umbrella devices to close interatrial communications holes within the oval fossa. *Cardiol Young* 2000;10(5):519–526.

16. Masura J, et al. Transcatheter closure of secundum atrial septal defects using the new self-centering amplatzer septal occluder: Initial human experience. *Cathet Cardiovasc Diagn* 1997;42(4):388–393.

17. Chan KC, et al. Transcatheter closure of atrial septal defect and interatrial communications with a new self expanding nitinol double disc device (Amplatzer septal occluder): Multicentre UK experience. *Heart* 1999;82(3):300–306.

18. Mazic U, et al. The role of transesophageal echocardiography in transcatheter closure of secundum atrial septal defects by the Amplatzer septal occluder. *Am Heart J* 2001;142(3):482–488.

19. Cooke JC, et al. Echocardiologists' role in the deployment of the Amplatzer atrial septal occluder device in adults. *J Am Soc Echocardiogr* 2001;14(6):588–594.

20. Ewert P, et al. Transcatheter closure of atrial septal defects without fluoroscopy: Feasibility of a new method. *Circulation* 2000;101(8):847–849.

21. van den Bosch AE, et al. Characterization of atrial septal defect assessed by real-time 3-dimensional echocardiography. *J Am Soc Echocardiogr* 2006;19(6):815–821.

22. Maeno YV, et al. Impact of dynamic 3D transoesophageal echocardiography in the assessment of atrial septal defects and occlusion by the double-umbrella device (CardioSEAL). *Cardiol Young* 1998;8(3):368–378.

23. Franke A, et al. Quantitative analysis of the morphology of secundum-type atrial septal defects and their dynamic change using transesophageal three-dimensional echocardiography. *Circulation* 1997;96(9 Suppl):II-323–327.

24. Acar P, et al. Influence of atrial septal defect anatomy in patient selection and assessment of closure with the Cardioseal device; a three-dimensional transoesophageal echocardiographic reconstruction. *Eur Heart J* 2000;21(7):573–581.

25. Magni G, et al. Two- and three-dimensional transesophageal echocardiography in patient selection and assessment of atrial septal defect closure by the new DAS-Angel Wings device: Initial clinical experience. *Circulation* 1997;96(6):1722–1728.

26. Cao Q, et al. Transcatheter closure of multiple atrial septal defects. Initial results and value of two- and three-dimensional transoesophageal echocardiography. *Eur Heart J* 2000;21(11):941–947.

27. Podnar T, et al. Morphological variations of secundum-type atrial septal defects: Feasibility for percutaneous closure using Amplatzer septal occluders. *Catheter Cardiovasc Interv* 2001;53(3):386–391.

28. Amin Z. Transcatheter closure of secundum atrial septal defects. *Catheter Cardiovasc Interv* 2006;68(5):778–787.

29. Moore JW, et al. Results of the combined U.S. Multicenter Pivotal Study and the Continuing Access Study of the Nit-Occlud PDA device for percutaneous closure of patent ductus arteriosus. *JACC Cardiovasc Interv* 2014;7(12):1430–1436.

30. El-Said HG, Moore JW. Erosion by the Amplatzer septal occluder: Experienced operator opinions at odds with manufacturer recommendations? *Catheter Cardiovasc Interv* 2009;73(7):925–930.

31. Amin Z, et al. Erosion of Amplatzer septal occluder device after closure of secundum atrial septal defects: Review of registry of complications and recommendations to minimize future risk. *Catheter Cardiovasc Interv* 2004;63(4):496–502.

32. Divekar A, et al. Cardiac perforation after device closure of atrial septal defects with the Amplatzer septal occluder. *J Am Coll Cardiol* 2005;45(8):1213–1218.

33. Cooke JC, et al. Cobrahead malformation of the Amplatzer septal occluder device: An avoidable compilation of percutaneous ASD closure. *Catheter Cardiovasc Interv* 2001;52(1):83–85; discussion 86–87.

34. Cooke JC, et al. Chiari network entanglement and herniation into the left atrium by an atrial septal defect occluder device. *J Am Soc Echocardiogr* 1999;12(7):601–603.

35. Krumsdorf U, et al. Incidence and clinical course of thrombus formation on atrial septal defect and patient foramen ovale closure devices in 1,000 consecutive patients. *J Am Coll Cardiol* 2004;43(2):302–309.

36. Moore JW, Levi DS. Transcatheter closure of atrial shunts. Focus on a lingering issue. *J Am Coll Cardiol* 2004;43(2):310–312.

37. Varma C, et al. Clinical outcomes of patent foramen ovale closure for paradoxical emboli without echocardiographic guidance. *Catheter Cardiovasc Interv* 2004;62(4):519–525.

38. Wahl A, et al. Long-term results after fluoroscopy-guided closure of patent foramen ovale for secondary prevention of paradoxical embolism. *Heart* 2008;94(3):336–341.

39. Shishehbor MH, et al. Long-term results after PFO closure. *Heart* 2008;94(1):100; author reply 100–101.

40. Hildick-Smith D, et al. Patent foramen ovale closure without echocardiographic control: Use of "standby" intracardiac ultrasound. *JACC Cardiovasc Interv* 2008;1(4):387–391.

41. Balzer DT, et al. Transcatheter occlusion of baffle leaks following atrial switch procedures for transposition of the great vessels (d-TGV). *Catheter Cardiovasc Interv* 2004;61(2):259–263.

42. Daehnert I, et al. Interventions in leaks and obstructions of the interatrial baffle late after Mustard and Senning correction for transposition of the great arteries. *Catheter Cardiovasc Interv* 2005;66(3):400–407.

43. Ebeid MR, et al. Catheter management of occluded superior baffle after atrial switch procedures for transposition of great vessels. *Am J Cardiol* 2005;95(6):782–786.

44. Sharaf E, et al. Simultaneous transcatheter occlusion of two atrial baffle leaks and stent implantation for SVC obstruction in a patient after Mustard repair. *Catheter Cardiovasc Interv* 2001;54(1):72–76.

45. Bentham J, et al. Effect of transcatheter closure of baffle leaks following senning or mustard atrial redirection surgery on oxygen saturations and polycythaemia. *Am J Cardiol* 2012;110(7):1046–1050.

46. Masura J, et al. Percutaneous management of cyanosis in Fontan patients using Amplatzer occluders. *Catheter Cardiovasc Interv* 2008;71(6):843–849.

47. Crowley DI, Donnelly JP. Use of Amplatzer occlusion devices to occlude Fontan baffle leaks during fenestration closure procedures. *Catheter Cardiovasc Interv* 2008;71(2):244–249.

48. Hijazi ZM, et al. Transcatheter closure of single muscular ventricular septal defects using the amplatzer muscular VSD occluder: Initial results and technical considerations. *Catheter Cardiovasc Interv* 2000;49(2):167–172.

49. Butera G, et al. Percutaneous closure of ventricular septal defects. State of the art. *J Cardiovasc Med (Hagerstown)* 2007;8(1):39–45.

50. Acar P, et al. Assessment of muscular ventricular septal defect closure by transcatheter or surgical approach: A three-dimensional echocardiographic study. *Eur J Echocardiogr* 2002;3(3):185–191.

51. Lock JE, et al. Transcatheter closure of ventricular septal defects. *Circulation* 1988;78(2):361–368.

52. Holzer R, et al. Transcatheter closure of postinfarction ventricular septal defects using the new Amplatzer muscular VSD occluder: Results of a U.S. Registry. *Catheter Cardiovasc Interv* 2004;61(2):196–201.

53. Ahmed J, et al. Percutaneous closure of post-myocardial infarction ventricular septal defects: A single centre experience. *Heart Lung Circ* 2008;17(2):119–123.

54. Roelke M, et al. The technique and safety of transseptal left heart catheterization: The Massachusetts General Hospital experience with 1,279 procedures. *Cathet Cardiovasc Diagn* 1994;32(4):332–339.

55. Tucker KJ, et al. Transesophageal echocardiographic guidance of transseptal left heart catheterization during radiofrequency ablation of left-sided accessory pathways in humans. *Pacing Clin Electrophysiol* 1996;19(3):272–281.

56. Hahn K, et al. Transesophageal echocardiographically guided atrial transseptal catheterization in patients with normal-sized atria: Incidence of complications. *Clin Cardiol* 1995;18(4):217–220.

57. Clark J, et al. Use of three-dimensional catheter guidance and trans-esophageal echocardiography to eliminate fluoroscopy in catheter ablation of left-sided accessory pathways. *Pacing Clin Electrophysiol* 2008;31(3):283–289.

58. Kantoch MJ, et al. Use of transesophageal echocardiography in radiofrequency catheter ablation in children and adolescents. *Can J Cardiol* 1998;14(4):519–523.

59. El-Said HG, et al. 18-year experience with transseptal procedures through baffles, conduits, and other intra-atrial patches. *Catheter Cardiovasc Interv* 2000;50(4):434–439; discussion 440.

60. Chierchia GB, et al. First experience with real-time three-dimensional transoesophageal echocardiography-guided transseptal in patients undergoing atrial fibrillation ablation. *Europace* 2008;10(11):1325–1328.

61. Guarracino F, et al. Influence of transesophageal echocardiography on intraoperative decision making for toronto stentless prosthetic valve implantation. *J Heart Valve Dis* 2001;10(1):31–34.

62. Abraham TP, et al. Accuracy of transesophageal echocardiography in preoperative determination of aortic anulus size during valve replacement. *J Am Soc Echocardiogr* 1997;10(2):149–154.

63. Moss RR, et al. Role of echocardiography in percutaneous aortic valve implantation. *JACC Cardiovasc Imaging* 2008;1(1):15–24.

64. Pavlides GS, et al. The value of transesophageal echocardiography in predicting immediate and long-term outcome of balloon mitral valvuloplasty: Comparison with transthoracic echocardiography. *J Interv Cardiol* 1994;7(5):401–408.

65. Goldstein SA, et al. Feasibility of on-line transesophageal echocardiography during balloon mitral valvulotomy: Experience with 93 patients. *J Heart Valve Dis* 1994;3(2):136–148.

66. Park SH, et al. The advantages of on-line transesophageal echocardiography guide during percutaneous balloon mitral valvuloplasty. *J Am Soc Echocardiogr* 2000;13(1):26–34.

67. Feldman T, et al. Percutaneous mitral repair with the MitraClip system: Safety and midterm durability in the initial EVEREST (Endovascular Valve Edge-to-Edge REpair Study) cohort. *J Am Coll Cardiol* 2009;54(8):686–694.

68. Biaggi P, et al. Assessment of mitral valve area during percutaneous mitral valve repair using the MitraClip system: Comparison of different echocardiographic methods. *Circ Cardiovasc Imaging* 2013;6(6):1032–1040.

69. Ruiz CE, et al. Clinical outcomes in patients undergoing percutaneous closure of periprosthetic paravalvular leaks. *J Am Coll Cardiol* 2011;58(21):2210–2217.

70. Cortes M, et al. Usefulness of transesophageal echocardiography in percutaneous transcatheter repairs of paravalvular mitral regurgitation. *Am J Cardiol* 2008;101(3):382–386.

71. Shapira Y, et al. Percutaneous closure of perivalvular leaks with Amplatzer occluders: Feasibility, safety, and short-term results. *J Heart Valve Dis* 2007;16(3):305–313.

72. Pate GE, et al. Percutaneous closure of prosthetic paravalvular leaks: Case series and review. *Catheter Cardiovasc Interv* 2006;68(4):528–533.

73. Silvestry FE, et al. Echocardiographic guidance and assessment of percutaneous repair for mitral regurgitation with the Evalve MitraClip: Lessons learned from EVEREST I. *J Am Soc Echocardiogr* 2007;20(10):1131–1140.

42

Transcatheter aortic valve replacement

STÉPHANE NOBLE AND PETER WENAWESER

INTRODUCTION AND HISTORICAL PERSPECTIVE

Due to a constant increase in life expectancy, the number of patients with degenerative aortic stenosis (AS) is steadily increasing in Western countries. Advancing age exposes the heart to fibrosis and calcification, and degenerative AS is in Western countries the most common valvular heart disease (VHD) in the elderly, with a prevalence of up to 5% in subjects >85 years of age.[1] Patients with severe, symptomatic AS have a class I indication for valve replacement, as they face a high morbidity and mortality on medical treatment.[2,3] Similar to the pathogenesis of arteriosclerosis, shear stress, inflammation, and lipid accumulation play an important role in the development of AS.[4] Attempts to reduce the progression of aortic valve disease with drugs, such as lipid-lowering agents[5] or angiotensin-converting enzymes (ACE) inhibitors, have failed.[6] Surgical aortic valve replacement (SAVR) has been the standard therapy for many years based on its efficacy in improving symptoms and survival.[7,8] However, comorbidities, advanced age, and frailty led to undertreatment of many elderly patients with symptomatic severe AS, despite the poor prognosis of medical therapy alone.[9,10]

The combination of this unmet clinical need and the desire for a less-invasive treatment than SAVR has driven the development of the transcatheter approach.

The first interventional treatment of VHD goes back to 1953 when Rubio-Alvarez et al. reported the first intracardiac valvulotomy by means of a catheter.[11] In 1979, "balloon valvulotomy" of a congenital pulmonary stenosis was successfully performed,[12] and in the following decades, percutaneous balloon valvuloplasty for pulmonary valve stenosis became standard.[13] The technique of balloon valvuloplasty was adopted for rheumatic mitral valve stenosis[14] and degenerative AS.[15] After the first promising procedural results of balloon valvuloplasty for valvular AS,[15] the analysis of larger patient populations demonstrated disappointing short-term and poor long-term clinical outcomes.[16] Balloon valvuloplasty of heavily calcified degenerative AS provided an acute gain of the aortic orifice area by fracturing calcified nodules, separating fused commissures, and stretching of the aortic valve ring. However, as only microfractures were achieved, the rate of recurrent stenosis was high (50%) within the first months after intervention, and the procedure was limited by periprocedural morbidity (i.e., stroke: 2% within the first 24 hours) and mortality (3% within the first 24 hours).[17] As a consequence, balloon valvuloplasty for the treatment of severe AS is currently only considered in emergency cases as a bridge to valve replacement.[2]

In 1992, developmental efforts led to the first successful transluminal implantation of a balloon-expandable prosthesis in the ascending aorta of closed chest pigs.[18] In 2000, P. Bonhoeffer performed the first human pulmonary transcatheter valve replacement.[19] A decade later on April 16, 2002—after the first animal implants—Alain Cribier in Rouen, France, performed the first human transcatheter aortic valve replacement (TAVR) using a trileaflet bovine pericardial valve mounted on a stainless steel, balloon-expandable stent (Cribier-Edwards valve).[20] On July 12, 2004, Grube and Laborde[21] implanted the first self-expanding CoreValve Revalving System consisting of a trileaflet pericardial tissue valve that is sutured in a self-expanding nitinol frame. Both valves received the Conformité Européene (CE) mark in 2007 and were U.S. Food and Drug Administration (FDA) approved (in 2011 the Edwards valve and in 2014 the Medtronic CoreValve). In less than 10 years, TAVR has developed from an experimental procedure into a routine intervention with more than 200,000 procedures performed in more than 65 countries worldwide as of the first trimester in 2016.

ANATOMIC CONSIDERATIONS

AS represents the most common cause of left ventricular outflow tract (LVOT) obstruction and has three principal etiologies: congenital, rheumatic, and degenerative. The aortic valve is mostly tricuspid, rarely unicuspid (0.02%), bicuspid (1%–2%), or even quadricuspid (0.008%–0.043%).[22] Nontricuspid valves undergo degeneration that may provoke severe symptoms already in infancy or in early adulthood. A bicuspid aortic valve is the most common cardiac congenital anomaly, with an incidence of 1%–2% in the general population. Bicuspid aortic valves may degenerate very early in childhood due to turbulent flow inducing trauma to the leaflets, finally resulting in fibrosis and calcification of the valve. However, in the majority of patients, bicuspid valves typically show signs of sclerosis in the second decade of life and calcification in the fourth decade. The majority of patients with a bicuspid valve will develop stenosis or insufficiency around the age of 70 years.[23] Three different anatomic types of bicuspid aortic valve anatomy have been identified: type 0 without any raphe found in 7%, type 1 with one raphe found in 88% of bicuspid valves, and type II with two raphes in 5% (Figure 42.1).[24]

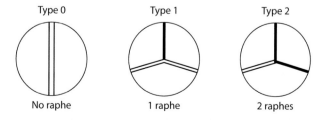

Figure 42.1 Different types of bicuspid valves. (Courtesy of chapter authors.)

Age-related degenerative AS, formerly called senile AS, is the most common cause of acquired AS, whereas rheumatic disease is rarely the cause in Western populations. The development of degenerative, calcific AS shares the risk factors of vascular atherosclerosis. Mechanical stress damages the endothelium of the leaflets, facilitating the subendothelial accumulation of oxidized low-density lipoprotein, the production of angiotensin II, and inflammation with T lymphocytes and macrophages.[4] Progressive calcification leads to severe obstruction.

A detailed assessment of the aortic valve, aortic root, and descending aorta, including the iliofemoral and subclavian axes, is warranted before attempting TAVR.[25] First, and of main interest, are the valvular anatomic details for estimating the amount and distribution of calcification, as well as the cusps. Second, the location of the orifices of the coronary arteries, usually within the two anterior sinuses of Valsalva, may vary. Of special interest with regard to transcatheter bioprostheses is the distance between the basal attachment of the leaflets and the corresponding orifice. In a morphometric and topographic study of the coronary ostia, the mean distances from the left and right coronary ostia to the bottom of the corresponding sinus were 12.6 ± 2.61 to 13.2 ± 2.64 mm, respectively.[26] The width of the sinuses of Valsalva is also an important parameter; the narrower, the higher is the risk of coronary obstruction at the time of TAVR.

The ascending and descending aorta, and the iliofemoral and the subclavian arteries need to be assessed to evaluate the feasibility of introducing the transcatheter valve system. Critical parameters include minimal diameter, tortuosity, calcification, and extension of atherosclerosis at the iliofemoral level. Figure 42.2 summarizes the minimum vascular diameter required for the different CE-approved valves.

FUNDAMENTALS

Different access routes

At present, the procedure is performed through a retrograde transfemoral approach in approximately 70%–95% of cases.[27,28] The antegrade approach via a transfemoral vein route—a challenging route prone to complications and hemodynamic instability—is no longer used.[20] Alternative nontransfemoral approaches were developed to overcome the difficulties related to the size of first-generation devices (≥18-Fr) and to the presence of significant iliofemoral disease. The transapical approach, in which the device is inserted through the anterolateral wall of the left ventricle (LV), was introduced into clinical practice in 2005.[22] Subclavian access had already been developed in the early years of TAVR using the first generation of the CoreValve Revalving System.[29-32] More recently, the direct aortic approach has been reported,[33] and a small number of interventions have also been performed through carotid access.[34]

The majority of transfemoral and subclavian cases are performed in the cardiac catheterization laboratory, whereas direct aortic and transapical procedures should be

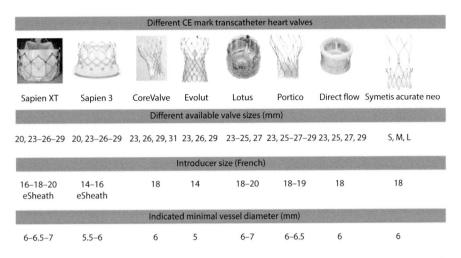

Different CE mark transcatheter heart valves							
Sapien XT	Sapien 3	CoreValve	Evolut	Lotus	Portico	Direct flow	Symetis acurate neo
Different available valve sizes (mm)							
20, 23–26–29	20, 23–26–29	23, 26, 29, 31	23, 26, 29	23–25, 27	23, 25–27–29	23, 25, 27, 29	S, M, L
Introducer size (French)							
16–18–20 eSheath	14–16 eSheath	18	14	18–20	18–19	18	18
Indicated minimal vessel diameter (mm)							
6–6.5–7	5.5–6	6	5	6–7	6–6.5	6	6

Figure 42.2 Minimum vascular diameter required for the different CE-approved devices. (Courtesy of chapter authors.)

preferentially performed in a hybrid operating room. The hybrid room should be large enough to accommodate multiple teams working together (i.e., the interventional cardiologists, echocardiographers, cardiac surgeons, anesthesiologists, perfusionists, and nurses), and it should be equipped with angiography equipment similar to that in a standard cardiac catheterization laboratory, a surgical table, and available connections for the cardiopulmonary bypass machine.

INDICATIONS

Patient selection and risk assessment

Patient selection plays a crucial role and needs to be performed in a systematic manner for every patient with a heart team approach. The heart team is composed of interventional cardiologists and cardiac surgeons. In addition, geriatricians, anesthesiologists, imaging specialists, neurologists, specialized nurses, and other specialists are included, if needed.

Patient selection is divided into three different steps. First, the diagnosis of severe AS is confirmed, and the indication for an intervention is validated according to current guidelines.[2,3] Second, patient frailty and concomitant disease are assessed in order to evaluate the risk of an SAVR. Third, the anatomical suitability for TAVR is evaluated using the different imaging options (multislice computed tomography [MSCT], angiography, and echocardiography).

Confirmation of aortic stenosis severity and indication for replacement

Doppler transthoracic echocardiogram (TTE) is the preferred technique for assessing AS severity, and classical criteria to define severe AS include a valve area of <1 cm² and <0.6 cm²/m², a mean transvalvular gradient of >40 mmHg, and a V_{max} (peak transvalvular velocity) of >4 m/s. The ideal way to quantify AS severity, from a theoretical point of view, is to measure the valve area.[3] However, the planimetry of the aortic valve remains challenging; therefore, the valve area is calculated using the continuity equation based on mean transvalvular gradient, peak transvalvular velocity, LVOT velocity, and diameter. In clinical practice, valve area assessment using TTE is operator-dependent and less robust than gradient/velocity estimates.

When TTE assessment is unequivocal, there is no need for invasive assessment of the AS severity, which requires crossing the valve with wires and catheters, potentially exposing patients to risk of cerebral emboli.[3,35] Simultaneous gradient measurement in the aorta and LV and cardiac output assessment should be considered for patients in atrial fibrillation with low gradient and low left ventricle ejection fraction (LVEF) or paradoxical low flow (<35 mL/m²), low gradient (<40 mmHg), but normal LVEF.[36] Furthermore, in cases with low gradient and low LVEF, low-dose dobutamine stress TTE or an invasive stress test is performed to differentiate between pseudo and true AS. A high calcium score using MSCT supports the relevance of AS.[37]

Risk assessment

The indication for TAVR is based largely on the estimation of the risk for conventional surgery. Multiple risk scores have been developed: The logistic Euro SCORE, Euro SCORE II, and the Society of Thoracic Surgeons (STS) risk score are the most widely used.[38–40] However, their predictive value in high-risk patients is limited. In particular, the Logistic Euro SCORE tends to overestimate the risk of mortality.[41] Since high-risk patients represented a small proportion of the patient population included in the models used to generate a score, the predictive reliability of these scores is limited. In addition, these scores do not take into account important aspects such as liver cirrhosis, hostile thorax (e.g., previous burns and radiation exposure), porcelain aorta, cognitive function, or frailty. Consequently, although these scores are taken into account, they do not define the therapeutic strategy.

Concomitant diseases and assessment of frailty are essential in elderly patients. Multidimensional geriatric assessment-based risk scores, including cognition, nutrition, mobility, activities of daily living, and frailty index, perform similarly to global risk scores in predicting all-cause mortality and major adverse cerebral and cardiovascular events at 30 days and 1 year after TAVR.[42] Recently, gait speed[43] and grip strength were introduced as more objective assessments of physical performance. Briefly, the gait speed test measures the time needed to walk 5 meters. If it is more than 6 seconds, 30-day mortality is increased fourfold. As this association is independent of the STS score, patients with high STS score and slow gait speed have the worst prognosis. Additional information on the general condition and physiological reserve of a patient can be provided by assessing recent weight loss, a history of recent falls, activity level, independence

in daily activities, and cognition using the Mini-Mental State Examination (MMSE).[44] Frailty is most often found in patients with significant concomitant diseases and often coexists with certain laboratory findings, such as low serum albumin, anemia, or elevated inflammatory markers.

Age is a major prognostic factor and is taken into account when selecting SAVR or TAVR. However, comorbidities and functional status have been shown to be better predictors of mortality than just age.[45,46] In octogenarians, the recovery period should be as short as possible for the patient to really benefit from the intervention, since these patients have already reached average life expectancy. Table 42.1 summarizes the risk factors assessed to select the best therapeutic option. Figure 42.3 summarizes the different risk categories according to the American College of Cardiology (ACC)/ American Heart Association (AHA) guidelines.[2]

Suitability and screening for transcatheter aortic valve replacement

An appropriate screening process is essential for a successful TAVR. The most important exams during the screening phase are echocardiography (TTE or transesophageal echocardiography [TEE]), MSCT and coronary angiogram, and ancillary tests, which are indicated in selected patients according to their history (such as a CT scan of the brain in patients with prior stroke).

TTE allows for the diagnosis of AS and the assessment of the mitral valve (i.e., to exclude associated severe mitral stenosis or regurgitation), LVEF, and right heart function, as well as an estimation of the systolic pulmonary artery pressure. Echocardiography also allows the exclusion of contraindications for TAVR, such as left ventricular thrombus, endocarditis,

Table 42.1 Risk assessment and tools

Risk factors	Measure
Comorbidities	Society of Thoracic Surgeons score
	Logistic EuroSCORE and EuroSCORE II
Weakness	Grip strength
	Recent falls
	Needing a wheelchair
Malnutrition	Serum albumin
	Weight loss
	Body mass index <20 kg/m²
Slowness	Gait speed test
Independence	Katz activities of daily living
	Nursing home resident
Cognitive aspect	Mini Mental State Evaluation score
Other	Porcelain aorta
	Hostile thorax
	Liver cirrhosis

	Low Risk (Must Meet ALL Criteria in This Column)	Intermediate Risk (Any 1 Criterion in This Column)	High Risk (Any 1 Criterion in This Column)	Prohibitive Risk (Any 1 Criterion in This Column)
STS PROM*	<4% AND	4%–8% OR	>8% OR	Predicted risk with surgery of death or major morbidity (all-cause) >50% at 1 y OR
Frailty†	None AND	1 Index (mild) OR	≥2 Indices (moderate to severe) OR	
Major organ system compromise not to be improved postoperatively‡	None AND	1 Organ system OR	No more than 2 organ systems OR	≥3 Organ systems OR
Procedure-specific impediment§	None	Possible procedure-specific impediment	Possible procedure-specific impediment	Severe procedure-specific impediment

*Use of the STS PROM to predict risk in a given institution with reasonable reliability is appropriate only if institutional outcomes are within 1 standard deviation of STS average observed/expected ratio for the procedure in question.

†Seven frailty indices: Katz Activities of Daily Living (independence in feeding, bathing, dressing, transferring, toileting, and urinary continence) and independence in ambulation (no walking aid or assist required or 5-meter walk in <6 s). Other scoring systems can be applied to calculate no, mild-, or moderate-to-severe frailty.

‡Examples of major organ system compromise: Cardiac—severe LV systolic or diastolic dysfunction or RV dysfunction, fixed pulmonary hypertension; CKD stage 3 or worse; pulmonary dysfunction with FEV1 <50% or DLCO₂ <50% of predicted; CNS dysfunction (dementia, Alzheimer's disease, Parkinson's disease, CVA with persistent physical limitation); GI dysfunction—Crohn's disease, ulcerative colitis, nutritional impairment, or serum albumin <3.0; cancer—active malignancy; and liver—any history of cirrhosis, variceal bleeding, or elevated INR in the absence of VKA therapy.

§Examples: tracheostomy present, heavily calcified ascending aorta, chest malformation, arterial coronary graft adherent to posterior chest wall, or radiation damage

CKD indicates chronic kidney disease; CNS, central nervous system; CVA, stroke; DLCO₂, diffusion capacity for carbon dioxide; FEV1, forced expiratory volume in 1 s; GI, gastrointestinal; INR, international normalized ratio; LV, left ventricular; PROM, predicted risk of mortality; RV, right ventricular; STS, Society of Thoracic Surgeons; and VKA, vitamin K antagonist.

Figure 42.3 Risk assessment combining Society of Thoracic Surgeons score, frailty, major organ system compromise, and procedure-specific impediment. (Reprinted from Nishimura, R.A., et al., *J. Am. Coll. Cardiol.*, 63, e57–e185, 2014. With permission.)

Table 42.2 Major exclusion criteria
in the PARTNER trial

Exclusion criteria in PARTNER trial

Anatomic Criteria
Bicuspid valve
Annulus size < 18 mm and > 25 mm

Patient Characteristics
Left ventricular ejection fraction <20%
Mitral regurgitation >3
Severe renal failure
Stroke within 6 months

or subvalvular stenosis. Coronary angiography is required to assess coronary artery disease. Coronary stenting may be performed in cases of severe stenosis in proximal segments of major vessels. MSCT is the exam of choice to assess the annulus size and vascular access. Figure 42.4 shows a typical case.

In the beginning of the TAVR experience, aortic annulus measurement was performed using echocardiography (TTE and TEE).[47] However, TTE provides only two-dimensional (2D) measurement, which is suboptimal because the annulus is commonly oval in shape as shown by three-dimensional (3D) assessment using MSCT analysis.[48-52] Many studies have shown differences in the dimensions of the annulus depending on the imaging modalities used for measurement.[48-54]

Most operators prefer to rely on 3D imaging provided by MSCT.[55,56] 3D TEE is a potential alternative when MSCT cannot be performed.[56] Importantly, dedicated centers are now able to image the heart and the vessels from the subclavian arteries down to the femoral arteries using an electrocardiographic (ECG)-gated MSCT with minimal use of contrast media (on average 60 cc). The manufacturers provide matrices for selecting the appropriate prosthesis size (Figure 42.5) based not only on maximum and minimum diameters but also on mean diameter, as well as annulus perimeter and area.[57] It has been shown that a difference between prosthesis size and annular size measured by MSCT was predictive of paravalvular aortic regurgitation (PAR).[58] Therefore, correct annulus sizing is critical in order to select the appropriate valve size. A large range of annulus size is now covered by the available devices (perimeter from 56.5 to 91.1 mm and diameter from 18 mm to 29 mm) (Figure 42.5).

If the diagnosis of severe symptomatic AS is clearly established by echocardiography, some operators start the assessment with a MSCT, followed by a coronary angiogram and right heart catheterization in order to assess the coronary arteries and the cardiac hemodynamics, including cardiac output. At the same time, angiography of the iliofemoral vessels is performed, although for some operators the assessment by MSCT is sufficient, especially in patients with renal insufficiency. An alternative strategy is to confirm the diagnosis of severe AS by a right and left heart catheterization using simultaneous pressure measurements in the LV and

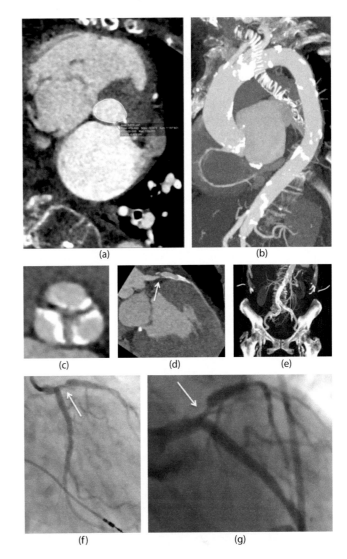

(a) (b)

(c) (d) (e)

(f) (g)

Figure 42.4 Typical case of transaortic valve implantation (TAVI) screening with multislice computed tomography (MSCT) performed with 60 cc of contrast and coronary angiography. (Courtesy of AL Hachulla, MD.) **(a)** MSCT with measurement of the aortic annulus performed with Osirix (perimeter: 64 mm, area: 3 cm²). **(b)** MSCT showing the view of the aortic arch showing the degree of calcification. **(c)** MSCT view showing that the valve is tricuspid and highly calcified. **(d)** Coro CT images showing a tight left anterior descending lesion (*arrow*) confirmed by the coronary angiography (**f** and **g**). **(e)** MSCT showing the iliofemoral vasculature down including the femoral bifurcation.

ascending aorta. Left catheterization may be especially useful if there are doubts on the severity of the stenosis at TTE. The MSCT or 3D TEE is then performed later to assess the annulus size. In this elderly population with decreased renal function, injections of contrast media should be as low as possible and ideally separated by several days.

Ad hoc TAVR procedures have been performed, thus highlighting that TAVR can be successfully performed without upfront CT scan.[59] In an emergency setting, balloon sizing has been promoted to help define the required valve size.[59,60]

Evolut R patient annulus range

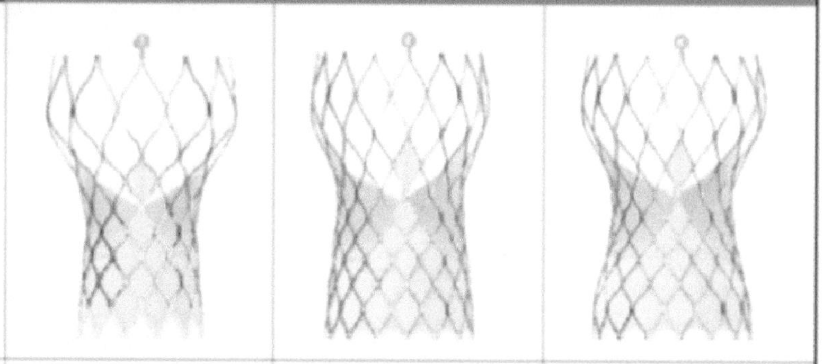

Valve size selection	Corevalve* Evolut™ R		
Size	23 mm	26 mm	29 mm
Annulus diameter	18–20 mm	20–23 mm	23–26 mm
Annulus perimeter*	56.5–62.8 mm	62.8–72.3 mm	72.3–81.7 mm
Sinus of valsalva diameter (mean)	≥25 mm	≥27 mm	≥29 mm
Sinus of valsalva height (mean)	≥15 mm	≥15 mm	≥15 mm
*Annulus perimeter = Annulus diameter xЛ			

(a)

Sapien 3 valve sizing: confirm THV size

Note:
Systolic measurements are recommended

3D Area-derived diameter (mm)		20.0	20.2	20.5	20.7	21.0	21.1	21.4	21.7	22.0	22.3	22.6	22.8	23.0	23.1	23.4	23.7	23.9	24.0	24.2	24.7
3D Annular area (mm²)		314	320	330	338	348	350	360	370	380	390	400	410	415	420	430	440	450	452	460	480
% Annular area over (+) or under (-) nominal by 3D CT	23 mm	29.3	26.9	23.0	20.1	17.3	16.0	12.8	9.7	6.8	4.0	1.5	–1.0	–2.2	–3.3	–5.6	–7.7	–9.8			
	26 mm											29.8	26.6	25.1	23.6	20.7	18.0	15.3	14.0	12.8	8.1
	29 mm																				

3D Area-derived diameter (mm)		25.0	25.2	25.5	25.7	26.0	26.2	26.4	26.5	26.7	26.9	27.2	27.4	27.6	27.9	28.0	28.1	28.3	28.5	28.8	29.0	29.2	29.4	29.5	29.6	29.9	30.1	30.3
3D Annular area (mm²)		490	500	510	520	530	540	546	550	560	570	580	590	600	610	615	620	630	640	650	660	670	680	683	690	700	710	720
% Annular area over (+) or under (–) nominal by 3D CT	23 mm																											
	26 mm	5.9	3.8	1.8	–0.2	–2.1	–3.9	–4.9	–5.6	–7.3	–8.5																	
	29 mm					29.8	27.3	24.8	22.5	20.2	18.9	18.0	15.9	13.9	11.9	10.0	8.2	6.4	5.5		3.0	1.4	–0.2	–1.7	–3.1	–4.6	–5.6	–5.9 –7.3 –8.6 –9.9

Note:
Bold = recommended sealing zones relate only to valves that are deployed with nominal volumes

Note:
All values presented are based on nominal/recommended inflation volumes

(b)

Figure 42.5 Matrix to select the valve size for (a) Evolut R and (b) SAPIEN 3. (Provided by Medtronic and Edwards.)

Indications for transcatheter aortic valve replacement according to guidelines

The latest European and American guidelines[2,3] recommend TAVR for symptomatic patients with a contraindication for surgery and a life expectancy >1 year. Compared with medical management, the results of cohort B in the PARTNER trial showed the superiority of TAVR in terms of 1-year mortality, with a number needed to treat of five. In this population, the recommendation for TAVR is class I indication, level of evidence B. In patients with high surgical risk, TAVR appears at least as effective as SAVR, according the Corevalve High Risk trial and the PARTNER A trial (class IIa indication, level B).[61,62] Most recently, the PARTNER 2 trial revealed superiority of the transfemoral TAVR approach over the conventional surgical approach in intermediate-risk patients.[63] Importantly, an experienced heart team is needed to provide optimal care for patients.

EQUIPMENT AND TECHNIQUE

Valves prostheses

Two devices encompass most of the clinical experience: the different generations of the Edwards transcatheter heart valve (THV) and the Medtronic CoreValve system. The latter is a self-expanding device with a supra-annular function, whereas the Edwards devices, until now, have been balloon-expandable valves. However, Edwards recently developed the Centera THV–14-Fr eSheath compatible, which consists of a nitinol self-expandable stent with treated bovine pericardial leaflets and polyethylene terephthalate (PET) fabric.

EDWARDS VALVES

Following the Edwards Cribier valve, the Edwards SAPIEN (used in the PARTNER trials and FDA-approved in November 2011) and the Edwards SAPIEN XT (implanted in the PARTNER II trial and FDA-approved in June 2014 for high-risk patients and in October 2015 for valve-in-valve [VIV] procedures) were the predecessors of the Edwards SAPIEN 3, which was first implanted in man in January 2012 and FDA-approved for high-risk patients in June 2015.[64] The latter is made from a cobalt chromium stent with trileaflet bovine pericardial tissue and has an increased height compared to former generations. Its profile has been further reduced and the delivery (e-Sheath) sheath for the 26 mm valve is 14-Fr equivalent corresponding to a true 18-Fr outer diameter, and to 24-Fr outer diameter when expanded. The inner part of the prosthesis is covered with a PET skirt, as previous generations, while an outer PET sealing cuff has been added in order to reduce PAR.

MEDTRONIC COREVALVE

The Medtronic CoreValve consists of a trileaflet porcine pericardial tissue valve that is sutured in a self-expanding nitinol frame. At present, the fifth generation, namely the Medtronic CoreValve Evolut R, is available in three sizes (23 mm, 26 mm, and 29 mm). The device was approved by the FDA in June 2015. As of June 2016, the 31 mm device still only exists in the fourth-generation model. The main new feature of the CoreValve Evolut R valve, compared with previous generations, is that it is repositionable. In addition, it has a shorter frame (by approximately 10 mm) at the level of its outflow with a paddle design, instead of the previously used tabs in order to facilitate the valve release from the delivery catheter, larger cell design to facilitate access to the coronary arteries, and a longer skirt to decrease PAR. Moreover, an alpha-amino oleic acid treatment of the leaflets was implemented in order to reduce short- and long-term calcific degeneration of the prosthesis.[65] The EnVeo R catheter has an InLine sheath—a 14-Fr equivalent corresponding to a true 18-Fr outer diameter—which allows the valve to be delivered without the requirement of a separate introducer sheath. Finally, in order to aid repositioning, the novel laser-cut nitinol-reinforced capsule is designed to enable the re-sheathing or recapture of the valve up to the point of 80% of maximal valve deployment.

Several companies have launched trials to assess the safety and efficacy of other devices, many with retrievable and repositionable features. Devices studied include the Lotus valve (Boston Scientific, first in man, June 2007, Siegburg, Germany[66]), which is a preloaded and stent-mounted valve; the Direct Flow valve (Direct Flow Medical, first in man in September 2007, Hamburg, Germany[67]), a nonmetallic bovine pericardial valve with a double-ring design; and the Portico device (St. Jude Medical, first in man in June 2011, Vancouver, Canada[68]), which is a self-expanding intra-annular valve. The ACCURATE TA device (Symetis SA, Ecublens, Switzerland, first in man in November 2009, Leipzig, Germany[69]) is a self-expandable nitinol stent with a three-leaflet porcine valve with the unique feature of self-positioning at a supra-annular level. Figure 42.6 shows the evolution of the available devices.

Implantation techniques

PROCEDURAL STEPS

The implantation techniques of a self-expanding and a balloon-expandable device are similar, except during deployment. For the balloon-expandable valve, it is essential to use rapid pacing at a rate of 180–220 beats per minute (bpm) in order to obtain a standstill heart for a safe and precise deployment. While routine rapid pacing is not required for the self-expanding device, pacing at approximately 120 bpm may be helpful to stabilize the delivery system during deployment in challenging and large anatomies (e.g., in cases of predominant aortic regurgitation [AR]).

Before the intervention, a temporary pacing lead should be inserted, preferably through a jugular vein, which enables rapid patient mobilization postprocedure. Usually, the lead is removed after 48 hours.

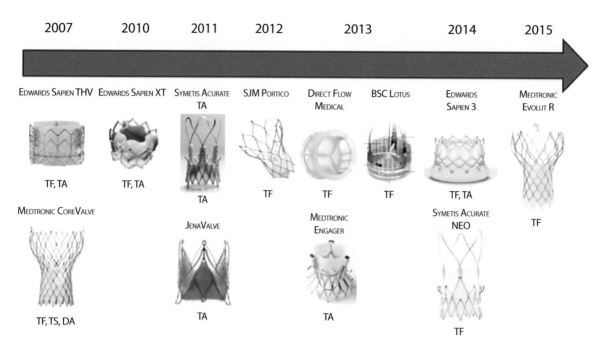

Figure 42.6 The evolution of the available devices. DA, direct aortic; TA, transapical; TF, transfemoral. (Courtesy of chapter authors.)

Transfemoral procedures can be safely performed under local anesthesia with sedation, although some centers prefer to perform the procedures under general anesthesia.[70] Most procedures are done under fluoroscopic guidance only, and periprocedural TEE is used in procedures done under general anesthesia (GA). Conversion from local anesthesia to GA is often needed in complicated cases (e.g., acute heart failure) or for patient comfort. GA avoids movements of the legs or the whole body due to discomfort and increases the level of comfort for the operators.[71] Benefits of local anesthesia include shorter procedural time and hospital stay, earlier recovery, and less hypotension requiring vasopressor support. Conversion from local to GA is required in approximately 5%–17% of procedures.[70,72,73]

The TAVR procedure can be summarized in three steps: access, valve deployment, and access closure. Transfemoral approach: the first step includes vascular access with the use of preclosing systems such as the Prostar XL or Perclose devices (Abbott vascular). The valve delivery sheath is inserted transfemorally over a stiff wire. From the contralateral femoral access site, a 5-Fr or 6-Fr pigtail is advanced into the ascending aorta and serves as a reference point (i.e., surrogate for cusps/annulus localization) and is used for dye injection. The stenotic valve is then crossed with a straight wire, most commonly a 5-Fr Amplatz Left (AL) 1 diagnostic catheter using the operator's preferred view (from right anterior oblique [RAO] 30° to left anterior oblique [LAO] 30 projection). The AL 1 is exchanged for a pigtail catheter over an exchange length 0.035-in in order to acquire, together with the other pigtail in the ascending aorta, simultaneous pressure tracing and mean aortic gradient and to safely place a stiff wire (i.e., Amplatz superstiff wire or a preshaped stiff wire [e.g., Medtronic Confida wire or Boston SAFARY

wire] for the CoreValve and Amplatz extrastiff wire for the Edwards THV) in the LV, usually using the RAO projection. The working view should be determined with the aim of aligning the three aortic leaflets on one plane. Some centers additionally use a dedicated software, such as the C-THV (Paieon Inc, Israel), 3mensio (Pie Medical Imaging, The Netherlands), or the Heart Navigator (Philips, Eindhoven, The Netherlands), which helps in the selection of the perpendicular view up front and may improve device positioning.[74] Without these tools, the optimal view may be determined—starting in a LAO 10° or 15° view—by performing low-volume aortographies (10 cc at 10 cc/s).

Subsequently, balloon aortic valvuloplasty (BAV) is performed using rapid pacing at a rate of 180–200 bpm. At the time of BAV, the valve should be ready for implantation in the event of acute severe AR, occurring in 1%–2% of cases.[75] The rate of BAV prior to device insertion has decreased over the last years but may still be required in cases of heavily calcified AS. Direct valve implantations are often performed, especially with self-expanding and repositionable devices.

Following BAV, the device is advanced to the aortic annulus. Self-expanding devices are slowly deployed under fluoroscopic guidance with repeated low-volume dye injections (usually three to six injections of 10 cc), whereas the balloon-expandable devices are deployed during a rapid pacing burst.

As soon as the bioprosthesis is released and deployed, a hemodynamic assessment is made with one pigtail in the aorta and one in the LV, which includes measurements of trans-aortic gradient, end-diastolic left ventricular pressure, and diastolic systemic pressure.[76,77] To assess a potential residual PAR, in addition to the hemodynamic assessment, aortography and/or TEE are performed. In patients who are not intubated in whom significant PAR is suspected, TTE may help to assess the degree and causes of PAR.

Finally, the procedure is finished by closing the entry site of the vascular access. The sutures of the pre-closing system are knotted while retrieving the large sheath. By using a crossover approach, a final angiography of the vascular access is performed to verify closure success. Failure of the Prostar XL device (Abbott Vascular) seems to be associated with obesity, small-diameter vessels with significant calcification, or a high puncture site.[78,79] In cases of closure failure or a major vascular complication (i.e., dissection, perforation, diffuse bleeding), a cross-over treatment with balloon inflation or covered stent implantation are successful in the majority of cases. Rarely, surgical repair is needed.

In the absence of puncture site complications, after 12 hours of compulsory bedrest, patients are mobilized. Standard antiplatelet treatment post TAVR consists of acetylsalicylic acid (ASA) 100 mg daily for life and Clopidogrel 75 mg daily for 1 to 6 months. For patients with an indication of oral anticoagulation, dual antiplatelet therapy (DAPT) can be omitted or combined with one antiplatelet agent depending on the risk of thrombotic complication versus bleeding events. Postmortem analysis of explanted THV at different time intervals showed that at 3 months, the initial fibrin coverage was already replaced by smooth muscle cells and endothelial cells, likely reducing the embolic potential.[80–82] Importantly, the distribution of the neointimal tissue conformed to the CoreValve design and covered most of the frame struts in contact with the aortic wall, but areas of high-velocity flow or not in contact with the aortic wall were not covered (Figure 42.7).[80] DAPT following TAVR is a source of debate, and there is no strong evidence for it to be prescribed.[83] Recently, a small series randomized 79 patients to aspirin alone or DAPT initiated the day before the procedure and maintained for 3 months. There was no increase of major cardiac or cerebrovascular adverse events with aspirin alone versus DAPT at 30 days (15% vs. 13%, $P = 0.71$) and 6 months (15% vs. 18%, $P = 0.85$).[84] There are two ongoing trials assessing the optimum antithrombotic regimen following TAVR: the AUREA study, which is evaluating the ability of double DAPT versus oral anticoagulation with a vitamin-K antagonist to reduce areas of cerebral injury, as assessed by magnetic resonance at 3 months; and the ARTE trial, which is designed to determine if DAPT versus aspirin alone may prevent major ischemic events (including myocardial infarction [MI], ischemic stroke, or death) without

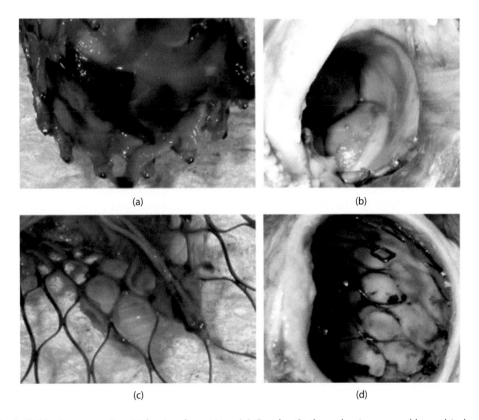

(a)   (b)

(c)   (d)

Figure 42.7 Endothelialization post CoreValve implantation. **(a)** On day 3, the valve is covered by a thin layer of tissue on the inner surface of the device. Small pieces of tissue in the cells on the inner surface near the valve suture areas on the stent. The tissue in microscopy corresponded to fibrin deposition and an inflammatory response. **(b)** At 3 months, the valve struts on the inflow part are completely covered by tissue. Distal spikes of the outflow part of the THV, but not the body of the device are covered by tissue corresponding to neo-intima with regression of the inflammatory response. **(c** and **d)** Gross photographs show coverage of the distal spikes but not the body of the device. Focal thrombus deposition is observed on the inner surface of the stent struts (black nodules in **[d]**). (Reprinted from Noble, S., et al., *EuroIntervention*, 5, 78–85, 2009. With permission.)

an increase in bleeding following TAVR using the Edwards THV.[83] In the PARTNER II trial, DAPT was prescribed for 1 month. Of note, if there is an indication for anticoagulation, aspirin for 1 month in addition to anti-vitamin-K medication can be considered or oral anticoagulation alone.

CLINICAL ASPECTS

Standardized endpoint definitions proposed by the Valve Academic Research Consortium (VARC) provide consistency and help to facilitate improved evaluation of TAVR.[85] This first consensus manuscript, published in January 2011, and which included surgeons, interventional and noninterventional cardiologists, imaging specialists, neurologists, geriatric specialists, clinical specialists, industry representatives, and the FDA, concentrated on two points: first, the selection of appropriate clinical endpoints reflecting device, procedure, and patient-related effectiveness; and second, safety and the standardization of definitions for single and composite clinical endpoints for TAVR clinical trials. Since October 2012, the VARC-II was created to adapt to emerging data and to expand understanding of patient risk stratification and selection.

Important clinical studies

INOPERABLE PATIENTS

PARTNER data. The pivotal PARTNER trial is the first randomized (1/1), controlled multicenter study assessing the effectiveness and safety of any THV in patients with severe, symptomatic AS who are considered inoperable (cohort B) or at high surgical risk (cohort A) using the second generation of the Edwards valve, the Edwards SAPIEN. The prosthesis was only available in 23 and 26 mm valve sizes for the transfemoral approach and required a 22-Fr or 24-Fr sheath, respectively, for the transfemoral route. The major exclusion criteria are summarized in Table 42.2. The primary endpoint was all-cause mortality with a follow-up of 5 years. Between May 2007 and March 2009, 358 patients who were not suitable candidates for SAVR were included in the PARTNER trial cohort B, and randomized either for TAVR (179 patients) or standard therapy (179 patients). The study was conducted in 21 sites from the United States, Canada, and Germany.[86-88] Results from this trial showed at 1 year that all-cause mortality was significantly lower with TAVR than with standard therapy including BAV in 84% of the cases (30.7% vs. 50.7%, $P < 0.001$). This 20% absolute risk reduction of all-cause mortality corresponds to a number needed to treat of only five patients to save one life at 1 year, which makes TAVR one of the most important advances in medicine over the last 15 years. As expected, major vascular complications (16.2% vs. 1.1%, $P < 0.001$) and major bleeding events (16.8% vs. 3.9%, $P < 0.001$) were more frequent following TAVR than with standard therapy, and there was an improvement in the quality of life in the TAVR arm as reflected by the improvement in the 6-minute walk distance test and New York Heart Association (NYHA) functional class. At 1 year, 74.8% of the surviving patients who had undergone TAVR were in functional class NYHA I or II, as compared to only 42% of the surviving patients in the standard therapy group ($P < 0.001$).

Subsequently, the results at 2- and 5-year follow-up were reported.[87-89] The rate of all-cause mortality at 2 years was 68% among patients in the standard therapy group, compared with 43.3% in the TAVR group ($P < 0.001$). The outcomes were unchanged when patients who had crossed over from standard therapy to TAVR were not excluded (67.6% vs. 43.4%, $P < 0.001$). The difference in death rate remained significant between the first and second year (18.2% in the TAVR group vs. 35.1% in the standard therapy group, $P = 0.02$). Similarly, the rate of cardiac death between the first and second year was significantly different between the TAVR and standard-therapy groups (13.2% vs. 32.1%, $P = 0.004$). The mortality benefit continues to increase in the 3-year survivors.

At 5 years follow-up, the only patient subgroup who did not benefit from TAVR corresponded to the patients with oxygen-dependent chronic obstructive pulmonary disease (COPD).[88] The echocardiographic analyses showed a sustained hemodynamic benefit from TAVR at 5 years. In summary, results from this trial showed that TAVR is superior to standard treatment (including BAV in 84% of the cases) at 1 year and up to the 5-year follow-up in patients with severe symptomatic AS who are not candidates for conventional SAVR.

INOPERABLE AND HIGH-RISK PATIENTS

The PARTNER cohort A trial randomized 699 patients with symptomatic severe AS considered at high surgical risk between SAVR and TAVR, either by transfemoral approach (244 transfemoral TAVR and 248 SAVR) when iliofemoral access was suitable, or transapical approach (104 transapical TAVR and 103 SAVR) when the iliofemoral arteries were too diseased or of too small a caliber.[61] After randomization, 8% of the surgical group refused the intervention, and 5% of the TAVR group never received the Edwards THV (conversion to open heart surgery in 2.6% and procedure aborted in 2.4%). The 30-day all-cause mortality was 3.4% in the TAVR group as compared to 6.5% in the surgical group ($P = .07$), thus inferior to the prediction of the risk score (mean STS score 11.8%). At 1-, 2-, and 5-year follow-up, there were no significant differences with respect to the all-cause mortality rates between the TAVR group (24.2%, 33.9%, and 67.8%, respectively) and the surgical group (26.8%, 35%, and 62.4%, respectively).[89,90] Results at 1, 2, and 5 years were also similar for cardiovascular mortality and all-cause mortality or stroke. Subgroup analysis showed that the transfemoral approach met the noninferiority criteria at 1-, 2-, and 5-year follow-up, whereas transapical approach did not. However, differences in baseline characteristics and the small number of transapical patients make the comparison between transfemoral and transapical groups unreliable.

SAVR and TAVR were associated with different complications. Following surgery, there were more new episodes of atrial fibrillation (16% vs. 8.6% in the TAVR group, $P < 0.01$)

and more major bleeding events (19.5% vs. 9.3%, $P < 0.01$). On the other hand, following TAVR there were more major vascular complications than after SAVR (11% vs. 3.2%, $P < 0.01$), and there were more strokes or transient ischemic attacks (TIAs) (5.5% vs. 2.4%, $P = 0.04$). Considering major stroke alone at 30 days, there were no significant differences (TAVR: 3.8% vs. SAVR 2.1%, $P = 0.20$), and for the combination of death or major stroke, the trend was reversed (TAVR: 6.9%, SAVR: 8.2%, $P = 0.52$). After the initial period postprocedure, there was no evidence of higher stroke rate in either group at 5-year follow-up. Moderate or severe PAR was more common after TAVR than surgery at 1, 2, and 5 years, and there was an association of PAR (mild, moderate, or severe versus none or trace) with increased late mortality. Finally, among survivors at 2 years, the mean NYHA functional class was similar in both groups (1.72 after TAVR vs. 1.70 after SAVR, $P = 0.87$), whereas at 30 days, more patients in the TAVR group than in the SAVR group had a reduction in symptoms to NYHA class ≤2. In summary, this clinical trial showed that TAVR is an alternative treatment with noninferior 1-year, 2-year, and 5-year outcomes when compared to conventional SAVR for surgical high-risk patients.

CoreValve data. The CoreValve U.S. pivotal trial had two arms: the extreme risk study, divided in the iliofemoral approach (500 patients) and the noniliofemoral approach (156 patients: 47% subclavian and 53% direct aortic access), and the patients at increased risk for SAVR that were randomized between TAVR and SAVR.

It was judged nonethical to randomize the extreme risk population to standard medical therapy in the light of the PARTNER IB results. Therefore, the outcomes of these patients were compared with a prespecified objective performance goal. Importantly, frailty assessment was included in this trial: 60% of the patients had a high Charlson score, 85% had a slow gait speed test result, and 27.6% were not independent in daily living activities. The classical risk scores revealed that the patients included were in the range of extreme risk patients (Logistic EuroSCORE 22.6 ± 17.1%, STS score 10.3 ± 5.5%). All-cause mortality at 1 year was 26%, and the comparison with the performance goal (43%) reached statistical significance. The rate of moderate or more PAR was favorable, with a rate of 10.5% at discharge that decreased to 4.1% at 1 year. Indeed, 80% of patients with moderate PAR at 1 month, who survived to 1 year, experienced a reduction of PAR over time. Only severe PAR significantly impacted 1-year mortality (85.7% vs. 23.8% for moderate PAR, 23.7% for mild PAR and 17.9% for none). The 2-year clinical outcome and hemodynamic valve performance remained favorable.[91] All-cause mortality increased from 24.3% at 1 year to 36.6% at 2 years, driven by comorbidities (coronary artery disease and STS PROM > 15%) and admission to an assisted living facility. The degree of PAR remained unchanged between 1- and 2-year follow-up.

The high-risk cohort randomized 795 patients between SAVR and TAVR either by iliofemoral approach (83%) or noniliofemoral approach (17%). The Logistic EuroSCORE and the STS score were lower (17.6 ± 13%, 7.3 ± 3%, respectively)

than in the PARTNER IA trial, but 80% of patients had a slow gait speed test result, not assessed in the PARTNER trial. This randomized study was the first to show a superiority of TAVR over SAVR with respect to mortality (1-year events 14.2% vs. 19.1%; $P = 0.04$). As expected, in the TAVR group there were more major vascular complications (5.9 vs. 1.7%, $P = 0.003$) and a higher rate of permanent pacemaker implantation (19.8% vs. 7.1%, $P < 0.001$). On the other hand, in the TAVR group there were fewer life-threatening bleeding events (13.6 vs. 35%, $P < 0.001$), new onset or worsening of atrial fibrillation (11.7% vs. 30.5%, $P < 0.001$), and acute kidney failure (6 vs. 15.1%, $P < 0.001$). Follow-up at 2 and 3 years showed an absolute difference in all-cause mortality between TAVR and SAVR of 4.8% at 1 year, 6.5% at 2 years, and 6.2% at 3 years (number needed to treat at any time point between 15 and 21).[92,93] At 3 years, this absolute difference was no longer statistically significant ($P = 0.068$). Stroke rate was not significantly different at 1 year, but at 2 and 3 years was in favor of TAVR (12.6% vs. 19% at 3 years, $P = 0.03$). Valve performance was maintained at 3 years.[92]

INTERMEDIATE-RISK PATIENTS

In Europe, and especially in Germany, TAVR has been performed in intermediate-risk patients (e.g., STS score ≤8) for several years.[94,95] In 2012, investigators from the German Heart Center in Munich observed a decline in complication rates in patients with lower surgical risk compared to high-risk patients.[95] In their series, the mean age, logistic EuroSCORE, and STS score decreased between quartiles 1 and 4 of enrollment, from 81 to 78 years, 25% to 17%, and 7% to 4%, respectively. The 30-day mortality decreased from 11.4% for the first quartile of their experience to 3.8% in the last quartile, which corresponds to a threefold reduction.[95] Similarly, 6-month mortality decreased from 23.5% to 12.4%, which corresponds to a twofold reduction. In a single-center experience, the same effect of more favorable outcome in intermediate-risk patients was observed,[94] and a three-center comparison of 1-year mortality between TAVR and SAVR using propensity score matching, demonstrated cumulative all-cause rates of mortality at 30 days and 1 year being comparable among the 405 matched pairs of TAVR and SAVR patients considered at intermediate risk.[96]

The Notion (Nordic and Aortic Valve Intervention) trial was the first to randomize 280 all-comer patients with AS, aged ≥70 years, between TAVR using the CoreValve device and SAVR in three Scandinavian centers from December 2009 and April 2013.[97] The mean age was 79.1 ± 4.8 years, and 82% had a STS-Prom score of <4, thus patients were considered at low surgical risk. The mean logistic EuroSCORE I and II were 8.6% and 2%, respectively. The primary outcome (composite of all-cause death, stroke, or MI at 1 year) showed no difference between both groups (13.1% for TAVR vs. 16.3% for SAVR, $P = 0.43$ for superiority). In *post hoc* analysis, using the same noninferiority margin as in PARTNER IA (7.5%), the noninferiority of TAVR compared with SAVR could be shown for the primary outcome. Individually, all-cause mortality, stroke, new-onset or worsening atrial fibrillation, and myocardial rates were not significantly different at 30 days but were numerically lower in

TAVR patients. However, major and life-threatening bleeding, cardiogenic shock, and acute kidney injury were significantly lower in the TAVR group compared with the surgical cohort. On the other hand, SAVR was associated with a significantly less need for permanent pacemaker at 30 days (1.6% vs. 34.1%, $P < 0.001$) and less moderate to severe PAR at 1 year (0.9% vs. 15.7%, $P < 0.001$). The high percentage of significant PAR may have been related to the absence of routine MSCT scanning for the annulus sizing. The difference in PAR may help explain the difference in the 1-year assessment of NYHA functional class, as TAVR patients more frequently were in NYHA class II or III (29.5% and 3% vs. 15% and 3.3%; $P = 0.01$).

Currently, two different randomized trials are targeting intermediate-risk patients: the SURTAVI (SUrgical Replacement and Transcatheter Aortic Valve Implantation) trial[98] and the PARTNER-II cohort A.

The SURTAVI trial is comparing TAVR using the Medtronic CoreValve and SAVR in moderate-risk patients (STS mortality risk score of ≥3% but ≤8%) with severe symptomatic AS. The study is being conducted in Europe, Canada, and the United States with a long-term follow-up of 5 years. Recruitment of 2,500 patients has been completed, and the results were released at the ACC meeting in 2017.

The PARTNER II cohort A, recently published, randomized 2,032 patients with a mean STS score of 5.8% between TAVR with the Edwards SAPIEN XT valve and SAVR.[63] The analysis showed that in intermediate-risk patients, the results of TAVR were noninferior to SAVR with respect to the primary endpoint of death or disabling stroke at 2 years (19.3% in the TAVR group vs. 21.1% in the SAVR group),

with a similar improvement of cardiac symptoms. The transfemoral approach even shows a potential superiority over SAVR, but it should be confirmed in a prospective and adequately powered evaluation. TAVR resulted in lower rates of acute kidney injury, severe bleeding, and new-onset atrial fibrillation, whereas surgery resulted in fewer major vascular complications and PAR. Furthermore, the improvement in gradients and aortic-valve areas were greater after TAVR. Even though these results are very positive, long-term data in this population are essential before promoting TAVR as the preferred approach in lower-risk patients.

Mortality rate

Mortality rate dramatically decreased over time with the growing experience of the operators, the improvement of the devices, and treatment of lower-risk patients. Figure 42.8 describes the 30-day mortality decrease over time in different trials. Table 42.3 summarizes mortality with the different CE marked devices.

Hemodynamic performance of transcatheter heart valves

The hemodynamic performance of THV was evaluated in different studies and compared to surgical bioprostheses.[61,99] Clavel et al. analyzed three groups of 50 patients implanted with an Edwards THV, a surgical stented Edwards Perimont Magna valve, or a surgical stentless Medtronic Freestyle valve. The THV provided superior hemodynamic performance at

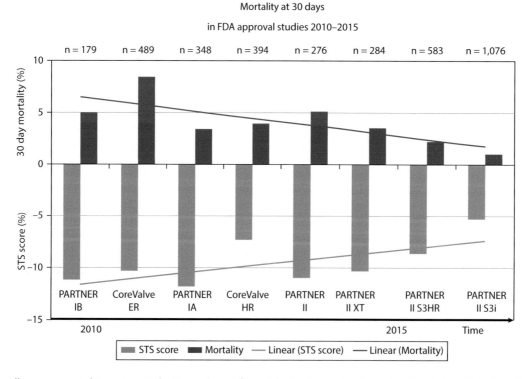

Figure 42.8 All-cause mortality as treated. (Reproduced from Pilgrim, T., and Windecker, S., *J. Am. Coll. Cardiol.*, 66, 1335–1338, 2015. With permission.) FDA, U.S. Food and Drug Administration; STS, Society of Thoracic Surgeons.

Table 42.3 Clinical outcomes with different CE marked devices[a]

Study	Number	MVC	PVL	PACE	Stroke					Mortality	
					All	Major	Minor	D	ND	All	CV
PARTNER IB[59]	179	16.2%	11.8%	3.4%	6.7%	5.0%	1.7%			5.0%	4.5%
PARTNER IA[60]	348	11%	12.2%	3.8%	4.7%	3.8%	0.9%			3.4%	3.2%
Surgery	351	3.2%	0.9%	3.6%	2.2%	2.1%	0.1%			6.5%	3.0%
PARTNER IIA[62]	1001	7.9%	3.7%	8.5%	5.5%			3.2%	2.3%	3.9%	3.3%
Surgery	1021	5.0%	0.6%	6.9%	6.1%			4.3%	1.8%	4.1%	3.2%
SAPIEN S3 CE[92] Mark	1076	5.3%	3.5%	13.3%	2.7%			0%	2.7%	2.1%	2.1%
CoreValve Extreme Risk[93]	506	8.2%	11.5%	21.6%	4.0%	2.3%	1.9%			1.1%	0.9%
CoreValve U.S. pivotal[94]	390	5.9%	9%	19.8%	4.9%	3.9%	1.0%			8.4%	8.4%
Surgery	357	1.7%	1%	7.1%	6.2%	3.1%	3.4%			4.5%	4.5%
EVOLUT CE Mark[26]	60	8.3%	3.4%	11.7%	0%					0%	0%
Lotus Reprise II[95]	120	2.5%	1%	28.6%	5.9%			1.7%	4.2%	4.2%	4.2%
Direct Flow Real world[96]	105	3.8%	1.9%	10%	1.9%					1.9%	NA
Portico multi-center[97]	222	5.9%	5.1%	13.1%				3.2%	2.3%	3.6%	3.6%

Note: CE, Conformité Européene; CV, cardiovascular; D, disabling; MVC, major vascular complication; ND, non-disabling; PVL, paravalvular leak.

[a] The following valves are FDA-approved as of June 2016: Medtronic CoreValve and Evolut R as well as the Edwards SAPIEN XT and S3.

discharge and follow-up compared with the surgical bioprostheses in terms of transprosthetic gradient (THV 10 ± 4 mmHg, stented valve 13 ± 5 mmHg, stentless valve 14 ± 6 mmHg) and prosthesis-patient mismatch, but was associated with a higher incidence of moderate or severe AR (8% with TVH vs. 0% for surgical bioprosthesis).[99]

In the PARTNER trials and CoreValve U.S. pivotal trials, greater valve area and lower postprocedural mean gradients compared to surgical valves were consistently found.

A Canadian multicenter study performed a direct hemodynamic comparison between the Edwards THV and Medtronic CoreValve.[100] A matched (for aortic annulus size, LVEF, body surface area and body mass index) comparison of 41 patients who received a 26 mm CoreValve or a 26 mm Edwards SAPIEN was performed. All echocardiographic assessments were performed by a core laboratory. The mean transprosthetic residual gradient was significantly lower in the CoreValve group than in the Edwards group (7.9 ± 3.2 mmHg vs. 9.7 ± 3.8 mmHg, $P = 0.024$), while no difference was observed in terms of effective orifice area (1.58 ± 0.31 cm^2 vs. 1.49 ± 0.24 cm^2, $P = 0.10$). However, the incidence of severe prosthesis-patient mismatch was similar for both prostheses (10%).

TRANSCATHETER AORTIC VALVE REPLACEMENT COMPLICATIONS

Vascular complications and bleeding

These complications dramatically decreased with the reduction of sheath size and better closure success using contralateral injection. Only major vascular complications are associated with an increase in 30-day mortality. Table 42.3 summarizes the vascular complications with the different CE marked devices.

Paravalvular aortic regurgitation

The newer generation of devices decreased the rate of PAR. Most studies, except the PARTNER IA trial, found that mild PAR did not influence mortality. Conversely, greater than moderate leaks were consistently associated with increased 1-year mortality.

Atrioventricular conduction disturbances and need of permanent pacemaker implantation

The risk of a need for permanent pacemaker implantation is associated with the depth of implantation and the device type.[27,28,101–103] As a general rule, the lower the implant into the LVOT, the higher the risk for atrioventricular (AV) conduction disorders and permanent pacemaker requirement. In the CE mark trial for the Edwards SAPIEN 3, the rate of pacemaker (14.6% for TF approach) was clearly higher than that observed in previous trials. As soon as the implantation technique was adapted and the devices were implanted higher, the rate decreased to 4% in a later series of 101 patients.[104,105]

With the Medtronic CoreValve, the rate of pacemaker implantation is consistently higher than with Edwards Sapien valves. However, it was also shown that a high CoreValve implant is associated with fewer conduction abnormalities. In a study on 134 patients, in which 85% of CoreValves were implanted between 0 and 6 mm below the annulus plane, the need for pacemaker implantation was 10.6%.[101] In the CE mark trial for the Evolut valve, the mean depth of implantation between the annulus plane and the noncoronary cusp for patients not requiring a permanent pacemaker was 3.3 + 2.5 mm, while the corresponding depth for patients who underwent permanent pacemaker implantation was 8.1 + 3.5 mm.[27] The rates of pacemaker implantation with the different CE marked devices are described in Table 42.3.

Stroke

Stroke is a feared complication of TAVR, SAVR, and BAV. Although rare, stroke significantly affects survival and quality of life. The dominant etiology likely consists of periprocedural, embolic events secondary to debris dislodgement from the native valve or aortic arch. As a foundation for this concept, Heyder et al. previously showed in a prospective randomized study that retrograde aortic valve catheterization in AS was associated with cerebral embolism in 22% of 101 cases when assessed by magnetic resonance imaging (MRI) the day before and within 48 hours postcatheterization.[35] By contrast, none of the group without retrograde valve catheterization or undergoing coronary angiography only had evidence of cerebral embolism at MRI assessment. With respect to TAVR procedures, MRI studies have identified new onset of clinically silent ischemic cerebral lesions in 68% to 91% of cases.[106–110] These new cerebral lesions were typically multiple and dispersed in hemispheres and vascular territories, a pattern strongly suggesting an embolic origin. Kahlert et al. compared 32 TAVR patients with a historical control group of 21 patients who underwent SAVR and found that new lesions were more frequent after TAVR than SAVR (84% vs. 48%, P = 0.011), but the total volume of these lesions was significantly smaller after TAVR than after SAVR (77 vs. 224 mm^3, P < 0.001).[108]

In order to understand the potential mechanisms for the embolic lesions and their relationship with the procedural steps of TAVR (i.e., trauma to the calcified valve during valve passage with semirigid and large-size delivery catheters, balloon valvuloplasty, valve deployment, and crushing of the native leaflet by the stent), studies using transcranial Doppler ultrasound were performed to detect and quantify, noninvasively and in real-time, high-intensity transient signals (HITS).[111,112] Indeed, HITS represent solid or gaseous cerebral microemboli passing the middle cerebral artery. In two studies, including 44 and 83 patients, all patients presented HITS during the procedure, which were symmetrically distributed between left and right middle cerebral arteries. HITS were predominantly observed during stent valve positioning and implantation. Neither study identified a difference in HITS load between transfemoral or transapical approaches.

Despite the high incidence of new clinically silent peri-interventional cerebral embolic lesions, the incidence of persistent neurological impairment is rather low, and the impact of silent cerebral injury on long-term outcome, especially on development/acceleration of vascular dementia, remains to be elucidated. Ghanem et al. suggested in a study including 22 patients that these silent embolic events had no detrimental influence on patients' self-sufficiency and survival within the first 12 months post TAVR.[110] However, more data are needed to understand the short- and long-term impact of these silent embolic events.

Similar to SAVR data, stroke is associated with a higher 30-day mortality following TAVR. In the PARTNER cohort A, stroke significantly increased the risk of death with both therapeutic options. In the Eggebrecht meta-analysis including more than 10,000 TAVRs, 30-day mortality was increased by 3.5-fold in patients who suffered from a stroke compared to those with no stroke (30-day mortality after stroke 25.5 ± 21.9% vs. 6.9 ± 4.2% in patients with no stroke diagnosed at 30 days).[113] In the Bern experience, stroke was associated with an increased mortality (42.3% vs. 5.1%, P < 0.001) compared with patients without stroke at 30-day follow-up.[114] In this latter study, the most important independent predictive factor for periprocedural stroke was repeated device implantation attempts, with an eightfold increased risk of periprocedural cerebrovascular events. Other predictors of stroke after TAVR were identified, such as COPD, body mass index <25 kg/m^2, advanced age, aortic arch atheroma, new onset of atrial fibrillation, smaller aortic valve area index, balloon postdilatation attempts, and valve dislodgment/embolization.[114–118] Not surprisingly, predictors of stroke after 30 days are more patient-related than procedure-related. Indeed, in a multicenter study, predictors of cerebrovascular events occurring after 30 days for up to 1 year after TAVR were chronic atrial fibrillation and peripheral and prior cerebrovascular disease.[116]

The availability of fully repositionable valves, smaller-size delivery catheters, and the use of embolic protection devices (under current clinical investigation)—which either filter or divert thromboembolic debris during TAVR—may play a role in reducing the risk of cerebral embolism and stroke.

LIMITATIONS

Before an extension of the indication to younger and lower-risk patients, more data are needed on the long-term durability (i.e., beyond 10 years) of the valves and their platforms. The goal is to further decrease vascular complications and reduce the need for permanent pacemakers. All efforts should be made also to reduce the occurrence of stroke.

Specific anatomic features also represent limitations for TAVR in general, or for specific devices. For example, infected valves are better treated with a conventional SAVR which allows for removal of the infected tissue. Similarly, in dilated ascending aorta, the 2014 European Society of Cardiology (ESC) guidelines recommend replacement of the ascending aorta for a diameter of >45 mm when concomitant aortic valve surgery is required, while TAVR is contraindicated in operable patients with dilated ascending aorta.[119]

Finally, the absence of calcification in selected cases of rheumatic AS or stenosis after radiotherapy represent a contraindication for a balloon-expandable valve. A tubular ascending aorta with a very narrow sinus of Valsalva represents a contraindication for the CoreValve device because of the risk of coronary occlusion. The height of the takeoff of the coronary ostia is also an important parameter to be considered before implanting an Edwards valve because of the associated risk of coronary occlusion.

SPECIAL ISSUES AND FURTHER DEVELOPMENT

Following the growing worldwide experience with TAVR in severe AS, several off-label indications have been developed for TAVR, such as treatment of pure severe native AR, bicuspid valves, or degenerated surgical bioprosthesis.

Pure aortic regurgitation

Data regarding pure and severe, native AR without AS are limited.[120,121] The JenaValve (JenaValve Technology, Munich Germany, first in man in May 2010, Leipzig, Germany[122]) is the only approved device; it received CE mark approval in September 2013 for the treatment of patients with pure AR, while no device has so far received FDA approval. This transapical self-expanding device allows for the capture of the aortic valve leaflets thanks to specific clips in order to minimize the risk of PAR and valve embolization.

The largest series is a worldwide registry from 14 centers that reported the results of 43 nonoperable patients with a pure severe native AR treated with a Medtronic CoreValve.[57] Technically, the procedure is challenging, especially in cases without valve calcification (90% of the patients in the registry had mild or no valve calcification) because of the absence of fluoroscopic landmarks to indicate the annulus plane and also because of the increased risk of valve instability during deployment. Two techniques may be of interest to facilitate the procedure in the absence of calcification. First, the use of two pigtails (in the noncoronary and left coronary cusps) permits visualization of the annulus plane despite the absence of calcification. Second, pacing at a rate of 100–120 bpm may improve valve stability and decrease the risk of valve migration during the first two-thirds of valve deployment. In the registry, 90% of patients had degeneration of the valve leaflets without aortic root dilatation. Almost 80% of patients had a final residual regurgitation grade of ≤1. During the index procedure, a second valve was required in 18.6% of patients due to residual AR; no patient had valve calcification. The 30-day mortality was 9.3%, while the need for a second valve was not associated with increased mortality. Interestingly, the patients with an aneurysm of the ascending aorta had a poor outcome (three of four patients died within the first 6 months postprocedure due to arrhythmia, cardiac failure, and perforated gastric ulcer), and the authors suggested that native aortic valve regurgitation associated with aneurysmal aortic dilatation should be considered a contraindication to TAVR. Overall, TAVR with the Medtronic CoreValve in pure native AR is feasible, but technically challenging and associated with a higher risk of requiring two valves and of significant residual PAR. Table 42.4 summarizes the available studies of TAVR for AR.[57,123,124–128]

Bicuspid valve

Bicuspid aortic valves are considered a relative contraindication to TAVR despite the fact that the first in-man case performed by Cribier involved a bicuspid valve.[20] The reason not to perform TAVR in bicuspid valves is the presumed risk of poor valve seating or PAR due to severe distortion of the native leaflets. Three Canadian centers reported a series of 11 patients treated with the Edwards SAPIEN valve.[129] Valves were successfully implanted in all patients, and 10 patients had significant symptomatic and hemodynamic improvement. In one patient, an undersized, suboptimally positioned, unstable valve required late conversion to open surgery followed by death and two patients had moderate PAR. This series suggests that a bicuspid valve does not necessarily prevent symmetric expansion of the Edwards balloon-expandable valve. The first series reported with bicuspid AS treated with the Medtronic CoreValve is a single-center experience from Paris involving 15 patients.[130]

Table 42.4 Available studies reporting TAVR series for pure aortic regurgitation

Register report	No. of patients	Device type	30-day mortality %	Residual AR ≥ II%
Sarkar 2012[114]	4	CoreValve	0	0
Roy 2013[55]	43	CoreValve	9	21
Testa 2014[115]	26	CoreValve	23	23
Seiffert 2013[116]	5	JenaValve[a]	0	0
Seiffert 2014[117]	31	JenaValve	13	0
Schlingloff 2014[119]	10	JenaValve	30	0
Wendt 2014[118]	8	Symetis Acurate	0	0

Note: None of these devices are FDA-approved for this indication. AR, aortic regurgitation; CE, Conformité Européene; FDA, U.S. Food and Drug Administration.

[a] The JenaValve is the only device to receive a CE mark approval for pure acute aortic regurgitation.

In one patient, the valve was implanted too low and surgical conversion was required, but the patient died. The remaining 14 patients had hemodynamic and clinical improvement despite asymmetric expansion of the CoreValve at the level of the native annulus. The function was satisfactory with no PAR >2 and most PAR ≤1 (13/14), and mean gradient ranging from 5 to 18 mmHg.

The largest series (139 patients, 34% Edwards SAPIEN and 66% CoreValve) was reported by Mylotte et al. and showed a procedural mortality of 3.6%, valve embolization in 2.2%, and conversion to surgery in 2.2%.[131] This study emphasizes the importance of MSCT before the procedure to assess the annulus diameter, since MSCT assessment was associated with less PAR on multivariate analysis compared with the use of TEE for annulus sizing. Table 42.5 summarizes the available studies on TAVR for bicuspid AS.[129,131–136]

Valve-in-valve

Longer life expectancy and increased use of bioprosthetic valves has led to an increase in elderly and high-risk patients with degenerated surgical bioprosthesis. In 2007, Wenaweser et al. reported the first implantation of a Medtronic CoreValve into a degenerated surgical aortic bioprosthesis.[137] Since this first report, different series have reported the successful use of both Edwards devices and Medtronic CoreValve for TAVR in both stentless and stented degenerated surgical aortic bioprosthesis.[138–140] Dvir et al. first reported the Global Valve-in-Valve Registry—an international registry with a cohort of 202 patients (124 Medtronic CoreValve and 78 Edwards THV) involving 38 international centers—which showed a 30-day mortality of 8.4% without any difference between both THV groups, and clinical results were sustained at 1-year follow-up.[141] Overall, mean postprocedural gradient decreased to 15.9 ± .6 mmHg, while mean postprocedural gradients were 5 mmHg higher in the Edwards SAPIEN group than in the CoreValve group ($P < 0.0001$). Interestingly, there was a significant difference in the incidence of mean postprocedural gradient of >20 mmHg between the Edwards SAPIEN/XT group (58.8%) compared to the CoreValve group (20%) when the procedure was performed in small surgical bioprostheses (<20 mm, $n = 50$). The difference in postprocedural gradients is probably in relation with the intra-annular versus supra-annular leaflet location of the Edwards SAPIEN/XT and CoreValve prosthesis, respectively. In 2014, Dvir subsequently reported the results of 459 patients in 55 centers treated with VIV.[142] While the overall 30-day mortality rate was 7.2%, patients with stenotic degeneration had higher mortality (10.5%) than those presenting with AR. No differences between Edwards THV and CoreValve devices in terms of strokes and mortality rates were observed. The Edwards group had more major/life-threatening bleeding and more kidney injury events, while the CoreValve group required more permanent pacemaker implantation. The incidence of patient prosthesis mismatch was higher in patients who received an Edwards device versus a CoreValve (43.8%–15.2%), but 1-year survival was not affected. The overall 1-year survival rate was 83.2%. One-year survival was worse in patients with AS (76.6%) than in individuals with AR (91.2%) as well as in patients with small, degenerated prosthetic valves (<23 mm). Early mortality was related to small surgical bioprosthesis size.

A concern when performing VIV for failed surgical bioprostheses is the risk of ostial coronary occlusion, especially if the leaflets of the bioprosthetic valve are mounted to the exterior of the valve frame (e.g., Mitroflow valve, Sorin Group, BC, Canada) or in selected stentless prostheses (e.g., Freedom Stentless valves, Sorin Group). Indeed, in the Global Valve-in-Valve Registry, there was an ostial coronary obstruction rate of 7.7% of the Mitroflow cases (more than in other stented valves, $P = .049$) and in 50%

Table 42.5 Available series reporting bicuspid valve treatment

Register report	No. of patients	Device type		30-day mortality %
Wijesinghe 2010[121]	11	Edwards		18
Himbert 2012[122]	15	CoreValve		7
Hayashida 2013[123]	21	Edwards	52%	5
		CoreValve	48%	
Bauer 2014[124]	38	Edwards	32%	11
		CoreValve	68%	
Kochman 2014[125]	28	Edwards	18%	4
		CoreValve	82%	
Costopoulos 2014[126]	21	Edwards	38%	14
		CoreValve	62%	
Mylotte 2014[127]	139	Edwards	34%	5
		CoreValve	66%	
Yousef 2015[128]	108	Edwards	57%	8
		CoreValve	43%	

Note: None of these devices are FDA-approved for this indication.
FDA, U.S. Food and Drug Administration.

of the Freedom stentless valves (more than in other stentless valves, P = .02).[141] Supravalvular implantation of the surgical bioprosthesis, short distance between the coronary ostia and the bioprosthesis, and extensive pannus formation seem to increase the risk for ostial coronary occlusion.[143] The second concern is the relatively high rate of THV malpositioning (15.3%), which could be related to the relative lack of valvular calcification and difficulty in certain cases to define the optimal target for implantation on fluoroscopy, particularly in procedures involving stentless valves.

Understanding the different dimensions of surgical bioprosthesis is crucial for procedural success of VIV interventions. The manufacturer's labeled valve size does not correspond to the inner base ring diameter; in addition, pannus and calcification can lead to a discrepancy between expected and measured inner stent diameters. Reference tables for the different surgical valves are available and provide the inner diameter. Nevertheless, measurement with MSCT for size selection of the THV is of value, especially in restenotic valves to exclude thrombus as cause of the failure. Valve thrombosis or infective endocarditis are obvious contraindications for VIV procedures and need to be excluded before a VIV intervention. Moreover, paravalvular leakage as a cause of insufficient surgical bioprosthesis has to be ruled out using TEE as the preferred imaging technique for this purpose. Technical feasibility of VIV procedures has been shown, but a substantial proportion of procedures are technically demanding due to the large variety of surgical bioprosthesis. Major safety concerns include higher risk of device malpositioning, coronary obstruction, as well as accelerated valve degeneration.

Finally, some transcatheter aortic valve devices have been used in nonaortic position for the treatment of degenerated pulmonary conduits, degenerated mitral or tricuspid valve bioprostheses, as well as for failed mitral and tricuspid rings. Even in native calcified mitral stenosis, TAVI devices can be used via the transseptal or transapical approach, which opens up another field for the transcatheter valve technology.[138]

CONCLUSIONS

TAVR is to be considered one of the most important advances in medicine over the last 15 years. It already represents the standard therapeutic option for inoperable and high-risk patients with severe AS. Recently published clinical data of TAVR in intermediate-risk patients suggest the superiority of transfemoral TAVR compared to SAVR. Other studies, such as the SURTAVI trial, will provide further data for this risk class. For the time-being, SAVR is the standard of care for severe AS in low-risk patients. At present, a variety of CE marked devices are available, while FDA approval is limited to the Medtronic CoreValve and Evolut R, as well as the Edwards SAPIEN XT and S3. The improvements in design—in order to allow true repositioning, recapture, and retrieval—should contribute to an improvement in the safety and efficacy of this technique, as well as to the continuous expansion of this approach. Future innovational developments need to focus on technologies specifically designed for the treatment of aortic regurgitation, bicuspid aortic valves, and degenerated surgical valves.

REFERENCES

1. Supino PG, et al. The epidemiology of valvular heart disease: A growing public health problem. *Heart Fail Clin.* 2006; **2**(4): 379–93.
2. Nishimura RA, et al. 2014 AHA/ACC guideline for the management of patients with valvular heart disease: A report of the American College of Cardiology/American Heart Association Task Force on Practice Guidelines. *J Am Coll Cardiol.* 2014; **63**(22): e57–185.
3. Vahanian A, et al. Guidelines on the management of valvular heart disease (version 2012): The Joint Task Force on the Management of Valvular Heart Disease of the European Society of Cardiology (ESC) and the European Association for Cardio-Thoracic Surgery (EACTS). *Eur Heart J.* 2012; **33**(19): 2451–96.
4. Otto CM. Calcific aortic stenosis—Time to look more closely at the valve. *N Engl J Med.* 2008; **359**(82): 2111–15.
5. Rossebo AB, et al. Intensive lipid lowering with simvastatin and ezetimibe in aortic stenosis. *N Engl J Med.* 2008; **359**: 1343–56.
6. Rosenhek R, et al. Statins but not angiotensin—Converting enzyme inhibitors delay progression of aortic stenosis. *Circulation.* 2004; **110**: 1291–5.
7. Carabello BA. Aortic valve replacement should be operated on before symptom onset. *Circulation.* 2012; **126**(1): 112–17.
8. Selzer A. Changing aspects of the natural history of valvular aortic stenosis. *N Engl J Med.* 1987; **317**: 91–8.
9. Bouma BJ, et al. To operate or not on elderly patients with aortic stenosis: The decision and its consequences. *Heart.* 1999; **82**: 143–8.
10. Iung B, et al. Decision-making in elderly patients with severe aortic stenosis: Why are so many denied surgery? *Eur Heart J.* 2005; **26**: 2714–20.
11. Rubio-Alvarez V. Intracardiac valvulotomy by means of a catheter. *Arch Inst Cardiol Mex.* 1953; **23**: 183–92.
12. Semb BK, et al. Balloon valvulotomy of congenital pulmonary valve stenosis with tricuspid valve insufficiency. *Cardiovasc Radiol.* 1979; **2**: 239–41.
13. Chen CR, et al. Percutaneous balloon valvuloplasty for pulmonic stenosis in adolescents and adults. *N Engl J Med.* 1996; **335**: 21–5.
14. Inoue K, et al. Clinical application of transvenous mitral commissurotomy by a new balloon catheter. *J Thorac Cardiovasc Surg.* 1984; **87**: 394–402.
15. Cribier A, et al. Percutaneous transluminal valvuloplasty of acquired aortic stenosis in elderly patients: An alternative to valve replacement? *Lancet.* 1986; **1**: 63–7.
16. Otto CM, et al. Three-year outcome after balloon aortic valvuloplasty. Insights into prognosis of valvular aortic stenosis. *Circulation.* 1994; **89**: 642–50.
17. Participants NBVR. Percutaneous balloon aortic valvuloplasty. Acute and 30-day follow-up results in 674 patients from the NHLBI Balloon Valvuloplasty Registry. *Circulation.* 1991; **84**(6): 2383–97.

18. Andersen HR, Hasenkam JM. Transluminal implantation of artificial heart valves. Description of a new expandable aortic valve and initial results with implantation by catheter technique in closed-chest pigs. *Eur Heart J.* 1992; **13**: 704–8.

19. Bonhoeffer P, et al. Percutaneous replacement of pulmonary valve in a right-ventricle to pulmonary-artery prosthetic conduit with valve dysfunction. *Lancet.* 2000; **356**: 1403–5.

20. Cribier A, et al. Percutaneous transcatheter implantation of an aortic valve prosthesis for calcific aortic stenosis: First human case description. *Circulation.* 2002; **106**(24): 3006–8.

21. Grube E, et al. First report on a human percutaneous transluminal implantation of a self-expanding valve prosthesis for interventional treatment of aortic valve stenosis. *Catheter Cardiovasc Interv.* 2005; **66**(4): 465–9.

22. Roberts WC, Ko JM. Frequency by decades of unicuspid, bicuspid, and tricuspid aortic valves in adults having isolated aortic valve replacement for aortic stenosis, with or without associated aortic regurgitation. *Circulation.* 2005; **111**(7): 920–5.

23. Borger MA, David TE. Management of the valve and ascending aorta in adults with bicuspid aortic valve disease. *Semin Thorac Cardiovasc Surg.* 2005; **17**(2): 143–7.

24. Sievers HH, Schmidtke C. A classification system for the bicuspid aortic valve from 304 surgical specimens. *J Thorac Cardiovasc Surg.* 2007; **133**(5): 1226–33.

25. Piazza N, et al. Anatomy of the aortic valvar complex and its implications for transcatheter implantation of the aortic valve. *Circ Cardiovasc Interv.* 2008; **1**(1): 74–81.

26. Cavalcanti JS, et al. Morphometric and topographic study of coronary ostia. *Arq Bras Cardiol.* 2003; **81**: 359–62.

27. Manoharan G, et al. Treatment of symptomatic severe aortic stenosis with a novel resheathable supra-annular self-expanding transcatheter aortic valve system. *JACC Cardiovasc Interv.* 2015; **8**(10): 1359–67.

28. Gilard M, et al. Registry of transcatheter aortic-valve implantation in high-risk patients. *N Engl J Med.* 2012; **366**(18): 1705–15.

29. Grube E, et al. Percutaneous aortic valve replacement for severe aortic stenosis in high-risk patients using the second- and current third-generation self-expanding CoreValve prosthesis: Device success and 30-day clinical outcome. *J Am Coll Cardiol.* 2007; **50**(1): 69–76.

30. Lichtenstein SV, et al. Transapical transcatheter aortic valve implantation in humans: Initial clinical experience. *Circulation.* 2006; **114**(6): 591–6.

31. Walther T, et al. Minimally invasive transapical beating heart aortic valve implantation—Proof of concept. *Eur J Cardiothorac Surg.* 2007; **31**(1): 9–15.

32. Walther T, et al. Transapical minimally invasive aortic valve implantation: Multicenter experience. *Circulation.* 2007; **116**(11 Suppl): I240–5.

33. Bruschi G, et al. Alternative approaches for trans-catheter self-expanding aortic bioprosthetic valves implantation: Single-center experience. *Eur J Cardiothorac Surg.* 2011; **39**(6): e151–8.

34. Modine T, et al. Transcutaneous aortic valve implantation using the left carotid access: Feasibility and early clinical outcomes. *Ann Thorac Surg.* 2012; **93**(5): 1489–94.

35. Omran H, et al. Silent and apparent cerebral embolism after retrograde catheterisation of the aortic valve in valvular stenosis: A prospective, randomised study. *Lancet.* 2003; **361**(9365): 1241–6.

36. Dumesnil JG, et al. Paradoxical low flow and/or low gradient severe aortic stenosis despite preserved left ventricular ejection fraction: Implications for diagnosis and treatment. *Eur Heart J.* 2010; **31**(3): 281–9.

37. Clavel MA, et al. Impact of aortic valve calcification, as measured by MDCT, on survival in patients with aortic stenosis: Results of an international registry study. *J Am Coll Cardiol.* 2014; **64**(12): 1202–13.

38. Nashef SA, et al. EuroSCORE II. *Eur J Cardiothorac Surg.* 2012; **4**: 734–44.

39. Roques F, et al. Risk factors and outcome in European cardiac surgery: Analysis of the EuroSCORE multinational database of 19030 patients. *Eur J Cardiothorac Surg.* 1999; **15**: 816–22.

40. Clark RE. Calculating risk and outcome: The Society of Thoracic Surgeons database. *Ann Thorac Surg.* 1996; **62**(5 Suppl): S2–5.

41. Piazza N, et al. Relationship between the logistic EuroSCORE and the Society of Thoracic Surgeons Predicted Risk of Mortality score in patients implanted with the CoreValve ReValving system—A Bern-Rotterdam Study. *Am Heart J.* 2010; **159**(2): 323–9.

42. Stortecky S, et al. Evaluation of multidimensional geriatric assessment as a predictor of mortality and cardiovascular events after transcatheter aortic valve implantation. *JACC Cardiovasc Interv.* 2012; **5**(5): 489–96.

43. Afilalo J, et al. Gait speed as an incremental predictor of mortality and major morbidity in elderly patients undergoing cardiac surgery. *J Am Coll Cardiol.* 2010; **56**(20): 1668–76.

44. Folstein MF, et al. "Mini-mental state". A practical method for grading the cognitive state of patients for the clinician. *J Psychiatr Res.* 1975; **12**(3): 189–98.

45. Lordos EF, et al. Comparative value of medical diagnosis versus physical functioning in predicting the 6-year survival of 1951 hospitalized old patients. *Rejuvenation Res.* 2008; **11**(4): 829–36.

46. Zekry D, et al. Prospective comparison of six co-morbidity indices as predictors of 5 years post hospital discharge survival in the elderly. *Rejuvenation Res.* 2010; **13**(6): 675–82.

47. Moss RR, et al. Role of echocardiography in percutaneous aortic valve implantation. *JACC Cardiovasc Imaging.* 2008; **1**(1): 15–24.

48. Tops LF, et al. Noninvasive evaluation of the aortic root with multislice computed tomography implications for transcatheter aortic valve replacement. *JACC Cardiovasc Imaging.* 2008; **1**(3): 321–30.

49. Wood DA, et al. Role of multislice computed tomography in transcatheter aortic valve replacement. *Am J Cardiol.* 2009; **103**(9): 1295–301.

50. Messika-Zeitoun D, et al. Multimodal assessment of the aortic annulus diameter: Implications for transcatheter aortic valve implantation. *J Am Coll Cardiol.* 2010; **55**(3): 186–94.

51. Tzikas A, et al. Assessment of the aortic annulus by multislice computed tomography, contrast aortography, and trans-thoracic echocardiography in patients referred for transcatheter aortic valve implantation. *Catheter Cardiovasc Interv.* 2011; **77**(6): 868–75.

52. Schultz CJ, et al. Three dimensional evaluation of the aortic annulus using multislice computer tomography: Are manufacturer's guidelines for sizing for percutaneous aortic valve replacement helpful? *Eur Heart J.* 2010; **31**(7): 849–56.

53. Tuzcu EM, et al. Multimodality quantitative imaging of aortic root for transcatheter aortic valve implantation: More complex than it appears. *J Am Coll Cardiol.* 2010; **55**(3): 195–7.

54. Gurvitch R, et al. Aortic annulus diameter determination by multidetector computed tomography: Reproducibility, applicability, and implications for transcatheter aortic valve implantation. *JACC Cardiovasc Interv.* 2011; **4**(11): 1235–45.

55. Jilaihawi H, et al. Source. Cross-sectional computed tomographic assessment improves accuracy of aortic annular sizing for transcatheter aortic valve replacement and reduces the incidence of paravalvular aortic regurgitation. *J Am Coll Cardiol.* 2012; **59**(14): 1275–86.

56. Jilaihawi H, et al. Aortic annular sizing for transcatheter aortic valve replacement using cross-sectional 3-dimensional transesophageal echocardiography. *J Am Coll Cardiol.* 2013; **61**(9): 908–16.

57. Roy DA, et al. Transcatheter aortic valve implantation for pure severe native aortic valve regurgitation. *J Am Coll Cardiol.* 2013; **61**(15): 1577–84.

58. Willson AB, et al. 3-dimensional aortic annular assessment by multidetector computed tomography predicts moderate or severe paravalvular regurgitation after transcatheter aortic valve replacement: A multicenter retrospective analysis. *J Am Coll Cardiol.* 2012; **59**(14): 1287–94.

59. Pilgrim T, et al. Outcome of patients with severe aortic stenosis undergoing ad hoc transcatheter aortic valve implantation without invasive pre-evaluation. *Cardiovasc Med.* 2014; **17**(12): 364–70.

60. Condado JF, et al. Balloon versus computed tomography sizing of the aortic annulus for transcatheter aortic valve replacement and the impact of left ventricular outflow tract calcification and morphology on sizing. *J invasive Cardiol.* 2016; 28(7): 295–304.

61. Craig R, et al. Transcatheter versus surgical aortic-valve replacement in high-risk patients. *N Engl J Med.* 2011; **364**(23): 2187–98.

62. Adams DH, et al. Transcatheter aortic-valve replacement with a self-expanding prosthesis. *N Engl J Med.* 2014; **370**(19): 1790–8.

63. Leon MB, et al. Transcatheter or surgical aortic-valve replacement in intermediate-risk patients. *N Engl J Med.* 2016; **374**: 1609–1620.

64. Binder RK, et al. Transcatheter aortic valve replacement with the SAPIEN 3: A new balloon-expandable transcatheter heart valve. *JACC Cardiovasc Interv.* 2013; **6**(3): 293–300.

65. Sinning JM, et al. Medtronic CoreValve Evolut valve. *EuroIntervention.* 2012; 8 Suppl Q: Q94–6.

66. Buellesfeld L, et al. Percutaneous implantation of the first repositionable aortic valve prosthesis in a patient with severe aortic stenosis. *Catheter Cardiovasc Interv.* 2008; **71**(5): 579–84.

67. Schofer J, et al. Retrograde transarterial implantation of a non-metallic aortic valve prosthesis in high-surgical-risk patients with severe aortic stenosis: A first-in-man feasibility and safety study. *Circ Cardiovasc Interv.* 2008; **1**(2): 126–33.

68. Willson AB, et al. Transcatheter aortic valve replacement with the St. Jude Medical Portico valve: First-in-human experience. *J Am Coll Cardiol.* 2012; **60**(7): 581–6.

69. Kempfert J, et al. Trans-apical aortic valve implantation using a new self-expandable bioprosthesis: Initial outcomes. *Eur J Cardiothorac Surg.* 2011; **40**(5): 1114–19.

70. Yamamoto M, et al. Effect of local anesthetic management with conscious sedation in patients undergoing transcatheter aortic valve implantation. *Am J Cardiol.* 2013; **111**(1): 94–9.

71. See Tho VY, et al. Anaesthesia for transcatheter aortic valve implantation. *Trends Anaesth Crit Care.* 2013; **3**(6): 293–356.

72. Bergmann L, et al. Transfemoral aortic valve implantation under sedation and monitored anaesthetic care—A feasibility study. *Anaesthesia.* 2011; **66**(11): 977–82.

73. Durand E, et al. Transfemoral aortic valve replacement with the Edwards SAPIEN and Edwards SAPIEN XT prosthesis using exclusively local anesthesia and fluoroscopic guidance: Feasibility and 30-day outcomes. *JACC Cardiovasc Interv.* 2012; **5**(5): 461–7.

74. Dvir D, Kornowski R. Percutaneous aortic valve implantation using novel imaging guidance. *Catheter Cardiovasc Interv.* 2010; **76**: 450–4.

75. Agatiello C, et al. Balloon aortic valvuloplasty in the adult. Immediate results and in-hospital complications in the latest series of 141 consecutive patients at the University Hospital of Rouen (2002–2005). *Arch Mal Coeur Vaiss.* 2006; **99**(3): 195–200.

76. Noble S, Roffi M. Pressure curve measurements during transcatheter aortic valve implantation: A useful tool to assess the severity of aortic regurgitation. *Ann Thorac Surg.* 2013; **95**(1): e21.

77. Sinning JM, et al. Aortic regurgitation index defines severity of peri-prosthetic regurgitation and predicts outcome in patients after transcatheter aortic valve implantation. *J Am Coll Cardiol.* 2012; **59**(13): 1134–41.

78. Cockburn J, et al. Large calibre arterial access device closure for percutaneous aortic valve interventions: Use of the Prostar system in 118 cases. *Catheter Cardiovasc Interv.* 2012; **79**(1): 143–9.

79. Genereux P, et al. Clinical outcomes using a new crossover balloon occlusion technique for percutaneous closure after transfemoral aortic valve implantation. *JACC Cardiovasc Interv.* 2011; **4**(8): 861–7.

80. Noble S, et al. Anatomo-pathological analysis after CoreValve Revalving system implantation. *EuroIntervention.* 2009; **5**(1): 78–85.

81. Virmani R, et al. Accumulation of worldwide experience with postmortem studies of transcatheter aortic valve implantation—What should we be avoiding. In P Serruys, N Piazza, A Cribier, J Webb, JC Laborde, P de Jaegere (eds.), *Transcatheter aortic valve implantation: Tips and tricks to avoid failure* (1st ed., pp. 18–39). Informa Healthcare, New York, NY, 2009.

82. Nietlispach F, et al. Pathology of transcatheter valve therapy. *JACC Cardiovasc Interv.* 2012; **5**(5): 582–90.

83. Lynch DJ, et al. Considerations in antithrombotic therapy among patients undergoing transcatheter aortic valve implantation. *J Thromb Thrombolysis.* 2013; **35**(4): 476–82.

84. Ussia GP, et al. Dual antiplatelet therapy versus aspirin alone in patients undergoing transcatheter aortic valve implantation. *Am J Cardiol.* 2011; **108**(12): 1772–6.

85. Leon MB, et al. Standardized endpoint definitions for transcatheter aortic valve implantation clinical trials: A consensus report from the Valve Academic Research Consortium. *Eur Heart J.* 2011; **32**(2): 205–17.

86. Leon MB, et al. Transcatheter aortic-valve implantation for aortic stenosis in patients who cannot undergo surgery. *N Engl J Med.* 2010; **363**(17): 1597–607.

87. Makkar RR, et al. Transcatheter aortic-valve replacement for inoperable severe aortic stenosis. *N Engl J Med.* 2012; **366**(18): 1696–704.

88. Kapadia SR, et al. 5-year outcomes of transcatheter aortic valve replacement compared with standard treatment for patients with inoperable aortic stenosis (PARTNER 1): A randomised controlled trial. *Lancet.* 2015; **385**(9986): 2485–91.

89. Mack MJ, et al. 5-year outcomes of transcatheter aortic valve replacement or surgical aortic valve replacement for high surgical risk patients with aortic stenosis (PARTNER 1): A randomised controlled trial. *Lancet.* 2015; **385**(9986): 2477–84.

90. Susheel K, et al. Two-year outcomes after transcatheter or surgical aortic-valve replacement. *N Engl J Med.* 2012; **366**(18): 1686–95.

91. Yakubov SJ, et al. 2-year outcomes after iliofemoral self-expanding transcatheter aortic valve replacement in patients with severe aortic stenosis seemed extreme risk for surgery. *J Am Coll Cardiol.* 2015; **66**(12): 1327–34.

92. Deeb GM, et al. 3-year outcomes in high-risk patients who underwent surgical or transcatheter aortic valve replacement. *J Am Coll Cardiol.* 2016; **67**(22): 2565–74.

93. Reardon MJ, et al. 2-year outcomes in patients undergoing surgical or self-expanding transcatheter aortic valve replacement. *J Am Coll Cardiol.* 2015; **66**(2): 113–21.

94. Wenaweser P, et al. Clinical outcomes of patients with estimated low or intermediate surgical risk undergoing transcatheter aortic valve implantation. *Eur Heart J.* 2013; **34**(25): 1894–905.

95. Lange R, et al. Improvements in transcatheter aortic valve implantation outcomes in lower surgical risk patients: A glimpse into the future. *J Am Coll Cardiol.* 2012; **59**(3): 280–7.

96. Piazza N, et al. A 3-center comparison of 1-year mortality outcomes between transcatheter aortic valve implantation and surgical aortic valve replacement on the basis of propensity score matching among intermediate-risk surgical patients. *JACC Cardiovasc Interv.* 2013; **6**(5): 443–51.

97. Thyregod HG, et al. Transcatheter versus surgical aortic valve replacement in patients with severe aortic valve stenosis: 1-year results from the all-comers NOTION randomized clinical trial. *J Am Coll Cardiol.* 2015; **65**(20): 2184–94.

98. van Mieghem NM, et al. The SURTAVI model: Proposal for a pragmatic risk stratification for patients with severe aortic stenosis. *EuroIntervention.* 2012; **8**(2): 258–66.

99. Clavel MA, et al. Comparison of the hemodynamic performance of percutaneous and surgical bioprostheses for the treatment of severe aortic stenosis. *J Am Coll Cardiol.* 2009; **53**(20): 1883–91.

100. Nombela-Franco L, et al. Comparison of hemodynamic performance of self-expandable CoreValve versus balloon-expandable Edwards SAPIEN aortic valves inserted by catheter for aortic stenosis. *Am J Cardiol.* 2013; **111**(7): 1026–33.

101. Tchetche D, et al. Update on the need for a permanent pacemaker after transcatheter aortic valve implantation using the CoreValve(R) Accutrak system. *EuroIntervention.* 2012; **8**(5): 556–62.

102. Popma JJ, et al. Transcatheter aortic valve replacement using a self-expanding bioprosthesis in patients with severe aortic stenosis at extreme risk for surgery. *J Am Coll Cardiol.* 2014; **63**(19): 1972–81.

103. Nuis RJ, et al. Timing and potential mechanisms of new conduction abnormalities during the implantation of the Medtronic CoreValve System in patients with aortic stenosis. *Eur Heart J.* 2011; **32**(16): 2067–74.

104. Kodali S, et al. Early clinical and echocardiographic outcomes after SAPIEN 3 transcatheter aortic valve replacement in inoperable, high-risk and intermediate-risk patients with aortic stenosis. *Eur Heart J.* 2016; **37**(28): 2252–62.

105. Vahanian A. *30-day outcomes of intermediate-risk patients with the new generation balloon-expandable transcatheter heart valve via the transfemoral approach.* EuroPCR, Paris, 2015.

106. Ghanem A, et al. Risk and fate of cerebral embolism after transfemoral aortic valve implantation: A prospective pilot study with diffusion-weighted magnetic resonance imaging. *J Am Coll Cardiol.* 2010; **55**(14): 1427–32.

107. Rodes-Cabau J, et al. Cerebral embolism following transcatheter aortic valve implantation: Comparison of transfemoral and transapical approaches. *J Am Coll Cardiol.* 2011; **57**(1): 18–28.

108. Kahlert P, et al. Silent and apparent cerebral ischemia after percutaneous transfemoral aortic valve implantation: A diffusion-weighted magnetic resonance imaging study. *Circulation.* 2010; **121**(7): 870–8.

109. Astarci P, et al. Magnetic resonance imaging evaluation of cerebral embolization during percutaneous aortic valve implantation: Comparison of transfemoral and transapical approaches using Edwards Sapiens valve. *Eur J Cardiothorac Surg.* 2011; **40**(2): 475–9.

110. Ghanem A, et al. Prognostic value of cerebral injury following transfemoral aortic valve implantation. *EuroIntervention.* 2013; **8**(11): 1296–306.

111. Erdoes G, et al. Transcranial Doppler-detected cerebral embolic load during transcatheter aortic valve implantation. *Eur J Cardiothorac Surg.* 2012; **41**(4): 778–83; discussion 83–4.

112. Kahlert P, et al. Cerebral embolization during transcatheter aortic valve implantation: A transcranial Doppler study. *Circulation.* 2012; **126**(10): 1245–55.

113. Eggebrecht H, et al. Risk of stroke after transcatheter aortic valve implantation (TAVI): A meta-analysis of 10,037 published patients. *EuroIntervention.* 2012; **8**(1): 129–38.

114. Stortecky S, et al. Cerebrovascular accidents complicating transcatheter aortic valve implantation: Frequency, timing and impact on outcomes. *EuroIntervention.* 2012; **8**(1): 62–70.

115. Miller DC, et al. Transcatheter (TAVR) versus surgical (AVR) aortic valve replacement: Occurrence, hazard, risk factors, and consequences of neurologic events in the PARTNER trial. *J Thorac Cardiovasc Surg.* 2012; **143**(4): 832–43.

116. Nombela-Franco L, et al. Timing, predictive factors, and prognostic value of cerebrovascular events in a large cohort of patients undergoing transcatheter aortic valve implantation. *Circulation.* 2012; **126**(25): 3041–53.

117. Fairbairn TA, et al. Diffusion-weighted MRI determined cerebral embolic infarction following transcatheter aortic valve implantation: Assessment of predictive risk factors and the relationship to subsequent health status. *Heart.* 2012; **98**(1): 18–23.

118. Amat-Santos IJ, et al. Incidence, predictive factors, and prognostic value of new-onset atrial fibrillation following transcatheter aortic valve implantation. *J Am Coll Cardiol.* 2012; **59**(2): 178–88.

119. Erbel R, et al. 2014 ESC Guidelines on the diagnosis and treatment of aortic diseases: Document covering acute and chronic aortic diseases of the thoracic and abdominal aorta of the adult. The Task Force for the Diagnosis and Treatment of Aortic Diseases of the European Society of Cardiology (ESC). *Eur Heart J.* 2014; **35**(41): 2873–926.

120. Dhillon PS, et al. Transcatheter aortic valve replacement for symptomatic severe aortic valve regurgitation. *Heart.* 2010; **96**(10): 810.

121. Krumsdorf U, et al. Technical challenge of transfemoral aortic valve implantation in a patient with severe aortic regurgitation. *Circ Cardiovasc Interv.* 2011; **4**(2): 210–11.

122. Kempfert J, et al. A new self-expanding transcatheter aortic valve for transapical implantation—First in man implantation of the JenaValve. *Eur J Cardiothorac Surg.* 2011; **40**(3): 761–3.

123. Sarkar K, et al. Transcatheter aortic valve implantation for severe regurgitation in native and degenerated bioprosthetic aortic valves. *Catheter Cardiovasc Interv.* 2013; **81**(5): 864–70.

124. Testa L, et al. CoreValve implantation for severe aortic regurgitation: A multicentre registry. *EuroIntervention.* 2014; **10**(6): 739–45.

125. Seiffert M, et al. Transapical implantation of a second-generation transcatheter heart valve in patients with noncalcified aortic regurgitation. *JACC Cardiovasc Interv.* 2013; **6**(6): 590–7.

126. Seiffert M, et al. Initial German experience with transapical implantation of a second-generation transcatheter heart valve for the treatment of aortic regurgitation. *JACC Cardiovasc Interv.* 2014; **7**(10): 1168–74.

127. Wendt D, et al. Transapical transcatheter aortic valve for severe aortic regurgitation: Expanding the limits. *JACC Cardiovasc Interv.* 2014; **7**(10): 1159–67.

128. Schlingloff F, et al. Transcatheter aortic valve implantation of a second-generation valve for pure aortic regurgitation: Procedural outcome, haemodynamic data and follow-up. *Interact Cardiovasc Thorac Surg.* 2014; **19**(3): 388–93.

129. Wijesinghe N, et al. Transcatheter aortic valve implantation in patients with bicuspid aortic valve stenosis. *JACC Cardiovasc Interv.* 2010; **3**(11): 1122–5.

130. Himbert D, et al. Feasibility and outcomes of transcatheter aortic valve implantation in high-risk patients with stenotic bicuspid aortic valves. *Am J Cardiol.* 2012; **110**(6): 877–83.

131. Mylotte D, et al. Transcatheter aortic valve replacement in bicuspid aortic valve disease. *J Am Coll Cardiol.* 2014; **64**(22): 2330–9.

132. Hayashida K, et al. Transcatheter aortic valve implantation for patients with severe bicuspid aortic valve stenosis. *Circ Cardiovasc Interv.* 2013; **6**(3): 284–91.

133. Bauer T, et al. Comparison of the effectiveness of transcatheter aortic valve implantation in patients with stenotic bicuspid versus tricuspid aortic valves (from the German TAVI Registry). *Am J Cardiol.* 2014; **113**(3): 518–21.

134. Kochman J, et al. Comparison of one- and 12-month outcomes of transcatheter aortic valve replacement in patients with severely stenotic bicuspid versus tricuspid aortic valves (results from a multicenter registry). *Am J Cardiol.* 2014; **114**(5): 757–62.

135. Costopoulos C, et al. Comparison of results of transcatheter aortic valve implantation in patients with severely stenotic bicuspid versus tricuspid or nonbicuspid valves. *Am J Cardiol.* 2014; **113**(8): 1390–3.

136. Yousef A, et al. Transcatheter aortic valve implantation in patients with bicuspid aortic valve: A patient level multicenter analysis. *Int J Cardiol.* 2015; **189**: 282–8.

137. Wenaweser P, et al. Percutaneous aortic valve replacement for severe aortic regurgitation in degenerated bioprosthesis: The first valve in valve procedure using the Corevalve Revalving system. *Catheter Cardiovasc Interv.* 2007; **70**(5): 760–4.

138. Piazza N, et al. Transcatheter aortic valve implantation for failing surgical aortic bioprosthetic valve: From concept to clinical application and evaluation (part 2). *JACC Cardiovasc Interv.* 2011; **4**(7): 733–42.

139. Descoutures F, et al. Transarterial medtronic CoreValve system implantation for degenerated surgically implanted aortic prostheses. *Circ Cardiovasc Interv.* 2011; **4**(5): 488–94.

140. Cerillo AG, et al. Transcatheter valve in valve implantation for failed mitral and tricuspid bioprosthesis. *Catheter Cardiovasc Interv.* 2011; **78**(7): 987–95.

141. Dvir D, et al. Transcatheter aortic valve replacement for degenerative bioprosthetic surgical valves: Results from the global valve-in-valve registry. *Circulation.* 2012; **126**(19): 2335–44.

142. Dvir D, et al. Transcatheter aortic valve implantation in failed bioprosthetic surgical valves. *JAMA.* 2014; **312**(2): 162–70.

143. Mylotte D, et al. Transcatheter heart valve implantation for failing surgical bioprostheses: Technical considerations and evidence for valve-in-valve procedures. *Heart.* 2013; **99**(13): 960–7.

43

Percutaneous therapies for mitral valve disease

AKHIL PARASHAR, E. MURAT TUZCU, AND SAMIR R. KAPADIA

INTRODUCTION

The prevalence of mitral valve disease, especially mitral regurgitation (MR), is increasing.[1] Despite significant gains in the eradication of rheumatic fever, rheumatic mitral stenosis (MS) remains a health-care concern in many developing countries.[2] Notably, in industrialized countries, the decrease in frequency of rheumatic heart diseases has been accompanied by an increase in degenerative valve diseases.[3] In Western countries, the incidence of MR in the general population and in individuals over 75 years of age is almost 1.7% and 10%, respectively.[1] Although surgery is currently the gold standard for the treatment of severe MR, the presence of severe comorbidities precludes surgical treatment in up to 50% of patients with this condition.[4] The emergence of new percutaneous technologies for mitral valve disease has generated great interest in the interventional community.[5] This chapter reviews the indications and techniques for percutaneous therapies for mitral valve disease.

PERCUTANEOUS TREATMENT OF MITRAL STENOSIS

Fundamentals and anatomic considerations

ETIOLOGY

The most common cause of MS is rheumatic heart disease. Less commonly, congenital MS may be detected in children. MS is rarely the result of collagen vascular disease, mucopolysaccharidoses or amyloid deposits, or is drug induced. In rheumatic mitral valve disease, fusion of the mitral valve apparatus may occur in the commissures, the cusps, or the chordae tendineae. Generally, the mitral cusps thicken at the edges and fuse at the commissures, while the chordae thicken, shorten, and fuse. This leads to a funnel-shaped valve with reduced leaflet mobility and a fish-mouth-shaped orifice.[6] If the commissures are predominantly involved, this leads mainly to MS. Isolated thickening and shortening of the chordae results mainly in MR; however, if the cusps are thickened and adherent so they cannot adequately open or close, a combination of MS and MR occurs.

PATHOPHYSIOLOGY AND DIAGNOSIS

Clinical manifestations of MS are caused by increased left atrial pressure (shortness of breath), atrial fibrillation (thromboembolism), or increased pulmonary pressures (fatigue). The presence of symptoms is the most important indication for intervention. Gradients or size of mitral valve should not be used to time intervention in asymptomatic patients with normal pulmonary artery (PA) pressures.[7] Exercise echocardiography may be very useful to document functional status and hemodynamic changes with exercise. Echocardiography is the cornerstone for diagnosis. Transthoracic echocardiography (TTE) is most useful to image the subvalvular apparatus. Transesophageal echocardiography (TEE), especially with three-dimensional (3D) reconstruction, is very helpful in identifying commissural fusion. However, in the majority of patients, TTE provides adequate information on commisural fusion. If the degree of MR severity is uncertain, TEE is very helpful. The mitral valve splittability score is the most common method of assessment for the suitability of balloon mitral valvotomy (BMV), although there are other validated methods.[4,8,9]

Indications

SYMPTOMATIC MITRAL STENOSIS: ACC/AHA GUIDELINES

According to the American College of Cardiology (ACC) and American Heart Association (AHA) guidelines,[10] percutaneous BMV is recommended for symptomatic patients with severe MS (mitral valve area ≤1.5 cm², stage D) and favorable valve morphology in the absence of left atrial thrombus or moderate-to-severe MR (class Ia). BMV is reasonable for asymptomatic patients with severe MS (mitral valve area ≤1 cm², stage C) and favorable valve morphology in the absence of left atrial thrombus or moderate-to-severe MR (class IIa). Asymptomatic patients with new-onset atrial fibrillation with favorable anatomy have a class IIb indication (BMV may be indicated). It is not appropriate to perform BMV in patients with nonrheumatic mitral valve disease and patients with prosthetic mitral valve stenosis.

SURGICAL MITRAL VALVE REPAIR OR REPLACEMENT VERSUS PERCUTANEOUS BALLOON MITRAL VALVULOPLASTY

Surgical options for MS include closed commissurotomy, open commissurotomy, and mitral valve replacement (MVR). Closed commissurotomy is rarely indicated or performed in developed countries.[11] In developing countries where BMV may be more expensive than surgery, closed commissurotomy can be considered for economic reasons if surgical expertise is available. Open commissurotomy is also rarely indicated because if the valve morphology is suitable for this procedure, it is suitable also for BMV. The outcomes of BMV are very comparable to surgical procedures even in randomized trials and with long follow-ups.[12] Figure 43.1 shows mitral valve area following mitral commissurotomy using different techniques. Valve replacement is reserved for patients who need mitral valve intervention but are not candidates for BMV or if BMV has failed. However, a special mention of degenerative mitral stenosis (DMS)—a distinct entity from rheumatic MS—needs to be emphasized here

(Figure 43.2). The mainstay of therapy in DMS patients is medical management with heart rate control and diuretic therapy.[13] Invasive management of DMS is challenging because of the presence of extensive calcification. Because the calcification is mainly at the base of leaflets without any associated commissural fusion, percutaneous mitral BMV and surgical commissurotomy have traditionally played little role in DMS management. Currently, no medical therapy is available to specifically prevent the progressive annular and leaflet calcification and to delay the time to valve replacement. Traditionally, surgical MVR has been the method of choice for treating patients with symptomatic DMS. There are some early reports of treating calcific MS with percutaneous valve replacement, although this treatment should be considered experimental at this stage.[14]

PROCEDURE

Currently, BMV is exclusively performed using the Inoue Balloon (Toray International America, Inc., Houston, TX) in the United States and most of the world (Figure 43.3). Although BMV can be performed with double balloons, this method is rarely used.[15] A special metal dilator, the Cribier's dilator, has been used to reduce costs, but because of technical challenges and a potential safety issue, it did not gain widespread acceptance.[16]

Patient selection is the most critical step in the success of the procedure. Patients with asymmetric commissural calcification, severe subvalvular scarring, significant MR, and significant tricuspid regurgitation are not ideal candidates for BMV. These parameters are quantified with the Wilkins scoring system on echocardiography.[8] Each item is graded from

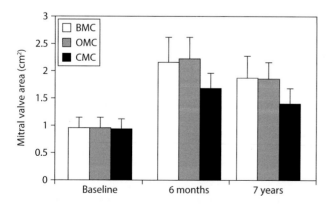

Figure 43.1 Mitral valve area following mitral commissurotomy by BMC, OMC, or CMC. BMC, balloon mitral commissurotomy; CMC, closed mitral commissurotomy; OMC, open mitral commissurotomy.

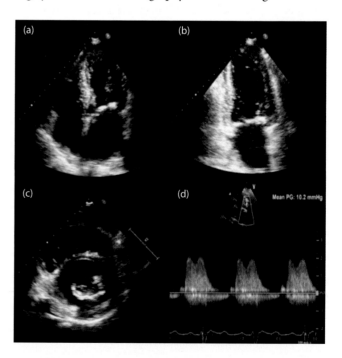

Figure 43.2 Severe degenerative mitral stenosis secondary to severe mitral annular calcification as seen on echocardiographic examination. (Adapted from Sud et al., *Circulation*, 2016;19;133(16):1594–604.)

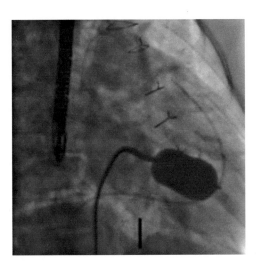

Figure 43.3 Fluoroscopic image of the Inoue balloon technique for mitral valvuloplasty. Note the simultaneous use of transesophageal echocardiography to guide balloon inflation.

1 (normal) to 4, which yield a total score ranging from 4 to 16. A score of 8 or less predicts a more favorable outcome than those with a higher score. However, a score higher than 8 does not exclude a patient from having BMV. The balloon size is selected by directly measuring the mitral annular diameter using two-dimensional (2D) echocardiography. Asymmetric commissural calcification is another important predictor for poor outcome after BMV. TEE is very helpful after each balloon inflation to make sure there is no left atrial clot and to assess the mechanism as well as severity of MR. 2D echocardiographic observations are performed after each dilatation. Assessment of MR and commissures with 3D TEE help to optimize BMV and hence help to improve procedural outcomes. Furthermore, TEE can also help in making transseptal puncture safer. TEE is typically performed in the catheterization laboratory without general anesthesia. It is important to note that many institutions perform BMV with transthoracic echo. This approach requires TEE to rule out a left atrial appendage (LAA) clot prior to BMV. Transseptal puncture can be performed with fluoroscopic guidance. However, in the current era of image-guided mitral interventions, the authors believe that TEE guidance can be considered state of the art.

It is standard procedure to perform BMV under the guidance of invasive hemodynamic monitoring, requiring two pressure transducers for simultaneous measurement of left atrial and left ventricular pressure. In addition, it is useful to monitor PA pressure and cardiac output during the procedure. The most straightforward configuration to begin the procedure includes an 8-Fr short, venous sheath in the left femoral vein; a 5-Fr arterial sheath in the left femoral artery or in the radial artery; and a 8-Fr short, venous sheath in the right femoral vein (RFV).

The left femoral or radial arterial sheath is used to perform diagnostic cardiac catheterization, if necessary, and to allow placement of a pigtail catheter into the noncoronary sinus. The pigtail catheter is useful in this position as a landmark to guide the transseptal puncture. If necessary for anatomic assessment prior to transseptal puncture, the left groin venous sheath can be used to introduce an NIH or pigtail catheter into the right atrium (RA) at the junction with the superior vena cava (SVC). A power injection at this location will opacify the RA and pulmonary vasculature during the dextro phase, followed by the pulmonary veins and left atrium (LA) during the levo phase. A PA catheter is always placed for PA pressure monitoring and assessment of cardiac output. The wedge position can be used to evaluate left atrial pressure and to monitor the ventricular wave (V wave).

The 8-Fr RFV sheath can be preclosed with one or two ProGlides and 14-Fr short sheath can be placed. Another option is to achieve hemostasis with manual pressure at the end and to perform the procedure without sheath or figure-of-eight stitch for hemostasis. An 8-Fr Mullins (Medtronic, Inc., Minneapolis, MN) sheath is advanced to the SVC (through a 14-Fr sheath or directly) over the wire, and then the wire is exchanged for the Brockenbrough needle (Medtronic, Inc., Minneapolis, MN). The sheath, dilator, and needle are slowly brought down within a clockwise rotation. Three drops are typically felt when the system crosses from SVC to RA, limbus, and aorta. The location is confirmed by anteroposterior (AP) and lateral views showing the needle on the right border of the spine in the AP view and facing posteriorly away from the aorta in the lateral view, just below the level of the noncoronary cusp. If there is good tactile pulsation of the LA, the needle is advanced across the septum, with the hemodynamic tracing showing a change from a right atrial waveform to a left atrial waveform without any loss of pressure. If there is a sudden drop in pressure during transit, this may indicate the needle has passed through the pericardial space; the needle should be withdrawn and the pericardium should be carefully investigated. If the passage is clean, the Mullins sheath can be advanced into the LA, and the dilator removed. Transseptal puncture is performed in the posterior and inferior part of the interatrial septum to achieve easy access to the mitral valve. Once the appropriate position of the sheath is confirmed, heparin (70 units/kg) may be administered. Following introduction of a coiled floppy Toray wire, the Mullins sheath is removed and the septum is dilated by multiple passages with a long 11-Fr dilator.

The Inoue balloon is sized according to the height of the patient. A 26-mm balloon is used for patients up to 170 cm, 28 mm balloons are for patients between 170 and 180 cm, and 30 mm balloons are for patients taller than 180 cm. Gradual dilatation in 1–2 mm increments should be used. Careful assessment of hemodynamics (LA pressure, gradient, V-wave, PA pressure), and TEE assessment of the valve (MR and MS) help one to decide how far to push. Commissural MR indicates that commissural splitting has been achieved. Sometimes a ventriculogram can help if the severity of MR remains questionable after TEE interrogation.

CLINICAL ASPECTS

The most important predictor of the long-term success of BMV is the procedural result. If mitral valve area after the procedure is >1.6 cm², the long-term outcome is excellent.[17,18] Some predictors of poor outcome include older age, presence of atrial fibrillation, and unfavorable valvular anatomy.[17,19–22] If the BMV is successful, PA and LA pressure will decrease immediately and cardiac output will improve. Patients also feel an immediate difference in their exercise tolerance.

Adequate control of heart rate and diuretic therapy are the cornerstone of medical management. It is also worthwhile to try and maintain sinus rhythm. Anticoagulation is imperative in patients with a history of thromboembolism or atrial fibrillation. Patients in sinus rhythm who have a large LA and are on beta blockers (which can predispose them to asymptomatic atrial fibrillation) should be strongly considered for oral anticoagulation. Follow-up with symptom review and echocardiogram is recommended.[7] Stress echocardiogram is helpful if there is any question about worsening symptoms. There is an unmet need for MVR among patients with DMS.[13] These patients are elderly with multiple comorbidities and are often high-risk candidates for surgery. With increasing life expectancy, more patients with DMS are likely to be encountered. Many patients are currently left untreated because of the presence of multiple comorbidities that significantly increase the risk of mortality with surgical MVR. A percutaneous or hybrid approach similar to transcatheter aortic valve replacement (TAVR) may provide an alternative treatment option for otherwise inoperable or high-risk cases. Although there are some reports of off-label use of TAVR devices for transcatheter mitral valve repair (TMVR) in this patient population, the field is in its infancy.[23]

LIMITATIONS

Patients with mixed MS and MR need MVR and cannot be treated with BMV. Severe MR following BMV is typically caused by a flail anterior mitral leaflet and usually requires surgery. Emergent surgery is rare (<1%) but should be available because BMV is usually performed in very young patients with otherwise excellent prognosis even with emergent surgery. Restenosis after BMV is 10%–30% at 5 years depending on the initial results.[24] A repeat procedure can be attempted depending on the cause of restenosis and anatomy.[25]

CONCLUSIONS

BMV is the treatment of choice for patients with severe symptomatic MS with favorable valvular anatomy. Procedural success determines long-term outcomes. Careful monitoring with TEE, fluoroscopy, and hemodynamics during the procedure makes this technique safe and effective.

PERCUTANEOUS TREATMENT OF MITRAL REGURGITATION

Introduction

Significant morbidity and mortality can be attributed to MR. This is true for patients with degenerative valve disease, as well as the growing population of patients with functional

and ischemic MR.[26] The most effective surgical approach for the treatment of severe ischemic MR remains controversial. In the past few years, the use of mitral valve repair has greatly exceeded the use of replacement. In a recently concluded Cardiothoracic Surgical Trials Network (CTSN) trial, the authors observed no significant difference in left ventricular reverse remodeling or survival at 12 months between patients who underwent mitral valve repair and those who underwent MVR.[27] There was higher recurrence of moderate or severe MR in the repair group (32.6% versus 2.3%, $P < 0.001$), but there was no significant between-group difference in clinical outcomes (Figure 43.4). However, the presence of severe comorbidities precludes surgical treatment in up to 50% of patients with severe MR.[28] Indeed, percutaneous mitral valve repair may be an alternative therapeutic option. Percutaneous repair of the mitral valve has the potential to provide decreased morbidity, improved recovery time, and shorter hospital stays compared with open heart surgery. These percutaneous techniques are predominantly based on existing surgical strategies, and each technique provides a different advantage based on the anatomical and functional characteristics of the MR. Proper patient selection will ultimately determine the success of these emerging technologies. In addition, imaging technologies inside and outside of the catheterization laboratory and integration of multiple imaging modalities will be important for the safety and efficacy of these percutaneous technologies.[29] Finally, evaluation of MR devices will be challenging as they will be compared with traditional surgical techniques, which may have different goals in patient management (e.g. need for repeat procedures and residual MR). These devices may possibly have a complementary role to surgery in the future. Of note, several percutaneous mitral valve repair technologies are being developed and are under investigation.[30] Furthermore, successful mitral valve repair with transcatheter aortic valve implantation (TAVI) prostheses have been performed in patients with degenerated surgical bioprostheses or with recurrent MR following annuloplasty.[14]

Fundamentals and anatomic considerations for percutaneous repair

MITRAL REGURGITATION, ETIOLOGY, DIAGNOSIS

Normal mitral valve closure depends on the appropriate anatomy and function of each component of the mitral valve, including the annulus, the anterior and posterior leaflets, the chordate tendineae, and the papillary muscles.[31] Primary mitral valve disease refers to myxomatous degeneration of the leaflets and chordae, resulting in chordal elongation or rupture, flail leaflet, or mitral valve prolapse. This is known as degenerative MR. Secondary valve disease (functional MR) is caused by disruption of the structural arrangement of the mitral apparatus, most commonly resulting from dilated cardiomyopathy, leading to ventricular dilatation, mitral annular dilation, and altered papillary

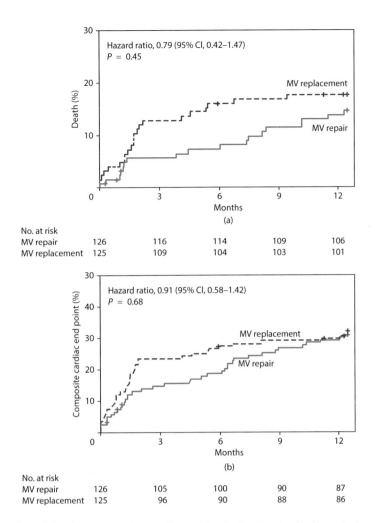

Figure 43.4 Rates of **(a)** death and **(b)** the composite cardiac endpoint in the Cardiothoracic Surgical Trials Network trial. The composite endpoint of the rate of major adverse cardiac or cerebrovascular events included death, stroke, subsequent mitral-valve (MV) surgery, hospitalization for heart failure, and an increase in the New York Heart Association class of 1 or more. Crosses indicate that patients' data were censored at that point.

muscle–leaflet interaction (Table 43.1). Moreover, ischemic cardiac disease may be associated with papillary muscle dysfunction or rupture, sometimes referred to as ischemic MR.[32] In this condition, changes in left ventricular geometry lead to leaflet "tenting" and anterior leaflet override, which prevents proper coaptation.[33]

In addition to the above categorization based on etiology and mechanism, a morphologic classification proposed by Carpentier's group is the mechanism of regurgitation according to leaflet pathophysiology.[34] This simplification has utility in terms of the surgical and percutaneous approach, as the goal of therapy may be to restore normal leaflet function but not necessarily normal valve anatomy (Figure 43.5). Various methods exist for quantification of MR, but echocardiography is considered the gold standard (Table 43.2). Direct measures, including regurgitant orifice area, regurgitant flow, or diameter of vena contracta, constitute the major quantitative parameters used in clinical trials. However, MR severity is judged after taking into account many other secondary effects like size and function of LA and left ventricle (LV), blunting of the pulmonary

venous flow, serial changes in all these parameters over time, and loading conditions. Furthermore, postprocedural MR is even harder to quantify at times because of anatomical distortion of the valve from various procedures, which may lead to very eccentric jets (e.g., after edge-to-edge repair). The design of medical devices aimed at treating MR should have different characteristics and goals on the basis of the underlying disease state. Hence, the complexity of MR should be recognized; the recommendations of the Mitral Valve Academic Research Consortium (MVARC) are particularly useful during the early development stage of transcatheter mitral devices.[29,30]

GENERAL INDICATIONS FOR INVASIVE TREATMENT OF MITRAL REGURGITATION

Per the 2014 guidelines released by the ACC/AHA, any patient with symptomatic, chronic, severe MR should undergo surgical valve repair or replacement especially if left ventricular ejection fraction (LVEF) is >30%.[10] When the patient is asymptomatic, the development of LV dysfunction (ejection fraction <60%) or dilation (LV end-systolic

Table 43.1 Causes of mitral regurgitation

Primary	Secondary (Functional)
Myxomatous degeneration • Mitral valve prolapse • Ehlers–Danlos syndrome • Osteogenesis Imperfecta	Mitral valve annular dilation • Ischemic cardiomyopathy • Dilated cardiomyopathy
Fibroelastic deficiency	Restricted leaflet motion • LA dilatation • LV dilation
Congenital mitral valve clefts • Mitral valve fenestrations • Parachute mitral valve abnormality • Double orifice mitral valve • Anomalous posterior leaflet rotation	Hypertrophic cardiomyopathy Aneurysmal dilation of LV
Systematic or inflammatory disease • Rheumatic heart disease • Systemic lupus erythematosus • Scleroderma • Amyloidosis • Still's disease • Endomyocardial fibrosis	Atrial fibrillation
Idiopathic causes	

Note: LA, left atrium; LV, left ventricle.

dimension >40 mm) indicates the need for surgical intervention. In surgical centers that are experienced in mitral repair, surgery can be considered in asymptomatic patients with less dilated LV and preserved systolic function, if repair is feasible. The development of atrial fibrillation or pulmonary hypertension in an asymptomatic patient can also be an indication for surgery. Among patients with primary valve disease and severe LV dilation or dysfunction, the role of surgery is controversial. In case of valve dysfunction secondary to LV dysfunction (functional MR), repair may be considered after medical optimization and more so if the patient has to undergo surgery for another indication.

Importantly, per the 2014 guidelines, *percutaneous* mitral valve repair may be considered for severely symptomatic patients (New York Heart Association [NYHA] class III to IV) with chronic severe primary MR; patients should have favorable anatomy for the procedure, a reasonable life expectancy, a prohibitive surgical risk because of severe comorbidities, and at the same time, remain severely symptomatic despite optimal medical therapy for heart failure. Per the 2012 European guidelines, the percutaneous edge-to-edge procedure may be considered in patients with symptomatic severe primary MR who fulfill the echo criteria of eligibility, are judged inoperable or at high surgical risk by a "heart team," and have a life expectancy greater than 1 year.[7] A similar level of recommendation exists for patients with symptomatic severe secondary MR despite optimal medical therapy (including CRT if indicated). Nevertheless, there are several caveats to these general guidelines, and individualization of therapy

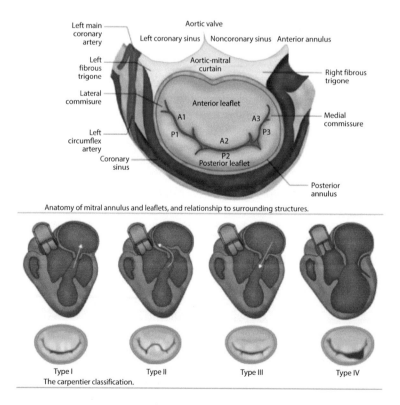

Anatomy of mitral annulus and leaflets, and relationship to surrounding structures.

The carpentier classification.

Figure 43.5 Anatomy of mitral annulus, leaflets and the Carpentier classification.

Table 43.2 Qualitative and quantitative parameters useful in grading mitral regurgitation severity

Parameter	Mild	Moderate	Severe
Structural Parameters			
LA size	Normal	Normal/dilated	Usually dilated
LV size	Normal	Normal/dilated	Usually dilated
Mitral leaflets/ support apparatus	Normal/abnormal	Normal/dilated	Abnormal/flail leaflet/ruptured papillary muscle
Doppler Parameters			
Color flow jet area	Small central jet (<4 cm² or <20% of LA area)	Variable	Large central jet (>10 cm² or >40%)or variable size wall impending jet swirling in LA
Mitral inflow-PW	A-wave dominant	Variable	E-wave dominant
Jet density-CW	Incomplete or faint	Dense	Dense
Jet contour-CW	Parabolic	Usually parabolic	Early peaking
Pulmonary vein inflow	Systolic dominance	Systolic blunting	Systolic flow reversal
Quantitative Parameters			
VC width (cm)	<0.3	0.3–0.69	≥0.7
R Vol (ml/beat)	<30	30–44 45–59	≥60
RF (%)	<30	30–39 40–49	≥50
EROA (cm²)	<0.20	0.20–0.29 0.30–0.39	≥0.40

Note: CW, continuous wave Doppler; EROA, effective regurgitant orifice area; LA, left atrium; LV, left ventricle; PW, pulsed wave Doppler; RF, regurgitant fraction; R Vol, regurgitant volume; VC, vena contracta.

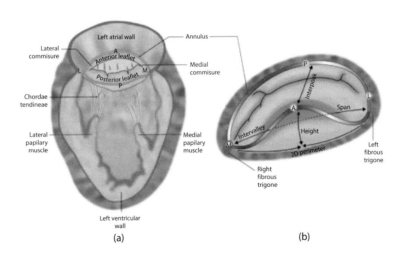

Figure 43.6 Anatomy of the **(a)** mitral valve and **(b)** complex mitral annulus.

is critical after considering functional status, anatomy of the mitral apparatus, LV function, as well as individual risk factors and preferences (Figure 43.6).

SURGICAL CONSIDERATIONS

Reviewing the surgical approaches to mitral valve repair is useful because the majority of percutaneous repair techniques attempt to mimic established surgical techniques.[35] Therefore, an understanding of the surgical approaches with their respective results and limitations is necessary to understand and evaluate emerging percutaneous techniques (Figure 43.7).

The most common methods of surgical repair are based on restricting the mobility of the posterior leaflet (and at times, prolapsing anterior leaflet) and reducing the size of annulus to achieve proper coaptation of leaflets. Therefore, these techniques address the leaflets and annulus at the same time. Annuloplasty is typically performed using a ring, although the choice of rings depends on the shape and stiffness, and the required extent of annular coverage remains controversial.[36] The classic leaflet repair techniques include triangular resection, quadrangular resection, sliding annuloplasty, or edge-to-edge repair.[37] Although techniques of annuloplasty and

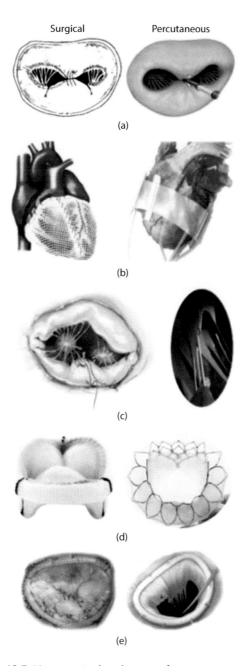

Surgical   Percutaneous

(a)

(b)

(c)

(d)

(e)

Figure 43.7 How surgical techniques for treating mitral regurgitation have inspired percutaneous counterparts. **(a)** A double orifice produced by the Alfieri stitch technique (L) and the MitraClip (R). **(b)** Left ventricular remodeling by the CorCap Cardiac Support Device (L) and the Extra-cardiac BACE (R). **(c)** Repairing chordae tendineae with surgical neochord placement (L) and the V-chordal device (R). **(d)** Replacing the mitral valve with a bioprosthetic mitral valve (L) and the TIARA mitral valve (R). **(e)** Annuloplasty of the mitral annulus surgically (L) and percutaneously (R). (L, left; R, right).

leaflet repair are usually combined when treating degenerative valve disease, isolated ring annuloplasty without leaflet repair is the dominant strategy for functional and ischemic MR.[38]

Annuloplasty for functional MR results in improvement in NYHA class, favorable LV remodeling, and decreased admissions for heart failure, but has failed to demonstrate a mortality benefit.[39] This may be in part due to the high recurrence rate of MR after isolated annuloplasty.[40] The combination of annuloplasty and leaflet repair (Carpentier's technique) for degenerative MR has shown the most favorable results in terms of mortality and recurrent MR. In experienced centers, Carpentier's technique has provided results that are better than with MVR, resulting in a mortality rate similar to that of the general population (86%–93% survival at 5 years).[41] The recurrence rate of severe MR (grade 3 or 4) after repair is 3.7% per year.[42]

CLASSES OF PERCUTANEOUS MITRAL VALVE REPAIR DEVICES

As a result of the variable anatomy and etiology of MR, a number of different approaches have been developed for percutaneous repair of the mitral valve (Tables 43.3 and 43.4). The goal of each approach is to bring the leaflets together to improve coaptation. The most advanced approach to date is edge-to-edge leaflet repair, based loosely on the surgical repair championed by Ottavio Alfieri.[43] Another approach takes advantage of the proximity of the coronary sinus (CS) to the mitral annulus to create favorable geometric changes in the annulus, moving the posterior leaflet closer to the anterior leaflet, improving coaptation. This approach is termed *indirect annuloplasty* or *CS reshaping*. Additionally, there are devices under investigation that perform a direct annular repair by plication from the left ventricular chamber. Other devices take a more direct approach to the annulus by applying suture-based plication systems. Cardiac chamber reshaping has been explored as a means to bring the leaflets into coaptation by decreasing the septal-to-lateral (SL) dimension of the ventricle or atrium. Finally, encouraging efforts are underway to develop and advance transcatheter MVR techniques.

CLINICAL AND ANATOMIC (IMAGING) SCREENING FOR EACH CLASS OF DEVICE

The dominant imaging modality for assessment of MR is echocardiography. 2D TTE is useful to evaluate valvular structure, the presence of calcifications, leaflet tethering, flail leaflet, or LV wall motion abnormalities (Figure 43.8). The severity of the regurgitation can be accurately quantified, as well as the specific hemodynamic consequences of the regurgitation. In most cases, a combination of clinical information and TTE data will establish the etiology of MR and define the anatomy of the mitral valve, the cornerstones of which are important in assessing candidacy for surgical or percutaneous intervention. TEE should be used to supplement the evaluation, often allowing greater definition of mitral valve structures and regurgitation severity. This can be particularly useful to determine if edge-to-edge valve repair is feasible, as valve anatomy characteristics, such as coaptation depth and annulus size, can be critical to assess clip feasibility.

Table 43.3 Percutaneous or minimally invasive mitral valve repair devices for functional mitral regurgitation

Device design		Developmental phase
Leaflet Techniques		
Edge-to-Edge Techniques		
MitraClip	Abbott labs, IL, USA	Approved; Ongoing COAPT and RESHAPE HF trials
Leaflet Space Occupiers		
Percu-Pro	Cardiosolutions, Stoughton, MA	First in man trial done
Annuloplasty		
Indirect		
CARILLON Mitral Contour System	Cardiac Dimensions, Kirkland, WA, USA	Two trials (Titan and Amadeus), Conformité Européenne approved
Direct		
Mitralign percutaneous annuloplasty system	Mitralign, Tewksbury, MA, USA	First in man, Conformité Européenne trial
GDS Accucinch annuloplasty system	GDS	First in man
Millipede percutaneous annuloplasty ring	MC3, Ann Arbor, MI, USA	Feasibility phase
Cardioband	Valtech Cardio Ltd, Or Yehuda, Israel	Preclinical phase
Adjustable annuloplasty ring	Mitral Solutions, Fort Lauderdale, FL, USA	Feasibility study over; post-market Conformité Européenne study
Dynamic annuloplasty ring	Micardia, Irvine, CA, USA	First in man
Left Ventricular Remodeling		
BACE device	Phoenix Cardiac Devices, Northbrook, IL, USA	First in man

Table 43.4 Percutaneous or minimally invasive mitral valve repair devices for degenerative mitral regurgitation

Device design		Developmental phase
Leaflet Techniques		
Edge-to-Edge Leaflet Repair		
MitraClip	Abbott Labs, IL, USA	Approved by U.S. Food and Drug Administration
Leaflet Space Occupiers		
Percu-Pro	CardioSolutions, Stoughton, MA	Phase I trials
Chordal Techniques		
NeoChord	NeoChord, Minnetonka, MN	Preclinical phase
V-chordal adjustable system	Valtech Cardio Lt, Or-Yehuda	Early clinical evaluation
Babic neochord		Preclinical phase

Other imaging modalities, including cardiac computed tomography (CT), cardiac magnetic resonance, and 3D TEE may be useful to determine which device may be appropriate for which patient.[44] In particular, indirect annuloplasty via the CS relies on proximity of the CS to the valve annulus. Cardiac CT is particularly well suited to assess this anatomical relationship, as well as proximity to the left circumflex artery, which can become obstructed by the placement of such devices. With cardiac MR, it is possible to obtain significant structural information regarding the geometry of the LV, mitral annulus and leaflets, and quantitative regurgitant volumes.[44] Finally, 3D TEE is becoming increasingly important in assessing valve characteristics and geometry, in addition to providing "real-time" guidance of percutaneous valve interventions.[29]

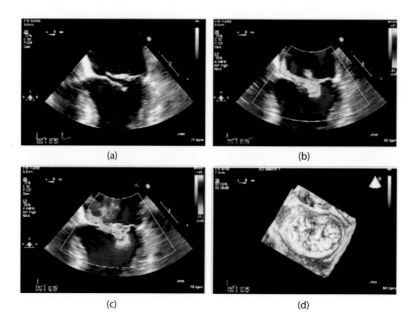

Figure 43.8 Echocardiographic diagnosis. **(a)** Posterior leaflet prolapse/flail. **(b and c)** Color Doppler showing anteriorly directed regurgitant jet. **(d)** Three-dimensional echo showing prolapse at P2 level.

Clinical aspects

Percutaneous valve repair technology shows promise for reducing the morbidity and mortality associated with traditional invasive surgical repair. The success of these techniques is dependent on proper selection of patients according to clinical presentation and anatomy, along with appropriate imaging of the valve before and at the time of procedure. The major advantage of a percutaneous approach, beyond its less invasive nature, is the ability to perform procedures on a beating heart, which allows for immediate evaluation of the hemodynamic and echocardiographic results of the valve intervention. If percutaneous technologies can be made simple and relatively safe, and preserve surgical options, they represent the future of valve intervention. Proper training of the interventionalists, not only in device manipulation but also in patient selection, imaging techniques, and catheter skills, will be necessary for wide application of these techniques with favorable results.[29]

Chordal techniques

Chordal rupture and chordal elongation are common findings in patients with degenerative MR. In the chordal techniques, defective chords can be replaced with artificial chords to achieve optimal leaflet coaptation. Most of these techniques are still under investigation.

NEOCHORD

The NeoChord (NeoChord Inc., St. Louis Park, MN) has been developed to treat ruptured chordae in degenerative MR. It involves a mini thoracotomy, off-pump, transapical access to implant the NeoChord, which stabilizes the prolapsing segments of the mitral valve. The technique was tested in the TACT (Transapical Artificial Chordae Tendinae) trial. Sixty-five patients with severe MR due to isolated Carpentier II prolapse of the posterior MV leaflet and no dilation were included. Those with anterior or bileaflet prolapse were excluded. Of the 30 patients enrolled, 26 (87%) had acute procedural success (APS). At 30 days, 65% had MR less than or equal to 2. Four patients with APS ultimately needed traditional mitral valve repair and MVR within 30 days.[45]

MITRAFLEX

With the MitraFlex (TransCardiac Therapeutics, Atlanta, GA) via a thoracoscopic transapical approach, the edge-to-edge clip repair is combined with neochordae replacement. An anchor is placed in the inner LV myocardium and another on the leaflet via a thoracoscopic transapical approach and connects the two with a synthetic chord; an edge-to-edge repair can also be performed at the same time.

V-CHORDAL SYSTEM

The V-Chordal system (Valtech Cardio Ltd., Or-Yehuda, Israel) is a modification of earlier chordal replacement techniques.[46] Unlike prior techniques, it allows adjustment of the neochordal length after the implant on the beating heart by direct vision through a mini-thoracotomy. A clip-attaching mechanism is being developed to allow transfemoral access.

BABIC NEOCHORD

The Babic NeoChord (from the name of the inventor, Uros Babic, MD) is a technique for leaflet repair in the beating heart. It uses a transseptal-transapical approach. The technique involves puncturing the mitral leaflet via the transapical approach and final anchoring of the leaflets with neochordae that are secured to the LV epicardial surface.

EDGE-TO-EDGE (DOUBLE-ORIFICE) LEAFLET REPAIR

An isolated edge-to-edge repair, championed by the Italian surgeon, Alfieri, has been shown in a small series to have reasonable long-term results.[43] This repair technique was the basis for one of the earliest applications of surgical repair techniques to percutaneous valve intervention. Like its surgical counterpart, the percutaneous edge-to-edge procedure produces a double-orifice and a fiber bridge segment without the development of significant MS.

MITRACLIP

The device with continued clinical activity is the MitraClip Endovascular Cardiovascular Valve Repair System (Abbott Laboratories, IL). This *v*-shaped clip device is delivered through a 24-Fr steerable guide catheter with a transseptal approach (Figure 43.9). The procedure is performed in the cardiac catheterization laboratory or hybrid operating room (OR) under general anesthesia with TEE guidance. TEE is used to guide transseptal access, steering and orientation of the clip delivery system and clip toward the mitral valve, and grasping of the leaflets to confirm placement of the device on the anterior and posterior leaflets of the mitral valve. Assessment of residual MR after clip deployment is complex. Pulmonary vein flow pattern, color Doppler assessment, systolic blood pressure, and mean left atrial pressure before and after clip deployments are all considered in the decision-making. Placement of a second clip may be necessary and the mitral valve area and mean gradients are evaluated prior to placement of a second clip. After this procedure, these patients are prescribed dual antiplatelet therapy (DAPT) for a minimum of 1–6 months. Anticoagulation with warfarin or xaban (XA) inhibitors is resumed if the patient was treated with these medications for other conditions like atrial fibrillation or thromboembolic venous disease. However, in the latter situations, there is no need for DAPT.

The initial experience with the MitraClip device consisted of 55 patients enrolled in the EVEREST (Endovascular Valve Edge-to-Edge Repair Study) phase I feasibility trial[47] and an additional 52 patients treated in the prerandomization start-up experience (roll-in phase) of the EVEREST II pivotal trial.[48] Patients were included if they were candidates for mitral valve repair or MVR surgery, had symptomatic moderate-to-severe (3+) or severe (4+) MR, or if they were asymptomatic and had an ejection fraction less than 60% or left ventricular end-systolic diameter of more than 45 mm (Figure 43.10). Of the 107 patients who underwent the MitraClip procedure, 70 (74%) achieved APS defined as a postprocedure reduction of MR to less than 2+. Of subjects who did not achieve APS, 17 (16%) had MitraClip implantation with acute MR grade more than 2+, and 11 (10%) had no MitraClip implanted with postprocedure MR more than 2+. At 12 months, not including crossover to surgery, 50 of 76 APS patients (66%) had echocardiographic follow-up and continued with MR less than 2+. A total of 32 patients underwent mitral valve surgery after a clip procedure, and when repair was planned, 84% were successfully repaired, demonstrating that mitral valve repair is feasible after prior MitraClip attempt or implantation. Freedom from death at up to 3 years follow-up was 90.1% and freedom from surgery was 76.3%. The majority of patients included had degenerative MR (79%), but patients with functional MR (21%) had similar acute results and durability. The EVEREST II[49] trial compared the MitraClip with MV surgery in patients with moderate-to-severe MR.[50] The study was a prospective, multicenter, randomized controlled trial with a 2:1 randomization to the study and control arms, respectively.[49] It was designed to show device safety superiority and noninferiority in efficacy compared to mitral surgery. A total of 279 patients with severe MR were randomized (184 to MitraClip and 85 to surgery), 73% of whom had degenerative MR and 27% had functional MR. Of the 184 patients assigned to the MitraClip, 178 underwent treatment, and APS was achieved in 137 (77%). The primary

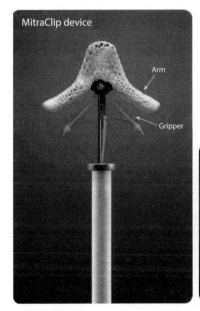
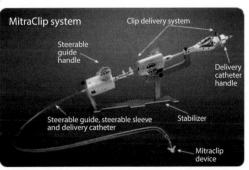

Figure 43.9 The percutaneous MitraClip system. (Adapted from Athappan, G., et al., *Interv. Cardiol. Clin.*, 5, 71–82, 2016.)

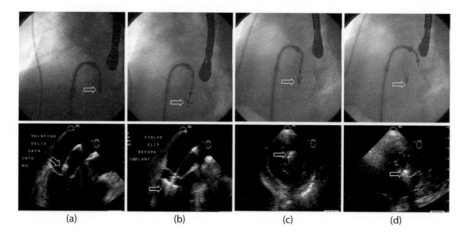

Figure 43.10 Fluoroscopic and corresponding transesophageal echocardiographic views of the MitraClip procedure. **(a)** Positioning of the MitraClip. **(b)** The MitraClip advanced into the left ventricle with the arms extended. **(c)** The mitral leaflets are grasped. **(d)** Final deployment. Arrows in the panels are depicting the MitraClip device. (Adapted from Yuksel, U.C., et al., *Curr. Cardiol. Rep.*, 13, 100–106, 2011.)

safety endpoint was major adverse events: a composite death, major stroke, reoperation of the mitral valve, urgent/emergent cardiovascular surgery, myocardial infarction (MI), renal failure, deep wound infection, ventilation more than 48 hours, new-onset permanent atrial fibrillation, septicemia, gastrointestinal complication requiring surgery, or transfusion >2 units. At 30 days, the primary safety endpoint was experienced by 9.6% of the percutaneous group and 57% of the "control" surgical group, though it should be noted that much of this difference was accounted for by the need for transfusions of more than two units in the surgical group (53.2% in surgical arm vs. 8.8% in MitraClip arm). Also notable, however, was the lack of death, major stroke, urgent or emergent surgery, or repeat mitral valve surgery in any of the 136 patients with MitraClip who achieved APS. An analysis of clinical effectiveness showed the MitraClip to be "noninferior" to surgery (72.4% vs. 87.8%; prespecified margin for noninferiority 31%). The 5-year follow-up included 154 patients from the device arm and 56 from the surgical arm.[50] The rate of the composite efficacy endpoint (freedom from death, mitral valve surgery, or 3+ or 4+ MR) in the as-treated population was lower in the percutaneous group, with no differences in the individual endpoint of mortality between the two groups. However, need for surgery or reoperation and 3+ or 4+ MR both were more frequent with percutaneous repair.

Efficacy of the MitraClip device is currently being evaluated in randomized controlled trials against best medical therapy in the COAPT (Clinical Outcomes Assessment of the MitraClip Percutaneous Therapy) and RESHAPE-HF (MitraClip Device in Heart Failure Patients with Clinically Significant Functional Mitral Regurgitation) trials. In a systematic review of 21 studies involving 6,463 patients, the pooled event rates for mortality and stroke (30 days after procedure) after MitraClip were 3% and 4.5%, respectively.[51] Notably, the MitraClip is the only U.S. Food and Drug Administration (FDA)-approved therapy for the transcatheter treatment of MR at this time, with a restricted indication for a small group of degenerative MR patients who are at prohibitive risk for surgery.

Indirect annuloplasty via coronary sinus

Annular dilation and shape are important contributors to the severity of functional MR.[52] Progressive dilation of the mitral annulus in dilated cardiomyopathy reduces coaptation of the leaflets leading to MR. The degree of MR has been found to be proportional to the increase in annular area. Indirect annuloplasty techniques have been developed to reshape the annulus by reducing its septolateral dimension by applying a constricting force through a device deployed in the CS. The close proximity of the CS to the annulus is exploited in indirect annuloplasty techniques.

CARILLON MITRAL CONTOUR SYSTEM

The CARILLON Mitral Contour System (developed by Cardiac Dimensions, Kirkland, WA) is a fixed-length, double-anchor device, which is advanced through a catheter and positioned in the CS.[53] After the device is deployed and locked into position, tension applied to the anchors of the device results in tissue plication and reduces the mitral valve annular diameter and MR (Figure 43.11). The procedure is performed percutaneously via internal jugular vein access, followed by distal CS cannulation with a 9-Fr catheter. A measuring catheter is used to determine the optimal positioning of the distal anchor in the CS. The nitinol annuloplasty device is advanced down the catheter to the target position in the CS. The distal anchor of the device is deployed by passive expansion and is locked into the fully expanded position by use of percutaneous treatment of the delivery catheter. Tension is placed on the delivery system, bringing the proximal anchor toward the CS ostium. The amount of tension can be manipulated, as needed, to optimize reduction in annular dimension (≈25%) and reduction in MR, which is verified by real-time echocardiography.

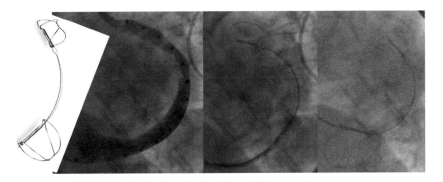

Figure 43.11 The Carillon Mitral contour system. (Courtesy of Samir Kapadia, Cleveland Clinic, Cleveland, Ohio, https://www.tctmd.com/sites/default/files/efs/public/2016-10/4441573.pdf.)

If the device position is considered to be optimal, the proximal anchor is deployed and locked into position in a similar fashion to the distal anchor. Importantly, if there is a concern about safety or efficacy, the device can be recaptured by advancing the delivery catheter over the device to collapse the anchors, and the apparatus can be adjusted or removed, as necessary. Clinical feasibility was evaluated in the prospective AMADEUS trial (CARILLON Mitral Annuloplasty Device European Union Study) using the next-generation CARILLON XE device in 48 patients with functional MR and LV systolic dysfunction.[54] The device was successfully implanted in 30 patients. At the 6-month follow-up, there was a durable and significant decrease in mitral annulus diameter (4.2–3.78 cm, 10%), MR (average reduction 23%), and NYHA class (2.9–0.8), as well as improvement in the quality-of-life score and 6-minute walk test (307–403 m). Of the remaining 18 patients, 5 did not receive implantation because of coronary sinus-related complications ($n = 3$) or fluoroscopic equipment failure ($n = 2$), and 13 patients had retrieval of the device after implantation because of either inadequate MR reduction or coronary compromise. With respect to safety, six patients (13%) experienced a total of seven complications within 30 days of the procedure: one patient died of multiorgan failure, three patients experienced MI, though none required percutaneous coronary intervention (PCI), and three patients experienced CS dissection or perforation. The complications were clustered early in the experience and resulted in changes to the implantation procedure, with the appearance of improvement in safety later in the study. On the basis of this early work, the CARILLON system has been granted the Conformité Européene (CE) mark of approval for use in Europe. Improvements to the device were evaluated in the follow-up TITAN (Tighten the Annulus Now) study, which enrolled 53 patients at eight centers across Europe.[55] An interim report at 6 months revealed successful implantation in 68% of patients; 15% did not receive implants because of transient coronary impingement. There was a 1.9% rate of major adverse cardiovascular events (MACEs), namely the death of a patient who did not receive an implant. At the 6-month follow-up, reduction in regurgitant fraction was 26%; there was a one-point reduction in NYHA class and 100 m improvement in 6-minute walk distance (MWD). More recently, the 2-year follow-up of the TITAN study was published. There was sustained benefit in 6-MWD and NYHA class. An enhanced version is being investigated in the TITAN II trial[56] that has finished enrolling patients. Preliminary data suggest improved safety with no device fractures. The device will also undergo testing in the single-center INTEGRAL trial in South America. The long-term safety and efficacy will be evaluated in the Percutaneous Repair in Functional Mitral Regurgitation (PRIME) study, a post-market European registry that is ongoing.

A clear limitation of the indirect annuloplasty approach relies on the progressive distance between the CS and the mitral plane following the enlargement of the atrium, the variable spatial relationship between the CS and mitral annulus, and the risk of circumflex artery compression. Thus, the annuloplasty approach will probably be appropriate for smaller atriums only.

Direct annuloplasty

Percutaneous direct annuloplasty via a retrograde transventricular approach is an exciting area of development. The obvious advantage to this approach is the ability to apply a repair directly to the annulus, where the pathologic mechanism of MR is frequently located. This approach eliminates the anatomic uncertainty about the left circumflex anatomy and the proximity of the CS to the mitral annulus, which plagues CS approaches; it also addresses the pathologic basis of functional MR, which may be missed with leaflet-only techniques.

MITRALIGN DIRECT ANNULOPLASTY SYSTEM

The Mitralign Direct Annuloplasty System (Mitralign, Tewksbury, MA) is based on the concept of direct suture annuloplasty. The system uses a device composed of three metal anchors connected by standard suture material. The anchors are placed in the mitral annulus, and the suture is cinched to perform the annuloplasty. The device is placed via retrograde ventricular access by using a unique translation catheter with a two-pronged "bi-dent" design for device delivery. The initial design used a magnetic-guiding catheter placed in the CS, but in the most recent iteration, the anchors are placed from the ventricular side using standard imaging techniques. The two anchors are positioned below the valve at the level of each posterior leaflet scallop and then deployed directly through the mitral annulus, remaining connected by suture material. The suture is then cinched, directly plicating the annulus, emulating the results of a surgical, suture-based annuloplasty.[57] The safety and performance data from the Mitralign Percutaneous Annuloplasty first in man study were recently reported.[58] Device success rate was 70.4% (n = 50 of 71). No intraprocedural deaths occurred. In patients receiving implants, four patients (8.9%) experienced cardiac tamponade. Thirty-day (n = 45) and 6-month (n = 41) rates for all-cause mortality, stroke, and MI were 4.4%, 4.4%, and 0% and 12.2%, 4.9%, and 0%, respectively. At 6 months, nonurgent mitral surgery was performed in one patient (2.4%) and nonurgent percutaneous repair in seven patients (17.1%).

GUIDED DELIVERY SYSTEMS ACCUCINCH ANNULOPLASTY SYSTEM

The Guided Delivery Systems (GDS) Accucinch Annuloplasty System (Santa Clara, CA) device provides for a catheter-based, transventricular approach to place anchors in the myocardium directly beneath the mitral annulus, yielding a plication annuloplasty. On the basis of encouraging studies in animal models, a first-in-human study was initiated in Europe. Preliminary feasibility and safety of the device were recently reported in 18 patients, five of whom had to be converted to open annuloplasty, but no acute deaths were reported.[59]

VALTECH CARDIOBAND

The Valtech Cardioband (Valtech Cardio, Or Yehuda, Israel) device is delivered via a transvenous, transseptal route and uses nitinol screws inserted into the atrial aspect of the mitral annulus in a commissure-to-commissure fashion. In a second step, the implant is cinched in order to reduce annular dimensions and MR. Recently, results of a multicenter feasibility study of Cardioband in 31 patients were reported.

All patients had functional (secondary) MR—33% with prior MI, 77% with atrial fibrillation. All patients had the Cardioband device implanted, but 29/31 patients had both a successful implant and technical performance of the device, defined as Cardioband reaching the posterior commissure with ability to reduce the implant size. MR reduction was achieved, with no severe MR at the end of the procedure in 29 patients, and 82% of the 27 patients followed for 30 days had ≤2+ MR by core lab assessment.[60]

Transcatheter mitral valve replacement

Transcatheter MVR is an attractive option as it targets the mitral valve complex as a whole, thereby eliminating the need for a combination of percutaneous approaches to achieve results on par with surgical repair/replacement (Table 43.5). However, the complex structural and functional anatomy of the mitral unit makes this a formidable challenge.[29] The challenges for mitral replacement are more complex than for the aortic valve, and it is clear that the testing of these devices will take more time than with TAVR (Figures 43.12 and 43.13). Device delivery and anchoring, and the large size and eccentric geometry of the mitral orifice, are the main complexities.[30]

BALLOON-EXPANDABLE VALVES USED IN MITRAL POSITION

Patients with mitral annular calcification (MAC) are an elderly high-risk patient population with multiple comorbidities even before they develop valvular dysfunction. There were isolated reports of successful TMVR with balloon-expandable valves in this patient population. The TMVR in the MAC Global Registry was established in 2013 to collect outcomes data of similar procedures performed worldwide to better understand its safety, and the results were recently reported from 64 patients across 32 centers worldwide.[14] SAPIEN valves (Edwards Lifesciences, Irvine, CA) were used in 7.8%, SAPIEN XT in 59.4%, SAPIEN 3 in 28.1%, and Inovare (Braile Biomedica, Brazil) in 4.7%. Access was

Table 43.5 Transcatheter mitral valve implantation: major devices with available and anticipated early human data

Device	Company	Developmental phase
The CardiAQ	Edwards Lifesciences, Irvine, CA	FIM studies complete; Early feasibility in USA
The Tendyne	Abbott Labs, IL, USA	FIM studies complete, Early feasibility
The Tiara	Neovasc Inc., Richmond, British Columbia, Canada	FIM studies complete, Early feasibility
The CardioValve	Valtech Cardio Ltd., Or Yehuda, Israel	Human clinical studies expected in early 2017
The Caisson valve	Caisson Interventional, USA	FIM studies complete, early feasibility
The Navigate TMVR	NCSI Inc., CA, USA	FIM studies completed
The Medtronic Intrepid	Medtronic, Minneapolis, MN, USA	FIM studies completed

Note: FIM, first in man; TMVR, transcatheter mitral valve repair.

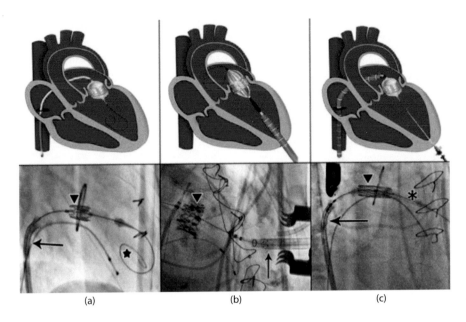

Figure 43.12 The different approaches for transcatheter aortic valve replacement: antegrade **(a)**, transapical **(b)**, and modified antegrade **(c)**. Arrowhead shows the prosthetic valve in the mitral position; long arrow points to the delivery sheath; the asterisk shows the externalized wire; and the star highlights the wire in the left ventricle. (Adapted from Sud et al., *Circulation*, 2016;133(16):1594-1604.)

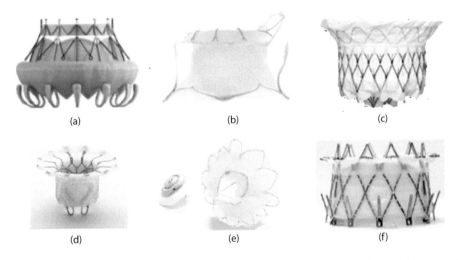

Figure 43.13 Transcatheter mitral valve implants: **(a)** the CardiAQ valve, **(b)** the Tiara valve, **(c)** the Intrepid valve, **(d)** the Fortis valve, **(e)** the Tendyne valve, and **(f)** the NaviGate valve. (Adapted from Krishnaswamy, A., et al., *Cleve. Clin. J. Med.*, 83, S10–S17, 2016.)

transatrial in 15.6%, transapical in 43.8%, and transseptal in 40.6%. Technical success according to Mitral Valve Academic Research Consortium criteria was achieved in 46 (72%) patients. Six (9.3%) had left ventricular tract obstruction with hemodynamic compromise. Mean mitral gradient postprocedure was 4 ± 2.2 mmHg; paravalvular regurgitation was mild or absent in all cases. Thirty-day, all-cause mortality was 29.7%, and 17.2% patients died of procedural complications. The authors concluded that TMVR with balloon-expandable valves is feasible in patients with severe MAC who are not candidates for standard mitral valve surgery, but it is associated with significant adverse events.

CARDIAQ VALVE

The CardiAQ valve (Edwards Lifesciences) is the first of its kind for the mitral valve. It is a transseptally delivered, trileaflet valve on a nitinol frame that self-anchors without the need of radial force. Results for 12 patients treated with the CardiaAQ transcatheter mitral valve under compassionate use were recently made available. There were two procedure-related deaths in this series—one due to interaction with a mechanical aortic valve, the other due to malpositioning related to subleaflet calcification. The U.S. early feasibility trial is now enrolling patients.[61]

TENDYNE

The Tendyne device (Abbott) consists of a *D*-shaped outer frame, a circular inner frame, and a porcine pericardial trileaflet valve that is deployed within the mitral annulus and tethered to the apex of the LV. The valve can be recaptured, repositioned, and if necessary, fully retrieved. The Tendyne Early Feasibility trial is a prospective, open-label, nonrandomized trial evaluating the device's safety and efficacy. A total of 37 cases have been reported with 32 early feasibility and 5 compassionate use implants. Detailed results from 12 patients (all males; age 75.3 + 3.4 years) have been published.[62] All patients had severe (4+) MR (11 secondary, 1 mixed pathology), and all were symptomatic (NYHA class II–IV). The LVEF was 40.2% + 11.8% (range 30%–61%), and the mean Society of Thoracic Surgeons (STS) score was 6.5 (range 2–16). In 11 patients, the device was deployed with no residual MR, no paravalvular leak, and no adverse events. In one patient, device deployment resulted in LV outflow obstruction and hypotension. It was removed without adverse sequelae. All patients were discharged alive with a length of stay ranging from 5 to 12 days.

TIARA VALVE

The Tiara valve (Neovasc Incorporation, Richmond, British Columbia, Canada) is a transapical self-expandable valve with biological tissue leaflets fixed to the frame. It has an atrial portion that hugs the mitral annulus, a ventricular portion with a covered skirt to prevent paravalvular leak, and a middle *D*-shaped orifice that matches the natural orifice of the mitral valve. Early results from group 1 (special access/compassionate use) and the currently enrolling group 2 (TIARA-I early feasibility clinical trial) cohorts of the implantation program are available. Of the 11 patients in which Tiara implantation was attempted, 8 had uneventful implantations, 2 died after being converted to urgent surgery, and a third patient died following erosion of septum at day 4. The early feasibility trial is now enrolling patients in the United States, Europe, and Canada.[61]

MEDTRONIC INTREPID VALVE

The Medtronic Intrepid valve (Medtronic, Minneapolis, MN) has a dual stent design with a conformable outer stent and circular inner stent housing a bovine pericardium valve. Early results showed that out of 11 patients, 9 patients achieved procedural success. Three patients died: one following unsuccessful device deployment, and the others at day 28 and day 54.[61]

CAISSON MITRAL VALVE IMPLANT

The Caisson mitral valve implant (Caisson Interventional, LLC, Austin, TX) is a transseptal device where the anchor is delivered first and then the valve is delivered inside of the anchor. The implant is fully repositionable and retrievable and only released after the function of the implant is fully assessed. The FDA recently approved the Investigational Device Exemption for this device under the PRELUDE study (Percutaneous Mitral Valve Replacement Evaluation Utilizing IDE Early Feasibility Study) for up to 20 patients in five centers. This valve has so far been used in three patients in the United States under this program.[63]

NAVIGATE TRANSCATHETER MITRAL VALVE REPLACEMENT

The Navigate TMVR (NCSI Inc., CA) is a self-expandable MVR device made of chemically preserved xenogenic pericardium, mounted on a nitinol frame and molded into a conical shape. Transatrial and transseptal approaches are present. Two patients have undergone this valve implantation.

CONCLUSION

Transcatheter-based techniques for the treatment of clinically significant MR have evolved tremendously in the past decade. These novel devices are primarily based on well-known surgical techniques that have subsequently progressed to less invasive approaches. The most advanced technique with the highest safety and efficacy, to date, is the edge-to-edge MitraClip repair system (Table 43.6). Current evidence suggests that the MitraClip is a valuable alternative to surgical mitral valve repair/MVR in selected high or prohibitive surgical risk patients with severe degenerative MR. The relative role of the MitraClip is under investigation for patients with functional MR. The ongoing COAPT and RESHAPE HF trials will provide more robust data upon completion. The majority of other catheter-based mitral valve repair devices are still at early human testing stages. It is important to emphasize that novel percutaneous techniques in the treatment of MR are not yet meant to replace surgical techniques in low-risk patients who are good candidates for surgery. Transcatheter MVR is promising as it targets the entire mitral apparatus unlike others that target individual components of the mitral valve complex. Efforts are already underway to gain the feasibility experience with ongoing enrollment in the United States for the Tendyne (Tendyne Holdings, Roseville, MN), CardiAQ (Edwards Lifesciences, Irvine, CA), and Tiara (Neovasc, Richmond, British Columbia, Canada) valve systems. The role of percutaneous repair/replacement will expand in the future with more novel device designs, advances in existing devices, improvements in imaging techniques, and operator experience. As percutaneous devices are more specifically tailored to the etiology of MR and the anatomy of the individual patient, the proper imaging and patient selection criteria for each device will have to be learned by interventionists.[29] Improvements in imaging techniques and the interpretation of these techniques with regard to percutaneous repair/replacement will also be necessary in preprocedural planning, in assessing intraprocedural efficacy and complications, and in postprocedural follow-up. Finally, it will be critical to continue the collegial interaction between the specialties of cardiac imaging, interventional cardiology, and cardiothoracic surgery (the "heart team approach") to achieve proper patient selection and clinical advancement in this burgeoning field.

Table 43.6 Major studies with MitraClip implantation

Studies	D	N	f/u	Age	EF	FMR	Euro	STS	Proce. success	30d mortality	All cause	Ische. stroke	Resid. ≥3+MR
High-Risk Patients													
TRAMI	R	1,064	80	75	-	61	23	12	95	5.9	11.8	1.4	3.9
ACCESS EU	R	567	365	75	-	56	23±18	-	91	3.4	17.3	1.1	8.8
REALISM	R	127	365	82	60	0	-	13±7	95	6.3	23.6	2.4	14.2
GRASP	R	117	410	72	38	-	12±14	-	100	0.8	16.2	0.9	9.8
MITRASWISS	R	100	365	77	48	56	19	-	85	4	16	1	21.8
Neu ss et al.	R	157	365	74	41	73	22±17	-	98	7	24	-	3
Trede et al.	R	202	365	75	44	65	36	-	92	-	10.4	-	-
Rudolph et al.	R	230	399	74	44	23	25	4.8	88	-	28	-	-
Low-Risk Patients													
EVEREST I	R	107	365	71	62	77	-	-	74	0.9	0.9	0	34.2
EVEREST II	RCT	184	1461	67	60	71	-	5±4	77	1.1	17.4	1.1	21.7
Versus Mitral Valve Surgery													
EVEREST II	"	184	1461	67	60	71	-	5±4	77	1.1	17.4	1.1	21.7
Con randi et al.	O	95	155	72	36	62	34±19	-	96	4.2	12.6	1.1	12
Paranskaya	O	24	365	78	58	33	8±6	4±4	92	0	8.3	4.2	0
Taramasso	O	52	255	65	28	100	22±16	-	98	-	11.1	-	9.6

Note: D, design; EF, ejection fraction; FMR, functional mitral regurgitation; f/u, follow up; MR; mitral regurgitation; N, number of patients; O, observational; R, registry; RCT, randomized control trial; STS, Society of Thoracic Surgeons score.

REFERENCES

1. Iung B, Vahanian A. Epidemiology of valvular heart disease in the adult. *Nat Rev Cardiol* 2011;8(3):162–172.
2. Kumar RK, Tandon R. Rheumatic fever & rheumatic heart disease: The last 50 years. *Indian J Med Res* 2013;137(4):643–658.
3. Vahanian A, et al. Changing demographics of valvular heart disease and impact on surgical and trans-catheter valve therapies. *Int J Cardiovasc Imaging* 2011;27(8):1115–1122.
4. Mueller UK, et al. Anterior mitral leaflet retraction—A new echocardiographic predictor of severe mitral regurgitation following balloon valvuloplasty by the Inoue technique. *Am J Cardiol* 1998;81(5):656–659.
5. Murat Tuzcu E, Kapadia SR. Percutaneous mitral valve repair and replacement: A new landmark for structural heart interventions. *Eur Heart J* 2016;37(10):828–836.
6. Martin RP. The fish mouth and three-dimensional echocardiography: New technology catches an old problem. *J Am Coll Cardiol* 2000;36(4):1362–1364.
7. Joint Task Force on the Management of Valvular Heart Disease of the European Society of Cardiology (ESC), et al. Guidelines on the management of valvular heart disease (version 2012). *Eur Heart J* 2012;33(19):2451–2496.
8. Wilkins GT, et al. Percutaneous balloon dilatation of the mitral valve: An analysis of echocardiographic variables related to outcome and the mechanism of dilatation. *Br Heart J* 1988;60(4):299–308.
9. Padial LR, et al. Echocardiography can predict the development of severe mitral regurgitation after percutaneous mitral valvuloplasty by the Inoue technique. *Am J Cardiol* 1999;83(8):1210–1213.
10. Nishimura RA, et al. 2014 AHA/ACC guideline for the management of patients with valvular heart disease: A report of the American College of Cardiology/American Heart Association Task Force on Practice Guidelines. *J Am Coll Cardiol* 2014;63(22):e57–e185.
11. Palacios IF, et al. Follow-up of patients undergoing percutaneous mitral balloon valvotomy. Analysis of factors determining restenosis. *Circulation* 1989;79(3):573–579.
12. Ben Farhat M, et al. Percutaneous balloon versus surgical closed and open mitral commissurotomy. Seven-year follow-up results of a randomized trial. *Circulation* 1998;97(3):245–250.
13. Sud K, et al. Degenerative mitral stenosis: Unmet need for percutaneous interventions. *Circulation* 2016;133(16):1594–1604.
14. Guerrero M, et al. Transcatheter mitral valve replacement in native mitral valve disease with severe mitral annular calcification. *JACC Cardiovasc Interv* 2016;9(13):1361–1371.
15. Stefanadis CI, et al. Retrograde nontransseptal balloon mitral valvuloplasty: Immediate results and intermediate long-term outcome in 441 cases—A multicenter experience. *J Am Coll Cardiol* 1998;32(4):1009–1016.
16. Cribier A, et al. Percutaneous mechanical mitral commissurotomy with a newly designed metallic valvulotome: Immediate results of the initial experience in 153 patients. *Circulation* 1999;99(6):793–799.
17. Hernandez R, et al. Long-term clinical and echocardiographic follow-up after percutaneous mitral valvuloplasty with the Inoue balloon. *Circulation* 1999;99(12):1580–1586.
18. Iung B, et al. Late results of percutaneous mitral commissurotomy in a series of 1024 patients. Analysis of late clinical deterioration: Frequency, anatomic findings, and predictive factors. *Circulation* 1999;99(25):3272–3278.

19. Meneveau N, et al. Predictors of event-free survival after percutaneous mitral commissurotomy. *Heart* 1998;80(4):359–364.

20. Lau KW, et al. Long-term (36–63 month) clinical and echocardiographic follow-up after Inoue balloon mitral commissurotomy. *Cathet Cardiovasc Diagn* 1998;43(1):33–38.

21. Langerveld J, et al. Predictors of clinical events or restenosis during follow-up after percutaneous mitral balloon valvotomy. *Eur Heart J* 1999;20(7):519–526.

22. Kang DH, et al. Long-term clinical and echocardiographic outcome of percutaneous mitral valvuloplasty: Randomized comparison of Inoue and double-balloon techniques. *J Am Coll Cardiol* 2000;35(1):169–175.

23. Kapadia SR, et al. Relationship of mitral valve annulus plane and circumflex-right coronary artery plane: Implications for transcatheter mitral valve implantation. *Catheter Cardiovasc Interv* 2017;89(5):932–943. doi:10.1002/ccd.26575.

24. Nunes MCP, et al. Update on percutaneous mitral commissurotomy. *Heart* 2016;102(7):500–507.

25. Tuzcu EM, Kapadia SR. Long-term efficacy of percutaneous mitral commissurotomy for recurrent mitral stenosis. *Heart* 2013;99(18):1307–1308.

26. Goel SS, et al. Prevalence and outcomes of unoperated patients with severe symptomatic mitral regurgitation and heart failure: Comprehensive analysis to determine the potential role of MitraClip for this unmet need. *J Am Coll Cardiol* 2014;63(2):185–186.

27. Acker MA, et al. Mitral-valve repair versus replacement for severe ischemic mitral regurgitation. *N Engl J Med* 2014;370(1):23–32.

28. Tuzcu EM, Kapadia SR. Percutaneous mitral valve repair and replacement: A new landmark for structural heart interventions. *Eur Heart J* 2016;37(10):826–828.

29. Stone GW, et al. Clinical trial design principles and endpoint definitions for transcatheter mitral valve repair and replacement: Part 1: Clinical trial design principles: A consensus document from the Mitral Valve Academic Research Consortium. *J Am Coll Cardiol* 2015;66(3):278–307.

30. Stone GW, et al. Clinical trial design principles and endpoint definitions for transcatheter mitral valve repair and replacement: Part 2: Endpoint definitions: A consensus document from the Mitral Valve Academic Research Consortium. *Eur Heart J* 2015;36(29):1878–1891.

31. Perloff JK, Roberts WC. The mitral apparatus. Functional anatomy of mitral regurgitation. *Circulation* 1972;46(2):227–239.

32. Cohn LH, et al. The effect of pathophysiology on the surgical treatment of ischemic mitral regurgitation: Operative and late risks of repair versus replacement. *Eur J Cardiothorac Surg* 1995;9(10):568–574.

33. Yousefzai R, et al. Outcomes of patients with ischemic mitral regurgitation undergoing percutaneous coronary intervention. *Am J Cardiol* 2014;114(7):1011–1017.

34. de Marchena E, et al. Respective prevalence of the different carpentier classes of mitral regurgitation: A stepping stone for future therapeutic research and development. *J Card Surg* 2011;26(4):385–392.

35. Feldman T, Young A. Percutaneous approaches to valve repair for mitral regurgitation. *J Am Coll Cardiol* 2014;63(20):2057–2068.

36. Nagy ZL, et al. Five-year experience with a suture annuloplasty for mitral valve repair. *Scand Cardiovasc J* 2000;34(5):528–532.

37. Aybek T, et al. Seven years' experience with suture annuloplasty for mitral valve repair. *J Thorac Cardiovasc Surg* 2006;131(1):99–106.

38. Bolling SF, et al. Intermediate-term outcome of mitral reconstruction in cardiomyopathy. *J Thorac Cardiovasc Surg* 1998;115(2):381–386.

39. Wu AH, et al. Impact of mitral valve annuloplasty on mortality risk in patients with mitral regurgitation and left ventricular systolic dysfunction. *J Am Coll Cardiol* 2005;45(3):381–387.

40. McGee EC, et al. Recurrent mitral regurgitation after annuloplasty for functional ischemic mitral regurgitation. *J Thorac Cardiovasc Surg* 2004;128(6):916–924.

41. Mohty D, et al. Very long-term survival and durability of mitral valve repair for mitral valve prolapse. *Circulation* 2001;104(12 Suppl 1):I1–I7.

42. Braunberger E, et al. Very long-term results (more than 20 years) of valve repair with carpentier's techniques in nonrheumatic mitral valve insufficiency. *Circulation* 2001;104(12 Suppl 1):I8–I11.

43. Alfieri O, et al. The double-orifice technique in mitral valve repair: A simple solution for complex problems. *J Thorac Cardiovasc Surg* 2001;122(4):674–681.

44. Natarajan N, et al. Peri-procedural imaging for transcatheter mitral valve replacement. *Cardiovasc Diagn Ther* 2016;6(2):144–159.

45. Seeburger J, et al. Off-pump transapical implantation of artificial neo-chordae to correct mitral regurgitation: The TACT Trial (Transapical Artificial Chordae Tendinae) proof of concept. *J Am Coll Cardiol* 2014;63(9):914–919.

46. Maisano F, et al. Beating-heart implantation of adjustable length mitral valve chordae: Acute and chronic experience in an animal model. *Eur J Cardiothorac Surg* 2011;40(4):840–847.

47. Feldman T, et al. Percutaneous mitral valve repair using the edge-to-edge technique: Six-month results of the EVEREST Phase I Clinical Trial. *J Am Coll Cardiol* 2005;46(11):2134–2140.

48. Feldman T, et al. Percutaneous mitral repair with the MitraClip system: Safety and midterm durability in the initial EVEREST (Endovascular Valve Edge-to-Edge REpair Study) cohort. *J Am Coll Cardiol* 2009;54(8):686–694.

49. Feldman T, et al. Percutaneous repair or surgery for mitral regurgitation. *N Engl J Med* 2011;364(15):1395–1406.

50. Feldman T, et al. Randomized comparison of percutaneous repair and surgery for mitral regurgitation: 5-year results of EVEREST II. *J Am Coll Cardiol* 2015;66(25):2844–2854.

51. Philip F, et al. MitraClip for severe symptomatic mitral regurgitation in patients at high surgical risk. *Catheter Cardiovasc Interv* 2014;84(4):581–590.

52. Popović ZB, et al. Mitral annulus size links ventricular dilatation to functional mitral regurgitation. *J Am Soc Echocardiogr* 2005;18(9):959–963.

53. Schofer J, et al. Percutaneous mitral annuloplasty for functional mitral regurgitation: Results of the CARILLON Mitral Annuloplasty Device European Union Study. *Circulation* 2009;120(4):326–333.

54. Siminiak T, et al. Effectiveness and safety of percutaneous coronary sinus-based mitral valve repair in patients with dilated cardiomyopathy (from the AMADEUS trial). *Am J Cardiol* 2009;104(4):565–570.

55. Siminiak T, et al. Treatment of functional mitral regurgitation by percutaneous annuloplasty: Results of the TITAN trial. *Eur J Heart Fail* 2012;14(8):931–938.

56. Lipiecki J, et al. Coronary sinus-based percutaneous annuloplasty as treatment for functional mitral regurgitation: The TITAN II trial. *Open Hear* 2016;3(2):e000411.

57. Kapadia SR, et al. Percutaneous direct annuloplasty: Lessons from an early feasibility trial. *J Am Coll Cardiol* 2016;67(25):2937–2940.

58. Nickenig G, et al. Treatment of chronic functional mitral valve regurgitation with a percutaneous annuloplasty system. *J Am Coll Cardiol* 2016;67(25):2927–2936.

59. Gooley RP, Meredith IT. The Accucinch transcatheter direct mitral valve annuloplasty system. *EuroIntervention* 2015;11 Suppl W:W60–W61.

60. Maisano F, et al. Cardioband, a transcatheter surgical-like direct mitral valve annuloplasty system: Early results of the feasibility trial. *Eur Heart J* 2015;37(10):817–825. doi:10.1093/eurheartj/ehv603.

61. Wood S. http://www.tctmd.com/show.aspx?id=133937.

62. Muller DWM, et al. The tendyne early feasibility trail of transcatheter mitral valve implantation. *J Am Coll Cardiol* 2016;67(13):32.

63. Caisson interventional. https://globenewswire.com/news-release/2016/09/16/872448/0/en/Caisson-Interventional-Completes-First-in-Human-Implants-of-Its-Transvascular-Mitral-Valve-Replacement.html.

44

Hypertrophic cardiomyopathy

SHIKHAR AGARWAL, SAMIR R. KAPADIA, AND E. MURAT TUZCU

INTRODUCTION

Hypertrophic cardiomyopathy (HCM) is a unique cardiovascular condition that may become symptomatic at any phase of life, from infancy to beyond 90 years of age.[1-6] The hallmark of the disease is myocardial hypertrophy that can lead to a variety of anatomic and clinical manifestations. Dynamic left ventricular outflow tract (LVOT) obstruction may or may not be present due to asymmetric hypertrophy of the basal interventricular septum. Following recent estimates suggesting that 1 in 500 individuals in the general adult population is affected by this autosomal dominant condition, HCM is to be considered one of the most common cardiac genetic disorders, and over 12 genes involved have been identified.[3,5,6] The genotypic foundation of HCM is directly related to abnormalities of the genes encoding sarcomeric proteins that regulate the contractile, regulatory, and structural functions of the myocardium. The consequent myocardial disarray and hypertrophy result in a complex pathophysiologic interplay among LVOT obstruction, diastolic dysfunction, myocardial ischemia, and mitral regurgitation. Depending on their particular phenotype, patients with HCM may have a wide spectrum of clinical and pathologic presentations ranging from exertional dyspnea, angina, palpitations, to syncope. The most fearsome and dramatic complication of HCM, sudden cardiac death, is one of the frequent causes of cardiovascular death among young people and the most common cause of mortality in competitive athletes.[7] Fortunately, HCM patients at high risk for sudden cardiac death constitute only a small proportion of the affected population (Table 44.1). Despite the widespread availability of genetic screening tests, the diagnosis of HCM remains primarily clinical and echocardiographic, based on symptoms and characteristic features, such as asymmetric septal hypertrophy, systolic anterior motion (SAM) of the mitral valve, and LVOT obstruction. Due to the relatively infrequent prevalence of patients with HCM, most cardiologists care for only a few HCM patients and may not be aware of the nuances of the contemporary management of this complex disease. This has led to an impetus for establishment of clinical programs of excellence, called "HCM Centers," which should be staffed with cardiologists, imagers, and cardiac surgeons familiar with the contemporary diagnostic and treatment options for HCM, including transthoracic echocardiography (TTE), cardiac magnetic resonance imaging (MRI), and both surgical septal myectomy and alcohol septal ablation, along with management of arrhythmias and implantation of implantable cardiac defibrillators (ICD), genetic testing, and counseling.

Given the heterogeneity of the disease process, clinical course and long-term outcomes may differ significantly in patients sharing the same mutation or even within the same family. HCM can be a dynamic disease process that can evolve with age, and the development of left ventricular hypertrophy has been observed at all ages.[8-10] Consequently, therapeutic interventions must take into consideration individual patient characteristics and preferences. Accordingly, management strategies range from medical therapy with close outpatient follow-up, to surgical or percutaneous remodeling of the myocardium. Medical therapy should be the initial therapeutic approach for the treatment of symptomatic patients with HCM. However, given the lack of randomized trials, current recommendations are based on expert opinion, clinical experience, and retrospective analyses. Beta-blocking agents, verapamil, and disopyramide (often titrated to high doses) have historically been utilized as first-line agents. In addition, limited data suggest that amiodarone may be another essential agent in HCM

704 Hypertrophic cardiomyopathy

Table 44.1 Risk factors for sudden cardiac death in hypertrophic cardiomyopathy

- Prior history of cardiac arrest
- Unexplained syncope (particularly if occurring with exertion)
- Spontaneous sustained ventricular tachycardia
- Abnormal response (particularly blood pressure) with stress testing
- Early onset of disease
- Family history of cardiac arrest or sudden cardiac death
- Nonsustained ventricular tachycardia on Holter monitoring
- Left ventricular thickness >30 mm
- Ischemia detected on perfusion testing (may be a result of microvascular circulation)
- Atrial fibrillation
- Concomitant severe aortic stenosis
- Concomitant congestive heart failure
- Other comorbidities, including pulmonary embolus and malignancy

patients, particularly in those with serious arrhythmias. Observational studies suggest that amiodarone reduces the risk of sudden cardiac death and improves survival in selected high-risk patients with nonsustained ventricular tachycardia.[11-13] Finally, a growing body of data suggest that ICD therapy is beneficial in patients who have survived sudden cardiac death (secondary prevention) or in selected individuals who are at high risk for such an event (primary prevention) (Table 44.1).[5,14-16]

Historically, the gold standard for the treatment of symptomatic HCM has been surgical septal myotomy. Evolved from the original septal myotomy first performed by Cleland[17] in the 1960s, the widely employed Morrow myectomy[18] consists of the resection of a variable amount of myocardial tissue from the septum extending from the base of the aortic valve to a region just distal to the mitral leaflets such that the LVOT is enlarged and the SAM of the mitral valve (and the resultant mitral regurgitation) is abolished.[19-21] Myectomy results in a durable reduction in outflow tract obstruction; a significant improvement in a patient's functional capacity, heart failure symptoms, and quality of life; and may offer a life expectancy similar to that of the general population.[19,22-25] The operative mortality rate for the modern day septal myectomy is approximately 1%–3% overall, but is <1% when performed in very experienced centers.[25-31]

Introduced by Sigwart in 1995, catheter-based alcohol septal ablation has become a widely utilized alternative treatment strategy to relieve outflow tract obstruction in symptomatic patients who are suboptimal surgical candidates due to comorbidities, personal preference, or who are located in areas lacking doctors with sufficient surgical expertise.[32] Given the less invasive nature and the promise of a significant reduction in recovery time, the procedure has seen a rapid adoption over the past decade and is now performed 15–20 times more frequently than surgical

myectomy, resulting in >5,000 ablations performed worldwide in total.[33,34] The septal ablation technique attempts to mimic the effect of myectomy by the infusion of 100% ethanol into either the first or second septal perforator artery supplying the septal bulge. This induces a controlled infarct in the basal portion of the hypertrophied interventricular septum, resulting in scarring, thinning, and akinesia. Under optimal conditions, the result is a reduction in the LVOT gradient as well as in the SAM of the mitral valvular apparatus.[25,32,35-40] Although long-term follow-up data and randomized trials are lacking, short-term observational studies suggest that ablation results in a significant reduction in LVOT gradient, improvement in limiting symptoms, and improved exercise tolerance, with a reported mortality equal to or less than that of surgery at 1%–4%.[3,35,37-39,41,42] Meta-analysis of 12 observational studies demonstrated similar short- and long-term mortality between patients treated using alcohol septal ablation or septal myectomy.[43] In addition, there were no significant differences in postintervention functional status as well as New York Heart Association (NYHA) functional class or ventricular arrhythmia occurrence. On the other hand, conduction abnormalities are more frequent and postintervention LVOT gradients are higher after alcohol ablation.[43] In one report, it has been suggested that alcohol septal ablation may reduce psychological distress and improve feelings of well-being at 3 months following the procedure.[44]

While randomized comparative studies are lacking, currently available data suggest that septal ablation and surgical myectomy have similar short- and mid-term success rates (Table 44.2). Postprocedurally, both modalities of septal reduction offer similar degrees of LVOT gradient reduction that appears to be durable up to 1 year after either procedure.[30,37,41,45-48] Furthermore, at 6- and 12-month follow-up, both treatment modalities were found to have similar and sustained improvements in NYHA functional class, Canadian cardiovascular angina class, and a reduction in the number of syncopal and presyncopal events.[30,41,49] However, both procedures have advantages as well as associated complications that further highlight the importance of clinical judgment during patient selection for either intervention. A retrospective analysis of 601 patients with severely symptomatic, drug refractory HCM referred to the Mayo Clinic for catheter ablation showed that alcohol septal

Table 44.2 Comparison of alcohol septal ablation and surgical myectomy

	Myectomy	Ablation
Mortality	<1–2%	1–2%
Symptoms	Decreased	Decreased
Gradient	Decreased to <10 mmHg	Decreased to <22 mmHg
Need for pacemaker	1–2%	5–10%
Sudden death risk	Low (long-term)	Low (mid-term)
Intramyocardial scar	Absent	Present

ablation offered a 4-year survival similar to that of age- and gender-matched patients who had undergone surgical myectomy, but were noted to have a complication rate that was significantly greater than that of myectomy.[50] These complications included new permanent pacemaker dependency (20.4%), cardiac tamponade (3.5%), urgent/emergent cardiac surgery (1.3%), death (1.4%), stroke (0.7%), and sustained ventricular tachycardia (0.7%). In summary, either surgical myectomy or alcohol ablation may be considered as a primary treatment modality in symptomatic patients with LVOT obstruction after careful consideration of the patient's clinical situation, anatomical characteristics, and institutional expertise. The current American College of Cardiology (ACC)/American Heart Association (AHA) guidelines recommend that septal reduction therapy should be performed in *eligible patients* with severe drug refractory symptoms and LVOT obstruction as defined by the following core criteria (all criteria must be fulfilled):[51]

- *Clinical*: Severe angina or dyspnea (NYHA class III/IV) or other symptoms like syncope or near syncope that interfere with activities of daily living or adversely affect quality of life despite adequate medical therapy
- *Hemodynamic*: Resting or provocable LVOT gradient more than 50 mmHg associated with septal hypertrophy and SAM of the mitral valve
- *Anatomic*: Targeted septal thickness sufficient to perform the procedure safely and effectively in the judgment of the individual operator

Septal reduction therapy should not be done for patients who are asymptomatic with normal exercise tolerance or whose symptoms are controlled by optimal medical therapy (class III).[51] Septal reduction therapies include septal myectomy and alcohol septal ablation. Although these are methodologically very different approaches and interventions, they have been treated similarly in ACC/AHA guidelines and

European guidelines[52] as they are both accepted methods for relief of symptoms in patients with LVOT obstruction.

ANATOMIC CONSIDERATIONS

In recognition of the fact that in current practice most patients with HCM are diagnosed noninvasively via echocardiography and many have not had invasive hemodynamic studies performed prior to presenting for ablation, most experienced operators will confirm the presence of significant LVOT obstruction by positioning an endhole catheter in the ventricular apex and recording a slow pullback under fluoroscopy. Alternatively, one may place a catheter in the ascending aorta and an endhole catheter in the in-flow portion of the left ventricle (LV) via transseptal puncture to provide simultaneous measurement of the ascending aortic and intracavitary pressures. If the operator has difficulty identifying an LVOT gradient under basal/resting conditions, provocation with either amyl nitrate or the strain phase of the Valsalva maneuver may be attempted.[53] Induction of a premature ventricular contraction with the pigtail catheter may also aid in the diagnosis, as it commonly results in the Brockenbrough–Braunwald phenomenon, which refers to diminished aortic pulse pressure and increased LVOT gradient secondary to a transient increase in obstruction (Figure 44.1). This maneuver can also be useful during the procedure, as it may isolate the appropriate septal perforator branch to intervene upon.[54] Balloon occlusion of the septal perforator followed by induction of the premature ventricular contraction might help demonstrate if the chosen septal perforator is the appropriate vessel to ablate during alcohol septal ablation. The left ventriculogram may have a variety of findings, including systolic cavity obliteration, varying degrees of mitral regurgitation, and occasionally, the hypertrophied septum prolapsing into the LVOT.

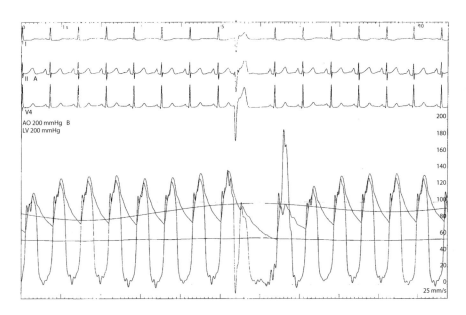

Figure 44.1 Brockenbrough–Braunwald phenomenon.

Standard diagnostic coronary angiography is performed as a first step to define coronary anatomy, identify the location and size of the septal perforator branches, and evaluate for the presence of concomitant coronary artery disease. Sometimes septal perforator branches originating from the left anterior descending (LAD) artery may be compressed during systole ("milking") due to contraction of the surrounding hypertrophied myocardium.[55] Similarly, systolic compression of the LAD artery resulting in a "sawfish" appearance has also been described.[56] In addition to evaluating for the presence of coronary artery disease, a critical component of the diagnostic angiogram is selection of the appropriate septal perforator branch through which the ablation will be performed (Figure 44.2).

The right anterior oblique (RAO) or posteroanterior (PA) cranial views usually provide the best view of the septal branches as they travel through the basal interventricular septum. There can often be substantial variation in the anatomy of the branches supplying the septum such that one subdivision runs along the left side of the septum while another runs along the right. The operator may gain a better understanding of this variation (i.e., on the right or left side) utilizing the left anterior oblique (LAO) cranial projection. To reduce the likelihood of inducing complete heart block during ethanol infusion, selection of the left-sided subdivision whenever possible is optimal for the ablation. This can be accomplished in the LAO view by avoiding the subdivision of the septal branch supplying the right side of the septum.

During angiographic assessment of the septal anatomy, a number of important factors must be considered with regard to proper vessel selection. It is critical that the operator pay close attention to vessel size, angulation, and the distribution of myocardial territories served by the given vessel. By virtue of the fact that larger vessels generally provide blood supply to a larger segment of myocardium, selection of septal branches with a diameter >2 mm may result in a large infarct; this should be taken into consideration when making the decision. Another often underappreciated consideration in vessel selection relates to the degree of angulation of the septal vessel with regard to its parent vessel.

The interventionalist should consider that septal vessels with a high degree of angulation and tortuosity might be a difficult target for the delivery of the angioplasty balloon since the coronary wire may often prolapse back into the LAD coronary artery (Figure 44.2).[53]

Substantial anatomic variation exists with regard to the vessel of origin as well as the distribution of blood flow supplied by the septal perforators in patients with HCM. Most commonly, septal perforator branches originate from the proximal LAD, although they may arise from virtually every major branch of the coronary tree, including the left main trunk, left circumflex coronary artery, ramus intermedius, diagonal branches, and, rarely, from branches of the right coronary artery.[53]

Previous work has demonstrated that the first septal perforator artery frequently provides blood flow to a substantially larger region of myocardium than might be expected. In addition, septal branches can exhibit marked variability in their course and provide blood flow to various regions of the myocardium—including the right ventricle (RV). Furthermore, cases in which both the first and second septal arteries provide blood supply to the basal septum have been described.[53,57] As a result, it is imperative that the operator have a thorough understanding of the distribution of blood flow supplied by the selected septal branch. This is imperative in order to target the correct area for ablation while avoiding infarction of an unanticipated region or damage of an oversized myocardial segment. To better delineate the area of myocardium subtended by the selected septal vessel prior to ethanol infusion, most operators will choose to perform a selective injection of echo-contrast during TTE imaging. Intracardiac echocardiography (ICE) may be utilized during this procedure to better visualize the hypertrophied septum and the course of the injected contrast material in selected patients (Figure 44.3).[58]

It is important to thoroughly evaluate for anatomical abnormalities that would require surgical management prior to proceeding with a catheter-based intervention. Such abnormalities include anomalous papillary muscle insertion into the mitral valve, anatomically abnormal mitral valve with a long anterior/posterior leaflet, coexistent coronary

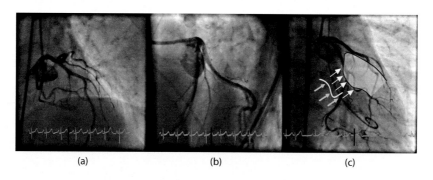

(a)　　　　　(b)　　　　　(c)

Figure 44.2 Diagnostic angiogram depicting the relationship of the first septal perforator to the plane of the aortic valve (*beneath*) and to the left ventricular cavity (**a** and **b**). (**c**) Simultaneous injection through both the guide and pigtail catheters, demonstrating the location of the interventricular septum (white arrows and shaded segment) in relation to the left ventricular cavity. The anterior leaflet of the mitral valve is outlined in the white line and green arrows.

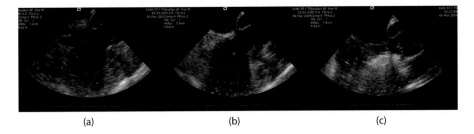

(a) (b) (c)

Figure 44.3 Intracardiac echocardiogram demonstrating the hypertrophied interventricular septum prior to **(a)** and after ethanol infusion **(b and c)**. Note the increased echogenicity of the basal septum following injection.

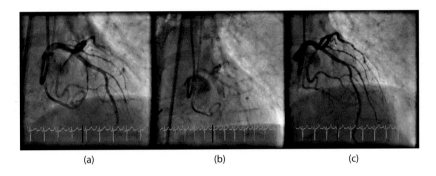

(a) (b) (c)

Figure 44.4 Angiogram depicting **(a)** the course of the left anterior descending artery and a septal perforator appropriate for ablation of basal-most portion of the septum. **(b)** A 0.014-in extra support coronary wire in the selected septal vessel with subsequent inflation of an over-the-wire–style angioplasty balloon prior to infusion of ethanol. **(c)** Angiogram documenting the integrity of the left anterior descending coronary artery and total occlusion of the recently injected septal branch.

artery disease, primary valvular disease (aortic or mitral), or subaortic membrane or pannus—none of which can be adequately addressed by septal ablation (Figure 44.4).[5,53] Furthermore, a subset of patients may be found to have an abnormal elongation and myomatous degeneration of the anterior mitral leaflet, resulting in an anterior displacement of the line of coaptation with resultant outflow tract obstruction. These gene-positive HCM patients have dynamic LVOT obstruction from papillary muscle orientation independent of septal hypertrophy.[59,60] These patients will require surgical consultation for consideration of myectomy with mitral valve plication and should not be considered for catheter-based therapy.[61] In addition, results of alcohol ablation in patients with severe hypertrophy (i.e., >3 cm) are inconsistent, and these patients are frequently referred for surgical correction.

PROCEDURAL TECHNIQUE AND EQUIPMENT

Placement of a prophylactic temporary transvenous pacemaker prior to beginning the procedure is an essential initial step, given the high incidence of complete heart block during, or in the days following, ablation. To reduce the possibility of dislodgment during the procedure or in patient transport, some operators place a screw-in–type pacing lead (rather than the blunt-tip models) into the right ventricular apex via the right internal jugular vein under fluoroscopy.

After placing the transvenous pacemaker, arterial access is obtained using a 6- or 7-Fr short sheath by either femoral or radial approach, and intravenous (IV) unfractionated heparin (UFH) is administered with a target activated clotting time (ACT) of 250–300 seconds to prevent development of thrombus in the guiding catheters or on the wires.

A guiding catheter capable of providing sufficient support, such as the 6- or 7-Fr XB/EBU catheter, is usually selected and used to engage the left main coronary artery (Table 44.3). A 0.014-in extra-support wire with a soft tip is subsequently advanced into the preselected septal perforator branch (Figure 44.4). The wire is usually preloaded in an over-the-wire (OTW) angioplasty balloon, usually a 1.5–2 mm × 8–12 mm, which is advanced over the guidewire into the proximal aspect of the septal vessel. Given that septal vessels often have an acute angle at their origin from the LAD, the operator may occasionally encounter difficulty in advancing the balloon to the target. In these situations, the coronary wire may be exchanged for a stiffer one over a microcatheter in order to provide the necessary support for balloon placement.[53] It is critical for the operator to ensure that the balloon is situated deeply enough (~5 mm) into the septal vessel to prevent the infused ethanol from accidentally refluxing into the LAD. The balloon should not be placed too distally in order to avoid the ethanol infusion, missing the basal-most portion of the septum and resulting in a suboptimal gradient reduction.

Table 44.3 Equipment for alcohol septal ablation

Equipment	Specific type	Comments
Guide	7-Fr XB/EBU, JL4, Amplatz	Provide better support
Catheter wire	0.014-in extrasupport wire with a soft tip	Standard interventional wire, though may require stiffer wire due to acute angulation of many septa
	1.5–2 mm × 8–12 mm	
Echocontrast	1–2 cc with balloon inflated	Check placement and for reflux into left anterior descending artery proper. Diluted 1:5 or 1:10
Alcohol	1–3 cc desiccated ethanol	Smaller volumes equally efficacious

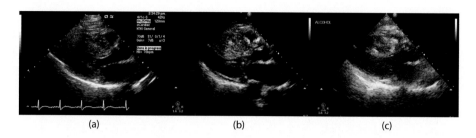

(a)   (b)   (c)

Figure 44.5 Transthoracic echocardiogram (parasternal long axis) demonstrating the grossly hypertrophied basal interventricular septum of a patient affected by hypertrophic cardiomyopathy prior to contrast injection (a). Note the increased echogenicity of the basal septum following infusion of contrast (b) and the echolucency immediately after ethanol infusion (c).

Prior to proceeding further, it is critical to assess the amount and location of myocardium supplied by the selected septal vessel. This is typically accomplished through the use of both echocardiographic and angiographic techniques. Following optimal placement, the balloon is inflated to approximately 10–12 atmospheres (atm) to occlude the septal vessel, and 1–2 cc of contrast are slowly injected through the distal end of the balloon to assess the full extent of myocardium supplied. While slowly infusing the contrast material to simulate the forthcoming ethanol injection, it is imperative for the operator to confirm that the balloon occlusion is sufficient to prevent any of the infused contrast from refluxing backward into the LAD. If even a very small amount of alcohol leaks into the major epicardial vessels, diffuse myocardial necrosis may result in severe LV dysfunction and death.

Contrast echocardiography, utilizing a transthoracic approach during contrast injection as just described, is the second commonly employed method of verifying the myocardial distribution supplied by the septal vessel. Following a complete examination of the morphology of the interventricular septum, most commonly in the parasternal short axis and apical three- and four-chamber views, 1–2 cc of echocardiographic contrast material is infused through the balloon into the septal branch through a tuberculin-type syringe. We find that many of the currently available contrast agents are too concentrated, and their infusion may result in echocardiographic "shadowing" from the opacified ventricles. To avoid this problem, the protocol in our laboratory is to open the contrast vials 10–15 minutes prior to the time of expected use and to further dilute the agent with a

sterile saline solution in a 1:5 or 1:10 mixture at the time of injection. It is also our standard practice to utilize pulsed-wave Doppler when employing the newly diluted contrast so as to avoid destruction of the microbubbles with the higher-frequency, continuous wave ultrasound. Given that the basal portion of septum is responsible for the greatest extent of septal to mitral contact and therefore the LVOT obstruction, the optimal septal vessel will deliver contrast material filling to this region alone (Figure 44.5).

Given the extensive variability of the septal anatomy, the operator should verify that the chosen vessel primarily supplies the proximal interventricular septum and does not provide blood flow to portions of the inferior wall (as in the presence of an occlusion of the right coronary artery), left ventricular papillary musculature, or the right ventricular free wall.[49] Should it be noted that the selected septal vessel provides flow to the distal septum or other regions of myocardium, ethanol infusion is contraindicated as proceeding could result in infarction of an undesired territory or of unanticipated size. Given that it has been demonstrated that a rapid reduction in gradient can be observed with balloon occlusion of a septal perforator branch in many but not all patients, documenting a reduction in LVOT gradient (generally >30%) during balloon inflation is another method to verify that the correct septal distribution has been targeted for ablation (Figure 44.5).[53] In addition, it is also important to check if there was any increase in the degree of mitral regurgitation during this maneuver.

At this point, confirmation of balloon placement and appropriate function of the temporary pacemaker must again be verified. The balloon can migrate during the above process, so another 1–2 cc contrast injection under fluoroscopy will ensure proper placement. Ethanol injection into the selected septal perforator may now be performed. In most cases, 1–3 cc of desiccated ethanol is sufficient—although the necessary volume can vary on the basis of the patient's septal anatomy and the behavior of contrast during the test infusion as performed earlier (Table 44.3).[35,37,45,53,62] If rapid washout of the contrast was observed due to collateral flow, standard practice is to reduce the volume and rate of ethanol injection to ensure that other areas of myocardium are not inadvertently damaged via these branches.[53,63] Accordingly, it should be the goal of the operator to use as little ethanol as possible during the procedure to avoid excessive or unintended myocardial necrosis. Importantly, it has been demonstrated that smaller volumes of ethanol are equally effective with regard to mid-term gradient reduction while significantly reducing the rate of complications.[64] Furthermore, the volume of alcohol used in the procedure has also been shown to be an independent predictor of survival—the lower, the better—in a single center study over 10 years of follow-up.[65]

With the balloon still inflated, the ethanol is injected into the septal branch over a period of 1–5 minutes. It is important that, prior to balloon deflation, the operator adequately flush the catheter with normal saline following ethanol infusion to ensure complete delivery of the agent and to prevent reflux at the time of balloon deflation. To provide maximal contact between ethanol and myocardium, many operators will continue balloon inflation for up to 5–10 additional minutes. This maneuver also helps to ensure that no reflux of ethanol into the LAD following balloon deflation will occur. During ethanol infusion, the resting LVOT gradient should be continuously monitored to gauge the relative success of the procedure. A successful procedure is generally regarded as one in which the resting LVOT gradient is reduced from >50 mmHg to <30 mmHg, or in which the provocable gradient is reduced by >50%.[37,53]

The balloon catheter is then removed. Some operators place the guidewire into the septal perforator before removing the balloon catheter in order to maintain access to the coronary artery in case of the need for re-instrumentation. A cine-angiogram should then be performed to document the integrity of the left main trunk and LAD. Although total occlusion of the recently injected septal branch is most commonly observed and some phasic flow may persist immediately following ablation (Figure 44.4).

Prior studies have demonstrated that patients with HCM have a reduction in coronary flow reserve—either due to a reversible adaptive response to systolic contraction overloading or from a chronic remodeling process of the coronary microcirculation. However, recent work suggests there is an immediate improvement in coronary flow reserve following alcohol septal ablation, suggesting that the dynamic response to the pressure overload from the LVOT obstruction is a critical component of this pathophysiology.[66]

Given the potential for serious intra- and periprocedural complications, observation of the patient in a coronary intensive care or intermediate care unit that is experienced with the nuances of the postprocedural care of such patients is advisable for 24–48 hours. Serum levels of creatinine phosphokinase (CPK) often reach levels between 800 and 1,200 U/L following ethanol injection, though variation in the observed value is dependent on the caliber of the injected vessel and volume of ethanol applied.[4,34,35,45,64] If telemetry monitoring reveals no episodes of heart block or progressive prolongation of PR interval, or bradyarrhythmias after 24–48 hours, the temporary pacemaker can safely be removed. Development of complete heart block in patients with no underlying conduction abnormalities is infrequent, but if it does occur, the presence of a temporary pacemaker is lifesaving. In most experienced centers, the patient is then generally observed on a regular nursing floor an additional 48–72 hours prior to discharge. Patients who had a transient episode of high-grade atrioventricular (AV) block during or after the procedure should be watched carefully.

Follow-up of patients after the procedure remains important, with attention to recurrence of symptoms and arrhythmias. When sustained ventricular arrhythmias are present, implantation of an ICD should be considered. Regular assessment of functional capacity with exercise testing is warranted. For patients in whom symptoms recur and another septal perforator branch is identified as a potential target, a repeat ethanol injection can be performed. Prior studies have shown this to be necessary in 5%–10% of cases. In the absence of a second target, patients are still eligible for surgical myectomy.[48] These patients carry a higher incidence of postoperative heart block following myectomy compared with those treated with myectomy only.[67] The reason is that, as mentioned, following alcohol ablation, patients frequently have also right bundle branch block, while isolated left bundle branch block is common after myectomy.

INDICATIONS

A number of patients will continue to experience lifestyle-modifying symptoms despite optimal medical therapy. A small but definite percentage of these patients (~5%–10%) may be candidates for either surgical myectomy or septal alcohol ablation. As it has been stressed previously, it is of critical importance that a careful screening process be in place to identify which patients are appropriate for a septal-modifying procedure and which type of procedure is best suited to the individual patient. Furthermore, it should be underscored that any form of septal modification is not a curative, but rather a symptom-reducing intervention. The clinical circumstances in which a surgical septal-modifying procedure may be considered have been outlined in the updated ACC/European Society of Cardiology (ESC) consensus statement and includes patients with severe septal hypertrophy (i.e., >18 mm), resting/basal or inducible LVOT obstruction with gradient >50 mmHg, and severely limiting heart failure symptoms (i.e., NYHA functional class III–IV) *despite* optimal medical therapy (Table 44.4).[4,23,25,27,53,68,69] Therefore, patients meeting these objective criteria may be considered for alcohol

Table 44.4 Selection criteria for alcohol septal ablation

- New York Heart Association heart failure symptoms (Classes III and IV) despite maximal medical therapy
- Left ventricular outflow tract gradient >30 mmHg at rest or >50 mmHg with provocation
- Absence of mitral valve or papillary muscle abnormalities
- Septal thickness >16–18 mm
- Compatible anatomy of septal branches
- Absence of significant coronary artery disease

Table 44.5 Conditions in which surgical correction of hypertrophic cardiomyopathy should be considered

- Coexistent coronary artery disease not amenable to percutaneous intervention
- Primary valvular disease (aortic or mitral)
- Anomalous papillary muscle insertion into the mitral valve
- Anatomically abnormal mitral valve with a long anterior/posterior leaflet
- Subaortic membrane or pannus
- Abnormal elongation and myomatous degeneration of the anterior mitral leaflet (resulting in an anterior displacement of the line of coaptation with resultant outflow tract obstruction)
- Patients with severe hypertrophy (i.e., >3.0 cm)

septal ablation if they are compliant with optimal medical therapy–and ineligible for surgical myectomy–but continue to experience significant functional limitation due to symptoms of chest pain, exertional dyspnea, or recurrent syncope.

CLINICAL ASPECTS

It is of critical importance that the clinicians thoroughly evaluate the patient for anatomical abnormalities that would require surgical management prior to proceeding with a catheter-based intervention. These abnormalities would include anomalous papillary muscle insertion into the mitral valve, anatomically abnormal mitral valve with a long anterior/posterior leaflet, coexistent coronary artery disease, primary valvular disease (aortic or mitral), or subaortic membrane or pannus—none of which can be adequately addressed with septal ablation.[4,53] In addition, outflow tract obstruction resulting from abnormal elongation and/or myomatous degeneration of the anterior mitral leaflet is a rare but important discovery that would not be readily amenable to a percutaneous solution. Therefore, these patients will require surgical consultation for consideration of myectomy with mitral valve plication and should not be considered for catheter-based therapy (Table 44.5).[61]

A thorough patient history, including a detailed assessment of functional status, is essential for appropriate patient selection. Regardless of the magnitude of the resting or dynamic LVOT gradient, it is inadvisable to perform either surgical or percutaneous septal modification in patients without significant symptoms (or symptoms that are easily controlled with medications), given the short-term risks inherent to these procedures and the paucity of data suggesting that the long-term outcome of untreated patients is *worse* than those undergoing the procedure. Therefore, given that both forms of septal reduction can have potentially serious complications, the risk of either form of procedure may well outweigh any possible benefit in a minimally symptomatic patient. In addition, it should be stressed that these procedures should be performed at experienced centers as there is a significant learning curve that impacts the odds of a successful outcome and the amelioration of symptoms.[70]

LIMITATIONS

Complications following ethanol septal ablation are infrequent and comparable to those following myectomy.

Although a left bundle branch block is often observed following septal myectomy (~47%),[71] a right bundle branch block (albeit transient) is observed in up to 80% of patients following septal ablation.[4,36,37,53] The incidence of complete heart block exists and ranges widely across the literature (anywhere from 5% to 40%), with an average value of 12%–15% at high-volume centers.[4,30,37,39,53,72] High-degree AV block requiring permanent pacemaker implantation following the procedure has been correlated with preexisting left bundle branch block and rapid injection of ethanol during the procedure.[72] As discussed previously, special care must be taken to ensure no ethanol spills into the LAD. When this occurs, it is a catastrophic event, often resulting in a large mid- to distal anterior wall myocardial infarction, with an associated increase in mortality. Rare cases of coronary dissection related to the use of an extra-support guidewire or guide catheter trauma have been reported in the literature. Cardiac tamponade is another rare complication, most commonly the result of perforation through the right ventricular apex during temporary pacemaker insertion. Another infrequent complication following the ablation is ventricular septal rupture, which can occur when an excess of ethanol is injected, resulting in an extensive area of infarction.[53] Ventricular arrhythmias following the procedure are rare in the first 48 hours and can usually be managed conservatively while on telemetry observation. It has been speculated that the intramyocardial scar that forms following septal ablation may predispose patients to late ventricular arrhythmias. However, this has so far not been convincingly demonstrated in the literature.[4,37,62,73] A recent prospective study on 123 patients has demonstrated a reduced number of ICD discharges in patients with HCM following alcohol septal ablation, arguing against the assumption that the procedure is proarrhythmic.[74]

SPECIAL ISSUES/CONSIDERATIONS

As with any specialized procedure, local expertise must be considered when deciding between surgical myectomy and alcohol septal ablation. To treat this condition successfully, the interventionalist should not only be technically skilled but also ensure appropriate clinical follow-up and management postprocedure. Each patient is unique, and his or her individual anatomy, symptoms, and risk of surgery will impact the decision to perform alcohol septal ablation versus surgical myectomy.

Although not a must for diagnosis, advances in cardiac MRI have improved diagnosis of the condition and give valuable information regarding location of papillary muscle insertion. Local expertise in this field is therefore also important. Given the risk of high-degree AV block and the potential need for permanent pacemaker implantation, centers with adequate electrophysiology support are also preferable. Recall that right bundle branch block is more common with alcohol septal ablation, which differs from surgical myectomy, in which left bundle branch block is more common. When surgical myectomy must be performed following failed alcohol septal ablation, the risk of requiring a permanent pacemaker increases further.

CONCLUSIONS

HCM is a unique cardiovascular condition associated with many different genetic mutations that result in a variety of phenotypes and variable clinical presentations at any age. Present in a minority of this patient population, outflow tract obstruction may vary significantly depending on physiological loading conditions, adrenergic state, and specific medications. Despite rapid advances in genetic screening, imaging modalities such as echocardiography and MRI remain the primary methods of diagnosis. Given the substantial variation in this population of patients, therapeutic interventions must take into consideration individual patient characteristics and preferences. Accordingly, management strategies range from medical therapy with close outpatient follow-up to surgical or percutaneous remodeling of the myocardium. While the initial intervention for symptomatic patients should be medical therapy, patients at high risk for sudden cardiac death should be considered for ICD therapy. In the setting of symptoms refractory to optimal medical management, surgical myectomy continues to be the gold standard therapy for HCM in appropriately risk-stratified patients in areas where an experienced team and facility are available. Alcohol septal ablation provides an excellent alternative treatment modality when performed in appropriately selected patients in an experienced center.

ACKNOWLEDGMENTS

The authors would like to acknowledge Casey Becker and Gus Theodos for previous versions of this chapter.

REFERENCES

1. Braunwald E, et al. Idiopathic Hypertrophic Subaortic Stenosis. I. A description of the disease based upon an analysis of 64 patients. *Circulation* 1964;30(suppl 4):3–119.

2. Cecchi F, et al. Hypertrophic cardiomyopathy in Tuscany: Clinical course and outcome in an unselected regional population. *J Am Coll Cardiol* 1995;26(6):1529–1536.

3. Maron BJ. Hypertrophic cardiomyopathy: A systematic review. *JAMA* 2002;287(10):1308–1320.

4. Maron BJ, et al. American College of Cardiology/European Society of Cardiology clinical expert consensus document on hypertrophic cardiomyopathy. A report of the American College of Cardiology Foundation Task Force on Clinical Expert Consensus Documents and the European Society of Cardiology Committee for Practice Guidelines. *J Am Coll Cardiol* 2003;42(9):1687–1713.

5. Maron BJ, et al. Hypertrophic cardiomyopathy. *JAMA* 1999;282(24):2302–2303.

6. Spirito P, et al. Clinical course and prognosis of hypertrophic cardiomyopathy in an outpatient population. *N Engl J Med* 1989;320(12):749–755.

7. Maron BJ, et al. Sudden death in young competitive athletes. Clinical, demographic, and pathological profiles. *JAMA* 1996;276(3):199–204.

8. Lewis JF, Maron BJ. Clinical and morphologic expression of hypertrophic cardiomyopathy in patients > or = 65 years of age. *Am J Cardiol* 1994;73(15):1105–1111.

9. Olivotto I, et al. Gender-related differences in the clinical presentation and outcome of hypertrophic cardiomyopathy. *J Am Coll Cardiol* 2005;46(3):480–487.

10. Spirito P, Maron BJ. Absence of progression of left ventricular hypertrophy in adult patients with hypertrophic cardiomyopathy. *J Am Coll Cardiol* 1987;9(5):1013–1017.

11. McKenna WJ. Does treatment influence the natural history of patients with hypertrophic cardiomyopathy? *Drugs* 1985;29(suppl 3):53–56.

12. McKenna WJ, Kleinebenne A. [Arrhythmias in hypertrophic cardiomyopathy. Significance and therapeutic consequences]. *Herz* 1985;10(2):91–101.

13. McKenna WJ, et al. Improved survival with amiodarone in patients with hypertrophic cardiomyopathy and ventricular tachycardia. *Br Heart J* 1985;53(4):412–416.

14. Boriani G, et al. Prevention of sudden death in hypertrophic cardiomyopathy: But which defibrillator for which patient? *Circulation* 2004;110(15):e438–e442.

15. Epstein AE, et al. ACC/AHA/HRS 2008 Guidelines for Device-Based Therapy of Cardiac Rhythm Abnormalities: A report of the American College of Cardiology/American Heart Association Task Force on Practice Guidelines (Writing Committee to Revise the ACC/AHA/NASPE 2002 Guideline Update for Implantation of Cardiac Pacemakers and Antiarrhythmia Devices) developed in collaboration with the American Association for Thoracic Surgery and Society of Thoracic Surgeons. *J Am Coll Cardiol* 2008;51(21):e1–e62.

16. Maron BJ, et al. Implantable cardioverter-defibrillators and prevention of sudden cardiac death in hypertrophic cardiomyopathy. *JAMA* 2007;298(4):405–412.

17. Cleland WP. The surgical management of obstructive cardiomyopathy. *J Cardiovasc Surg (Torino)* 1963;4:489–491.

18. Morrow AG. Hypertrophic subaortic stenosis. Operative methods utilized to relieve left ventricular outflow obstruction. *J Thorac Cardiovasc Surg* 1978;76(4):423–430.

19. Maron BJ, et al. The case for surgery in obstructive hypertrophic cardiomyopathy. *J Am Coll Cardiol* 2004;44(10):2044–2053.

20. Maron BJ, et al. Systolic anterior motion of the posterior mitral leaflet: A previously unrecognized cause of dynamic subaortic obstruction in patients with hypertrophic cardiomyopathy. *Circulation* 1983;68(2):282–293.

21. Spirito P, Maron BJ. Significance of left ventricular outflow tract cross-sectional area in hypertrophic cardiomyopathy: A two-dimensional echocardiographic assessment. *Circulation* 1983;67(5):1100–1108.

22. Krajcer Z, et al. Mitral valve replacement and septal myomectomy in hypertrophic cardiomyopathy. Ten-year follow-up in 80 patients. *Circulation* 1988;78(3 Pt 2):I35–I43.

23. Maron BJ, et al. Long-term clinical course and symptomatic status of patients after operation for hypertrophic subaortic stenosis. *Circulation* 1978;57(6):1205–1213.

24. Ommen SR. The effect of surgical myectomy on survival of patients with hypertrophic cardiomyopathy. *J Am Coll Cardiol* 2004;43(suppl A):215A.

25. Spirito P, et al. The management of hypertrophic cardiomyopathy. *N Engl J Med* 1997;336(11):775–785.

26. Heric B, et al. Surgical management of hypertrophic obstructive cardiomyopathy. Early and late results. *J Thorac Cardiovasc Surg* 1995;110(1):195–206; discussion 206–208.

27. McCully RB, et al. Extent of clinical improvement after surgical treatment of hypertrophic obstructive cardiomyopathy. *Circulation* 1996;94(3):467–471.

28. Merrill WH, et al. Long-lasting improvement after septal myectomy for hypertrophic obstructive cardiomyopathy. *Ann Thorac Surg* 2000;69(6):1732–1735; discussion 1735–1736.

29. Mohr R, et al. The outcome of surgical treatment of hypertrophic obstructive cardiomyopathy. Experience over 15 years. *J Thorac Cardiovasc Surg* 1989;97(5):666–674.

30. Qin JX, et al. Outcome of patients with hypertrophic obstructive cardiomyopathy after percutaneous transluminal septal myocardial ablation and septal myectomy surgery. *J Am Coll Cardiol* 2001;38(7):1994–2000.

31. Schulte HD, et al. Management of symptomatic hypertrophic obstructive cardiomyopathy—Long-term results after surgical therapy. *Thorac Cardiovasc Surg* 1999;47(4):213–218.

32. Sigwart U. Non-surgical myocardial reduction for hypertrophic obstructive cardiomyopathy. *Lancet* 1995;346(8969):211–214.

33. Maron BJ. Role of alcohol septal ablation in treatment of obstructive hypertrophic cardiomyopathy. *Lancet* 2000;355(9202):425–426.

34. Roberts R, Sigwart U. Current concepts of the pathogenesis and treatment of hypertrophic cardiomyopathy. *Circulation* 2005;112(2):293–296.

35. Faber L, et al. Percutaneous transluminal septal myocardial ablation for hypertrophic obstructive cardiomyopathy: Long term follow up of the first series of 25 patients. *Heart* 2000;83(3):326–331.

36. Flores-Ramirez R, et al. Echocardiographic insights into the mechanisms of relief of left ventricular outflow tract obstruction after nonsurgical septal reduction therapy in patients with hypertrophic obstructive cardiomyopathy. *J Am Coll Cardiol* 2001;37(1):208–214.

37. Gietzen FH, et al. Acute and long-term results after transcoronary ablation of septal hypertrophy (TASH). Catheter interventional treatment for hypertrophic obstructive cardiomyopathy. *Eur Heart J* 1999;20(18):1342–1354.

38. Knight C, et al. Nonsurgical septal reduction for hypertrophic obstructive cardiomyopathy: Outcome in the first series of patients. *Circulation* 1997;95(8):2075–2081.

39. Lakkis NM, et al. Nonsurgical septal reduction therapy for hypertrophic obstructive cardiomyopathy: One-year follow-up. *J Am Coll Cardiol* 2000;36(3):852–855.

40. Lakkis NM, et al. Echocardiography-guided ethanol septal reduction for hypertrophic obstructive cardiomyopathy. *Circulation* 1998;98(17):1750–1755.

41. Firoozi S, et al. Septal myotomy-myectomy and transcoronary septal alcohol ablation in hypertrophic obstructive cardiomyopathy. A comparison of clinical, haemodynamic and exercise outcomes. *Eur Heart J* 2002;23(20):1617–1624.

42. Ruzyllo W, et al. Left ventricular outflow tract gradient decrease with non-surgical myocardial reduction improves exercise capacity in patients with hypertrophic obstructive cardiomyopathy. *Eur Heart J* 2000;21(9):770–777.

43. Agarwal S, et al. Updated meta analysis of septal alcohol ablation versus myectomy for hypertrophic cardiomyopathy. *J Am Coll Cardiol* 2010;55(8):823–834.

44. Serber ER, et al. Depression, anxiety, and quality of life in patients with obstructive hypertrophic cardiomyopathy three months after alcohol septal ablation. *Am J Cardiol* 2007;100(10):1592–1597.

45. Boekstegers P, et al. Pressure-guided nonsurgical myocardial reduction induced by small septal infarctions in hypertrophic obstructive cardiomyopathy. *J Am Coll Cardiol* 2001;38(3):846–853.

46. van Dockum WG, et al. Early onset and progression of left ventricular remodeling after alcohol septal ablation in hypertrophic obstructive cardiomyopathy. *Circulation* 2005;111(19):2503–2508.

47. Nagueh SF, et al. Comparison of ethanol septal reduction therapy with surgical myectomy for the treatment of hypertrophic obstructive cardiomyopathy. *J Am Coll Cardiol* 2001;38(6):1701–1706.

48. Ralph-Edwards A, et al. Hypertrophic obstructive cardiomyopathy: Comparison of outcomes after myectomy or alcohol ablation adjusted by propensity score. *J Thorac Cardiovasc Surg* 2005;129(2):351–358.

49. Nagueh SF, et al. Role of myocardial contrast echocardiography during nonsurgical septal reduction therapy for hypertrophic obstructive cardiomyopathy. *J Am Coll Cardiol* 1998;32(1):225–229.

50. Sorajja P, et al. Outcome of alcohol septal ablation for obstructive hypertrophic cardiomyopathy. *Circulation* 2008;118(2):131–139.

51. Gersh BJ, et al. American College of Cardiology Foundation/American Heart Association Task Force on Practice Guidelines. 2011 ACCF/AHA Guideline for the Diagnosis and Treatment of Hypertrophic Cardiomyopathy: A report of the American College of Cardiology Foundation/American Heart Association Task Force on Practice Guidelines. Developed in collaboration with the American Association for Thoracic Surgery, American Society of Echocardiography, American Society of Nuclear Cardiology, Heart Failure Society of America, Heart Rhythm Society, Society for Cardiovascular Angiography and Interventions, and Society of Thoracic Surgeons. *J Am Coll Cardiol* 2011;58(25):e212–e260.

52. Maron BJ, et al. American College of Cardiology Foundation Task Force on Clinical Expert Consensus Documents; European Society of Cardiology Committee for Practice Guidelines. American College of Cardiology/European Society of Cardiology Clinical Expert Consensus Document on Hypertrophic Cardiomyopathy. A report of the American College of Cardiology Foundation Task Force on Clinical Expert Consensus Documents and the European Society of Cardiology Committee for Practice Guidelines. *Eur Heart J* 2003;24(21):1965–1991.

53. Holmes DR Jr, et al. Alcohol septal ablation for hypertrophic cardiomyopathy: Indications and technique. *Catheter Cardiovasc Interv* 2005;66(3):375–389.

54. Soon CY, Buergler JM. Alcohol septal ablation and the Brockenbrough-Braunwald phenomenon. *Catheter Cardiovasc Interv* 2008;72(7):1016–1024.

55. Pichard AD, et al. Septal perforator compression (narrowing) in idiopathic hypertrophic subaortic stenosis. *Am J Cardiol* 1977;40(3):310–314.

56. Brugada P, et al. "Sawfish" systolic narrowing of the left anterior descending coronary artery: An angiographic sign of hypertrophic cardiomyopathy. *Circulation* 1982;66(4):800–803.

57. Singh M, et al. Anatomy of the first septal perforating artery: A study with implications for ablation therapy for hypertrophic cardiomyopathy. *Mayo Clin Proc* 2001;76(8):799–802.

58. Alfonso F, et al. Intracardiac echocardiography guidance for alcohol septal ablation in hypertrophic obstructive cardiomyopathy. *J Invasive Cardiol* 2007;19(5):E134–E136.

59. Austin BA, et al. Abnormally thickened papillary muscle resulting in dynamic left ventricular outflow tract obstruction: An unusual presentation of hypertrophic cardiomyopathy. *J Am Soc Echocardiogr* 2009;22(1):105.e5–e6.

60. Kwon DH, et al. Abnormal papillary muscle morphology is independently associated with increased left ventricular outflow tract obstruction in hypertrophic cardiomyopathy. *Heart* 2008;94(10):1295–1301.

61. Klues HG, et al. Diversity of structural mitral valve alterations in hypertrophic cardiomyopathy. *Circulation* 1992;85(5):1651–1660.

62. Kuhn H, et al. Transcoronary ablation of septal hypertrophy (TASH): A new treatment option for hypertrophic obstructive cardiomyopathy. *Z Kardiol* 2000;89(suppl 4):IV41–IV54.

63. Faber L, et al. Percutaneous transluminal septal myocardial ablation in hypertrophic obstructive cardiomyopathy: Results with respect to intraprocedural myocardial contrast echocardiography. *Circulation* 1998;98(22):2415–2421.

64. Veselka J, et al. Effects of varying ethanol dosing in percutaneous septal ablation for obstructive hypertrophic cardiomyopathy on early hemodynamic changes. *Am J Cardiol* 2005;95(5):675–678.

65. Kuhn H, et al. Survival after transcoronary ablation of septal hypertrophy in hypertrophic obstructive cardiomyopathy (TASH): A 10-year experience. *Clin Res Cardiol* 2008;97(4):234–243.

66. Jaber WA, et al. Immediate improvement in coronary flow reserve after alcohol septal ablation in patients with hypertrophic obstructive cardiomyopathy. *Heart* 2009;95(7):564–569.

67. Nagueh SF, et al. Outcome of surgical myectomy after unsuccessful alcohol septal ablation for the treatment of patients with hypertrophic obstructive cardiomyopathy. *J Am Coll Cardiol* 2007;50(8):795–798.

68. Maron MS, et al. Effect of left ventricular outflow tract obstruction on clinical outcome in hypertrophic cardiomyopathy. *N Engl J Med* 2003;348(4):295–303.

69. Robbins RC, Stinson EB. Long-term results of left ventricular myotomy and myectomy for obstructive hypertrophic cardiomyopathy. *J Thorac Cardiovasc Surg* 1996;111(3):586–594.

70. van der Lee C, et al. Usefulness of clinical, echocardiographic, and procedural characteristics to predict outcome after percutaneous transluminal septal myocardial ablation. *Am J Cardiol* 2008;101(9):1315–1320.

71. Wang S, et al. A retrospective clinical study of transaortic extended septal myectomy for obstructive hypertrophic cardiomyopathy in China. *Eur J Cardiothoracic Surg* 2013;43:534–540.

72. Chang SM, et al. Complete heart block: Determinants and clinical impact in patients with hypertrophic obstructive cardiomyopathy undergoing nonsurgical septal reduction therapy. *J Am Coll Cardiol* 2003;42(2):296–300.

73. Maron BJ, et al. Efficacy of implantable cardioverter-defibrillators for the prevention of sudden death in patients with hypertrophic cardiomyopathy. *N Engl J Med* 2000;342(6):365–373.

74. Cuoco FA, et al. Implantable cardioverter defibrillator therapy for primary prevention of sudden death after alcohol septal ablation of hypertrophic cardiomyopathy. *J Am Coll Cardiol* 2008;52(21):1718–1723.

45

Left atrial appendage exclusion

BASIL ALKHATIB, ATHANASIOS SMYRLIS, AND SRIHARI S. NAIDU

INTRODUCTION

Stroke is the most feared complication in patients surviving a cardiovascular event and occurs with an incidence of approximately 780,000 cases per year in the United States (90% of them being ischemic strokes).[1] In Western countries, stroke is the third most common cause of mortality and a leading cause of disability; this condition accounts for approximately $60 billion in annual costs in the United States. The impact of stroke on a patient and family cannot be overemphasized because of the associated loss of independence and function. Accordingly, because of these issues, attempts at stroke prevention have received considerable emphasis.

Atrial fibrillation (AF) is the most common sustained cardiac arrhythmia and is increasing in frequency as the population ages.[2–11] In individuals over 40 years old, the lifetime risk of AF is one in four. The relationship between increasing age, AF, and stroke has been studied intensively. Stroke occurs at an annual rate of 5% in patients with AF, and this rate increases with age. In patients >80 years of age, AF is the cause of approximately 25% of all strokes. Accordingly, as life expectancy increases, there will be increased need for strategies to prevent stroke in AF.

Although multiple randomized trials have documented the effectiveness of warfarin therapy for stroke prevention in the setting of AF compared with placebo, aspirin alone, or aspirin in combination with clopidogrel, only approximately 50% of high-risk patients with AF are treated with warfarin.[12–27] This is a result of the narrow therapeutic index associated with warfarin, poor patient compliance, the presence of absolute or relative contraindications—particularly related to the potential for bleeding—and the wide variability in dosing schedules that make treatment difficult and inconvenient.[27] Although new agents (the so-called non-vitamin K antagonist oral anticoagulants [NOACs]) are being evaluated and have been approved, the lifetime use may be limited by costs, compliance issues, as well as bleeding risk.[28,29]

Multiple sources of data, including pathological and echocardiographic studies, have documented that the left atrial appendage (LAA) is the site of thrombus formation in approximately 90% of patients with nonvalvular AF (Figure 45.1).[30] Recent trials have shown that exclusion of LAA from the rest of the left atrium (LA) reduces the risk of stroke without the need for concomitant long-term anticoagulation. In the past few years, multiple devices or techniques, both surgical and percutaneous, have been developed to exclude the LAA from the systemic circulation (see Table 45.1). The advent of these devices coincides with advancements in the ability to image and approach the appendage. Namely, two- and three-dimensional transesophageal echocardiography (TEE) has been extremely helpful and has allowed for a better assessment of LAA anatomy and its suitability for closure, as well as to guide the closure procedure itself and assess the completeness of closure. Recently, cardiac computed tomography (CT) is gaining attention as an imaging modality to plan the closure.

ANATOMIC CONSIDERATIONS

The application and potential role of these approaches require understanding of the anatomy of the LAA.[31-33] The LAA is a diverticulum that arises from the LA and lies within the pericardium superior to the left ventricular (LV) free wall and next to the superior and lateral aspect of the main pulmonary artery (PA). It varies significantly in structure, volume, and three-dimensional configuration (Figure 45.2).[34] Veinot et al.[33] evaluated 500 normal autopsy hearts. This series included 25 male and 25 female subjects from each decade of life for a total of 10 decades. A striking finding was that 54% of specimens had two lobes of the LAA, while only 20% of specimens had a single lobe. These lobes were found to lie in multiple planes and have a variable distance from ostium to the distal tip. More recent data from the SPARC study also found that approximately 50% of patients have multiple lobes.[35,36] In addition to wide variability in number of lobes, the volume and dimensions also vary. In an autopsy study of 220 cases with resin casts of the LAA, volume varied widely, from 0.7 mL up to 19.2 mL, and the length ranged from 16 to 51 mm.[35]

This extreme variability in dimensions has significant implications for approaches aimed at LAA exclusion. The approach with the best chance to most completely and reliably abolish stroke will require the ability to fully cover the ostium of all lobes as well as the origin of the LAA. Exclusion of that portion of the LAA that contains pectinate muscles may also be important as thrombus could potentially develop between adjacent muscles. Importantly, residual flow into a patient lobe after incomplete exclusion may actually result in an increased incidence of stroke at follow-up. The length of the LAA and shape are also important, as any implantable device must be able to fit into the body of the LAA without protruding out into the body of the LA itself.

Assessment of the specific details of LAA anatomy is essential for patient selection and procedural performance. TEE is the most commonly used approach but CT is used with increasing frequency (Figure 45.3). The purpose of the imaging work-up is threefold:

1. *Identifying the presence or absence of thrombus.* If a thrombus is present as a filling defect or is suspected because of the presence of a dense cloud of echoes (smoke), then percutaneous approaches should be avoided because of the potential for clot embolization during the procedure. In this setting, warfarin should be administered and repeat imaging performed to document either persistence or disappearance of the thrombus. Only if thrombus disappearance is documented can device implantation be performed.
2. *Dimensions of the LAA and relationship to the pulmonary veins.* Budge et al.[31] compared LAA morphology in 53 patients with atrial fibrillation using TEE, planar CT, and segmented three-dimensional CT. They measured maximal LAA orifice diameter, width, and depth with each modality. In addition, they assessed the relationship of the LAA to the

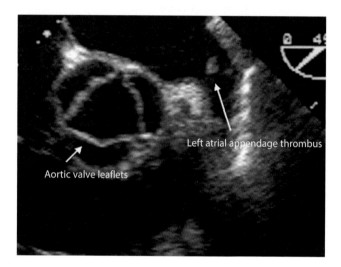

Figure 45.1 Echocardiography documenting thrombus within the left atrial appendage.

Table 45.1 Left atrial appendage closure devices

Device	Deployment	Sizes	Antithrombotic treatment post-procedure
PLAATO (ev3 endovascular)	Endovascular	15–32 mm	N/A
WATCHMAN (Boston Scientific)	Endovascular	21, 24, 27, 30, and 30 mm	Yes, warfarin for 45 days, then aspirin and clopidogrel for first 6 months
LARIAT (SentreHEART)	Endo-epicardial	Max. target size: W40 mm × H2O mm × L70 mm; Min. access size: 4.3 mm	Some patients may require AC because they may develop early or late reopening (No standard practice)
ACP AMULET (St. Jude Medical)	Endovascular	16–34 mm	Aspirin and clopidogrel for first 3 months, then aspirin only
AtriClip (Atricure inc)	Epicardial	35, 40, 45, and 50 mm	Aspirin only

Note: AC, anticoagulation; L, length; N/A, not applicable; W, width.

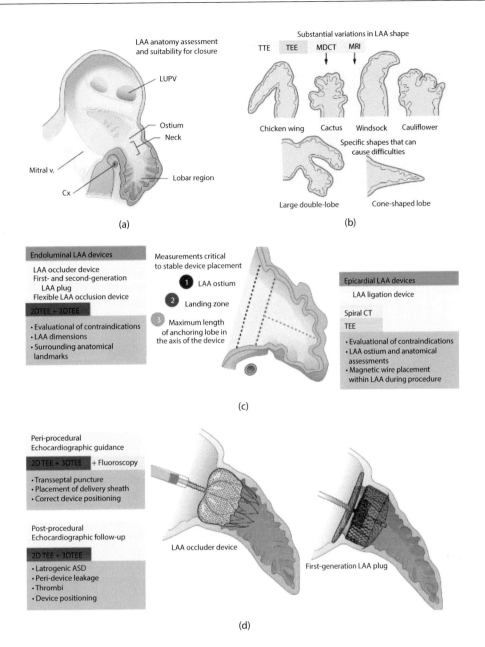

Figure 45.2 Imaging approach to LAA closure, an overview. **(a)** A cross-section of the left atrium and the orientation of the left atrial appendage (LAA), left circumflex coronary artery, mitral valve, as well as the left upper pulmonary vein. **(b)** The various LAA morphologies and shapes. **(c)** The critical locations where measurements need to be made for optimal sizing of the LAA occlusion device. **(d)** The optimal placement of LAA occluder device and first-generation LAA plug for LAA occlusion. 2D, two-dimensional; 3D, three-dimensional; ASD, atrial septal defect; CT, computed tomography; Cx, circumflex coronary artery; LAA, left atrial appendage; LUPV, left upper pulmonary vein; MDCT, multidetector computed tomography; MRI, magnetic resonance imaging; TEE, transesophageal echocardiography; TTE, transthoracic echocardiography. (With permission from Wunderlich, N.C., et al., *JACC Cardiovasc. Imaging*, 8(4), 472–488, 2015.)

left pulmonary veins. There were quantitative differences in measurements depending on which modality was used (Table 45.2). In general, the orifice diameter values measured by TEE and planar CT were similar, while values obtained using segmented CT reconstruction were greater. This has important implications for device sizing, because with current endovascular devices, the size depends on the orifice diameter. There were also differences in the mean LAA depth, which ranged from 25.1 mm with planar CT to 35.9 mm with TEE. This measurement also has important implications for device selection and size. Early generation devices were relatively long; more recent devices are shorter and can fit in most anatomic situations. Of importance is the fact that in the Budge et al.[31] study, in contrast to the pathology series, the majority of appendages studied were single-lobed. The presence of multiple lobes can complicate device placement. In some patients, not all lobes can be covered and therefore should not undergo percutaneous occlusion, while in others, to cover the ostium adequately, one of the lobes must be entered deeply for device placement. If the angulation between lobes is large, this can create problems trying to achieve a stable position.

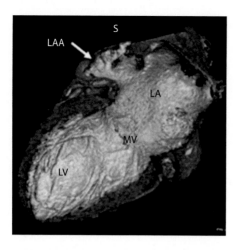

Figure 45.3 CT imaging documenting the relationship between the left atrial appendage (LAA), left atrium (LA), mitral valve (MV), and left ventricle (LV). Note the angulation into the LA, which may complicate device placement.

Table 45.2 Comparison of left atrial appendage anatomy depending on specific imaging modality in 53 patients with atrial fibrillation

No. of LAA lobes	TEE (±SD)	CTp (±SD)	CTsg (±SD)
LAA — short axis (mm)	1.21 ± 0.41	1.11 ± 0.32	1.08 ± 0.27
LAA — long axis (mm)	26.1 ± 6.4	26.2 ± 4.1	28.5 ± 4.5
LAA depth (mm)	35.9 ± 6.2	25.1 ± 6.3	29.2 ± 5.7
LAA width (mm)	23.0 ± 5.8	23.5 ± 4.2	
LAA volume (mL)			9.8 ± 4.2
LAA volume (mL)			111.6 ± 30.4

Note: CTp, planar computed tomography; CTsg, segmented computed tomography; LAA, left atrial appendage; SD, standard deviation; TEE, transesophageal echocardiography.

3. *The relationship between the LAA and pulmonary veins.* Budge et al.[31] found that the superior aspect of the plane of the LAA was typically located in the mid-portion of the left superior pulmonary vein, while the inferior aspect was high relative to the plane of the left inferior pulmonary vein. These relationships may have important implications for accessing the LAA as well as for device placement. Depending on the amount of protrusion into the LA by a device, it is possible to impinge on the orifice of one of the left pulmonary veins, thereby impeding normal flow.

PROCEDURAL APPROACHES

Approaches to closure of the LAA include endovascular approach via transseptal puncture to plug the appendage, and epicardial approaches, either surgical or percutaneous. Although several devices have been evaluated for LAA occlusion,[37–45] the WATCHMAN device from Boston

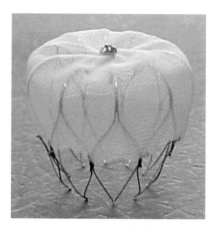

Figure 45.4 The WATCHMAN (Boston Scientific) implant is a composite device with a self-expanding nitinol frame with a permeable polyester fabric on the atrial-facing surface of the device. Fixation barbs help to anchor the device in position.

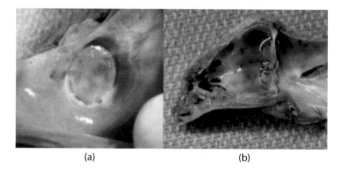

(a)   (b)

Figure 45.5 Experimental animal preparation documenting placement of the WATCHMAN (Boston Scientific) device at the origin of the left atrial appendage **(b)** and endothelialization of the atrial surface **(a)**.

Scientific (Figure 45.4),[41] which is a self-expanding nitinol frame structure with fixation barbs and a permeable polyethylene membrane, is currently the only U.S. Food and Drug Administration (FDA)-approved device indicated for the reduction of thromboembolism in patients with nonvalvular AF.[40,41,43,44] This device is available in diameters ranging from 21 mm to 33 mm to accommodate variations in LAA anatomy. The device is implanted through the endovascular approach using a transseptal puncture and a catheter-based delivery system to cover the ostium of the LAA (Figure 45.5). Device implantation is guided by fluoroscopy as well as TEE or intracardiac echocardiography (ICE) to verify proper position and stability.

ENDOVASCULAR TECHNIQUE

If the endovascular procedure is performed under ICE guidance, three vascular access sheaths are placed; these include two femoral venous sheaths, one for the appendage occlusion device itself and one for ICE, while the third is for arterial access. The arterial access sheath should be small (e.g., 4-Fr); this sheath allows placement of a pigtail catheter to identify the level of the aortic valve for optimizing the transseptal procedure as well as for monitoring aortic pressure. The venous sheaths placed need to accommodate the intracardiac ultrasound catheter using an 8- to 10-Fr device, as well as the occlusion device. The venous access for the occlusion device should be from the right femoral vein as this trajectory facilitates transseptal puncture. The site should be prepared so that eventually a 14-Fr sheath can be placed. The other two sheaths are usually placed on the contralateral left femoral side.

Approaches to the transseptal catheterization vary considerably and have evolved over time. The goal for left appendix exclusion is to cross the atrial septum at the level of the fossa ovalis. In many laboratories, biplane fluoroscopic imaging is used with orthogonal views, either anteroposterior (AP) and lateral or 30° RAO/60° LAO. The most important complication to avoid is entry into the ascending aorta. While entry with the Brockenbrough needle into the aorta does not necessarily lead to catastrophic bleeding, if high pressure is identified with needle puncture, it is essential to avoid placement of a larger dilator and sheath, as this results in major hemorrhage. More recently, intracardiac ultrasound has been used more extensively for guidance of transseptal catheterization. With this approach, the needle can be visualized within the right atrium (RA) and the details of septal anatomy can be characterized. In some patients, particularly those who have had prior transseptal procedures, the atrial septum may be fibrotic and the needle may slide cranially, leading to a puncture site that is too superior. Similarly, a fatty limbus may impact the entrance site. With ICE or TEE, the needle can be visualized as it enters the LA using injection of saline or contrast. The level of puncture of the interatrial septum is of importance because it impacts the ability to optimize a guiding sheath into the LAA. If the LAA angulates quickly caudally, then a lower septal puncture helps so that the guiding sheath can be placed more coaxially into the appendage. The development and subsequent wide use of steerable guiding sheaths will help to minimize this issue. In addition, radiofrequency ablation needles (Baylis, Inc.) may provide improved safety by avoiding the sliding of the needles during forward pressure, avoiding posterior wall puncture in aneurismal or floppy septums, and ensuring proper septal position prior to puncture.

Once safe access to the LA is accomplished, heparin is administered. Typically, an activated clotting time (ACT) is measured with a goal of approximately 250 seconds. It is important to administer heparin promptly because thrombus can form in the long sheaths and can embolize during the procedure. The next goal of the procedure is safe access into the LAA once a sheath has been placed into the LA. Knowledge of the detailed anatomy is important, particularly the relationship between the LAA and pulmonary veins. The large 14-Fr sheath for device delivery can easily damage the left atrial wall, particularly the dome, or the LAA itself. Although several approaches can be used, the current recommended approach is to engage the LAA with a pigtail catheter. This approach minimizes the potential for trauma that can result in perforation of the thin-walled LAA. Once the LAA is entered with the pigtail catheter, the sheath is advanced gently over the pigtail to the ostium of the appendage where a stable position is obtained and documented by angiography.

The current sheath has marker bands at its distal tip that facilitate placement of the device. The device is selected on the basis of the dimension of the orifice determined by contrast angiography as well as TEE, although as previously mentioned, CT image analysis prior to the procedure may be helpful in selecting the optimal device size (Figure 45.3). The device is then advanced, being careful to minimize the chance for entrapment of air. Avoidance of trapping air is best accomplished by a high-pressure saline line that infuses saline during advancement of the device. Once the device is positioned in the LAA and confirmation has been obtained that there is no damage to the LAA, the sheath is withdrawn leaving the occlusion device in place. If the device is positioned too deeply in the LAA, giving incomplete protection against clot formation, it can be recaptured and withdrawn to a more ideal position. If the device is positioned so that it protrudes too far into the LA, then the device needs to be completely removed because of the risk of embolization and a different size device placed (Figure 45.6). Identifying the orientation of the device with the ostium of the LAA is best achieved using echocardiography. If a satisfactory axial position has been secured, angiography is performed to document that there has been compression of the device, with a goal of compression of the dimensions of the unconstrained device by 10%–20%. Angiography through the sheath is used to assess the degree of obliteration of LAA flow. Finally, a "tug test" is performed during which the operator places manual traction on the device to ensure that it is stable. During this time, TEE can document that the LAA wall invaginates during device traction. Following this, the device is released and the sheath withdrawn.

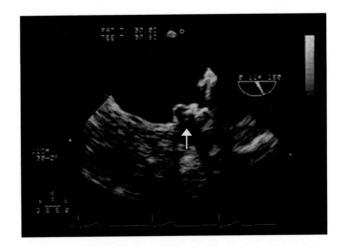

Figure 45.6 Echocardiography at implantation documenting that the device (WATCHMAN, Boston Scientific) is positioned suboptimally and protrudes into the left atrium. Recapture and deployment of another device is indicated.

Following the procedure with the WATCHMAN (the only FDA-approved device), patients are treated with aspirin and warfarin for 45 days until a scheduled echocardiographic (TEE) follow-up. If that follow-up echocardiogram documents successful exclusion of the LAA, the regimen is changed to aspirin and clopidogrel. After 6 months, the clopidogrel can be discontinued if the clinical condition is satisfactory.

PLAATO

The PLAATO[39,46] occluder (Figure 45.7) was the first device designed and FDA-approved for percutaneous LAA occlusion, but it has since been taken off the market. This device was a self-expandable nitinol cage that was covered with an impermeable expanded polytetrafluoroethylene (e-PTFE) membrane. It had anchors to prevent embolization and came in different sizes ranging from 20 to 32 mm to ensure optimal sealing. This device was also delivered by a transseptal approach as described above using a special 12-Fr sheath. Although this device is no longer marketed, there are important data available regarding the patient population in which it was used and its outcome.

Ostermayer et al.[46] reported on the outcome of two international multicenter feasibility trials that included 111 patients. All of these patients had a contraindication for anticoagulant therapy and were at risk for stroke. Implantation of the PLAATO device was successful in 108 patients. Three patients required pericardiocentesis for hemopericardium, and one patient required urgent cardiovascular surgery and subsequently died of neurologic causes. The primary endpoint for these registries was the incidence of major adverse events defined as a composite of stroke, death, myocardial infarction (MI), or need for procedural-related cardiovascular surgery during follow-up. All of these patients received aspirin and clopidogrel initially but no warfarin. Long-term treatment varied but at a minimum consisted of aspirin administered indefinitely. During follow-up that averaged 9.8 months, there were six deaths (5.4%) and the observed annual stroke rate was 2.2%.

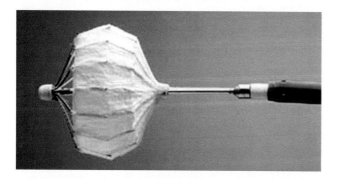

Figure 45.7 The PLAATO device (no longer manufactured) is a self-expanding nitinol cage that, in contrast to the WATCHMAN device, has an occlusive polytetrafluoroethylene membrane. It also has small anchors to prevent embolization.

On the basis of the baseline CHADS-2 score, this 2.2% event rate appeared improved compared with the predicted 6.3% rate. In a larger experience of 210 patients treated with the PLAATO device worldwide,[37] device implantation success was also high at 97.6%. In this group, during a follow-up of 258 patient-years, only five patients had a stroke that was again less than predicted by the baseline CHADS-2 score.

WATCHMAN

The initial worldwide experience with this specific device included 75 patients, while in 66 of them (88%) the procedure could be successfully implanted.[44] The most common reason for failure to implant the device was the fact that LAA anatomy was not suitable. Out of the 75 patients, pericardial effusions were documented in 2 (2.6%), and in both cases, the effusion was thought to be related to the transseptal procedure. Two devices embolized during implantation and were retrieved percutaneously. Mean follow-up was available for 740 ± 341 days. During this time, 91.7% of patients were able to discontinue warfarin, and there were no ischemic strokes or systemic embolizations. Two patients had a transient ischemic attack.

The multicenter PROTECT AF study (Watchman Left Atrial Appendage System for Embolic Protection in Patients with Atrial Fibrillation) was subsequently conducted to determine whether percutaneous LAA closure with a filter device (WATCHMAN) was noninferior to warfarin for stroke prevention in nonvalvular AF.[41,47] A total of 707 patients with AF and at least one risk factor (age >75 years, hypertension, heart failure, diabetes, or prior stroke/transient ischemic attack) were randomized to either the WATCHMAN device ($n = 463$) or continued warfarin ($n = 244$) in a 2:1 ratio. The composite primary efficacy endpoint included stroke, systemic embolism, and cardiovascular death, and primary analysis was by intention to treat. After a mean follow-up of 2.3 ± 1.1 years, the primary efficacy event rates were 3% and 4.3% in the WATCHMAN and warfarin groups, respectively, meeting the criteria for noninferiority. The PROTECT AF trial, for the first time, proved the role the LAA plays in the pathogenesis of stroke in AF. However, with regard to primary safety endpoint, this endpoint included serious adverse events related to excessive major bleeding (e.g., intracranial or gastrointestinal bleeding) or procedure-related complications (e.g., serious pericardial effusion, device embolization, and procedure-related stroke). The outcome rate was higher in the LAA closure group (5.5% per year) than in the control group (3.6% per year), driven by early periprocedural events.

Due to the higher rate of adverse outcomes in patients undergoing WATCHMAN device implantation in PROTECT AF, a subsequent randomized study, the PREVAIL trial, was designed to further assess the efficacy and safety of the WATCHMAN device as procedural experience grew.[48] Patients were randomly assigned (in a 2:1 ratio) to undergo LAA occlusion and subsequent discontinuation of warfarin (intervention group, $n = 269$) or receive chronic warfarin therapy (control group, n = 138). Early safety events, defined as device embolization, arteriovenous fistula (AVF), cardiac perforation, cardiac tamponade, and major bleeding requiring transfusion occurred in 2.2% of the WATCHMAN arm, significantly lower than in PROTECT AF, satisfying the pre-specified safety performance goal. Despite using a broader, more inclusive definition of adverse events, these were lower in the PREVAIL trial than in PROTECT AF (4.2% vs. 8.7%; P = 0.004). The PREVAIL trial thereby provided additional data that LAA occlusion is a reasonable alternative to warfarin therapy for stroke prevention in patients with nonvalvular AF, leading to FDA approval.

The amount of long-term data on patients with LAA closure with the WATCHMAN device is now growing. In a recently released series of 102 patients, outcomes of percutaneous LAA closure with the WATCHMAN device were reported up to 5 years.[49] Mean age was 71.6 ± 8.8 years, and mean CHA_2DS_2-VASc Score was 4.3 ± 1.7. During a mean follow-up period of 3 ± 1.6 years, a low adverse event rate was demonstrated. Specifically, the annual rates of transient ischemic attack, stroke, intracranial hemorrhage, and death were 0.7%, 0.7%, 1.1%, and 3.5%, respectively.

AMPLATZER OCCLUSION DEVICES

Amplatzer atrial septal occluder devices have historically been used "off-label" to occlude the LAA (Figure 45.8).[38,43] In initial experience in two small trials enrolling 16 patients and 27 patients (43 patients total), respectively, there were six device embolizations, three of which required surgery for retrieval. At the time of publication, no patient experienced a stroke during 30 patient-years of follow-up.

The Amplatzer device has since been modified for optimizing placement in the LAA. This new device developed by St. Jude Medical is called the Amplatzer Amulet LAA

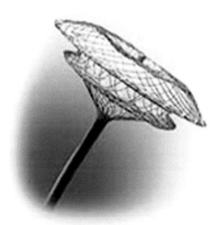

Figure 45.8 Amplatzer septal occlusion devices (St. Jude Medical) have also been used "off-label" to occlude the left atrial appendage. Typically, the distal disk is deployed within the left atrial appendage and the proximal disk is deployed just at the ostium.

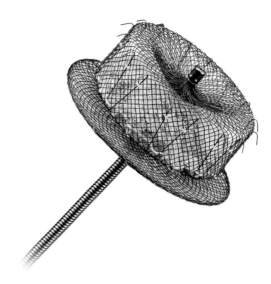

Figure 45.9 AMPLATZER Amulet Left Atrial Appendage Occluder (investigational). (AMPLATZER, Amulet and St. Jude Medical are trademarks of St. Jude Medical, Inc. or its related companies. Reprinted with permission of St. Jude Medical, ©2016. All rights reserved.)

occluder (Figure 45.9). This device is made of a flexible nitinol braid, and its design was built on existing Amplatzer technology. Instead of two discs as in the septal occluder, the Amulet has one disc (sits outside the appendage to be flush with the left atrial wall) and a plug (sits in the appendage). This design allows it to completely seal a wide range of LAA anatomy, with landing zones (i.e., orifice diameter) ranging from 11 to 31 mm in size.

The Amulet device was studied in a prospective single-center study of 25 patients undergoing percutaneous LAA occlusion.[50] The implantation of the device was successful in 24 patients (96%) without any procedural stroke, pericardial effusion, or device embolization. Patients who underwent device implantation were placed on dual antiplatelet therapy for the first month and then continued on aspirin only for next 5 months. At 3-month follow-up, none of the patients presented with clinical events. Follow-up TEE showed complete LAA sealing in all patients with no residual leak, but one patient (4.1%) was found to have asymptomatic thrombus apposition on the device. Larger randomized clinical trials are now ongoing to further evaluate the effectiveness and safety of the Amulet compared with oral anticoagulation.

EPICARDIAL APPROACHES

Surgical ligation of the LAA was first performed by Madden in 1949. Today, it is a procedure performed in selected patients undergoing cardiac valve surgery or as an adjunct to the Maze procedure.[51–53] Surgical techniques for LAA occlusion include simple neck ligation, surgical staplers, purse string techniques, and endocardial suturing. However, amputation of the LAA has proven to be challenging because of its thin, fragile, and delicate wall and close proximity to vital structures, such as coronary arteries. Complications are not infrequent and include bleeding and myocardial ischemia. Therefore, reinforcement with autologous pericardium has been implemented to make LAA amputation safer. Another method for LAA occlusion described by Hernandez-Estefania is invagination of the LAA and ligation with a purse-string suture and a second-running suture.[54] Following LAA invagination, the base of the appendage is tied by the purse-string suture delineating the LAA rim and is subsequently sealed with a running suture along the long axis of the LAA.

The AtriClip (Atricure, Inc., Westchester, OH) is a promising LAA exclusion clip that can safely and atraumatically exclude the LAA during open cardiac surgery.[53,55–57] In addition, the LigaSure Vessel Sealing System (LVSS; Tyco Healthcare, Valleylab, Boulder, CO), which can be applied during both on- and off-pump procedures, has been described by Jayakar et al. with acceptable results. The LVSS uses radiofrequency energy to create tissue fusion of the LAA lumen. Following histological amalgamation, the appendage is ready to be excised and a distal running suture is used as a backup.[58]

THORACOSCOPIC LIGATION

An additional surgical approach includes thorascopic extracardiac obliteration. An initial experience with 15 patients was reported by Blackshear et al.[59] With this approach, a double-lumen intratracheal tube is used. Selective intubation and ventilation of the right lung result in reduction in the volume of the left lung. Using video-assisted thorascopic instruments, the pericardium is opened and the tip of the LAA can be grasped. A loop is then manipulated to position it at the base of the appendage where it is cinched to occlude the appendage. In this small series, success was achieved in 14 of 15 patients; one patient developed bleeding and was converted to open thoracotomy. In all patients, there was a contraindication to anticoagulant therapy.

Patients were followed up for a mean of 42 ± 14 months. One fatal stroke occurred 55 months after surgery and one nondisabling stroke 3 months after surgery. There were two other deaths. In a subgroup of 11 patients with a history of prior thromboembolism, there was an annualized rate of stroke of 5.2% per year, which compared with a historical control rate of 13% per year for similar aspirin-treated patients from the Stroke Prevention in Atrial Fibrillation trials.

PERCUTANEOUS EPICARDIAL EXCLUSION

The Lariat suture delivery device (SentreHEART, Inc., Palo Alto, CA), which is FDA-approved for delivery of sutures for soft tissue closure, is being used off-label for LAA ligation. This is a closed-chest, percutaneous, epicardial catheter-based LAA ligation technique utilizing a pre-tied suture contained on a closure snare.[60] The technique involves the use of magnet-tipped wires that are advanced under fluoroscopic

guidance at both sides of the LAA (from lumen and surface). Accordingly, there is an intracardiac wire placement after standard transvenous access and transseptal puncture, and an epicardial wire via percutaneous subxiphoid intrapericardial access. A balloon is then placed at the ostium of the LAA to mark it. Subsequently, the LARIAT device is guided through the epicardial catheter over the LAA in order to close the LAA by suture ligation.[52,55,60] The position of the snare at the LAA ostium is guided by the balloon catheter positioned inside the ostium of the LAA and confirmed by TEE. Following placement verification, the snare is closed and tightened using the suture tightener. A repeat left atriogram is performed to ensure complete LAA closure. In the initial report, 10 of the 11 patients successfully underwent acute LAA ligation using this novel approach (9 with percutaneous epicardial access and 2 with simultaneous open surgical mitral valve (MV) replacement).[60]

An advantage of this approach is the lack of need for anticoagulation immediately following the procedure. Unlike some intracardiac implants that require anticoagulation to protect against thrombus formation while endothelialization occurs, the LARIAT snare device can offer immediate LAA closure without implantation of a foreign body inside the LA. In addition, it has some advantages compared with implantable devices in terms of complications, such as cardiac perforation, and device migration and embolization. The main procedural limitation of this approach is the need for epicardial access—a technique that is not familiar to the majority of operators. Finally, epicardial access is often not possible in patients with prior cardiac surgery and/or pericardial adhesions. There are also anatomical considerations, such as large LAA, posteriorly rotation of LAA, superiorly orientated LAA lobes, and posteriorly rotated hearts that may challenge successful ligation of the LAA using the LARIAT snare device.[51–53,55,60] Pericarditis and pain are common postprocedure.

Recently, concern was raised regarding off-label use of the LARIAT for LAA exclusion in the manner herein described with significant complications, including death and urgent surgery reported in the FDA Manufacturer and User Facility Device Experience (MAUDE) database.[61] A subsequent multicenter observational study also found similar complication rates, as well as an increased incidence of pericarditis. These complications were mitigated by micropuncture needle–based pericardial access and short-term use of colchicine, respectively.[62] Nonetheless, with the FDA approval of the WATCHMAN device, LARIAT utilization has declined recently.

CONCLUSIONS

Stroke is one of the most feared complications among survivors of a cardiovascular event because of the associated morbidity and mortality. Accordingly, prevention of stroke has received great attention. The relationship between stroke, AF, and increasing age has been clearly identified. Multiple series have documented that, in the setting of nonvalvular AF, thrombus originates in the LAA in the vast majority of patients. Given the constellation of stroke, AF, and LAA thrombogenicity, multiple efforts are currently aimed at exclusion of the latter structure. Complete LAA exclusion is now documented to be safe and effective in preventing subsequent strokes, leading to one FDA approval in the WATCHMAN device, with others sure to follow. It is anticipated that this approach will be widely used in patients who cannot take long-term oral anticoagulation. Further studies are needed to determine if current- or next-generation devices may obviate the need for even short-term warfarin, and whether such devices can replace warfarin for the majority of AF patients.

REFERENCES

1. Rosamond W, et al. Heart disease and stroke statistics—2008 update: A report from the American Heart Association Statistics Committee and Stroke Statistics Subcommittee. *Circulation* 2008;117(4):e25–e146.
2. Benjamin EJ, et al. Independent risk factors for atrial fibrillation in a population-based cohort. The Framingham Heart Study. *JAMA* 1994;271(11):840–844.
3. Garcia DA, Hylek E. Reducing the risk for stroke in patients who have atrial fibrillation. *Cardiol Clin* 2008;26(2):267–275, vii.
4. Lin HJ, et al. Stroke severity in atrial fibrillation. The Framingham Study. *Stroke* 1996;27(10):1760–1764.
5. Lloyd-Jones DM, et al. Lifetime risk for development of atrial fibrillation: The Framingham Heart Study. *Circulation* 2004;110(9):1042–1046.
6. Miyasaka Y, et al. Secular trends in incidence of atrial fibrillation in Olmsted County, Minnesota, 1980 to 2000, and implications on the projections for future prevalence. *Circulation* 2006;114(2):119–125.
7. Onalan O, Crystal E. Left atrial appendage exclusion for stroke prevention in patients with nonrheumatic atrial fibrillation. *Stroke* 2007;38(2 Suppl):624–630.
8. Psaty BM, et al. Incidence of and risk factors for atrial fibrillation in older adults. *Circulation* 1997;96(7):2455–2461.
9. Rulgomez A, et al. Incidence of chronic atrial fibrillation in general practice and its treatment pattern. *J Clin Epidemiol* 2002;55(4):358–363.
10. Stewart S, et al. Population prevalence, incidence, and predictors of atrial fibrillation in the Renfrew/Paisley study. *Heart* 2001;86(5):516–521.
11. Wolf PA, et al. Atrial fibrillation as an independent risk factor for stroke: The Framingham Study. *Stroke* 1991;22(8):983–988.
12. The effect of low-dose warfarin on the risk of stroke in patients with nonrheumatic atrial fibrillation. The Boston Area Anticoagulation Trial for Atrial Fibrillation Investigators. *N Engl J Med* 1990;323(22):1505–1511.
13. Stroke Prevention in Atrial Fibrillation Study. Final results. *Circulation* 1991;84(2):527–539.
14. Optimal oral anticoagulant therapy in patients with non-rheumatic atrial fibrillation and recent cerebral ischemia. The European Atrial Fibrillation Trial Study Group. *N Engl J Med* 1995;333(1):5–10.
15. Bungard TJ, et al. Why do patients with atrial fibrillation not receive warfarin? *Arch Intern Med* 2000;160(1):41–46.
16. ACTIVE Writing Group of the ACTIVE Investigators, et al. Clopidogrel plus aspirin versus oral anticoagulation for atrial fibrillation in the atrial fibrillation Clopidogrel Trial with Irbesartan for prevention of Vascular Events (ACTIVE W): A randomised controlled trial. *Lancet* 2006;367(9526):1903–1912.
17. Connolly SJ, et al. Canadian Atrial Fibrillation Anticoagulation (CAFA) Study. *J Am Coll Cardiol* 1991;18(2):349–355.
18. Ezekowitz MD, et al. Warfarin in the prevention of stroke associated with nonrheumatic atrial fibrillation. Veterans Affairs Stroke Prevention in Nonrheumatic Atrial Fibrillation Investigators. *N Engl J Med* 1992;327(20):1406–1412.
19. Fang MC, et al. Age and the risk of warfarin-associated hemorrhage: The anticoagulation and risk factors in atrial fibrillation study. *J Am Geriatr Soc* 2006;54(8):1231–1236.
20. Gage BF, et al. Adverse outcomes and predictors of underuse of antithrombotic therapy in medicare beneficiaries with chronic atrial fibrillation. *Stroke* 2000;31(4):822–827.
21. Gage BF, et al. Selecting patients with atrial fibrillation for anticoagulation: Stroke risk stratification in patients taking aspirin. *Circulation* 2004;110(16):2287–2292.
22. Go AS, et al. Warfarin use among ambulatory patients with nonvalvular atrial fibrillation: The anti-coagulation and risk factors in atrial fibrillation (ATRIA) study. *Ann Intern Med* 1999;131(12):927–934.
23. Go AS, et al. Anticoagulation therapy for stroke prevention in atrial fibrillation: How well do randomized trials translate into clinical practice? *JAMA* 2003;290(20):2685–2692.
24. Hart RG, et al. Meta-analysis: Antithrombotic therapy to prevent stroke in patients who have nonvalvular atrial fibrillation. *Ann Intern Med* 2007;146(12):857–867.
25. Hylek EM, et al. Major hemorrhage and tolerability of warfarin in the first year of therapy among elderly patients with atrial fibrillation. *Circulation* 2007;115(21):2689–2696.
26. Petersen P, et al. Placebo-controlled, randomised trial of warfarin and aspirin for prevention of thromboembolic complications in chronic atrial fibrillation. The Copenhagen AFASAK study. *Lancet* 1989;1(8631):175–179.
27. Waldo AL, et al. Hospitalized patients with atrial fibrillation and a high risk of stroke are not being provided with adequate anticoagulation. *J Am Coll Cardiol* 2005;46(9):1729–1736.
28. Albers GW, et al. Ximelagatran vs. warfarin for stroke prevention in patients with nonvalvular atrial fibrillation: A randomized trial. *JAMA* 2005;293(6):690–698.
29. Olsson SB, Executive Steering Committee of the SPORTIF III Investigators. Stroke prevention with the oral direct thrombin inhibitor ximelagatran compared with warfarin in patients with non-valvular atrial fibrillation (SPORTIF III): Randomised controlled trial. *Lancet* 2003;362(9397):1691–1698.
30. Blackshear JL, Odell JA. Appendage obliteration to reduce stroke in cardiac surgical patients with atrial fibrillation. *Ann Thorac Surg* 1996;61(2):755–759.

31. Budge LP, et al. Analysis of in vivo left atrial appendage morphology in patients with atrial fibrillation: A direct comparison of transesophageal echocardiography, planar cardiac CT, and segmented three-dimensional cardiac CT. *J Interv Card Electrophysiol* 2008;23(2):87–93.

32. Ernst G, et al. Morphology of the left atrial appendage. *Anat Rec* 1995;242(2):553–561.

33. Veinot JP, et al. Anatomy of the normal left atrial appendage: A quantitative study of age-related changes in 500 autopsy hearts: Implications for echocardiographic examination. *Circulation* 1997;96(9):3112–3115.

34. Wunderlich NC, et al. Percutaneous interventions for left atrial appendage exclusion: Options, assessment, and imaging using 2D and 3D echocardiography. *JACC Cardiovasc Imaging* 2015;8(4):472–488.

35. Kerut EK. Anatomy of the left atrial appendage. *Echocardiography* 2008;25(6):669–673.

36. Meissner I, et al. Prevalence of potential risk factors for stroke assessed by transesophageal echocardiography and carotid ultrasonography: The SPARC study. Stroke Prevention: Assessment of Risk in a Community. *Mayo Clin Proc* 1999;74(9):862–869.

37. Bayard YL, et al. Percutaneous devices for stroke prevention. *Cardiovasc Revasc Med* 2007;8(3):216–225.

38. Cruz-Gonzalez I, et al. Left atrial appendage exclusion using an Amplatzer device. *Int J Cardiol* 2009;134(1):e1–e3.

39. El-Chami MF, et al. Clinical outcomes three years after PLAATO implantation. *Catheter Cardiovasc Interv* 2007;69(5):704–707.

40. Fountain R, et al. Potential applicability and utilization of left atrial appendage occlusion devices in patients with atrial fibrillation. *Am Heart J* 2006;152(4):720–723.

41. Fountain RB, et al. The PROTECT AF (WATCHMAN Left Atrial Appendage System for Embolic PROTECTion in Patients with Atrial Fibrillation) trial. *Am Heart J* 2006;151(5):956–961.

42. Gage BF, et al. Validation of clinical classification schemes for predicting stroke: Results from the National Registry of Atrial Fibrillation. *JAMA* 2001;285(22):2864–2870.

43. Meier B, et al. Transcatheter left atrial appendage occlusion with Amplatzer devices to obviate anticoagulation in patients with atrial fibrillation. *Catheter Cardiovasc Interv* 2003;60(3):417–422.

44. Sick PB, et al. Initial worldwide experience with the WATCHMAN left atrial appendage system for stroke prevention in atrial fibrillation. *J Am Coll Cardiol* 2007;49(13):1490–1495.

45. Sievert H, et al. Percutaneous left atrial appendage transcatheter occlusion to prevent stroke in high-risk patients with atrial fibrillation: Early clinical experience. *Circulation* 2002;105(16):1887–1889.

46. Ostermayer SH, et al. Percutaneous left atrial appendage transcatheter occlusion (PLAATO system) to prevent stroke in high-risk patients with non-rheumatic atrial fibrillation: Results from the international multi-center feasibility trials. *J Am Coll Cardiol* 2005;46(1):9–14.

47. Reddy VY, et al. Percutaneous left atrial appendage closure for stroke prophylaxis in patients with atrial fibrillation. 2.3-year follow-up of the PROTECT AF trial. *Circulation* 2013;127(6):720–729.

48. Holmes DR Jr, et al. Prospective randomized evaluation of the Watchman Left Atrial Appendage Closure device in patients with atrial fibrillation versus long-term warfarin therapy: The PREVAIL trial. *J Am Coll Cardiol* 2014;64(1):1–12.

49. Wiebe J, et al. Percutaneous left atrial appendage closure with the Watchman device: Long-term results up to 5 years. *J Am Coll Cardiol* 2015;8(15):1915–1921.

50. Feixa X, et al. Left atrial appendage occlusion: Initial experience with the Amplatzer™ Amulet™. *Int J Cardiol* 2014;174(3):492–496.

51. Singh IM, Holmes D. Left atrial appendage closure. *Curr Cardiol Rep* 2010;12(5):413–421.

52. Aryana A, et al. Left atrial appendage occlusion and ligation devices: What is available, how to implement them, and how to manage and avoid complications. *Curr Treat Options Cardiovasc Med* 2012;14(5):503–519.

53. Sakellaridis T, et al. Left atrial appendage exclusion—Where do we stand? *J Thorac Dis* 2014;6(Suppl 1):S70–S77.

54. Hernandez-Estefania R, et al. Left atrial appendage occlusion by invagination and double suture technique. *Eur J Cardiothorac Surg* 2012;41(1):134–136.

55. Apostolakis E, et al. Surgical strategies and devices for surgical exclusion of the left atrial appendage: A word of caution. *J Card Surg* 2013;28(2):199–206.

56. Hanke T, et al. Surgical closure of the left atrial appendage in patients with atrial fibrillation. Indications, techniques and results. *Herzschrittmacherther Elektrophysiol* 2013;24(1):53–57.

57. Starck CT, et al. Epicardial left atrial appendage clip occlusion also provides the electrical isolation of the left atrial appendage. *Interact Cardiovasc Thorac Surg* 2012;15(3):416–418.

58. Jayakar D, et al. Use of tissue welding technology to obliterate left atrial appendage—Novel use of Ligasure. *Interact Cardiovasc Thorac Surg* 2005;4(4):372–373.

59. Blackshear JL, et al. Thoracoscopic extracardiac obliteration of the left atrial appendage for stroke risk reduction in atrial fibrillation. *J Am Coll Cardiol* 2003;42(7):1249–1252.

60. Bartus K, et al. Percutaneous left atrial appendage suture ligation using the LARIAT device in patients with atrial fibrillation: Initial clinical experience. *J Am Coll Cardiol* 2013;62(2):108–118.

61. Chatterjee S, et al. Safety and procedural success of left atrial appendage exclusion with the lariat device: A systematic review of published reports and analytic review of the FDA MAUDE Database. *JAMA Intern Med* 2015;175(7):1104–1109.

62. Lakkireddy D, et al. Short and long-term outcomes of percutaneous left atrial appendage suture ligation: Results from a US multicenter evaluation. *Heart Rhythm* 2016;13(5):1030–1036.

46

Percutaneous closure of atrial septal defect and patent foramen ovale

FABIAN NIETLISPACH AND BERNHARD MEIER*

INTRODUCTION

Percutaneous closures of atrial communications are often simple and safe procedures, but in some patients they can be rather intricate. Indications for closure are prevention of paradoxical embolism or arrhythmia, or prevention and treatment of heart failure. Further indications may be considered case by case (e.g. migraine relief and treatment of sleep apnea syndrome), but they currently represent only a small minority of indications. Percutaneous closures of atrial septal defects (ASDs) and patent foramen ovale (PFO) are most likely underused considering that effective and low-risk closure techniques exist and the treatment can make a big difference for patients.

ATRIAL SEPTAL DEFECTS

Two years before Andreas Güntzig's first percutaneous coronary balloon angioplasty, King and Mills performed the first percutaneous ASD closures in 1975.[1] They used the King–Mills double-umbrella device, consisting of a stainless steel umbrella covered with Dacron. Implantation principles were similar to current techniques, including balloon-sizing of the ASD, device oversizing, retraction of the deployed left atrial disc to lean against the atrial septum, followed by release of the right atrial disc, locking of the discs, and detachment from the delivery cable. The pioneers reported very late follow-up of these patients, confirming the effectiveness and safety of the procedure.[2]

Embryology and classification

The fetal single atrium is divided into a right and left atrium (RA and LA) by the formation of the *septum primum* (SP). The SP grows from the atrial roof caudal to the endocardial cushion and leaves a communication between the RA and LA above the endocardial cushion—the *foramen primum*. The foramen primum is slowly overgrown and closes, while more cranially, a second foramen forms inside the SP, the *foramen secundum*. Later, from the right atrial roof, the *septum secundum* (SS) extends caudally to the SP, covering the *foramen secundum*. A slit-like opening remains between the SP and the SS, named the *foramen ovale*. The foramen ovale closes after birth in the majority of people, but remains patent in 20%–25% of adults (patent foramen ovale, PFO). The region of the foramen ovale is called the *fossa ovalis*.

* Please note that Fabian Nietlispach and Bernhard Meier are consultants for Abbott.

Atrial septal defects can be classified according to their location:

- *Ostium secundum ASD*: in the region of the fossa ovalis
- *Ostium primum ASD*: in the region of the foramen primum, adjacent to the atrioventricular valves
- *Sinus venosus ASD (SV-ASD)*:
  - Superior vena cava SV-ASD: in the region of the superior vena cava (SVC) and the upper right pulmonary vein
  - Inferior vena cava SV-ASD: in the region of the inferior vena cava (IVC)
- *Coronary sinus ASD*: fenestration of the coronary sinus into the LA; most often associated with persistent left SVC

Associated anomalies are mitral valve prolapse (associated with ostium secundum ASD), mitral stenosis, and anomalous pulmonary venous return (APVR) into the RA (associated with SVC SV-ASD).

The ostium primum ASD is a complex defect, which involves the atrioventricular canal and is associated with mitral valve malformations and coarctation of the aorta. Complex ostium primum ASDs are treated surgically.

The pathophysiology of ASDs does involve left-to-right shunting and the risk for paradoxical embolism (occasional right-to-left shunt). This can result in arrhythmias, heart failure, pulmonary hypertension, and arterial embolism (stroke, myocardial infarction [MI], or other arterial occlusions). Patients with an ASD are not necessarily at higher risk for endocarditis and they do not require endocarditis prophylaxis if the defect remains unclosed. Yet, a possible endocarditis risk might arise from turbulences at the pulmonary valve due to the high right ventricular volume output. These turbulences are documented by the systolic murmur in patients with ASD.

Indications for percutaneous closure

- Large ASD with significant left-to-right shunt ($Qp/Qs \geq 1.5$), or documented right ventricular or atrial enlargements to prevent heart failure and arrhythmias (surgical closure indicated if percutaneous closure not possible)
- Small ASD to prevent paradoxical embolism and reduce volume load

While the first indication is generally accepted, the second is debatable. Most operators would agree to close small ASDs in case a bidirectional shunt is discovered, which is, however, almost always the case (e.g., if the patient performs a Valsalva maneuver). Moreover, closing a small ASD, like closing a PFO, yields almost 100% success without complication.

In the exquisitely rare patients with long-standing severe and fixed pulmonary hypertension and consecutive permanent right-to-left shunt (Eisenmenger syndrome), closure of the ASD is not recommended, since it could result in acute right ventricular failure. However, successful cases of ASD closure in this clinical setting have been described, but most patients required aggressive pulmonary vasodilation, temporary extracorporeal circulation, and long intensive care unit stays.

In patients with large ASDs and long-standing left-to-right shunt, percutaneous closure is generally advisable, although intermittent aggravation of pre-existing left ventricular failure may occur and may require higher doses of diuretics.

In these settings, some operators prefer implantation of fenestrated ASD closure devices (see below), which allows for partial reduction of the ASD. Other operators recommend monitoring pulmonary pressure for 15 minutes after closure of the ASD and before final release of the device.

Devices

Figure 46.1 depicts a selection of the most frequently used devices for ASD closure.

The market leader is the AMPLATZER septal occluder (Abbott, [formerly, St. Jude Medical] St. Paul, MN), designed and developed by Kurt Amplatz.[3] The device consists of two discs and a connecting waist made out of braided 0.005-in nitinol wires and is filled with polyester to enhance fibrin deposition, thereby enhancing effective closure and endocardialization. Its properties include self-centering and repositionability. The size of the occluder is given by the diameter of the waist and ranges from 4 to 40 mm. The right atrial disc extends the waist by 8–10 mm, and the left atrial disc is 12–16 mm. The devices require a 6-Fr to 12-Fr sheath, which typically comes with a 45° angulation. In some cases, differently shaped sheaths are used (e.g., 45° × 45° sheath). The device is further available in a fenestrated version to only partially close the ASD, leaving the option for a second intervention for gradual closure of the communication, thereby allowing the heart to progressively adapt to the new hemodynamic situation.

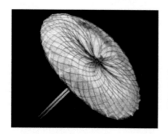 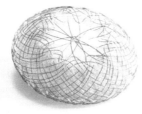 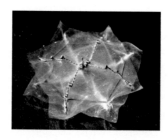 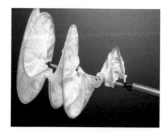

Figure 46.1 Four of the clinically used devices for percutaneous atrial septal defect closure (left to right): the AMPLATZER septal occluder (Abbott, St. Paul, MN), the Occlutech Figulla Flex II ASD device (Occlutech, Helsingborg, Sweden), the BioSTAR (discontinued, NMT Medical Inc, Boston, MA), and the Helex/Gore septal occluder (W.L. Gore & Associates Inc., Flagstaff, AZ).

For Swiss cheese–type ASDs (multiple small ASDs), a purpose-specific device was designed—the AMPLATZER Cribriform occluder. This device consists of two discs and a small connector. Both discs are of equal size and range from 18 to 40 mm, requiring an 8-Fr to 10-Fr sheath.

The Occlutech Figulla Flex II ASD device (Occlutech, Helsingborg, Sweden) is a derivative of the AMPLATZER septal occluder covering the same range of ASD sizes. Opposed to the AMPLATZER device, there is no hub on the left atrial disc and the device is filled with polyethylene terephthalate.

A different but discontinued device line was the BioSTAR (NMT Medical Inc, Boston, MA), succeeding the STARFlex, the CardioSEAL, and the RASHKIND devices. In the BioSTAR device, two pairs of nonferrous alloy arms were hinged by a spring and an absorbable collagen matrix covered each pair of arms. Over time, the collagen matrix was absorbed by the replacing tissue and only the arms were left behind in the interatrial septum.

The Helex/Gore septal occluder (W.L. Gore & Associates Inc., Flagstaff, AZ) is a polytetrafluorethylene (PTFE)-based device. The PTFE membrane is wound up on a nitinol wire, which forms a disc on each side of the ASD after deployment. The device comes in sizes ranging from 15 to 35 mm. This device is better suited for small- and medium-sized ASDs than for large ASDs.

Closure techniques

Before the procedure, a transesophageal echocardiography (TEE) is performed to define the anatomy of the defect (e.g. type of ASD) and to exclude associated anomalies. Furthermore, TEE can define the extent of the rims that margin the ASD. It is particularly an insufficient, inferior rim (<3 mm) that increases the risk of an unstable device position and will raise the operator's attention during the procedure. Some operators would exclude a patient to undergo attempt of percutaneous ASD closure solely based on the presence of deficient rims. Since there is still a high chance for successful ASD closure in these situations, many operators—including the authors of this chapter—would not exclude a patient in advance for such a reason, but oversize the device more than usual and pay particular attention to device stability before release.

The procedures can be performed under general anesthesia and using TEE and fluoroscopic guidance, or under local anesthesia with intracardiac echocardiographic (ICE) and fluoroscopic guidance, or under local anesthesia with fluoroscopic guidance alone.

Atrial septal defect closure using an AMPLATZER or AMPLATZER-like device

At the commencement of the procedure, 5,000 units of heparin are given, followed by venous puncture and crossing of the defect with a standard 0.035-in wire. If the wire does not cross the ASD spontaneously, it may be necessary to guide the wire through the defect by using a multipurpose or Judkins right catheter. Over the standard wire, a "sizing balloon" is advanced and placed inside the defect and slowly inflated. Indentations on the sizing balloon will be recognized, indicating proper stretching of the ASD. A fluoroscopic image should be obtained in an angle perpendicular to the sizing balloon for measurement of the defect (Figure 46.2). A properly sized device is chosen: we recommend to generously oversize the device (20%–30% if the balloon sits stably in the ASD and more if it continues to slip in and out), which will make implantation easier and reduce the risk for device embolization. In cases guided by echocardiography, the stop-flow technique is recommended.[4] It measures the ASD using the balloon diameter the moment the Doppler flow around the growing balloon stops. This avoids overstretching and tearing of the atrial septum.

The sizing balloon is removed and the delivery sheath is introduced to the LA, and the wire and the sheath introducer are subsequently removed. Particular attention must be paid to always keep the outside end of the sheath low in order to avoid air embolism. The sheath is then carefully de-aired.

The device is introduced through the sheath and the proper attachment to the delivery gear is checked before it is advanced out of the sheath. The left atrial disc, the waist, and part of the right atrial disc are deployed in the LA (Figure 46.3). The sheath–device assembly is then retracted to the interatrial septum. Partial deployment of the right atrial disc in the LA will ensure that the device self-centers within the ASD. The right atrial disc is pulled into the RA and released. A vigorous pull-and-push test, as well as contrast medium injections in a projection showing the device in perfect profile without any overlay of the discs will confirm a stable and correct device position (Figure 46.4). We recommend acquiring cine images not only during contrast medium injection to the RA, but also after recirculation of the contrast medium to the LA (levophase).

The device is then detached from the delivery cable. It is possible that the device will move considerably after detachment, except if a delivery cable with a movable core wire is used,[5] which allows to release the tension on the device before detachment (currently only available from

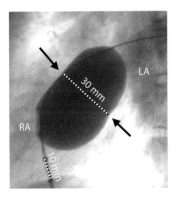

Figure 46.2 Sizing balloon: indentations on the balloon indicate the borders of the defect. LA, left atrium; RA, right atrium.

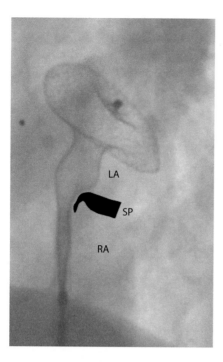

Figure 46.3 Technique of percutaneous atrial septal defect (ASD) closure: the disc meant for the right atrium (RA) is partially deployed in the left atrium (LA) and pulled back into the ASD. This technique enhances the self-centering properties of the device. The indentation caused by the septum primum (SP) indicates that the correct position is not yet reached and the device needs to be pulled down more.

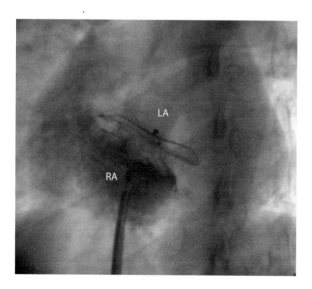

Figure 46.4 Contrast medium injection into the right atrium (RA) in a perpendicular view confirms proper position of the device. LA, left atrium.

Comed B.V., Bolsward, Netherlands). An additional contrast medium injection after detachment is typically performed, unless the patient suffers from severe kidney failure.

Postprocedural care involves brief bed rest (with the patient pressing the groin when getting up as the pressure in the femoral vein abruptly increases from about 8 mmHg to 60 mmHg because of the blood column head to groin when erect) and a transthoracic echocardiogram the next day or, in case of an outpatient procedure, a couple of hours after the procedure. The patient is discharged without any physical restrictions. Antiplatelet therapy consists of acetylsalicylic acid for 3–6 months (unless another indication for indefinite acetylsalicylic acid therapy exists) and clopidogrel for 1–6 months. After 3–6 months, a follow-up TEE is performed to ensure complete closure of the ASD and to rule out device thrombus. Prophylaxis against endocarditis is usually recommended for a few months. Palpitations due to harmless atrial arrhythmia are common for several weeks. Delayed device embolizations are rare and almost unheard of after the initial mobilization of the patient. Erosion of a free atrial wall is the only significant late complication. It occurs, however, in less than 1% and is usually heralded in time by chest pain.

Pitfalls

- Balloon not stable during balloon sizing
- Possible solution (Figure 46.5):
  - Use a support wire (e.g., Meier Backup wire, Boston Scientific, Marlborough, MA).
  - Pre-curve the support wire.
- Enlargement of the ASD during balloon sizing or during deployment of device.
  - Possible solution:
    - If the enlarged defect is <35 mm → deploy a larger device.
    - If the enlarged defect is >35 mm → send for surgical correction.
- Device embolization

- Possible solution (Figure 46.6):
  - Snare device and externalize through a larger sheath or bevel the tip of the sheath to enlarge the opening to accommodate for the nonaxial approach of the screw.
  - Stabilize device using a biotome, then snare and externalize the device.

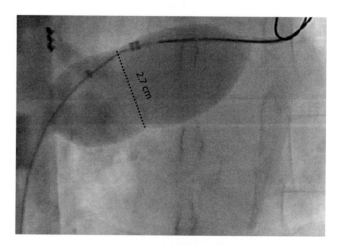

Figure 46.5 Use of a manually shaped support wire enhances stability of the sizing balloon.

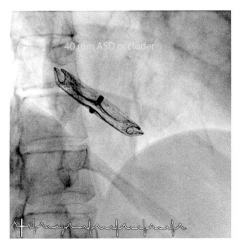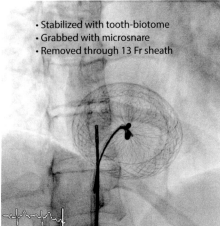

• Stabilized with tooth-biotome
• Grabbed with microsnare
• Removed through 13 Fr sheath

Figure 46.6 If the embolized and freely floating device (left) cannot be snared by a Gooseneck snare, it can be stabilized using a biotome, making subsequent snaring easier (right).

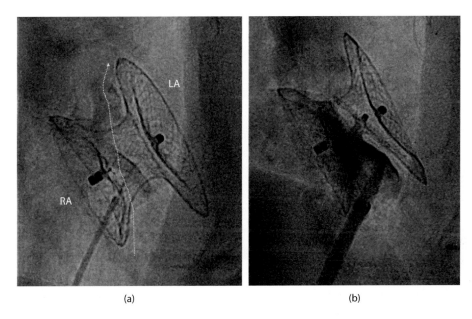

(a)   (b)

Figure 46.7 A residual shunt (**a**, arrow) 5 months after initial atrial septal defect (ASD) closure is treated with a second device (**b**, 18 mm AMPLATZER PFO occluder).

- Residual leak on follow-up TEE
  - Possible solution (Figure 46.7):
    – Implant an additional device.
- Device thrombus on follow-up TEE
  - Possible solution:
    – Prescribe 6–12 weeks of oral anticoagulation.
    – Thereafter, repeat TEE, if thrombus resolved, replace oral anticoagulation with acetylsalicylic acid.

Special considerations

- Percutaneous repair of SVC SV-ASD with anomalous pulmonary venous return[6]
  - Although for a long time SV-ASD was considered to be contraindicated for percutaneous repair, feasibility was recently shown in a 65-year-old woman who refused open heart surgery. The ASD was closed with an AMPLATZER

ASD occluder and the anomalous pulmonary vein draining into the SVC was occluded with an AMPLATZER ventricular septal defect occluder, after waiting for 15 minutes before its detachment, during which the awake and unsedated patient felt perfectly fine. Occlusion of the pulmonary vein remained asymptomatic and double-shunt closure resulted in sustained disappearance of the patient's symptoms.[7]
  - Concomitant ASD closure and primary preventive left atrial appendage (LAA) occlusion (Figure 46.8)
  - Patients suffering from large ASDs with marked dilatation of the atria may still be in sinus rhythm. However, they are at very high risk for the development of atrial fibrillation during follow-up. If such a patient undergoes ASD closure, the risk of atrial fibrillation increases temporarily because of the irritation by the ASD closure device and remains high despite the fact that the atria usually decrease in size after shunt closure.

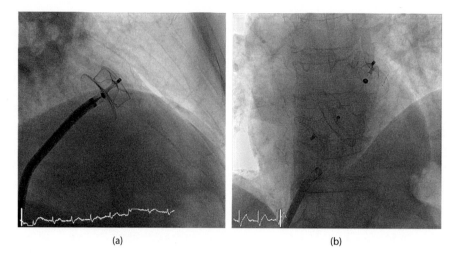

(a)   (b)

Figure 46.8 Primary (before the occurrence of atrial fibrillation) preventive left atrial appendage closure **(a)** in a patient undergoing closure of a large atrial septal defect **(b)**.

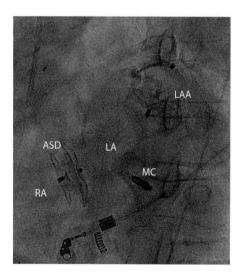

Figure 46.9 Closure of an iatrogenic atrial septal defect (ASD) after mitral valve intervention with a MitraClip (MC, Abbott Vascular, Santa Clara, CA) and left atrial appendage (LAA) occlusion. LA, left atrium; RA, right atrium.

- Furthermore, it may be difficult, if not impossible, to perform percutaneous LAA occlusion with a large ASD occluder completely barring the transseptal passage. Therefore, concomitant LAA occlusion may be a good indication in such patients who typically have not yet suffered a cerebrovascular accident or a bleeding problem (primary prevention) and who have had no atrial fibrillation so far (primary prevention).
- Closure of iatrogenic ASDs[8]
  - Transseptal access has become more frequently used for a variety of structural interventions: LAA occlusion, mitral balloon valvuloplasty, percutaneous mitral valve repair, and percutaneous mitral valve implantation.
  - Mitral valve interventions, in particular, create large iatrogenic ASDs. Indication for closure is not well defined; however, preliminary data indicate that persistent iatrogenic ASDs may be associated with worse outcome.[7]

- Many operators perform ASD closure in this setting, in case bidirectional shunting across the ASD is present. In such situations, the patient is at risk for paradoxical embolism, and the shunt may worsen heart failure symptoms.
- The size of such ASDs is typically 8–10 mm and can be closed with a 12 mm AMPLATZER ASD occluder (Figure 46.9).

PATENT FORAMEN OVALE

Embryology and classification

A PFO is a consequence of the absence of fusion of the SS and the SP in the region of the foramen ovale. The PFO is a slit-like tunnel that allows for right-left and rarely left-right shunting. Right-to-left shunting or embolism through the PFO can lead to different symptoms:

- Arterial thromboembolism → stroke, MI, peripheral arterial occlusions
- Serotonin and other neurotransmitters → migraine
- Nitrogen bubbles → decompression incidents
- Air or fat embolism → surgical complications

Besides these diseases, other different pathologies are associated with a PFO, although the pathophysiology of the association is not yet fully understood: sleep apnea syndrome,[9] high-altitude pulmonary edema,[10] and platypnea orthodeoxia syndrome.[11]

PFOs can be classified according to their anatomy as follows:

- PFO with right-left shunt
- PFO with bidirectional shunt
- PFO with atrial septal aneurysm (mobile and flaccid SP with protrusion of ≥10 mm into the RA or LA, also a reason for a PFO)

- PFO with eustachian valve or Chiari network (membranes in the RA at the junction with the IVC that direct the blood toward the foramen ovale, also reasons for a PFO)

The amount of shunting through the PFO can be graded semiquantitatively according to the amount of bubbles crossing the interatrial septum during a single frame of a contrast echocardiogram with Valsalva maneuver:

- Grade 0: none (no bubbles)
- Grade 1: minimal (1–5 bubbles)
- Grade 2: moderate (6–20 bubbles)
- Grade 3: severe (>20 bubbles)

Indications for closure

So far, evidence for PFO closure comes from trials on secondary prevention of stroke and on patients suffering from migraine. This does not, however, imply that PFO closure is only justified in these settings. Evidence suggests performing PFO closure for secondary stroke prevention is the most compelling indication. There is no evidence on how to deal with a PFO that was incidentally found (e.g. during right heart catheterization or during a routine echocardiogram).[12]

Patent foramen ovale closure for secondary stroke prevention

Three randomized controlled trials have been conducted so far, comparing medical therapy (vitamin-K-antagonists [VKA] or antiplatelet agents) and percutaneous PFO closure in patients with previous cryptogenic stroke: the CLOSURE-1 trial (Evaluation of the STARFlex Septal Closure System in Patients with a Stroke and/or Transient Ischemic Attack due to Presumed Paradoxical Embolism through a Patent Foramen Ovale),[13] the PC trial (Percutaneous Closure of Patent Foramen Ovale in Cryptogenic Embolism),[14] and the RESPECT trial (Randomized Evaluation of Recurrent Stroke Comparing PFO Closure to Established Current Standard of Care Treatment).[15] After 2–4 years of follow-up, all three trials did not meet statistical significance for the superiority of PFO closure for death or secondary prevention of stroke in the intention-to-treat analyses, thereby suggesting that both therapies (PFO closure and medical therapy) are equally effective. As-treated analyses, meta-analyses, and longer follow-up analyses, however, found clear evidence of superiority of PFO closure over medical therapy.[16] One prospective, nonrandomized study with follow-up of up to 10 years even found a significant reduction in mortality after PFO closure compared to medical therapy.[17]

In summary, all three randomized trials pointed in the same direction with less events in the PFO closure arm, which became a significant benefit when looking at as-treated or per-protocol analyses or with longer follow-up. PFO closure therefore appears to be the therapy of choice for secondary stroke prevention in patients with cryptogenic stroke.

Migraine

The prevalence of migraines are higher in patients with a PFO (up to 25%), particularly, the incidence of severe migraine with aura. The majority of patients who underwent PFO closure had an improvement in their migraine intensity or frequency and about one-third of these patients were even cured after PFO closure in an observational study.[18] The randomized PRIMA (Percutaneous Closure of Patent Foramen Ovale in Migraine with Aura) trial showed similar findings with a significant reduction of migraine with aura days and freedom from migraine in 10% of patients.[19] Therefore, PFO closure may be advocated in patients suffering from severe migraines, since they have a high chance of reduction of their symptoms and as a "collateral benefit," may get protected from future paradoxical embolism.

Other indications

PFO closure for primary prevention and in patients without migraines is still controversial, since it is a field with evidence not yet considered unequivocal. Therefore, these indications should be thoroughly discussed with the patient, and the patient should be aware that there is no decisive evidence that would guide physicians in decision-making.

Such indications for PFO closure include the following:
- Diseases associated with PFO
  - Migraines
  - High-altitude edema
  - Decompression incident
  - Exercise desaturation
  - Sleep apnea
  - Platypnea orthodeoxia
- Incidental finding of a PFO in high-risk situations
  - "High-risk PFOs" in the presence of conditions associated with an increased risk of stroke (atrial septal aneurysm, eustachian valve, Chiari network)
  - High-risk activities (deep-sea divers, mountain climbers, brass musicians, pilots)
  - Patients at high risk for venous thrombosis (thrombophilia, recurrent deep vein thrombosis, intracardiac electrode carrier)

Devices

The most frequently used devices are the AMPLATZER PFO occluder (St. Jude Medical, St. Paul, MN)[20] or AMPLATZER-like devices (e.g., Occlutech Figulla Flex II PFO device, Occlutech, Helsingborg, Sweden; Hyperion PFO occluder, Comed B.V., Bolsward, Netherlands). Another frequently used device is the Helex/Gore septal occluder (W.L. Gore & Associates Inc., Flagstaff, AZ).

When comparing the randomized trials (CLOSURE-1 using the obsolete StarFLEX Device, PC and RESPECT using AMPLATZER devices), it seems that the AMPLATZER devices have slight advantages over the StarFLEX device, with less thrombus on the device, resulting in less new-onset atrial fibrillation, as well as higher closure rates (>90%). In fact, adverse events in the PC and RESPECT trials were not different in the PFO closure group when compared with patients randomized to medical therapy. These findings were confirmed in a randomized trial comparing the AMPLATZER to the Helex/Gore and the obsolete CardioSEAL devices, where the embolization rate was highest when the Helex/Gore occluder was used, whereas the CardioSEAL occluder showed the most device thrombi and new-onset atrial fibrillation.[21] Overall, PFO closure could be safely performed with all three devices.

Closure techniques

PFO closure is technically the simplest procedure in interventional cardiology. A single operator can safely and effectively perform the procedure under local anesthesia and with fluoroscopic guidance alone. Some operators prefer to sedate the patient and perform the procedure with additional TEE guidance or using ICE. The additional imaging modalities come at the price of making the procedure more intricate, time-consuming, costly, and add some small risks associated with general anesthesia, esophageal intubation, or additional venous access.

After application of 5,000 units of heparin intravenously, the femoral vein is punctured followed by insertion of a standard 0.035-in wire. As with ASD closure, the wire may cross the PFO upon insertion, while in other cases, the wire has to be guided through the PFO with the help of a curved (e.g., Multipurpose) catheter.

The properly sized sheath is then advanced over the standard wire into the LA. The wire and the introducer are removed, holding the end of the sheath low to prevent air embolism. Back-bleeding is observed to make sure the sheath is de-aired. The device is crimped into the introducer under water or flushed vigorously and then advanced into the sheath. The left atrial disc is deployed, the device and the sheath pulled back to the septum (in a left anterior oblique view which best shows when the disc gets aligned to the septum), and under light tension the right disc is deployed. While the device is still attached to the pusher cable, a stable and correct device position is confirmed:

- Pacman sign (Figure 46.10)
  - The two discs are separated more cranially by the thicker SS than caudally by the thin SP.
- Push-and-pull test
  - The device can be pushed and pulled without embolizing either into the RA or LA.
- Contrast medium injections (Figure 46.11)
  - In a projection showing the device in perfect profile with no overlapping of the discs, a 10–20 mL contrast medium injection through the sheath is performed. Direct injection will confirm the right disc completely being in the RA, whereas the levophase will confirm the left disc being completely in the LA.

Once a stable device position is confirmed, the device is unscrewed from the delivery cable.

Postinterventional care involves bed rest for up to 2 hours with slight compression of the groin (e.g., by the patient's hand). Thereafter, normal physical activities without

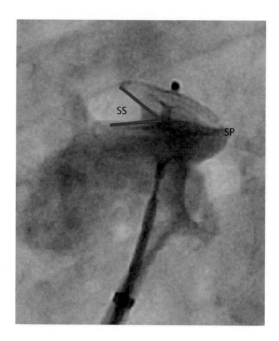

Figure 46.10 The Pacman sign indicates a correct position of the patent foramen ovale occluder: the two discs are more separated by the thicker septum secundum (SS) than by the membranous septum primum (SP).

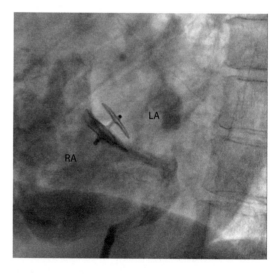

Figure 46.11 Contrast medium injections in a perpendicular view to the device confirms correct device position. LA, left atrium; RA, right atrium.

restrictions are possible. Medication involves acetylsalicylic acid for 5–6 months (unless another indication is present) and clopidogrel for 1–6 months, during which a TEE should be performed to confirm complete closure and to exclude thrombus on the device.

Pitfalls

- If the sheath does not easily advance through the groin:
  - If insertion of the sheath causes a lot of pain or a lot of resistance, in spite of the usual screwing motion, is encountered, it is wise to depict the sheath on fluoroscopy.

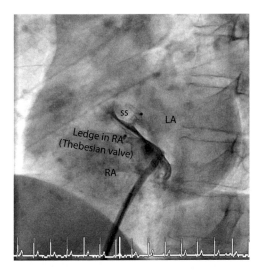

Figure 46.12 After release of the AMPLATZER PFO occluder, the right disc looks to be partially in the left atrium. This is, however, misjudged because of an injection below the Thebesian vein, which is keeping the contrast medium away from the septum. Observing the levophase or repositioning of the sheath for a reinjection confirms a correct device position. LA, left atrium; RA, right atrium; SS, septum secundum.

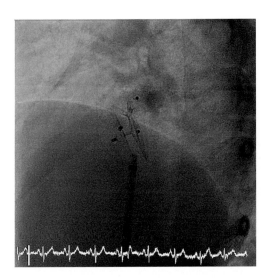

Figure 46.13 Closure of a residual leak through the AMPLATZER PFO occluder: a second AMPLATZER PFO occluder is deployed.

- If the only problem is too big a resistance of the soft tissue in spite of adequate skin incision, the sheath can invariably be screwed into the vein (turn the entire sheath around its own axis rather than just half-turns left and right). Alternatively, the standard wire can be replaced by a support wire (which is rarely needed).
- If the tip of the sheath kinked the wire and progressed into the soft tissue, the sheath should be pulled back and the kinked wire needs to be partially advanced or retracted or replaced by a new wire, preferably the support type.

- If there is no back-bleeding through the sheath upon removal of the wire and the introducer:
  - Most likely, the sheath is too far into the LA and is wedged against the atrial wall. If the sheath is withdrawn 2 cm, back-bleeding usually can be observed.
- Injections before releasing the device confirmed a correct device position. Upon injection after release, the right disc seems to have migrated to the LA (Figure 46.12):
  - The most likely cause is a contrast medium injection below the Thebesian ledge, directing the contrast medium away from the septum.
  - The device position is most likely correct and can be confirmed by observing the levophase or by placing the sheath higher up in the RA and closer to the device and repeating the contrast medium injection.
- How to proceed if a leak is detected during a follow-up TEE:
  - The patient can either remain on antiplatelet therapy for another 3–6 months, during which the TEE is repeated. However, the chances for complete late closure during follow-up are low.
  - A second device (18 or 25 PFO occluder or vascular plug) can be implanted, which will close the residual shunt in a vast majority of patients (Figure 46.13).
- What to do if a device thrombus is detected during follow-up TEE:
  - Oral anticoagulation for 4–6 weeks, during which the TEE is repeated. If the thrombus resolved, acetylsalicylic acid is given for a few months.

REFERENCES

1. King TD, et al. Secundum atrial septal defect. Nonoperative closure during cardiac catheterization. *JAMA* 1976;235(23):2506–2509.
2. Mills NL, King TD. Late follow-up of nonoperative closure of secundum atrial septal defects using the King-Mills double-umbrella device. *Am J Cardiol* 2003;92(3):353–355.
3. Sharafuddin MJ, et al. Transvenous closure of secundum atrial septal defects: Preliminary results with a new self-expanding nitinol prosthesis in a swine model. *Circulation* 1997;95(8):2162–2168.
4. Carlson KM, et al. Transcatheter atrial septa defect closure: Modified balloon sizing technique to avoid overstretching the defect and oversizing the Amplatzer septal occluder. *Catheter Cardiovasc Interv* 2005;66(3):390–396.
5. Meier B. Catheter-based atrial shunt occlusion, when the going gets even tougher: Editorial comment to use of a straight, side-hole (SSH), delivery sheath for improved delivery of AMPLATZER ASD occluder. *Catheter Cardiovasc Interv* 2007;69(1):21–22.
6. Meier B. Sinus venous defect, new important indication for structural interventional cardiology. *Catheter Cardiovasc Interv* 2014;84(3):478.
7. Meier B, et al. Percutaneous repair of sinus venosus defect with anomalous pulmonary venous return. *Eur Heart J* 2014;35(20):1352.
8. Schueler R, et al. Persistence of iatrogenic atrial septal defect after interventional mitral valve repair with the MitraClip system: A note of caution. *JACC Cardiovasc Interv* 2015;8(3):450–459.

9. Rimoldi SF, et al. Effect of patent foramen ovale closure on obstructive sleep apnea. *J Am Coll Cardiol* 2015;65(20):2257–2258.

10. Allemann Y, et al. Patent foramen ovale and high-altitude pulmonary edema. *JAMA* 2006;296(24):2954–2958.

11. Devendra GP, et al. Provoked exercise desaturation in patent foramen ovale and impact of percutaneous closure. *JACC Cardiovasc Interv* 2012;5(4):416–419.

12. Nietlispach F, Meier B. Percutaneous closure of patent foramen ovale: An underutilized prevention? *Eur Heart J* 2015;37(26):2023–2028.

13. Furlan AJ, et al. Closure or medical therapy for cryptogenic stroke with patent foramen ovale. *N Engl J Med* 2012;366(11):991–999.

14. Meier B, et al. Percutaneous closure of patent foramen ovale in cryptogenic embolism. *N Engl J Med* 2013;368(12):1083–1091.

15. Carroll JD, et al. Closure of patent foramen ovale versus medical therapy after cryptogenic stroke. *N Engl J Med* 2013;368(12):1092–1100.

16. Kent DM, et al. Device closure of patent foramen ovale after stroke: Pooled analysis of completed randomized trials. *J Am Coll Cardiol* 2016;67(8):907–917.

17. Wahl A, et al. Long-term propensity score-matched comparison of percutaneous closure of patent foramen ovale with medical treatment after paradoxical embolism. *Circulation* 2012;125(6):803–812.

18. Wahl A, et al. Improvement of migraine headaches after percutaneous closure of patent foramen ovale for secondary prevention of paradoxical embolism. *Heart* 2010;96(12):967–973.

19. Mattle HP, et al. Percutaneous closure of patent foramen ovale in migraine with aura, a randomized controlled trial. *Eur Heart J* 2016;37(26):2029–2036.

20. Han YM, et al. New self-expanding patent foramen ovale occlusion device. *Catheter Cardiovasc Interv* 1999;47(3):370–376.

21. Hornung M, et al. Long-term results of a randomized trial comparing three different devices for percutaneous closure of a patent foramen ovale. *Eur Heart J* 2013;34(43):3362–3369.

47

Pediatric and adult congenital cardiac interventions

SAWSAN M. AWAD, QI-LING CAO, AND ZIYAD M. HIJAZI

INTRODUCTION

Interventional cardiology is a rapidly progressing field that has seen major growth in the last three decades. Interventional therapy has become an acceptable alternative treatment to cardiac surgery and a standard of care for many pediatric and adult patients with congenital heart disease. In cases where conventional interventional therapy is not feasible due to limited access or associated conditions that may require surgical repair, a hybrid approach has been increasingly implemented with obvious advantages to the patient. This concept involves direct exposure of the heart via a median sternotomy performed by the surgeon, followed by an interventional procedure performed by the interventional cardiology team without subjecting the patient to cardiopulmonary bypass.

While atrial septal defect (ASD) and patent foramen ovale (PFO) are covered in Chapter 46, in this chapter, we discuss additional congenital cardiovascular conditions for which interventional therapy has been established as the preferred management strategy, including ventricular septal defect (VSD) device closure, semilunar valvuloplasty for congenital aortic and pulmonary valve stenosis, and right ventricular outflow tract (RVOT) stent in tetralogy of Fallot (TOF). In addition, we summarize the value of interventional therapies for selected adult congenital cardiac lesions, such as coarctation of the aorta (COA), pulmonary artery

stenosis (PAS), coronary artery fistula, aortopulmonary collaterals (APCs), pulmonary arteriovenous fistula (AVF), and finally, the established percutaneous pulmonary valve implantation (PPVI) for patients with severe pulmonary insufficiency and/or stenosis.

GENERAL PRINCIPLES OF TREATMENT AND EQUIPMENT

The performance of interventional cardiac catheterization procedures for congenital heart disease (CHD), both in adult and pediatric patients, requires well-trained cardiologists and a well-equipped cardiac catheterization laboratory. A description of training requirements for interventionalists performing the procedures is beyond the scope of this chapter. General anesthesia is used most of the time in the pediatric age group for interventional procedures. Conscious sedation may be used in adolescents and young adults in some cases of ASD closure. Transesophageal echocardiogram (TEE) is used for interventional procedure guidance. It provides continuous monitoring of cardiac function and is valuable in guidance for certain procedures such as ASD device closure and atrial septal puncture. TEE neonatal probe can be used in patients weighing 1.7–3 kg. Pediatric TEE probe, on the other hand, can be used in patients with a weight between 3.5 and 15 kg. Intracardiac echocardiography (ICE) is an important tool in the direct imaging of internal cardiac structures. ICE use decreases the discomfort level produced by TEE. While using ICE, several interventional procedures can be performed under conscious sedation without the need for general anesthesia. It may also lead to decreased radiation exposure by decreasing the need for frequent fluoroscopy use to guide the procedure. The development of smaller ICE catheters allowed utilization of this technique in smaller children without major vascular complications and similar success procedural rates compared with adults.[1] Biplane fluoroscopy imaging is preferred as it allows a better understanding of the anatomy and location of the defect and minimizes the amount of contrast agent administered. Surgical backup and extracorporeal membrane oxygenator (ECMO) support capabilities are mandatory in any institution planning to have an interventional program for CHD. An interventional procedure for CHD should never fail due to lack of proper equipment. Therefore, multiple types of wires, catheters, balloons, retrieval catheters or snares, and other devices should be readily available.

INTERVENTIONS

ASD and PFO closures are detailed in Chapter 46 and not discussed in the present chapter.

Percutaneous ventricular septal defect closure

ANATOMY/EMBRYOLOGY CONSIDERATIONS

VSDs are the most common cardiac abnormalities found in children, accounting for approximately 30% of all defects.[2,3]

VSDs may be located in four different positions according to the Kirklin classification.[4] Membranous VSDs are the most common (representing 75%), followed by the muscular type, which represents 10%–15%. Rare acquired causes of VSD include a defect following traumatic injury to the chest or myocardial infarction (MI). Acquired VSDs are encountered in 0.2% of all MI patients.

Approximately 70% of muscular VSDs and 30% of membranous VSDs close spontaneously within 5 years after initial diagnosis. Patients with large defects (as big as the aortic valve) may present with signs and symptoms of congestive heart failure (CHF) or failure to thrive. All VSDs can be repaired surgically with the exception of apical defects and the Swiss cheese–type of VSD, characterized by multiple apical muscular VSDs. The overall risk for VSD surgical repair is <5%. Mortality and morbidity rates increase with multiple VSDs, pulmonary hypertension, residual VSD, and complex associated anomalies. Morbidities include complete heart block immediately after surgery that occurs in <1% of patients. Late-onset complete heart block is a rare problem, encountered especially in patients with postoperative complete right bundle branch block (RBBB) and/or left anterior hemiblock.

Lock et al.[5] performed the first percutaneous VSD device closure in 1987, and since then, many devices have been used for this purpose. The most widely used device

in the United States and Europe is the Amplatzer muscular VSD occluder device (AGA Medical, Plymouth, MN). It is specifically designed for the ventricular septum and is made of 0.004–0.005-in nitinol wire. Holzer and colleagues reported on the use of this device in a U.S. registry with favorable results.[6] In that registry, a total of 75 patients were enrolled in 14 cardiac centers in the United States. The median age of patients was 1.4 years (range 0.1–54.1 years). The median size of the primary VSD was 7 mm (range 3–16 mm). Implantation of multiple devices was required in 20.5% of the procedures. The complete closure rate immediately after the procedure was 47.2%, increasing to 69.6% at 6 months, and 92.3% at 12-month follow-up. Major complications occurred in 10.7% of patients, while 2.7% of patients died. The percutaneous closure approach is preferred over surgery, if the anatomy is suitable, for children weighing more than 5 kg. Even if the patient's weight is <5 kg or if the septal anatomy precludes a percutaneous approach (e.g., transposition of the great arteries, double-outlet right ventricle [RV]), or if the venous access is not present, a hybrid approach has been advocated as an alternative to surgery with cardiopulmonary bypass.[7] For single muscular VSD, the procedure can be safely performed without TEE guidance as angiographic/fluoroscopic images are satisfactory for guidance. However, for multiple defects/Swiss cheese septum, it is advisable to perform the procedure under TEE guidance. The closure steps are demonstrated in Figure 47.1. The femoral artery and vein are accessed routinely. If the VSD is located in the mid, posterior, or apical septum, the right internal jugular vein is also accessed. The patient is heparinized to achieve an activated clotting time (ACT) of >200 seconds at the time of device placement. Routine right and left heart catheterization is performed to assess the degree of shunting and to evaluate the pulmonary vascular resistance. Angiography in single plane (35° left anterior oblique [LAO]/35° cranial) is performed to define the location, size, and number of VSDs. This projection profiles the muscular septum. A complete TEE study is performed. Specific attention is paid to the characterization of the VSDs and nearby structures, including the papillary muscles, moderator band, and the chordae tendineae. The atrioventricular (AV) valves are interrogated at baseline for any regurgitation. The appropriate Amplatzer VSD device size is chosen to be 1–2 mm larger than the VSD size as assessed by TEE or angiography at end diastole (the bigger of the two diameters). The authors of this chapter depend mainly on echocardiographic and/or angiographic sizing of the defect, while others rely on balloon sizing. A long venous sheath (6- to 8-Fr) is then placed across the VSD. This is accomplished in a variety of ways. The most common approach used for midmuscular VSDs is to advance a curved 4-Fr end-hole catheter (Judkins right or Cobra) from left ventricle (LV) across the VSD into the RV. An exchange-length 0.035-in J-tipped guidewire is advanced through the VSD and the RV into either pulmonary artery (PA) branch. This wire is then snared and exteriorized through the right internal jugular vein. This provides a

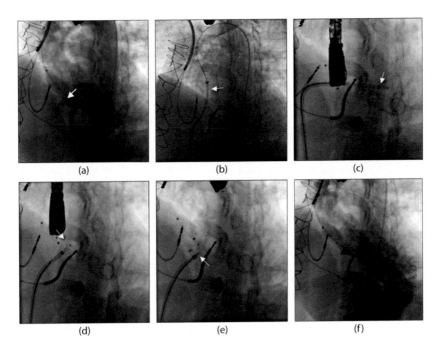

Figure 47.1 Cinefluoroscopic images during ventricular septal defect (VSD) closure. **(a)** Angiogram in the left ventricle in the long axial oblique view demonstrating the presence of high muscular VSD (*arrow*). **(b)** Cine fluoroscopy after the defect has been crossed and the wire was exteriorized from the right femoral vein and the delivery sheath (*arrow*) was positioned in the left ventricle. Note the arteriovenous loop is still established. **(c)** The delivery sheath with the Amplatzer device (*arrow*) is in mid-left ventricle. **(d)** Deployment of the left desk (*arrow*) in the left side of the defect. **(e)** The device was released from the cable (*arrow*). **(f)** Final left ventricle angiogram showing complete closure of the defect.

stable arteriovenous loop and allows a 6- to 8-Fr–long Mullins-type sheath (AGA Medical) to be advanced from the jugular vein to the RV and positioned into the LV. The approach from the jugular vein provides a straight course for mid, apical, or posterior defects. Some larger midmuscular or apical VSDs can be easily crossed from the RV side. However, care should be exercised not to go through the trabeculae in the RV. Once a catheter crosses into the LV, an exchange-length guidewire is positioned into the LV apex and a 6- to 8-Fr–long Mullins type-sheath is advanced over this wire and positioned into the body of the LV. On occasion, after removal of the dilator and wire from the long sheath, kinking of the distal part of the sheath (at the ventricular septum) is encountered. In such circumstances, a 0.018-in J-tipped glidewire is advanced through the dilator and left inside the sheath while advancing the device beside it. This helps minimize kinking of the sheath. Once the device approaches the tip of the sheath, this wire is removed and the device is deployed in the usual fashion. TEE and angiography using a pigtail catheter positioned in the LV are very helpful imaging techniques in guiding device position. The LV disk is deployed in the middle of the LV, and the entire assembly (cable/sheath) is pulled into the VSD with further retraction of the sheath to expand the waist inside the septum. Repeat TEE and angiography to confirm optimal device position prior to deployment of the RV disk is of great importance. Once position is confirmed, further retraction of the sheath to expand the RV disk is performed. Again, prior to device release, repeat TEE and

angiography are performed. If device position is satisfactory, the device is released by counterclockwise rotation of the cable using the pin vise.

For anterior muscular VSDs, we prefer the femoral vein approach as it is an easier course for the delivery sheath. Once the wire crosses the VSD into the PA, it is snared and exteriorized out into the femoral vein. The delivery sheath is then placed over this wire into the LV apex. The remaining steps are similar to the above. After device release, a brief complete TEE study is performed with additional imaging in multiple planes to confirm device placement and to assess for residual shunting or any obstruction or regurgitation induced by the device. The device orientation commonly changes slightly to align with the septum as it is released from the delivery cable and all tension on the device is eliminated. Additional VSDs are then occluded in the same fashion. Repeat LV angiogram in 35° LAO/35° cranial view is performed 10 minutes after final device release to assess the result. Complete closure was achieved in near 100% of cases in two small series.[8,9] Significant residual shunts can be managed by additional devices at the same or subsequent sessions. Patients receive a dose of an appropriate antibiotic (commonly Cefazolin at 20 mg/kg) during the catheterization procedure and two further doses at 8-h intervals. The patients are recovered in an appropriate setting (usually intensive care unit) and are routinely discharged home the following day. Observation for subacute bacterial endocarditis prophylaxis is recommended for 6 months or until complete closure is obtained. Patients are instructed to avoid contact sports for 1 month. Follow-up includes TEE, chest radiograph, and electrocardiogram at 6 months post-closure and yearly thereafter.

Congenital aortic stenosis/pulmonary stenosis

VALVULAR AORTIC STENOSIS

Valvular aortic stenosis (AS) occurs in approximately 3%–6% of patients with CHD.[3] The stenotic valve is usually secondary to aortic valve maldevelopment with increased thickening and rigidity of the valve tissue and variable degrees of commissural fusion. Compensatory LV hypertrophy is proportional to the degree of obstruction. With severe hypertrophy and valvular obstruction, myocardial ischemia may result from the combination of limited cardiac output, reduced coronary perfusion, and increased myocardial oxygen consumption.

In neonatal critical AS, CHF and shock occur around the time of natural patent ductus arteriosus (PDA) closure. In older children and adolescents, the presentation could be the systolic ejection murmur characteristic for valvar AS.

Balloon aortic valvuloplasty is a safe initial treatment in most patients with congenital aortic valve stenosis (see Figure 47.2). Patients with severely dysplastic valves may have less favorable results with balloon aortic valvuloplasty, but in most patients, the results are similar to those obtained with surgical valvotomy.[10,11] The overall goal, especially in neonates and infants, is to relieve the aortic valve obstruction to a degree sufficient to normalize LV systolic function without inducing significant valve insufficiency. Achievement of this goal typically entails performing a conservative balloon valvuloplasty by reducing the peak-to-peak systolic gradient by 50%. Balloon diameters are usually 85%–90% of the aortic valve annulus dimension measured via aortic angiography. If an unsatisfactory result is encountered and no significant increase in aortic regurgitation is noticed, additional valvuloplasty is performed with larger balloon size. In critically ill patients, surgical backup and circulatory support in the form of an ECMO should be available.

Right and left heart catheterization assessment is indicated prior to valvuloplasty to evaluate the right-sided pressure and the LV end-diastolic pressure. It is best to measure the gradient across the valve by placing a catheter above the valve and another one in the LV simultaneously. In symptomatic patients, this condition may be treated by valvuloplasty even in the presence of a lower gradient. In asymptomatic patients, a peak-to-peak gradient of over 55 mmHg is an indication to proceed. However, often under general anesthesia, the gradient is lower than under normal conditions. Therefore, prior assessment by echocardiography or the administration of dobutamine during catheterization will unmask significant obstruction. Patients with a peak-to-peak aortic gradient <55 mmHg should be followed medically unless they become symptomatic.

Retrograde crossing of the aortic valve via the femoral artery is preferred; however, in neonates, a carotid cut-down is employed by many interventionalists to allow crossing of the valve. Transseptal approach is another technique to cross the valve in an antegrade fashion that was reported to decrease the risk of silent cerebral embolism frequently seen with the retrograde approach. Accordingly, in a series

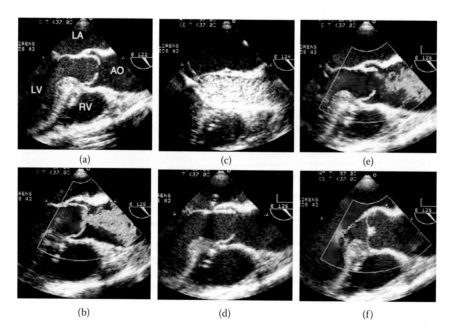

(a) (c) (e)

(b) (d) (f)

Figure 47.2 Transesophageal echocardiographic images during balloon aortic valvuloplasty in a teenage boy. **(a)** Longitudinal view demonstrating the domed stenotic aortic valve; **(b)** same view as **(a)** with color Doppler showing the stenotic mosaic color jet; **(c)** balloon inflation; **(d)** after the valvuloplasty showing complete opening of the valve; **(e)** with color during systole showing improved opening of valve; and **(f)** diastolic frame showing no aortic insufficiency. AO, aorta; LA, left atrium; LV, left ventricle; RV, right ventricle.

of 101 patients, the rate of asymptomatic lesion on magnetic resonance imaging (MRI) was 22%.[12]

Left ventriculography demonstrates the stenotic valve orifice. It is also helpful in evaluating the subaortic and supra-aortic areas for the presence of an additional level of stenosis.

Selection of the balloon size depends on the orifice size measured during angiographic assessment.

ISOLATED VALVULAR PULMONARY STENOSIS

Isolated valvular pulmonary stenosis (PS) represents 8%–10% of all patients with CHD. The stenotic valve is usually dome-shaped with diffuse thickening and commissural fusion. Patients with mild PS are usually asymptomatic. The diagnosis is usually made during routine physical examination with audible ejection systolic murmur. Patients with moderate or severe degrees of PS may have mild exertional dyspnea. Adults may be asymptomatic irrespective of the severity of their obstruction. Patients with severe PS may present with signs of CHF and cyanosis due to shunting of blood across the PFO or ASD. Treatment is indicated in asymptomatic patients with severe PS (peak-to-peak gradient >55 mmHg) or in symptomatic patients with evidence of RV dysfunction irrespective of the gradient.

Balloon pulmonary valvuloplasty was initially described by Kan et al.[13] The overall success rates are excellent (85%) for children with classical PS; however, for patients with dysplastic valves or supravalvular and/or subvalvular PS, the success rate is low (35%–65%).

In selected infants with membranous pulmonary atresia and adequate size RV, perforation of the membrane with either a stiff end of a wire or radiofrequency perforation catheter followed by balloon dilation has been successful in creating an open RVOT.[14–17]

Femoral venous access and right heart catheterization to assess the hemodynamics are performed. Femoral artery access is rarely needed. In neonatal critical PS, umbilical vein access may be used. Right ventricular angiography is performed in both anteroposterior and lateral projections to identify the pulmonary valve and measure the annular size (between the hinge points). The balloon size is selected to be no more than 1.2 times the diameter of the valve annulus. A balloon endhole catheter is advanced to the distal right or left PA. A stiff exchange-length guidewire is then placed in the branch PA. We prefer to insert the balloon via a sheath. This, we believe, minimizes access vessel injury. The balloon is introduced over the guidewire and is centered at the pulmonary valve. Adjustment of the balloon position may be performed by repeated small pressure inflations and waist verification. The balloon is inflated rapidly until the waist disappears and then it is deflated immediately. If suboptimal results with significant residual gradient across the valve are obtained, repositioning of the balloon and repeating the previous steps may be done. Larger balloon size may be used for the second inflation if optimal results are not achieved and no pulmonary regurgitation is observed.

Stenting right ventricular outflow tract in patients with tetralogy of Fallot

TOF is the most common congenital cyanotic heart disease. In certain groups of TOF patients, significant narrowing of the RVOT and pulmonary valve impair adequate oxygenation in the newborn period and dictate an early intervention to establish acceptable pulmonary blood flow. Neonatal corrective surgery might not be feasible due to low weight, associated syndromes, or other comorbidities. Palliative stenting of the RVOT and pulmonary valve, either via a percutaneous approach or a hybrid approach, becomes handy and valuable in this group of patients. Castleberry et al. reported their experience in RVOT stenting. All their five patients showed significant improvement of both oxygenation and pulmonary tree diameter. The result of RVOT stenting was greatly comparable to surgical Blalock–Taussig shunt palliation.[18]

Femoral vein access was established followed by right ventriculography in cranially angulated anteroposterior and lateral projections to measure the PV annulus, RVOT, and PA branches. Wire passage through pulmonary valve was facilitated by a right coronary catheter with a 1.5 or 2 cm curve (Judkins, Merit Medical OEM, South Jordan, UT). Directing the wire into the right PA provided secure wire position for the subsequent balloon dilation and stenting. Balloon angioplasty of the pulmonary valve is usually performed first, followed by stent deployment into the RVOT. Please refer to detailed step-by-step balloon pulmonary valvuloplasty discussed earlier in this chapter. Stent selection depends on the size and length of RVOT. A premounted ParaMount Mini GPS (EV3, Polymouth, MN) or coronary balloon expandable stent are usually used. Stent diameter should be 1–2 mm greater than the annular dimension of the RVOT.

ADDITIONAL INTERVENTIONS IN ADULTS WITH CONGENITAL HEART DISEASE

Coarctation of the aorta

COA is a relatively common defect that accounts for 5%–8% of all CHDs. COA occurs as an isolated lesion or in association with other congenital heart defects, the most common of which are bicuspid aortic valve and VSD. Coarctation almost always occurs in the thoracic aorta distal to the origin of the left subclavian artery. Neonates with critical COA may present with shock-like symptoms around the time of ductal closure. Less severe COA may not be detected until later in childhood or even in adulthood. One of the most common late presentations is systemic hypertension. Murmur may be another late presentation sign secondary to the presence of a well-developed collateral arterial system.

Indications for COA treatment are basically the same as those for surgery and include hypertension proximal to the coarctation with a resting systolic pressure gradient across the narrowed segment >20 mmHg or angiographically

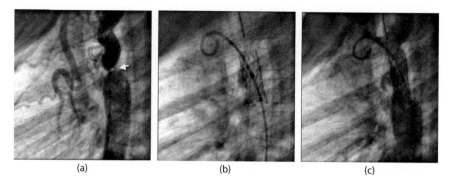

Figure 47.3 Cinefluoroscopic images in straight lateral projection in a patient with coarctation of the aorta. (a) Angiogram in the ascending aorta showing severe coarctation of the aorta (*arrow*) and presence of collaterals. (b) Cine frame showing the stent that was implanted at the site of coarctation. (c) Final angiogram showing good stent position, no residual obstruction. The distal end of the stent is not fully apposed to the wall of the aorta.

severe coarctation with extensive collaterals.[19] Coarctation angioplasty requires femoral venous and arterial access (Figure 47.3). The patient is heparinized to achieve an ACT of >200 seconds. Retrograde approach is the most commonly used technique; however, on occasions in severe coarctation or if there is acquired atresia, crossing from above (transseptal or left subclavian artery) is indicated. Right and left heart catheterization with hemodynamic assessment is performed. Biplane aortography is performed. The narrowest area of the coarctation is measured, as well as the proximal, distal, and the aorta at the level of the diaphragm. Balloon size selection depends on the nature of the coarctation. In native coarctation, the balloon size is selected to be equal to the aorta at the isthmus. In postoperative coarctation, the balloon is chosen to be around 2.5 to 3 times the diameter of the narrowest coarctation area but not more than the area immediately distal to the coarctation (poststenotic dilatation).

The selected balloon is centered at the coarctation area. The balloon is inflated until the waist disappears and then deflated immediately. Simultaneous pressure measurement between the ascending and descending aorta pressures is obtained. Angiography is performed after balloon inflation to determine the effect of angioplasty on the coarctation area. Tears or dissection of the aorta may also be detected. If optimal results are not achieved with the presence of significant residual gradient across the coarctation area, a larger balloon may be used for a second inflation. Temporary chest pain during balloon inflation is acceptable. If chest pain persists after balloon deflation, dissection may be present. It is important to note that at no time should the freshly dilated area be crossed with a catheter. Therefore, once a guidewire is left in place and is used for the angioplasty, all catheter manipulations are performed over this wire to prevent disruption of the freshly dilated area.

In the adult patient, stent angioplasty is currently preferred over balloon angioplasty for both native and recurrent coarctation. Stent placement eliminates the elastic recoil of aortic tissue observed after balloon angioplasty. It also allows the use of smaller balloon size, minimizing the risks of using large balloons. Stent placement was noticed to

have less residual gradient and better opening of the coarctation segment. Covered stents should be available in any catheterization laboratory engaged in balloon/stent angioplasty of coarctation. We routinely use covered stents for appropriate coarctation in any patient with an adult-size aorta (around 18–20 mm). Covered stents can be used as a primary tool or as bailout therapy after angioplasty to treat dissections or aneurysms.

Pulmonary artery stenosis

PAS accounts for 2%–3% of all CHD. PAS may be isolated (Williams syndrome, Alagille syndrome) or associated with more complex CHD, such as TOF or transposition of the great arteries. PAS may be also central, peripheral, intermediate, unilateral, or bilateral. Gay et al. established four PAS classes according to the anatomic location of the narrowing. Type I includes single constriction of varying length confined to the main pulmonary artery (MPA), the right pulmonary artery (RPA), or the left pulmonary artery (LPA) (types IA, IB, and IC, respectively). Type II includes bifurcation stenosis where the constriction involves the distal end of the MPA, RPA, and LPA. This type is further subdivided into IIA, where the narrowing segment is short and localized, and IIB, where the narrowing segment is long. Type III includes multiple peripheral stenosis, and type IV includes combined central and peripheral stenosis.[20]

Patients with mild to moderate arterial obstruction are usually asymptomatic. Cases with severe stenosis may have dyspnea on exertion, easy fatigability, and occasional right-sided heart failure. Treatment of PAS depends on the site of the stenotic segment. Percutaneous pulmonary angioplasty is suitable for distal lesions unreachable by surgery, and surgical pulmonary arterioplasty is feasible for more proximal lesions.

Variable modalities of percutaneous techniques include balloon pulmonary angioplasty using high-pressure balloons (Figure 47.4), cutting balloon angioplasty, and intravascular stent placement. Despite advances in balloon types and pressure achieved, around one-third of vessels, more often distal, are resistant to angioplasty. The use of cutting balloons is an effective treatment for small lobar PAS

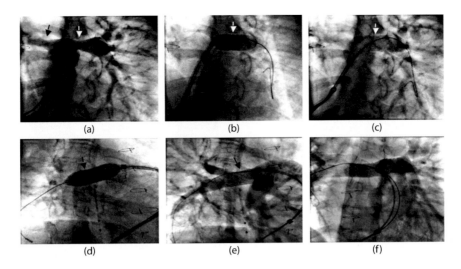

Figure 47.4 Cinefluoroscopic views in a patient with bilateral branch pulmonary artery stenosis at their origin.
(a) Angiogram in the main pulmonary artery showing the narrowing at the origin of each branch (*white* and *black arrows*).
(b) Stent deployment in the left pulmonary artery (*arrow*). **(c)** Angiogram in the left pulmonary artery after the stent deployment showing expansion of the area with good result. **(d)** Stent deployment in the right pulmonary artery (*arrow*). **(e)** Angiogram in the right pulmonary artery showing expansion of the area and good result. **(f)** Final angiogram showing elimination of the narrowing.

refractory to balloon angioplasty.[21] Stenting of branch pulmonary arteries is frequently used in children with PAS and/or hypoplasia.[22-24] Because of the higher immediate success and less incidence of restenosis, stenting of pulmonary arteries may be a reasonable first-line therapy.

The most commonly used access is the femoral vein. Right heart catheterization with hemodynamic assessment is performed first. PA angiography is then performed to localize the affected segment(s). Selective injection to the lung and the lobe affected is highly recommended. Before starting the balloon dilation procedure, a stiff exchange-length wire should be placed in a large vessel distal to the stenotic branch. The selected balloon diameter should be two to four times the diameter of the narrow segment but not more than two times the diameter of the normal vessel on either side of the lesion.[25] The balloon is inflated until the waist disappears. After dilation, the area is reassessed by pressure recording across the dilated area and angiography. Successful dilation results in improved diameter of the segment, increase in distal pressure, and/or a decrease of >20% in systolic RV to aortic pressure ratio.

Cutting balloons may be used for vessels resistant to conventional balloon angioplasty. Initially, the vessel is dilated with the cutting balloon and then a high-pressure balloon is employed to open up the vessel to a larger diameter. One limiting factor about cutting balloons is the lack of availability of large sizes since the largest cutting balloon available is 8 mm. Therefore, cutting balloon angioplasty is good for vessels up to 8 mm in diameter.

Stent placement of the affected area will avoid the recoil nature encountered after balloon angioplasty. However, stent placement is technically more challenging and could potentially have more complications and commit the patient to repeat interventions, especially if continued growth of the

patient is expected. Intraoperative intravascular stent placement is a hybrid technique that could be used in difficult situations. It is suitable in the early postoperative period, with difficult vascular anatomy, in bilateral stenosis requiring simultaneous stent implantation, with short proximal segment stenosis (too short for the shortest stent available), with marginal hemodynamics, severe bilateral branch stenosis, in patients on ECMO, and in patients with other cardiac lesions requiring concomitant surgery.[26]

Coronary artery fistula

Coronary artery fistula (CAF) is a connection between one or more of the coronary arteries and a cardiac chamber or great vessel, bypassing the myocardial capillary bed. The abnormality is rare—the exact incidence is unknown—and usually occurs as an isolated finding. The fistulas originate from the right coronary artery in more than half of the cases. The left anterior descending coronary artery is the next most frequently involved, in approximately one-third of cases, followed by the circumflex coronary artery.[27] Most of the fistulas from either coronary artery drain into the right side of the heart. The RV is the most common site for drainage followed by the right atrium (RA), coronary sinus, and lastly, the PA trunk.

Most patients with CAF are asymptomatic. Diagnosis is usually suspected when a continuous murmur is detected during a routine visit or examination for other reasons. Symptoms depend on the size of the fistula, which is usually small, and the pressure difference between the two sides of the fistula. Rarely, CHF occurs. CAFs usually are small in size and close spontaneously by the second decade of life. If not closed, complications may be the first presenting symptom. Reported complications include steal from the adjacent myocardium causing myocardial ischemia, thrombosis and embolism, cardiac failure, atrial fibrillation (AF), rupture, endocarditis/endarteritis, and arrhythmias.[27–30] Other reported rare complications include thrombosis within the fistula, leading to acute MI; atrial or ventricular arrhythmias; and spontaneous rupture of the aneurysmal fistula causing hemopericardium.[31,32]

Cardiac catheterization is the main diagnostic technique. Cardiac catheterization is needed initially to assess the hemodynamic significance of the fistula and to provide detailed anatomy, including size, origin, course, presence of any stenosis, and the drainage site.

The main goal of treatment of CAF is complete occlusion with no residual fistulae. Catheter closure of the fistulas is now considered to be a safe and effective alternative to surgery. Catheter closure should be as distal to the endpoint of the fistula as possible to avoid possible occlusion of branches to the normal myocardium.

Selective coronary angiography is needed to confirm the diagnosis and the detailed anatomy of the fistula. Detailed angiographic views in multiple projections are essential to the successful treatment of these fistulas.

Access is usually obtained in both femoral arteries and one femoral vein (Figure 47.5). One arterial access is used for angiographic assessment and the other for the actual closure of the fistula. We use a coaxial system to manage these fistulas. A coronary guide catheter of proper size and shape is advanced to the ostium of the involved coronary artery. The fistula is crossed with the proper coronary exchange-length wire. Then a Berman endhole balloon catheter is passed over this wire inside the guide catheter, and the balloon is positioned distal to the last viable myocardial branch and inflated with contrast to temporarily occlude the vessel for 5–10 minutes to assess the risk of ischemia with fistula occlusion. If no detectable ischemic changes are noted, then the choice of technique is based on the size of the fistula and on the available equipment. Coils or devices (Amplatzer PDA device, Amplatzer vascular plug, Amplatzer VSD devices) can be used to close the fistula. If coils are chosen, they are usually deployed retrograde (going from the guide catheter inside the delivery catheter, positioned distal), and if devices are chosen, the wire is usually snared and exteriorized from either the femoral or jugular vein and the proper size sheath is advanced into the fistula; then the device is advanced from the vein to the fistula. The guide catheter is used for selective injections to guide the deployment site and to look for other feeding vessels.[33]

Complete occlusion of the fistula may be achieved in >95% of patients. The remaining patients may be managed conservatively if the residual fistulas are small, or further procedures may be required.

Complications of the procedure are rare and include coil embolization, transient ischemic changes, transient bundle branch block, and MI.[34] Postclosure, we recommend the use of antiplatelet agents (if fistulas are small) or

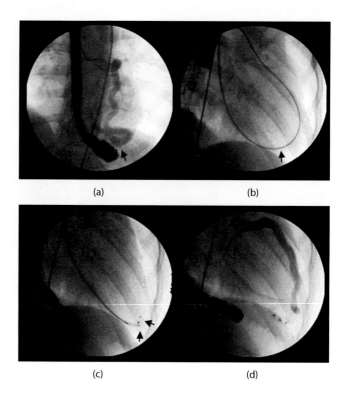

(a)

(b)

(c)

(d)

Figure 47.5 Cine fluoroscopic images in a patient with left anterior descending coronary artery to right ventricle fistula. **(a)** Selective left main coronary angiogram showing the distal end of the fistula draining into the right ventricle. **(b)** The fistula was crossed (*arrow*) retrograde and the wire was exteriorized from the right internal jugular vein. **(c)** Deployment of the second Amplatzer vascular plug from the right internal jugular vein to the distal end of the fistula, note the two plugs (*arrows*). **(d)** Final angiogram showing complete closure of the fistula.

anticoagulation (if large) to prevent thrombosis and closure of the larger main coronary artery.

Aortopulmonary collaterals

Collateral vessels occur in a wide variety of conditions, including pulmonary atresia with VSD, TOF, scimitar syndrome, and in hearts undergoing Fontan-type reconstruction. They may be arterial or venous and may shunt left-to-right or right-to-left. APCs typically originate from the descending aorta and connect with true pulmonary arteries at different levels. The potential disadvantage of APCs in patients with univentricular physiology include left-to-right shunts causing volume overload on the ventricle and unwanted blood return on the operative field during cardiopulmonary bypass. The increased pulmonary blood flow also raises the PA pressure. Ventricular volume overload and elevated PA pressure have been identified as risk factors for the Fontan operation. Hemoptysis from rupture of thin-walled vessels may also occur as one of the adverse effects of APCs.

Before an APC artery is embolized, the presence of dual blood supply from the true pulmonary arteries to the affected segment of the lung should be determined. Embolization should only be performed if true pulmonary arteries supply the same territories as the collateral vessel.

Various agents or devices are used for embolization of APCs, including tissue adhesives, Gelfoam, detachable balloons, and coils. Sharma et al. reported on APC occlusions in one of the largest series in this field of 56 patients.[35] Indications for occlusion in this study were hemoptysis, intractable cardiac failure, and routine preoperative procedure in most of the patients. Complete occlusion was achieved in 76% of cases with an 8% failure rate secondary to migration of the coils to the distal pulmonary arteries.

The technique of closure is similar to the techniques used in CAF embolization and other extracardiac vascular abnormalities. Coil migration is still one of the most common complications, and use of detachable coils leads to a marked decrease in the risk of coil migration.

Pulmonary arteriovenous fistula

Pulmonary AVF is an abnormal communication between pulmonary arteries and pulmonary veins. It can be either congenital (most of the cases) or sometimes acquired, especially in patients after bidirectional Glenn anastomosis for single ventricle. The clinical presentation varies from no symptoms to severe illness. The most common clinical presentation includes epistaxis, dyspnea, and hemoptysis. Cyanosis may occur from the right-to-left shunt between the pulmonary arteries and pulmonary veins. The resultant shunt may lead to paradoxical embolus, resulting in stroke or transient ischemic attack (TIA). Acquired fistula is seen in patients after cavopulmonary anastomosis and less in patients after Fontan surgery. Transcatheter embolization of pulmonary AVF is considered the mainstay of treatment of this abnormality.[36–39] The technique of embolization is not different from closure of the other extracardiac vascular anomalies (CAFs and APCs). The most commonly used device is the Gianturco coils. Embolization of the entire nidus of the malformation is important to prevent recanalization. All feeding vessels should be identified and embolized. The risk of coil migration through the malformation into systemic circulation has been eliminated with detachable coils. Detachable balloons are reserved for malformations with larger feeding vessels >1 cm in diameter.

Percutaneous pulmonary valve implantation

The presence of severe pulmonary insufficiency may lead to RV enlargement and dysfunction. Surgical placement of a competent valve between the RV and pulmonary arteries to treat this condition requires cardiopulmonary bypass, which may aggravate an already compromised RV. Bonhoeffer was the first to place a valve in this position percutaneously[40] and since then, thousands of patients have benefited from his technique.[41] Currently, two valves are being evaluated for the percutaneous management of patients with severe conduit failure due to regurgitation and/or stenosis. The Medtronic Melody valve developed by Bonhoeffer (Figure 47.6) consists of a bovine jugular vein

with a valve inside sewn into a Platinum Cheatham stent. The Edwards SAPIEN THV[42] is made of bovine pericardial leaflets sewn inside a stainless steel stent. Both valves are balloon expandable and require a large delivery system for deployment (up to 22- to 24-Fr).

Current indications for PPVI include patients with moderate to severe pulmonary regurgitation who are symptomatic. In the absence of symptoms, we rely on objective parameters obtained by MRI, including indexed right ventricular end-diastolic volume (RVEDV) of 150 mL/m^2, RV dysfunction (right ventricular ejection fraction [RVEF] of 40%, or less), pulmonary regurgitant fraction of 40%, or more. Finally, electrocardiographic prolongation of QRS duration of 180 ms or more, which oftentimes is associated with malignant ventricular arrhythmias.

Technical considerations for percutaneous pulmonary valve implantation

Transcatheter pulmonary valve replacement is usually performed under general anesthesia with biplane fluoroscopic guidance.[43] Femoral or jugular access can be performed. Jugular access is usually preferred to provide a more favorable anatomic curvature for valve delivery. Right heart catheterization is initially performed to assess pressures and saturations with special attention to any relevant pulmonary branch stenosis. The balloon-tipped catheter is then replaced with a ultrastiff guidewire (0.035-in Lunderquist ultra stiff [Cook, Bloomington, IN]) and positioned into a distal branch PA, preferably the left lower branch, given its vertical orientation, to provide adequate support to advance the delivery system. Biplane RVOT angiography is performed to assess the proposed site for device implantation and measurement of the PA trunk where the valve will be implanted. Simultaneous coronary angiography should be performed during full balloon inflation in the RVOT to assess the course and proximity of the coronary arteries to the RVOT due to the risk of compression with RVOT expansion. We believe this is a crucial step in the procedure and should be performed in all patients, especially when the coronary arteries are close to the RVOT.

Presenting of the conduit with a bare-metal or covered stent, if available, has several advantages. It is required in almost all cases (for the Edwards valve due to the short length of the valve) to provide a landing zone for the stented valve, and to reduce the risk of stent fracture (for Melody valve). The stent is typically deployed on a BiB (balloon-in-balloon) catheter (NuMED Inc., Hopkinton, NY) to a diameter of up to 2 mm less than the original conduit size in stenotic conduits or slightly larger in conduits without stenosis. We typically use the balloon-expandable IntraStent (ev3, Plymouth, MN) or the Palmaz XL stents. Covered stents, when available, can be alternatively used if there are concerns of conduit rupture. This is important in heavily calcified conduits. Postdilatation of the stent using a noncompliant balloon may be needed to achieve the intended final diameter. Pressure measurements after stenting should document no to minimal residual

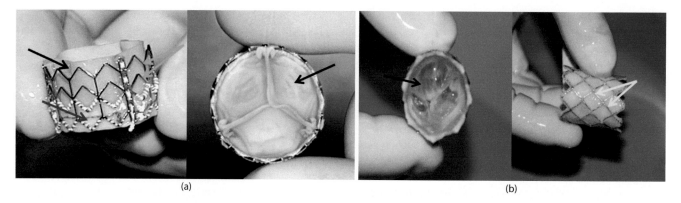

Figure 47.6 **(a)** The Edwards SAPIEN Pulmonic Transcatheter Heart Valve (PHV). It is a bovine pericardium valve (*black arrows*) with a radiopaque, stainless steel balloon-expandable support structure (frame) (*blue arrows*), and a polyethylene terephthalate fabric cuff (*red arrow*). **(b)** The Melody valve. This is a bovine jugular vein valve (*black arrow*) sutured within a platinum iridium stent (*yellow arrows*). The valve leaflets are thin and compliant and open fully and close readily with minimum of pressure.

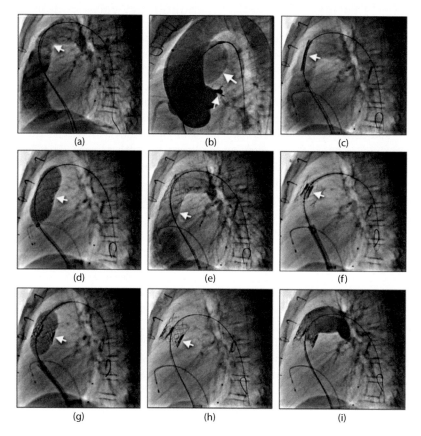

Figure 47.7 Steps of SAPIEN valve placement. **(a)** Pulmonary homograft angiography demonstrates severe pulmonic regurgitation. **(b)** Conduit balloon sizing with simultaneous aortic root angiography. Large arrow shows the balloon inflation in the conduit; small arrow demonstrates left coronary artery with an acceptable distance from the conduit. **(c)** Bare-metal stent placement in conduit with hand injection angiography to delineate stent position. **(d)** Balloon stent deployment. **(e)** Angiography post-stent deployment demonstrating no conduit stenosis with free pulmonary regurgitation. **(f)** SAPIEN valve positioned in the middle of the stent. **(g)** Balloon deployment of the valve. **(h)** Excellent valve position inside the stent. **(i)** Final angiography in conduit demonstrating no significant pulmonary regurgitation.

gradient across the outflow tract prior to proceeding with device implantation. The appropriate device size is then selected based on the diameter of the balloon at full inflation during prestenting. For the Melody valve, the choice of Ensemble delivery system depends on the size of the conduit.

As for the SAPIEN valve, prosthesis size is determined based on the degree of conduit stenosis.

After appropriate device selection, the delivery system is advanced over the guidewire, bringing the valve into the implantation site (Figures 47.7 and 47.8). A maneuver that

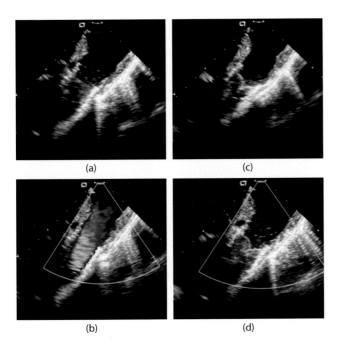

Figure 47.8 Intracardiac echocardiography (ICE) images during SAPIEN valve placement. **(a)** Two-dimensional ICE in systole demonstrating complete opening of SAPIEN valve leaflets. **(b)** Color Doppler in systole demonstrating no narrowing passing SAPIEN valve. **(c)** Two-dimensional ICE in diastole demonstrates complete valve closure. **(d)** Color Doppler in diastole demonstrates trivial pulmonary regurgitation.

can facilitate advancing the delivery system when it is at the entrance of the conduit is looping (buckling) the system within the RA. This generates a forward force aiding passage into the conduit. Once the Melody valve is in the appropriate position, it is unsheathed, followed by gradual inflation of the inner then the outer balloons. Slow inflation allows time to adjust the position in the event of device slippage. Similarly, the SAPIEN valve is inflated on a single balloon slowly. Repeat angiography and pressure measurements are made to confirm a positive outcome. Occasionally, the implanted valves may require postdilatation with a noncompliant balloon.

In patients with RVOT larger than the maximum size of available percutaneous valves, a hybrid approach can be implemented where a full median sternotomy is performed; plication of the PA to the designated size and a stab incision on the anterior surface of the proximal RVOT just proximal to the infundibulum/infundibular patch is created. This approach is done on a beating heart with a shorter recovery/hospital stay time. A newly developed tissue valve mounted on a self-expanding stent, the No-React Injectable BioPulmonic (BioIntegral Surgical Inc., Toronto, Canada), is then introduced.[44] For young TOF patients who meet the criteria for valve placement but their small body surface area/vessel size will not accommodate the large delivery system, another hybrid approach can be performed. This approach involves a subxiphoid incision and a delivery sheath to implant the valve, inserted into the RV.[45]

New large valves for patients with native outflow tract (post-transannular patch repair) are being developed. One such valve is the Venus P, which is made of a self-expandable nitinol stent and a porcine pericardial valve leaflet.[46]

CONCLUSIONS

This chapter has summarized interventional techniques used for treating CHDs in the catheterization laboratory. Adult CHD is a growing field and requires skilled personnel trained in both adult and pediatric CHDs who understand the physiology and anatomy of the cardiac lesion. The practice of interventional cardiology for CHD also requires a fully equipped catheterization laboratory to help minimize the risks of such procedures. Anesthesia, as well as surgical backup, are crucial in any institution practicing congenital cardiac intervention. Last, cardiac intervention is a rapidly growing and expanding field that now involves, at its far end, percutaneous valve placement and valve repair.

REFERENCES

1. Patel A, et al. Intracardiac echocardiography to guide closure of atrial septal defects in children less than 15 kilograms. *Catheter Cardiovasc Interv* 2006;68:287–291.
2. Lewis DA, et al. Descriptive epidemiology of membranous and muscular ventricular septal defects in the Baltimore-Washington Infant Study. *Cardiol Young* 1996;6(4):281–290.
3. Miyague NI, et al. Epidemiological study of congenital heart defects in children and adolescents. Analysis of 4,538 cases. *Arq Bras Cardiol* 2003;80(3):269–278.
4. Kirklin JW, Barrat-Boyes BG. Cardiac surgery: Morphology, diagnostic criteria, natural history, techniques, results and indications. In: Kirklin JW, Barrat-Boyes BG, eds. *Ventricular Septal Defects*. New York: Churchill Livingstone, 1985:749–824.
5. Lock JE, et al. Transcatheter closure of ventricular septal defects. *Circulation* 1988;78(2):361–368.
6. Holzer R, et al. Device closure of muscular ventricular septal defects using the Amplatzer muscular ventricular septal defect occluder: Immediate and mid-term results of a U.S. registry. *J Am Coll Cardiol* 2004;43(7):1257–1263.
7. Bacha EA, et al. Multicenter experience with perventricular device closure of muscular ventricular septal defects. *Pediatr Cardiol* 2005;26(2):169–175.
8. Amin Z, et al. Intraoperative closure of muscular ventricular septal defect in a canine model and applicability of the technique in a baby. *J Thorac Cardiovasc Surg* 1998;115:1374–1376.
9. Hijazi ZM, et al. Transcatheter closure of single muscular ventricular septal defects using the amplatzer muscular VSD occluder: Initial results and technical considerations. *Cathet Cardiovasc Interv* 2000;49:167–172.
10. Moore P, et al. Midterm results of balloon dilation of congenital aortic stenosis: Predictors of success. *J Am Coll Cardiol* 1996;27(5):1257–1263.
11. Pedra CA, et al. Outcomes after balloon dilation of congenital aortic stenosis in children and adolescents. *Cardiol Young* 2004;14(3):315–321.

12. Omran H, et al. Silent and apparent cerebral embolism after retrograde catheterisation of the aortic valve in valvular stenosis: A prospective, randomised study. *Lancet* 2003;361(9365):1241–1246.

13. Kan JS, et al. Percutaneous transluminal balloon valvuloplasty for pulmonary valve stenosis. *Circulation* 1984;69(3):554–560.

14. Alwi M, et al. Pulmonary atresia with intact ventricular septum percutaneous radiofrequency-assisted valvotomy and balloon dilation versus surgical valvotomy and Blalock Taussig shunt. *J Am Coll Cardiol* 2000;35(2):468–476.

15. Hausdorf G, et al. Catheter creation of an open outflow tract in previously atretic right ventricular outflow tract associated with ventricular septal defect. *Am J Cardiol* 1993;72(3):354–356.

16. Hijazi ZM, et al. Transcatheter retrograde radio- frequency perforation of the pulmonic valve in pulmonary atresia with intact ventricular septum, using a 2 French catheter. *Cathet Cardiovasc Diagn* 1998;45(2):151–154.

17. Humpl T, et al. Percutaneous balloon valvotomy in pulmonary atresia with intact ventricular septum: Impact on patient care. *Circulation* 2003;108(7):826–832.

18. Castleberry CD, et al. Stenting of the right ventricular outflow tract in the high-risk infant with cyanotic teratology of Fallot. *Pediatr Cardiol* 2014;35(3):423–430.

19. Allen HD, et al. Pediatric therapeutic cardiac catheterization: A statement for healthcare professionals from the Council on Cardiovascular Disease in the Young, American Heart Association. *Circulation* 1998;97(6):609–625.

20. Gay BB Jr, et al. The roentgenologic features of single and multiple coarctations of the pulmonary artery and branches. *Am J Roentgenol Radium Ther Nucl Med* 1963;90:599–613.

21. Bergersen L, et al. Follow-up results of cutting balloon angioplasty used to relieve stenoses in small pulmonary arteries. *Cardiol Young* 2005;15(6):605–610.

22. Fogelman R, et al. Endovascular stents in the pulmonary circulation. Clinical impact on management and medium-term follow-up. *Circulation* 1995;92(4):881–885.

23. O'Laughlin MP, et al. Use of endovascular stents in congenital heart disease. *Circulation* 1991;83(6):1923–1939.

24. O'Laughlin MP, et al. Implantation and intermediate-term follow-up of stents in congenital heart disease. *Circulation* 1993;88(2):605–614.

25. Rao PS, et al. Five- to nine-year follow-up results of balloon angioplasty of native aortic coarctation in infants and children. *J Am Coll Cardiol* 1996;27(2):462–470.

26. Ing FF. Delivery of stents to target lesions: Techniques of intra- operative stent implantation and intraoperative angiograms. *Pediatr Cardiol* 2005;6(3):260–266.

27. McNamara JJ, Gross RE. Congenital coronary artery fistula. *Surgery* 1969;65(1):59–69.

28. Alkhulaifi AM, et al. Coronary artery fistulas presenting with bacterial endocarditis. *Ann Thorac Surg* 1995;60(1):202–204.

29. Skimming JW, Walls JT. Congenital coronary artery fistula suggesting a "steal phenomenon" in a neonate. *Pediatr Cardiol* 1993;14(3):174–175.

30. Wilde P, Watt I. Congenital coronary artery fistulae: Six new cases with a collective review. *Clin Radiol* 1980;31(3):301–311.

31. Bauer HH, et al. Congenital coronary arteriovenous fistula: Spontaneous rupture and cardiac tamponade. *Ann Thorac Surg* 1996;62(5):1521–1523.

32. Ramo OJ, et al. Thrombosed coronary artery fistula as a cause of paroxysmal atrial fibrillation and ventricular arrhythmia. *Cardiovasc Surg* 1994;2(6):720–722.

33. Qureshi SA. Coronary arterial fistulas. *Orphanet J Rare Dis* 2006;1:51.

34. Kharouf R, et al. Transcatheter closure of coronary artery fistula complicated by myocardial infarction. *J Invasive Cardiol* 2007;19(5):E146–E149.

35. Sharma S, et al. Systemic-to-pulmonary artery collateral vessels and surgical shunts in patients with cyanotic congenital heart disease: Perioperative treatment by transcatheter embolization. *AJR Am J Roentgenol* 1995;164(6):1505–1510.

36. Dutton JA, et al. Pulmonary arteriovenous malformations: Results of treatment with coil embolization in 53 patients. *AJR Am J Roentgenol* 1995;165(5):1119–1125.

37. Lee DW, et al. Embolotherapy of large pulmonary arteriovenous malformations: Long-term results. *Ann Thorac Surg* 1997;64(4):930–939; discussion 939–940.

38. Mager JJ, et al. Embolotherapy of pulmonary arteriovenous malformations: Long-term results in 112 patients. *J Vasc Interv Radiol* 2004;15(5):451–456.

39. White RI Jr, et al. Pulmonary arteriovenous malformations: Techniques and long-term outcome of embolotherapy. *Radiology* 1988;169(3):663–669.

40. Bonhoeffer P, et al. Percutaneous replacement of pulmonary valve in a right-ventricle to pulmonary-artery prosthetic conduit with valve dysfunction. *Lancet* 2000;356(9239):1403–1405.

41. Lurz P, et al. Percutaneous pulmonary valve implantation: Impact of evolving technology and learning curve on clinical outcome. *Circulation* 2008;117(15):1964–1972.

42. Garay F, et al. Percutaneous replacement of pulmonary valve using the Edwards-Cribier percutaneous heart valve: First report in a human patient. *Catheter Cardiovasc Interv* 2006;67(5):659–662.

43. Suradi HS, Hijazi ZM. Percutaneous pulmonary valve implantation. *Glob Cardiol Sci Pract* 2015;2015(2):23.

44. Suleiman T, et al. Recent development in pulmonary valve replacement after tetralogy of fallot repair: The emergence of hybrid approaches. *Front Surg* 2015;2:22.

45. Holoshitz N, et al. Perventricular melody valve implantation in a 12 kg child. *Catheter Cardiovasc Interv* 2013;82(5):824–827.

46. Cao QL, et al. Early clinical experience with a novel self-expanding percutaneous stent-valve in the native right ventricular outflow tract. *Catheter Cardiovasc Interv* 2014;84(7):1131–1137.

48

Embolization for fistulas and arteriovenous malformations

NICHOLAS KIPSHIDZE, ROBERT J. ROSEN, AND IRAKLI GOGORISHVILI

PERIPHERAL ARTERIOVENOUS MALFORMATIONS

Introduction

An arteriovenous fistula is an abnormal connection between an artery and a vein. As a consequence, the blood bypasses the capillary bed. The majority of arteriovenous malformations (AVMs) are congenital, but some can be acquired due to trauma, infection, or malignancy. An arteriovenous fistula (AVF) may be the result of a vascular catheter insertion or may be created surgically to provide access for hemodialysis in patients with end-stage kidney failure. AVMs can occur anywhere in the body, including the central nervous system. Congenital AVMs are present at birth, and although they may be asymptomatic, they always persist and do not involute,[1,2] unlike true hemangiomas. AVMs may become symptomatic with age, sometimes at puberty in female patients, during pregnancy, or after trauma. Of special interest are pulmonary AVMs, mostly related to hereditary hemorrhagic telangiectasia (Osler-Weber-Rendu syndrome), a condition that is discussed later in the chapter.

Anatomic considerations

Vascular malformations are divided into low- and high-flow lesions. Low-flow malformations are venous, lymphatic, or mixed and therefore cause congestion of either type.

High-flow lesions contain an arterial component and determine left-to-right shunt.

AVMs types differ with respect to clinical course and treatment options. High-flow malformations are less common, more difficult to treat, and prone to recurrence. High-flow AVMs result in a similar pathophysiology to AVFs and may result in:

1. Compressive and erosive effects
2. Venous stasis
3. Ischemia due to peripheral steal phenomenon
4. And high-output heart failure

Although AVMs can occur anywhere in the body, the pelvis and the extremities are the most common locations for peripheral AVMs.

Clinical aspects

Pelvic AVMs (Figure 48.1) may produce pain, pelvic venous congestion, sexual dysfunction, and, occasionally, high-output cardiac failure and hemorrhage. With respect to hemorrhage, this is generally a lower gastrointestinal bleed or hematuria, while hemorrhage in the abdominal cavity is extremely rare. Although the most frequent blood supply of pelvic AVMs arises from the hypogastric arteries, there may also be multiple feeding branches from the inferior mesenteric artery, middle sacral artery, lumbar artery, and femoral arteries.[3] Extremity AVM (Figure 48.2) symptoms

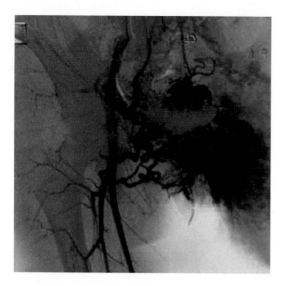

Figure 48.1 Pelvic AVM. AVM, arteriovenous malformation.

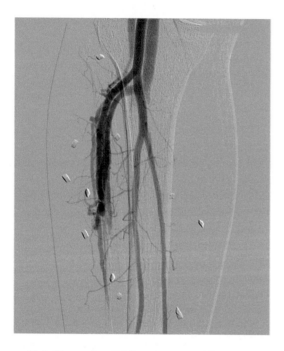

Figure 48.2 Extremity AVM. A 23-year-old soldier with traumatic arteriovenous fistula treated later with stent graft. AVM, arteriovenous malformation. (Courtesy of Kipshidze University Hospital.)

range from mild swelling or soft tissue mass, extremity overgrowth or growth retardation, bleeding, ulceration, gangrene, or rarely, congestive heart failure.

Indications for treatment

Treatment of AVMs, especially high-flow AVMs, is challenging and not always successful regardless of the type of procedure chosen (percutaneous, surgical, or combined). Treatment should therefore be undertaken only when clinically indicated.[3] Asymptomatic lesions that are discovered

Table 48.1 Indications for treatment in arteriovenous malformations

Absolute indications for treatment
- Hemorrhage, major or recurrent minor
- Gangrene or ulcer of arterial, venous, or combined origin
- Ischemic complication of acute and/or chronic arterial insufficiency
- Progressive venous complication of chronic venous insufficiency with venous hypertension
- High-output cardiac failure (clinical and/or laboratory)
- Lesion located at life-threatening vital areas that compromises vision, hearing, eating, or breathing

Relative indications for treatment
- Various symptoms and signs affecting the quality of life; disabling pain and/or functional impairment
- Lesions with a potentially high risk of complications (e.g., hemarthrosis) and/or limb-threatening location
- Lesions causing limb length discrepancy
- Cosmetically severe deformity with or without functional disability

incidentally generally do not require treatment. Absolute and relative indications for treatment are listed in Table 48.1.

Principles of treatment

The mainstay of treatment of high-flow AVMs is permanently closing or eliminating the vascular nidus where arterial blood is shunted to the veins.

Historically, surgical treatment alone proved to be inadequate or even disastrous, often leading to extensive damage to adjacent structures with high recurrence rates or major amputation.[4,5] The reason for failure is that it is rarely possible to completely resect the nidus, which can be large or supplied by multiple collaterals. Proximal ligation of feeding arterial branches is ineffective as aggressive recruitment of new feeding collaterals is common.[6,7]

Disappointing results of surgical treatment stimulated the development of alternative approaches. The introduction of embolotherapy in the early 1970s[8,9] and advancements in catheter technology made it possible to treat AVMs less invasively. Although AVMs are uncommon, data about interventions and follow-up are increasing.[10–15] Some centers document very promising results with interventional treatment. However, several reports have documented worsening of symptoms after embolization.[16] This is why most authors recommend intervention only for patients with significant symptoms.[11,13]

Embolization technique

The goal of treatment is to occlude the nidus of the malformation through selective catheterization and embolization of feeding branches (Figure 48.3).

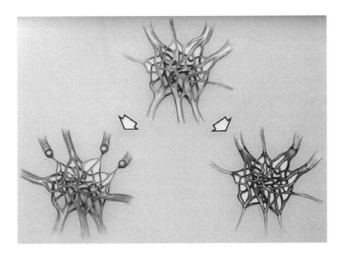

Figure 48.3 AVM "nidus" showing that only complete occlusion of all feeding branches will result in complete AVM elimination. AVM, arteriovenous malformation.

Embolization of the nidus of an AVM often requires super-selective catheterization of numerous arterial feeding branches. This is facilitated by use of coaxial microcatheter systems. A 2- to 3-Fr microcatheter is coaxially introduced through a 4- to 5-Fr selective catheter and can be manipulated into the terminal feeding artery. Embolic agents are then delivered via the microcatheter, an ideal tool for the delivery of liquid agents, particles, and small coils.

Embolic agents for high-flow lesions

Use of the proper embolic agent (Table 48.2) is critical when treating AVMs, as the wrong agent may not only fail to treat the lesion, but may also interfere with future attempts at treatment. In most cases, the goal is penetration and eradication of the nidus of the lesion. Fibered coils (Figure 48.4) have been the material of choice for vessel occlusion since

Table 48.2 Embolic agents

- Metallic coils
- Detachable balloons
- Covered stents
- Particulate agents
  - Polyvinyl alcohol particles
  - Trisacryl gelatin microspheres (Embosphere)
  - Ytrium-90 glass radioactive microspheres (TheraSphere)
  - Embogold
  - Gelfoam
  - N-butyl 2-cyanoacrylate
  - Onyx
- Liquid sclerosing agents
  - Ethanol or absolute alcohol
  - Hypertonic dextrose
  - Sotradecol
  - Ethibloc

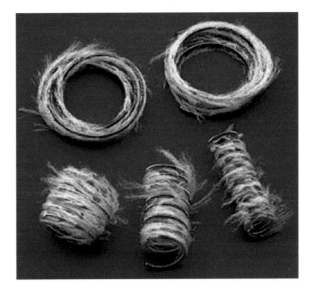

Figure 48.4 Nester coils (Cook Inc., Bloomington, IN).

their introduction 30 years ago.[17] However, their value in treating AVMs is limited as they result in proximal occlusion, which is functionally equivalent to surgical ligation. Therefore, fibered coils are appropriate only in lesions with a fistula-like architecture.

The basic fibered coil consists of a length of guidewire with multiple polyester threads attached transversely along most of its length. Fibered coil emboli are preshaped into a variety of different configurations and then stretched out in a cartridge for delivery into a catheter. Coils are made of steel and platinum with spring sizes 0.035- to 0.038-in and 0.018-in. Selecting the correct coil size is extremely important for the success of the procedure. The coils should be slightly oversized relative to the diameter of the target vessel, allowing them to grip the vessel wall and be closely packed. Significantly oversized coils tend to pass through the vessel like a guidewire and may elongate to a feeding branch rather than coiling up. Undersized coils may fail to lodge and migrate, causing unintended embolization into other vessels.

Guglielmi detachable coils without fibers were introduced for controlled and safer embolization. But their high cost and limited thrombogenicity confine their use to treatment of intracerebral aneurysms.

Detachable balloons were used to occlude large arteriovenous communications, but their complexity and cost remain significant drawbacks. In addition, they are not commercially available in the United States at this time.

Polyvinyl alcohol particles ranging from <100 to >1000 mm in size are used for permanent vessel embolization. The particles wedge in vessels of corresponding diameter and produce a permanent occlusion by thrombosis and subsequent fibrosis. The particle-contrast suspension is injected slowly in small aliquots under continuous fluoroscopic control once the delivery catheter is positioned in the desired location. While the particles themselves are permanent, the effect on the malformation is often temporary, with collateral recruitment and recanalization around the particles.

Liquid occlusive agents, including sclerosants and glue, are very attractive for AVM nidus occlusion (Figure 48.5). Absolute ethanol is a very potent sclerosant and should be used with great care. Although good long-term results have been reported, intra-arterial ethanol injection carries a significant risk of damage to normal tissues if nontarget embolization occurs.

Glue or tissue adhesives, such as *N*-butyl cyanoacrylate (n-BCA) and isobutyl cyanoacrylate, are another category of liquid embolic agents that polymerize on contact with an ionic environment, such as blood. In experienced hands, these are very effective for AVM occlusion, but require frequent, time-consuming catheter exchanges, and as with ethanol, great care should be taken to avoid nontarget embolization.

Complications

Embolotherapy, although minimally invasive and relatively safe, is not without complications. Therefore, patients need to be fully informed of the potential risks of the treatment. The most common complication is probably ischemia due to nontarget embolization or distal migration of the embolic agent. Sometimes, superficial tissue necrosis occurs, and extensive lesions may require skin grafting.

Postembolization syndrome caused by tissue necrosis may be encountered after embolotherapy. The symptoms of pain, fever, leukocytosis, and nausea arise shortly after embolotherapy and usually resolve within a few days; however, they may persist up to a week. Compared to tumor embolization and organ embolotherapy, postembolization syndrome occurs less frequently after the treatment of AVMs.

PULMONARY ARTERIOVENOUS MALFORMATIONS

Pulmonary arteriovenous malformations (PAVMs) are discussed separately because of their unique pathologic mechanisms, associated risk factors, and different treatment approaches. Like other AVF malformations, PAVMs consist of a congenital connection between a pulmonary artery and vein without normal capillary beds. Unlike other AVMs, the shunt is from right to left. This carries significant implications in terms of clinical presentation and treatment. Approximately 70% of PAVMs are congenital and multiple[19,20] and 60%–90% of them are associated with hereditary hemorrhagic telangiectasia, also called Osler-Weber-Rendu syndrome. The remainder are isolated lesions in otherwise healthy patients with no family history. Rarely, PAVMs are acquired and related to cirrhosis, congenital heart disease (Glenn and Fontan shunts), tumors, trauma, and infection.

Anatomic considerations and clinical aspects

PAVMs are classified as *simple* (80%–90% of cases) when they are supplied by an artery contained within one

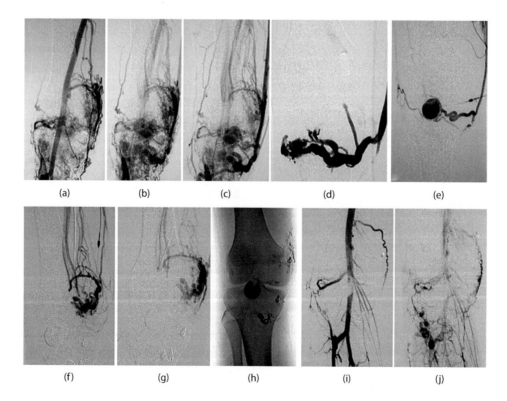

(a)   (b)   (c)   (d)   (e)

(f)   (g)   (h)   (i)   (j)

Figure 48.5 Arteriovenous malformation involving the right leg of a teenage boy. (**a–d**) Preintervention angiography. The steps for primary embolization using permanent liquid agents (**e,f**)—direct injection—and placing adjunctive coils (**g,h**) are shown. The patient had an excellent result after four embolizations carried out in two hospital visits, and he is now symptom free. (From Rutherford, R.B., (ed.), *Vascular Surgery*, 6th ed., Saunders, Philadelphia, PA, 2005.)

pulmonary segment, or *complex* when they are fed by arteries from more than one pulmonary segment (Figures 48.6 and 48.7). Approximately 65% of the lesions are located in lower lobes.[22] PAVMs vary in size from tiny, angiographically invisible structures to giant malformations occupying an entire lobe (Figure 48.8).

Up to 55% of PAVMs are asymptomatic and are discovered incidentally. Those that are symptomatic can present in a variety of ways.[23] The most common presentations are dyspnea, cyanosis, easy fatigability, clubbing, hemoptysis, or hemothorax. Pathologic mechanisms related to PAVM are hypoxemia due to right-to-left shunt, rupture and

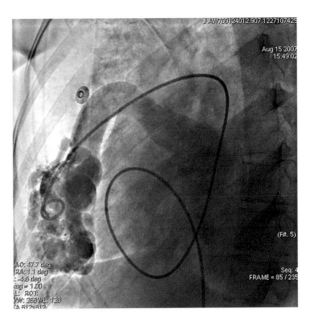

Figure 48.8 Angiography in left anterior oblique projection demonstrating a huge PAVM in the right lung of a 24-year-old woman. PAVM, pulmonary arteriovenous malformation. (Reprinted from *Journal of Vascular and Interventional Radiology*, 7, Robert I. White, Jeffrey S. Pollak, and Joel A. Wirth. Pulmonary arteriovenous malformations: Diagnosis and transcatheter embolotherapy. 787–804, Copyright 1996. With permission from Elsevier.)

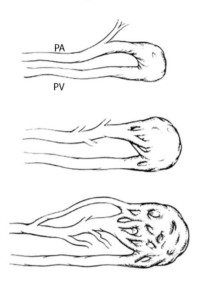

Figure 48.6 Simple PAVMs (supplied with only one feeding artery). The nidus on the lower two panels consists of a network of small branches and septations. PA, pulmonary artery; PAVM, pulmonary arteriovenous malformation; PV, pulmonary vein. (Reprinted from *Journal of Vascular and Interventional Radiology*, 7, Robert I. White, Jeffrey S. Pollak, and Joel A. Wirth. Pulmonary arteriovenous malformations: Diagnosis and transcatheter embolotherapy. 787–804, Copyright 1996. With permission from Elsevier.)

bleeding of pathologic vessels, and paradoxical embolism due to loss of lung-filtering function. Paradoxical embolism is the main complication associated with PAVMs. It is estimated that in patients with PAVMs, the lifetime probability of transient ischemic attack or stroke is 25% and of cerebral abscess is 10%.[23,24] For this reason, PAVMs tend to be treated more aggressively than other lesions, even when asymptomatic.

Indications for pulmonary arteriovenous malformation treatment

A PAVM with a >3 mm feeding artery is generally considered an indication for intervention. Diagnostic tests for pulmonary vascular malformation include pulse oximetry (platypnea orthodeoxia may be seen), chest X-ray, contrast echocardiography (high sensitivity >90%), computed tomographic (CT) angiography, magnetic resonance imaging (MRI), and finally pulmonary angiography—considered the gold standard for diagnosis. In recent years, the availability of multidetector CT scanning has allowed for noninvasive diagnosis and high-resolution reconstruction of pathologic anatomy.[25]

Treatment considerations

The initial treatment for PAVMs was surgical, including vascular ligation, lobectomy, or pneumonectomy, and was associated with up to 10% recurrence and serious morbidity.

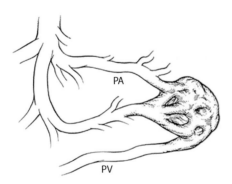

Figure 48.7 Complex pulmonary arteriovenous malformation. PA, pulmonary artery; PV, pulmonary vein. (Reprinted from *Journal of Vascular and Interventional Radiology*, 7, Robert I. White, Jeffrey S. Pollak, and Joel A. Wirth. Pulmonary arteriovenous malformations: Diagnosis and transcatheter embolotherapy. 787–804, Copyright 1996. With permission from Elsevier.)

In 1977, Porstmann performed the first PAVM embolization and over time, this has become the standard of treatment.

The embolization procedure is generally performed from a femoral approach using 6- to 7-Fr guiding catheters positioned in the feeding artery. Embolization is performed using one of a variety of macroscopic devices, including coils, microcoils, detachable plugs, and detachable balloons.

During the procedure, the patient is anticoagulated, commonly with 5,000 units of heparin, and meticulous care must be taken to avoid air bubble injection, which can result in procedure-related stroke.

The most popular embolization devices for PAVMs today are coils. There are several techniques for deploying different types of coils (Figures 48.9 through 48.11). Usually, the

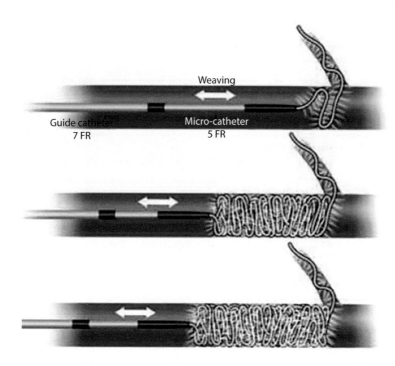

Figure 48.9 Anchor technique. The guide catheter maintains position in the artery and the first 1–2 cm of coil is placed in the side branch. The remaining coil is deposited as a tight coil mass. (Courtesy of Cook, Inc.)

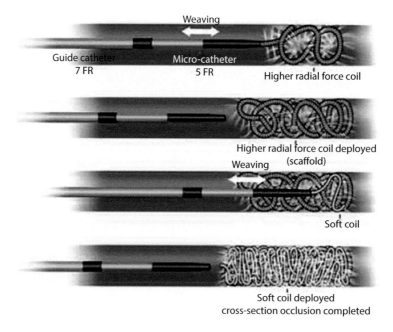

Figure 48.10 Scaffold technique. Deployment of first higher radial force coil began the formation of a "nidus" or "endo-skeleton" for placement of additional coils. (Courtesy of Cook, Inc.)

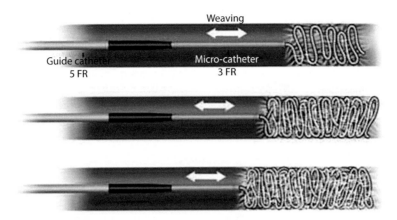

Figure 48.11 Coaxial technique to prevent coil elongation. To achieve permanent occlusion with fibered coils, it is useful to have a guide catheter, proximal in the artery, and use a smaller coaxial catheter to tightly pack (nest) the coils and achieve cross-sectional occlusion. (Courtesy of Cook, Inc.)

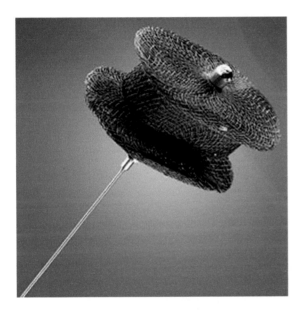

Figure 48.12 Amplatzer vascular plug (AGA Medical, Golden Valley, MN).

first coil selected has a diameter at least 20% larger than the vessel to be occluded. Cross-sectional occlusion is the goal to minimize the chance of future recanalization. It is important to perform the embolization with coils placed as distally as possible in the feeding vessel. This technique avoids the occlusion of branches to normal lung and reduces the risk of pleuritic pain or pulmonary infarction. Detachable balloons have the advantage of flow guidance but have largely been replaced by detachable coils and plugs that are easier to use. Amplatzer vascular plugs, which are made of tightly woven nitinol mesh, can be repositioned prior to detachment and have provided excellent results (Figure 48.12). Recently it was demonstrated that for small or tortuous AVMs, MVP-7Q and MVP-9Q microvascular plugs (Medtronic) are most effective. Those plugs can be delivered through 4- and 5-Fr catheters, respectively. Figure 48.13 shows two examples of complex PAVMs treated with coils.

Procedural success in recent studies is 85%–95%.[26,27] Although overall results during follow-up have been satisfactory, in patients with diffuse PAVMs[29], improvement of dyspnea, oxygenation, and shunt fraction may not be

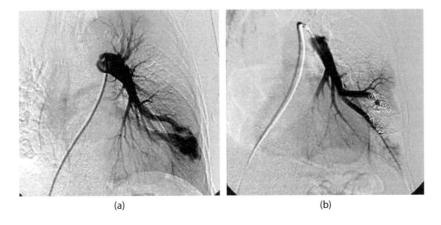

(a)   (b)

Figure 48.13 Two complex PAVMs (a) successfully treated with coils (b). PAVMs, pulmonary arteriovenous malformations.

complete.[28] Major neurologic complications such as cerebral abscess, transient ischemic attack, or stroke related to reperfused or newly perfused PAVMs also have been reported.[27] On the basis of this experience, helical CT scans at 6 and 12 months and then every 3–5 years afterward are recommended. Complications of the procedure are uncommon and include device migration (1%) and air embolism (up to 4%). The most frequent symptom postprocedure is pleuritic pain (13%), which usually resolves within 24 hours.

LOW-FLOW VASCULAR MALFORMATIONS

Low-flow malformations include venous and lymphatic lesions. Venous malformations are the most common type of congenital lesion encountered clinically. They may occur anywhere in the body but have a predilection for the lower extremities. Venous malformations may be of the cavernous type (sometimes incorrectly referred to as cavernous hemangiomas) or consist of abnormal venous channels. In some patients, such as those with Klippel–Trenaunay syndrome, there may be a combination of both types of lesion.

Presenting symptoms may include pain, swelling, cutaneous lesions causing bleeding, venous hypertension, and spontaneous thrombosis. Some of the venous syndromes may be associated orthopedic or growth disturbances. Evaluation is by ultrasound, CT, and MRI, where they are particularly well demonstrated.

Conservative treatment may be effective in mild cases, with measures such as elevation and elastic support. For larger or more symptomatic lesions, embolization techniques can be highly effective. Since these are by definition venous lesions, embolizing the arterial supply to the area is generally ineffective. Direct injection of sclerosing agents is the mainstay of treatment, using agents such as ethanol and sodium tetradecyl sulfate (Sotradecol). These agents cause thrombosis of the venous spaces, followed by an inflammatory reaction, and finally shrinkage and fibrosis. While multiple treatments may be required, clinical improvement or resolution of symptoms can be achieved in most patients.

Lymphatic malformations are less common and more difficult to treat. They range from large cystic lesions (cystic hygroma) to cutaneous lesions with vesicle formation. One of the distinguishing characteristics of lymphatic malformations is their tendency for infection. The presence of infection in a vascular malformation nearly always indicates presence of a lymphatic component.

Treatment varies according to the type of lesion. Large cystic lesions can be treated surgically or by percutaneous drainage followed by sclerotherapy. Agents shown to be particularly effective in lymphatic lesions include OK-432, bleomycin, and doxycycline. Superficial lesions are particularly difficult to manage and may require surgical resection and/or laser therapy.

CONCLUSIONS

Over the past two decades, catheter-based embolization has assumed a primary role in the management of AVMs. With improvements in technology, procedures have become increasingly safe and effective. While peripheral AVMs are usually treated only in the presence of symptoms, PAVMs may be treated in asymptomatic patients to prevent ischemic neurologic events or cerebral abscesses.

REFERENCES

1. Belov S. Anatomopathological classification of congenital vascular defects. *Semin Vasc Surg* 1993;6(4):219–224.
2. Mulliken JB, Glowacki J. Classification of pediatric vascular lesions. *Plast Reconstr Surg* 1982;70(1):120–121.
3. Zhou W, et al. Embolotherapy of peripheral arteriovenous malformations. *Endovasc Today* 2005:85–91.
4. Coursley G, et al. Congenital arteriovenous fistulas in the extremities; an analysis of sixty-nine cases. *Angiology* 1956;7(3):201–217.
5. Gomes MM, Bernatz PE. Arteriovenous fistulas: A review and ten-year experience at the Mayo Clinic. *Mayo Clin Proc* 1970;45(2):81–102.
6. Malan E. Surgical problems in the treatment of congenital arteriovenous fistulae. *J Cardiovasc Surg (Torino)* 1965;5(6):Suppl:251–255.
7. Tille JC, Pepper MS. Hereditary vascular anomalies: New insights into their pathogenesis. *Arterioscler Thromb Vasc Biol* 2004;24(9):1578–1590.
8. Grace DM, et al. Vascular embolization and occlusion by angiographic techniques as an aid or alternative to operation. *Surg Gynecol Obstet* 1976;143(3):469–482.
9. Yazaki T, et al. Congenital renal arteriovenous fistula: Case report, review of Japanese literature and description of non-radical treatment. *J Urol* 1976;116(4):415–418.
10. Jacobowitz GR, et al. Transcatheter embolization of complex pelvic vascular malformations: Results and long-term follow-up. *J Vasc Surg* 2001;33(1):51–55.
11. Rockman CB, et al. Transcatheter embolization of extremity vascular malformations: The long-term success of multiple interventions. *Ann Vasc Surg* 2003;17(4):417–423.
12. Sofocleous CT, et al. Congenital vascular malformations in the hand and forearm. *J Endovasc Ther* 2001;8(5):484–494.
13. Tan KT, et al. Peripheral high-flow arteriovenous vascular malformations: A single-center experience. *J Vasc Interv Radiol* 2004;15(10):1071–1080.
14. Upton J, et al. Vascular malformations of the upper limb: A review of 270 patients. *J Hand Surg Am* 1999;24(5):1019–1035.
15. White RI Jr, et al. Long-term outcome of embolotherapy and surgery for high-flow extremity arteriovenous malformations. *J Vasc Interv Radiol* 2000;11(10):1285–1295.
16. Dickey KW, et al. Management of large high-flow arteriovenous malformations of the shoulder and upper extremity with transcatheter embolotherapy. *J Vasc Interv Radiol* 1995;6(5):765–773.
17. Gianturco C, et al. Mechanical devices for arterial occlusion. *Am J Roentgenol Radium Ther Nucl Med* 1975;124(3):428–435.

18. Rutherford RB, ed. *Vascular Surgery*. 6th edn. Philadelphia, PA: Saunders, 2005.

19. Gossage JR, Kanj G. Pulmonary arteriovenous malformations. *A state of the art review. Am J Respir Crit Care Med* 1998;158(2):643–661.

20. Shovlin CL, Letarte M. Hereditary haemorrhagic telangiectasia and pulmonary arteriovenous malformations: Issues in clinical management and review of pathogenic mechanisms. *Thorax* 1999;54(8):714–729.

21. White RI Jr, et al. Pulmonary arteriovenous malformations: Diagnosis and transcatheter embolotherapy. *J Vasc Interv Radiol* 1996;7(6):787–804.

22. McWilliams J, Gandhi RT. Treating pulmonary arteriovenous malformations. *Endovasc Today* 2016;15(4):52–55.

23. White RI Jr, et al. Angioarchitecture of pulmonary arteriovenous malformations: An important consideration before embolotherapy. *AJR Am J Roentgenol* 1983;140(4):681–686.

24. Shovlin CL, et al. Diagnostic criteria for hereditary hemorrhagic telangiectasia (Rendu-Osler-Weber syndrome). *Am J Med Genet* 2000;91(1):66–67.

25. White RI Jr. Recanalization after embolotherapy of pulmonary arteriovenous malformations: Significance? outcome? *AJR Am J Roentgenol* 1998;171(6):1704–1705.

26. Remy J, et al. Pulmonary arteriovenous malformations: Evaluation with CT of the chest before and after treatment. *Radiology* 1992;182(3):809–816.

27. Mager JJ, et al. Embolotherapy of pulmonary arteriovenous malformations: Long-term results in 112 patients. *J Vasc Interv Radiol* 2004;15(5):451–456.

28. Remy-Jardin M, et al. Transcatheter occlusion of pulmonary arterial circulation and collateral supply: Failures, incidents, and complications. *Radiology* 1991;180(3):699–705.

29. Faughnan ME, et al. Diffuse pulmonary arteriovenous malformations: Characteristics and prognosis. *Chest* 2000;117(1):31–38.

PART 9

Peripheral interventional procedures

49

Peripheral arterial intervention (lower and upper extremity)

M. RIZWAN SARDAR AND J. DAWN ABBOTT

BACKGROUND AND EPIDEMIOLOGY

Atherosclerotic peripheral arterial disease (PAD) is highly prevalent and estimated to be in 8–12 million adults living in the United States.[1] As the population continues to age, the incidence will undoubtedly increase. The prevalence of PAD depends on the age of the studied population and underlying risk factors for atherosclerotic disease, with a range of 3%–10%. The true prevalence, however, is unknown as greater than 50% of patients with lower extremity PAD may remain undiagnosed.[1-7] Most epidemiological surveys have used intermittent claudication (IC) as a marker of symptomatic disease and an abnormal noninvasive ankle-brachial index (ABI) to diagnose and target treatment for asymptomatic PAD. However, clinical history, particularly in the absence of routine screening of at-risk individuals, may underestimate the true burden of lower extremity PAD.[8]

PAD can have a major impact on quality of life and remains a significant source of morbidity and mortality. Because atherosclerosis is a systemic process, patients with PAD are at a high risk of coronary and cerebrovascular ischemic events, and thus the diagnosis has strong prognostic implications. Over the last 10–20 years, there has been an exponential growth in the number of endovascular revascularization procedures for lower extremity claudication and critical limb ischemia (CLI). The procedures have grown in several subspecialties, including cardiology, vascular surgery, and interventional radiology. Advances in technology have led to the development of more effective endovascular approaches that have prompted a swing away from open surgical repair. While the endovascular first approach is widely accepted, we must continue to recognize the risks and advantages of revascularization modalities to assure the lowest-risk procedure and most durable outcome for the individual patient.

PATIENT SELECTION

Screening and diagnostic tests

ANKLE BRACHIAL INDEX

ABI is a ratio of the blood pressure in the ankle (dorsalis pedis or posterior tibial artery, whichever is higher) and blood pressure in the higher of the brachial arteries. At baseline, it should be measured in both lower limbs. PAD is typically defined as an ABI of <0.9, with values from 0.9 to 1 considered as borderline abnormal. An ABI of >1 and <1.4 is normal.[9] An ABI of >1.4 is generally consistent with calcified, noncompressible atherosclerotic vessels, which is associated with an increased cardiovascular risk and limits the ability to identify obstructive PAD.[10] The ABI is usually the initial diagnostic test for screening patients who exhibit signs and symptoms suggestive of PAD; it is one of the most cost-effective, reproducible, and inexpensive tests. A resting ABI of <0.9 is usually associated with greater than 50% angiographic stenosis of a major lower extremity vessel with high sensitivity and specificity.[4] An ABI at rest in the range of 0.9–0.4 is suggestive of moderate disease, and an ABI less than 0.4 is highly consistent with critical disease. Patients with clinically suspected PAD and artificially high resting ABI should get a toe-brachial index (TBI) with an abnormal value defined as <0.7. Exercise ABIs are helpful in unclear cases, with discordance between clinical symptoms and resting ABI. A decrease of at least 15 mmHg in the ankle systolic pressure following exercise is considered abnormal.

PULSE VOLUME RECORDING

Pulse volume recording (PVR) is performed with pressure cuffs inflated to 60 mmHg at various segments of the lower extremities. In conjunction with ABI, PVRs are a reasonable first step to establish PAD diagnosis and are very helpful in localizing stenosis. A normal PVR tracing will have a rapid upstroke and downstroke in the presence of a dicrotic notch. Depending on the severity of PAD, PVR findings can demonstrate a waveform with attenuated upstrokes and downstrokes and widened arterial waveform, or a flat and nonpulsatile waveform.

SEGMENTAL BLOOD PRESSURE CUFFS

Segmental blood pressure cuffs are placed at the level of thigh, calf, ankle, foot, and big toe. The cuffs are sequentially inflated to 20 mmHg above the systolic pressure in that segment. Cuff pressures are slowly released, and continuous wave-Doppler pulse measures pressure at each segment. A pressure drop of ≥30 mmHg between two consecutive levels indicates the presence of stenosis in the segment proximal to the blood pressure cuff.

NONINVASIVE IMAGING

Procedural planning can be optimized by diagnostic noninvasive imaging tests like duplex ultrasound (dUS), high-resolution computed tomography angiography (CTA), and magnetic resonance angiography (MRA). These tests provide a detailed assessment of lesion severity and complexity, patency of previously treated segments, appropriate selection of interventional equipment, and arterial access choice. These insights help to minimize procedural time, radiation dose, and use of contrast. The choice of noninvasive study is usually institution and physician specific; however, certain elements favor one study over another.

dUS avoids radiation and contrast but requires a trained technician and reader to provide consistent, accurate readings. Ultrasound is also helpful in detecting pseudoaneurysms and iatrogenic traumatic lesions, and guiding thrombin injection. A limitation of dUS is that it may overestimate residual stenosis following endovascular revascularization; nevertheless, it is recommended for routine surveillance after bypass revascularization (femoral-popliteal or femoral-tibial-pedal) and generally

used post-endovascular intervention. Usual frequencies of assessment intervals are approximately 3, 6, and 12 months and then yearly after graft placement.[11] CTA is faster and provides a detailed assessment of lesion characteristics (inside the lumen) and vessel wall, but risks radiation exposure. MRA is without radiation risk, but as a luminogram, can only provide information about intravascular lesions. Both CTA and MRA are relatively contraindicated in patients with advanced chronic kidney disease (CKD) with the use of iodinated contrast agents for CTA and gadolinium for MRA.

At the present time, there is no guideline or outcome data concerning the choice of preprocedural imaging. Selection of preprocedural imaging is dictated by local availability, expertise of physicians and technicians, and specific patient characteristics (CKD and the presence of magnetic resonance imaging (MRI)-incompatible devices).

Clinical presentation and initial management

All patients diagnosed with PAD require antiplatelet and statin therapy, risk factor control, and lifestyle modification. Asymptomatic patients should be monitored for symptom development but have no indication for revascularization.[12,13] Symptomatic patients may present with typical symptoms of IC, such as leg cramping with exertion and relief with rest; however atypical symptoms like leg fatigue, numbness, or tingling are also found. For symptomatic patients, supervised exercise programs improve outcomes and are recommended but are not readily available. Another alternative is home-based exercise for patients who cannot go or do not want to undergo a supervised exercise program, but this method is not as beneficial.[14] Cilostazol is the only approved medication for IC; it improves walking distance and time to symptoms onset. However, the side effect profile, including diarrhea and dyspnea and contraindication in patients with heart failure, limits its use.[15] In contrast to more severe forms of PAD, IC does not pose a threat to limb viability; therefore, need and timing of revascularization are dictated by the degree of lifestyle or vocational limitation. Lesions that are responsible for IC comprise femoral-popliteal arteries in 60%–70%, aorto-iliac arteries in 20%–30% and are rarely due to isolated tibial lesions.[16] Severity of IC is usually classified by Rutherford–Baker or Fontaine classification schemes (Table 49.1).[13,17,18] Patients presenting with CLI have a high 6-month risk of amputation and mortality, and urgent revascularization is generally advocated. Acute limb ischemia (ALI) is a medical emergency that requires emergent treatment to salvage life and limb.

INTERVENTIONAL FUNDAMENTALS

The basic fundamentals for performing endovascular repair, once indications have been satisfied, begin with an in-depth understanding of vascular anatomy, collateral supply, and the ability to perform an imaging work-up, allowing for

Table 49.1 Rutherford–Baker or Fontaine classification of chronic peripheral arterial disease severity

Symptoms	Rutherford–Baker class	Fontaine class
Asymptomatic	Stage 0	Stage I
Mild claudication	Stage 1	Stage IIa (symptoms with >200 m distance)
Moderate claudication	Stage 2	Stage IIb (symptoms with <200 m distance)
Severe claudication	Stage 3	
Rest pain	Stage 4	Stage III
Ischemic ulceration (limited to digits)	Stage 5	Stage IV
Severe ischemic ulceration or frank gangrene	Stage 6	

detailed planning of the intervention. There are pathways to gain clinical competence, either through a dedicated training program or physician experience tract. Comprehensive knowledge of the equipment available is another vital component of a successful endovascular program. Unlike coronary equipment, peripheral interventional devices may be 0.014-, 0.018-, or 0.035-in guidewire compatible and may require varying sheath and guide diameters. In addition, the working length of devices may range from 70 to 150 cm.

LOWER EXTREMITY ENDOVASCULAR REVASCULARIZATION

Revascularization is usually required in one of three scenarios: (1) lifestyle limiting IC with failure of medical and exercise therapy, (2) CLI, or (3) ALI. The decision to perform a revascularization procedure—surgical or endovascular—cannot be made exclusively on anatomic considerations. Patients should be selected on the basis of the severity of the symptoms, disability as assessed by the patient and physician, failure of medical therapy, and a favorable risk/benefit ratio of intervention, including procedural success and long-term patency. In patients with lifestyle or vocational limiting IC or those who progress to ischemic rest pain, ulceration, or gangrene, revascularization attempts are warranted. Guidelines for the performance of endovascular revascularization (ERV) for claudication have been published by a joint American College of Cardiology (ACC)/American Heart Association (AHA) task force.[4] In general, endovascular repair is most successful when utilized in larger inflow arteries with discrete lesions. Less favorable long-term outcomes are associated with endovascular repair of diffuse disease in smaller outflow and runoff vessels. Comorbid conditions also play a role in the decision process with more aggressive endovascular approaches being accepted in patients at higher risk for open surgical repair or without venous conduits. More recently, the Society for Cardiac Angiography and Interventions (SCAI) developed expert consensus statements on the appropriate use of femoral-popliteal arterial and aorto-iliac arterial interventions.[19,20]

Over the past decade, there has been tremendous growth of endovascular equipment, which has enabled endovascular treatment of complex lesions that were historically treated by surgery. While the technical feasibility of ERV is high in all lesion types and locations, there are anatomic subgroups that deserve special consideration. The following sections discuss the outcomes for ERV strategies according to arterial location.

Aorto-iliac intervention

COMPARISON WITH MEDICAL THERAPY AND SURGERY

In patients with IC due to aortoiliac disease, stents improve symptoms, walking distance, ABI scores, and perfusion to the feet, compared to medical therapy alone. The Claudication: Exercise Versus Endoluminal Revascularization (CLEVER) Study compared treatment strategies for patients with IC due to aorto-iliac disease. This small randomized trial suggested that supervised exercise or stent revascularization were better than optimal medical therapy alone with respect to walking distance and quality of life.[21] These two strategies should be considered complementary rather than mutually exclusive. Historically, aortofemoral bypass surgery had been the gold standard for occlusive aorto-iliac disease with excellent long-term patency rates of around 90% at 5 years and 50%–60% at 20 years. The rates of intra-operative mortality of 3%–5% and major complications of surgery, in combination with improved safety and intermediate to long-term patency of stents, has led to the adoption of a percutaneous approach in most patients. Results from a Swedish randomized control trial, in which 37% patients had iliac artery disease, showed comparable results between the iliac artery stent group and surgery with patency of 90% in stent arm and 94% in surgical arm.[22] In practice, surgery is generally reserved for long total occlusion, including involvement of the aorta or in those patients with simultaneous infrarenal aneurysms. Current societal recommendations, however, are more conservative. Figure 49.1[23] and Table 49.2 summarize the Trans-Atlantic Inter-Society Consensus Document (TASC) classification and recommendations of the TASC working group for the appropriate revascularization strategy of iliac lesions. An endovascular procedure is the treatment of choice for type A, and surgery is the procedure of choice for type D. At present, endovascular treatment is more commonly used in type B lesions, and surgical treatment is more commonly used in type C lesions.

Type A lesions

• Unilateral or bilateral stenoses of CIA
• Unilateral or bilateral single short (≤3 cm) stenosis of EIA

Type B lesions

• Short (≤3 cm) stenosis of infrarenal aorta
• Unilateral CIA occlusion
• Single or multiple stenosis totaling 3–10 cm involving the
  EIA not extending into the CFA
• Unilateral EIA occlusion not involving the origins of
  internal iliac or CFA

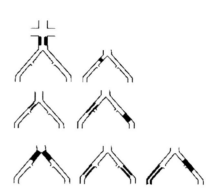

Type C lesions

• Bilateral CIA occlusions
• Bilateral EIA stenoses 3–10 cm long not extending into
  the CFA
• Unilateral EIA stenosis extending into the CFA
• Unilateral EIA occlusion that involves the origins of
  internal iliac and/or CFA
• Heavily calcified unilateral EIA occlusion with or without
  involvement of origins of internal iliac and/or CFA

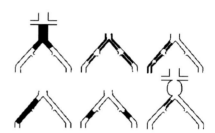

Type D lesions

• Infra-renal aorto iliac occlusion
• Diffuse disease involving the aorta and both iliac arteries
  requiring treatment
• Diffuse multiple stenoses involving the unilateral CIA,
  EIA, and CFA
• Unilateral occlusion of both CIA and EIA
• Bilateral occlusions of EIA
• Iliac stenoses in patients with AAA requiring treatment
  and not amenable to endograft placement or other
  lesions requiring open aortic or iliac surgery

Figure 49.1 Trans-Atlantic Inter-Society Consensus (TASC) document classification of aorto-iliac lesions. AAA, abdominal aortic aneurysm; CFA, common femoral artery; CIA, common iliac artery; EIA, external iliac artery. (Adapted from Norgren, L., et al., *Eur. J. Vasc. Endovasc. Surg.*, 33, S1–S75, 2007. With permission.)

Table 49.2 The recommendation of the Trans-Atlantic Inter-Society Consensus (TASC) working group for the revascularization strategy of aortoiliac femoropopliteal lesions

	Iliac lesion	Femoral lesions
TASC A	Single, <3 cm of CIA or EIA (unilateral/bilateral)	Single, ≤3 cm in length, does not involve the SFA or popliteal artery
TASC B	1. Single, 3–10 cm, not extending into the CFA 2. Two stenoses <5 cm long in the CIA and/or EIA, does not extend to the CFA 3. Unilateral CIA occlusion	1. Single stenosis or occlusion 3 to 5 cm long, does not involve the distal popliteal artery 2. Heavily calcified, ≤3 cm, or multiple stenosis or occlusions each <3 cm 3. Single or multiple lesions in the absence of patent tibial runoff
TASC C	1. Bilateral 5- to 10-cm stenosis of the CIA and/or EIA, does not extend to CFA 2. Unilateral EIA occlusion or stenosis, does not extend into the CFA 3. Bilateral CIA occlusion	1. Single stenosis/occlusion >5 cm 2. Multiple stenoses or occlusions 3–5 cm, with or without heavy calcification
TASC D	1. >10-cm lesions or diffuse, multiple, unilateral stenosis that involve the CIA, EIA, and CFA 2. Unilateral occlusion that involves both the CIA and EIA 3. Bilateral EIA occlusions 4. Diffuse disease involving the aorta and both iliac arteries or lesions in a patient that requires aortic or iliac surgery (AAA)	1. Complete CFA or SFA occlusions

Source: Modified from Dormandy, J.A., et al., *J. Vasc. Surg.*, 31(1 Pt 2), S1–S296, 2000.
Note: AAA, abdominal aortic aneurysm; CFA, common femoral artery; CIA, common iliac artery; EIA, external iliac artery; SFA, superficial femoral artery.

Evidence is insufficient to make firm recommendations, particularly in cases with types B and C lesions.

AORTO-ILIAC DEVICES AND TRIALS

For ERV of iliac disease, stenting is an acceptable default strategy. Although clinical trials have not demonstrated a clear patency benefit of routine stenting over balloon angioplasty with provisional stenting, there is a lower rate of complications with stenting.[24-27]

Overall, the procedural success for iliac artery lesion revascularization is greater than 90% and almost 100% for isolated focal iliac artery lesions. Patency rates for iliac stenting are approximately 85% at 1 year and 75% at 4 years but are influenced by several factors, including initial stenosis severity and length, procedural indication (IC vs. CLI), distal flow, and female sex.[4,28-30]

There is little available data comparing outcomes for balloon-expandable stainless steel and self-expanding nitinol stents in aorto-iliac disease. Given the lack of external compressive forces and the general nontortuous course of common iliac arteries, balloon-expandable stents are generally preferred due to greater radial strength and ability to deploy with precision, which is particularly relevant in aortic bifurcation lesions. In cases where there is long diffuse disease, tortuous vessels, or involvement of the external iliac artery, self-expanding stents should be used. Self-expanding stents provide better flexibility and may reduce the risk of vessel rupture and of stent deformity and fracture at flexion points. The Cordis Randomized Iliac Stent Project-United States (CRISP-US) trial compared a nitinol (S.M.A.R.T stent, Cordis Endovascular, Warren, NJ) and stainless steel (Wallstent, Boston Scientific, Natick, MA) self-expanding stent. There was higher acute procedural success with the nitinol stent; however, 1 year patency rates were similar (91.1% with the Wallstent and 94.7% with the S.M.A.R.T. stent).[31] Nitinol is the preferred alloy for self-expanding stents due to its elasticity and thermal shape memory, which results in resistance to external deformation.

Stent grafts, or covered stents, are also an option for iliac disease. Stent grafts designed with polytetrafluoroethylene (PTFE) or Dacron lining were introduced with an idea of providing a mechanical barrier to restenosis and neointimal hyperplasia from the contiguous wall. Stent grafts do not completely eliminate the risk of restenosis, but shift the pattern of restenosis from within the stent to the stent edge. Stent grafts are available as balloon expandable (Viabahn, Gore or Fluency, Bard) or self-expanding (Atrium, iCast). The Covered Versus Balloon-Expandable Stent Trial (COBEST) was a prospective randomized control, multicenter trial involving 125 patients and 168 iliac artery lesions, treated with either a covered balloon-expandable stent or bare-metal stent (BMS). Aorto-iliac lesions treated with the covered stent were significantly more likely to remain free from binary restenosis than those that were treated with a BMS (hazard ratio [HR], 0.35; 95% CI, 0.15–0.82; $P = 0.02$). In subgroup analysis, this benefit remained significant for TASC C and D lesions; however, stent types were equivalent in TASC B lesions.[32] The Dutch Iliac Stent Trial: Covered Balloon-Expandable Versus Uncovered Balloon-Expandable Stents in the Common Iliac Artery (DISCOVER) trial, a prospective, double-blind, controlled, multicenter trial of 174 total patients with common iliac artery occlusions or stenosis of >30 mm in length randomized to covered versus uncovered balloon-expandable stents is presently enrolling patients.[33] Balloon-expandable stent grafts can be considered as an alternative to BMSs in iliac lesions that are complex (TASC C/D) or that have a high risk of rupture due to calcification. Elective use of a stent graft should be avoided, if use will occlude a major side branch or collateral or compromise future access. Operators need to be familiar with guide compatibility and deployment of stents grafts for treatment of iliac perforations, which require emergent sealing to prevent fatal hemorrhage. All labs performing endovascular interventions need to keep a sufficient supply in inventory.

PROCEDURAL CONSIDERATIONS AORTO-ILIAC INTERVENTION

In patients with unilateral iliac stenosis without the involvement of the common femoral artery (CFA), ipsilateral access through CFA and retrograde percutaneous angioplasty is preferred as it provides direct access and coaxial alignment with the vessel and lesion. Contralateral access with the use of a crossover sheath is reserved for lesions that involve the distal external iliac and/or CFAs or when intervention on a more distal vessel in the same limb is required. In aortic bifurcation lesions, the bilateral retrograde approach is utilized to make alignment easy for simultaneous kissing stents and balloons. Brachial and radial accesses are also acceptable alternatives if the artery can accommodate the required sheath size and devices have adequate length for delivery.

Complications in aortoiliac interventions are seldom encountered and are usually related to the access site, including bleeding, hematomas, pseudoaneurysms, retroperitoneal bleed, and arteriovenous (AV) fistula formation. The most life-threatening complication is arterial perforation, and operators should be competent at management. Among all arteries suffering iatrogenic perforations, the external iliac artery has the highest incidence rate.[34,35] In most series, complication rates are in the range of 5%–6% with perforation in up to 2%.[34]

Common femoral artery intervention

The CFA is exposed to constant flexion and compression and is a common access site for endovascular procedures—factors that limit the use of stents in this vascular segment. Surgical endarterectomy carries a low procedural risk and high durability and for the majority of patients is the preferred approach. There are no randomized trials comparing surgical and endovascular therapy for CFA disease. Observational data, primarily from single centers, have shown acceptable 1-year outcomes for CFA balloon angioplasty with provisional stenting, particularly in high-risk surgical patients with a procedural indication of limb salvage.[36] Debulking technologies like atherectomy combined with drug-coated balloons (DCBs) may improve ERV outcomes and lower the risk of bail-out stenting; however, flow limiting dissections, extensive calcification, and arterial recoil may limit such an approach.[37] For patients who develop restenosis after surgical endarterectomy, percutaneous transluminal angioplasty (PTA) can be performed.

Femoropopliteal intervention

The superficial femoral artery (SFA) is a long artery with few side branches and is uniquely positioned to face complex external mechanical stress forces including torsion, flexion, and compression. The distal SFA traverses the adductor canal, which further increases susceptibility to compression during flexion of the knee joint. The femoropopliteal segment is the most common site of occlusive disease causing IC. The historically poor primary patency rates of EVR in this region, which likely result from the forces described in combination with very long occlusions, have challenged the field. Surgery with autologous vein femoropopliteal bypass has a primary graft patency of up to 80% at 5 years and may be preferred over EVR in certain patients, such as those who have low surgical risk.[30] Operative mortality varies from 1.3% to 6.3% and is related to cardiovascular risk. Surgery with synthetic conduits or more distal arterial targets, however, has significantly lower patency.

Primary patency for femoropopliteal EVR depends on several factors, including occlusion length and adequacy of runoff, but the importance of device strategy should be considered. Stent technology has improved over time with use of metal alloys with superelastic properties, greater radial strength, and lower risk for fracture. In addition, paclitaxel-eluting self-expanding stents and DCBs reduce intimal hyperplasia and lower restenosis. Debulking techniques, such as atherectomy, may obviate the need for stenting or improve stent expansion. Considering the low morbidity and mortality associated with EVR and the higher patency rates observed with contemporary therapy, an endovascular approach is generally preferred over surgery in the majority of patients. Societal recommendations have been relatively conservative with respect to the lesion types recommended for EVR (Table 49.2). Femoropopliteal lesions appropriate to consider for EVR include (1) less than 10 cm in length; (2) multiple stenosis less than 5 cm, not involving the trifurcation; (3) a single lesion less than 15 cm, not involving trifurcation; and (4) prior to surgery in patients with no continuous tibial runoffs in order to improve inflow for surgical bypass. In practice, more complex disease is often treated by EVR and the choice rests on careful consideration of the risks and benefits.

FEMOROPOPLITEAL DEVICES AND TRIALS

The optimal approach to femoropopliteal EVR remains controversial. In no other vascular territory are there so many devices to choose from, and yet no clear algorithm to guide clinicians. PTA with provisional stenting for suboptimal results (residual diameter >50% stenosis, persistent translesional gradient, and evidence of flow limiting dissection) has long been the default strategy. Adjunctive therapy, including directional atherectomy or cutting/scoring balloons, has been used in an attempt to improve on PTA patency and avoid stenting. Self-expanding nitinol stents offer an advantage over PTA in long lesions (>10 cm) and improvements in stent design have decreased stent fracture and restenosis. More recently, approved therapies, including paclitaxel drug-eluting stents (DES) and DCBs, have further improved patency of *de novo* lesions, and laser atherectomy and DCB are used to treat restenosis. For very long lesions, including those due to restenosis, with sufficient runoff, self-expanding stent grafts, such as Viabahn, are also an option.

SELF-EXPANDING STENTS

The Vienna randomized trial, a small trial of 106 patients, showed superior patency of a self-expanding stent compared to balloon angioplasty alone with better walking capacity.[38] Another small study involving 73 patients confirmed primary stenting with a self-expanding nitinol stent for treatment of intermediate-length SFA lesions resulted in superior clinical midterm results compared with balloon angioplasty with bailout stenting.[39] The Randomized Study Comparing the Edwards Self-Expanding LifeStent Versus Angioplasty Alone in Lesions Involving the SFA and/or Proximal Popliteal Artery (RESILIENT) also showed improved outcomes with primary stenting using a self-expanding stent compared to balloon angioplasty, with 1 year primary lesion patency of 87.5% vs. 45.3%. There was a 40.5% crossover rate to stenting from the angioplasty group.[40] There is some conflicting data on the superiority of stenting for femoropopliteal lesions, which is likely due to nonuniformity of stent design and the lesions enrolled with regard to the percent of total occlusions, lesions length, and degree of calcification. The Femoral Artery Stenting Trial (FAST) failed to demonstrate superiority of self-expanding nitinol stents over balloon angioplasty in patients with shorter SFA lesions (<10 cm),[41] likely due to less complex lesions enrolled and small sample size. This was further validated in post hoc analysis of the RESILIENT study, which showed no benefit of stenting over PTA in shorter lesions.[38] Mwipatayi et al., in a meta-analysis of 934 patients, concluded that stenting in occlusive femoropopliteal disease does not show higher patency over balloon angioplasty at 1 year.[32] Schillinger et al. randomized patients with occlusive femoropopliteal disease to self-expanding platform or balloon angioplasty with provisional stenting, and showed superior patency of stent when used for SFA lesions of >10 cm at 6 and 12 months. Based on the above studies, PTA alone is not recommended for SFA lesions longer than 10 cm due to dismal patency. Self-expanding stents can be considered in this circumstance along with other strategies.

All stents, especially in regions of high mechanical stress like the SFA, can suffer mechanical fracture, which can lead to in-stent restenosis and thrombosis. The stent design, length, and stent overlap are factors that can influence the risk of mechanical disruption. Limiting stent length and avoiding the use of more than two stents with adequate overlap between stents is generally recommended.[42,43] Newer stent designs, including the Supera and Complete stents, have lesser stent deformation secondary to mechanical stress. The Complete Self-Expanding trial that used a new nitinol self-expanding stent to treat femoropopliteal disease demonstrated a low rate of target lesion revascularization (TLR) (8.4%) and no stent fractures at 12 months.[44] The Supera Interwoven Nitinol Stent Outcomes in Above-Knee Interventions (SAKE) study used the novel interwoven-wire Supera stent and showed high rates of patency at 6 and 12 months and no incidence of stent fractures.[45] Similar results were achieved using Supera stents in the Leipzing SUPERA popliteal artery stent registry with primary patency rates as high as 94.6% at 6 and 12 months and no incidence of stent fracture.[46]

DRUG-ELUTING STENTS

In-stent restenosis has remained an Achilles heel for SFA lesions, particularly in long lesions, which naturally led to the development of DES. The Sirolimus Coated Cordis SMART Nitinol Self-Expandable Stent for the Treatment of SFA Disease (SIROCCO I and II trials) studied Sirolimus stents versus bare-metal nitinol stents for SFA disease. Despite early promising results of SIROCCO I, later time points failed to demonstrate any significant advantage with this particular stent platform with 24-month restenosis rates in the sirolimus group slightly higher than in the BMS group (22.9% vs. 21.1%, $P > 0.05$).[47,48] High rates of stent fracture were observed in both arms (31% of all patients), which may have contributed to the unfavorable outcomes. Dake et al. evaluated the Zilver PTX paclitaxel-eluting stent (Cook Medical), which is a polymer-free, paclitaxel-coated, nitinol DES compared to BMS platform for femoropopliteal occlusive diseases. The DES group showed superior 12-month primary patency (83.1% vs. 32.8%, $P < 0.001$) and event-free survival (90.4% vs. 82.6%, $P = 0.004$).[49,50] The paclitaxel-eluting stent superiority over BMS was sustained at 2 years, based on which the U.S. Food and Drug Administration (FDA) approved Zilver PTX as the first and only DES for SFA lesions. Subgroup analysis showed that the benefit of DES was also seen in complex lesions, long lesions of >7 cm, and high-risk patients, including those with diabetes mellitus or CLI (Rutherford class 4–6). Cost-effectiveness data for a DES strategy are not available in the United States. A French study, however, showed that despite the higher cost of the Zilver PTX DES, there was a potential net saving of $7,445,715.06 over 5 years by reducing the need for future interventions compared to PTA.[51] The duration of dual antiplatelet agents after DES peripheral artery revascularization is debatable and needs further evidence, but 6 months is recommended.

COVERED SELF-EXPANDING STENTS

The use of covered self-expanding stents is theoretically intriguing as it may confer a lower risk of restenosis due to the barrier to neointimal hyperplasia. A small randomized trial comparing the Viabahn expandable PTFE nitinol stent versus balloon angioplasty for symptomatic SFA disease revealed better ultrasound proven primary patency in the stent group (65% vs. 40%). This trial led to the FDA approval of the Viabahn stent for SFA disease.[52] The Viabahn Endoprosthesis Versus Bare Nitinol Stent in the Treatment of Long Lesion Superficial Femoral Artery Occlusive Disease (VIBRANT) trial randomized patients to the Viabahn covered stent versus a self-expanding BMS for symptomatic SFA disease and showed low primary stent patency in both groups (53% vs. 58% at 12 months and 24.2% vs. 25.9% at 36 months) and higher stent fracture in BMS group (50% vs. 2%).[53] The Viabahn was redesigned to reduce the occurrence of thrombosis, and subsequent studies showed more favorable outcomes. The Viabahn Endoprosthesis with heparin bioactive surface was studied in a registry as well as a randomized trial; both showed higher primary patency rates of 78.1% vs. 53.5%, $P = 0.009$ compared to BMS without increased stent thrombosis.[54] The single-arm Viabahn Endoprosthesis with Heparin Bioactive Surface in the Treatment of Superficial Femoral Artery Obstructive Disease (VIPER) trial used the latest iteration of the Viabahn with a redesigned proximal edge to reduce inflow compromise. Primary patency was 73% with secondary patency of 92% with stent oversizing implicated as a cause of reduced patency.[55] Long-term data regarding restenosis and late stent thrombosis are still lacking (Figures 49.2 and 49.3). The Viabahn stent is used to cover SFA perforation and in-stent restenosis of bifurcating aorto-iliac disease.

Some special considerations are required before deciding to use a covered stent to treat SFA disease. Although in-stent restenosis may be lower compared to other stent platforms and does not seem to be associated with long lesion length, stent edge dissection or stenosis can still occur partly due to oversizing and sometimes due to stent deployment in an unhealthy segment of the vessel. Covered stents can cover collateral circulation as well and may lead to acute thigh pain and less improvement in symptoms secondary to impingement of collaterals. Due to the same mechanism, it can be hypothesized that ALI may occur rapidly in the setting of covered stent in-stent thrombosis, as collateral supply is jeopardized. In addition, use of covered stents is cautioned in patients with single vessel or poor runoff due to increased risk of thrombosis. There are no head-to-head comparisons of the Viabahn stent to approaches other than BMS; comparison to DES and DCB are lacking.

DRUG-COATED BALLOON

In-stent restenosis is the most frequently encountered complication after lower extremity stents, and DCB is an attractive alternative for treatment of *de novo* stenosis. In most cases, a permanent metal implant and accompanying

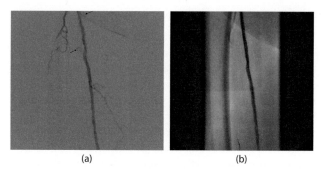

Figure 49.2 **(a)** SFA perforation (arrows) post balloon angioplasty with 4 × 100 mm² balloon and **(b)** post 6 × 150 mm² Viabahn stent fully covering lesion and perforation. SFA, superficial femoral artery.

complications can be avoided. Preclinical studies have shown that homogenous drug delivery and distribution can be achieved with DCBs;[56] however, DCBs do face the challenge of a lack of mechanical scaffold to address elastic recoil and the potential for inadequate delivery of the drug in highly calcified or tortuous arterial segments. DCBs have also been studied for the treatment of BMS restenosis.

In the Local Taxan with Short Exposure for Reduction of Restenosis in Distal Arteries (THUNDER) trial, the paclitaxel DCB reduced TLR at 6 and 12 months compared to PTA in *de novo* femoropopliteal disease (37% in the control group, 4% in the group treated with paclitaxel-coated balloons, $P < 0.001$). At 6 months, the mean late lumen loss was 1.7 ± 1.8 mm in the control group, as compared with 0.4 ± 1.2 mm ($P < 0.001$) in the DCB group.[57] Similar results were seen in the Paclitaxel-Coated Balloons in Femoral Indication to Defeat Restenosis (PACIFIER) trial, showing improved primary outcomes at 12 months.[58] The Drug-Eluting Balloon Evaluation for Lower Limb Multilevel Treatment (DEBELLUM) trial randomized 50 patients and 122 lesions (75.4% femoropopliteal and 24.6% below the knee) with IC or CLI to paclitaxel-eluting balloons versus traditional PTA. Late lumen loss, TLR, and adverse events were significantly lower and ABI and Fontaine class higher in the DCB arm at 12 months.[59] The Lutonix Paclitaxel-Coated Balloon for the Prevention of femoropopliteal Restenosis Trial (LEVANT I) evaluated the safety and efficacy of Lutonix DCB, which is coated with low-dose 2 µg/mm² paclitaxel and a polysorbate-sorbitol carrier for treatment of femoropopliteal artery lesions. At 6 months, late lumen loss was 58% lower for the Lutonix DCB group than for the control group (0.46 ± 1.13 mm vs. 1.09 ± 1.07 mm; $P = 0.016$). The Lutonix DCB showed benefit when used as balloon angioplasty alone or with stenting.[37] Similar results were found in the Drug-Eluting Balloon in Peripheral Intervention for The Superficial Femoral Artery (DEBATE-SFA) trial where upfront DCB or PTA followed by stent was performed.[60]

INFRAPOPLITEAL INTERVENTIONS

Isolated infrapopliteal disease is rarely the cause of IC, and EVR is not a first-line treatment.[4] (See Figure 49.4 for popliteal intervention.) Tibioperoneal angioplasty is limited due

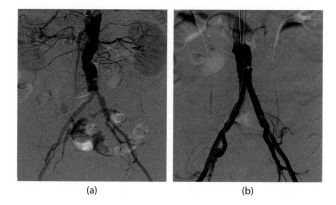

Figure 49.3 **(a)** Bilateral iliac artery disease with 80% in-stent restenosis of the previously placed stent in the right common iliac artery and 50% in-stent restenosis in the previously placed stent in the left common iliac. Resting gradient of 34 mmHg on the right side with hyperemic response gradients increased to 55 mmHg. **(b)** Successful bilateral common iliac artery stenting with deployment of two kissing 8 × 40 mm iCAST covered stents and resolution of the pressure gradient across the stenosis and excellent angiographic results.

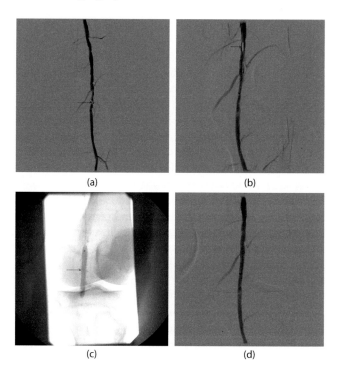

Figure 49.4 **(a)** High-grade stenosis of the popliteal artery; **(b)** postatherectomy with 2.25 Diamondback catheters in the popliteal artery (*arrow*); **(c)** drug-coated balloon inflation after Diamondback atherectomy of the popliteal artery (*arrow*); **(d)** final result after Diamondback atherectomy.

to anatomical challenges including long occlusions, calcification, and small-diameter vessels. Historically, the main limitations of infrapopliteal EVR were acute technical failure, complications, and poor long-term patency. However, with new technology in the hands of experienced operators and a meticulous approach in carefully selected patients, acute procedural success rates are 95% (98% for stenosis and 86% for total occlusion) and can be achieved with a 1% complication rate.[28,61–63] Nevertheless, patency remains an issue, and there is a concern that infrapopliteal EVR could accelerate progression to CLI. Due to lack of the outcome data on infrapopliteal EVR for IC, the risks and benefits of revascularization should be clearly assessed.

ACCESS FOR FEMOROPOPLITEAL AND INFRAPOPLITEAL INTERVENTIONS

Access is usually obtained from the contralateral CFA using crossover sheaths that can be positioned in the distal external iliac, CFA, or SFA, depending on the target lesion location. This approach provides excellent support and is generally preferred but in some instances cannot be used, such as in the presence of contralateral CFA disease or CFA stent, narrow angle calcified aorto-iliac bifurcations, prior bifurcation common iliac stents extending into the aorto- or prior aorto-bifemoral bypass. Alternative access sites include the brachial artery, antegrade CFA, retrograde popliteal or pedal (Figure 49.5). The risk of access site complications with alternative access is higher and consideration should be given to the use of ultrasound guidance in addition to fluoroscopic landmarks. The antegrade approach provides strong support for crossing total occlusions and calcified stenosis, but the proximal SFA must be free of significant disease. Antegrade ipsilateral access is mostly utilized for infrapopliteal EVR. Although it requires expertise to minimize complications, the straight-line approach to the lesion allows shorter length sheaths or balloon shafts, better torque control for wires, and pushability of revascularization instruments to cross occlusive or stenotic lesions. Brachial access suffers from the inability to reach distal lesions due to the working length of most catheters but may be possible in patients with short stature or proximal SFA

disease. A popliteal artery approach can be employed to cross an occluded SFA from below the knee but has many disadvantages.[64] It requires a patent popliteal artery, prone positioning, has increased operator radiation exposure, cannot treat concomitant infrapopliteal disease, potential for compartment syndrome, risk of bleeding and AV fistulae, and can be occlusive and cause distal limb ischemia. Lesions that are uncrossable antegrade are usually successfully crossed from a retrograde approach. Pedal access (via anterior, posterior tibial arteries and rarely peroneal artery) is a potential option in limb salvage situations where the occlusion cannot be crossed antegrade. Potential advantages include a supine patient position allowing simultaneous attempts from above and below, higher procedural success, low risk of bleeding without affecting distal targets for potential future bypass surgery, and the interventionalist may have less radiation exposure. In circumstances where both above the knee and below knee interventions are required, initial revascularization of tibioperoneal vessel will improve outflow and may lower the risk of peripheral embolization and maintain viable surgical bail-out options.

Revascularization for critical limb ischemia

CLI is defined as the presence of chronic ischemic resting pain, gangrene, or ulceration caused by chronic diminished perfusion due to occlusive PAD, which is associated with ABI < 0.4 and toe pressure <30 mmHg. The incidence of CLI is rising due to longer life expectancy and an increasing prevalence of diabetes mellitus. Mortality is high for CLI patients, 25% at 12 months, and 50% of untreated patients eventually require amputation within the same time frame.[65,66] Despite improvements in endovascular and surgical techniques, over 200,000 amputations are performed annually worldwide as a result of CLI.[67] Major amputation of a limb is always associated with loss of mobility and

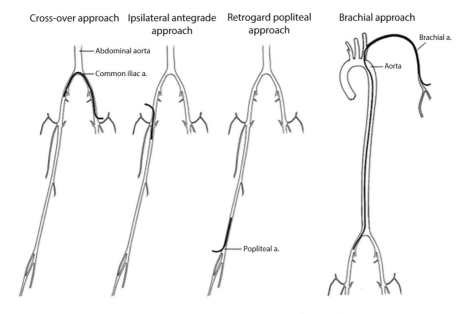

Figure 49.5 Common access sites and approaches to lower extremity endovascular intervention.

independence, and strategies that can minimize the extent of amputation (defined as below the ankle including a digital, ray, or transmetatarsal amputation) can maintain limb function without the need of a prosthesis. Patients with CLI have multiple comorbidities and are therefore at high risk for surgical interventions; this is where less invasive endovascular options can be useful.

The Angioplasty in Severe Ischemia of the Leg (BASIL) trial is the only trial available that randomized patients with CLI to either bypass surgery (75% with autologous saphenous vein) or balloon angioplasty and showed comparable results at 6 months (amputation-free survival 48 vs. 60 patients; unadjusted hazard ratio 1.07, 95% CI 0.72–1.6; adjusted hazard ratio 0.73, 0.49–1.07).[68] Longer-term follow-up showed better outcomes in the surgical group; however, this trial had several limitations including lack of patency endpoints and use of PTA alone. A Cochrane Review of bypass surgery versus PTA for chronic lower extremity ischemia (IC and CLI) found no difference between the revascularization strategies in mortality and amputation rates. Bypass was associated with a higher rate of complications but greater primary patency at 12 months; however, this benefit was lost by 4 years.[69] Until more contemporary trials are available, an endovascular first approach to CLI is reasonable in the majority of patients with surgery reserved for those with low surgical risk, long life expectancy, venous conduits, and suitable distal anatomic targets. Currently, the Best Endovascular versus Best Surgical Therapy in Patients With Critical Limb Ischemia (BEST-CLI) trial is enrolling and will provide needed data in this high-risk patient subset (ClinicalTrials.gov, Identifier NCT02060630).

Lesions at multiple anatomical levels cause CLI. Diabetes and end-stage renal disease are associated with more below-the-knee disease and tend to be diffuse, complex, and calcified, usually resulting in poor outcomes.[70] In comparison, patients without these risk factors have more focal lesions. In general, the aim is to establish in-line flow to the ischemic zone. A recent meta-analysis showed an angiosome-targeted revascularization strategy is superior to indirect revascularization of an ischemic zone for wound healing and limb salvage.[71] The need for an angiosome-targeted revascularization, however, remains controversial, and performing the most complete revascularization possible in the setting of CLI is recommended.

AORTO-ILIAC AND FEMOROPOPLITEAL REVASCULARIZATION FOR CRITICAL LIMB ISCHEMIA

Hybrid surgical and endovascular therapy for multilevel peripheral TASC D lesions, involving both the aorto-iliac and/or superficial femoral and CFAs, was studied in a small case series of 21 lower limbs in 20 patients with IC and CLI. The average ABI significantly increased from 0.50 ± 0.32 to 0.79 ± 0.24 (P = 0.002). Overall, primary patency rates were 94%, 70%, and 70% at 6, 12, and 24 months, respectively, with 100% limb salvage at 24 months.[72] Small series

have shown that SFA stenting is feasible for CLI and that primary patency rates at 30 months can equal that of the IC patient population.[73-75] The DEBATE-SFA randomized trial enrolled 110 femoropopliteal lesions (IC and CLI) into DCB + BMS and PTA + BMS groups and showed a significant reduction in 12-month binary restenosis and a trend toward lower TLR with DCB, and there were no major amputations.[60] Similar results were seen in the DEBELLUM trial, where DCB showed significantly lower TLR; however, only a trend toward reduction in the incidence of amputation was observed.[59]

INFRAPOPLITEAL BALLOON ANGIOPLASTY FOR CRITICAL LIMB ISCHEMIA

Almost 30% of CLI patients have popliteal and infrapopliteal disease. Surgical options are limited due to poor distal targets, comorbidities, and lack of autologous veins. The case series from Dorros et al. demonstrated high acute procedural success with tibioperoneal vessel angioplasty and showed that shorter lesions (less than 10 cm), stenotic lesions, and visualized distal vessels are good prognostic factors for procedural success.[76] The largest U.S. experience prospectively assessed 284 patients with CLI, Fontaine stages III and IV, and showed tibioperoneal vessel angioplasty had a success rate of 98% for stenotic lesions, but only 73% for total occlusions.[77] A more recent series from Söder et al.[78] involved older and sicker patients, the majority with tissue loss and ineligible for bypass surgery due to inadequate runoff. Primary angiographic success was 84% in stenotic lesions and 61% in occlusive lesions and at 10 months restenosis rates were 32% and 52%, respectively. Clinical success, defined as improvement in claudication or avoidance of amputation, was achieved in 65% of patients, which is comparable to the outcomes from surgical registries.

DRUG-COATED BALLOONS FOR CRITICAL LIMB ISCHEMIA

The initial experience with DCBs for infrapopliteal CLI has been mixed. Using the In.Pact Amphirion paclitaxel balloon (Medtronic, Minneapolis, MN) in 109 limbs, rates of clinical improvement (91.2%), complete wound healing (74.2%), TLR (17.3%), and limb salvage (95.6%) at 12 months were favorable.[79] The Drug-Eluting Balloon in Peripheral Intervention for Below The Knee Angioplasty Evaluation (DEBATE-BTK) trial studied DCB in diabetic CLI patients with infrapopliteal lesions and showed significantly less restenosis, TLR, and better wound healing as compared to conventional balloon angioplasty.[80] Despite encouraging results, caution is warranted considering the results of IN.PACT DEEP, which was terminated prematurely due to safety concerns, as there was a trend toward more major amputation in the DCB arm (8.8% vs. 3.6%; P = 0.80).[81] Several trials outside the United States are currently underway to study safety of DCB in CLI due to infrapopliteal PAD. See Figure 49.6 for infrapopliteal angioplasty in a patient with CLI.

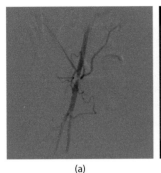 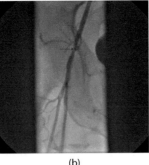

(a)   (b)

Figure 49.6 **(a)** Calcified high-grade CFA stenosis (*arrow*) and **(b)** postatherectomy using SilverHawk MS system. CFA, common femoral artery.

INFRAPOPLITEAL STENTING FOR CRITCAL LIMB ISCHEMIA

The expanding horizon of EVR for CLI has led to the use of coronary stents for tibioperoneal revascularization. Small single-center studies have shown reduced TLR and incidence of amputations with DES compared to BMS in CLI patients.[82,83] Rastan et al. investigated sirolimus DES versus BMS in a randomized double-blind trial for focal infrapopliteal *de novo* lesions. The event-free survival rate, defined as freedom from target limb amputation, target vessel revascularization (TVR), myocardial infarction (MI), and death was 65.8% in the DES group and 44.6% in the BMS group (log-rank $P = 0.02$). Amputation rates were 2.6% and 12.2% ($P = 0.03$), and TVR rates were 9.2% and 20% ($P = 0.06$), respectively.[84] In the CLI cohort of this trial, there was no significant difference in death or TVR. Rates of limb salvage were similarly high in both groups (97.4% vs. 87.1%; $P = 0.10$), although the rate of major or minor amputation was lower with DES (5.3% vs. 22.6%; $P = 0.04$).[84] The Drug-Eluting Stents in the Critically Ischemic Lower Leg (DESTINY) trial evaluated everolimus DES versus BMS for infrapopliteal CLI and found significantly improved primary patency and freedom from repeat revascularization at 12 months with DES, but no difference in rates of amputation between the two groups.[85] In the Comparing Angioplasty and Drug-Eluting Stents in the Treatment of Subjects with Ischemic Infrapopliteal Arterial Disease (ACHILLES) trial, DES, were compared with PTA, and although angiographic restenosis and vessel patency favored DES there was no difference in freedom from TLR and amputation.[86]

The available data suggest that DES offers less repeat revascularization compared to BMS for infrapopliteal revascularization; however, the benefits of routine use compared with PTA or balloon angioplasty with provisional stenting are less certain. Therefore, operators need to use judgment regarding the potential clinical efficacy of DES for infrapopliteal disease, particularly given the cost of DES. There is also a concern for stent thrombosis when DES is used in vessel with poor outflow, or when there is suboptimal expansion or stent edge dissections.

Acute limb ischemia

ALI is defined as an acute decrease in limb perfusion with eminent threat to limb viability and salvage. ALI may develop in a previous asymptomatic individual or in a patient with IC and carries a grave prognosis with high mortality (18%–25%) and rates of limb amputation (5%–30%).[87,88] The incidence of ALI in the general population is estimated to be 14 per 100,000 and is the indication for 10% of all endovascular procedures. The etiology of ALI can be embolism or *in situ* thrombosis. In the vast majority of cases, ALI is due to embolization from the heart, typically due to atrial fibrillation. Other mechanisms include iatrogenic from arterial catheterization, aneurysm-associated thrombus, bypass graft thrombosis, paradoxical embolism, trauma, or dissection of large vessels with distal progression. Emboli typically lodge at a branch point in the lower extremity circulation (aortoiliac, femoral bifurcation, tibial trifurcation); however, thrombotic ALI can occur anywhere in the arterial tree with SFA being the most common location. Patients with embolic ALI are more likely to die due to their underlying medical comorbidities; however, patients with thrombotic ALI are more likely to lose their limbs. Embolic ALI usually presents with acute onset of symptoms due to the lack of developed collateral circulation.

Despite advances in the endovascular, surgical, and pharmacological therapies for PAD over the past several decades, the incidence of ALI and poor prognosis has not changed. Once the diagnosis of ALI is made, the goal is to prevent thrombus propagation and worsening leg ischemia. Unless contraindicated, anticoagulation with heparin is required as a first step in management. For viable limbs (Fontaine class I and II), flow restoration by endovascular, open catheter-based embolectomy, or pharmacological reperfusion is paramount. In patients with a nonviable limb (Fontaine class III), unfortunately, amputation is the only option. See Table 49.3 for classification of ALI.

INTERVENTIONAL TREATMENT FOR ACUTE LIMB ISCHEMIA

In a study by Ouriel et al., patients with ALI of less than 7 days' duration were randomized to catheter-directed thrombolysis (CDT) or surgical intervention. This study showed high mortality in the surgical arm (84% vs. 58%, $P = 0.01$) and comparable 12-month rates of limb amputation, 18%.[89] The Surgery versus Thrombolysis for Ischemia of the Lower Extremity (STILE) trial randomized patients with ALI (<14 days in duration) to surgery versus CDT. Endovascular treatment significantly improved limb salvage rates.[90] The Thrombolysis or Peripheral Arterial Surgery (TOPAS) trial randomized ALI due to native arterial or bypass occlusion (<14 days of in duration) into CDT or surgical arm. The rates of amputation-free survival at 12 months were comparable (65% vs. 69.9%; $P = 0.23$), although major hemorrhagic complications were more common in the thrombolysis

Table 49.3 Stages of acute limb ischemia

Category	Description	Findings	Doppler
I	Viable	No sensory of muscle weakness	Audible arterial and venous
IIa	Threatened (slightly)	Minimal	Frequently inaudible arterial, audible venous
IIb	Threatened (imminent)	Mild to moderate, associated with pain	Frequently inaudible arterial, audible venous
III	Irreversible	Profound deficit	No signals

Source: Modified from Weaver, F.A., et al., *J. Vasc. Surg.*, 24(4), 513–521, 1996.

Table 49.4 Recommended doses of antiplatelet, antithrombotic, and thrombolytic medications for management of acute limb ischemia

Medication	Route	Dosage	Laboratory
Aspirin	PO/PR	325 mg	None
Clopidogrel	PO	300–600 mg loading, 75 mg maintenance dose	None
Heparin	IV	600 U/kg bolus then 12 U/Kg/hr	aPTT, platelet, HCT
Mannitol	IV	12.5–25 g	Creatinine
Plasminogen activator	IA	Depends on agent[a]	FSP, HCT, fibrinogen
Urokinase	IA	80–200,000 U/h tapering infusion	FSP, HCT, fibrinogen

Source: Modified from Rajagopalan, S., et al., (eds.), *Manual of Vascular Diseases*, Lippincott, Wilkins & Williams, Philadelphia, PA, 2004, p. 92.

Note: aPTT, activated partial thromboplastin time; FSP, fibrin split products; HCT, hematocrit; IA, intraarterial; IV, intravenous; PO, oral; PR, per rectum.

[a] Depends on thrombolytic (retaplase 0.25–1.0 U/hr; alteplase 0.2–1.0 mg/h; tenecteplase 0.25–0.5 mg/h).

group (12.5% vs. 5.5%; $P = 0.005$). On the basis of these trials, CDT is the most effective therapy for the treatment of viable limbs and is less invasive and causes less morbidity and mortality compared to surgery. Contraindications to thrombolytic therapy should be weighed prior to administration. See Table 49.4 for recommended medications and doses of thrombolytic therapy.

RHEOLYTIC THROMBECTOMY

An alternative nonsurgical treatment for ALI is thrombectomy. Although the FDA has approved many mechanical thrombectomy devices for use in thrombosed hemodialysis grafts, only the AngioJet LF140 (Possis Medical, Inc., Minneapolis, MN) is currently approved for use in peripheral arterial occlusive disease.[91] The Angiojet rheolytic thrombectomy system has been shown to be effective in the treatment of acutely occluded infra-aortic native arteries and bypass grafts, with the majority of acute thrombotic material being removed. The rheolytic catheter has been used successfully in conjunction with CDT in one series of 86 patients with acute and subacute limb-threatening ischemia. After primary rheolytic thrombectomy was performed, secondary CDT was performed in 50 patients, yielding a high acute success rate with a reported 6-month patency rate of 79%.[91] Additional evidence has been reported in a retrospective analysis by Ansel et al., in which 99 consecutive patients underwent rheolytic therapy for thrombotic occlusions in

80 native arteries or 19 bypass grafts. Complete thrombus removal was accomplished in 71% of patients and partial in 22%. Mortality and amputation rates at 30 days were 7.1% and 4%, respectively.[92] Although the Angiojet system likely provides a more forceful and complete thrombus aspiration, other simpler devices are available; Pronto V3 extraction catheter (Vascular Solutions, Minneapolis, MN), Export XT catheter (Medtronic Vascular, Santa Rosa, CA), Fetch (Possis Medical, Inc.), and the Diver CE (ev3, Plymouth, MN). Similarly, simple straight endhole catheters can be used for thrombus aspiration. Aspiration thrombectomy, however, has not been validated in comparison to CDT and surgery, and the role of thrombectomy as part of a hybrid revascularization strategy in CLI is unclear.

Adjunctive devices for peripheral intervention

With the growing use of EVR for a broad range of patients with PAD, there is an accompanying expectation of procedural success, even in patient and lesion subsets not studied in clinical trials. Many patients have complex disease, heavily calcified vessels, and long chronic total occlusions (CTOs), where traditional techniques have poor outcomes. In order to overcome these challenges several adjunctive devices are manufactured, facilitating wire crossing and plaque modification.

DEBULKING DEVICES

Atherectomy has been used to treat PAD in the past with mixed results. More recently, there has been renewed interest in debulking devices with the development of the SilverHawk (Fox Hollow Technologies, Redwood City, CA) excisional atherectomy system, and the Diamondback 360 Orbital Atherectomy System (Cardiovascular System Inc., St. Paul, MN). Both devices are FDA approved. Although there are no randomized trials comparing excisional atherectomy to balloon angioplasty or stenting, there are several registries and single-center experiences with the SilverHawk system. The Treating Peripherals with SilverHawk: Outcomes Collection (TALON) Registry enrolled 601 consecutive patients at 19 institutions. A total of 1,258 symptomatic lower extremity atherosclerotic lesions were treated with a mean lesion length of 63 mm above the knee and 69 mm below the knee. The primary endpoint of the study was TLR at 6 and 12 months. Procedural success was 98%, and the 6- and 12-month freedoms of TLR rates were 90% and 80%, respectively. Predictors of TLR were a history of MI or coronary revascularization, increasing Rutherford category, and lesion length. Multiple single-center series have also reported good initial success with similar mid- and long-term outcomes with this device within the femoropopliteal and infrapopliteal vessels.[93–96] The most recent prospective directional atherectomy registry, the Determination of Effectiveness of the SilverHawk Peripheral Plaque Excision System for the Treatment of Infrainguinal vessels/Lower Extremities (DEFINITIVE LE), enrolled 800 subjects from multiple centers. The 12-month primary patency rate was high (78% in IC), and in CLI patients, freedom from major unplanned amputation of the target limb was 95%. The rate of bail-out stenting was low at 3.2%. Periprocedural adverse events were uncommon but included embolization and perforation in 3.8% and 5.3% of patients, respectively.[97]

The advantage of the Silver-Hawk system is the ability to remove plaque with or without the performance of adjunctive angioplasty. This treatment may be particularly useful for locations where stenting should be avoided such as the distal SFA, popliteal, and CFA. The system comes in various sizes, allowing treatment from the CFA to the tibial vessels.

Limitations to the device have been its inability to cut calcified plaques, needing to use more than one device if treating varying size vessels in the same patient, and the risk of distal embolization requiring distal protection, especially for patients with limited patent runoff vessels. Figure 49.6 shows postatherectomy results of CFA using the SilverHawk MS system.

The Diamondback 360 Orbital Atherectomy System is a promising new device for treating lower extremity symptomatic PAD. The device differs from other atherectomy technologies by its unique orbital action to remove plaque and the ability to increase treatment diameter by increasing orbital speed. The Orbital Atherectomy System for Treating Peripheral vascular Stenosis (OASIS), a prospective multicenter clinical study, was conducted to evaluate the efficacy and safety of this system. In 2,207 patients, more than 350 cases with the Diamondback were documented. Results revealed low rates of dissection (2%), perforation (2.3%), and embolism (2%). Advantages for this device over the SilverHawk are its ability to cut through calcified lesions and the ability to increase cutting size by increasing rotational speed, thus potentially limiting the number of catheters needed per case.[98] The device is hampered by the inability to cut soft plaque and its tendency for distal embolization without the potential for distal protection given its need for a dedicated wire. Figure 49.7 shows the result of Diamondback atherectomy in infrapopliteal artery revascularization.

Excimer laser–assisted angioplasty (ELA) for the treatment of PAD has been commercially available in Europe since 1994. The technique is based on intense bursts of ultraviolet light in short pulse durations. The advantage of ELA lay in its ability to break molecular bonds directly by photochemicals rather than by pure heat, which limits continuous-wave hot-tip lasers. ELA is most applicable in the treatment of long complex lesions, calcified or noncalcified, and to facilitate crossing of CTO. The most advanced system used is the TURBO elite laser system (Spectranetics, Colorado Springs, CO). When combined with the TURBO-Booster guiding catheter, the elite laser can be used to create larger lumens for infrainguinal arteries. Scheinert and

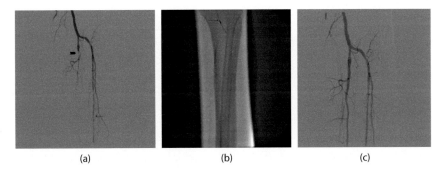

(a)   (b)   (c)

Figure 49.7 **(a)** Bifurcation of the popliteal artery into the anterior tibial artery and tibioperoneal (TP) trunk revealing a totally occluded TP trunk (*arrowhead*) and severe disease in the AT (*arrow*); **(b)** 1.25 Diamondback catheter advanced for multiple runs in the AT; **(c)** final result in the PT trunk and AT after atherectomy and low-atmosphere balloon inflation. AT, anterior tibial; PT, posterior tibial.

colleagues analyzed data from 318 consecutive patients who underwent ELA of 411 SFA with chronic occlusions averaging 19.4 ± 6 cm in length. Initial and secondary crossing success was 82% and 90.5%, respectively. The primary patency at 1 year was 33.6% with the 1-year assisted primary and secondary patency rates being 65.1% and 75.9%, respectively.[99,100] In the Laser Angioplasty for Critical Limb Ischemia (LACI) trial, a prospective registry at 14 sites in the United States and Germany, 145 patients with 155 critically ischemic limbs were enrolled. At 6-month follow-up, limb salvage was achieved in 92% of surviving patients.[99]

DEVICES TO CROSS CHRONIC TOTAL OCCLUSION

The Frontrunner XP CTO Catheter (Cordis) enables controlled crossing of CTO lesions using blunt microdissection to create a channel and facilitate wire placement. The device features a crossing profile of 0.039-in with an actuating jaw that opens to 2.3 mm. The shapeable distal tip and effective torque control enhance maneuverability while supported by a 4.5-Fr microguide catheter. Once the lesion is crossed, the microguide catheter is advanced into the true lumen, and the Frontrunner is removed and replaced with a guidewire up to 0.035-in. Mossop et al. prospectively evaluated the technical success and safety of controlled blunt microdissection for the treatment of resistant peripheral CTO. They enrolled 36 patients with 44 symptomatic CTOs (2 terminal aortic, 24 iliac, 16 femoral, and 2 popliteal), which had previously failed conventional percutaneous revascularization. Procedural success was achieved in 91% of the 44 CTOs.[101] This device is most helpful when the proximal cap of a CTO is refractory to initial guidewire penetration.

The CROSSER (FlowCardia, Inc., Sunnyvale, CA) is a novel CTO device that delivers vibrational energy to facilitate the crossing of occluded arteries. The CROSSER system has been proven safe and feasible in occluded coronary arteries with a procedure success rate of 73%,[102] but there is no available outcome data for peripheral arteries. The peripheral system is advanced over a 0.018-in guidewire until it reaches the proximal cap, and the wire is then retracted within the Crosser catheter. Once the catheter crosses the length of the lesion and reenters the true lumen, the wire is then reintroduced into the true lumen and the catheter removed, making

way for advancement of interventional equipment. This device relies on remaining within the true lumen and, therefore, may not be effective in long total occlusions, but it can aid in the initial crossing of heavily calcified caps. The Turbo Elite catheter (Spectranetics) delivers pulses of ultraviolet energy to able atherosclerotic tissue and thrombus and has been investigated in the Laser-assisted Angioplasty for Critical Ischemia international registry with a success rate of crossing the lesion in 86% of cases.[99] There are several other specialty catheters available like Wildcat, Ocelot, Kittycat, Kittycat2, and Avinger; however, they all lack formal outcome data.

There are two FDA-approved reentry devices for use in peripheral arteries. The Pioneer (Volcano) catheter uses ultrasound to guide reentry from the subintimal space into the true lumen, and the Outback LTD (Cordis) relies solely on fluoroscopic guidance.[103] In a small study, the devices were successful in achieving true lumen reentry in all cases, and the time to reentry was routinely less than 10 minutes.[104] The Outback LTD device can be delivered through a 6-Fr sheath and has a smaller crossing profile than the Pioneer catheter, which requires a 7-Fr sheath.

DEVICES ASSISTING DISTAL LUMEN REENTRY

In the presence of a CTO, there are various techniques and devices at the operator's disposal. For long occlusions, subintimal angioplasty has become a standard approach to revascularization. A stiff hydrophilic wire is advanced into the proximal cap with the aid of a backup catheter. The wire is then used to probe the cap until a small loop is formed in the subintimal space. The backup catheter is then advanced forward, keeping the wire loop as small as possible, limiting the size of the dissection plane. Maintaining the smallest dissection plane possible will increase the likelihood of reentering the true lumen with the guidewire. Once the distal cap is reached, the wire is then retracted into the catheter and redirected without the loop in attempt to cross back into the true lumen (Figure 49.8). Typically, reentry into the true lumen is the most time consuming and tedious aspect of treating a CTO. Reentry catheters, such as the Outback or Pioneer, have shown remarkable success if reentry into the true lumen is not possible with standard catheter and guidewire technique. Once across the distal cap, angioplasty of

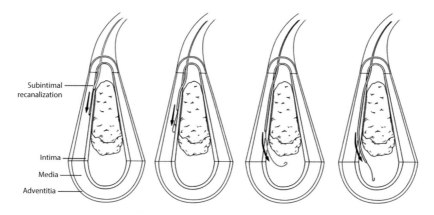

Figure 49.8 Subintimal dissection of CTO. CTO, chronic total occluded vessel.

Table 49.5 Devices for use in CTO endovascular intervention

	Minimal sheath (Fr)	Wire	RX/ OTW
CTO Crossing Devices			
Frontrunner (Cordis)	6	NA	NA
Crosser 14S (Flow Cardia)	5	0.014	RX
Crosser 18 (Flow Cardia)	6	0.018	RX
Reentry Devices			
Pioneer (Medtronic)	7	0.014[a]	RX
Outback LTD (Cordis)	6	0.014[a]	RX

Note: CTO, chronic total occlusion; OTW, over the wire; RX, monorail.

[a] Ironman or Grandslam wire.

the involved segment is performed, typically followed by self-expanding stent implantation. CTO equipment and compatibility are listed in Table 49.5.

EMBOLIC PROTECTION DEVICES FOR LOWER EXTREMITY REVASCULARIZATION

Since the initial introduction of distal protection during carotid stenting, embolic protection devices (EPDs) are now routinely used in coronary vein graft intervention as well as carotid artery stenting. These devices are either balloon-based, GuardWire Plus (Medtronic Vascular), or filter-based, like the AngioGuard (Cordis), FilterWireEX (Boston Scientific), NeuroShield (MedNova, Galway, Ireland), and the Spider (ev3, Plymouth). Although there are no randomized trials currently accessing EPDs for lower extremity revascularization, there have been studies that suggest these devices may be efficacious.[105–107] The use of these devices is limited in the lower extremity by their micropores—which are designed to retain cholesterol particles—and their susceptibility to becoming overwhelmed with fibrinous debris.[108] Although routine use of EPDs for lower extremity interventions is not recommended, there are specific cases in which protection may be efficacious. Consideration should be given for EPDs for any lesion proximal to a single-vessel runoff, SilverHawk atherectomy in heavily calcified lesions, and prior to rheolytic thrombectomy.

Surveillance after percutaneous interventions

There are no specific guidelines available on optimal timing and frequency of clinical and imaging surveillance.[75] The anatomic location and baseline clinical indication can serve as a guide with more frequent evaluation in CLI patients and long lesions, particularly those treated with stent grafts. Since there are no randomized studies, most recommendations are based on expert opinion. Routine ABI shortly after intervention is acceptable to establish a baseline to guide future surveillance. In cases of revascularization in high-risk patients or lesions, we suggest to have the first clinical

follow-up in 1–3 months, then 6 months, 1 year, and then annually. ABI surveillance is cost effective and can give good predictive value for hemodynamically significant restenosis in the presence of consistent exams and history. These surveillance intervals can be lengthened for interventions at low-risk of restenosis, such as isolated iliac stenting.

UPPER EXTREMITY ENDOVASCULAR INTERVENTION

In contrast to lower extremity disease, upper extremity vascular disease is uncommon and usually manifests with arm claudication, rest pain, and ischemic ulcerations. Rare manifestations of a subclavian stenosis are vertebrobasilar insufficiency if the contralateral vertebral artery is diseased or occluded, and angina in a patient with previous mammary artery used as a conduit for coronary artery bypass graft (CABG). The most common cause of large artery disease of the upper extremity is atherosclerosis. The involvement is typically limited to the proximal segments of the innominate and subclavian arteries, while more distal lesions are rare. Less common causes of occlusive disease are vasculitis, postradiation, and external compression.[109] Goals of revascularization in the upper extremity include relief from claudication, prevention of digit or limb loss, reversal of vascular steal from the internal mammary artery, or compromise of arterial-venous shunts for hemodialysis. Historically, upper extremity ischemic disease involving the large vessels was managed surgically using bypass or endarterectomy techniques. Currently, endovascular repair is the most accepted modality of treatment with data to support the lack of difference in long-term patency rates compared to surgery. More recently, Bates et al. reported a success rate of 97% and 1-year patency of 96% in 89 patients who underwent subclavian artery stenting.[110]

Anatomic considerations

The primary anatomical consideration when stenting the proximal left subclavian artery is the location of the left vertebral artery. Appropriate angulations should be performed to see the true ostium of the vertebral artery prior to stent implantation. The majority of cases will allow a landing zone prior to the vertebral origin. When there is no landing zone prior to the vertebral artery, the operator must be aware of the consequences of jailing or shifting plaque into the vertebral artery. In this case, to avoid compromise of a dominant or sole vertebral artery, angiography of both vertebral arteries, including intracranial views, is recommended.

When approaching the right system, the operator must adequately visualize the bifurcation of the right common carotid and right vertebral arteries when repairing the innominate and right subclavian artery, respectively. Typically, the bifurcation of the right common carotid and innominate artery is best seen in the right anterior oblique (RAO) projection. In the setting of significant atherosclerotic burden, distal protection within the vertebral system has been advocated by some, although the risk of stroke is small, potentially due to delayed reversal of vertebral artery blood flow from retrograde to antegrade following angioplasty of the subclavian artery.[111,112] Similarly, distal protection within the right internal carotid artery during repair of the right innominate may be considered for bulky atherosclerotic lesions.

Access and technique

Access for endovascular repair of the innominate or subclavian artery can be via the common femoral, brachial, or radial arteries. The CFA approach will permit the use of either a sheath or guide catheter. When using a sheath, the operator can either wire the lesion through a diagnostic catheter and replace the entire system with a sheath (usually 6- to 7-Fr and 90 cm in length) or more simply telescope the diagnostic catheter through the sheath, and once wired, advance the sheath into the appropriate location over the diagnostic catheter. Guiding catheters are limited by their smaller internal diameter when compared to that of similar-sized sheath. Sheaths are routinely used during brachial (6- to 7-Fr, 45 cm) and radial (6-Fr, 65–90 cm) access. Once the lesion has successfully been crossed with a standard 0.035-in wire, balloon predilatation can be used to gauge size and length prior to stent implantation. Subclavian arteries usually accommodate 7–10 mm diameter stents, while innominate arteries may require larger devices. Balloon-expandable stents are primarily used for their radial strength and precise placement. If the lesion is located aorto-ostially, the stent should protrude 1–2 mm into the aorta to have complete coverage of the lesion. Although most investigators believe that no distal protection of the vertebral artery is required at the time of proximal upper extremity intervention, thoughtful consideration must be given to protecting the right internal carotid for bulky innominate lesions. Protection of the right internal carotid can be accomplished via access and deployment of the protection device through an additional sheath in the right brachial or radial artery while primarily working through a sheath from the CFA to repair the innominate.

SECONDARY PREVENTION

After peripheral revascularization, blood pressure control, smoking cessation, statin therapy, and exercise are key secondary prevention tools to reduce future cardiovascular events. Lifelong aspirin or clopidogrel monotherapy is generally acceptable after all endovascular revascularizations. There are limited data on dual antiplatelet therapy (DAPT); nonetheless, the BMS trials for femoral intervention have used DAPT for 1–3 months. DAPT for 6 months is suggested in patients treated with DES or stent grafts. Antiplatelet therapy can be individualized based on a patient's disease status, risk of restenosis, and bleeding risk.[113] Data for Cilostazol reducing in-stent restenosis and TVR are limited to the Japanese population and may be related to genetic differences.[114–116] The antiplatelet agent vorapaxar

(protease-activated receptor [PAR]-1 antagonist) was examined in patients with PAD. Compared to placebo, vorapaxar reduced the risk of ALI and peripheral revascularization at the expense of increased bleeding. The rate of ALI was 1.3% per year, and more than 50% of events were due to surgical graft thrombosis with a quarter from in situ thrombosis and the remainder due to stent thrombosis or thromboembolism.[117] The algorithm for which patients should be treated with vorapaxar, as opposed to other antiplatelet agents, such as ticagrelor, is unclear. Ongoing studies to address the optimal antiplatelet and antithrombin therapy in PAD patients include A Study Comparing Cardiovascular Effects of Ticagrelor and Clopidogrel in Patients With Peripheral Artery Disease (EUCLID) (ClinicalTrials.gov Identifier: NCT01732822) and Efficacy and Safety of Rivaroxaban in Reducing the Risk of Major Thrombotic Vascular Events in Subjects With Peripheral Artery Disease Undergoing Peripheral Revascularization Procedures of the Lower Extremities (VOYAGER PAD) (ClinicalTrials.govIdentifier: NCT02504216).

MISCELLANEOUS CONDITIONS

Peripheral aneurysms

Aneurysms are primarily due to atherosclerosis; however, they can be familial or due to hypertension or connective tissue diseases. They are usually asymptomatic and often found bilaterally at the same level. Complications include rupture, embolization, and infection. Iliac artery aneurysms are also associated with obstructive uropathies and iliac vein obstruction. Traditionally, surgical resection is indicated in symptomatic patients or a size of >3 cm in diameter. Endovascular procedures with coiling and stent grafts have been employed with encouraging safety results, but long-term patency data compared to surgery are lacking.[118] Endovascular data for femoral artery aneurysms are limited to case reports only. Popliteal artery aneurysms are bilateral in 50% of the cases and can be diagnosed by ultrasound; however, contrast angiography is usually required before surgical excision or planned endovascular procedure. Endovascular covered stents are a viable option for popliteal aneurysms with encouraging early results. Ultrasound should be performed to appropriately size the neck and distal part of aneurysm (Figure 49.9).

May-Thurner syndrome

May-Thurner syndrome (MTS) is an extrinsic compression of the left common iliac vein at the level of crossover position of the right common iliac artery against bony structures, subsequently causing venous stenosis and outflow obstruction of the ipsilateral limb. MTS is more common in females, usually in their third or fourth decades of life, with an incidence of 2%–5% of all lower extremity venous swellings.[119] The majority of MTS patients are asymptomatic; however, patients can have varied presentation including acute swelling and pain of left lower extremity, acute

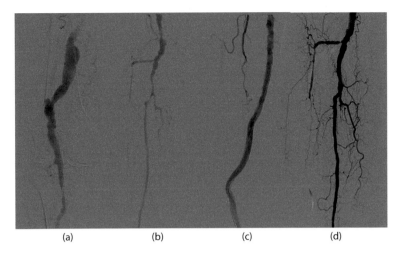

(a) (b) (c) (d)

Figure 49.9 **(a)** Right-sided femoropopliteal aneurysm. It is evaluated by IVUS to approximate neck and distal landing zone for a covered stent. **(b)** Careful assessment of distal run-off vessel is established and balloon angioplasty is performed to improve below-the-knee circulation prior to placement of a covered stent. **(c** and **d)** Post Viabahn stent placement angiogram showing complete apposition of stent to the neck of aneurysm and good distal flow. IVUS, intravascular ultrasound.

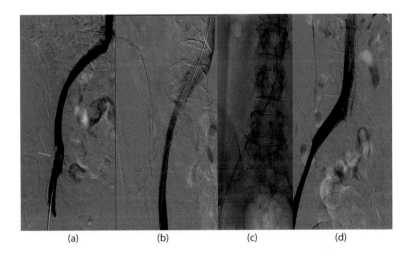

(a) (b) (c) (d)

Figure 49.10 **(a)** Venographic pictures are taken in prone position. Yellow mark indicates acute iliofemoral vein DVT. **(b)** Compression of left iliac vein by right iliac artery, yellow mark. **(c** and **d)** Stent of the ostial left common iliac vein utilizing a 16 mm diameter × 60 mm Boston Scientific Wall stent, a self-expanding stainless steel stent with successful reduction of left common iliac vein ostial stenosis from 85% stenosis to a less than 10% residual. DVT, deep vein thrombosis.

deep venous thrombosis, chronic venous insufficiency, lipodermatosclerosis, superficial venous thrombophlebitis, and even pulmonary embolism. The initial diagnostic test is ultrasound but ultimately a CT scan with venous phase or magnetic resonance venography may be required. The morphology of the lesion spur within the common iliac vein is seen best with an intravascular ultrasound (IVUS), which is not only useful in evaluating stenosis but also calibrating the size of vessels prior to stents (Figure 49.10).

CONCLUSION

The past two decades have seen an exponential increase in EVR therapies to treat upper and lower extremity PAD. Although there is a clear shift in the approach toward treating PAD with an endovascular first approach, the long-term safety and patency should be considered when deciding on the appropriate revascularization strategy in an individual patient. With the promise of several technologies on the horizon, we do expect similar growth trends in the field of peripheral revascularization for years to come.

REFERENCES

1. Selvin E, Erlinger TP. Prevalence of and risk factors for peripheral arterial disease in the United States: Results from the National Health and Nutrition Examination Survey, 1999–2000. *Circulation* 2004;110(6):738–743.
2. Dormandy JA, Rutherford RB. Management of peripheral arterial disease (PAD). TASC Working Group. Trans Atlantic Inter-Society Consensus (TASC). *J Vasc Surg* 2000;31(1 Pt 2):S1–S296.

3. Fowkes FG, et al. Edinburgh Artery Study: Prevalence of asymptomatic and symptomatic peripheral arterial disease in the general population. *Int J Epidemiol* 1991;20(2):384–392.

4. Hirsch AT, et al. ACC/AHA 2005 Practice Guidelines for the management of patients with peripheral arterial disease (lower extremity, renal, mesenteric, and abdominal aortic): A collaborative report from the American Association for Vascular Surgery/Society for Vascular Surgery, Society for Cardiovascular Angiography and Interventions, Society for Vascular Medicine and Biology, Society of Interventional Radiology, and the ACC/AHA Task Force on Practice Guidelines (Writing Committee to Develop Guidelines for the Management of Patients With Peripheral Arterial Disease): Endorsed by the American Association of Cardiovascular and Pulmonary Rehabilitation; National Heart, Lung, and Blood Institute; Society for Vascular Nursing; TransAtlantic Inter-Society Consensus; and Vascular Disease Foundation. *Circulation* 2006;113(11):e463–e654.

5. Hirsch AT, et al. The Minnesota Regional Peripheral Arterial Disease Screening Program: Toward a definition of community standards of care. *Vasc Med Lond Engl* 2001;6(2):87–96.

6. Management of peripheral arterial disease (PAD). TransAtlantic Inter-Society Consensus (TASC). Section D: Chronic critical limb ischaemia. *Eur J Vasc Endovasc Surg* 2000;19 Suppl A:S144–S243.

7. Willigendael EM, et al. Peripheral arterial disease: Public and patient awareness in The Netherlands. *Eur J Vasc Endovasc Surg* 2004;27(6):622–628.

8. Criqui MH, et al. The prevalence of peripheral arterial disease in a defined population. *Circulation* 1985;71(3):510–515.

9. Aboyans V, et al. Measurement and interpretation of the ankle-brachial index: A scientific statement from the American Heart Association. *Circulation* 2012;126(24):2890–2909.

10. Abbott JD, et al. Ankle-brachial index and cardiovascular outcomes in the Bypass Angioplasty Revascularization Investigation 2 Diabetes trial. *Am Heart J* 2012;164(4):585–590.e4.

11. Anderson JL, et al. Management of patients with peripheral artery disease (compilation of 2005 and 2011 ACCF/AHA guideline recommendations): A report of the American College of Cardiology Foundation/American Heart Association Task Force on Practice Guidelines. *Circulation* 2013;127(13):1425–1443.

12. 2011 WRITING GROUP MEMBERS, et al. 2011 ACCF/AHA Focused Update of the Guideline for the Management of patients with peripheral artery disease (Updating the 2005 Guideline): A report of the American College of Cardiology Foundation/American Heart Association Task Force on practice guidelines. *Circulation* 2011;124(18):2020–2045.

13. Norgren L, et al. Inter-society consensus for the management of peripheral arterial disease. *J Vasc Surg* 2007;26(2):81–157.

14. McDermott MM, et al. Home-based walking exercise intervention in peripheral artery disease: A randomized clinical trial. *JAMA* 2013;310(1):57–65.

15. Pande RL, et al. A pooled analysis of the durability and predictors of treatment response of cilostazol in patients with intermittent claudication. *Vasc Med Lond Engl* 2010;15(3):181–188.

16. Zeller T. Current state of endovascular treatment of femoro-popliteal artery disease. *Vasc Med* 2007;12(3):223–234.

17. Fontaine R, et al. [Surgical treatment of peripheral circulation disorders]. *Helv Chir Acta* 1954;21(5–6):499–533.

18. Rutherford RB, et al. Recommended standards for reports dealing with lower extremity ischemia: Revised version. *J Vasc Surg* 1997;26(3):517–538.

19. Klein AJ, et al. SCAI expert consensus statement for aorto-iliac arterial intervention appropriate use. *Catheter Cardiovasc Interv* 2014;84(4):520–528.

20. Klein AJ, et al. SCAI expert consensus statement for femoral-popliteal arterial intervention appropriate use. *Catheter Cardiovasc Interv* 2014;84(4):529–538.

21. Murphy TP, et al. Supervised exercise versus primary stenting for claudication resulting from aortoiliac peripheral artery disease: Six-month outcomes from the claudication: Exercise versus endoluminal revascularization (CLEVER) study. *Circulation* 2012;125(1):130–139.

22. Connors G, et al. Percutaneous revascularization of long femoral artery lesions for claudication: Patency over 2.5 years and impact of systematic surveillance. *Catheter Cardiovasc Interv* 2011;77(7):1055–1062.

23. Norgren L, et al. Inter-society consensus for the management of peripheral arterial disease (TASC II). *J Vasc Surg* 2007;45 Suppl S:S5–S67.

24. Bosch JL, Hunink MG. Meta-analysis of the results of percutaneous transluminal angioplasty and stent placement for aortoiliac occlusive disease. *Radiology* 1997;204(1):87–96.

25. Klein WM, et al. Dutch iliac stent trial: Long-term results in patients randomized for primary or selective stent placement. *Radiology* 2006;238(2):734–744.

26. Tetteroo E, et al. Randomised comparison of primary stent placement versus primary angioplasty followed by selective stent placement in patients with iliac-artery occlusive disease. Dutch Iliac Stent Trial Study Group. *Lancet* 1998;351(9110):1153–1159.

27. Whyman MR, et al. Randomised controlled trial of percutaneous transluminal angioplasty for intermittent claudication. *Eur J Vasc Endovasc Surg* 1996;12(2):167–172.

28. Management of peripheral arterial disease (PAD). TransAtlantic Inter-Society Consensus (TASC). *Int Angiol* 2000;19(1 Suppl 1):I–XXIV, 1–304.

29. Sacks D, et al. Reporting standards for clinical evaluation of new peripheral arterial revascularization devices. Technology Assessment Committee. *J Vasc Interv Radiol* 1997;8(1 Pt 1):137–149.

30. Taylor LM, Porter JM. Clinical and anatomic considerations for surgery in femoropopliteal disease and the results of surgery. *Circulation* 1991;83(2 Suppl):I63–I69.

31. Ponec D, et al. The Nitinol SMART stent vs Wallstent for suboptimal iliac artery angioplasty: CRISP-US trial results. *J Vasc Interv Radiol* 2004;15(9):911–918.

32. Mwipatayi BP, et al. A comparison of covered vs bare expandable stents for the treatment of aortoiliac occlusive disease. *J Vasc Surg* 2011;54(6):1561–1570.

33. Bekken JA, et al. DISCOVER: Dutch Iliac Stent trial: COVERed balloon-expandable versus uncovered balloon-expandable stents in the common iliac artery: Study protocol for a randomized controlled trial. *Trials* 2012;13:215.

34. Ballard JL, et al. Complications of iliac artery stent deployment. *J Vasc Surg* 1996;24(4):545–553.

35. Creasy TS, et al. Is percutaneous transluminal angioplasty better than exercise for claudication? Preliminary results from a prospective randomised trial. *Eur J Vasc Surg* 1990;4(2):135–140.

36. Bonvini RF, et al. Endovascular treatment of common femoral artery disease: Medium-term outcomes of 360 consecutive procedures. *J Am Coll Cardiol* 2011;58(8):792–798.

37. Scheinert D, et al. The LEVANT I (Lutonix paclitaxel-coated balloon for the prevention of femoropopliteal restenosis) trial for femoropopliteal revascularization: First-in-human randomized trial of low-dose drug-coated balloon versus uncoated balloon angioplasty. *JACC Cardiovasc Interv* 2014;7(1):10–19.

38. Schillinger M, et al. Balloon angioplasty versus implantation of nitinol stents in the superficial femoral artery. *N Engl J Med* 2006;354(18):1879–1888.

39. Dick P, et al. Balloon angioplasty versus stenting with nitinol stents in intermediate length superficial femoral artery lesions. *Catheter Cardiovasc Interv* 2009;74(7):1090–1095.

40. Laird JR, et al. Nitinol stent implantation vs. balloon angioplasty for lesions in the superficial femoral and proximal popliteal arteries of patients with claudication: Three-year follow-up from the RESILIENT randomized trial. *J Endovasc Ther* 2012;19(1):1–9.

41. Krankenberg H, et al. Nitinol stent implantation versus percutaneous transluminal angioplasty in superficial femoral artery lesions up to 10 cm in length: The femoral artery stenting trial (FAST). *Circulation* 2007;116(3):285–292.

42. Scheinert D, et al. Prevalence and clinical impact of stent fractures after femoropopliteal stenting. *J Am Coll Cardiol* 2005;45(2):312–315.

43. Schlager O, et al. Long-segment SFA stenting—The dark sides: In-stent restenosis, clinical deterioration, and stent fractures. *J Endovasc Ther* 2005;12(6):676–684.

44. Laird JR, et al. Nitinol stent implantation in the superficial femoral artery and proximal popliteal artery: Twelve-month results from the complete SE multicenter trial. *J Endovasc Ther* 2014;21(2):202–212.

45. George JC, et al. SUPERA interwoven nitinol Stent Outcomes in Above-Knee IntErventions (SAKE) study. *J Vasc Interv Radiol* 2014;25(6):954–961.

46. Scheinert D, et al. Treatment of complex atherosclerotic popliteal artery disease with a new self-expanding interwoven nitinol stent: 12-month results of the Leipzig SUPERA popliteal artery stent registry. *JACC Cardiovasc Interv* 2013;6(1):65–71.

47. Duda SH, et al. Sirolimus-eluting versus bare nitinol stent for obstructive superficial femoral artery disease: The SIROCCO II trial. *J Vasc Interv Radiol* 2005;16(3):331–338.

48. Duda SH, et al. Sirolimus-eluting stents for the treatment of obstructive superficial femoral artery disease: Six-month results. *Circulation* 2002;106(12):1505–1509.

49. Dake MD, et al. Sustained safety and effectiveness of paclitaxel-eluting stents for femoropopliteal lesions: 2-year follow-up from the Zilver PTX randomized and single-arm clinical studies. *J Am Coll Cardiol* 2013;61(24):2417–2427.

50. Dake MD, et al. Paclitaxel-eluting stents show superiority to balloon angioplasty and bare metal stents in femoropopliteal disease: Twelve-month Zilver PTX randomized study results. *Circ Cardiovasc Interv* 2011;4(5):495–504.

51. De Cock E, et al. A budget impact model for paclitaxel-eluting stent in femoropopliteal disease in France. *Cardiovasc Intervent Radiol* 2013;36(2):362–370.

52. Saxon RR, et al. Randomized, multicenter study comparing expanded polytetrafluoroethylene-covered endoprosthesis placement with percutaneous transluminal angioplasty in the treatment of superficial femoral artery occlusive disease. *J Vasc Interv Radiol* 2008;19(6):823–832.

53. Geraghty PJ, et al. Three-year results of the VIBRANT trial of VIABAHN endoprosthesis versus bare nitinol stent implantation for complex superficial femoral artery occlusive disease. *J Vasc Surg* 2013;58(2):386–395.e4.

54. Lammer J, et al. Heparin-bonded covered stents versus bare-metal stents for complex femoropopliteal artery lesions: The randomized VIASTAR trial (Viabahn endoprosthesis with PROPATEN bioactive surface [VIA] versus bare nitinol stent in the treatment of long lesions in superficial femoral artery occlusive disease). *J Am Coll Cardiol* 2013;62(15):1320–1327.

55. Saxon RR, et al. Heparin-bonded, expanded polytetrafluoroethylene-lined stent graft in the treatment of femoropopliteal artery disease: 1-year results of the VIPER (Viabahn Endoprosthesis with Heparin Bioactive Surface in the Treatment of Superficial Femoral Artery Obstructive Disease) trial. *J Vasc Interv Radiol* 2013;24(2):165–173; quiz 174.

56. Speck U, et al. Neointima inhibition: Comparison of effectiveness of non-stent-based local drug delivery and a drug-eluting stent in porcine coronary arteries. *Radiology* 2006;240(2):411–418.

57. Tepe G, et al. Local delivery of paclitaxel to inhibit restenosis during angioplasty of the leg. *N Engl J Med* 2008;358(7):689–699.

58. Werk M, et al. Paclitaxel-coated balloons reduce restenosis after femoro-popliteal angioplasty: Evidence from the randomized PACIFIER trial. *Circ Cardiovasc Interv* 2012;5(6):831–840.

59. Fanelli F, et al. The "DEBELLUM"—Lower limb multilevel treatment with drug eluting balloon—Randomized trial: 1-year results. *J Cardiovasc Surg (Torino)* 2014;55(2):207–216.

60. Liistro F, et al. Drug-eluting balloon in peripheral intervention for the superficial femoral artery: The DEBATE-SFA randomized trial (drug eluting balloon in peripheral intervention for the superficial femoral artery). *JACC Cardiovasc Interv* 2013;6(12):1295–1302.

61. Ljungman C, et al. A multivariate analysis of factors affecting patency of femoropopliteal and femorodistal bypass grafting. *Vasa* 2000;29(3):215–220.

62. Matsi P. Percutaneous transluminal angioplasty in critical limb ischaemia. *Ann Chir Gynaecol* 1995;84(4):359–362.

63. Muradin GS, et al. Balloon dilation and stent implantation for treatment of femoropopliteal arterial disease: Meta-analysis. *Radiology* 2001;221(1):137–145.

64. Saha S, et al. Early results of retrograde transpopliteal angioplasty of iliofemoral lesions. *Cardiovasc Intervent Radiol* 2001;24(6):378–382.

65. Lepäntalo M, Mätzke S. Outcome of unreconstructed chronic critical leg ischaemia. *Eur J Vasc Endovasc Surg* 1996;11(2):153–157.

66. Wolfe JH, Wyatt MG. Critical and subcritical ischaemia. *Eur J Vasc Endovasc Surg* 1997;13(6):578–582.

67. Allie DE, et al. Critical limb ischemia: A global epidemic. A critical analysis of current treatment unmasks the clinical and economic costs of CLI. *EuroIntervention* 2005;1(1):75–84.

68. Adam DJ, et al. Bypass versus angioplasty in severe ischaemia of the leg (BASIL): Multicentre, randomised controlled trial. *Lancet* 2005;366(9501):1925–1934.

69. Fowkes F, Leng GC. Bypass surgery for chronic lower limb ischaemia. *Cochrane Database Syst Rev* 2008;2:CD002000.

70. Kawarada O, et al. Predictors of adverse clinical outcomes after successful infrapopliteal intervention. *Catheter Cardiovasc Interv* 2012;80(5):861–871.

71. Biancari F, Juvonen T. Angiosome-targeted lower limb revascularization for ischemic foot wounds: Systematic review and meta-analysis. *Eur J Vasc Endovasc Surg* 2014;47(5):517–522.

72. Nishibe T, et al. Hybrid surgical and endovascular therapy in multifocal peripheral TASC D lesions: Up to three-year follow-up. *J Cardiovasc Surg (Torino)* 2009;50(4):493–499.

73. Hu H, et al. Endovascular nitinol stenting for long occlusive disease of the superficial femoral artery in critical limb ischemia: A single-center, mid-term result. *Ann Vasc Surg* 2011;25(2):210–216.

74. Lichtenberg M, et al. Superficial femoral artery TASC D Registry: Twelve-month effectiveness analysis of the Pulsar-18 SE nitinol stent in patients with critical limb ischemia. *J Cardiovasc Surg (Torino)* 2013;54(4):433–439.

75. Todoran TM, et al. Femoral artery percutaneous revascularization for patients with critical limb ischemia: Outcomes compared to patients with claudication over 2.5 years. *Vasc Med* 2012;17(3):138–144.

76. Dorros G, et al. The acute outcome of tibioperoneal vessel angioplasty in 417 cases with claudication and critical limb ischemia. *Cathet Cardiovasc Diagn* 1998;45(3):251–256.

77. Dorros G, et al. Tibioperoneal (outflow lesion) angioplasty can be used as primary treatment in 235 patients with critical limb ischemia: Five-year follow-up. *Circulation* 2001;104(17):2057–2062.

78. Söder HK, et al. Prospective trial of infrapopliteal artery balloon angioplasty for critical limb ischemia: Angiographic and clinical results. *J Vasc Interv Radiol* 2000;11(8):1021–1031.

79. Schmidt A, et al. First experience with drug-eluting balloons in infrapopliteal arteries: Restenosis rate and clinical outcome. *J Am Coll Cardiol* 2011;58(11):1105–1109.

80. Liistro F, et al. Drug-eluting balloon in peripheral intervention for below the knee angioplasty evaluation (DEBATE-BTK): A randomized trial in diabetic patients with critical limb ischemia. *Circulation* 2013;128(6):615–621.

81. Zeller T, et al. Drug-eluting balloon versus standard balloon angioplasty for infrapopliteal arterial revascularization in critical limb ischemia: 12-month results from the IN.PACT DEEP randomized trial. *J Am Coll Cardiol* 2014;64(15):1568–1576.

82. Scheinert D, et al. Comparison of sirolimus-eluting vs. bare-metal stents for the treatment of infrapopliteal obstructions. *EuroIntervention* 2006;2(2):169–174.

83. Siablis D, et al. Sirolimus-eluting versus bare stents after suboptimal infrapopliteal angioplasty for critical limb ischemia: Enduring 1-year angiographic and clinical benefit. *J Endovasc Ther* 2007;14(2):241–250.

84. Rastan A, et al. Sirolimus-eluting stents for treatment of infrapopliteal arteries reduce clinical event rate compared to bare-metal stents: Long-term results from a randomized trial. *J Am Coll Cardiol* 2012;60(7):587–591.

85. Bosiers M, et al. Randomized comparison of everolimus-eluting versus bare-metal stents in patients with critical limb ischemia and infrapopliteal arterial occlusive disease. *J Vasc Surg* 2012;55(2):390–398.

86. Scheinert D, et al. A prospective randomized multicenter comparison of balloon angioplasty and infrapopliteal stenting with the sirolimus-eluting stent in patients with ischemic peripheral arterial disease: 1-year results from the ACHILLES trial. *J Am Coll Cardiol* 2012;60(22):2290–2295.

87. Earnshaw JJ, et al. National Audit of Thrombolysis for Acute Leg Ischemia (NATALI): Clinical factors associated with early outcome. *J Vasc Surg* 2004;39(5):1018–1025.

88. Eliason JL, et al. A national and single institutional experience in the contemporary treatment of acute lower extremity ischemia. *Ann Surg* 2003;238(3):389–390.

89. Ouriel K, et al. A comparison of thrombolytic therapy with operative revascularization in the initial treatment of acute peripheral arterial ischemia. *J Vasc Surg* 1994;19(6):1021–1030.

90. Weaver FA, et al. Surgical revascularization versus thrombolysis for nonembolic lower extremity native artery occlusions: Results of a prospective randomized trial. The STILE Investigators. Surgery versus Thrombolysis for Ischemia of the Lower Extremity. *J Vasc Surg* 1996;24(4):513–521.

91. Kasirajan K, et al. Rheolytic thrombectomy in the management of acute and subacute limb-threatening ischemia. *J Vasc Interv Radiol* 2001;12(4):413–421.

92. Ansel GM, et al. Rheolytic thrombectomy in the management of limb ischemia: 30-day results from a multicenter registry. *J Endovasc Ther* 2002;9(4):395–402.

93. Kandzari DE, et al. Procedural and clinical outcomes with catheter-based plaque excision in critical limb ischemia. *J Endovasc Ther* 2006;13(1):12–22.

94. Matsi PJ, et al. Femoropopliteal angioplasty in patients with claudication: Primary and secondary patency in 140 limbs with 1-3-year follow-up. *Radiology* 1994;191(3):727–733.

95. Zeller T, et al. Long-term results after directional atherectomy of femoro-popliteal lesions. *J Am Coll Cardiol* 2006;48(8):1573–1578.

96. Zeller T, et al. Midterm results after atherectomy-assisted angioplasty of below-knee arteries with use of the Silverhawk device. *J Vasc Interv Radiol* 2004;15(12):1391–1397.

97. McKinsey JF, et al. Lower extremity revascularization using directional atherectomy: 12-month prospective results of the DEFINITIVE LE study. *JACC Cardiovasc Interv* 2014;7(8):923–933.

98. Safian RD, et al. Orbital atherectomy for infrapopliteal disease: Device concept and outcome data for the OASIS trial. *Catheter Cardiovasc Interv* 2009;73(3):406–412.

99. Laird JR, et al. Limb salvage following laser-assisted angioplasty for critical limb ischemia: Results of the LACI multicenter trial. *J Endovasc Ther* 2006;13(1):1–11.

100. Scheinert D, et al. Excimer laser-assisted recanalization of long, chronic superficial femoral artery occlusions. *J Endovasc Ther* 2001;8(2):156–166.

101. Mossop P, et al. First case reports of controlled blunt microdissection for percutaneous transluminal angioplasty of chronic total occlusions in peripheral arteries. *Catheter Cardiovasc Interv* 2003;59(2):255–258.

102. Melzi G, et al. A novel approach to chronic total occlusions: The crosser system. *Catheter Cardiovasc Interv* 2006;68(1):29–35.

103. Saket RR, et al. Novel intravascular ultrasound-guided method to create transintimal arterial communications: Initial experience in peripheral occlusive disease and aortic dissection. *J Endovasc Ther* 2004;11(3):274–280.

104. Jacobs DL, et al. True lumen re-entry devices facilitate subintimal angioplasty and stenting of total chronic occlusions: Initial report. *J Vasc Surg* 2006;43(6):1291–1296.

105. Siablis D, et al. Outflow protection filters during percutaneous recanalization of lower extremities' arterial occlusions: A pilot study. *Eur J Radiol* 2005;55(2):243–249.

106. Suri R, et al. Distal embolic protection during femoropopliteal atherectomy. *Catheter Cardiovasc Interv* 2006;67(3):417–422.

107. Wholey MH, et al. Early experience in the application of distal protection devices in treatment of peripheral vascular disease of the lower extremities. *Catheter Cardiovasc Interv* 2005;64(2):227–235.

108. König CW, et al. Frequent embolization in peripheral angioplasty: Detection with an embolism protection device (AngioGuard) and electron microscopy. *Cardiovasc Intervent Radiol* 2003;26(4):334–339.

109. Rodriguez-Lopez JA, et al. Stenting for atherosclerotic occlusive disease of the subclavian artery. *Ann Vasc Surg* 1999;13(3):254–260.

110. Bates MC, et al. Subclavian artery stenting: Factors influencing long-term outcome. *Catheter Cardiovasc Interv* 2004;61(1):5–11.

111. Nasim A, et al. Protection against vertebral artery embolisation during proximal subclavian artery angioplasty. *Eur J Vasc Surg* 1994;8(3):362–363.

112. Ringelstein EB, Zeumer H. Delayed reversal of vertebral artery blood flow following percutaneous transluminal angioplasty for subclavian steal syndrome. *Neuroradiology* 1984;26(3):189–198.

113. Schillinger M, et al. Sustained benefit at 2 years of primary femoropopliteal stenting compared with balloon angioplasty with optional stenting. *Circulation* 2007;115(21):2745–2749.

114. Soga Y, et al. Initial and 3-year results after subintimal versus intraluminal approach for long femoropopliteal occlusion treated with a self-expandable nitinol stent. *J Vasc Surg* 2013;58(6):1547–1555.

115. Soga Y, et al. Restenosis after stent implantation for superficial femoral artery disease in patients treated with cilostazol. *Catheter Cardiovasc Interv* 2012;79(4):541–548.

116. Soga Y, et al. Impact of cilostazol on angiographic restenosis after balloon angioplasty for infrapopliteal artery disease in patients with critical limb ischemia. *Eur J Vasc Endovasc Surg* 2012;44(6):577–581.

117. Bonaca MP, et al. Acute limb ischemia and outcomes with vorapaxar in patients with peripheral artery disease: Results from the trial to assess the effects of vorapaxar in preventing heart attack and stroke in patients with atherosclerosis-thrombolysis in myocardial infarction 50 (TRA2°P-TIMI 50). *Circulation* 2016;133(10):997–1005.

118. Working Party on Thrombolysis in the Management of Limb Ischemia. Thrombolysis in the management of lower limb peripheral arterial occlusion—A consensus document. *J Vasc Interv Radiol* 2003;14(9 Pt 2):S337–S349.

119. Hassell DR, et al. Unilateral left leg edema: A variation of the May-Thurner syndrome. *Cardiovasc Intervent Radiol* 1987;10(2):89–91.

50

Renal and mesenteric artery interventions

SUMIT BARAL, ROBERT A. LOOKSTEIN, AND JOHN H. RUNDBACK

INTRODUCTION

Little has changed in the last decade regarding our understanding of renal artery stenosis (RAS) and the role of renal artery interventions. Emerging data from the U.S. Registry for Fibromuscular Dysplasia (FMD)[1] continue to provide insights into the genetic, epidemiologic, and clinical science of this unique arteriopathy. FMD predominantly affects women in their sixth decade of life—older than previously thought—and is associated with a high rate of both familial and personal histories of cerebrovascular symptoms.[2] Dissections and aneurysms are recognized in more than 20% of these patients, mandating a thorough evaluation of both the presence and extent of renal and extrarenal (predominantly cervical carotid) involvement. Percutaneous transluminal renal angioplasty (PTRA) alone provides satisfactory and durable clinical results in the majority of patients (Figure 50.1), although renal stenting has been described as a bailout for angiographic failures or dissection after PTRA.

Atherosclerotic renal artery stenosis (ARAS), generally due to aortic atheroma impinging on the renal artery ostia, remains the predominant cause of RAS, affecting an older and more frequently male demographic. Autopsy studies have shown ARAS as a common but often incidental finding.[3] Although there has been an association between both the presence and severity of ARAS and subsequent cardiac events,[4,5] the relevance of this finding in the era of modern data is uncertain. Prospective, randomized core-lab adjudicated results from the completed ASTRAL (Angioplasty and Stenting for Renal Artery Lesions, n = 806)[6] and CORAL (Cardiovascular Outcomes in Renal Artery Lesions, n = 947)[7] studies did not demonstrate a benefit for renal artery stenting (RAST) compared with medical therapy alone for systolic or diastolic blood pressure (BP), renal function, myocardial infarction (MI), heart failure, or stroke. Both an independent prospective trial of 84 patients[8] and a MRI substudy from ASTRAL (21 RAST patients, 23 medically treated patients)[9] found no difference in cardiac function or morphology in patients undergoing RAST. Finally, a meta-analysis of seven trials, including ASTRAL and CORAL, with a total of 1,916 patients (937 with revascularization, 979 with medication alone) found no relevant difference in any measured clinical outcome.[10] A subsequent post hoc analysis of data from CORAL has suggested potential clinical improvements in a subset of patients with minimal or no proteinuria.

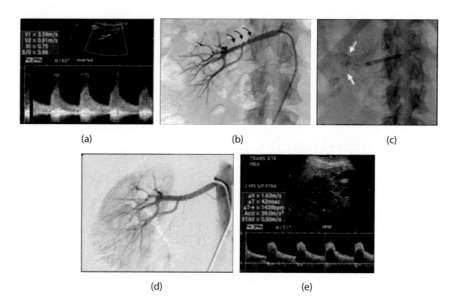

(a)   (b)   (c)

(d)   (e)

Figure 50.1 Renal fibromuscular dysplasia (FMD) in a 42-year-old woman. Initial duplex sonography **(a)** shows a peak systolic velocity (PSV) of 359 cm/s in the mid renal artery consistent with severe FMD. Angiography confirms medial fibroplasia with a "string of beads" appearance in the mid to distal renal artery **(b)**. Percutaneous transluminal renal angioplasty (PTRA) was performed with a 5 mm balloon over a pressure-sensing wire and exchange wire **(c)** with complete resolution of webs and stenosis on angiography completion **(d)**. The patient became normotensive, and follow-up renal duplex sonography 2 years later showed persistent, normalized Doppler waveforms in the renal artery **(e)**.

Murphy identified a baseline urinary albumin to creatinine ratio of ≤22.5 mg/g that was associated with a significantly better, event-free survival for the composite of attributable coronary and renal events, cardiac/renal death, overall survival, and worsening renal insufficiency.[11]

Observational data

The results from these randomized studies are to some extent discordant with a long prior history of observational data regarding the role of RAST (Tables 50.1 and 50.2).[12–29] Revascularization in most of these series resulted in reproducible and sustainable reductions in both systolic and diastolic BP. In the largest published registry series to date, Dorros et al.[13] reported on 1,058 successfully stented patients, including 901 (85%) who were treated for poorly controlled hypertension. Follow-up data demonstrated a durable and statistically significant improvement in BP control (at 4 years: systolic, 168 ± 27 to 147 ± 21 mmHg; diastolic 84 ± 15 to 78 ± 12 mmHg; $P < 0.05$), as well as a significant decrease in the number of antihypertensive medications (2.4 ± 1.1 to 1.8 ± 0.9 at 3 years; $P < 0.05$). Two core laboratory adjudicated industry-sponsored prospective trials support these findings. In the ASPIRE-2 study,[18] systolic/diastolic BP was reduced from 168 ± 25/82 ± 13 mmHg at baseline to 149 ± 25/77 ± 12 mmHg at 2 years ($P < 0.001$) in 208 patients.[30] The number of antihypertensive medications was changed from 2.8 ± 0.9 at baseline to 2.3 ± 1.3 at follow-up ($P < 0.001$). The RENAISSANCE study[21] evaluated 100 patients for up to 3 years. Average systolic BP was noted to be reduced by 15 ± 28 mmHg ($P = 0.0003$), with diastolic pressure lowered by 4 ± 15 mmHg ($P = 0.0510$).

Cohort series have also shown that the majority of patients undergoing RAST for renal insufficiency will have functional benefit, defined either as stabilization or improvement in either serum creatinine or calculated glomerular filtration rate (GFR) (Table 50.2).[14,17,20,23–26,31–44] Overall, between 50% and 90% of patients in these reports have seen clinical benefit following RAST. Studies evaluating single kidney or total GFR after RAST have consistently demonstrated incremental positively directed changes when plotting the change in slope of inverse serum creatinine curves prior to and following intervention.[35] Predictors of benefit include an absence of diabetes or proteinuria, bilateral disease, recent rapid declines in renal function, and lower baseline serum creatinine. However, none of these are absolute, and benefit may still be observed in patients with measurable proteinuria,[38] diabetes, and advanced renal insufficiency. Recent reports have even described renal recovery for dialysis-dependent patients after RAST.[43]

Critical analysis of randomized studies

There have been several critical reviews of the ASTRAL and CORAL trials that have sought to identify reasons inherent in their study designs to explain the lack of effect of RAST.[44–46] Notably, the ASTRAL study design was limited in its randomization of patients in whom the anticipated benefit of stenting compared to medical therapy was uncertain, thus raising concern that patients with overt cardiorenal syndromes and RAS may have been excluded from the trial. The CORAL trial did not have this limitation as it did consider potential therapeutic equipoise in the randomization scheme. However, reasons for nonenrollment include

Table 50.1 Hypertension outcomes after renal artery stenting

Author	N	Follow-up (mo)	Systolic BP (millimeters of mercury)			Diastolic BP (millimeters of mercury)			Comments
			Baseline	Postprocedure	Change	Baseline	Postprocedure	Change	
Dangas, 2001[12]	131	Mean 15 ± 9 (n ¼ 118)	170 ± 25	145 ± 20	–	84 ± 14	74 ± 12	–	48% improved
Dorros, 2002[13]	1,058	12	168 ± 27	146 ± 24	–	84 ± 15	75 ± 12	–	
Zeller, 2004[15]	340	6 (n ¼ 278)	144 ± 19	136 ± 15	–	79 ± 11	72 ± 9	–	
		12 (n ¼ 211)		133 ± 15	–		75 ± 10	–	
Sapoval, 2005[16]	52	6 (n ¼ 46)	172	152	–	92	85	–	5% cure, 61% improved
Tsao, 2005[17]	34	6 (n ¼ 33)	148 ± 4	130 ± 2	–	78 ± 3	70 ± 2	–	85% cure/improved
Rocha-Singh, 2005[18]	208	9 (n ¼ 178)	168 ± 25	149 ± 24	–	82 ± 13	77 ± 12	–	
Ruchin, 2007[19]	89	Mean: 28	161.7 ± 29.5	138.7 ± 17.9	–	78.4 ± 13.8	76.7 ± 10.8	–	
Goncalves, 2007[20]	46	Median: 23	177 ± 30	135 ± 28	42.11 ± 37.85	98 ± 17	83 ± 8	15	43% improved
Rocha-Singh, 2008[21]	100	Mean: 24.5 ± 15.2 9 (n ¼ 92)	156 ± 18	148 ± 22	9 ± 24	75 ± 12	75 ± 9	–	
		36		141 ± 22	16 ± 29		71 ± 9	4 ± 15	

BP, blood pressure.

Table 50.2 Renal function outcomes after renal artery stenting

First author, year	n	Follow-up (mo)	Mean serum creatinine (mg/dL)			Categorical outcomes (%)[a]	
			Baseline	Follow-up	p	Improved	Stabilized
Dorros, 2002[13]	1,058		1.7 ± 1.1	1.3 ± 0.8	<0.05	–	–
Rocha-Singh, 2002[21]	51		2.3 ± 0.9	1.7 ± 0.7	<0.001	–	–
Zeller, 2003[23]	215	12	1.21	1.1	0.047	51	–
Zeller, 2004[15]	354	34	–	–	–	10	39
Ramos, 2003[24]	105		1.7 ± 0.9	1.4 ± 0.7	<0.0001	–	–
Gill, 2003[25]	100	25	–	–	–	31	42
Ilkay, 2004[26]	13		2.6 ± 0.9	1.8 ± 0.6	<0.001	–	–
Rivolta, 2005[27]	52	24	2.9 ± 1.8	–	–	16	60
Rocha-Singh, 2005 (ASPIRE-2 Study)[18]	63[b]	9	–	–	–	91	
Kashyap, 2007[28]	125	12	2.2 ± 0.9	2.4 ± 1.5	0.1	42	25
Bates, 2008[29]	111[b]	36	–	–	–	23	52
Rocha-Singh, 2008 (RENAISSANCE Trial)[21]	100	36	1.3 ± 0.4	1.4 ± 0.6	0.1		

[a] Definitions for improvement and stabilization vary by report.
[b] Cohort of study patients with baseline serum creatinine 2:1.5 mg/dL.

patient preference in 17%, physician preference in 4%, and other unspecified reasons in 23%.[47] The impact of this potentially selective enrollment is difficult to ascertain, but somewhat slow recruitment resulted in an easing of the eligibility criteria during the course of the trial—the initial requirement that patients have refractory hypertension despite adequate antihypertensive therapy was changed to include patients with controlled BP. In addition, a requirement for trans-stenotic pressure measurements was removed early in the study.

A principal criticism of CORAL is that it did not by design include patients who could potentially benefit most from renal intervention, notably those with the highest level of baseline BP, severe stenosis, and lesions with measurable trans-stenotic gradients of at least 20 mmHg. The CORAL study included 85 stented patients and 58 medically treated patients with ≥80% stenosis by core lab analysis (198 stented patients and 166 medically treated patients with ≥80% RAS by site reported data), 151 stented and 142 medical patients with systolic BP ≥160 mmHg, and 110 stents/102 medical patients with ≥20 mmHg gradient (including 68 RAST and 38 medical patients having a greater than 40 mmHg gradient). However, in a post hoc analysis of patients with these specific characteristics, there was no statistically measurable difference in renal or cardiac endpoints.[47] Although these comparisons were not prespecified or well powered, the 199 patients with measured lesional gradients represent the largest dataset of this kind.

Microcirculatory disturbances can potentially mitigate any response to remediation of a proximal renal artery stenosis. Scoble et al., in 1999, postulated the concept of "atherosclerotic nephropathy," describing the "downstream" intrarenal effects of ARAS in the main renal artery due to cholesterol emboli, inflammation, and cytokine responses.[48] In support of this concept, an elevated renal resistive index (RRI), a measure of microcirculatory disturbance, has repeatedly been shown to correlate with a poor response to RAST.[49–51] Similarly, the identification of RAS may occur after substantial morphologic injury has already occurred in the kidney, impacting potential recovery with intervention. Albuminuria is negatively correlated with benefit from RAST in multiple series including CORAL,[38,52–54] and may be a marker of unrecoverable renal tubulointerstitial fibrosis.

It is notable that improvements in pharmacotherapy may have impacted the negative findings of CORAL. The medications used in CORAL were remarkably effective and included candesartan, a thiazide, amlodipine, and atorvastatin. Arguably, these or similar medications within each class, now represent the current standard of medical care for patients with RAS. A recent survey of 872 patients evaluated at a single institution over the time period from 1986 to 2014 (prior to early trials, through to post ASTRAL and CORAL) showed incrementally increased utilization of angiotensin-converting enzyme (ACE) inhibitors and angiotensin receptor blockers (ARBs), statins, and beta-blockers. Although patients in the most contemporary time period had higher cardiovascular comorbidities, there were progressively less proteinuria, renal insufficiency, and cardiovascular events.[55] Misra et al., in a retrospective evaluation of 1,052 patients following RAST, found ACE/ARB predictive of a decreased risk of renal failure, and statins to be associated with lower all-cause mortality.[56]

Perhaps the greatest reason that the randomized trials failed to show a benefit from RAST is that physiologically relevant RAS is either substantially less common than the anatomic presence of disease or that it is discovered too late. As such, the clinical identification of patients who will be helped from stenting remains uniquely elusive. There is emerging evidence that RAS results in a variable and chronic renal adaptive response to recurrent ischemic injury. In the future, advanced magnetic resonance imaging (MRI) techniques, such as perfusion imaging, diffusion-weighted imaging (DWI), diffusion tensor imaging, and blood oxygen level dependent (BOLD) renal imaging may identify patients with clinical disease and a potentially physiologic "penumbra" to predict the response to revascularization.[30]

CURRENT INDICATIONS FOR RENAL INTERVENTION

Given the current landscape of data for renal angioplasty and stenting in ARAS, all indications for intervention are relative, and further clinical trials will be necessary to definitively define which patients will best benefit from therapy. Despite this, there are several individual cohorts for whom RAST may be warranted based upon the existing knowledge base.

Acute renal failure

The rate of decline prior to RAST has been demonstrated in multiple series to be a strong predictor of renal improvement.[33,34,57,58] In a series of 125 patients undergoing RAST for chronic kidney disease (CKD),[58] 53 (42%) were considered "responders" (eGFR improved more than 20% from baseline) and an additional 31 (25%) experienced stabilized renal function (eGFR ±20% of baseline). Responders had statistically significant differences in the slope of renal decline in the 6 months prior to intervention. Modrall et al. identified a threshold of 0.46%/week reduction in preprocedural eGFR to have a sensitivity of 0.88 and negative predictive value of 0.94 for predicting outcomes of RAST in a small population of patients with renal insufficiency.[59] However, specificity and positive predictive value were relatively low, suggesting that utilization of a strict cutoff value may limit the potential of benefit for some patients with more gradual onset of disease. A benefit from intervention is notable, since responders are more likely to avoid or substantially delay the onset of renal replacement therapy.[58] Although the influence of successful RAST on overall mortality has not been proven, two studies have suggested improved survival in patients who regain renal function after undergoing intervention.[60,61]

Predialytic renal failure

Two recent reports have affirmed that RAST may be uniquely valuable in patients with predialytic (CKD stage 3–5) renal failure.[62,63] In a prospective review of 908 patients undergoing RAST for advanced kidney disease, Kalra et al. reported an odds ratio for improvement in GFR of at least 20% 1 year after intervention to be 2.69 (1.55–4.68) for patients with eGFR ≤60 mL/min/1.73 m² (stage 3 CKD), and 6.72 (3.59–12.56) for eGFR under 30 mL/min/1.73 m² (stage 4–5 CKD). Both of these observations had strong

statistical significance.[62] Further data from the 251 patient ODORI registry noted 12-month increases of 12.9 mL/min/1.73 m² mean eGFR in patients with baseline stage 4 CKD (P = 0.04); similar but nonstatistically significant trends were noted in other CKD subsets. In contrast, significant decreases in eGFR were observed in patients with eFGR ≥60 mL/min/1.73 m².[63] These findings of potential renal recovery warrant further investigation of RAS screening and treatment paradigm in patients being audited for initial renal replacement therapy.

Complete removal of patients from renal replacement therapy following RAST has also been reported.[43] A recent series by Thatipelli et al.[43] described the cessation of hemodialysis in 8 of 16 patients with both chronic and acute renal failure as the cause for renal replacement therapy. Renal size and absence of proteinuria have been found to be associated with dialysis cessation.[64]

Heart failure

RAS is associated with left ventricular (LV) dysfunction, including reduced diastolic compliance (measured as LV end diastolic volume), that can result in recurrent episodes of heart failure (HF) or otherwise unexplainable "flash" pulmonary edema despite a normal systolic ejection fraction.[65,66] A contemporary trial by Kane et al. compared medical therapy alone versus renal revascularization in patients with RAS and recurrent HF. Revascularization in this series produced substantial and positive differences in subsequent HF severity, proportion of follow-up hospital admissions for HF, and time to first HF hospitalization.[67] The CORAL trial did not find this same association.[66] A history of HF was present in 12% (n = 69) and 15% (n = 54) of the stented and medical arms, respectively. There was no difference in either congestive heart failure (CHF) admission (20% vs. 26%, P = 0.112) or cardiovascular death (16% vs. 17%, P > 0.99) between the groups.[68] However, it is important to note that only 8% of the CORAL cohort had *active* CHF, limiting the assessment in this subgroup.

Severely refractory hypertension

In a study of 149 patients undergoing RAST,[59] one-third of patients were determined to benefit from intervention. Responders were noted to have four predictive criteria: ≥4 antihypertensive medications, clonidine use, and a baseline diastolic BP of ≥90 mmHg. A larger renal size measured by cross-sectional ultrasound volume was an additional discriminator of favorable outcome. A trend toward better outcomes in patients treated for bilateral RAS was also observed. Interestingly, responders as a group had lower baseline GFR than nonresponders.

In addition to being a drug-sparing procedure in most cases, percutaneous transluminal renal stenting (PTRS) has the important advantage of improving BP medication flexibility, particularly in patients with concomitant coronary artery disease requiring ACE inhibitors.[69]

TECHNIQUES AND TECHNICAL OUTCOMES

For ARAS, primary or direct stenting is generally performed. Despite the fact that ostial calcification is often present, lesions are effaceable with direct stent implantation in almost all cases. Stents should be implanted so as to completely cover the culprit lesion, with 1–3 mm extension into the aorta in most cases (Figure 50.2). In scenarios in which remodeling of the aortorenal ostium proximal to the ARAS results in different medial positions of the upper and lower edges of the renal artery origin, complete stent coverage across the most medial edge is necessary.

Positioning of renal artery stents requires that the treated renal artery origin is seen in complete profile. Computed tomography (CT) studies demonstrate that the right renal artery is often best imaged from a straight anteroposterior (AP) image. The left renal usually arises obliquely from the aorta and is best visualized with a 20°–40° left anterior oblique (LAO) image.[70] To accommodate these differences, initial angiographic imaging is often performed in the 15° LAO position. Review of prior CT or magnetic resonance angiography (MRA) images will often allow precise identification of the optimal imaging angulation needed for stenting.

Multiple renal arteries occur in up to 25% of patients. In patients with accessory RAS, the use of smaller profile devices is preferred. Early evidence suggests that drug-eluting stents may play a role for the treatment of arteries <5 mm in diameter due to the higher restenosis rate of these lesions.[71]

Renal interventions are most commonly performed via the common femoral artery approach using shaped guides (advanced through a sheath) or guide sheaths (containing an inner introducer and integrated hemostatic valve). A variety of guide shapes can be utilized, with common shapes including the renal double curve, internal mammary, and multipurpose designs, with the objective of having a sheath tip that is directed toward and aligns with the angulation of the renal artery origin. The renal arteries can, on occasion, have a sharp caudal angulation. In cases in which this precludes successful lesion crossing or results in inadequate guide support for stenting, alternative approaches such as a brachial or radial puncture can be used. These techniques have been facilitated by the routine use of low-profile stent systems that can be placed through smaller sheath introducers. Procedures may also be facilitated in the most challenging cases using deflectable sheaths, or robotic assistance with specialized systems.

There are three critical steps involved in PTRA and PTRS: lesion traversal, treatment selection decision-making

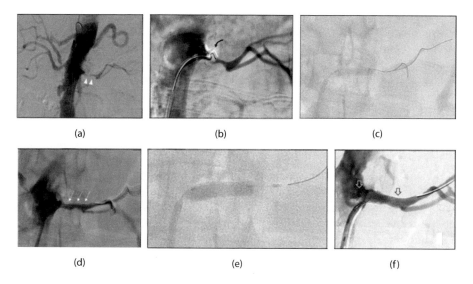

(a)   (b)   (c)

(d)   (e)   (f)

Figure 50.2 Left renal artery stenosis in a 60-year-old male with poorly controlled hypertension. Initial angiography **(a)** shows a patent and proximally bifurcated right renal artery, and a high-grade para-ostial and main renal artery stenosis on the left (*arrowheads*). Selective positioning of a renal double-curve guide sheath at the left renal artery ostium better demonstrates the stenosis and initial attempts at crossing the lesion with a floppy tipped 0.014-in guidewire **(b**, *curved arrow*). After placing the exchange wire and pressure-sensing wire for both a buddy wire technique (to stabilize sheath position) and to allow hemodynamic measurements, initial percutaneous transluminal renal angioplasty (PTRA) was performed with a 5 mm balloon **(c)**. Although unusual, primary balloon angioplasty was performed due the extension of the renal artery stenosis to the renal branches. Angiography after initial PTRA demonstrated an unsatisfactory residual stenosis **(d**, *short arrows*). This was treated with placement of a 5 mm diameter by 16 mm long Formula 414 stent (Cook, Bloomington, IN); note the horizontal orientation of the balloon during stent deployment which is achieved by "spooling out" or carefully advancing the balloon after it initially engages the vessel wall **(e)**. This prevents disruption of the aortorenal ostium. Completion angiography **(f)** shows complete resolution of the stenosis with preserved branch flow (stent margins marked with open arrows).

(including determination of transstenotic pressures), and balloon/stent positioning and deployment. Patients are routinely anticoagulated prior to treatment with either heparin or bivalirudin.

Lesion traversal

Crossing the lesion is often the most difficult component of percutaneous renal revascularization, particularly in cases of severe stenosis or occlusion. The selected guide should have sufficient breadth in its secondary curve to abut the contralateral aortic wall so that there is sufficient support for controlling and advancing the renal crossing wire. For horizontally oriented renal arteries, the guide is initially positioned immediately at or just above the renal artery. A floppy-tipped wire with a gentle curve on the tip is then directed toward the angiographically demonstrated remaining renal artery lumen; imaging is performed using small contrast injections through the sheath sidearm. Gently rotating the guide and/or wire tip may allow engagement of the true lumen when crossing eccentric lesions. With a properly shaped guide, primary lesion crossing is usually performed using a 2 cm floppy-tipped 0.014- or 0.018-in guidewire. Care must be taken to avoid excessive pushing if there is resistance to wire advancement, and it is important that the wire remain visualized with its tip in first- or second-order branches during all phases of the procedure. Wires advanced too distally can result in cortical perforation and retroperitoneal hemorrhage.[72] After crossing, the stiff portion of the guidewire should extend across the aortorenal angle to allow subsequent balloon and stent passage. For more caudally directed renal arteries, the use of a reverse curve catheter (e.g., Sos Omni, AngioDynamics, Queensbury, NY) can often be useful. With this technique, the reverse catheter is formed using a floppy-tipped 0.035-in guidewire either in the aorta below the renal arteries or at the thoracic aortic arch. The catheter is initially positioned below the renal artery, with the tip facing the side to be treated. With approximately 5 mm of wire protruding from the catheter tip, the catheter is gently advanced cranially. When the renal artery is engaged, there will be a visible "quick flip" of the wire. The wire is then advanced into the artery while simultaneously retracting the reverse curve catheter across the lesion. The renal guide is then gently advanced and rotated until it engages the renal ostium, and exchange is made through the catheter for a stiffer stenting wire. The catheter is then removed and angioplasty or stenting performed.

"Don't touch" technique

This technique minimizes manipulation in the perirenal aorta, theoretically reducing the risk of plaque or cholesterol embolization into the kidney during lesion crossing. There are several different don't touch techniques. The most commonly described method is to advance a "J" wire beyond the guide tip into the suprarenal aorta. This pushes the guide tip away from the aortic wall, preventing plaque disruption. A second curved 0.014-in floppy tip wire is then used to cross the RAS, before removing the J wire, allowing the guide to engage the renal artery ostium, and proceeding with the procedure.

"Buddy wire" technique

Although not a method for lesion crossing, the buddy wire technique represents a useful strategy, allowing for successful procedure completion in cases when the severity of the RAS impedes balloon or stent placement. After initial lesion crossing, the guide is aligned with the renal artery ostium, and a second short transition 0.014-in guidewire is passed into the renal artery (Figures 50.1 and 50.2). Balloon or stent advancement is then performed over the stiffer wire, with the buddy wire serving to stabilize the guide and allow more directed translation of pushing forces across the artery without recoiling the guide.

Selecting the interventional strategy

Uncomplicated FMD (without associated dissection) is treated with PTRA first, whereas ostial ARAS is usually approached with an intent to stent. Truncal or nonostial ARAS may be managed with an initial attempt at PTRA alone. In these cases, the plaque causing the stenosis is not in direct contiguity with the aorta, and there is a resulting proximal "normal" renal artery segment. Balloons and stents are sized to the normal diameter of the renal artery, either proximal to the stenosis or beyond any area of post-stenotic dilatation. The contralateral renal artery may also be used for vessel sizing if necessary. Renal artery diameters are usually 5–6 mm in women, and 6–7 mm in men.

Intervention is not warranted for a <50% RAS. For stenoses causing 60%–80% narrowing, determination of the transstenotic pressure gradient is recommended.[73] After crossing the lesion, simultaneous dual-channel pressure measurements are obtained from the renal artery distal to the stenosis and from the aortic sheath. Renal pressures may be recorded either through a 4-Fr catheter or, more recently, by using a pressure-sensing wire.[74] The latter has the advantage of preventing obturation of the renal artery resulting in speciously low-pressure measurements. Although there is no absolute gradient that is hemodynamically significant, a trans-stenotic gradient exceeding 20 mmHg and a >10% peak aortic systolic gradient ([aortic-renal]/aortic <0.90) are two criteria frequently utilized to indicate a stenosis warranting intervention. Fractional flow reserve can also be obtained to determine stenosis severity prior to PTRS.

Balloon and stent positioning

The selected balloon should be limited to just slightly longer than the RAS treated. Dilatation more than 1 cm beyond the stenosis should be avoided to prevent distal dissection. Balloon inflation is performed over 20–30 seconds.

After engaging the stenosis with partial balloon inflation, the balloon catheter shaft should be advanced slightly forward so that the balloon assumes a more horizontal course at the renal ostium; sharp downward angulation of the balloon at the aorta can result in an aortic tear.[75] For ostial ARAS, the shortest possible stent that will completely cover the lesion and extend 1–3 mm into aorta should be used. When there is uncertainty as to the exact location of the ostium due to extensive aortic plaque, it is preferred to have complete coverage by assuring that a small amount of stent projects into the aorta.

Distal embolic protection

Cholesterol, platelet, and plaque embolization occur in almost all cases of renal intervention.[36] In *ex vivo* models, embolic debris has been recorded during each phase of the procedure, including wire traversal, balloon dilation, stent insertion, and stent deployment.[76] One recent study suggested a high preponderance of platelet-rich embolic debris and suggested a role for a dual strategy of distal embolic protection (DEP) and intravenous glycoprotein IIB/IIIA receptor antagonism.[77] Several different types of DEP have been used in the renal artery.[78–81] There are several technical and anatomic considerations that are unique to renal DEPs. Principal among technical issues are device rigidity and crossing profile, which can affect the ability to position the DEP beyond the stenosis without injury, and characteristics of the landing zone (position of filter positioning), which may limit filter positioning or the ability for vessel wall apposition and complete protection. The use of DEPs imposes other anatomic considerations. CT studies have demonstrated a relatively short average length of the renal artery from origin to its first bifurcation, particularly on the left side (distance to bifurcation of 43 ± 15 mm in the right and 33 ± 14 mm in the left renal artery).[71] This has a considerable impact on DEP selection, since the distance of many filters from cone to base may leave insufficient space for stent positioning within the renal artery. Similarly, determinations of arterial diameter in the DEP "landing zone" can exceed the diameter of the protection device, rendering it ineffective, or necessitating a partial (segmental) protection strategy.[71]

COMPLICATIONS OF RENAL INTERVENTION

Renal intervention is generally safely performed. Risks of the procedure are related to puncture site complications, contrast-induced nephropathy, aortic or renal embolization, including cholesterol embolization syndrome, and injury to the renal artery during lesion crossing, angioplasty, or stent placement. General procedural risks include periprocedural cardiac events and mortality, although both of these are distinctly uncommon. Complications may be either clinically relevant (e.g., major complications) or procedurally occurring events without anticipated clinical sequelae.

Nonclinically important procedural events that increase the time or complexity of the procedure are termed *technical-procedural complications*[82] and would include small groin hematomas not increasing the level of care, minor arterial dissections, and suboptimal stent positioning or need for a second stent placement. This last event is minimized by optimal profiling of ostial lesions before stent deployment.

The Society of Interventional Radiology has established guidelines delineating thresholds for major complications.[83] On the basis of review of large meta-analyses, these established thresholds are 30-day mortality of 1%, periprocedural renal failure or exacerbation of 2%–5%, access site hematoma requiring intervention of 5%, and symptomatic embolization or procedure-related renal artery occlusion of approximately 5%.[83] Overall, major complications occur in approximately 5%.[84,85] As noted earlier, renal embolic events may be minimized with the routine administration of antiplatelet agents and the use of distal embolic devices in selected cases.

Postprocedural care

All patients undergoing renal intervention should be maintained on antiplatelet therapy for at least several months. While the optimal antiplatelet regimen has not been established, clopidogrel is the most commonly used agent and the *de facto* standard of care. Some investigators apply the coronary principle of dual antiplatelet therapy (DAPT) with aspirin and clopidogrel for 1 month followed by long-term aspirin alone, although this may be associated with a higher hemorrhagic risk. No additional anticoagulation is necessary postprocedurally. For patients with FMD, antihypertensive medication may be withheld following the procedure and BP closely monitored to determine the need for reinstitution of therapy. Since BP in this scenario is frequently renin mediated, ACE inhibitors or ARB II are preferred. For patients with ARAS, blood pressure medications should be considered, although the most recently added or increased drug may sometimes be held pending an evaluation of clinical results. Abrupt hypotension is uncommon, and antihypertensive therapy should otherwise be performed according to best medical care. In patients with renal insufficiency, serum creatinine and GFR should be measured within 1 week of intervention as well as at other clinical follow-up appointments.

Due to the recognized risk of restenosis after stenting (Figure 50.3), duplex surveillance is recommended.[21] Baseline studies obtained within 1–2 weeks of intervention provide a comparison for subsequent studies performed at 3–6 months, then annually for 3–5 years. Recurrent clinical events, particularly declining renal function or accelerated hypertension, warrant prompt evaluation. Since duplex criteria for restenosis within stents may be different than for *de novo* RAS,[86] particularly in patients with aortic endografts,[87] standards need to be developed and validated at local vascular laboratories. In questionable cases, CT angiography may be valuable for detecting in-stent restenosis.[88]

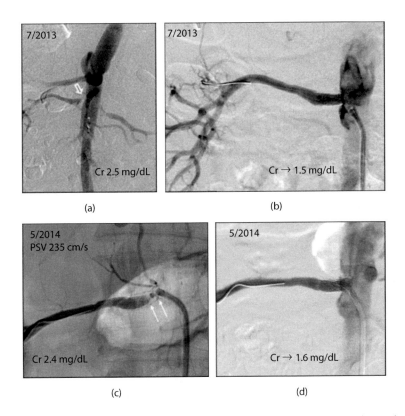

Figure 50.3 Recurrent RAS and ischemic nephropathy. Initial angiography in July 2013 **(a)** showed a high-grade ostial right RAS (*open arrow*) and moderate left RAS. Baseline serum creatinine (Cr) was 2.5 mg/dL. Following successful RAST **(b)**, there is no residual stenosis and the patient's creatinine normalized. Ten months later, azotemia again occurred, and renal duplex showed a recurrent in-stent RAS on the right side (PSV 235-cm/s), which was confirmed with selective angiography (*arrows*, **c**). This was treated by placement of a short stent-graft **(d)** with restored renal artery patency and quick return to baseline renal function. Of note, although the left renal artery was only mildly stenotic, there was presumably intrinsic disease on this side which made the patient functionally uninephric. The right RAS was nephroprotective on this side, allowing a good physiologic response to revascularization. PSV, peak systolic velocity; RAS, renal artery stenosis; RAST, renal artery stenting.

CONCLUSION

RAS is a common clinical problem. The safety of renal interventions has improved with evolving techniques, and there is strong, albeit predominantly observational data, supporting clinical value for the treatment of associated hypertension, renal failure, or pulmonary edema. Demonstration of a cardiovascular survival benefit will be a critical determinant of long-term acceptability and is currently the subject of a large, international multicenter prospective trial. Currently, the only class I indication for RAST is in patients with hemodynamically significant RAS with recurrent, unexplained HF or sudden unexplained episodes of "flash" pulmonary edema.[89] Patients with accelerated or resistant hypertension (defined as failure of ≥3 maximally tolerated medications including a diuretic), global renal ischemia (bilateral RAS or severe RAS in a solitary functioning kidney), or hypertension with medication intolerance also generally benefit from RAST after a trial of optimal medical therapy, and are considered class IIa indications for stenting.[90]

CHRONIC MESENTERIC ISCHEMIA

Introduction

Chronic mesenteric ischemia (CMI) or mesenteric angina is an uncommon, but not rare form of peripheral vascular disease. It is a diagnosis of exclusion, made after eliminating more common possibilities. The disease usually develops after the age of 60 and is three- to fourfold more common in women than men. Patients commonly have prior vascular disease affecting the lower extremities, coronary arteries, renal arteries, or cerebral arteries.[91] The etiology of CMI is often multifactorial, with atherosclerosis the most common cause. Thus, risk factors for atherosclerosis, including cigarette smoking, hypertension, and diabetes mellitus, are common. The classic symptomatic triad—which typically occurs with advanced disease—is postprandial pain, fear of eating, and involuntary weight loss, although patients rarely present with all three. The characteristic pain is chronic and dull, begins 15–30 minutes after meals, and persists for 1–4 hours thereafter.[92] As the disease progresses, the pain becomes progressively more severe and longer lasting and occurs after eating smaller amounts of food.

Due to its low prevalence and nonspecific presentation, a high index of suspicion is paramount in accurately diagnosing CMI. Physical examination often reveals an abdominal bruit.[91] Signs of weight loss and malnutrition, such as temporal wasting, are common. Many patients have evidence of peripheral vascular disease, such as absent distal pulses and trophic changes in the feet, and of coronary artery disease, such as electrocardiographic abnormalities.[92]

Anatomic considerations

The abdominal viscera are supplied by the celiac axis, superior mesenteric artery (SMA), and inferior mesenteric artery (IMA). The occlusive disease progresses slowly in CMI, permitting collaterals to develop to prevent bowel infarction. The celiac artery and SMA communicate by anastomoses between the superior pancreaticoduodenal branch of the gastroduodenal artery, which arises from the hepatic artery, and the inferior pancreaticoduodenal artery, which arises from the first part of the SMA (Figure 50.4a). When the celiac artery is stenosed or occluded, blood flows from the SMA to branches of the celiac artery, and when the proximal SMA is occluded or stenosed, blood flows in the reverse direction. An anastomosis may also occur between the ascending division of the left colic branch of the IMA and the left division of the middle colic branch of the SMA in response to stenosis or occlusion of either the IMA or proximal SMA. This anastomosis is called the arc of Riolan or mesenteric meandering artery (Figure 50.4b).[93] Additionally, an anastomosis between the terminal branches of the SMA and IMA may form an arcade along the inner border of the colon called the marginal artery

of Drummond. Occasionally, the IMA, which is usually small, may become enlarged and supply the entire abdominal viscera.[94,95] Because of this rich collateral network, at least two of the three major mesenteric vessels are usually diseased before symptoms of CMI occur.[96]

Indications

The goals of revascularization in patients with symptomatic CMI are to improve symptoms and nutritional status and prevent intestinal infarction and perforation.[97] Prophylactic mesenteric revascularization is rarely performed in the asymptomatic patient undergoing an aortic procedure for other indications.[98]

Fundamentals and equipment

Both upper extremity and femoral approaches have been utilized in mesenteric angioplasty and stenting. Upper extremity access, including radial and brachial approaches, appears to have a slight advantage in cases of acute angulation at the mesenteric vessel origin off the aorta. While a brachial approach was traditionally used, radial access is increasingly becoming the principal choice in many institutions due to its lower complication rate and improved patient comfort.[99–103] A 6-Fr sheath is inserted via the access vessel. If the radial or brachial artery has been accessed, then early heparinization is advised to prevent thrombosis at the sheath insertion site. A pigtail catheter is advanced through the sheath into the abdominal aorta, and a diagnostic arteriogram is performed, first in the anteroposterior direction to assess the SMA and celiac branches, and then in the lateral projection

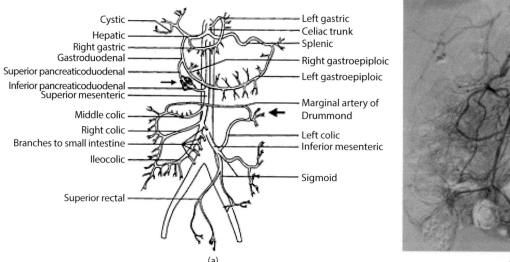
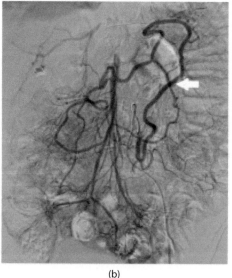

(a) (b)

Figure 50.4 Schematic and conventional angiogram of arterial supply to the viscera illustrates the intrinsic collateral pathways seen in chronic mesenteric ischemia. The major collateral pathway between the celiac and superior mesenteric artery is the anastomosis between the superior and inferior pancreaticoduodenal arteries (*thin black arrow*). The major pathways between the superior and inferior mesenteric arteries are the marginal artery of Drummond (*thick black arrow*) and Arc of Riolan (*white arrow*).

to assess the arterial orifices and confirm the presence and severity of stenosis. The pigtail is subsequently exchanged for a selective catheter. Our preference is to use a reverse curve catheter during femoral access and an angled multipurpose catheter during a radial or brachial approach (Figure 50.5). The catheter is navigated into the abdominal aorta and engages the target vessel, either celiac or SMA. If not already given, heparin (usually 5,000 units) should be administered at that point. The lesion can then be crossed with a 0.035-in guidewire. Alternatively, a 0.014-in wire can be used if one plans to use a rapid exchange system. A 6- or 7-Fr guiding catheter or sheath is then placed just proximal to the lesion and the balloon and/or stent is delivered to the lesion. Angiography through the guiding system is obtained to pinpoint the stenosis, and the angioplasty or stent placement follows. Alternatively, a no-touch technique has been described and can be used if the origin of the target vessel is very calcified or ulcerated. With this technique, the guide catheter is positioned in the aorta and is maintained straight by means of a 0.035-in wire that keeps the catheter from engaging the takeoff of the target vessel. A 0.014-in wire is then inserted in the guiding catheter, the 0.035-in wire is removed, and the lesion is crossed with the finer 0.014-in wire.[104] The guiding catheter can at this point be advanced to engage the lesion and the intervention follows. After the procedure, and if a stent has been deployed, the patient stays on clopidogrel and aspirin for at least 6 months.

The question of primary versus selective stenting has not been resolved. It appears to be a general consensus that an unsatisfactory result after angioplasty alone as evidenced by residual stenosis of >30% or >15 mmHg pressure gradient across the lesion, calcified ostial or high-grade eccentric stenoses, chronic occlusions, or the presence of dissection after angioplasty all constitute indications for stent placement. Balloon-expandable stents that offer precise placement are favored by most authors. Placement with a 1–2 mm protrusion into the aortic lumen is advised. Oderich et al.[105] compared covered stents versus bare-metal stents (BMS) in 225 patients with CMI and found covered stents associated with higher freedom from restenoses, symptom recurrence, and reintervention compared to BMS. Postdilation is performed, and depending on the angiographic result, the pressure gradient across the lesion may be measured.

Complications

Access complications are by far the most common and can take the form of either hemorrhage or thrombosis. Hemorrhage is common in femoral and high brachial or axillary approaches. Bleeding into the axillary sheath has the potential to permanently compromise nerve function; therefore, early diagnosis and prompt evacuation are essential to minimize morbidity. Careful technique that involves an ultrasound-guided stick using a micropuncture needle is of paramount importance to prevent this complication. The radial artery, due its relatively superficial route, allows for easier compression and monitoring of possible hematomas or hemorrhages. It also decreases possible complications such as arteriovenous fistulas (AVFs) and neuropathy due to the absence of adjacent major venous structures or nerves. Thrombosis occurs almost exclusively in the radial or brachial artery that is small in size and can be totally occluded by interventional sheaths. Rapid heparinization after sheath insertion is usually an adequate preventive measure. The status of the radial and ulnar circulation should be documented preoperatively before attempting any upper extremity access. Radial access should be avoided in patients with abnormal or poor hand perfusion (abnormal Barbeau test), history of Reynaud's phenomenon, physical examination suggesting the radial artery is too small for sheath insertion,

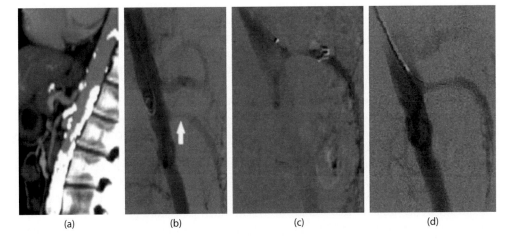

(a)　　　　(b)　　　　(c)　　　　(d)

Figure 50.5 Chronic mesenteric ischemia. A 72-year-old female with 8 months of progressive postprandial pain and 30-pound weight loss. Computed tomography and conventional angiograms demonstrate high-grade stenosis of the superior mesenteric artery (**b**, *white arrow*). Also note extensive atherosclerosis of the infrarenal aorta with complete occlusion of the inferior mesenteric artery. From a radial approach, the superior mesenteric artery is selectively catheterized and a balloon-expandable stent is delivered into the ostium (**c**) with excellent angiographic result (**d**). The patient remains symptom-free at 36-month follow-up.

or ipsilateral hemodialysis fistula or shunt. In the case of brachial access, any evidence of hand vascular compromise after the completion of the endovascular procedure should be aggressively treated with thromboembolectomy of the brachial artery to avoid permanent ischemic sequelae.

Entering a subintimal plane while trying to cross a high-grade stenosis or occlusion causes dissection, which necessitates stent placement to avoid distal propagation and arterial occlusion. If reentry to the true lumen and successful wire advancement through the lesion are not possible, then conversion to an open operation may be necessary. Bowel ischemia is a related but infrequent complication that develops in cases of underestimated dissection after percutaneous transluminal angioplasty or as a result of distal embolization after crossing long occlusions. If intestinal malperfusion is suspected intraoperatively and confirmed angiographically, then standard catheter-based salvage techniques are available and should be implemented immediately. When these are not successful, or if abdominal symptoms from presumed intestinal ischemia have been established, abdominal exploration with bowel inspection and thromboembolectomy is indicated. Other complications that are common to all the endovascular procedures, such as renal failure and anaphylactic reaction, may also infrequently occur. One recognized pitfall of endovascular therapy of CMI is a relatively high restenosis and reintervention rate (Table 50.3).[105–112] This fact has led to our institution initiating an aggressive duplex surveillance protocol following mesenteric revascularization procedures to improve the primary patency of these procedures.

SPECIAL CONSIDERATIONS

Acute mesenteric ischemia

The role of endovascular therapy in acute mesenteric ischemia (AMI) remains uncertain, although the proportion of patients undergoing endovascular intervention versus open surgery increased from 11.9% in 2005 to 30% in 2009.[113] In cases of AMI, assessment of intestinal viability is crucial and is best achieved by abdominal exploration and direct bowel inspection. General consensus is that endovascular treatment is an appropriate alternative for the occasional patient who is at prohibitive operative risk and does not have frank peritoneal signs on physical examination, as well as for those patients who have a contaminated peritoneal cavity and lack an autogenous conduit for the performance of a mesenteric or celiac bypass. Accordingly, Boley et al.[114] used arteriography and subsequent catheter-based interventions or transcatheter vasodilator therapy as the initial or sole therapy of AMI. Raupach et al.[115] retrospectively evaluated 37 patients over 12 years who underwent transcatheter embolus aspiration of the SMA and found a technical success rate of 92%, a subsequent laparotomy rate of 73%, and 30-day mortality of 27%; primary endovascular therapy with on-demand laparotomy is their recommended algorithm to treat acute embolic SMA occlusion. Similarly, our institution had

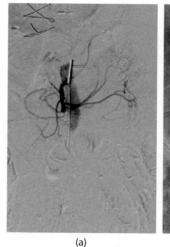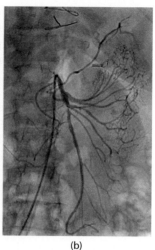

(a)   (b)

Figure 50.6 Acute mesenteric ischemia. 84-year-old female with new-onset atrial fibrillation presents with acute abdominal pain and CTA findings of super mesenteric artery embolus. DSA **(a)** demonstrates abrupt cutoff of contrast in the proximal SMA. Penumbra catheter was used for embolus aspiration. Postprocedural angiogram **(b)** demonstrates restored flow through the SMA and its branches. CTA, computed tomography angiography; DSA, digital subtraction angiography; SMA, superior mesenteric artery.

a recent case of SMA embolus causing AMI, which was successfully treated with thrombectomy via Penumbra aspiration catheter (Figure 50.6). Catheter-directed thrombolysis,[116,117] as well as percutaneous angioplasty,[118] has also been used with good results in the treatment of acute mesenteric embolism. Demirpolat et al.[119] reported three patients with increasing abdominal pain but without peritoneal findings who were treated percutaneously with good outcome. Last, Lim and colleagues[120,121] have reported the use of an endovascular approach in surgically unfit patients with good result. All these authors emphasized the importance of performing endovascular treatment in the absence of peritoneal signs and only when bowel viability can be assessed either clinically or with imaging techniques.

Total occlusions

The presence of total occlusion implies a more demanding technical procedure, but it does not constitute a contraindication for endovascular intervention. Only a few attempts to cross occlusions were seen in the early studies, and Kasirajan et al.[122] noted that it was more common for their group to use an open procedure to treat patients with occluded vessels. A major concern at the time was the potential for plaque fragmentation, with subsequent distal embolization. This, however, has not been confirmed by authors who crossed and treated occluded mesenteric vessels.[120] The length of the occlusion correlates with plaque burden and seems to be an important predictor of the likelihood for distal embolization; however, given the few patients studied, this has not been statistically confirmed. Low-profile systems and evolving expertise have now made successful treatment of occluded vessels feasible. A retrospective review of 47 patients with chronic total occlusions of the SMA treated enodvascularly[123] revealed 87% technical success; 100% immediate clinical improvement; 95% and 78% freedom from symptomatic recurrence at 1- and 2-year follow-up, respectively; and 7% and 0% minor and major complication rates, respectively. Several studies[108,124,125] have shown that endovascular treatment of total mesenteric occlusion has technical success, clinical success, and follow-up patency rates similar to endovascular treatment of stenotic vessels; notably, Sarac et al.[108] retrospectively compared occluded and stenotic mesenteric vessels and found endovascular therapy to have indistinguishable outcomes between the two types of lesions.

In principle, treatment of SMA lesions takes priority over treatment of lesions in the celiac axis or the IMA. Even this rule, however, has an exception. In a study by Matsumoto et al.,[126] four patients with occluded SMA had only their IMAs treated and remained asymptomatic in long-term follow-up. A patent meandering artery can assure collateral circulation in the event of a difficult-to-treat SMA occlusion. The feeding vessel of such important collateral should be visualized in detail, and any stenotic lesions found should be treated aggressively.

Comparison of endovascular with open surgical technique

Surgical intervention for mesenteric occlusive disease has traditionally been the treatment of choice. Open surgical techniques (bypass grafting, transaortic or local endarterectomy, patch angioplasty, and reimplantation) have achieved an immediate clinical success that approaches 100% in a number of different series.[127–131] The number of vessels revascularized has often been reported to influence the long-term outcome. However, it has been noted that revascularization of the SMA is of paramount importance and provides optimal long-term symptomatic relief, even if revascularization of other compromised arteries is not possible.[119,132]

While long-term patency rates appear to be superior with the open technique, 1-, 2-, 3-, and 5-year survival rates between the two treatment options are the same.[133–136] The endovascular approach, however, is associated with lower mortality and morbidity rates as well as shorter hospital stay, while maintaining high technical and immediate clinical success (Table 50.3). A recent systematic literature review performed by Pecoraro et al.[134] revealed perioperative mortality to be 3.6% (range 0–5%) for endovascular treatment versus 7.2% (range 0–15%) in open revascularization. Similarly, perioperative morbidity was found to be 13.2% (range 0–15%) and 33.1% (range 0–53%) in endovascular versus open surgical approaches, respectively. The mean hospital stay for open surgical revascularization has been reported to be 12 days, compared to 3 days for endovascular treatment.[133]

There is no randomized study comparing open versus endovascular intervention, and given the rarity of this condition, structuring such a study would be a challenging task. Although open surgical revascularization has traditionally been considered the gold standard of therapy, there is a current trend toward utilizing endovascular intervention as first-line therapy. During the 1990–1999 decade, only 17% of patients with CMI underwent endovascular therapy, compared to 83% treated with surgical revascularization. From 2000 to 2009, the two treatment approaches were nearly evenly numbered.[134] An endovascular approach is increasingly being used as initial treatment for patients who have poor life expectancy, especially high-risk and older patients with suitable anatomy, or for the individual patient with unclear symptomatology and questionable diagnosis. Open surgery should be considered in patients with good nutritional status and few comorbidities.

Median arcuate ligament syndrome

Median arcuate ligament (MAL) syndrome results from compression of the celiac artery by the MAL. Compression by the adjacent sympathetic plexus may also contribute to the celiac axis compression. Most patients are asymptomatic. Symptoms, when present, mimic the clinical picture of CMI.

Table 50.3 Outcomes of recent series of endovascular treatment for chronic mesenteric ischemia

Author (year)	No. patients	No. vessels	Technical success (%)	Complications (%)	30-day mortality (%)	Initial symptom relief (%)	Mean follow-up (months)	Reintervention (%)
Silva (2006)	59	79	96	3	2	85	38	17
Atkins (2007)	31	43	97	29	3	87	15	16
Sarac (2008)	65	87	94	31	8	85	12	11
Lee (2008)	31	41	98	6	13	71	26	13
Dias (2010)	43	49	96	23	0	95	43	33
Peck (2010)	49	66	88	16	2	90	37	29
Fioole (2010)	51	60	93	4	0	78	25	25
Olderich (2013)	42	42	98	12	0	98	19	10
Total	371	467	95	14	3	86	27	19

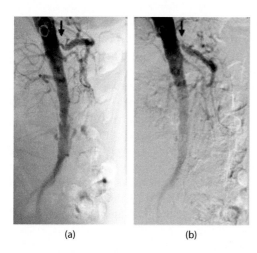

(a)   (b)

Figure 50.7 Median arcuate ligament syndrome. Images from a lateral aortogram in a patient with symptoms of chronic mesenteric ischemia. At expiration, there is an extrinsic compression on the superior wall of the celiac artery (**a**, *small arrow*) from the anterior crus of the diaphragm. At inspiration, the compression is relieved (**b**, *large arrow*). There is moderate atherosclerotic plaque in this vessel, as well as the superior mesenteric artery.

Because of the extrinsic nature of the lesion, angioplasty or stenting in these patients is associated with high failure rates and is not recommended by most authors.[106,120] The typical angiographic finding is that of a nonostial, eccentric, anterior, and superior lesion of the celiac artery that becomes more pronounced during deep expiration (Figure 50.7).[137] In the occasional patient with unclear symptomatology for whom relief of symptoms after percutaneous transluminal angiography or stenting predicts a good response to operative intervention, and for the high-risk, malnourished patient who will not be able to tolerate an open surgical procedure, the endovascular approach can be of benefit.

CONCLUSION

Endovascular management of patients with CMI offers a number of significant advantages to the traditional open techniques of revascularization while maintaining similar long-term survival. It is associated with shorter hospital stay and low morbidity and mortality rates. Percutaneous endovascular treatment of intestinal arterial stenosis currently is indicated in patients with chronic intestinal ischemia as a class I recommendation.[138] Perioperative use of heparin, postoperative administration of antiplatelet agents, more liberal use of stents, improvement in the skill level, and more careful patient selection, with increased awareness of the MAL syndrome, all have the potential to improve technical and short- and long-term clinical success rates. Patient anatomy, age, comorbidities, life expectancy, nutritional status, and center expertise should all be considered when deciding between endovascular therapy and open revascularization.

REFERENCES

1. Olin JW, et al. The United States Registry for Fibromuscular Dysplasia: Results in the first 447 patients. *Circulation* 2012;125(25):3182–3190.
2. Kadian-Dodov D, et al. Dissection and Aneurysm in Patients with Fibromuscular Dysplasia: Findings From the U.S. Registry for FMD. *J Am Coll Cardiol* 2016;68(2):176–185.
3. Schwartz CJ, White TA. Stenosis of renal artery: An unselected necropsy study. *Br Med J* 1964;2(5422):1415–1421.
4. Conlon PJ, et al. Severity of renal vascular disease predicts mortality in patients undergoing coronary angiography. *Kidney Int* 2001;60(4):1490–1497.
5. Mui KW, Sleeswijk M, et al. Incidental renal artery stenosis is an independent predictor of mortality in patients with peripheral vascular disease. *J Am Soc Nephrol* 2006;17(7):2069–2074.
6. ASTRAL Investigators, et al. Revascularization versus medical therapy for renal-artery stenosis. *N Engl J Med* 2009;361(20):1953–1962.
7. Cooper CJ, et al. Stenting and medical therapy for atherosclerotic renal-artery stenosis. *N Engl J Med* 2014;370(1):13–22.
8. Marcantoni C, et al. Effect of renal artery stenting on left ventricular mass: A randomized clinical trial. *Am J Kidney Dis* 2012;60(1):39–46.
9. Ritchie J, et al. Effect of renal artery revascularization upon cardiac structure and function in atherosclerotic renal artery stenosis: Cardiac magnetic resonance sub-study of the ASTRAL trial. *Nephrol Dial Transplant* 2016. doi: 10.1093/ndt/gfw107
10. Zhu Y, et al. Percutaneous revascularization for atherosclerotic renal artery stenosis: A meta-analysis of randomized controlled trials. *Ann Vasc Surg* 2015;29(7):1457–1467.
11. Murphy T, et al. Relationship of albuminuria and renal artery stent outcomes in the CORAL study. *J Vasc Interv Radiol* 2016;27(3):S70–S71.
12. Dangas G, et al. Intravascular ultrasound-guided renal artery stenting. *J Endovasc Ther* 2001;8(3):238–247.
13. Dorros G, et al. Multicenter Palmaz stent renal artery stenosis revascularization registry report: Four-year follow-up of 1,058 successful patients. *Catheter Cardiovasc Interv* 2002;55(2):182–188.
14. Dorros G, et al. Four-year follow-up of Palmaz-Schatz stent revascularization as treatment for atherosclerotic renal artery stenosis. *Circulation* 1998;98(7):642–647.
15. Zeller T, et al. Stent-supported angioplasty of severe atherosclerotic renal artery stenosis preserves renal function and improves blood pressure control: Long-term results from a prospective registry of 456 lesions. *J Endovasc Ther* 2004;11(2):95–106.
16. Sapoval M, et al. Low-profile stent system for treatment of atherosclerotic renal artery stenosis: The GREAT trial. *J Vasc Interv Radiol* 2005;16(9):1195–1202.
17. Tsao CR, et al. Delicate percutaneous renal artery stenting minimizes postoperative renal injury and protects kidney in patients with severe atherosclerotic renal artery stenosis and impaired renal function. *Int Heart J* 2005;46(6):1061–1072.

18. Rocha-Singh K, et al. Evaluation of the safety and effectiveness of renal artery stenting after unsuccessful balloon angioplasty: The ASPIRE-2 study. *J Am Coll Cardiol* 2005;46(5):776–783.

19. Ruchin PE, et al. Long-term follow-up of renal artery stenting in an Australian population. *Heart Lung Circ* 2007;16(2):79–84.

20. Goncalves JA, et al. Clinical efficacy of percutaneous renal revascularization with stent placement in atherosclerotic renovascular disease. *Arq Bras Cardiol* 2007;88(1):85–90.

21. Rocha-Singh K, et al. Renal artery stenting with noninvasive duplex ultrasound follow-up: 3-year results from the RENAISSANCE renal stent trial. *Catheter Cardiovasc Interv* 2008;72(6):853–862.

22. Rocha-Singh KJ, et al. Long-term renal function preservation after renal artery stenting in patients with progressive ischemic nephropathy. *Catheter Cardiovasc Interv* 2002;57(2):135–141.

23. Zeller T, et al. Stent angioplasty of severe atherosclerotic ostial renal artery stenosis in patients with diabetes mellitus and nephrosclerosis. *Catheter Cardiovasc Interv* 2003;58(4):510–515.

24. Ramos F, et al. Renal function and outcome of PTRA and stenting for atherosclerotic renal artery stenosis. *Kidney Int* 2003;63(1):276–282.

25. Gill KS, Fowler RC. Atherosclerotic renal arterial stenosis: Clinical outcomes of stent placement for hypertension and renal failure. *Radiology* 2003;226(3):821–826.

26. Ilkay E, et al. Effect of renal artery stenting on renal function in patients with ischemic nephropathy. *Jpn Heart J* 2004;45(4):637–645.

27. Rivolta R, et al. Stenting of renal artery stenosis: Is it beneficial in chronic renal failure? *J Nephrol* 2005;18(6):749–754.

28. Kashyap VS, et al. The management of renal artery atherosclerosis for renal salvage: Does stenting help? *J Vasc Surg* 2007;45(1):101–108; discussion 108–109.

29. Bates MC, et al. Serum creatinine stabilization following renal artery stenting. *Vasc Endovascular Surg* 2008;42(1):40–46.

30. Sag AA, et al. Atherosclerotic renal artery stenosis in the post-CORAL era part 1: The renal penumbra concept and next-generation functional diagnostic imaging. *J Am Soc Hypertens* 2016;10(4):360–367.

31. Dubel GJ, Murphy TP. The role of percutaneous revascularization for renal artery stenosis. *Vasc Med* 2008;13(2):141–156.

32. Radermacher J, et al. Use of Doppler ultrasonography to predict the outcome of therapy for renal-artery stenosis. *N Engl J Med* 2001;344(6):410–417.

33. Harden PN, et al. Effect of renal-artery stenting on progression of renovascular renal failure. *Lancet* 1997;349(9059):1133–1136.

34. Pattynama PM, et al. Percutaneous angioplasty for atherosclerotic renal artery disease: Effect on renal function in azotemic patients. *Cardiovasc Intervent Radiol* 1994;17(3):143–146.

35. Watson PS, et al. Effect of renal artery stenting on renal function and size in patients with atherosclerotic renovascular disease. *Circulation* 2000;102(14):1671–1677.

36. Muray S, et al. Rapid decline in renal function reflects reversibility and predicts the outcome after angioplasty in renal artery stenosis. *Am J Kidney Dis* 2002;39(1):60–66.

37. Safian RD, Textor SC. Renal-artery stenosis. *N Engl J Med* 2001;344(6):431–442.

38. Halimi JM, et al. Albuminuria predicts renal functional outcome after intervention in atheromatous renovascular disease. *J Hypertens* 1995;13(11):1335–1342.

39. Beutler JJ, et al. Long-term effects of arterial stenting on kidney function for patients with ostial atherosclerotic renal artery stenosis and renal insufficiency. *J Am Soc Nephrol* 2001;12(7):1475–1481.

40. Rundback JH, et al. Balloon angioplasty or stent placement in patients with azotemic renovascular disease: A retrospective comparison of clinical outcomes. *Heart Dis (Hagerstown, Md.)* 1999;1(3):121–125.

41. Bali HK, Jha V. Nephrotic syndrome and recurrent pulmonary oedema in bilateral atherosclerotic renal artery stenosis: Resolution following renal angioplasty and stenting. *Natl Med J India* 2006;19(5):253–254.

42. Zuccala A, et al. Renovascular disease in diabetes mellitus: Treatment by percutaneous transluminal renal angioplasty. *Nephrol Dial Transplant* 1998;13 Suppl 8:26–29.

43. Thatipelli M, et al. Renal artery stent placement for restoration of renal function in hemodialysis recipients with renal artery stenosis. *J Vasc Interv Radiol* 2008;19(11):1563–1568.

44. Ritchie J, et al. Where now in the management of renal artery stenosis? Implications of the ASTRAL and CORAL trials. *Curr Opin Nephrol Hypertens* 2014;23(6):525–532.

45. White CJ. The "chicken little" of renal stent trials: The CORAL trial in perspective. *JACC Cardiovasc Interv* 2014;7(1):111–113.

46. Luft FC, et al. Gunfight at O.K. CORAL. *J Am Soc Hypertens* 2014;8(4):276–280.

47. Murphy TP, et al. Renal artery stent outcomes: Effect of baseline blood pressure, stenosis severity, and translesional pressure gradient. *J Am Coll Cardiol* 2015;66(22):2487–2494.

48. Scoble JE. Atherosclerotic nephropathy. *Kidney Internat Suppl* 1999;56 Suppl 71:S106–S109.

49. Brouwers JJ, et al. The use of intrarenal Doppler ultrasonography as predictor for positive outcome after renal artery revascularization. *Vascular* 2016;25(1):63–73.

50. Limbourg F, et al. 1D.07: Long-term outcome after angioplasty in patients with renal artery stenosis and high resistive index. *J Hypertens* 2015;33 Suppl 1:e16.

51. Bruno RM, et al. Predictive role of renal resistive index for clinical outcome after revascularization in hypertensive patients with atherosclerotic renal artery stenosis: A monocentric observational study. *Cardiovasc Ultrasound* 2014;12:9–11.

52. Cianci R, et al. Ischemic nephropathy: Proteinuria and renal resistance index could suggest if revascularization is recommended. *Ren Fail* 2010;32(10):1167–1171.

53. Keddis MT, et al. Ischaemic nephropathy secondary to atherosclerotic renal artery stenosis: Clinical and histopathological correlates. *Nephrol Dial Transplant* 2010;25(11):3615–3622.

54. Tuttle KR, et al. Effects of stenting for atherosclerotic renal artery stenosis on eGFR and predictors of clinical events in the CORAL trial. *Clin J Am Soc Nephrol* 2016;11(7):1180–1188.

55. Vassallo D, et al. Three decades of atherosclerotic reno-vascular disease management—Changing outcomes in an observational study. *Kidney Blood Press Res* 2016;41(3):325–334.

55. Misra S, et al. Mortality and renal replacement therapy after renal artery stent placement for atherosclerotic renovascular disease. *J Vasc Interv Radiol* 2016;27(8):1215–1224.

57. Arthurs Z, et al. Renal artery stenting slows the rate of renal function decline. *J Vasc Surg* 2007;45(4):726–732.

58. Valluri A, et al. Do patients undergoing renal revascularization outside of the ASTRAL trial show any benefit? Results of a single centre observational study. *Nephrol Dial Transplant* 2012;27(2):734–738.

59. Modrall JG, et al. Clinical and kidney morphologic predictors of outcome for renal artery stenting: Data to inform patient selection. *J Vasc Surg* 2011;53(5):1282–1289.

60. Kennedy DJ, et al. Renal insufficiency as a predictor of adverse events and mortality after renal artery stent placement. *Am J Kidney Dis* 2003;42(5):926–935.

61. Pizzolo F, et al. Renovascular disease: Effect of ACE gene deletion polymorphism and endovascular revascularization. *J Vasc Surg* 2004;39(1):140–147.

62. Kalra PA, et al. The benefits of renal artery stenting in patients with atheromatous renovascular disease and advanced chronic kidney disease. *Catheter Cardiovasc Interv* 2010;75(1):1–10.

63. Sapoval M, et al. One year clinical outcomes of renal artery stenting: The results of the ODORI registry. *Cardiovasc Intervent Radiol* 2010;33(3):475–483.

64. Korsakas S, et al. Delay of dialysis in end-stage renal failure: Prospective study on percutaneous renal artery interventions. *Kidney Int* 2004;65(1):251–258.

65. Rzeznik D, et al. Effect of renal artery revascularization on left ventricular hypertrophy, diastolic function, blood pressure, and the one-year outcome. *J Vasc Surg* 2011;53(3):692–697.

66. Wright JR, et al. Progression of cardiac dysfunction in patients with atherosclerotic renovascular disease. *QJM* 2009;102(10):695–704.

67. Kane GC, et al. Renal artery revascularization improves heart failure control in patients with atherosclerotic renal artery stenosis. *Nephrol Dial Transplant* 2010;25(3):813–820.

68. Yu S, et al. 4A.02: Stenting of atherosclerotic renal artery stenosis does not improve clinical outcomes in patients presenting with congestive heart failure, an analysis of the CORAL trial. *J Hypertens* 2015;33 Suppl 1:e49.

69. Gross CM, et al. Ostial renal artery stent placement for atherosclerotic renal artery stenosis in patients with coronary artery disease. *Cathet Cardiovasc Diag* 1998;45(1):1–8.

70. Beregi JP, et al. Anatomic variation in the origin of the main renal arteries: Spiral CTA evaluation. *Eur Radiol* 1999;9(7):1330–1334.

71. Misra S, et al. Preliminary study of the use of drug-eluting stents in atherosclerotic renal artery stenoses 4 mm in diameter or smaller. *J Vasc Interv Radiol* 2008;19(6):833–839.

72. Olteanu B, et al. Embolization of a perforation of a cortical renal artery occurring during percutaneous renal angioplasty. *Eur Radiol* 2000;10(8):1357.

73. De Bruyne B, et al. Assessment of renal artery stenosis severity by pressure gradient measurements. *J Am Coll Cardiol* 2006;48(9):1851–1855.

74. Colyer WR Jr, et al. Utility of a 0.014@ pressure-sensing guidewire to assess renal artery translesional systolic pressure gradients. *Catheter Cardiovasc Interv* 2003;59(3):372–377.

75. Rasmus M, et al. Extensive iatrogenic aortic dissection during renal angioplasty: Successful treatment with a covered stent-graft. *Cardiovasc Intervent Radiol* 2007;30(3):497–500.

76. Hiramoto J, et al. Atheroemboli during renal artery angioplasty: An ex vivo study. *J Vasc Surg* 2005;41(6):1026–1030.

77. Cooper CJ, et al. Embolic protection and platelet inhibition during renal artery stenting. *Circulation* 2008;117(21):2752–2760.

78. Hagspiel KD, et al. Renal angioplasty and stent placement with distal protection: Preliminary experience with the FilterWire EX. *J Vasc Interv Radiol* 2005;16(1):125–131.

79. Henry M, et al. Renal angioplasty and stenting under protection: The way for the future? *Catheter Cardiovasc Interv* 2003;60(3):299–312.

80. Holden A, et al. Renal artery stent revascularization with embolic protection in patients with ischemic nephropathy. *Kidney Int* 2006;70(5):948–955.

81. Edwards MS, et al. Distal embolic protection during renal artery angioplasty and stenting. *J Vasc Surg* 2006;44(1):128–135.

82. Beek FJ, et al. Complications during renal artery stent placement for atherosclerotic ostial stenosis. *Cardiovasc Intervent Radiol* 1997;20(3):184–190.

83. Martin LG, et al. Quality improvement guidelines for angiography, angioplasty, and stent placement in the diagnosis and treatment of renal artery stenosis in adults. *J Vasc Interv Radiol* 2002;13(11):1069–1083.

84. Crea GA, et al. Managing complications of renovascular interventions. *Tech Vasc Interv Radiol* 1999;2(2):98–106.

85. Novick AC. Complications during renal artery stent placement for atherosclerotic ostial stenosis. *J Urol* 1998;159(6):2245–2246.

86. Chi YW, et al. Ultrasound velocity criteria for renal in-stent restenosis. *J Vasc Surg* 2009;50(1):119–123.

87. Mohabbat W, et al. Revised duplex criteria and outcomes for renal stents and stent grafts following endovascular repair of juxtarenal and thoracoabdominal aneurysms. *J Vasc Surg* 2009;49(4):827–837; discussion 837.

88. Raza SA, et al. Multislice CT angiography in renal artery stent evaluation: Prospective comparison with intra-arterial digital subtraction angiography. *Cardiovasc Intervent Radiol* 2004;27(1):9–15.

89. Parikh SA, et al. SCAI expert consensus statement for renal artery stenting appropriate use. *Catheter Cardiovas Intervent* 2014;84(7):1163–1171.

90. Hirsch AT, et al. ACC/AHA 2005 Guidelines for the management of patients with peripheral arterial disease (Lower extremity, renal, mesenteric, and abdominal aortic): Executive summary a collaborative report from the American Association for Vascular Surgery/Society for Vascular Surgery, Society for Cardiovascular Angiograpy and Interventions Society for Vascular Medicine and Biology, Society of Interventional Radiology, and the ACC/AHA Task Force on Practice Guidelines (Writing Committee to Develop Guidelines for the Management of Patients with Peripheral Arterial Disease): Endorsed by the American Association of Cardiovascular and Pulmonary Rehabilitation; National Heart, Lung, and Blood Institute; Society for Vascular Nursing; TransAtlantic Inter-Society Consensus; and Vascular Disease Foundation. *Circulation* 2006;113(11):e463–654.

91. Rheudasil JM, et al. Surgical treatment of chronic mesenteric arterial insufficiency. *J Vasc Surg* 1988;8(4):495–500.

92. Geelkerken RH, et al. Chronic mesenteric vascular syndrome. Results of reconstructive surgery. *Arch Surg* 1991;126(9):1101–1106.

93. Harward TR, et al. Multiple organ dysfunction after mesenteric artery revascularization. *J Vasc Surg* 1993;18(3):459–469; discussion 467–469.

94. Moawad J, Gewertz BL. Chronic mesenteric ischemia. Clinical presentation and diagnosis. *Surg Clin North Am* 1997;77(2):357–369.

95. Connolly JE, Kwaan JH. Management of chronic visceral ischemia. *Surg Clin North Am* 1982;62(3):345–356.

96. Allen RC, et al. Mesenteric angioplasty in the treatment of chronic intestinal ischemia. *J Vasc Surg* 1996;24(3):415–421; discussion 421–423.

97. Morris GC Jr, et al. Abdominal angina. *Surg Clin North Am* 1966;46(4):919–930.

98. Cunningham CG, et al. Chronic visceral ischemia. *Surg Clin North Am* 1992;72(1):231–244.

99. Louvard Y, et al. Coronary angiography through the radial or the femoral approach: The CARAFE study. *Catheter Cardiovasc Interv* 2001;52(2):181–187.

100. Rao SV, et al. Trends in the prevalence and outcomes of radial and femoral approaches to percutaneous coronary intervention: A report from the National Cardiovascular Data Registry. *JACC Cardiovasc Interv* 2008;1(4):379–386.

101. Jolly SS, et al. Radial versus femoral access for coronary angiography or intervention and the impact on major bleeding and ischemic events: A systematic review and meta-analysis of randomized trials. *Am Heart J* 2009;157(1):132–140.

102. Agostoni P, et al. Radial versus femoral approach for percutaneous coronary diagnostic and interventional procedures; Systematic overview and meta-analysis of randomized trials. *J Am Coll Cardiol* 2004;44(2):349–356.

103. Jolly SS, et al. Radial versus femoral access for coronary angiography and intervention in patients with acute coronary syndromes (RIVAL): A randomized, parallel group, multicentre trial. *Lancet* 2011;377(9775):1409–1420.

104. Rose SC, et al. Revascularization for chronic mesenteric ischemia: Comparison of operative arterial bypass grafting and percutaneous transluminal angioplasty. *J Vasc Interv Radiol* 1995;6(3):339–349.

105. Oderich GS, et al. Comparison of covered stents versus bare metal stents for treatment of chronic atherosclerotic mesenteric arterial disease. *J Vasc Surg* 2013;58(5):1316–1323.

106. Silva JA, et al. Endovascular therapy for chronic mesenteric ischemia. *J Am Coll Cardiol* 2006;47(5):944–950.

107. Atkins MD, et al. Surgical revascularization versus endovascular therapy for chronic mesenteric ischemia: A comparative experience. *J Vasc Surg* 2007;45(6):1162–1171.

108. Sarac TP, et al. Endovascular treatment of stenotic and occluded visceral arteries for chronic mesenteric ischemia. *J Vasc Surg* 2008;47(3):485–491.

109. Lee RW, et al. Long-term outcomes of endoluminal therapy for chronic atherosclerotic occlusive mesenteric disease. *Ann Vasc Surg* 2008;22(4):541–546.

110. Dias NV, et al. Mid-term outcome of endovascular revascularization for chronic mesenteric ischaemia. *Br J Surg* 2010;97(2):195–201.

111. Peck MA, et al. Intermediate-term outcomes of endovascular treatment for symptomatic chronic mesenteric ischemia. *J Vasc Surg* 2010;51(1):140–147.e1–e2.

112. Fioole B, et al. Percutaneous transluminal angioplasty and stenting as first-choice treatment in patients with chronic mesenteric ischemia. *J Vasc Surg* 2010;51(2):386–391.

113. Beaulieu RJ, et al. Comparison of open and endovascular treatment of acute mesenteric ischemia. *J Vasc Surg* 2014;59(1):159–164.

114. Boley SJ, et al. Initial results from an aggressive roentgenological and surgical approach to acute mesenteric ischemia. *Surgery* 1977;82(6):848–855.

115. Raupach J, et al. Endovascular management of acute embolic occlusion of the superior mesenteric artery: A 12-year single-centre experience. *Cardiovasc Intervent Radiol* 2016;39(2):195–203.

116. McBride KD, Gaines PA. Thrombolysis of a partially occluding superior mesenteric artery thromboembolus by infusion of streptokinase. *Cardiovasc Intervent Radiol* 1994;17(3):164–166.

117. Gallego AM, et al. Role of urokinase in the superior mesenteric artery embolism. *Surgery* 1996;120(1):111–113.

118. VanDeinse WH, et al. Treatment of acute mesenteric ischemia by percutaneous transluminal angioplasty. *Gastroenterology* 1986;91(2):475–478.

119. Demirpolat G, et al. Acute mesenteric ischemia: Endovascular therapy. *Abdom Imaging* 2007;32(3):299–303.

120. Lim RP, et al. Endovascular treatment of arterial mesenteric ischaemia: A retrospective review. *Australas Radiol* 2005;49(6):467–475.

121. Lim RP, et al. Angioplasty and stenting of the superior mesenteric artery in acute mesenteric ischaemia. *Australas Radiol* 2004;48(3):426–429.

122. Kasirajan K, et al. Chronic mesenteric ischemia: Open surgery versus percutaneous angioplasty and stenting. *J Vasc Surg* 2001;33(1):63–71.

123. Grilli CJ, et al. Recanalization of chronic total occlusions of the superior mesenteric artery in patients with chronic mesenteric ischemia: Technical and clinical outcomes. *J Vasc Interv Radiol* 2014;25(10):1515–1522.

124. Landis MS, et al. Percutaneous management of chronic mesenteric ischemia: Outcomes after intervention. *J Vasc Interv Radiol* 2005;16(10):1319–1325.

125. Sharafuddin MJ, et al. Endovascular recanalization of total occlusions of the mesenteric and celiac arteries. *J Vasc Surg* 2012;55(6):1674–1681.

126. Matsumoto AH, et al. Percutaneous transluminal angioplasty and stenting in the treatment of chronic mesenteric ischemia: Results and longterm followup. *J Am Coll Surg* 2002;194 Suppl 1:S22–S31.

127. Gentile AT, et al. Isolated bypass to the superior mesenteric artery for intestinal ischemia. *Arch Surg* 1994;129(9):926–931; discussion 931–932.

128. McAfee MK, et al. Influence of complete revascularization on chronic mesenteric ischemia. *Am J Surg* 1992;164(3):220–224.

129. Foley MI, et al. Revascularization of the superior mesenteric artery alone for treatment of intestinal ischemia. *J Vasc Surg* 2000;32(1):37–47.

130. Johnston KW, et al. Mesenteric arterial bypass grafts: Early and late results and suggested surgical approach for chronic and acute mesenteric ischemia. *Surgery* 1995;118(1):1–7.

131. Mateo RB, et al. Elective surgical treatment of symptomatic chronic mesenteric occlusive disease: Early results and late outcomes. *J Vasc Surg* 1999;29(5):821–831; discussion 832.

132. Park WM, et al. Current results of open revascularization for chronic mesenteric ischemia: A standard for comparison. *J Vasc Surg* 2002;35(5):853–859.

133. Kougias P, et al. Clinical outcomes of mesenteric artery stenting versus surgical revascularization in chronic mesenteric ischemia. *Int Angiol* 2009;28(2):132–137.

134. Pecoraro F, et al. Chronic mesenteric ischemia: Critical review and guidelines for management. *Ann Vasc Surg* 2013;27(1):113–122.

135. Schermerhorn ML, et al. Mesenteric revascularization: Management and outcomes in the United States, 1988–2006. *J Vasc Surg* 2009;50(2):341–348.e1.

136. Gupta PK, et al. Chronic mesenteric ischemia: Endovascular versus open revascularization. *J Endovasc Ther* 2010;17(4):540–549.

137. Reuter SR. Accentuation of celiac compression by the median arcuate ligament of the diaphragm during deep expiration. *Radiology* 1971;98(3):561.

138. Hirsch AT, et al. ACC/AHA 2005 guidelines for the management of patients with peripheral arterial disease (lower extremity, renal, mesenteric, and abdominal aortic): Executive summary a collaborative report from the American Association for Vascular Surgery/Society for Vascular Surgery, Society for Cardiovascular Angiography and Interventions, Society for Vascular Medicine and Biology, Society of Interventional Radiology, and the ACC/AHA Task Force on Practice Guidelines (Writing Committee to Develop Guidelines for the Management of Patients With Peripheral Arterial Disease) endorsed by the American Association of Cardiovascular and Pulmonary Rehabilitation; National Heart, Lung, and Blood Institute; Society for Vascular Nursing; TransAtlantic Inter-Society Consensus; and Vascular Disease Foundation. *Circulation* 2006;113(11):e463–654.

51

Carotid and vertebral artery interventions

PIERO MONTORSI, STEFANO GALLI, AND MARCO ROFFI

INTRODUCTION

In Western countries, stroke is the third most common cause of death behind cardiac disease and cancer, and is the number one condition associated with serious, long-term disability.[1] The yearly incidence of stroke approaches 0.2% of the Western population and the number of stroke-related deaths is expected to double over the next 30 years. In the United States, each year approximately 800,000 people experience a new or recurrent stroke and between 2011 and 2012, the estimated direct and indirect cost of stroke was $33 billion.[1] A stenosis of the internal carotid artery (ICA) is the underlying condition of 10%–20% of patients presenting with ischemic stroke.[2]

Large-scale randomized clinical trials have established the superiority of carotid endarterectomy (CEA) over medical management in patients with high-grade carotid stenosis, particularly in the presence of symptoms. However, these results were obtained by high-volume surgeons on selected patients and therefore may not be reproducible in clinical practice.

Although balloon angioplasty of carotid stenosis has been performed since the early 1980s, the use of stents in the mid-1990s, and of emboli protection devices (EPDs) around the year 2000, have led to an exponential growth of carotid artery stenting (CAS) procedures performed worldwide. However, a nationwide survey including over 450,000 patients later showed a 30% decrease in the annual rates of carotid revascularization in the period between 2002–2010 in the United States.[3] This was mainly due to a decrease in the number of CEAs. Numbers deeply varied across U.S. regions. Despite payer-based attempts to limit utilization of CAS and controversies about its safety and efficacy compared to CEA and medical therapy alone, rates of CAS showed a slight increase over time in the United States. The majority of CAS procedures were performed by cardiologists (49% of all CAS cases), followed by vascular surgeons (36%), and radiologists (15%) (Figure 51.1).

A stenosis of the vertebral artery (VA) rarely causes symptoms, and revascularization is seldom required. While surgery is not considered a viable option for VA stenosis in most centers,

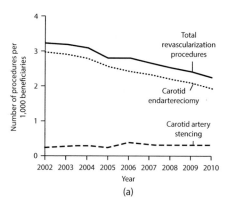
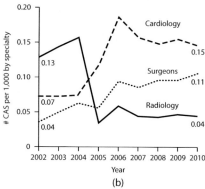

Figure 51.1 Annual rates of carotid revascularization per 1,000 Medicare beneficiaries, 2002–2010 **(a)**. Annual number of carotid artery stents (CAS) placed by cardiologists, surgeons, and radiologists per 1,000 Medicare beneficiaries from 2002 to 2010 **(b)**. The change in rate from 2002 to 2010 was statistically significant for each specialty ($P < 0.001$ for each). (From Wallaert, J.B., et al., *J. Vasc. Surg.*, 63, 89–97, 2016. With permission.)

the number of endovascular vertebral procedures remains limited compared with CAS procedures. Although the main focus of the chapter is on carotid artery interventions, the specifics of vertebral interventions will be mentioned.

ANATOMIC CONSIDERATIONS AND ANGIOGRAPHY

Aortic arch and carotid arteries

The details of carotid and cerebral angiography are described in detail in Chapter 26. The present section recalls just the anatomic notions critical for the planning and the performance of CAS. The vertebral circulation, not covered elsewhere in the book, is addressed in more detail. Acquired abnormalities of the aortic arch are common and may increase the difficulty of carotid cannulation. Commonly, all three great vessels (i.e., brachiocephalic trunk [or innominate artery], left common carotid artery [LCCA], and left subclavian artery [SCA]) arise from the apex of the aortic arch so that a horizontal line drawn perpendicular to the long axis of the human body at the apex of the arch will intersect the origin of all three vessels (type I arch) (Figure 51.2). However, elongation and rostral migration of the distal aortic arch with increasing age, atherosclerotic burden, and hypertension, may lead to a change in the relative positions of the great vessels: the origins of the LCCA and the left SCA migrate rostrally along with the distal arch, which takes on a narrowed and peaked appearance rather than a smooth convex shape. This leads to the brachiocephalic trunk arising "lower," as if it would originate from a prolongation of the ascending aorta, followed by the LCCA and then the left SCA. This constellation makes cannulation of the brachiocephalic trunk and LCCA difficult, if not impossible (type III arch) (Figure 51.2). The cannulation of the LCCA may also be challenging in the presence of the *bovine arch*. In this configuration, only the brachiocephalic trunk and the left SCA arteries arise from the arch, while the LCCA either shares a common origin with the brachiocephalic trunk (type 1) or originates from the brachiocephalic trunk itself (type 2) (Figure 51.2).

Once the CCA is cannulated, it is important to clearly differentiate the ICA from the external carotid artery (ECA). The most important difference between the two is that the ICA has no branches in its extracranial portion, while the ECA—usually smaller in caliber—has extensive early branching. Subsequently, baseline intracranial imaging of the carotid artery territory needs to be performed to assess the presence of collaterals, as described in Chapter 26, and have a baseline angiographic status.

Cerebral angiography

The fundamentals of cerebral angiography are reported in Chapter 26. Prior to CAS, noninvasive assessment of extracranial and intracranial circulation by either computed tomography angiography (CTA) or magnetic resonance angiography (MRA) is recommended. Cerebral angiography, defined as the selective engagement of both CCA and the nonselective engagement of at least one VA, is rarely needed for diagnostic purposes (e.g., in the presence of extensive disease and suboptimal visualization with noninvasive imaging). The complication rates of diagnostic angiography have significantly decreased over the last two decades, likely due to improvements in equipment and operators' skills. Important measures to increase safety include periprocedural anticoagulation and monitoring of the catheter-tip pressure throughout the procedure in order to prevent plaque dislodgement during catheter manipulation or dye injection. A prospective series of almost 3,000 diagnostic cerebral angiographies showed astonishing low rates of neurologic complications with 0.3% transient ischemic attacks (TIAs) and no permanent deficit.[4] Similarly, an analysis of over 19,000 consecutive patients detected a permanent neurologic deficit rate following cerebral angiography of 0.14%.[5]

Vertebral artery anatomy

The VA is usually the first branch off the SCA artery. On rare occasions, the left VA arises directly from the aortic

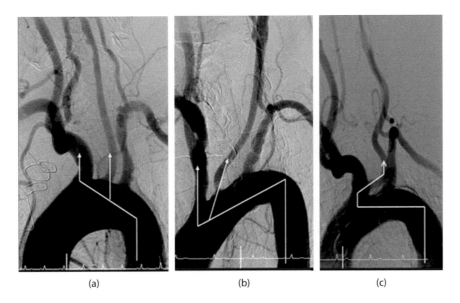

Figure 51.2 Aortic arch configurations as demonstrated on aortic arch angiography in 40° left anterior oblique projection. **(a)** Favorable angles to be overcome in order to cannulate the common carotid arteries (CCA) in a type I arch. **(b)** A type III arch configuration makes the cannulation of the CCA more challenging. **(c)** A "bovine" arch configuration makes the cannulation of the left CCA from a femoral approach more difficult.

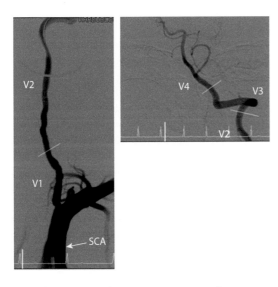

Figure 51.3 Digital subtraction angiography in posteroanterior view showing the four segments of the left vertebral artery (V1 to V2 in the left panel and V2 to V4 in the right panel). SCA, subclavian artery.

- The V1 segment extends from the VA origin to the transverse foramen of the sixth cervical (C6) vertebra; it has no branches.
- The V2 segment extends from the transverse foramen of C6–C1; it gives off the meningeal, muscular, and radicular arteries.
- The V3 segment extends from the transverse foramen of C1 to the foramen magnum, where it penetrates the dura; it provides small meningeal branches.
- The V4 segment extends from the entrance of the VA through the dura to the level of medullopontine junction, where it joins the other VA to form the basilar artery (BA); the major branches are the anterior and posterior spinal arteries as well as the largest branch of the VA.

The circulation at the level of the circle of Willis is detailed in Chapter 26. With respect to the posterior circulation, the most common variants are hypoplastic or absent posterior communicating artery (PCom) unilaterally or bilaterally occurring in 25%–33%. In the other common variant, the *fetal posterior cerebral artery* (PCA) defines the persistence of a large PCom that feeds the entire PCA having no (or a rudimental) connection with the BA; this occurs in 30% of cases. In this variant, the PCA is a branch of the ICA.

Vertebral artery angiograhy

As for carotid angiography, the procedure is usually performed in local anesthesia and using a femoral approach. The administration of an anticoagulant—commonly unfractionated heparin (UFH)—prior to cannulation of the supra-aortic vessels is recommended, particularly if a complete cerebral angiogram is planned. With respect to VA angiography, in order to delineate the intracranial circulation, the injection of one VA—the dominant—is sufficient. Since cannulation of the VA might be associated with

arch, between the LCCA and left SCA or distally to the left SCA. The diameter of the VA is 3–5 mm, and in the same patient, the caliber may vary to a great extent between the left and the right side. The left and the right VA are dominant in over 50% and 25% of cases, respectively. In the remaining cases, the two vessels have similar caliber. In approximately 15% of the population, one VA is atretic—that is, it has a diameter <2 mm—and supplies only the posterior inferior cerebellar artery (PICA) or gives only minimal contribution to the basilar system. The VA is divided into four segments (Figure 51.3):

higher complication rates than CCA cannulation, selective VA angiography is not routinely performed. Subselective VA opacification with the catheter placed in the SCA is usually sufficient for diagnostic purposes. In order to improve the quality of the subselective injection, we recommend the inflation of a blood pressure cuff at the ipsilateral arm at suprasystolic pressure.

The left SCA and the brachiocephalic trunk are usually easily accessible with a variety of diagnostic catheters, including Judkins right 4, vertebral/Bernstein, or headhunter. In more complex arches, the brachiocephalic trunk may be cannulated using catheter shapes such as Benson, Simmons/Sidewinder, or Vitek. A road map is than performed, and the catheter is advanced over a steerable 0.035-in wire in the SCA.

Selective VA angiography requires gentle manipulation and for that purpose, simple-shaped diagnostic catheters—such as the vertebral, Judkins right, or headhunter—are preferred. Frequently, positioning the catheter at the ostium may allow selective angiography. If this is not the case and selective angiography is required, a steerable floppy 0.035-in guidewire is positioned at the mid-distal third of the V2 segment, avoiding hooking in small branches, and then the catheter is advanced in the VA over the wire. For diagnostic purposes, the catheter should be kept in the V1 segment. In difficult anatomical situations, the selective catheterization of the VA should be discouraged because of the associated dissection risk. Vessel wall injury may be the result of catheter manipulations or forced contrast injection.

INDICATIONS FOR ENDOVASCULAR REVASCULARIZATION

Carotid artery stenting

The presence of a carotid bruit is neither sensitive nor specific for the presence of a significant stenosis of the ICA. The initial imaging modality of choice in patients with suspected carotid stenosis is duplex ultrasound (DUS).[6] If a significant stenosis of the ICA is detected, the finding should be confirmed either by CTA or MRA. At the same time, the brain should be imaged for the detection of silent ischemic lesions and to rule out associated intracranial pathologies, such as brain tumors, arteriovenous malformations, or vascular aneurysms. The combination of DUS and CTA is currently the favorite strategy in many centers and has been found to be the more cost-effective than DUS plus MRA in patients with either TIA or minor stroke in the setting of 70%–99% carotid stenosis.[7] A cardiothoracic radiologist or a neuroradiologist should be part of the CAS team due to the large experience of assessing vascular anomalies relevant to CAS.[8] Notably, studies from surgical groups have shown that an additional imaging technique following DUS, either CTA or MRA, modified the CAS strategy (i.e., change in CAS technique, type of stent and vascular approach, or even CAS decline) in up to 37% of patients scheduled for CAS.[9,10]

CAS is an appealing alternative to CEA because it is less invasive and it can potentially address lesions that may not be treated surgically. With respect to the degree of stenosis to be treated in asymptomatic and symptomatic patients, CAS and CEA share the same indications. The widely accepted guidelines of the American Heart Association (AHA)[11–13] support CEA as the treatment of choice for symptomatic patients (i.e., TIA or ischemic stroke within the past 6 months) with ipsilateral 70%–99% carotid artery stenosis as documented by noninvasive imaging if the perioperative morbidity and mortality risk is estimated to be <6% (class I; level of evidence A). For patients with 50%–69% carotid stenosis as documented by catheter-based imaging or two noninvasive imaging modalities (commonly DUS plus CTA or DUS plus MRA), CEA is recommended depending on patient-specific factors, such as age, sex, and comorbidities, if the perioperative morbidity and mortality risk is estimated to be <6% (class I; level of evidence B). CAS is indicated as an alternative to CEA for symptomatic patients at average or low risk of complications associated with endovascular intervention when the diameter of the lumen of the ICA is reduced by >70% by noninvasive imaging, or >50% by catheter-based imaging or noninvasive imaging with corroboration, and the anticipated rate of periprocedural stroke or death is <6% (class IIa; level of evidence B). According to trial results, CEA is recommended for asymptomatic patients with >60% carotid stenosis as long as the estimated perioperative death or stroke is <3% and life expectancy is 5 years. In this setting, CAS might be considered in highly selected asymptomatic patients with >60% stenosis by angiography or >70% by validated Doppler ultrasound, but its effectiveness compared to best medical treatment alone has not been established (class IIb, level of evidence B).

However, due to the usually benign course of asymptomatic carotid disease, in clinical practice, asymptomatic stenosis is usually treated in 75%–80% by noninvasive assessment or if one or more characteristics associated with increased stroke risk is identified, such as ipsilateral silent infarction on CT/MRI, fast stenosis progression, hypoechoic plaques or Doppler ultrasound grey scale median (GSM) <15, irregular plaques or micro-ulceration using three-dimensional (3D) ultrasound, impaired cerebral vascular reserve, spontaneous embolization on transcranial Doppler, intraplaque hemorrhage in MRI, carotid plaque area >80 mm^2 and a juxtaluminal black area >10 mm.[2,14] Finally, failure to appropriately control patient risk factors or poor patient compliance to both lifestyle modifications and medical treatment might be considered as a reason for endovascular/surgical treatment of an asymptomatic carotid artery stenosis.

Once the indication for revascularization is established, further steps in decision-making should be based on the surgical and endovascular risk of the patient and on the locally available CAS expertise (Figure 51.4). Importantly, the conditions associated with poor outcomes for CEA and CAS do differ. Accordingly, while the outcomes of CEA are greatly influenced by the comorbidities of the patient, poor outcomes with CAS are related to challenging anatomies at

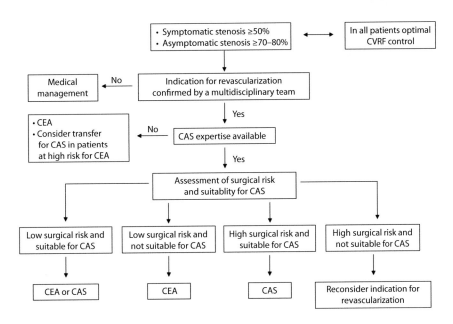

Figure 51.4 Management algorithm for patients requiring carotid revascularization. CAS, carotid artery stenting; CEA, carotid endarterectomy; CVRF; cardiovascular risk factor; EPD, embolic protection devices. (From Roffi, M., et al., *Heart*, 2010;96(8):636–642. With permission.)

Table 51.1 Pros and cons of carotid revascularization procedures

	CEA	CAS
Pros	Widely available	Outcome less influenced by comorbidities
	Excellent results for high-volume surgeons/ hospital in low-risk patients	Local anesthesia
		No neck incision/scar
		Usually next day discharge
Cons	Outcome influenced by comorbidities	Fewer experienced operators
	Frequently performed in general anesthesia	Procedure risk may increase in patients with:
		• severe PAD
		• severely calcified, tortuous/steep aortic arch
		• severe calcification/tortuosity of cervico-cranial vessels
	Neck incision/scar	Femoral access site complications
	Neck complications, cranial nerve palsies	
	Not suitable for high or low carotids	
	Longer hospital stay	

Note: CAS, carotid artery stenting; CEA, carotid endarterectomy; PAD, peripheral artery disease.

the level of the aortic arch and of the carotid arteries. While advantages and disadvantages of CEA and CAS are listed in Table 51.1, the (relative) contraindications to CAS are reported in Table 51.2.

The greatest advantage of CAS over CEA appears to be in patients with restenosis post CEA, following neck radiation or neck dissection, contralateral carotid occlusion, or poorly surgically accessible carotid lesions (hostile neck). CAS may also be considered for patients who recently underwent coronary drug-eluting stent (DES) implantation, as any surgical procedure including CEA—even if performed under dual antiplatelet therapy (DAPT) with aspirin and clopidogrel—may be associated with an increased risk of coronary stent thrombosis.

Surgery should be preferred in the presence of severe peripheral arterial disease not allowing for femoral arterial access. Although CAS can be performed via the brachial or

radial approach, this technique is time consuming, technically demanding, and requires a steep learning curve. Another challenging setting for CAS is the steep aortic arch with or without severe tortuosity of the common or ICA (Figure 51.2). As a general rule, if unexpected difficulties are encountered during engagement of the CCA because of (underestimated) anatomic challenges, it is preferable to abort the procedure and to consider surgery. The inability to use an EPD, a rare occurrence based on the multiple devices available, should also be considered a relative contraindication to CAS. Additional relative contraindications to CAS include severe circumferential calcification of the carotid bulb >3 mm in width, especially if deep, which may limit the ability to dilate the lesion; extreme ICA tortuosity with ≥2 angles >90° within 5 cm of the lesion, including the takeoff of the ICA from CCA; and thrombus-containing

Table 51.2 Conditions associated with increased procedural risk and contraindications for CAS

Increased Risk

Age ≥80 years

Symptomatic ICA lesion

Severe renal insufficiency

Severely disease and/or type II-III aortic arch

Severely diseased and/or tortuous distal ICA

Severely diseased and/or tortuous CCA

Severe stenosis with distal ICA collapse

Poor femoral access

Major stroke within 4–6 weeks

Vascular encephalopathy

Contraindications

Intolerance to aspirin and/or clopidogrel (R)

Circumferential ICA calcification (R)

Intraluminal thrombus (R)

Intracranial aneurysm or AVM requiring treatment (R)

Chronic ICA occlusion (A)

Note: A, absolute; AVM, arteriovenous malformation; CAS, carotid artery stenting; CCA, common carotid artery; ICA, internal carotid artery; R, relative.

lesions that may increase the risk of distal embolization. Moreover, patients with renal insufficiency or a history of allergic reactions to angiographic contrast may not be appropriate candidates for CAS. It has to be said that most of these complications were reported in the early phase of CAS. In high-volume centers, technological advantages and operator expertise over time made it possible to also treat patients with those characteristics with endovascular techniques with favorable results. Finally, for patients who cannot tolerate DAPT with aspirin and clopidogrel (e.g., in the presence of bleeding diathesis, intracerebral hemorrhage or cerebral arteriovenous malformation, documented intolerance to one of the agents, or noncompliance), surgery might be preferred.

The locally available surgical and endovascular expertise is also an important parameter in decision-making. The indication for and modality of revascularization should be discussed within a multidisciplinary team involving interventionalists, surgeons, and neurologists. Centers performing CAS should have documented CAS expertise with a track record of complications within the guideline's limits, and implement prospective quality control programs.

Reimbursement issues influence the practice of CAS. While in Europe, CAS is reimbursed in most but not all countries, in the United States, the Centers for Medicare and Medicaid Services (CMS) have concluded that CAS with EPD is reasonable and appropriate for symptomatic patients with carotid stenosis >70% at high risk for surgery[15] using U.S. Food and Drug Administration (FDA)–approved or FDA-cleared CAS systems and stents, with FDA-approved or FDA-cleared EPD in CMS-approved institutions. If performed within clinical trials or CAS postapproval studies, the procedure may be performed in high-risk symptomatic patients with 50%–70% stenosis as well as in high-risk asymptomatic individuals with stenosis >80%. Carotid stenting is considered appropriate if performed in facilities and by operators complying with the set standards.[15,16]

Vertebral artery stenting

Treatment of atherosclerotic extracranial VA occlusive disease can consist of medical, surgical, or endovascular therapies. While the optimal antithrombotic therapy—aspirin, clopidogrel, or warfarin—in VA stenosis has not been defined, most patients are treated with low-dose aspirin. Surgery—including vertebral endarterectomy and bypass operations—is technically challenging and is not considered a viable option in most centers.

The most recent AHA stroke prevention guidelines state that endovascular treatment of patients with symptomatic extracranial vertebral stenosis may be considered when patients remain symptomatic despite optimal medical management (class IIb, level of evidence C).[10–12] As with any interventional procedure, the risk of the intervention must be outweighed by the potential benefits of revascularization. The need to intervene is tempered by the fact that the posterior circulation is supplied by the confluence of the two VA and a large proportion of patients remain asymptomatic despite occlusion of one VA. However, this anatomic characteristic does not protect the posterior circulation from embolic events.

Patients with isolated stenosis of the extracranial VA >50% confirmed on angiography and symptoms attributed to vertebrobasilar ischemia, despite optimal medical treatment, may benefit from stenting, especially if the vessel is dominant or the contralateral site occluded. The majority of patients with asymptomatic extracranial VA disease do not require treatment. On a case-by-case decision, stenting of an asymptomatic high-grade (>80%) stenosis may be considered if the severity of the lesion is progressive and the affected VA is the dominant or the only patent one.

EQUIPMENT FOR CAROTID ARTERY STENTING

In addition to an appropriate angiography suite with digital subtraction and road-map/overlay capabilities, the equipment required for CAS includes diagnostic catheters, sheath systems, guiding catheters, guidewires, EPD, balloons catheters, and stents. Since for every device manipulation there is a learning curve, it is recommended at the beginning of the CAS experience to be familiar with a limited basic armamentarium, which can be subsequently expanded (Table 51.3). The basic equipment should include few diagnostic catheters, a 6- or 8-Fr guiding catheter or 90-cm-long sheath, three 0.035-in wires (steerable, hydrophilic stiff, and stiff in exchange length), one balloon catheter type, one nitinol open and one closed-cell design stent, and one or

Table 51.3 Minimal equipment to start carotid artery stenting (CAS)

Angiographic suite with DSA and road-mapping capabilities
Diagnostic catheters (4–5 Fr)
• JR4, internal mammary, vertebral, Headhunter, Vitek or Simmons/Sidewinder 1,2 Multipurpose 125 cm long
Guidewires (0.035-in)
• Steerable, hydrophilic stiff, and stiff (exchange length)
Guiding catheters (6–8 Fr) and sheaths (5–6 Fr, 90 cm long)
• Headhunter, Multipurpose, JR, Hockey stick
• Shuttle, Pinnacole Destination, Penumbra
Balloon catheter, 0.014-in, rapid exchange, approved for CAS
Self-expanding stent, rapid exchange and coronary balloon-expandable stent
Coronary aspiration catheters
Femoral closure devices

Note: DSA, digital subtracted angiography; JR, Judkins right.

two filter-based EPD systems. If a 8-Fr guiding catheter is used, we encourage advancing it over a 5-Fr, 125-cm-long diagnostic catheter with Judkins right or multipurpose shapes (telescoping technique). Rarely, the filter EPD may get clogged during the procedure as a consequence of distal embolization, with subsequent no flow in the ICA. In these circumstances, a coronary aspiration catheter such as the 6- or 7-Fr Export (Medtronic, Santa Rosa, CA) or Eliminate (Terumo) should be used to aspirate the blood column in the internal carotid prior to EPD removal. With increasing CAS experience, the goal should be to tailor the equipment to the patient and the lesion. To prevent femoral access bleeding in those patients aggressively anticoagulated, we encourage the use of femoral closure devices.

Sheath systems

Several sheath systems, usually 90 cm long, are available to access the CCA. Important features include kinking resistance and flexibility, a radiopaque band at the tip of the sheath to allow for accurate positioning, an atraumatic soft tip to reduce vessel trauma during engagement, and hydrophilic coating for enhanced trackability. Frequently used devices include the Cook Shuttle sheath (Cook Inc., Bloomington, IN), the Penumbra sheath (Penumbra Inc, Alameda, CA), and the Pinnacle Destination guiding sheath (Terumo Medical Corporation, Somerset, NJ). We recommend the use of the 6-Fr sheath despite the fact that some of the stent systems may be 5-Fr sheath compatible. Accordingly, a tight fit of the stent system in the sheath bears the risk of air entrapment at the time of device advancement with subsequent embolization.

Guiding catheters

Guiding catheters may be used to cannulate the CCA as alternative to long sheaths. The most frequently used shapes are the headhunter (H1, Cordis, Paolo Alto, CA, or Cook), the multipurpose, and the Judkins right. In order to avoid air entrapment/embolization and to allow for angiographic control of stent positioning, we recommend the use of 8-Fr guiding catheters, although some 5-Fr compatible stents may be delivered through 6-Fr guiding catheters. The choice of performing CAS using a long sheath or a guiding catheter is a matter of personal preference and the patient's anatomy. Overall, guiding catheters provide better torque control and stability and have a lower probability of kinking but require larger access size. In addition, during advancement of the guiding catheter over a 0.035-in guidewire, the abrupt transition at the tip may predispose to scraping the vessel wall with subsequent distal embolization. Therefore, we recommend to always advance a 6-Fr and 8-Fr guiding catheter over a 125-cm long 4- or 5-Fr diagnostic catheter (coaxial or telescoping technique), respectively. As a general rule, the more complex the anatomy at the level of the aortic arch and origin of the supra-aortic vessels, the more advantageous may be the use of a guiding catheter over a sheath.

Guidewires

Several 0.035-in guidewires are available for selective CCA cannulation for diagnostic and interventional purposes, including steerable guidewires with soft tip such as the Emerald (Cordis) wires, or hydrophilic wires such as the Radiofocus (Terumo, Westwood, MA). For excessively tortuous arteries and challenging aortic arches, a stiff hydrophilic wire (e.g., stiff Radiofocus, Terumo) may be used to advance the diagnostic catheter. If the initial wire needs to be exchanged (over the diagnostic catheter) for a stiff one to allow for the advancement of a long sheath in challenging anatomies, then the options include the Supracore (Abbott Vascular, Redwood City, CA), the Magic Torque (Boston Scientific, Natick, MA), and the Amplatz guidewires (Boston Scientific or Cook) in exchange length. Typically, a 5-Fr diagnostic catheter is advanced in the ECA over a soft wire and the latter is then exchanged for a stiffer one. Once cannulation of the CCA with the guiding catheter or long sheath is completed, the CAS procedure is continued over a 0.014-in guidewire, usually incorporated in the EPD. For cases performed with proximal occlusion EPD or with filter systems that allow use of separate preferred guidewires, a variety of 0.014-in coronary guidewires may be used, such as the Balanced Middle Weight or Balanced Heavy Weight (Abbott) and the Choice PT (Boston Scientific). The same wires can also be used as additional "buddy wires" in the presence of excessive tortuosity of the ICA to straighten up the artery, allowing for the positioning of a filter device. However, the buddy wire technique may induce a vessel "accordion effect," worsening rather than facilitating EPD advancement. Unprotected CAS (not recommended) may also be performed over 0.018-in peripheral guidewires such as Steelcore (Abbott), V18 Control (Boston Scientific), Roadrunner (Cook), and SV (Cordis).

Emboli protection devices

Two types of EPD are commonly used for CAS: distal protection with filter and proximal protection (±flow reversal) (Figure 51.5). Additional details on EPD are provided in Chapter 37. A large prospective registry reported that

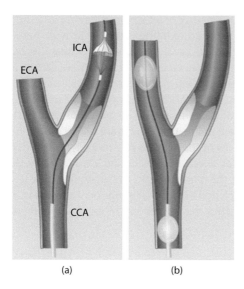

ICA
ECA
CCA
(a)   (b)

Figure 51.5 Strategies for emboli protection in carotid artery stenting. **(a)** A filter device. **(b)** A proximal occlusive device. Filter devices incorporate an angioplasty guidewire with a filter that expands and is placed distal to the lesion to capture and retrieve embolic debris that should get detached during the intervention. At the end of the procedure, the filter is collapsed and removed from the artery. The principle of proximal occlusion devices **(a)** is based on simultaneous occlusion of the external carotid artery (ECA) and of the common carotid artery (CCA). Depending on the devices used during the stenting procedure, the flow in the internal carotid artery (ICA) is arrested and then aspirated or actively reversed through a filtration system connected to a sheath draining into the venous system (MO.MA, Medtronic, Santa Rosa, CA).

filter-based EPD is the currently the preferred method of emboli protection for CAS in clinical practice, and both filter-based and distal occlusion EPD seem to be equally effective.[17] Advantages and disadvantages of the different device types are reported in Table 51.4. Filter-based EPD usually incorporates a 0.014-in guidewire with a filter that expands and is placed distal to the target lesion to capture and retrieve embolic debris that may get detached during balloon angioplasty and stenting. The filtering is performed by a polyurethane membrane with laser-drilled holes or a nitinol mesh (Figure 51.6). At the end of the procedure, the filter is collapsed, trapping the embolic debris, and is removed from the artery. The major advantage of filter EPD is that the perfusion is maintained throughout the procedure. A variety of filter-based EPDs are currently on the market, and the technical details are reported in Table 51.5. In the majority of the devices, the filter EPD is mounted directly on a wire (wire-dependent). Few of them, such as the Emboshield Pro (Abbott) or Spider (Medtronic), allow for the advancement of a wire followed by the device (wire-independent). This may be of advantage for complex lesions (Table 51.4).

Another approach for EPD is proximal protection. The concept is to arrest (no flow condition) or invert (reverse flow condition) the blood flow into the target ICA during CAS by a simultaneous balloon occlusion of both ECA and CCA. The endovascular occlusion, mimicking surgical clamping during CEA, is supposed to prevent brain embolization of debris throughout all CAS phases, including lesion crossing. The proximal balloon occlusion system Mo.Ma Ultra (Medtronic, Santa Rosa, CA) received FDA approval. There is still debate regarding the optimal way to protect CAS from distal embolization. The available data on proximal protected CAS with Mo.Ma were summarized in a meta-analysis of five multicenter registries and one single-center registry including a total of 2,397 patients (31% symptomatic), and reporting a stroke/death and MI rate at 30 days of 2.25% and a stroke rate of 1.7%.[18] A randomized study enrolled 53 patients with high-risk plaque

Table 51.4 Pros and cons of embolic protection devices

Device type	Pros	Cons
Filters	Preserve antegrade flow throughout the procedure	May not capture debris smaller than pore size
	Optimal visualization of the lesion	Not as steerable as coronary wires[a]
	Lesion crossing with guidewire of choice possible (with wire-independent systems)	May cause spasm/dissection in ICA
		Difficult to place in tortuous distal ICA
	Can be deployed and captured rapidly	Arterial wall apposition suboptimal in tortuous ICA
	Easy to use	Unprotected lesion crossing
Proximal balloon occlusion ± flow reversal	All CAS step protected	Potential intolerance to flow arrest[b]
	Lesion crossing with guidewire of choice	No lesion visualization with CM injection during all CAS phases
	Protection possible also in tortuous ICA	Handling more demanding than filter
	Protection independent of particle size	Larger size required (8–9 Fr)
		Balloon-induced dissection or spasm of both ECA and ICA

Note: CAS, carotid artery stenting; CM, contrast medium; ECA, external carotid artery; ICA, internal carotid artery.
[a] Does not apply to wire-independent systems.
[b] Problematic in patients with severe stenosis/occlusion of the contralateral ICA.

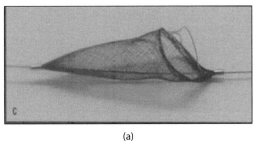
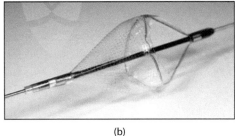

(a)   (b)

Figure 51.6 Two examples of filter emboli protection devices. **(a** and **b)** The SpiderRx (ev3, Plymouth, MN) and the Emboshield Pro (Abbott Vascular, Redwood City, CA), respectively.

Table 51.5 Comparison of selected distal embolic protection filters

Characteristic	Spider	Filterwire	Angioguard	Accunet	Emboshield Pro	Interceptor
Manufacturer	ev3	BSC	CJJ	GDT	ABT	MDT
Material	N	N, PU	N, PU	N, PU	N, PU	N
Guidewire (in.)	0.014	0.014	0.014	0.014	0.014	0.014
RX	Yes	Yes	Yes	Yes	Yes	Yes
Independent wire	Yes	No	No	No	Yes	No
Sheath (Fr)	6	6	6	6	6	6
Vessel size (mm)	3.0–7.0	3.5–5.5	4.0–8.0	4.5–7.5	4.0–7.0	4.5–6.5
Profile (Fr)	3.2	3.2	3.2–3.9	3.5–3.7	3.2	2.7
Pore size (m)	167–209	110	100	150	140	100
FDA approval	Yes	Yes	Yes	Yes	Yes	Yes

Source: From National Coverage Determination (NCD) for Percutaneous Transluminal Angioplasty (PTA) (20.7), (cited 31 July 2015), http://www.cms.gov/medicare-coverage-database/Details.

Note: ABT, Abbott Medical Corporation; BSC, Boston Scientific Corporation; CJJ, Cordis/Johnson & Johnson Inc.; ev3, Covidien/Medtronic; FDA, United States Food and Drug Administration; Fr, French; GDT, Guidant Corporation; MDT, Medtronic Corporation; N, nitinol; PU, polyurethane; RX, rapid exchange.

characteristics to CAS with distal or proximal protection using transcranial micro-embolic signals (MES) count as surrogate of cerebral microembolization.[19] The carotid Wallstent was used in all cases. The Mo.Ma group showed a significantly lower number of MES as compared to the filter group, especially in the phases of the procedures known to be associated with MES (i.e., predilation, stent crossing/deployment, and stent postdilation). Notably, proximal protection was the only independent predictor of lower MES number. A recent meta-analysis supported the notion of superiority of Mo.Ma over filter EPD in the number of post CAS new ischemic lesions detected by MR imaging.[20] Recently, a device allowing CAS under flow reversal using a transcervical approach, the ENROUTE transcarotid Neuroprotection system (ENROUTE TNS, Silk Road Medical), has also received FDA approval. Preliminary results in 141 patients enrolled into the pivotal phase of the Roadster trial showed a 99% technical success with a death/stroke/MI rate of 3.5%.[21]

Balloon catheters

As a general rule, the balloon catheter used for predilation (optional) should be greatly undersized, and the one chosen for postdilatation (mandatory) should be shorter than the stent and also slightly undersized. To minimize the risk of distal embolization, a residual stenosis of up to 30% following postdilatation of the stent is commonly accepted. Typically, balloon catheters 3–4 mm in diameter and 20 mm in length are used for predilatation, while the balloon size for postdilatation of the stent is usually 5–5.5 mm in diameter and 20 mm in length. The use of 0.014-in rapid exchange balloon catheters is recommended.

Stents

In order to prevent stent crushing, the devices used in the carotid territory are all self-expanding (Figure 51.7). With the exception of the stainless steel Carotid Wallstent (Boston Scientific), all the devices are based on nitinol, an alloy allowing for excellent flexibility, conformability, and crush resistance. The properties of some of the carotid stents on the market are listed in Table 51.6. With respect to stent design, the most important differentiation is between open- and closed-cell designs. Closed-cell stents are characterized by fully connecting struts and may offer greater plaque coverage than open-cell stents—with both connecting and nonconnecting struts—potentially reducing the risk of delayed embolism due to plaque protrusion. Therefore, this

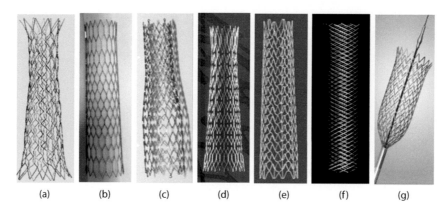

Figure 51.7 Self-expading nitinol carotid stents available in the U.S. market. **(a)** Nexstent (BSI); **(b)** X-act stent (Abbott), **(c)** Protegeé Rx stent (Medtronic); **(d)** Viveex stent (Bard); **(e)** Acculink (Abbott); **(f)** Carotid Wallstent (BSI); and **(g)** PrecisePro (Cordis).

Table 51.6 Design and brand names of commonly used stents

Stent type	Name	Company	FDA approval
Open-cell nitinol	Acculink	Abbott	Yes
	Exponent	Medtronic	Yes
	Precise Pro	Cordis	Yes
	ProtegèeRx	Medtronic	Yes
	Viveex	Bard	Yes
Closed-cell nitinol	Next stent	Boston Scientific	Yes
	X-act[a]	Abbott	Yes
Hybrid[b]	Cristallo Ideale	Medtronic	Yes
Stainless steel	Carotid Wallstent	Boston Scientific	Yes

Note: FDA, Food and Drug Administration.
[a] X-act stent: closed-cell area in the central part of the stent. The two edges have an open cell area design.
[b] Cristallo Ideale: the closed-cell design in the middle third of the stent, whereas both proximal and distal third do have an open-cell design.

type of stent may be preferred for soft or ulcerated plaques with high embolic potential. Finally, closed-cell stents have higher radial strength, an important feature in severely calcified lesions. Open-cell stents are more flexible, conform better to the artery, and result in better wall apposition. Therefore, the latter stent type may be preferred in tortuous arteries and in lesions extending into the CCA.

Recently a new class of stents has been put on the market, namely, the double-layer mesh stent. The defining characteristic of these stents is a second mesh made either of nitinol or polytetraethylene (PTE)/polytetrafluoroethylene (PTFE) material that is attached (either inside or outside) to the main stent strut. The second mesh, with a very small free cell area (360 microns) (Figure 51.8), is supposed to increase the plaque containment capacity of the device and, as a consequence, reduce the risk of both peri- and postprocedural cerebral embolization due to plaque prolapse through the stent struts. Preliminary studies showed encouraging results compared with historical series using the FDA-approved Roadsaver nitinol stent (Terumo).[22,23] Although differences in stent designs are interesting from a conceptual standpoint, their clinical impacts remain to be demonstrated.

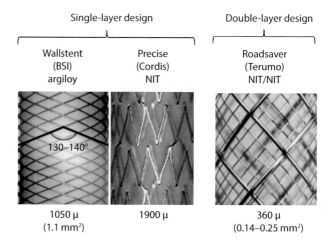

Figure 51.8 Close-up of three carotid stents. The Carotid Wallstent (closed-cell design) and the Precise Rx stent (open-cell design) are single-layer devices, whereas the Roadsaver stent is a double mesh device that is not yet approved by the FDA. The stent free cell area is reported below each stent frame. In the Roadsaver stent, the free cell area refers to the inner stent mesh. NIT, nitinol.

EQUIPMENT FOR VERTEBRAL INTERVENTIONS

Most vertebral interventions can be performed with coronary equipment using a 6-Fr guiding catheter, a medium or extra support 0.014-in coronary guidewire, and a balloon-expandable coronary or peripheral stent.[24] Guiding catheter shapes frequently used includes the Judkins right and the vertebral. Since the lesions are frequently in ostial location, coronary stents with good radial strength are preferred. There are no specific recommendations in regards to distal protection in vertebral interventions due to the lack of data, as well as the limited size of the artery that is prone to complications such as dissection and spasm.[25]

PROCEDURAL ASPECTS OF CAROTID ARTERY STENTING

Pre-, peri-, and postoperative medical and fluid management

Patients scheduled for CAS should receive overnight hydration (e.g., 1 mL/kg/h), and antihypertensive drugs should be withdrawn the morning of the procedure. This approach is suggested to mitigate the hypotension/bradycardia response that usually occurs after stent postdilation due to carotid bulb receptor stimulation. Atropine, 0.5 to 1 mg IV, is routinely administered prior to stent postdilation to counteract the vagal activation. To gain the most of the atropine effect, it may be useful to wait with postdilatation until heart rate increases by >10% of the baseline value as a proof of sympathetic system activation. Although randomized outcome data on optimal antithrombotic treatment during CAS are lacking, DAPT with aspirin and clopidogrel should be administered preferably at least 10 days before and for at least 30 days after CAS, followed by ASA lifelong. Alternatively, a loading dose of 300–600 mg of clopidogrel may be given the day before the procedure. Patients not on chronic aspirin require 250 mg of aspirin administered orally or intravenously prior to the procedure. In patients not on statins, a high-dose atorvastatin load (80 + 40 mg) 12 hours before the procedure, associated with 600 mg clopidogrel load (in clopidogrel-naïve patients) 6 hours before the procedure has been found to provide better neuroprotection, as demonstrated by a lower rate of new ischemic lesions at diffusion weighted (DW)-MRI.[26] While documented aspirin or clopidogrel allergy may be considered a relative contraindication for CAS, switch to indobufen or prasugrel or desensitization to both drugs have been reported to be a safe and effective alternative treatment.[27,28]

Intraprocedural anticoagulation is obtained by UFH (5,000 units IV bolus and subsequent heparin doses as needed) to achieve an activated clotting time (ACT) of 250–300 seconds. The ACT time should be rechecked after 30 minutes. Alternatively, bivalirudin has been used as anticoagulant for peripheral interventions including CAS.[29,30] To allow for assessment of alertness, speech, and communication, periprocedural sedation should be limited to low-dose benzodiazepines to alleviate anxiety, if necessary.

Techinques

Intubation of the CCA may be achieved with a variety of diagnostic catheters. In the presence of a "friendly" aortic arch, CCA engagement can be achieved with catheter shapes such as the Judkins right coronary or the vertebral/Bernstein catheters. Alternatively, the headhunter or the Benson diagnostic catheters can be used. For more steep/tortuous aortic arches, shapes such as the Vitek or the Simmons/Sidewinder or the Benson may be used. The handling of these catheters is more challenging and may be associated with an increased risk of cerebral microembolization.

Particularly in the early phase of the learning curve, CAS should be performed in a standardized way using limited and familiar equipment (Table 51.3). Lesion length and vessel size to guide equipment choice are usually estimated visually. A step-by-step description of the procedure is summarized in Table 51.7. Over a 0.035-in long steerable wire, a 125 cm 5-Fr diagnostic catheter is inserted inside an 8-Fr guiding catheter or a 90 cm, 6-Fr sheath. The origin of the LCCA or the brachiocephalic trunk is cannulated with the diagnostic catheter. Under "road-map" or "overlay" functions, a steerable 0.035-in guidewire is advanced into the distal CCA or, if necessary, into the ECA. The diagnostic catheter is advanced over the guidewire into the distal CCA. Subsequently, the 8-Fr guiding catheter or the 6-Fr sheath is advanced over the diagnostic catheter. This step should be performed under lower magnification in order to have control of both the guidewire in the distal CCA or ECA and the catheter advancement in the aortic arch.

As an alternative to the telescoping technique, the steerable 0.035-in guidewire such as Wholey (Mallinckrodt), Magic Torque (Boston Scientific), or Glidewire (Terumo) can be advanced under road map into the ECA and then the diagnostic 5-Fr catheter can be advanced over the wire into the ECA. Subsequently, the steerable guidewire is exchanged for a stiff 0.035-in guidewire such as the Supracore (Abbott) or the Amplatz superstiff (Boston Scientific). With the stiff guidewire in place in the ECA, the short 5-Fr sheath is exchanged for a 90 cm, 6-Fr sheath, which is advanced into the distal CCA. This type of engagement is applicable in the presence of a friendly anatomy of the aortic arch and the CCAm and has the advantage of requiring a smaller femoral access. However, it may not be used in the presence of severe ECA or distal CCA disease. In patients with bovine arch, direct intubation of the LCCA with a guiding catheter (e.g., AL1 8-Fr) may be considered.

Following intubation of the CCA with the guiding catheter or sheath, the lesion, usually located at the origin of the ICA, is crossed under road map with the filter EPD. The device should be placed in a straight segment of the ICA and filter apposition to the vessel wall should be verified by angiography. On rare occasions, primary crossing

Table 51.7 Carotid artery stenting protocol using telescoping technique, filter-based distal emboli protection, and unfractionated heparin as anticoagulant

- Patient pretreated with aspirin and clopidogrel
- Common femoral arterial access in local anesthesia with a 5-Fr sheath
- Intravenous unfractionated heparin to achieve activated clotting time 250–300 seconds
- 5-Fr pigtail catheter for aortic arch angiography (LAO 45°)
- Insert a 125-cm, 5-Fr diagnostic catheter (e.g., JR4) inside a 100-cm, 8-Fr guide catheter (e.g., H1)
- Intubation of the CCA with the diagnostic catheter
- Under roadmap, 0.035-in guidewire is advanced into the distal CCA or ECA, then the diagnostic catheter is advanced into the distal CCA, then the 8-Fr guide catheter is advanced over the diagnostic catheter into the mid/distal CCA
- Diagnostic catheter and 0.035-in guidewire are retrieved
- DSA angiography of the carotid bifurcation and of the intracranial circulation
- ICA lesion passed with filter EPD under roadmap, filter deployed
- 0.5–1.0 mg of IV atropine
- Balloon predilation (if required) with a 3.0–4.0 × 20-mm, 0.014-in rapid exchange balloon catheter
- Stenting with a nitinol, self-expanding, rapid exchange, 8.0–9.0 × 30–40-mm stent
- Postdilation (always) with a 5.0–5.5 × 20-mm, 0.014-in rapid exchange balloon catheter
- Filter retrieved
- DSA angiography of the carotid bifurcation and intracranial circulation
- Non-DSA angiography of the CCA during retrieval of guiding catheter/sheath
- Femoral closure device if patient is hemodynamically stable

Note: CCA, common carotid artery; DSA, digital subtraction angiography; ECA, external carotid; EPD, embolic protection device; IV, intravenous; LAO, left anterior oblique projection.

of the lesion with the EPD may not be possible because of lesion complexity. In these cases, a wire-independent EPD system or a proximal occlusion type of EPD should be considered. Alternatively, a buddy wire or pre-predilation with an undersized balloon (e.g., 1.5–2 mm) may be used in order to be able to advance the EPD. However, since this maneuver may increase the risk of distal embolization, it should be avoided whenever possible. Balloon predilation should be considered when it is anticipated that advancement of the stent may be problematic, and in particular, in the presence of a high-grade and/or severely calcified stenosis. Advancement of the stent within the guiding catheter should be performed slowly, as air may get entrapped during this maneuver. A "de-bubbling" of the system should be performed before crossing the lesion and deploying the stent. This may take some time depending on the clearance between the guiding catheter internal lumen and the stent. The clearance of air in the system is particularly important if angiography is performed to check stent positioning. In this respect, the use of road-map or overlay functions is preferred. However, it has to be taken into account that the rigidity of the stent may change the anatomy of the vessel. With respect to stent length, it is recommended to be generous, since the whole diseased segment should be covered and, unlike in the coronary arteries, restenosis is a minor concern in CAS. As a consequence, almost invariably the stent will/should cover the carotid bifurcation (Figure 51.9). Even if the ECA seems compromised following ICA stenting, patients do not have related symptoms and the ECA stenosis does not need to be treated. Postdilation of the stent is mandatory, aiming to obtain at least a residual stenosis <30%. In case of near optimal angiographic result soon after

stent deployment (as in case of very soft plaque) postdilation may be skipped to avoid plaque debris embolization. Finally, the EPD is retrieved using the dedicated retrieval sheath. Should the flow be compromised during the procedure because of filling of the filter EPD with debris, then the blood column in the ICA should be aspirated with an aspiration catheter, such as the Export (Medtronic) or Eliminate (Terumo) catheter, prior to EPD removal to prevent distal embolization.

If a proximal balloon occlusion system is used (i.e., MO. MA Ultra system), then the device is advanced over a stiff guidewire previously placed in the ECA. Once in position, the system mandrel is removed while the stiff wire is left in place. The optimal positioning of the ECA balloon (as close as possible to the ECA ostium in order to exclude all collaterals) is checked by angiography and, if fine, the balloon is inflated. Stiff wire is then removed. After double-checking the blood pressure transducer "zero" level, the CCA balloon is inflated. Patient tolerance should be assessed for 30 seconds and average back pressure should be recorded. A value >40 mmHg has been found to be an independent predictor of patient tolerance.[31] Angiography may be taken at this time to confirm flow arrest and as a road map to facilitate wire/stent crossing and positioning. No further injections of contrast should be done during the remaining CAS phases. After stent postdilation, aspiration of 60 mL (3 syringes, 20 mL each) of blood is performed and then to check for debris, the blood is filtered into three separated baskets. If no debris is found in the last basket then blood flow may be restored by deflating the ECA balloon first followed by the CCA balloon deflation (Figure 51.10). The handling of occlusive EPD is technically more demanding than the one of filters EPD and should be

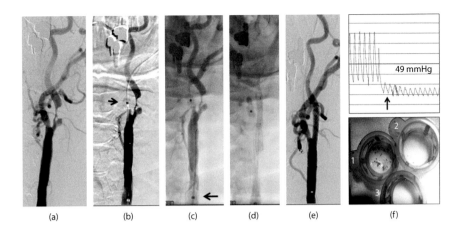

Figure 51.9 CAS with proximal protection in a patient with left hemispheric TIA. Severe, soft-ulcerated LICA stenosis **(a)**; Positioning of the 8-Fr Mo.Ma system through a 0.035-in stiff wire in the ECA. The Mo.Ma balloon in the ECA is inflated (*black arrow*) and contrast medium is injected to confirm ECA exclusion (a small superior tyroid artery is left unoccluded because it is too close to the ostium) **(b)**. Full endovascular occlusion is achieved by CCA balloon inflation (*black arrow*) **(c)**. Stent depoyment and postdilation **(d)**. Final angiographic results after Mo.Ma removal **(e)**. Back pressure (49 mmHg) at the time of full endovascular occlusion (*black arrow*) **(f, *upper frame*)**. Debris collected during aspiration at the end of the procedure. No debris are collected into the third basket allowing defletion of both balloons **(f, *lower frame*)**. CAS, carotid artery stenting; CCA, common carotid artery; ECA, external carotid artery; LICA, left internal carotid artery; TIA, transient ischemic attack.

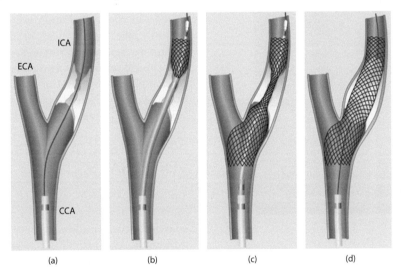

Figure 51.10 Carotid artery stenting procedure. Following engagement of the common carotid artery (CCA) with a guiding catheter or long sheath, the lesion in the internal carotid artery (ICA) is passed with the filter emboli protection device **(a)**. Subsequently, a self-expanding stent is deployed, usually covering the carotid bifurcation **(b and c)**. Thereafter, a balloon postdilation is performed to achieve a good stent expansion **(d)**. ECA, external carotid artery. (From Roffi, M., et al., *Eur Heart J* 2009;30(22):2693-2704. With permission.)

introduced later in the CAS learning curve. The Mo.Ma system is available in a 8- and 9-Fr version and also in a mono-balloon version indicated in case of ECA occlusion.

Following retrieval of the EPD, the patient is examined on the catheterization table to detect major neurologic deficits and final DSA angiography of the carotid bifurcation and the intracranial vasculature are performed (Figure 51.11). In the absence of neurologic or angiographic abnormalities, the guiding catheter/sheath is retrieved into the descending aorta at the time of contrast injection to exclude complications at the level of the CCA such as catheter-induced dissections. If the patient is hemodynamically stable, the

sheath may be removed and hemostasis may be achieved with a femoral closure device such as Starclose or Perclose (Abbott) or Angioseal (St. Jude Medical, St. Paul, MN). Alternatively, the sheath can be pulled a few hours following the procedure to allow for the effect of heparin to dissipate, and hemostasis can be achieved by manual compression.

Transradial access

Carotid stenting through unconventional vascular approach has been proposed in specific anatomic settings, such as bovine aortic arch associated with a left internal carotid artery (LICA) stenosis, type II–III aortic arch and right internal carotid artery (RICA) stenosis, aortic arch atherosclerotic disease, and lack of peripheral accesses (Figure 51.12). These anatomies have been found to be associated with high risk of cerebral embolization following CAS from the standard femoral route.[32,33] A pre-intervention CTA is of paramount importance in this specific setting. Right radial catheterization should be the first option in every patient, according to the standardized protocol for transradial coronary interventions. Alternatively, the right ulnar, left radial, or right brachial arteries may be utilized. Target vessel cannulation strictly depends on the vessel anatomy. 5 or 6-Fr diagnostic Judkins right or internal mammary catheters are indicated for cannulation of both the right common carotid artery (RCCA) and LCCA in the presence of a bovine arch. A Simmons-1 or -2 catheter should be the first choice in acute (<45°) RCCA takeoff and in all cases of LCCA originating from the aorta. Stent deployments are performed through either 6-Fr guiding catheters using 5-Fr compatible stents—such as Carotid Wallstent 7 mm (Boston Scientific) and PrecisePro 8 mm (Cordis)—or 6-Fr sheaths allowing all stent sizes. Embolic distal protection is obtained with standard filters.

Despite equipment similarity with what is used for transfemoral CAS, transradial access requires dedicated techniques and has a steep learning curve. Advantages of transradial access may include: avoidance (full or partial) of catheter navigation into the aortic arch, reduced bleeding/hemorrhage rate from the artery entry point, early ambulation, reduced hospital length of stay, and overall patient preference. A series enrolling 382 patients in two centers reported favorable 30-day clinical results (stroke/death/myocardial infarction (MI) rate: 1.7%) with a crossover rate to femoral approach of 9%.[34] A randomized study assessed the safety and efficacy of transradial ($n = 130$) versus transfemoral CAS ($n = 130$) patients.[35] No difference was observed in access site complication or in major adverse cardiac or cerebrovascular events between the radial and the femoral approach, while a 10% crossover rate was confirmed. Moreover, radiation exposure was increased by 29% in transradial approach versus femoral approach, basically reflecting the steep learning curve of the new CAS technique. Recently, a single-center series reported favorable clinical results (stroke/death/MI rate 1.9%) and vascular complications (1.9%) of CAS through the transradial/brachial approach in 214 patients, including 60 patients in whom the 8-Fr proximal protection was used.[36]

PROCEDURAL ASPECTS OF VERTEBRAL STENTING

Similar to CAS, endovascular treatment of extracranial VA stenosis is usually performed under local anesthesia and conscious sedation allowing for early detection of neurologic symptoms. After arterial access is obtained, UFH is administered to achieve an ACT of 250–300 seconds. Access is usually obtained at the common femoral artery. Occasionally, the radial or brachial artery access may be preferred based on an unfavorable anatomy at the level of the aortic arch or

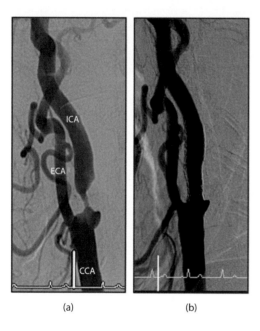

(a)   (b)

Figure 51.11 Digital subtraction angiography of the carotid bifurcation showing **(a)** a severe stenosis of the internal carotid artery (ICA) and **(b)** the result following stenting. CCA, common carotid artery; ECA, external carotid artery.

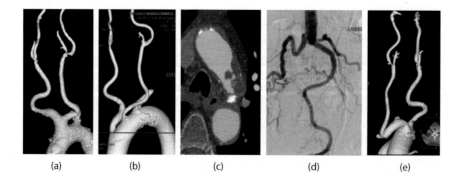

(a)   (b)   (c)   (d)   (e)

Figure 51.12 CT angiography volume rendering images of patients with indication for transradial CAS **(a)** Bovine aortic arch configuration with LICA stenosis. **(b)** Type III aortic arch with RICA stenosis. **(c)** Aortic arch atherosclerosis. **(d)** Peripheral arterial disease. **(e)** "Plongeant" brachiocephalic trunk with RICA stenosis. CAS, carotid artery stenting; CT, computed tomography; LICA, left internal carotid artery; RICA, right internal carotid artery.

in the presence of excessive angulation between the subclavian and the vertebral arteries. A 6-Fr guiding catheter is advanced over a 0.035-in wire to obtain a stable position in the SCA. Usual curves include the vertebral, Judkins right, and the multipurpose one. If additional stability is needed, the use of a 7-Fr guiding catheter or 6-Fr, 90 cm sheath may be helpful because it allows the advancement of 0.014- or 0.018-in buddy wire into the distal SCA. If the long sheath approach is chosen, then a 0.035-in exchange length wire is advanced over a diagnostic catheter positioned in the SCA in the axillary artery and the long sheath is then advanced over the wire. Angiographic runs are performed to visualize the extracranial and intracranial VA and to obtain accurate views defining the VA lesions and its relation to the SCA.

The use of EPD for VA stenosis is controversial. The smaller caliber of the VA, the frequently marked angulation between the VA origin and the SCA, the tortuosity of the proximal VA segments, and the tendency to develop spasms are all factors that may cause difficulties in the advancement of the EPD device. In addition, recovery of the system may also be difficult in the presence of spasms or unfavorable angulation of the VA origin, angulation that may be more pronounced following stent deployment. The use of EPD may be considered for VA with diameters exceeding 3.5 mm, favorable geometric orientation of the VA origin, and the presence of with ulcerated target lesions.[37]

Under road-map guidance, the VA lesion is crossed with a 0.014-in medium-support or extra-support coronary wire. In order to obtain stable guiding catheter position, the wire should be positioned far enough distally in the VA. The tip of the wire should be visualized during the entire procedure to reduce the risk of perforation. Stent selection (either self-expanding or balloon mounted) is based mainly on lesion location. Ostial VA lesions—by far the most frequent site of obstruction—are treated preferably

with balloon-expandable coronary stents because of high radial force, lack of foreshortening, and low crossing profile. For true ostial lesions, the stent should protrude 1–2 mm into the SCA to allow for optimal lesion coverage, and a second balloon inflation at high pressure should be performed following partial balloon retrieval to optimize the apposition of the stent struts at the vessel wall, the so-called "flaring of the ostium." Self-expanding stents are reserved for nonostial lesions in vessels with larger diameters (i.e., >5.5 mm).[37] In the presence of a severe or calcified lesion, balloon dilatation prior to stenting may be appropriate. The balloon selected should be undersized and shorter than the intended stent (Figure 51.13).

RANDOMIZED DATA ON CAROTID ARTERY STENTING

Seven major—that is, including over 300 patients each—randomized trials have compared endovascular and surgical carotid revascularization. While the SAPPHIRE (Stenting and Angioplasty with Protection in Patients at HIgh Risk for Endarterectomy) trial[38] focused on patients—both symptomatic and asymptomatic—at high risk for surgery, CAVATAS (CArotid and Vertebral Artery Transluminal Angioplasty Study),[39] SPACE (Stent-protected Percutaneous Angioplasty of the Carotid artery vs. Endarterectomy),[40] EVA-3S (Endarterectomy vs. Angioplasty in patients with Symptomatic Severe carotid Stenosis),[41] and ICSS (International Carotid Stenting Study),[42] enrolled exclusively symptomatic patients. CREST (Carotid Revascularization Endarterectomy vs. Stenting Trial) enrolled both symptomatic and asymptomatic patients.[43] Finally, ACT (Asymptomatic Carotid Trial)-I enrolled only asymptomatic patients.[44]

The CAVATAS, performed in the late 1990s, randomized 504 symptomatic patients at low to moderate risk for surgery to CEA or carotid angioplasty.[39] The incidence of death or stroke at 30 days was 10% and 9.9% in the endovascular and surgical group, respectively. The outcomes between the two groups remained comparable at 3 years. The SAPPHIRE study is the only randomized trial comparing CEA and CAS performed with the systematic use of EPD.[38] The trial included symptomatic and asymptomatic patients at high risk for surgery and was designed to prove the noninferiority of the endovascular approach. The study was terminated prematurely because of slow enrollment due to competing CAS registries. Among the 334 patients randomized (29% of them being symptomatic), major adverse events at 1 year occurred in 12.2% in the CAS group and in 20.1% in the CEA group ($P = 0.053$). In the actual treatment analysis, the observed difference reached statistical significance ($P = 0.048$). The difference was mainly driven by a reduction in the rate of MI (at 30 days 0.6% in the CAS group versus 4.3% in the CEA group; $P = 0.04$). No cranial nerve injury was observed in the CAS group, while this complication occurred in 5.3% of the CEA patients ($P < 0.01$). The durability of CAS was documented by a comparable cumulative

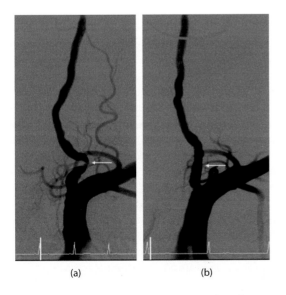

Figure 51.13 Digital subtraction angiography of a proximal stenosis in the left vertebral artery **(a)** treated with a balloon-expandable coronary stent **(b)**.

percentage of major (1.3% for CAS vs. 3.3% for CEA) and minor (6.1% for CAS vs. 3% for CEA) ipsilateral strokes at 3 years, as well as by a low rate of repeat revascularization during the same period of time (3% for CAS vs. 7.1% for CEA).[45]

The SPACE study sought to prove the noninferiority of CAS compared with CEA among symptomatic patients.[40] The use of EPD in the CAS arm was left at the discretion of the treating physician and was used in 27% of cases. Although the required sample size based on interim analysis was >2,400 patients, the trial had to be terminated following the inclusion of 1,200 patients because of slow enrollment and lack of funding. The incidence of ipsilateral stroke or death at 30 days was the primary endpoint of the study and did not differ between the groups, occurring in 6.8% of cases in the endovascular group and in 6.3% of patients in the surgical arm. At 2-year follow-up, no difference in adverse events between the two groups could be detected.[46]

The EVA-3S was a randomized noninferiority trial comparing CAS with CEA in patients with a >60% symptomatic carotid artery stenosis.[41] The primary endpoint was the cumulative incidence of any stroke or death within 30 days after treatment. The protocol did not mandate the use of EPD. The performance of CAS without EPD protection in the study was rapidly halted following the observation that 4/15 patients treated without protection suffered a stroke, while the proportion of patients treated with protection was 5/58 (OR 3.9; 95% CI, 0.9–16.7).[27] The entire trial was then stopped prematurely after the inclusion of 527 patients because of significant increased event rates in the CAS arm (death or stroke 9.6% in the CAS arm and 3.9% in the CEA arm; $P < 0.01$).[47] At 6 months, the incidence of any stroke or death was 11.7% in the CAS group and 6.1% in the CEA group ($P = 0.02$). At 4-year follow-up, the death or stroke rate still favored CEA, driven by the 30-day events. Beyond 30 days, no difference was observed.[47,48]

The ICSS randomized 1,710 symptomatic patients to CAS or CEA.[42] The primary endpoint is the long-term survival free of disabling stroke. The use of EPD was not mandatory. The 30-day incidence of death, stroke, or periprocedural MI was 8.5% in the CAS group and 5.1% in the CEA group ($P = 0.004$). No difference was observed in the survival free of disabling stroke at 120 days. At follow-up, the number of fatal or disabling strokes and cumulative 5-year risk did not differ significantly between the stenting and endarterectomy groups (6.4% vs. 6.5%; hazard ratio [HR] 1.06, 95% CI 0.72–1.57, $P = 0.77$). Any stroke was more frequent in the stenting group than in the endarterectomy group (119 vs. 72 events; ITT population, 5-year cumulative risk 15.2% vs. 9.4%, HR 1.71, 95% CI 1.28–2.30, $P < 0.001$; per-protocol population, 5-year cumulative risk 8.9% vs. 5.8%, 1.53, 1.02–2.31, $P = 0.04$), but were mainly nondisabling strokes.[49]

CREST randomized 2,502 symptomatic and asymptomatic patients to CAS vs. CEA. The primary composite endpoint was stroke, MI, and death from any cause during the periprocedural period or any ipsilateral stroke within 4 years after randomization.[43] At 30 days, there was no

difference in stroke, MI, and death (5.2% in CAS vs. 4.5% in CEA group, $P = 0.38$). CAS patients had more minor strokes (2.9% vs. 1.4%, $P = 0.009$), whereas CEA patients had more MI (2.3% vs. 1.1%, $P = 0.03$). Over 10 years of follow-up, there was no difference in the rate of the primary composite endpoint between the stenting group (11.8%; 95% CI, 9.1–14.8) and the endarterectomy group (9.9%; 95% CI, 7.9–12.2) (hazard ratio, 1.10; 95% CI, 0.83–1.44).[50] No significant between-group differences with respect to either endpoint were detected when symptomatic patients and asymptomatic patients were analyzed separately.[51]

A meta-analysis of 13 randomized controlled trials was then published, including 3,723 CEA and 3,754 CAS patients (Figure 51.14). Regarding short-term outcomes, CAS was associated with elevated risk for stroke and "death or stroke." CAS also exhibited a marginal trend toward higher death and "death or disabling stroke" rates. CEA was associated with higher rates of MI and cranial nerve injury (Figure 51.12). Concerning long-term outcomes, CAS was associated with higher rates of stroke (pooled OR, 1.37; 95% CI, 1.13–1.65) and "death or stroke" (pooled OR, 1.25; 95% CI, 1.06–1.48).[52]

ACT-1, published after the mentioned meta-analysis, enrolled asymptomatic patients at standard surgical risk and randomized them 3:1 to CAS with EPD vs. CEA. The study was prematurely stopped after inclusion of 1,453 of the 1,658 planned patients (88%) because of slow enrollment (over 8 years). CAS was noninferior to CEA endarterectomy with regard to the primary composite endpoint of death, stroke, or MI within 30 days after the procedure or ipsilateral stroke within 1 year (event rate, 3.8% and 3.4%, respectively; $P = 0.01$ for noninferiority). The rate of stroke or death within 30 days did not differ (2.9% in the CAS group and 1.7% in the CEA group ($P = 0.33$). The cumulative 5-year rate of stroke-free survival was 93.1% in the stenting group and 94.7% in the endarterectomy group ($P = 0.44$).[44]

Limitations of the carotid artery stenting versus carotid endarterectomy randomized trials

Current randomized data comparing CAS and CEA have several limitations. First, the minimal endovascular experience required per protocol was, in most of the trials, incredibly low and five out of seven large randomized trials (i.e., enrolling over 300 patients) allowed endovascular treatment in the presence of a tutor for interventionalists with insufficient experience (Table 51.8). It has to be underscored that tutors were usually only allowed to give suggestions and comments to the operators during the procedure and not to perform the procedure themselves. Other than SAPPHIRE, none of the randomized trials would have satisfied the minimum recommended endovascular experience according to a multispecialty CAS clinical competence statement.[50,53] Second, the use of EPD was mandatory in three trials only.[38,43,44] When adopted, the type of EPD varied from a single type of filter for all patients[38,43] to seven different distal protection systems.[41]

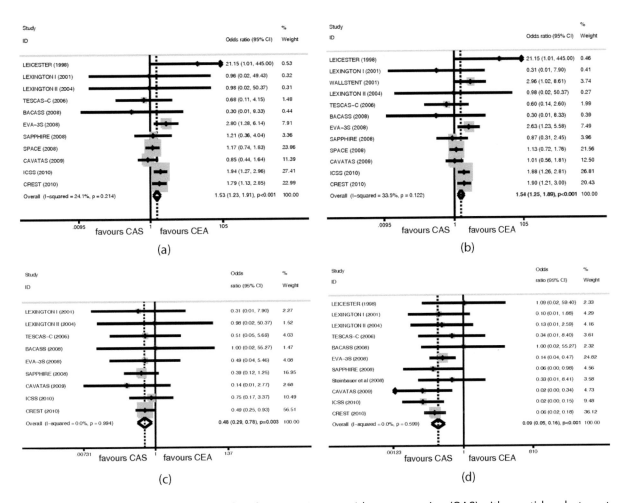

Figure 51.14 Meta-analysis of the randomized trials comparing carotid artery stenting (CAS) with carotid endarterectomy (CEA). Fore plot of short-term ORs for **(a)** stroke, **(b)** death or stroke, **(c)** myocardial infarction, and **(d)** cranial nerve injury. OR, odds ratio. (From Konstantinos, P., et al., *Stroke*, 42, 687–692, 2011. With permission.)

Table 51.8 Minimal requirements in terms of endovascular expertise in large-scale CAS vs. endarterectomy randomized trials

CAVATAS (39)	Training in neuroradiology and angioplasty (but not necessarily in the carotid artery) required. Tutor-assisted procedures allowed.
SAPPHIRE (38)	Procedures submitted to an executive review committee; CAS periprocedural death or stroke rate had to be <6%. No tutor-assisted procedures allowed.
SPACE (40)	25 successful CAS or assistance of a tutor for interventionalists having performed at least 10 CAS.
EVA-3S (41)	12 CAS cases or ≥5 CAS and >30 cases of endovascular treatment of supra-aortic trunks. Tutor-assisted CAS allowed for centers not fulfilling minimal requirements.
ICSS (42)	A minimum of 50 total stenting procedures, of which at least 10 should be in the carotid artery. Tutor-assisted procedures allowed for interventionalists with insufficient experience.
CREST (43)	A minimum of 20 CAS in the previous year. If <20, tutor-assisted CAS during the lead-in phase.
ACT-1 (44)	>25 CAS/CEA procedures for each investigator. Lead-in phase during which sites were required to show proficiency with the study devices in at least 2 cases before they could treat randomly assigned patients.

Source: Modified with permission from Roffi, M., et al. *Eur Heart J* 2009;30(22):2693-2704.
Note: CAS, carotid artery stenting; CEA, carotid endarterectomy.

Notably, proximal protection was never used. Finally, several types of stents have been used. While no randomized studies have been published comparing safety and efficacy of different carotid stents, closed-cell design stents have been associated with lower cerebral embolization rates, especially in symptomatic patients.[54,55]

Third, the data on asymptomatic patients are limited since only one trial included exclusively asymptomatic patients. Fourth, none of the trials mandated imaging of the aortic arch/supra-aortic trunks prior to randomization. Therefore, we do not know whether patients undergoing CAS in the trials had favorable anatomy for the procedure or not.

Fifth, while MI rate has been found to be significantly higher in CEA as compared to CAS, this variable was considered as a component of the primary endpoint in only a few studies.[38,43] However, recent evidence supports a systematic preoperative coronary angiography eventually followed by coronary interventions or bypass surgery as a strategy to lower myocardial ischemic complications.[56,57]

Finally, the trials missed the main purpose of randomized testing of a new procedure, namely, to show that the novel therapy is efficacious in the hands of the most skilled operators on selected (favorable) patients. In this respect, early testing of CEA against medical therapy was properly conducted. In the ACAS trial, for example, patients at high risk for surgery were excluded from the trial and both the centers and the individual surgeons had to demonstrate a 30-day death or stroke rate of <3% to be able to enroll. In addition, during the study, the surgeons were audited in the presence of more than one complication and were allowed to continue enrollment only if no operator-related problem was observed.[58]

Large-scale carotid artery stenting registries

The results of seven CAS registries enrolling over 1,000 patients have been published, for a total of 21,405 patients (Table 51.9). All but two were performed in the United States, included patients at high risk for surgery, and the majority of patients included were asymptomatic. The good quality of the studies is demonstrated by the high proportion of mandatory neurologic assessment pre- and postprocedure (5/8) and clinical event committee adjudication of adverse events (5/8). The use of EPD was mandatory in six studies and used in the majority of patients in the remaining two.

The PRO-CAS registry enrolled in German patients with variable risk for surgery and reported an in-hospital death or stroke rate of 3.6%.[59] Symptomatic and asymptomatic patients had an event rate of 4.3% and 2.7%, respectively. In the CAPTURE registry, the 30-day stroke/mortality rate was 5.7% among 3,500 patients, with symptomatic individuals experiencing a stroke rate of 8.9% and asymptomatic patients a rate of 4.1%.[60] The CASES-PMS registry recorded outcomes in 1,493 high-risk patients treated with CAS utilizing EPD reported a stroke/mortality rate of 4.5%, with a stroke rate of 5.3% in symptomatic patients and 3.4% in asymptomatic individuals.[61] The SAPPHIRE Worldwide registry reported a 30-day stroke or death rate of 4% in 2001 among high-risk patients, with higher event rates in symptomatic compared to asymptomatic patients (adjusted OR 2.4).[62]

The SVS registry reported 30-day outcomes among 1,450 patients who underwent CAS and 1,368 patients treated with surgery.[63] In this analysis, the CAS group had significantly higher event rates than CEA (death, stroke, or MI rate 6.4% vs. 2.6%). This analysis was limited by the marked imbalances among the groups, the <50% collection of 30-day events, the lack of systematic neurologic assessment

and event adjudication, as well as the different definition of MI among the centers.

The results of two large-scale registries enrolling patients at high risk for surgery, the EXACT (N = 2145) and the CAPTURE 2 (N = 4175) studies were recently reported.[64] The overall 30-day death and stroke rates in the two studies were 4.1% and 3.4%, respectively. In the population comparable to AHA guidelines (age <80 years), the pooled analysis of the two registries denoted a death or stroke rate within current recommendations for CEA, namely, 5.3% for symptomatic patients and 2.9% for asymptomatic patients. In patients ≥80 years of age, the death and stroke rates in symptomatic and asymptomatic patients were 10.5% and 4.4%, respectively.

Finally, the proximal endovascular occlusion registry enrolled 1,300 patients (50% high surgical risk, 28% symptomatic) who underwent CAS with proximal protection in all (MO.MA Ultra system). Technical success was achieved in 99.7% of patients. Death and any stroke at 30-day interval occurred in 1.38% of all patients and in 3.04%, 0.82%, and 1.88% of symptomatic, asymptomatic, and high surgical risk patients, respectively. No MI occurred.[65]

To investigate further the discrepancy between the CAS suboptimal results shown in the major controlled randomized trials and the favorable results of large industry-funded registries on CAS in the everyday clinical practice, a recent systematic review assessed the stroke/rate death of CEA vs. CAS in contemporary administrative dataset registries (2008–2015).[66] Twenty-one registries involving more than 1,500,000 procedures in both symptomatic and asymptomatic patients at "high or average risk for CEA" were evaluated. Stroke/death rate was significantly higher after CAS than after CEA in 52% and 61% of registries involving "average risk of CEA" in asymptomatic and symptomatic patients, respectively. Moreover, CAS stroke/death rate exceeded the AHA-recommended thresholds in 43% and 72% of the registries involving "average risk of CEA" asymptomatic and symptomatic patients, respectively. Inappropriate patient selection, poor interventional expertise, and the involvement of multiple specialties were potential reasons to explain CAS performance rate. Interestingly, in a study involving 186 University Health System Consortium hospitals, the stroke/death rate among 17,716 asymptomatic patients was 1.5% vs. 4% in CEA and CAS, respectively. Notably, the median number of CAS procedures per operator was only 1.5 (IQR 1–3) and per hospital per year was 4.4 (IQR 0–10). Furthermore, vascular surgeons performed the higher number of CAS with a 4.1% stroke/death rate as compared with 2.6% rates obtained by cardiologists and 6% by radiologists.[67]

DATA ON VERTEBRAL INTERVENTIONS

The data on vertebral interventions are virtually limited to single-center series, most of them retrospective.[68–77] Table 51.10 reports the results of the larger series with at least 50 patients. In most series, the technical success is greater than 95%, the

Table 51.9 Thirty-day event rate in carotid artery stenting registries enrolling over 1,000 patients

Name	Year	N	Industry sponsored	Surgical high-risk	EPD	Sympt patients (%)	Neurologist[a]	CEC adjud. (%)	D/S	D/S/ MI (%)	D/S sympt (%)	D/S asymp (%)
CAPTURE (60)	2007	3500	Yes	Yes	Mandatory	14	Yes	Yes	5.7	6.3	10.6	4.9
CASES PMS (61)	2007	1493	Yes	Yes	Mandatory	22	Yes	Yes	4.5	5.0	NA	NA
PRO-CAS (59)	2008	5341	No	No	75	55	70	No	3.6[b]	NA	4.3[b]	2.7[b]
SAPPHIRE –W (62)	2009	2001	Yes	Yes	Mandatory	28	No[c]	Yes	4.0	4.4	NA	NA
SVS (63)	2009	1450	No	Yes	95	45	No	No	NA	5.7	NA	NA
EXACT (64)	2009	2145	Yes	Yes	Mandatory	10	Yes	Yes	4.1	NA	7.0	3.7
CAPTURE 2 (64)	2009	4175	Yes	Yes	Mandatory	13	Yes	Yes	3.4	NA	6.2	3.0
PROXIMAL ENDOVASCULAR PROTECTION (65)	2010	1300	No	Yes	Mandatory	28	Yes	No	1.4	1.4	3.0	0.8

Source: Modified from Roffi, M., et al. *Eur Heart J* 2009;30(22):2693–2704.

Note: asympt, asymptomatic; CEC adjud., clinical event committee adjudication; D, death; MI, myocardial infarction; S, stroke; sympt, symptomatic.

a Neurologist, independent pre- and postprocedural assessment by a neurologist.
b Refers to in-hospital events; EPD ¼ emboli protection devices.
c Neurologic assessment performed by stroke scale certified staff member.

Table 51.10 Series of stenting of the extracranial vertebral artery including at least 50 procedures

Series	Year	Vessel treated (N)	Type of stent (%)	Technical success (%)[a]	Periprocedural stroke (%)	Follow-up (months)	Significant restenosis (%)[b]
Chastain, et al. (68)	1999	55	BMS 100	98	0	6	10
Lin, et al. (69)	2004	67	BMS 100	100	4.1	11	25
Hatano T, et al. (70)	2005	101	BMS 100	99	0	6	9.5
Taylor, et al. (71)	2009	77	BMS 100	99	3.9[d]	8	48
Vajda, et al. (72)	2009	52	DES 100	100	0	7	12
Jenkins, et al. (76)	2010	112	BMS 86	100	0	29	13.1[c]
Song L, et al. (77)	2012	148	BMS 46	100	0	26	19.2
		156	DES 54	98.7	0	19	4.83
Edgell R, et al. (73)	2013	148	BMS 38	100	0.8	7	15.5
			DES 57				
Mohammadian, et al. (74)	2013	239	BMS 89	97.6	0	13	15.9
Radak, et al. (75)	2014	73	BMS 68	93	0	44	10

Note: BMS, bare-metal stent; DES, drug-eluting stent.
[a] Usually defined as stent successfully placed and residual stenosis <50%.
[b] Usually defined as >50% diameter stenosis on angiography (as % of patients who underwent f/u).
[c] Target lesion revascularization.
[d] Related to other lesions treated at the same time.

occurrence of periprocedural stroke is a rare event, and a balloon-expandable stent was the most frequently implanted device. While the major issue with vertebral intervention is restenosis, the true incidence is unknown because the follow-up of most series was not systematic and the reported results varied considerably (between 3% and 52%).

Two systematic reviews summarized the safety and the efficacy of endovascular treatment of extracranial VA stenosis.[78,79] The first paper focused on proximal VA stenosis (the most frequent involved site).[78] Forty-two selected studies (from 1966 to 2011) reporting endovascular treatment of 1,117 vertebral arteries in 1,099 patients were assessed. Vertebral artery stenting was performed through the femoral approach in 92% of patients using BMS and DES in 79% and 21%, of patients, respectively. The weighted mean technical success rate was 97% (range 36%–100%). Periprocedural TIA occurred in 17 patients (1.5%). The combined stroke and death rate was 1.1%. Recurrent symptoms of vertebrobasilar insufficiency developed in 65 of 967 patients (8%) within a reported follow-up of 6–54 months. Restenosis developed in 183 of 789 patients (23%) who underwent follow-up imaging (range 0%–58%). Reintervention for recurrent disease during follow-up occurred in 86 patients (9%; range 0%–35%). A lower in-stent restenosis at 24-month follow-up has been reported in lesions treated with DES as compared to bare-metal stents (BMS) (11% vs. 30%). A recent meta-analysis on five studies compared DES ($n = 156$) vs. BMS ($n = 148$) in the treatment of symptomatic vertebral artery stenosis. There were no differences in technical success, clinical success, and periprocedural complications between groups. At follow-up, treatment with DES showed a significantly lower rate of restenosis (15% vs. 33%), recurrent symptoms (2.7% vs. 11.2%; OR = 3.3, $P = 0.011$) and repeat revascularization (4.8% vs. 19.1%; OR = 4.09, $P = 0.001$) in favor of DES.[80]

LIMITATIONS AND COMPLICATIONS OF CAROTID ARTERY STENTING

In addition to the limitation of the randomized comparison against CEA just described, the main limitation of CAS is that it has not been studied prospectively in specific patient populations. For surgical high-risk patients with asymptomatic carotid disease (e.g., SAPPHIRE population), it remains to be demonstrated that carotid revascularization (both stenting and surgery) is of benefit over best medical management. As previously mentioned, adequately powered randomized trials in vertebral revascularization are lacking. Complications of endovascular procedures not specific to carotid or vertebral interventions include access site vascular compromise, bleeding events, allergic reactions to contrast, heart failure, contrast-induced nephropathy, and atheroembolism. While less data are available on the complications related to vertebral revascularization—mainly distal embolization with the associated neurologic symptoms, spasms, or dissections—the complications related to CAS are described in detail.

Bradycardia and hypotension

Hemodynamic instability, characterized by hypotension and bradycardia, is fairly common during CAS.[81] A dysfunction of adventitial stretch baroreceptors in the carotid sinus following balloon catheter dilatation and stent deployment, leading to sympathetic fibers inhibition and parasympathetic pathway stimulation, has been postulated as the trigger mechanism.[82] Although benign, this hemodynamic response may rarely lead to asystole or profound hypotension. While in the early days of the procedure, a temporary transvenous pacemaker was inserted to prevent bradycardia, this rhythm disturbance can be effectively prevented with atropine (0.5–1 mg intravenously) administered routinely prior to stent postdilation. To treat hypotension, large volumes of normal saline and, at times, vasopressors (e.g., noradrenaline 5–10 mcg as repeated bolus and, if needed, 1–5 mcg/min as an infusion or dopamine IV) may be required. Prolonged hypotension and persistent hemodynamic instability have been found to be independently associated with periprocedural major clinical events and stroke.[82] These hemodynamic disturbances have been found more frequently in heavily calcified lesions, female gender, and elderly patients. Post CEA restenosis as well as carotid lesion far away from the carotid bulb showed far less vagal effect during stent postdilation.

Hypertension and hyperperfusion syndrome

Rarely, patients may be hypertensive following CAS. Strict blood pressure control is mandatory because severe hypertension following carotid revascularization (both with CEA and with CAS) may be associated with hyperperfusion syndrome.[83] The clinical presentation is characterized by headache, alteration of consciousness, or seizure. The pathophysiologic mechanism underlying hyperperfusion syndrome is an alteration of the blood-brain barrier with fluid extravasation and cerebral edema. This is the result of an impaired cerebral vessel autoregulation secondary to the long-standing compensatory vasodilation. The more severe forms may lead to intracranial hemorrhage. Therefore, any persistent severe headache post CAS should be investigated with an emergent CT scan. High-risk features associated with the development of hyperperfusion syndrome include peri- and postprocedural hypertension and the revascularization of a severe stenosis supplying a poorly collateralized cerebral area (e.g., isolated hemisphere) or the revascularization of a stenosis in the presence of a contralateral severe carotid stenosis or occlusion.[84]

Intracranial hemorrhage may occur in <1% of carotid revascularization cases (both with CEA and CAS) and is associated with high morbidity and mortality. In addition to hyperperfusion syndrome, bleeding may be the result of hemorrhagic conversion of a previously infarcted region or of severe small vessel intracranial disease and is favored by DAPT and periprocedural anticoagulation. Patients with hyperperfusion syndrome and intracranial hemorrhage should be monitored in an intensive care unit with neurologic or neurosurgical evaluation, careful fluid and blood pressure management, and mannitol or hyperventilation for treatment of increased intracranial pressure. Arterial blood pressure should be maintained <140/80 mmHg with intravenous (IV) clonidine and labetalol as the preferred drugs that reduce blood pressure values without increasing cerebral blood flow. Nitrates, nifedipine, and ACE inhibitors should not be routinely used in this situation.[85]

Spasm, dissection, and slow-flow/no-flow

Some degree of spasm of the ICA may be frequently observed at the level of the placement of the filter EPD. Since most of the currently available filters are fixed to the wire, any movement of the wire translates to a movement of the filter, potentially triggering distal ICA spasm. Spasms are usually asymptomatic, do not compromise flow, and resolve mostly spontaneously. If needed, nitroglycerin 50–200 mcg may be administered in the CCA through the guiding catheter or sheath. However, patients are frequently hypotensive during the procedure, and whenever possible, spontaneous resolution of the spasms should be awaited in order not to exacerbate hypotension. Vessel dissection is a rare event in CAS. It can happen in the ICA distally to the treated area, as propagation of a previously unrecognized dissection following angioplasty or as an injury occurring at the time of stent postdilation. Measures to prevent dissection include the use of undersized balloons for predilation, the coverage of the lesion with a nitinol stent having a safety margin of several millimeters distally and proximally to the lesion, and more importantly, the performance of postdilation prevented by avoiding pushing in case of difficult advancement, and by advancement of the guiding catheter over a diagnostic catheter (telescoping technique) or over the introducer if a sheath is used. In order to detect injuries to the CCA, it is recommended to perform a final angiogram while retrieving the guiding catheter or sheath. In the presence of dissection of the CCA, an additional nitinol self-expanding stent should be used to cover it.

A temporary slow-flow or no-flow condition in the target ICA may be due to filter-induced spasm, unseen dissection, intravascular thrombosis due to suboptimal anticoagulation, and filter obstruction due to embolized debris. An angiography should be required to identify the potential mechanism of obstruction focusing on filter area and intracranial circulation. While ACT value should be checked first, aspiration of the ICA blood column with an aspiration catheter such as Export (Medtronic) or Eliminate (Terumo) should be carefully performed in all cases. EPD should be removed if the cause of obstruction is a filter basket full of debris. In this situation, a partial recapture of the EPD within the recovery system is recommended to avoid "squeezing" of embolic material into the cerebral circulation.

Periprocedural stroke

In patients with periprocedural neurologic deficits occurring during CAS, the presumptive diagnosis is ischemic stroke and not intracranial hemorrhage. Therefore, these patients should not be primarily transferred for CT scan but instead should receive emergent cerebral angiogram (to be compared with pre-CAS angiography). If a patient develops neurologic symptoms during the procedure, it is generally best to complete the intervention, retrieve the EPD, and reassess the patient clinically and angiographically. Once problems at the level of the ICA, such as spasms or dissections are excluded, the intracranial angiogram should be carefully examined and compared with the baseline images. Findings suggestive of distal embolization include vessel-filling defects or cutoffs and delayed vessel filling.

The decision to perform neurorescue should be based on the in-house expertise with intracranial interventions, the localization of the vessel closure, and the clinical course of the patient. According to the recent evidence of the efficacy of mechanical thrombectomy in the treatment of large stroke due to major vessel occlusion (M1-M2, basilar artery), thrombus aspiration and retrieval through specific devices should be tried first.[86,87] The use of adjunctive pharmacologics (i.e., with glycoprotein IIb/IIIa receptor inhibitors or local or systemic fibrinolytic agents) should be left for selected patients with minor strokes in a distal vessel, after discussion of pros and cons (notably the risk of bleeding) with a stroke neurologist. Attention should be paid to "push" on antithrombotic treatment in a patient on full heparinization and double antiplatelet treatment. A hemorrhagic complication following rescue may be far more devastating than the ischemic stroke one intended to treat.

SPECIAL ISSUES AND CONSIDERATIONS WITH CAROTID ARTERY STENTING

There are three groups of patients at high risk for whom the best approach (CAS vs. CEA) remains to be determined. The first group includes patients with evidence of thrombus in a symptomatic carotid lesion. An angiography thrombus appears as intraluminal filling defect, although the differentiation with a severe but focal calcification or a ruptured eccentric plaque may not always be possible. In the North American Symptomatic Carotid Endarterectomy Trial (NASCET), these patients carried an 18%–22% risk of perioperative stroke.[88] With respect to CAS, such patients have been excluded from the trials, but it is generally agreed that the stroke risk is also high with the endovascular treatment. In these patients, a short period of anticoagulation in addition to aspirin may be considered, followed by CEA or CAS once the thrombus resolves. In patients experiencing ongoing ischemia despite anticoagulation, endovascular therapy may be an option if it can be performed with flow reversal/ blockage to prevent embolization during EPD placement.

Similarly, the best revascularization strategy for patients over the age of 80 years remains undefined. Octogenarians were excluded from the CEA randomized trials but are known to have a higher perioperative complication rate than younger patients. In the CREST lead-in phase in octogenarians, the 30-day stroke and death rate among octogenarians was 12.2%.[89] In the more recent CAPTURE registry, the 30-day event rate in octogenarians ranged according to the level of expertise of the treating interventionalists, which ranged between 6.3% and 10.3%.[54] The role of CAS with proximal protection in octogenarians was tested in 198 consecutive patients (39% symptomatic). Technical success was 100% and the rate of stroke/death was 2.52%.[90] Since the benefit from revascularization of asymptomatic patients

becomes evident at 5 years, routine carotid revascularization of asymptomatic patients older than 80 years of age should be carefully assessed.

The third group of patients for whom the best strategy needs to be defined includes those with recent (<6 weeks), large, and disabling strokes. These patients were also excluded from both the CEA and the CAS randomized trials. The primary concern is that in patients with stroke, especially large strokes, revascularization predisposes to intracerebral hemorrhage due to the cerebral hyperperfusion syndrome. This complication is well-described after CEA but has also been reported following CAS.[82] Predisposing conditions for cerebral hyperperfusion syndrome include recent ischemia, perioperative hypertension, revascularization of a severe stenosis with poor collateral blood flow, and the presence of bilateral severe stenoses or contralateral occlusion. In this setting, intracerebral hemorrhage may have devastating consequences and carries nearly 80% mortality rate. Therefore, if only a small territory of viable cortex fed by the symptomatic carotid remains at risk of ischemia, the risk of revascularization—both in terms of periprocedural ischemic stroke and intracerebral hemorrhage—should be weighed against the risk of recurrent ischemia, which may be as high as 10%–14% over 4–6 weeks. If it is decided to proceed to revascularization, then periprocedural strict blood pressure control is mandatory. If periprocedural hypertension can be aggressively controlled, then revascularization may be considered.[85]

CONCLUSIONS

CAS has emerged as a less invasive alternative to surgery for patients with stenosis of the ICA. In patients at high risk for surgery, CAS is equivalent to CEA. In symptomatic patients, a meta-analysis suggests that CAS is inferior to CEA in terms of 30-day death or stroke rate, while beyond 30 days current evidence supports the equivalence of both revascularization strategies in stroke prevention. As a limitation, the majority of the randomized studies had inadequate requirements in terms of endovascular expertise, did not mandate the use of EPD or include the proximal embolic protection, and no closed-cell design stent was systematically used. In asymptomatic patients, the randomized data are limited but no difference between CAS and CEA could be detected. Contrary to the randomized data, large-scale high-quality registries have reported CAS results in the range of current recommendations, for CEA, even in patients at high risk for surgery. Until further data become available, the performance of CAS should be limited to experienced CAS centers. Independently of the revascularization strategy used, patients with carotid artery stenosis remain at risk of cardiovascular events and require aggressive secondary cardiovascular prevention. With respect to vertebral revascularization, data remain limited. Surgery is in most centers not considered a viable option. Percutaneous revascularization, currently reserved to symptomatic patients refractory to medical treatment, appears to be associated with high technical success and low complication rates, but in-stent restenosis remains a concern. Preliminary data on DES appear promising. Also, in patients with VA stenosis, the focus of treatment should be the global reduction of vascular risk, including pharmacologic prevention of stroke and MI.

REFERENCES

1. Writing Group Members, et al. Executive summary: Heart Disease and Stroke Statistics—2016 update: A report from the American heart association. *Circulation* 2016;133:447–454.
2. Fairhead JF, Rothwell PM. The need for urgency in identification and treatment of symptomatic carotid stenosis is already established. *Cerebrovasc Dis* 2005;19:355–358.
3. Wallaert JB, et al. Physician specialty and variation in carotid revascularization technique selected for Medicare patients. *J Vasc Surg* 2016;63:89–97.
4. Dawkins AA, et al. Complications of cerebral angiography: A prospective analysis of 2,924 consecutive procedures. *Neuroradiology* 2007;49:753–759.
5. Kaufmann TJ, et al. Complications of diagnostic cerebral angiography: Evaluation of 19,826 consecutive patients. *Radiology* 2007;243:812–819.
6. Grant EG. Carotid artery stenosis: Gray-scale and Doppler US diagnosis—Society of radiologists in ultrasound consensus conference. *Radiology* 2003;229:340–346.
7. Tholen AT, et al. Suspected carotid artery stenosis: Cost-effectiveness of CT angiography in work-up of patients with recent TIA or minor ischemic stroke. *Radiology* 2010;256:585–597.
8. Berko NS, et al. Variants and anomalies of thoracic vasculature on computed tomographic angiography in adults. *J Computed Assist Tomogr* 2009;33:523–528.
9. Timaran CH, et al. Accuracy and utility of three-dimensional contrast-enhanced magnetic resonance angiography in planning carotid stenting. *J Vasc Surg* 2007;46:257–264.
10. Wyers MC, et al. The value of 3D-CT angiographic assessment prior to carotid stenting. *J Vasc Surg* 2009;49:614–622.
11. Kernan WN et al. Guidelines for the prevention of stroke in patients with stroke and transient ischemic attack: A guideline for healthcare professionals from the American Heart association/American stroke association. *Stroke* 2011;42:e420.
12. Kernan WN, et al. Guidelines for the prevention of stroke in patients with stroke and transient ischemic attack: A guideline for healthcare professionals from the American Heart association/American stroke association. *Stroke* 2014;45:2160.
13. Roffi M. Current evidence for carotid endarterectomy and carotid artery stenting. *Stroke* 2014;45:2160.
14. Naylor AR, et al. Clinical and imaging features associated with an increased risk of late stroke in patients with asymptomatic carotid disease. *Eur J Vasc Endovasc Surg* 2014;48:633–640.
15. National Coverage Determination (NCD) for Percutaneous Transluminal Angioplasty(PTA) (20.7). (cited 31 July 2015). http://www.cms.gov/medicare-coverage-database/Details

16. Safian RD. Carotid artery stenting: Payment, politics, and equipose. *J Am Coll Cardiol* 2012;59:1390–1391.
17. Zahn R, et al. Embolic protection devices for carotid artery stenting: Is there a difference between filter and distal occlusive devices? *J Am Coll Cardiol* 2005;45:1769–1774.
18. Bersin RM, et al. A meta-analysis of proximal occlusion device outcomes in carotid artery stenting. *Catheter Cardiovasc Interv* 2012;80(7):1072–1078.
19. Montorsi P, et al. Microembolization during carotid artery stenting in patients with high-risk lipid plaque: A randomized trial of proximal versus distal cerebral protection. *J Am Coll Cardiol* 2011;58:1656–1663.
20. Stabile E, et al. Cerebral embolic lesions detected with diffusion-weighted magnetic resonance imaging following carotid artery stenting: A meta-analysis of 8 studies comparing filter cerebral protection and proximal balloon occlusion. *JACC Cardiovasc Interv* 2014;7:1177–1183.
21. Kwolek CJ, et al. Results of the ROADSTER multicenter trial of transcarotid stenting with dynamic flow reversal. *J Vasc Surg* 2015;62:1227–1235.
22. Nerla R, et al. Carotid artery stenting with a new-generation double-mesh stent in three high-volume Italian centres: Clinical results of a multidisciplinary approach. *EuroIntervention* 2016;12(5):e677–e683.
23. Bosiers M, et al. The CLEAR-ROAD study: Evaluation of a new dual layer micromesh stent system for the carotid artery. *EuroIntervention* 2016;12:e671–e676.
24. Mukherjee D, et al. Percutaneous intervention for symptomatic vertebral artery stenosis using coronary stents. *J Invasive Cardiol* 2001;13:363–366.
25. Canyigit M, et al. Distal embolization after stenting of the vertebral artery: Diffusion-weighted magnetic resonance imaging findings. *Cardiovasc Intervent Radiol* 2007;30:189–195.
26. Patti G, et al. Strategies of clopidogrel load and atorvastatin reload to prevent ischemic cerebral events in patients undergoing protected carotid stenting. Results of the randomized ARMYDA-9 CAROTID (Clopidogrel and Atorvastatin Treatment During Carotid Artery Stenting) study. *J Am Coll Cardiol* 2013;61(13):1379–1387.
27. Bianco M, et al. Efficacy and safety of available protocols for aspirin hypersensitivity for patients undergoing percutaneous coronary intervention: A survey and systematic review. *Circ Cardiovasc Interv* 2016;9(1):e002896.
28. Fernando SL, Assaad NN. Rapid and sequential desensitization to both aspirin and clopidogrel. *Intern Med J* 2010;40(8):596–599.
29. Kimmelstiel C, et al. Bivalirudin is associated with improved in-hospital outcomes compared with heparin in percutaneous vascular interventions: Observational, propensity-matched analysis from the Premier Hospital database. *Circ Cardiovasc Interv* 2016;9(1):e002823.
30. Stabile E, et al. Heparin versus bivalirudin for carotid artery stenting using proximal endovascular clamping for neuroprotection. Results from a prospective randomized trial. *J Vasc Surg* 2010;52:1505–1510.
31. Giugliano G, et al. Predictors of carotid occlusion intolerance during proximal protected carotid artery stenting. *JACC Cardiovasc Interv* 2014;7(11):1237–1244.
32. Faggioli GL, et al. Aortic arch anomalies are associated with increased risk of neurological events in carotid stent procedures. *Eur J Vasc Endovasc Surg* 2007;33:436–441.

33. Werner M, et al. Anatomic variables contributing to a higher periprocedural incidence of stroke and TIA in carotid artery stenting: Single center experience of 833 consecutive cases. *Catheter Cardiovasc Interv* 2012;80:321–328.

34. Etxegoien N, et al. The transradial approach for carotid artery stenting. *Catheter Cardiovasc Interv* 2012;80:1081–1087.

35. Ruzsa Z, et al. A randomized comparison of transradial and transfemoral approach for carotid artery stenting: The RADACAR study. *Eurointervention* 2014;10:381–391.

36. Montorsi P, et al. Carotid artery stenting with proximal embolic protection via a transradial or transbrachial approach: Pushing the boundaries of the technique while maintaining safety and efficacy. *J Endovasc Ther* 2016;23:549–560.

37. Wehman JC, et al. Atherosclerotic occlusive extracranial vertebral artery disease: Indications for intervention, endovascular techniques, short-term and long-term results. *J Interv Cardiol* 2004;17:219–232.

38. Yadav JS, et al. Protected carotid-artery stenting versus endarterectomy in high-risk patients. *N Engl J Med* 2004;351:1493–1501.

39. CAVATAS Investigators. Endovascular versus surgical treatment in patients with carotid stenosis in the Carotid and Vertebral Artery Transluminal Angioplasty Study (CAVATAS): A randomised trial. *Lancet* 2001;357:1729–1737.

40. Ringleb PA, et al. 30 day results from the SPACE trial of stent-protected angioplasty versus carotid endarterectomy in symptomatic patients: A randomised non-inferiority trial. *Lancet* 2006;368:1239–1247.

41. Mas JL, et al. Endarterectomy versus stenting in patients with symptomatic severe carotid stenosis. *N Engl J Med* 2006;355:1660–1671.

42. Ederle J, et al. Carotid artery stenting compared with endarterectomy in patients with symptomatic carotid stenosis International Carotid Stenting Study: An interim analysis of a randomised controlled trial. *Lancet* 2010;375(9719):985–997.

43. Brott TG (for the CREST investigators). Stenting versus Endarterectomy for treatment of carotid-artery stenosis. *N Engl J Med* 2010;363:11–23.

44. Rosenfield K (for the ACS I investigators). Randomized study of stent versus surgery for asymptomatic carotid stenosis. *N Engl J Med* 2016;374:1011–1020.

45. Gurm HS, et al. Long-term results of carotid stenting versus endarterectomy in high-risk patients. *N Engl J Med* 2008;358:1572–1579.

46. Eckstein HH, et al. Results of the Stent Protected Angioplasty versus Carotid Endarterectomy (SPACE) study to treat symptomatic stenoses at 2 years: A multinational, prospective, randomised trial. *Lancet Neurol* 2008;7:893–902.

47. Mas JL, et al. Carotid angioplasty and stenting with and without cerebral protection: Clinical alert from the Endarterectomy versus Angioplasty in patients with symptomatic severe carotis stenosis (EVA-3S) trial. *Stroke* 2004;35:e18–e20.

48. Mas JL, et al. Endarterectomy versus Angioplasty in patients with symptomatic severe carotid stenosis (EVA-3S) trial: Results up to 4 years from a randomised, multicentre trial. *Lancet Neurol* 2008;7:885–892.

49. Bonati LH, et al. Long-term outcomes after stenting versus endarterectomy for treatment of symptomatic carotid stenosis: The International Carotid Stenting Study (ICSS) randomised trial. *Lancet* 2015;385(9967):529–538.

50. ACAS Investigators. Endarterectomy for asymptomatic carotid artery stenosis. Executive Committee for the Asymptomatic Carotid Atherosclerosis Study. *JAMA* 1995;273:1421–1428.

51. Brott GT, et al. Long-term results of stenting versus endarterectomy for carotid-artery stenosis. *N Engl J Med* 2016;374:1021–1031.

52. Konstantinos P, et al. Carotid artery stenting versus carotid endarterectomy: A comprehensive meta-analysis of short-term and long-term outcomes. *Stroke* 2011;42:687–692.

53. Aronow HD, et al. SCAI/SVM expert consensus statement on carotid stenting: Training and credentialing for carotid stenting. *Cath Cardiovasc Int* 2016;87:188–199.

54. Schnaudigel S, et al. New brain lesions after carotid stenting versus carotid endarterectomy: A systematic review of the literature. *Stroke* 2008;39:1011–1119.

55. Bosier M, et al. Does free cell area influence the outcome in carotid artery stenting? *Eur J Vasc Endovasc Surg* 2007;33:135–141.

56. Illuminati G, et al. Systematic preoperative coronary angiography and stenting improved postoperative results of carotid endarterectomy in patients with asymptomatic coronary artery disease: A randomized controlled trial. *Eur J Vasc Endovasc Surg* 2010;39:139–145.

57. Illuminati G, et al. Long-term results of a randomized controlled trial analyzing the role of systematic preoperative coronary angiography before electibe carotid endarterectomy in patients with asymptomatic coronary artery disease. *Eur J Vasc Endovasc Surg* 2015;49366–49374.

58. ACAS Investigators. Study design for randomized prospective trial of carotid endarterectomy for asymptomatic atherosclerosis. *Stroke* 1989;20:844–849.

59. Theiss W, et al. Predictors of death and stroke after carotid angioplasty and stenting: A subgroup analysis of the Pro-CAS data. *Stroke* 2008;39:2325–2330.

60. Gray WA, et al. The CAPTURE registry: Results of carotid stenting with embolic protection in the post approval setting. *Catheter Cardiovasc Interv* 2007;69:341–348.

61. Katzen BT, et al. Carotid artery stenting with emboli protection surveillance study: Thirty-day results of the CASES-PMS study. *Catheter Cardiovasc Interv* 2007;70:316–323.

62. Massop D, et al. Stenting and angioplasty with protection in patients at high-risk for endarterectomy: SAPPHIRE Worldwide Registry first 2,001 patients. *Catheter Cardiovasc Interv* 2009;73:129–136.

63. Sidawy AN, et al. Risk-adjusted 30-day outcomes of carotid stenting and endarterectomy: Results from the SVS Vascular Registry. *J Vasc Surg* 2009;49:71–79.

64. Gray WA, et al. 30-Day outcomes for carotid artery stenting in 6320 patients from two prospective, multicenter, high surgical risk registries. *Circ Cardiovasc Interv* 2009;2:159–166.

65. Stabile E, et al. Proximal endovascular occlusion for carotid artery stenting: results from a prospective registry of 1,300 patients. *J Am Coll Cardiol* 2010;55(16):1661–1667.

66. Praskevas KI, et al. Stroke/death rates following carotid artery stenting and carotid endarterectomy in contemporary administrative dataset registries: A systematic review. *Eur J Vasc Endovasc Surg* 2016;51:3–12.

67. Choi JC, et al. Early outcomes after carotid artery stenting compared to endarterectomy for asymptomatic carotid stenosis. *Stroke* 2015;46:120–125.

68. Chastain HD, et al. Extracranial vertebral artery stent placement: In-hospital and follow-up results. *J Neurosurg* 1999;91:547–552.

69. Lin YH, et al. Symptomatic ostial vertebral artery stenosis treated with tubular coronary stents: Clinical results and restenosis analysis. *J Endovasc Ther* 2004;11:719–726.

70. Hatano T, et al. Stenting for vertebrobasikar artery stenosis. *Acta Neurochir* 2005;94:137–141.

71. Taylor RA, et al. Vertebral artery ostial stent placement for atherosclerotic stenosis in 72 consecutive patients: Clinical outcomes and follow-up results. *Neuroradiology* 2009;51:531–539.

72. Vajda Z, et al. Treatment of stenoses of vertebral artery origin using short drug-eluting coronary stents: Improved follow-up results. *Am J Neuroradiol* 2009;30:1653–1656.

73. Edgell RA, et al. Multicenter study of safety in stenting for symptomatic vertebral artery origin stenosis: Results from the society of vascular and interventional neurology research consortium. *J Neuroimag* 2013;23:170–1674.

74. Mohammadian R, et al. Angioplasty and stenting of symptomatic vertebral artery stenosis. Clinical and angiographic follow-up in 206 cases from northwest Iran. *Neuroradiol J* 2013;26:454–463.

75. Radak D, et al. Endovascular treatment of symptomatic high-grade vertebral artery stenosis. *J Vasc Surg* 2014;60:92.

76. Jenkins JS, et al. Endovascular stenting for vertebral artery stenosis. *J Am Coll Cardiol* 2010;55:538–542.

77. Song L, et al. Drug-eluting vs. bare metal stent for symptomatic vertebral stenosis. *J Endovas Ther* 2012;19(2):231–238.

78. Antoniou AG, et al. Percutaneous transluminal angioplasty and stenting in patients with proximal vertebral artery stenosis. *J Vasc Surg* 2012;55:1167–1177.

79. Stayman AN, et al. A systematic review of stenting and angioplasty of symptomatic extracranial vertebral artery stenosis. *Stroke* 2011;42:2212–2216.

80. Tank V, et al. Drug eluting stents versus bare metal stents for the treatment of extracranial vertebral artery disease: A meta-analysis. *J NeuroIntervent Surg* 2015;0:1–5.

81. Mlekusch W, et al. Hypotension and bradycardia after elective carotid stenting: Frequency and risk factors. *J Endovasc Ther* 2003;10:851–859.

82. Bagshaw RJ, Barrer SJ. Effects of angioplasty upon carotid sinus mechanical properties and blood pressure control in the dog. *Neurosurgery* 1987;21:324–330.

83. Abou-Chebl A, et al. Intracranial hemorrhage and hyperperfusion syndrome following carotid artery stenting: Risk factors, prevention, and treatment. *J Am Coll Cardiol* 2004;43:1596–1601.

84. Lieb M, et al. Cerebral hyperperfusion syndrome after carotid interventions: A review. *Cardiol Rev* 2012;20:84–89.

85. Abou-Chebl A, et al. Intensive treatment of hypertension decreases the risk of hyperperfusion and intracerebral hemorrhage following carotid artery stenting. *Catheter Cardiovasc Interv* 2007;69:690–696.

86. Berkhemer OA, et al. MR CLEAN Investigators. A randomized trial of intra-arterial treatment for acute ischemic stroke. *N Engl J Med* 2015;372:11–20.

87. Goyal M, et al. The ESCAPE trial investigators. Randomized assessment of rapid endovascular treatment of ischemic stroke. *N Engl J Med* 2015;372:1009–1018.

88. North American Symptomatic Carotid Endarterectomy Trial Collaborators. Beneficial effect of carotid endarterectomy in symptomatic patients with high-grade stenosis. *N Engl J Med* 1991;325:445–453.

89. Hobson RW, et al. Carotid artery stenting is associated with increased complications in octogenarians: 30-day stroke and death rates in the CREST lead-in phase. *J Vasc Surg* 2004;40:1106–1111.

90. Micari A, et al. Carotid artery stenting in octogenarians using a proximal endovascular occlusion cerebral protection device: A multicenter registry. *Catheter Cardiovasc Interv* 2010;76:9–15.

52

Treatment of intracranial arterial disease

ALBERTO MAUD AND GUSTAVO J. RODRIGUEZ

INTRODUCTION

Intracranial arterial disease is a heterogeneous group of diseases that encompasses atherosclerotic to inflammatory and degenerative arteriopathies. Intracranial arteries are divided into two categories: large and small. The term *intracranial arterial disease* refers to involvement of the large intracranial arteries. The small cerebral arteries are affected by long-standing, uncontrolled arterial hypertension, and they are grouped under the term *small vessel disease* (cerebral microangiopathy). They typically cause small, subcortical infarcts, also known as lacunar infarctions. The second most common complication of small vessel disease is hypertensive basoganglionic intracerebral hemorrhage. Small vessel disease is the main cause of vascular dementia in North America. Vascular dementia is a preventable form of dementia.

Brain arterial embolism is the most common cause of occlusion of a large intracranial artery. Acute embolic occlusion of a large, proximal intracranial artery is a treatable condition in the first hours of an ischemic stroke. The treatment implies a combination of intravenous thrombolytic infusion, plus adjunctive mechanical embolectomy with retrieval stents.[1]

In situ disease of a large intracranial artery can be caused by different arterial diseases, including atherosclerosis, vasculitis (autoimmune, infectious, and postinfectious), dissection, moyamoya disease (MMD), cerebral vasoconstriction syndrome, delayed radiation-induced arteriopathy, cerebral amyloid angiopathy, and other less defined entities, like transient cerebral arteriopathy, intracranial fibromuscular dysplasia, and dolichoectasia. Intracranial atherosclerotic disease (ICAD) is the most common disease that affects the large intracranial arteries, and it will be the focus of this chapter.

ICAD is a focal and segmentary disease that affects specific arterial segments of the large intracranial arteries.[2] In a simple sense, ICAD is just a cerebral manifestation of systemic atherosclerotic disease. It shares similar patterns with atherosclerotic coronary arterial disease.[3] However, there are other unique characteristics of the intracranial arteries (anatomic and physiologic), epidemiologic features (particular predilection of ICAD in Asian population), mechanism of infarction, response to treatment, including antithrombotic medications and lowering cholesterol medications, and invasive interventions that are unique to the atherosclerosis in this particular location that will be discussed in this chapter.

ANATOMY AND PATHOPHYSIOLOGY

The vessels of the circle of Willis, which are the vessels that are most often associated with intracranial atherosclerosis, are comparable in size to the coronary arteries. The vessels include the:

- Paired intracranial internal carotid arteries (ICA, 3–4 mm)
- Middle cerebral arteries (MCA, 2–3 mm)
- Anterior cerebral arteries (ACA, 1.5–2 mm)

- Intracranial vertebral arteries (VA, 2–3 mm)
- Posterior cerebral arteries (PCA, 1.5–2 mm)
- Singular basilar artery (BA, 2.75–3.5 mm)
- Anterior inferior, posterior inferior, and superior cerebellar arteries

There are major differences between the intracranial and coronary arteries and other muscular arteries. The cerebral vessels have no external elastic lamina, and they have a thinner tunica media and trivial adventitia; this makes these vessels quite fragile. They also differ from the coronary arteries in being partly (i.e., the petrous and cavernous carotids) surrounded by bone or rigid and fibrous tissue (i.e., the dura mater). Combined with significant tortuosity in their proximal segments, this makes the navigation of endovascular devices to the intracranial vessels more challenging, which greatly increases the risk of vessel injury and perforation during endovascular therapy. The most tortuous and rigid segments of the artery are the petrous and cavernous segments of the ICA. As a consequence, access to the MCA may be difficult. A quite unique anatomical characteristic of the cerebral vasculature is the circle of Willis. This potentially robust source of collateral blood flow can completely restore flow to the territory of an occluded ICA or VA. The circle of Willis consists of the two posterior communicating (PCom) arteries connecting the terminal ICAs and the PCA and the anterior communicating artery connecting the two ACAs. Unfortunately, the circle of Willis is fully developed in only 25% of humans, and anatomical variants are numerous. The circle of Willis is an important source of collateral circulation between both cerebral hemispheres through the anterior communicating artery and between the anterior and posterior circulations through the PCom arteries. Pial collaterals, connections between the distal branches of the MCA, ACA, and PCA, and the cerebellar arteries over the surface of the brain, are less robust potential collaterals. Interventionists must also be aware of the presence of multiple small perforating branches from both the MCA and BA, which originate superiorly and posteriorly, respectively, to avoid inadvertent cannulation. These are end arteries that have poor collaterals. Their ostia can be occluded by angioplasty and stenting, leading to ischemia. Other essential branches to be aware of are the ophthalmic artery arising anteriorly from the cavernous ICA, the PCom arising posteriorly from the carotid siphon, and the very small anterior choroidal artery arising just distal to the PCom. Occlusion of this vessel causes infarction of the internal capsule with a resultant severe contralateral hemiplegia. The VA has several muscular branches in its distal cervical segments, and the posterior inferior cerebellar artery (PICA) can often arise extracranially at the C1 level. Intracranially, the VA gives off the PICA dorsally, and just before the vertebrobasilar junction, each VA gives off the very small anterior spinal artery to the spinal cord dorsomedially.

Atherosclerosis is a progressive disease that starts early in life and is manifested clinically as coronary heart disease (CHD), a cerebrovascular disorder, or peripheral arterial disease. This disease can be hidden in the human body for many years and can ultimately lead to vascular remodeling. Atherosclerosis is a dynamic disease that combines a genetic predisposition and several epigenetic factors that lead to the formation and growth of atherosclerotic arterial plaque.[4] Hyperlipidemia is the most common factor related to the development of atherosclerotic plaque, and inflammation is a common finding associated with complication of a plaque.[5] The atherosclerotic plaque formation is a dynamic process, and remodeling of the brain arteries in response to the atherogenic risk factors and response to the medical and invasive treatments are currently active areas of research. Traditionally, the diagnosis of ICAD depended on the stenosis measured by cerebral angiography and by noninvasive diagnostic methods, like computerized tomography (CT) and magnetic resonance angiography (MRA) as well as transcranial Doppler (TCD). Schwarze et al. had found that intracranial arterial stenosis is a dynamic lesion, and that it can evolve and cause further reductions of the arterial diameters after relatively short periods of time. They observed a group of patients with a mean follow-up of 21 months.[6] Ten (35%) arteries with lesions had TCD evidence of progression. Wong et al. observed 143 patients with symptomatic MCA stenosis or occlusion.[7] They repeated TCD examinations 6 months after the initial examinations and recorded any stroke or coronary events during this period. The changes of MCA flow velocities were categorized as normalized artery, stable artery, and progressed artery, which were determined according to the changes of MCA velocities at 6 months. By analyzing both the initial and repeated TCD findings, there were 42 patients (29%) in the normalized group, 88 patients (62%) in the stable group, and 13 patients (9%) in the progressed group. For clinical events during the 6-month period, 18 (12.6%) of the patients had further documented vascular events, including ten recurrent strokes (nine ischemic strokes and one hemorrhagic stroke), five transient ischemic attacks (TIAs), and three acute coronary syndromes.

Progression of MCA occlusive disease is associated with an increased risk of vascular events. It became clear that intracranial artery stenosis is a process of dynamic change. The speed of progress is different for each case. Through the prospective study, it is found that lesions may progress, improve, or not change at all over a period of time. The proportion of progression is about 9%–12% for 6 months. The possibility of the progression depends on the time, and it may be greater as time goes on. The progression of stenosis may lead to increased risk of vascular events.[8] However, lumen narrowing is a poor indicator of plaque burden when vessels accommodate plaque formation by compensatory remodeling. Outward remodeling of the coronary artery can preserve the lumen at plaque burdens as high as 40% of the vessel area, whereas ICA remodeling has been shown to preserve the lumen at even higher plaque burdens approximating 62%. Remodeling can also be inward with a constricting vessel area during plaque formation and hastening stenosis. Understanding a vessel's pattern of remodeling might provide insight into our ability to detect plaque by angiography and better characterize its risk. For example, although outward remodeling limits the hemodynamic impact, coronary plaques with outward remodeling may be associated with increased plaque vulnerability, clinical symptoms, and poor clinical outcome after coronary intervention.

High-resolution black blood magnetic resonance imaging (BBMRI) has been used to characterize arterial remodeling in extracranial vessels. Recently, this technique has been optimized as a three-dimensional (3D) sequence for imaging the walls of intracranial arteries, enabling reliable measurements of the thickness and burden of ICAD. Using BBMRI, Qiao et al.[9] studied the ability and extent of the intracranial arteries to remodel and its relation with ischemic events. They found that intracranial arteries of the posterior circulation (intracranial vertebral arteries [ICVAs] and BA) had the greater capacity to accommodate the plaque formation (eccentric plaque also known as positive remodeling) without reducing the arterial lumen. Intracranial arterial dolichoectasia, a term to refer to intracranial arteries that are wider and longer than normal, is a relatively common angiographic finding in a patient with cerebrovascular disease. However, its specific significance and the relevance of intracranial arterial dolichoectasia is not established. Dolichoectasia also has a predilection for the posterior circulation suggesting that it could share a common pathogenesis with positive remodeling. Unfortunately, they studied a very selective population with symptomatic intracranial atherosclerotic stenosis, and more similar studies of this kind in the asymptomatic population are needed to further elucidate the natural history of the disease.

Intracranial vessel wall imaging (IVWI) is changing our understanding of the natural history of ICAD. Studies have suggested that plaques with positive remodeling (outer wall remodeling) are more frequently symptomatic than negative remodeling plaques. Plaque signal characteristic evaluation is helpful in assessing plaque composition. The T2 hyperintense fibrous cap overlies the lipid-rich necrotic core (LRNC), which is isointense on T1-weighted imaging and on fat-saturated T2-weighted imaging.[10] Increased volume of the LRNC has been associated with higher rates of rupture. Intraplaque hemorrhage (IPH) has proved to be an important risk factor for plaque vulnerability with increased rates of plaque complications and stroke. IPH will appear as an intraplaque T1 hyperintensity >150% of the signal intensity of internal reference muscle tissue. Additionally, ischemic infarcts are associated with upstream eccentric enhancing plaques within the first 4 weeks after the stroke, and over time, the degree of enhancement progressively diminishes. In patients with multifocal disease, culprit lesions enhance, and they do so more avidly than nonculprit lesions, which enhance inconsistently. The typical appearance of ICAD on IVWI is an eccentric, heterogeneous mild to moderately enhancing, outward remodeling lesion with heterogeneous T2 signal and juxtaluminal T2 hyperintensity that typically involves proximal intracranial branches or bifurcation points, which is distinctive in appearance from other vasculopathies described below.[11] The radial location of plaques along the MCA has been shown to be important for predicting symptoms and stroke type. For example, plaques along the superior wall of the MCA have been associated with deep infarcts, presumably owing to ostial stenosis/occlusion at the origins of lenticulostriate perforators.

Mechanism of stroke

Stroke associated with ICAD occurs in association with various stroke mechanisms such as *in situ* thrombotic occlusion, artery-to-artery embolism, hemodynamic insufficiency, and branch occlusion. Patients with unstable intracranial plaque may show large territorial lesions via sudden thrombotic occlusion. Artery-to-artery embolism, which commonly causes multiple corticosubcortical infarcts, can be detected by performing transcranial duplex monitoring. Branch occlusive disease (BOD) is one of the main stroke mechanisms of ICAD, which can be characterized by a milder degree of stenosis and comma-shaped infarcts extending to the basal surface of the parent artery. Patients with symptomatic (vs. asymptomatic) and non-BOD type (vs. BOD) ICAD have characteristic changes in (1) the wall area (larger plaques), (2) plaque signals (eccentric enhancement and heterogeneous signal intensity suggesting unstable plaque), and (3) remodeling patterns (positive remodeling suggesting outward expansion of the vessel wall). On the contrary, superiorly located MCA plaques (near to the orifices of penetrating arteries) are associated with BOD-type ICAD.[12]

EPIDEMIOLOGY

The importance of ICAD as a cause of stroke is underscored as compared to that of extracranial carotid stenosis and nonvalvular atrial fibrillation (AF). There have been several studies with long-term follow-up data and randomized clinical trials in extracranial carotid stenosis and nonvalvular AF; the risk of stroke and treatment effects were evaluated separately in both asymptomatic (stroke-free) and symptomatic patients. On the contrary, ICAD was not considered or was lumped with extracranial carotid stenosis as an atherosclerotic stroke subtype in most clinical trials. The reason for this negligence was, in part, due to the difficulties related with imaging the intracranial arteries. The diagnosis of extracranial carotid stenosis or nonvalvular AF can easily be done with a carotid Doppler ultrasound or electrocardiogram. Until recently, the catheter cerebral angiogram was the only available technique to image the intracranial arteries. In recent years, the availability of noninvasive imaging modalities like CT, MRA, and transcranial ultrasound, have increased our awareness of ICAD during the workup of patients with acute ischemic stroke. However, until today, there are no studies addressing the incidence of ICAD in the general population. There is very limited information about the natural history of asymptomatic ICAD.[13] It is suspected that ICAD might be as prevalent as extracranial atherosclerotic disease.

Based on the heterogeneity in vascular anatomy and physiology of the intracranial arteries as describe above, it is expected that intracranial atherosclerosis might have a distinct course compared to the atherosclerosis involving the cervical arteries, and herein lies the importance of differentiating these two entities when studying the natural history of this condition.

The population-based Rotterdam study has evaluated the prevalence of intracranial ICA calcification, a marker of intracranial atherosclerosis, and observed it in over 80% of older, white subjects.[14] In addition, a TCD study showed that the prevalence of asymptomatic MCA stenosis ranged from 7.2% to 30% of Asian patients who had vascular risk factors without a history of stroke or TIA. ICAD causes 30%–50% of strokes in Asia, and 8%–10% of strokes in North America, making it one of the most common causes of stroke worldwide. ICAD is more prevalent in Asians than in Westerners; the reason for this higher prevalence in Asians is unknown. Possible explanations include inherited susceptibility of intracranial vessels to atherosclerosis, acquired differences in the prevalence of risk factors, and differential responses to the same risk factors.

Lifestyle may play a role in the racial-ethnic differences: the pattern of ischemic stroke is changing in Asian patients. With the Westernized lifestyle, the incidence of extracranial cervical disease is rising. Last, it is also possible that patients with adult-onset MMD are misclassified as having ICAD, which may partly explain the high prevalence of intracranial atherosclerosis in Asians. Ring finger 213 (RNF213) was recently identified as the strongest susceptibility gene for MMD in East Asian people by a genome-wide linkage analysis and an exome analysis. The number of patients with MMD was estimated to be more than 53,800 in East Asian populations.[15] The prevalence of MMD has recently increased with more careful consideration of the disease and better diagnostic techniques; many patients may have been misclassified as having ICAD.[16]

Asymptomatic intracranial atherosclerotic disease

It is presumed that the risk of stroke associated with asymptomatic ICAD is relatively low. The factors involved in the transition between an asymptomatic to a symptomatic status are unknown. Metabolic syndrome is a cluster of cardiovascular disease risk factors and metabolic alterations associated with excess fat. There is an association between ICAD and metabolic syndrome. Risk factors, components of metabolic syndrome, elevated serum insulin, and adipokines secreted from adipocytes, all cause oxidative stress and endothelial dysfunction. Adults with the metabolic syndrome have suboptimal concentrations of several antioxidants, and intracranial arteries may become susceptible to oxidative stress. Oxidative stress leads to the attenuation of endothelial function through decreased production of nitric oxide (NO) and increased destruction of NO by superoxide.[17] The Asymptomatic Intracranial Atherosclerosis

(AsIA) study showed that asymmetric-dimethylarginine (ADMA, an endogenous inhibitor of endothelial NO) was associated with ICAD.[18] In addition, a recent report evaluating the circulating endothelial microparticle pattern in stroke patients showed that ICAD and extracranial atherosclerosis (ECAS) may have different pathophysiologies. It was speculated that the endothelial activation is related to plaque instability in patients with extracranial arterial stenosis, and endothelial apoptosis is related to vascular narrowing in patients with ICAD.

In an observational study of 50 patients with asymptomatic ICAD in the MCA by Kremer et al., none of the patients suffered from ischemic stroke during the follow-up; only one suffered from a transient ischemic attack (TIA). Patients were followed for periods of 12 months and were found to have an asymptomatic atherosclerotic stenosis in the MCA by TCD examination.[19] Kern et al. compared the incidence of stroke and recurrent stroke after diagnosis of an atherosclerotic stenosis. The incidence of stroke went from 12% to 3% per year in symptomatic versus asymptomatic subjects, confirming the important differences between asymptomatic versus symptomatic status at the time of assessing future risk. Overall, the annual incidence of ipsilateral stroke per year for patients with asymptomatic stenosis appears to be much lower than patients with symptomatic stenosis.[20]

Aggressive medical management including dual antiplatelet regimen is the mainstay treatment after a TIA or ischemic stroke associated with ICAD. The benefit of aggressive medical management for asymptomatic ICAD is not yet established.

Symptomatic intracranial atherosclerotic disease

Patients with symptomatic ICAD present most of the time with established infarctions or TIAs in the arterial territory corresponding to the culprit stenotic artery. It is not uncommon to have multiple episodes of stereotyped TIAs ("flurry of TIAs") that can precede a cerebral infarction. Stereotyped TIAs can be often misinterpreted as partial seizures. Cerebral infarcts due to ICAD can adopt different presentations from a shower of multiple small cortical emboli to internal (deep) or cortical (superficial) border zone infarcts (watershed infarctions). Occasionally, an isolated small subcortical (lacunar infarct) ischemic lesion in the basal ganglia, corona radiate, or pons can be the presentation of a severe intracranial atherosclerotic stenosis. A percentage of patients with ICAD present with symptoms of an acute ischemic stroke within the first 3 hours after symptoms onset may be amenable for intravenous (IV) thrombolysis. A particularly challenging situation is a patient with ICAD presenting with acute ischemic stroke symptoms and occlusion of a proximal large intracranial artery. The role of mechanical embolectomy with the use of intracranial retrieval stents in the context of an acute embolic emergent large vessel occlusion is well-supported by multiple randomized clinical trials and meta-analyses. The role of endovascular treatment in acute ischemic stroke associated to an atherosclerotic occlusion of a proximal large ICAD is not well-established.

The recurrence of ischemic events, including TIAs and ischemic stroke, associated with an intracranial atherosclerotic stenosis higher than 50% is significant. Compared with other stroke subtypes (cardioembolism and extracranial atherosclerotic arterial disease), ICAD portended a high risk of recurrence despite medical treatment. In the Warfarin-Aspirin Symptomatic Intracranial Disease trial (WASID) conducted more than a decade ago, the risk of stroke or death in the first year after a stroke attributed to ICAD (50%–99% stenosis) was 15% and 17%, respectively, when treated by aspirin and warfarin.[21] In the recent Clopidogrel in High-risk patients with Acute Non-disabling Cerebrovascular Events (CHANCE) study, among patients with noncardioembolic minor stroke or TIA, those with ICAD had significantly higher rates of recurrent stroke at 90 days than those without (12.5% vs. 5.4%; $P < 0.0001$), irrespective of the antiplatelet regimen assigned.[22] Patients with a high-grade (70%–99%) symptomatic ICAD stenosis experienced an even higher risk of recurrence. In the Stenting and Aggressive Medical Management for Preventing Recurrent Stroke in Intracranial Stenosis (SAMMPRIS) trial, patients in the medical arm had a stroke or death risk of 15% at 1 year, despite aggressive medical treatment.[23]

The location of the diseased vessel may affect prognosis and treatment. The prognosis after an ischemic stroke related to ICAD appears to be worse in the patients with severe stenosis in the posterior circulation as opposed to the MCA or the intracranial ICA. A series of reports from the Center Posterior Circulation registry helps us better understand stroke in the posterior circulation. The overall 30-day mortality was 3.6%. Embolic mechanism, distal territory location, and BA-occlusive disease carried the poorest prognosis. The best outcome was in patients who had multiple arterial occlusive sites; they had position-sensitive TIAs for months to years. For patients with moderate to severe BA occlusive disease, the mortality rate was 2.3%, and 62 patients (almost 75%) had minor or no deficits at follow-up.[24] For patients with bilateral ICVA occlusive disease, the short- and long-term (mean length of follow-up was 31.4 months) outcomes were usually favorable, but patients with bilateral ICVA and BA-occlusive lesions often had poor outcomes. Patients with distal territory infarcts due to emboli from the ICVA had the worst outcome.[25] Qureshi et al. published a retrospective multicenter study.[26] A total of 102 patients were included and accepted the mean follow-up period of 15 months. Fourteen patients experienced recurrent stroke (arbitrary territory of artery). Eight patients experienced stroke in the territory of vertebrobasilar artery. Twenty-one patients died during follow-up, and among them, 16 patients died of fatal stroke. These results suggested that overall incidence of stroke was 11%, annual incidence of stroke in the territory of vertebrobasilar artery was 6.3%, and overall annual mortality was 6.3%. The Kaplan-Meier analysis revealed that stroke-free survival of patients was 76% at 12 months and 48% at 5 years. This suggested that most patients with symptomatic intracranial stenosis, in the 5 years after the initial onset, would suffer recurrent stroke or death. In this analysis, age and lack of antiplatelet or anticoagulant therapy were independent predictors of poor prognosis. On the other hand, the atherosclerotic stenosis of the MCA appears to have a lower incidence of recurrent ischemic event, but even more importantly, a lower associated mortality when compared to BA stenosis. Furthermore, the incidence of cardiac complication, including acute myocardial infarction (MI), appears to be higher in patients with symptomatic vertebrobasilar atherosclerotic stenosis compared to MCA stenosis. Acute MI is an important contributor for mortality in the short term after a symptomatic ischemic event related to atherosclerotic stenosis of the BA. Arenillas et al. screened for consecutive TIA or stroke patients, and 40 of them entered the study, which was confirmed by TCD and cerebral angiography MCA stenosis. During the mean follow-up period of 26.5 months, eight patients (20%) had a cerebral ischemic event in the territory of stenotic MCA (six TIAs and two stokes), annual incidence of ipsilateral TIA was 6.8%, and annual incidence of ipsilateral stroke was 2.3%. Progression of stenosis was an independent predictor of stroke recurrence.[27] The benefit of aggressive medical management and lifestyle modification on the recurrence of ischemic events in patients with symptomatic ICAD was assessed in the medical arm of the SAMMPRIS trial. Up to 17% of the patients with a symptomatic severe (more than 70%) atherosclerotic stenosis of an intracranial artery had recurrent ischemic stroke in spite of aggressive medical management. The majority of them carried atherosclerotic lesions in the MCA.

MEDICAL MANAGEMENT

Antiplatelets versus anticoagulants

The WASID trial investigated the effects of oral vitamin K antagonist warfarin (with a target international normalized ratio of 2–3) vs. aspirin in patients with recent ischemic stroke or TIA attributed to 50%–99% stenosis of a major intracranial artery. Patient recruitment in WASID was prematurely stopped at 569 patients, owing to safety concerns of patients treated by warfarin. Warfarin and aspirin showed comparable effects in preventing the composite primary endpoint (ischemic stroke, brain hemorrhage, or vascular death) in a mean follow-up of 1.8 years (21.8% vs. 22.1%, $P = 0.83$). However, long-term usage of warfarin significantly increased the rates of major adverse events, including death (9.7% vs. 4.3%, $P = 0.02$) and major hemorrhage (8.3% vs. 3.2%, $P = 0.01$).[21] Post-hoc subgroup analyses showed a beneficial effect of warfarin over aspirin (16% vs. 33%, $P = 0.04$) in preventing the primary endpoint in patients with stroke attributed to BA stenosis, but there was no significant difference in recurrent vertebrobasilar ischemic stroke between the two groups.[28] The Fraxiparine in Ischemic Stroke (FISS-tris) study randomized 603 patients and compared the safety and efficacy of anticoagulation (subcutaneous low-molecular-weight heparin [LWMH, nadroparin calcium] for 10 days followed by aspirin for 6 months) vs. aspirin only for 6 months. Among the 353 patients who had large artery occlusive disease, 300 had ICAD only, 11 had extracranial disease only, and 42 had both.[29] Post-hoc analysis indicated that the early use of LWMH in patients with large artery occlusive disease may reduce early neurological deterioration within 10 days after stroke, although the primary endpoint of the trial (favorable functional outcome at 6 months with a Barthel index e85) did not differ between the LWMH and aspirin groups. There was no significant difference in the risks of recurrent stroke from Day 10 to 6 months (4% vs. 5%, $P = 0.74$) or death within 6 months (5% vs. 5%, $P = 0.88$) in the two groups, either. Subgroup analyses suggested a more favorable functional outcome in patients with vertebrobasilar territory stroke treated with LWMH (OR 5.76, 95% CI 2–16.56; $P = 0.001$).[30] Therefore, warfarin or short-term subcutaneous LWMH, are not superior to aspirin in preventing stroke in symptomatic ICAD.

Combined antiplatelets (dual antiplatelet regimen)

In the medical groups of SAMMPRIS[31] and the Vitesse Intracranial Stent Study for Ischemic Stroke Therapy (VISSIT) trial,[32] patients with a recent ischemic stroke or TIA due to 70%–99% stenosis of a major intracranial artery received dual antiplatelet of aspirin and clopidogrel for 3 months followed by aspirin alone, coupled with lifestyle modification and a stringent control of vascular risk factors. In the medical arm of SAMMPRIS, the risks of stroke or death within 30 days (5.8%) or stroke recurrence within 1 year (12.2%) were much lower than that in WASID (10.7% and 25%, respectively). A similar trend was also observed in the medical arm of VISSIT, as well as in a recent study using similar aggressive medical regimen in Chinese ICAD patients with 70%–99% stenosis, in which the stroke risk in the first year was 14%. This study also revealed a higher frequency of ICAD regression by stringent risk factor management compared with a study conducted in the WASID era.[33] The risk of stroke in medical groups of SAMMPRIS and VISSIT dramatically diminished 6 months after the index stroke, which can potentially be attributed to plaque stabilization and a lower risk of artery-to-artery embolism. This is concordant with the findings in the CLAIR study (Clopidogrel plus Aspirin for Infarct Reduction in acute stroke/TIA patients with large artery stenosis and microembolic signal), where aspirin plus clopidogrel for 7 days significantly reduced microembolic signals by TCD on Day 7, compared with aspirin alone.[34] These findings support strict risk factor control and the short-term use of dual antiplatelets (aspirin and clopidogrel) followed by aspirin alone for ICAD patients with 70%–99% stenosis. So far, no major clinical trial has specifically studied the effects of dual antiplatelet therapy (DAPT) by aspirin and clopidogrel vs. aspirin alone in preventing recurrent stroke in ICAD

patients with 50% stenosis, although a post-hoc subgroup analysis of the CHANCE trial may provide a clue. In this large, multicenter randomized controlled trial conducted in China, patients with acute minor stroke or moderate-to-high-risk TIA (ABCD2 score 4) were randomly assigned to two groups: dual antiplatelet group (clopidogrel plus aspirin for the first 21 days followed by clopidogrel alone between 22 and 90 days) and the mono antiplatelet group (aspirin alone for 90 days).[35] In the image subgroup analysis of CHANCE, dual antiplatelet was neither significantly more effective than aspirin alone in preventing stroke recurrence (11.3% vs. 13.6%), nor significantly more hazardous in causing severe or moderate bleeding events (0% vs. 0.4%) within 90 days of enrollment.[22] Therefore, short-term use of DAPT by aspirin and clopidogrel may be a choice in minor stroke or moderate-to-high-risk TIA patients with symptomatic ICAD (50% stenosis). But such inference needs further investigation. The Trial of cilOstazol in Symptomatic intracranial arterial Stenosis (TOSS) and TOSS-2 conducted in East Asian populations tested another combination of DAPT (i.e., cilostazol plus aspirin) in symptomatic ICAD patients with mild to severe stenosis or occlusion.[36,37] Both studies used imaging endpoint (i.e., progression of the symptomatic ICAD lesion on magnetic resonance imaging [MRI]) instead of clinical events as the primary endpoint. In TOSS (135 patients), cilostazol plus aspirin was associated with less progression of symptomatic ICAD at 6 months compared with aspirin alone; yet the small number of clinical events did not allow statistical analysis. In TOSS-2, when cilostazol plus aspirin was compared with clopidogrel plus aspirin in 457 patients, no significant difference was found between the two regimens in terms of the frequencies of progression of symptomatic ICAD, new ischemic lesions, or major hemorrhage in 7 months.

Interventional approach

Angioplasty and/or stenting aims to restore the luminal patency and improve cerebral perfusion in a minimally invasive approach. SAMMPRIS and VISSIT were two multicenter randomized controlled trials comparing early adjunctive PTAS and medical therapy in high-grade (70%–99%) symptomatic ICAD patients. SAMMPRIS studied the safety and efficacy of aggressive medical management alone vs. aggressive medical management plus perutaneous transluminal angioplasty and stenting (PTAS) (by Wingspan, a self-expanding stent system) within 30 days from an index ischemic stroke or TIA attributed to a 70%–99% stenosis of a major intracranial artery. Aggressive medical management included dual antiplatelet (aspirin and clopidogrel) for 3 months followed by aspirin alone, strict control of vascular risk factors, and lifestyle modification. The enrollment was prematurely terminated at 451 patients (224 in PTAS group and 227 in medical group), due to a significantly higher 30-day rate of stroke or death in the stent arm (14.7% vs. 5.8%, $P = 0.002$).[31] The periprocedural event rate in SAMMPRIS was higher than that in previous reports (typically less than 10%), mostly based on retrospective studies or post-hoc analysis of prospective studies. Final results of SAMMPRIS indicated a lower rate of primary endpoint in the medical arm throughout the follow-up period: 12.6% vs. 19.7% at 1 year ($P = 0.0428$), 14.1% vs. 20.6% at 2 years ($P = 0.07$), and 14.9% vs. 23.9% at 3 years ($P = 0.0193$). SAMMPRIS concluded that PTAS with the Wingspan stent system, in addition to aggressive medical therapy, was inferior to aggressive medical therapy alone in the study population, owing to the high risk of periprocedural complications in patients treated by PTAS. Moreover, no additional benefit of PTAS was observed beyond the first 30 days after the procedure.

VISSIT started soon after SAMMPRIS with a similar study design, but testing the safety and efficacy of a balloon-expandable stent, PHAROS Vitesse, in patients with 70%–99% symptomatic intracranial stenosis. The medical management of VISSIT was comparable to SAMMPRIS, but relatively less aggressive in risk factor control or lifestyle coaching.[32] Again, PTAS in VISSIT, although by a different device, was shown to be inferior to medical treatment. The primary endpoints of any stroke in the same territory within 1 year, or hard TIA in the same territory between 2 days and 1 year, were 15.1% and 36.2% in the medical and PTAS groups, respectively. Periprocedural events (any stroke or death within 30 days, or hard TIA within 2–30 days) occurred in 24.1% of patients receiving PTAS.

In a single-center randomized study in China of a similar design but limited to patients with high-grade MCA stenosis, the PTAS group showed a 30-day rate of stroke or death as low as 2.8% (by several types of intracranial stents); yet, this was not superior to medical treatment.[38] The interventional procedures were conducted in a comprehensive stroke center with a high patient load by four highly experienced neurointerventionalists with a combined experience of >500 intracranial stenting prior to the trial enrollment. The impact of experience and credentialing of neurointerventionists remained controversial. A post-hoc analysis of SAMMPRIS opined that operators with less experience in Wingspan were not responsible for the high periprocedural complications in SAMMPRIS. Nevertheless, it was suggested that a lead-in phase of training and credentialing may reduce the risk of periprocedural events in future stenting trials for ICAD.[39]

So far, patient selection for PTAS in clinical practice or trial recruitment has relied on the severity of the symptomatic stenosis lesion (i.e., 70%–99% stenosis) that was shown to independently predict stroke recurrence. But an increasing body of evidence has pinpointed the importance of collateral circulation that may alter the pathophysiology of symptomatic ICAD lesions and the subsequent relapse, notably among WASID and SAMMPRIS subjects.[40] Furthermore, there are several other factors that could influence the periprocedural event rate of intracranial stenting. For instance, a long (>5 mm), eccentric, or tortuous lesion under Mori classification is known to be associated with a higher rate of procedural complication and in-stent restenosis. In patients who have perforator occlusion from atheromatous branch disease, stenting not only cannot revascularize the occluded perforators, but may exacerbate perforator occlusion as a result of a "snow plowing" effect. However, SAMMPRIS and VISSIT did not address these lesion characteristics upon subject recruitment.

In a recent multicenter prospective Chinese trial of stent placement in patients with symptomatic high-grade intracranial stenosis using the Wingspan stent, the overall 30-day rate of stroke and death was just 2% (95% CI 0.2%–7%). Only high-volume centers and patients with distal hypoperfusion and or cortical involvement were included. Patients with perforating artery ischemic stroke were explicitly excluded. The results of this prospective multicenter study demonstrated the outcome with safety in patients treated with a Wingspan stent within 30 days, which suggested operators' experience at high-volume sites and strict patient selection are critical in reducing periprocedural complications and events.

In a recent small retrospective study by Lee et al., 30 patients with symptomatic ICAD underwent intracranial stent placement using the Enterprise self-expanding balloon followed by an undersized angioplasty. They found an excellent performance of the Enterprise stent regarding technical feasibility and safety. The frequency of periprocedural complications at 30 days was 10% due to one case of in-stent thrombosis and reocclusion, postop hyperperfusion intracerebral hemorrhage, and a perforator stroke.[41] Even though it is a small retrospective experience, it gives a new perspective of the experience using a different stent and a different technique beyond the Wingspan stent.

The China Angioplasty and Stenting for Symptomatic Intracranial Severe Stenosis trial has been initiated and is an ongoing, prospective, multicenter randomized trial, which is being conducted in eight sites intending to recruit 380 subjects (stent placement, 190; medical treatment alone, 190).[42] The study aims to demonstrate a 10.7% absolute reduction in ipsilateral stroke and/or death during 12 months (assuming an event rate of 18% for medically treated patients and 7.3% for stent-treated patients). The sample size provides 80% power with a two-sided test at the 5% level of significance and provides a 20% rate of lost follow-up. Because many of the periprocedural complications of the intracranial stent placement are related to the stent itself, some investigators are also testing the feasibility and impact of primary intracranial angioplasty (alone) for prevention of recurrent ischemic event in patients with symptomatic severe ICAD compared to aggressive medical management.

In a retrospective cohort from Japan, Okada et al. described a total of 47 patients with symptomatic severe (more than 70%) stenosis of the MCA refractory to medical treatment. They found an acceptable rate of complications at 30 days postprocedure around 6%. Even though approximately one-quarter of the patients suffered from restenosis in the follow-up, only 10% were symptomatic at 52 months at the latest follow-up.[43]

Dumont et al. published a prospective phase 1 study assessing submaximal angioplasty (only) for symptomatic intracranial atherosclerosis. They enrolled a total of 24 patients with symptomatic severe (70%–99%) intracranial atherosclerotic stenosis during a period of 3 years.[44] All procedures were performed under moderate sedation and patients underwent a submaximal angioplasty (Gateway balloon size matched 50%–70% of the nondiseased segment of the vessel). They found an excellent rate of periprocedural complication. At day 30, only one patient suffered from a TIA without further implications, and at 1 year, from the 18 patients available for follow-up, only one patient suffered from a recurrent ischemic stroke associated with a reocclusion of the angioplastied artery that required reintervention and stent placement.

Primary intracranial angioplasty (alone) is an attractive endovascular technique for patients with symptomatic severe ICAD that recurs with relapsing cerebrovascular ischemic event in spite of aggressive medical treatment (Figure 52.1). The lower complexity of primary intracranial angioplasty compared to intracranial stent placement and the lack of in-stent thrombosis, stenosis, and occlusion as potential periprocedural complications, makes it a very attractive area of research. However, its applicability and effectiveness compared to aggressive medical management and intracranial stent placement are still unproven. The latest guideline from the American Heart Association/American Stroke Association does not support PTAS as an initial treatment in ICAD patients. The U.S. Food and Drug Administration (FDA) currently limits the indication of Wingspan stent to those with two or more strokes despite aggressive medical treatment.

Endovascular treatment for acute proximal large intracranial arterial occlusion due to atherosclerotic disease

The vast majority of patients presenting with an acute ischemic stroke and emergent large vessel occlusion of a proximal intracranial artery harbor a brain embolism from a proximal source. Endovascular treatment using stent retrievers is a proven adjunctive therapeutic modality combined with intravenous thrombolysis. However, it is estimated that approximately one-fifth of the acute large vessel occlusions are *in situ* atherosclerotic plaque as opposed to embolic occlusions. Similar to an acute coronary artery occlusions responsible for an ST-elevation myocardial infarction (STEMI), the atherosclerotic disease of an intracranial artery can result in acute plaque rupturing and the formation of occlusive superimposed thrombi.

The performance of stent retrievers in treating intracranial large vessel occlusion due to atherosclerotic disease is not well-established. Unfortunately, in the acute scenario of an acute ischemic stroke due to an emergent large vessel occlusion, it might be challenging to establish with certainty that *in situ* atherosclerosis (as opposed to brain embolism) is the underlying mechanism of intracranial occlusion (Figure 52.2). In a retrospective study by Lee et al.,[45] a total of nine patients presented with acute ischemic stroke due to a large vessel occlusion caused by ICAD (two in the BA and the rest in the stent of the MCA). All patients underwent mechanical embolectomy using a retrieval stent (Solitaire FR device) as the first-line method. The median number of stent retriever passes was two. In all patients, the occlusion was successfully crossed and the transient flow restoration was achieved after deployment of stent. However, after the

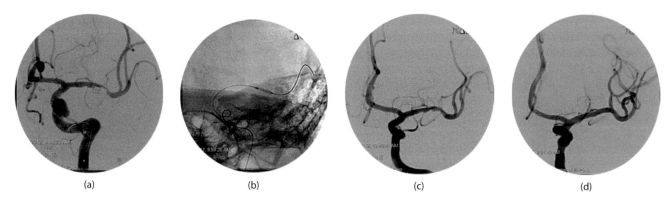

(a)   (b)   (c)   (d)

Figure 52.1 A 56-year-old man with a symptomatic severe stenosis in the left middle cerebral artery refractory to aggressive medical management came with repetitive episodes of transient ischemic attacks and minor strokes in the distribution of the left middle cerebral artery. The stenosis measured 90% by WASID criteria. Patient underwent a primary single subnominal balloon angioplasty of the left middle cerebral artery using a 2 × 15 mm Gateway balloon. Residual stenosis at the final of the procedure measured less than 50% by WASID criteria. Patient was kept on aggressive medical treatment and a follow-up cerebral angiogram at 6 months showed further improvement of the lesion with total normalization of the lumen diameter. **(a)** Cerebral angiogram anterior-posterior view of the left middle cerebral artery. The injection is done through a 6-Fr guide catheter in the left internal carotid artery. **(b)** Primary single submaximal balloon angioplasty. **(c)** Postprocedure angiographic run showing less than 50% residual stenosis. **(d)** Follow-up cerebral angiogram months after the original balloon angioplasty showing a significant improvement of the angioplasty segment with almost complete angiographic regression of the atherosclerotic plaque. (Image courtesy of Drs. Alberto Maud and Gustavo Rodriguez.)

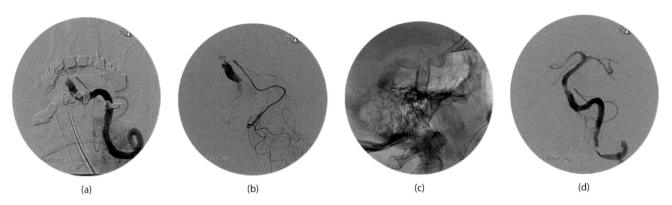

(a) (b) (c) (d)

Figure 52.2 A 55-year-old man with hypertension, coronary artery disease, and cigarette smoking developed transient ischemic attacks in the posterior circulation and was found to have a >90% atherosclerotic stenosis in the midbasilar artery. He was placed on aggressive medical management with excellent adherence to the lifestyle modification. Four months later, he returned after 45 minutes of an abrupt onset of dysarthria, dysphagia, diplopia, and facial palsy. After head computed tomography ruled out intracerebral hemorrhage, intravenous recombinant tissue plasminogen activator (rtPA) was administered 90 minutes after symptom onset. During the intravenous infusion of the thrombolytic he deteriorated his neurologic exam and went into a coma, and he was emergently intubated. Computed tomography angiogram showed interval occlusion of the basilar artery. He was emergently taken to the neuroangiography suite, and he underwent an emergent basilar artery angioplasty (2.5 × 9 mm Gateway noncompliant balloon) followed by stent placement (3.5 × 15 mm Wingspan stent). The final residual stenosis was less than 30%, and he had a complete neurologic recovery. The mRS at 90 days was less than 2, and he remained free of recurrent ischemic event for the next 12 months. **(a)** Cerebral angiogram anterior-posterior view of the basilar artery. The injection is done through a 6-Fr guide catheter in the left vertebral artery. **(b)** Microcatheter injection confirming complete occlusion of the midbasilar artery immediately above the origin of the left anterior inferior cerebellar artery. **(c)** Balloon angioplasty followed by stent placement. **(d)** Postprocedure angiographic run showing acute recanalization of the basilar artery and mild residual stenosis. (Image courtesy of Drs. Alberto Maud and Gustavo Rodriguez.)

stent was removed, the target artery reoccluded. Transient recanalization of the lesion was achieved, and small debris was extracted (plaque vs. superimposed thrombus "peeling effect"). The most common rescue endovascular treatment used primary acute intracranial angioplasty and super-selective intra-arterial infusion of glycoprotein 2b3a inhibitors. Overall, the majority of the patients achieved an incomplete recanalization (AOL score of 2) and only half of them achieved an independent life without significant disability at 3 months. This is a small cohort, and patients who never recanalized were excluded, which can overestimate the performance of the endovascular treatment. However, it appears that the stent retriever-based thrombectomy, in cases of atherosclerotic acute occlusion of an intracranial artery, might be safe to remove the superimposed *in situ* thrombosis. The effectiveness might be more disappointing because of the frequent use of rescuing additional endovascular methods, particularly primary intracranial angioplasty and potent antiplatelet intrathrombus infusion.

Seo et al. published their experience on acute intracranial stent placement for patients presenting with acute ischemic stroke due to a symptomatic intracranial atherosclerotic lesion.[46] A total of 10 patients were identified within the first 6 hours with stroke in evolution due to a severe (75%–99%) atherosclerotic stenosis. Because of the presence of fluctuating neurologic symptoms, they underwent acute intracranial angioplasty followed by stent placement. In nine out of ten, the intracranial stenting was successfully placed. One patient suffered from hyperacute in-stent thrombotic occlusion and died. At 24 hours, six out of ten showed signs of neurologic stability and improvement. At 3 months, seven patients achieved a mRS less than 2. In the Stent-Assisted Recanalization in Acute Ischemic Stroke (SARIS) trial, recanalization with a Thrombolysis in MI score of 3 was achieved in 60% of patients within 8 hours after the onset of symptoms following an acute stroke. At 1 month, modified Rankin Scale (mRS) 0-3 was achieved in 60% of patients, and mRS 0-1 was noted in 45% of patients.[47] Kim et al. published the incidence of reocclusion after emergent intracranial angioplasty with or without stent placement as a rescue treatment for acute large vessel occlusion. From a total of 46 patients, 32 patients underwent angioplasty followed by stent placement, while 14 underwent only angioplasty.[48] All 46 patients were not pretreated before the intervention. All patients underwent a CT of the head immediately after the procedure. Only five patients were not treated with aspirin and clopidogrel immediately after the procedure because of the presence of hemorrhage in the CT. Six patients (13%) suffered from acute postprocedure reocclusion, and it was more frequent in the angioplasty alone group, and the most common predisposing factor was a suboptimal angioplasty (more than 50% stenosis at the end of the procedure). Finally, the best methods (stent retriever, primary acute angioplasty, stent placement for emergent revascularization, intra-arterial infusion of GP2b3a inhibitors) as well as performance and effectiveness of endovascular treatment in this acute intracranial atherosclerotic large vessel occlusion still need to be proven.

Periprocedural management

Periprocedural management, and in the intraoperative and early postoperative periods, hemodynamic management are of paramount importance during endovascular revascularization treatment of ICAD. Elective cases should be pretreated with at least 5 days of a combination of two antiplatelets, preferentially synergistic but with different mechanisms of action. The most common combination worldwide is 81–325 mg of daily aspirin, plus 75 mg of daily clopidogrel. In urgent cases, a loading dose of 600 mg of clopidogrel will affect the platelet function about 6 hours after the oral dosing. If the patient is known or suspected to have a genetic resistance to the antiplatelet effect of clopidogrel, genetic analysis is the only test that can prove that the patient is resistant or excessively sensitive to its effect. Cilostazol, tirofiban, prasugrel, and ticagrelor are alternatives to clopidogrel. In case of emergent endovascular treatment for acute proximal large intracranial arterial occlusion, pretreatment with antiplatelet medication is usually not possible. In this case, the presence and the size of established infarction and hemorrhagic complication, including hemorrhagic transformation of the ischemic stroke, as well as technical complication, including subarachnoid hemorrhage induced by microware perforation or vessel ruptured due to postangioplasty dissection, will mandate the promptness of DAPT initiation. If the procedure is finished without evident complication, it is recommended to perform a CT of the head without contrast, and if there are no hemorrhagic complications, it is advisable to start on a low dose of aspirin and between 300 and 600 mg of clopidogrel. The time and the intensity of the DAPT in the case of acute ischemic stroke will depend on the size of the evolving infarction. If during one of the steps of the endovascular procedure (immediately postangioplasty or after stent placement) a local thromboembolic complication happens, the available parenteral antiplatelet can be used. The most common parenteral antiplatelet is eptifibatide because of its short action and short half-life. A reduced bolus dosing is recommended for neurointerventional procedures (0.135 mcg/kg, which is approximately one-quarter of the cardiac bolus doses used in coronary reperfusion). The need of a maintenance dose of continuous intravenous infusion of GP2b3a inhibitors will depend on the timing for initiation of the oral antiplatelet medication.

Intraprocedural and postprocedural hemodynamic management is of extreme importance for the success of endovascular revascularization in patients with ICAD. Arterial blood pressure is a simple physiologic parameter that is always measured, can be modulated, and may affect outcome in certain circumstances.[49] For this type of complex procedure, we recommend systematically placing an arterial (preferable 4-Fr radial arterial sheath) access for continuous invasive blood pressure monitoring. The invasive blood pressure monitoring allows a more precise and stricter monitoring of the blood pressure in real-time, and it dissipates the potential discrepancies with noninvasive

(indirect measurement) blood pressure monitoring (oscillometric method). This is of particular importance in cases of endovascular treatment performed under general anesthesia. During anesthetic induction, hypotension is a common undesired consequence with potential harmful complications. It is advisable to stop vasodilators before the procedure, especially the long-acting ones, to avoid their superimposed long therapeutic effects during the procedure. Caution should be applied when stopping certain vasodilators (like beta-blockers and clonidine) that are known to cause rebound arterial hypertension after abrupt discontinuation. Vasodilators and vasoconstrictors should be readily available during the procedure to counteract the blood pressure contingencies. Potent, short-acting, and easy-to-titrate drugs are preferable. The most common vasoactive drug used in neurointerventional procedures is phenylephrine, and the most common vasodilator used is nicardipine. Esmolol and labetalol are also valid alternatives to nicardipine. Certain vasodilators, like nitroprusside, that cause venous cranial vasodilation should be avoided because they potentially increase intracranial pressure. The optimal management of arterial blood pressure and the exact blood pressure parameters to maintain during endovascular recanalization of steno-occlusive atherosclerotic disease of the cervical and intracranial arteries is not established. It has been proven that extreme arterial blood pressure variation affects the outcome. This is particularly true for intracranial atherosclerotic stenosis. ICAD is a focal and segmental disease, and inadequately low arterial blood pressure can affect cerebral perfusion in not only the target vessel but also in other distant steno-occlusive areas. Alternatively, inappropriately elevated blood pressure immediately after an intracranial artery is associated with reperfusion injury. This is an undesired complication that can result in acute neurologic symptoms (most commonly severe headache) and worsening of neurologic status (depressed level of consciousness) as a result of acute brain edema and occasionally hemorrhagic complication. Acute hypertensive response is a very common hemodynamic response in the acute phase of an ischemic stroke, intracerebral hemorrhage, and subarachnoid hemorrhage. It appears to be mediated by a central sympathetic response. However, its exact significance and its subsequent management are not yet established. In cases of acute ischemic stroke due to acute large vessel embolic occlusion, the acute hypertensive response is suspected to be responsible for maintenance of the perfusion pressure in the retrograde leptomeningeal collateral circulation. In cases of long-standing intracranial large steno-occlusive atherosclerotic arterial disease, we have to add to the equation another complex process.

Long-standing ICAD causes chronic ischemia in the distal arterial bed at the capillary level. The compensatory response (cerebrovascular reserve) implies vasodilation of the precapillary arterioles to adjust the diminished oxygen delivery to the neuronal demands. The cerebral tissue perfused under this ischemic condition is more prone to injury due to systemic blood pressure changes and to local blood flow and perfusion changes after revascularization.

Observational studies have found a *U*-shaped curve for the association between systolic blood pressure and outcomes in acute ischemic stroke.[50] Persistent low blood pressure during the acute phase of ischemic stroke is associated with worse outcome. In the same fashion, persistent severe elevation in the blood pressure and further increases in blood pressure during the subacute phase have been associated with worse outcomes. But a moderate hypertension, as defined by systolic blood pressure ranging from 140 to 150 mmHg, has been associated with the most favorable outcome. This is also reflected in retrospective and prospective observational studies that investigate the blood pressure and outcomes in acute ischemic stroke treated with intravenous thrombolysis in the first 3 hours after symptom onset.[51] During acute ischemic stroke reperfusion, we allowed an acute hypertensive response to set the blood pressure range to certain limits (185/105 mmHg). The goal of permissive hypertension is to optimize blood flow to the ischemic penumbra until IV thrombolytics can be administered, and intra-arterial recanalization therapies can be employed, or optimization of the collateral vasculature can occur. Even though the upper limit of the permissive hypertension is up to 185 mmHg for the systolic blood pressure number, the best outcome is found in the patient who presented with systolic blood pressure ranging from 140 to 160 mmHg. At the present time, there is a paucity of data on the impacts of pharmacologic elevation and reduction of blood pressure in the hyperacute and early acute settings. We need to develop clues to help identify subgroups that may benefit the most from aggressive blood pressure modulation depending on patient-specific factors such as location of the occlusion, status of the collateral circulation, blood pressure trends within the individual, and other medical comorbidities. Certainly, acute ischemic stroke due to large vessel occlusion and particularly large vessel occlusion due to intracranial arteriosclerotic steno-occlusive disease will be the subgroup to benefit the most from research on blood pressure modulation to improve final outcome.

Surgical treatment

Extracranial-intracranial (EC/IC) arterial bypass surgery was first attempted for cerebrovascular occlusive disease half a century ago. Nevertheless, the EC/IC bypass study that compared the procedure with medical treatment in stroke or TIA patients due to steno-occlusion of extracranial or intracranial ICA or MCA, failed to prove superiority of EC/IC bypass surgery over medical treatment among the 1,377 patients recruited. In those with severe MCA stenosis ($n = 109$), the risk of fatal or nonfatal stroke was substantially higher in the surgical group. The EC/IC bypass procedure was again futile in a subsequent study. The Carotid Occlusion Surgery Study (COSS) enrolled patients with atherosclerotic ICA occlusion coupled with significant hemodynamic failure confirmed by using oxygen extraction fraction in positron emission tomography.[52] However, COSS was terminated early after 194 subjects had been randomized, due to an analysis of the 139 subjects who had completed 2-year follow-up. Thus, EC/IC bypass surgery is no longer considered under most circumstances for patients with atherosclerotic cervicocerebral arterial stenosis or occlusion. Encephaloduroarteriosynangiosis (EDAS), an indirect surgical revascularization method, has recently been reported safe and possibly effective in selected ICAD patients with recurrent stroke despite best medical treatment. Thirty-six patients with symptomatic stenosis (>70%) or occlusion of intracranial ICA or MCA underwent EDAS in a single center. The rate of stroke or death during a median follow-up of 2 years was 5.6% lower than that in the medical or PTAS group in SAMMPRIS.[53] It was suggested that EDAS might prevent stroke by augmenting collateral circulation to the ischemic territory. Currently, the safety and efficacy of EDAS are being tested in a prospective, single-arm clinical trial, the EDAS (Surgical) Revascularization for Symptomatic Intracranial Arterial Stenosis trial.

Lifestyle modification and management of vascular risk factors

One of the most important lessons we learned from the SAMMPRIS trial was the potentially powerful impact of aggressive medical management on the secondary prevention of events (including recurrent TIA, ischemic stroke, MI, and death) in patients with symptomatic ICAD. The unexpected low incidence of ischemic events at 30 days in the medical arm set a new benchmark for the acceptable rates of complications for new alternate therapies. In prior randomized clinical trials of medical treatment for secondary prevention of recurrent ischemic events in patients with ICAD, the rate of recurrent ischemic events was higher than the medical arm of the SAMMPRIS. In the WASID trial, a prospective double-blind randomized clinical trial comparing the effectiveness of aspirin vs. warfarin for secondary prevention of patients with symptomatic severe ICAD was found at a much higher rate of recurrent ischemic events compared to the medical arm in SAMMPRIS (10.5% [95% CI 6.5%–16.9%] versus 5.8% [95% CI 3.4%–9.7%] at 30 days, respectively). Although the studies were performed at a different time (almost a decade apart), the population included in both studies was quite homogeneous except for more subjects taking statins at the time of randomization and more subjects having ischemic stroke (as opposed to TIA) as a qualifying event in the SAMMPRIS study. After adjusting for these last two confounders, it turned out that subjects in the medical arm of SAMMPRIS had a much lower incidence of recurrent event because of the aggressive medical management.[54] This new therapeutic approach (aggressive medical management) goes beyond the pharmacologic approach and implies a coached lifestyle with modification, including optimization of the body mass index and daily physical activity. When combined with dual antiplatelet regimen plus blood pressure medication, statins, and optimization of the glycemic control in diabetic subjects, a surprisingly low incidence of recurrent stroke resulted. This aggressive medical management and coached lifestyle modification is now the new landmark to achieve for secondary prevention in ICAD and probably a reference for other atherosclerotic diseases, including cervical carotid and vertebral artery atherosclerotic disease.

However, aggressive medical management leaves up to 15% of the patients unprotected, and they can continue having episodes of recurrent TIAs and ischemic strokes. The most important factors associated with the recurrence of ischemic events, in spite of aggressive medical management, were diabetes, female gender, not taking statin at the time of randomization, degree of stenosis higher than 80% by WASID criteria, and having ischemic stroke (as opposed to transient ischemic stroke) as a qualifying event. Research must continue to identify new therapeutic alternatives in this particular subgroup of patients who are refractory to aggressive medical management. The experience of aggressive medical management for symptomatic ICAD cannot, unfortunately,

be translated to the asymptomatic ICAD. This is particularly true for the pharmacologic component of the management, particularly the dual antiplatelet regimen. However, the benefit of coached lifestyle modification and daily physical activity are even beyond the ICAD, and it can be extended to the overall cardiovascular, respiratory, and neurocognitive and behavioral aspect of human health maintenance.

Clinical recommendations

Atherosclerotic stenosis of the intracranial arteries is an important cause of ischemic stroke, and effective therapies can modify/reduce risk:

- Optimal evidence-based medical therapy that includes antiplatelet and antihypertensive agents, statins, and lifestyle modification is recommended for every patient with intracranial stenosis (Table 52.1).
- DAPT with aspirin plus clopidogrel for 90 days, followed by antiplatelet monotherapy, might be reasonable for patients with recently symptomatic intracranial large artery disease.[55]

Table 52.1 Management algorithm for patients with suspected intracranial atherosclerosis

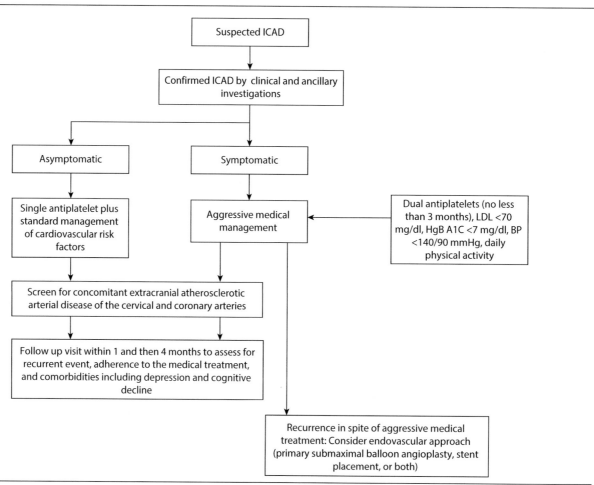

Source: Modified from Qureshi, A.I., et al., *Lancet*, 383(9921), 984–998, 2014. With permission.
Note: BP, blood pressure; Hgb A1C, glycosylated hemoglobin; ICAD, atherosclerotic intracranial disease; LDL, low density lipoproteins; dual antiplatelets refer to a combination of aspirin plus a second oral antiplatelet medication, including clopidogrel or others (cilostazol or ticagrelor).

- Although the benefits are uncertain, the use of endovascular therapy (primary balloon angioplasty and or intracranial stent placement) should be offered to a select population of patients after failure of aggressive medical management.
- The effectiveness of endovascular treatment for acute large vessel occlusion due to ICAD within the first hours of an acute ischemic stroke is unproven.

REFERENCES

1. Powers WJ, et al. 2015 American Heart Association/ American Stroke Association Focused Update of the 2013 Guidelines for the Early Management of Patients With Acute Ischemic Stroke Regarding Endovascular Treatment: A Guideline for Healthcare Professionals From the American Heart Association/American Stroke Association. *Stroke* 2015;46(10):3020–3035.

2. VanderLaan PA, et al. Site specificity of atherosclerosis: Site-selective responses to atherosclerotic modulators. *Arterioscler Thromb Vasc Biol* 2004;24(1):12–22.

3. Leng X, et al. The contemporary management of intracranial atherosclerotic disease. *Expert Rev Neurother* 2016;16(6):701–709.

4. Muka T, et al. The role of epigenetic modifications in cardiovascular disease: A systematic review. *Int J Cardiol* 2016;212:174–183.

5. Soeki T, Sata M. Inflammatory biomarkers and atherosclerosis. *Int Heart J* 2016;57(2):134–139.

6. Schwarze JJ, et al. Longitudinal monitoring of intracranial arterial stenoses with transcranial Doppler ultrasonography. *J Neuroimaging* 1994;4(4):182–187.

7. Wong KS, et al. Progression of middle cerebral artery occlusive disease and its relationship with further vascular events after stroke. *Stroke* 2002;33(2):532–536.

8. Jeon HW, Cha JK. Factors related to progression of middle cerebral artery stenosis determined using transcranial Doppler ultrasonograhy. *J Thromb Thrombolysis* 2008;25(3):265–269.

9. Qiao Y, et al. Patterns and implications of intracranial arterial remodeling in stroke patients. *Stroke* 2016;47(2):434–440.

10. Degnan AJ, et al. MR angiography and imaging for the evaluation of middle cerebral artery atherosclerotic disease. *AJNR Am J Neuroradiol* 2012;33(8):1427–1435.

11. Mossa-Basha M, et al. Vessel wall imaging for intracranial vascular disease evaluation. *J Neurointerv Surg* 2016;8(11):1154–1159.

12. Bang OY. Intracranial atherosclerosis: Current understanding and perspectives. *J Stroke* 2014;16(10):27–35.

13. Pu Y, et al. Natural history of intracranial atherosclerotic disease. *Front Neurol* 2014;5:125.

14. Bos D, et al. Intracranial carotid artery atherosclerosis: Prevalence and risk factors in the general population. *Stroke* 2012;43(70):1878–1884.

15. Liu W, et al. Distribution of moyamoya disease susceptibility polymorphism p.R4810K in RNF213 in East and Southeast Asian populations. *Neurol Med Chir (Tokyo)* 2012;52(5):299–303.

16. Im SH, et al. Prevalence and epidemiological features of moyamoya disease in Korea. *J Cerebrovasc Endovasc Neurosurg* 2012;14(2):75–78.

17. Anderson TJ. Assessment and treatment of endothelial dysfunction in humans. *J Am Coll Cardiol* 1999;34(3):631–638.

18. Lopez-Cancio E, et al. Biological signatures of asymptomatic extra- and intracranial atherosclerosis: The Barcelona-AsIA (Asymptomatic Intracranial Atherosclerosis) study. *Stroke* 2012;43(10):2712–2719.

19. Kremer C, et al. Prognosis of asymptomatic stenosis of the middle cerebral artery. *J Neurol Neurosurg Psychiatry* 2004;75:1300–1303.

20. Kern R, et al. Stroke recurrences in patients with symptomatic vs asymptomatic middle cerebral artery disease. *Neurology* 2005;65:859–864.

21. Chimowitz MI, et al. Comparison of warfarin and aspirin for symptomatic intracranial arterial stenosis. *N Engl J Med* 2005;352(13):1305–1316.

22. Liu L, et al. Dual antiplatelet therapy in stroke and ICAS: Subgroup analysis of CHANCE. *Neurology* 2015;85(13):1154–1162.

23. Waters MF, et al. Factors associated with recurrent ischemic stroke in the medical group of the SAMMPRIS trial. *JAMA Neurol* 2016;73(3):308–315.

24. Voetsch B, et al. Basilar artery occlusive disease in the New England Medical Center Posterior Circulation Registry. *Arch Neurol* 2004;61(4):496–504.

25. Tariq N, et al. Clinical outcome of patients with acute posterior circulation stroke and bilateral vertebral artery occlusion. *J Vasc Interv Neurol* 2011;4(2):9–14.

26. Qureshi AI, et al. Stroke-free survival and its determinants in patients with symptomatic vertebrobasilar stenosis: A multicenter study. *Neurosurgery* 2003;52(5):1033–1039; discussion 1039–1040.

27. Arenillas JF, et al. Progression and clinical recurrence of symptomatic middle cerebral artery stenosis: A long-term follow-up transcranial Doppler ultrasound study. *Stroke* 2001;32(12):2898–2904.

28. Kasner SE, et al. Warfarin vs aspirin for symptomatic intracranial stenosis: Subgroup analyses from WASID. *Neurology* 2006;67(7):1275–1278.

29. Wong KS, et al. Low-molecular-weight heparin compared with aspirin for the treatment of acute ischaemic stroke in Asian patients with large artery occlusive disease: A randomised study. *Lancet Neurol* 2007;6(5):407–413.

30. Wang QS, et al. Low-molecular-weight heparin versus aspirin for acute ischemic stroke with large artery occlusive disease: Subgroup analyses from the Fraxiparin in Stroke Study for the treatment of ischemic stroke (FISS-tris) study. *Stroke* 2012;43(2):346–349.

31. Chimowitz MI, et al. Stenting versus aggressive medical therapy for intracranial arterial stenosis. *N Engl J Med* 2011;365(11):993–1003.

32. Zaidat OO, et al. Effect of a balloon-expandable intracranial stent vs medical therapy on risk of stroke in patients with symptomatic intracranial stenosis: The VISSIT randomized clinical trial. *JAMA* 2015;313(12):1240–1248.

33. Leung TW, et al. Evolution of intracranial atherosclerotic disease under modern medical therapy. *Ann Neurol* 2015;77(3):478–486.

34. Wang X, et al. The effectiveness of dual antiplatelet treatment in acute ischemic stroke patients with intracranial arterial stenosis: A subgroup analysis of CLAIR study. *Int J Stroke* 2013;8(8):663–668.

35. Wang Y, et al. Clopidogrel with aspirin in acute minor stroke or transient ischemic attack. *N Engl J Med* 2013;369(1):11–19.

36. Kwon SU, et al. Cilostazol prevents the progression of the symptomatic intracranial arterial stenosis: The multi-center double-blind placebo-controlled trial of cilostazol in symptomatic intracranial arterial stenosis. *Stroke* 2005;36(4):782–786.

37. Kwon SU, et al. Efficacy and safety of combination antiplatelet therapies in patients with symptomatic intracranial atherosclerotic stenosis. *Stroke* 2011;42(10):2883–2890.

38. Miao Z, et al. Randomized controlled trial of symptomatic middle cerebral artery stenosis: Endovascular versus medical therapy in a Chinese population. *Stroke* 2012;43(12):3284–3290.

39. Zaidat OO, et al. Impact of SAMMPRIS on the future of intracranial atherosclerotic disease management: Polling results from the ICAD symposium at the International Stroke Conference. *J Neurointerv Surg* 2014;6(3):225–230.

40. Lopez-Cancio E, et al. Infarct patterns, collaterals and likely causative mechanisms of stroke in symptomatic intracranial atherosclerosis. *Cerebrovasc Dis* 2014;37(6):417–422.

41. Lee KY, et al. Undersized angioplasty and stenting of symptomatic intracranial tight stenosis with Enterprise: Evaluation of clinical and vascular outcome. *Interv Neuroradiol* 2016;22(2):187–195.

42. Gao P, et al. China Angioplasty and Stenting for Symptomatic Intracranial Severe Stenosis (CASSISS): A new, prospective, multicenter, randomized controlled trial in China. *Interv Neuroradiol* 2015;21(2):196–204.

43. Okada H, et al. Reappraisal of primary balloon angioplasty without stenting for patients with symptomatic middle cerebral artery stenosis. *Neurol Med Chir (Tokyo)* 2015;55(2):133–140.

44. Dumont TM, et al. Submaximal angioplasty for symptomatic intracranial atherosclerosis: A prospective Phase I study. *J Neurosurg* 2016;125(4):964–971.

45. Lee JS, et al. Primary stent retrieval for acute intracranial large artery occlusion due to atherosclerotic disease. *J Stroke* 2016;18(1):96–101.

46. Seo WK, et al. Intracranial stenting as a rescue therapy in patients with stroke-in-evolution. *J Stroke Cerebrovasc Dis* 2016;25(6):1411–1416.

47. Levy EI, et al. First Food and Drug Administration-approved prospective trial of primary intracranial stenting for acute stroke: SARIS (stent-assisted recanalization in acute ischemic stroke). *Stroke* 2009;40(11):3552–3556.

48. Kim GE, et al. Incidence and clinical significance of acute reocclusion after emergent angioplasty or stenting for underlying intracranial stenosis in patients with acute stroke. *AJNR Am J Neuroradiol* 2016;37(9):1690–1695.

49. McManus M, Liebeskind DS. Blood pressure in acute ischemic stroke. *J Clin Neurol* 2016;12(2):137–146.

50. Leonardi-Bee J, et al. Blood pressure and clinical outcomes in the International Stroke Trial. *Stroke* 2002;33(5):1315–1320.

51. Mazya M, et al. Predicting the risk of symptomatic intracerebral hemorrhage in ischemic stroke treated with intravenous alteplase: Safe Implementation of Treatments in Stroke (SITS) symptomatic intracerebral hemorrhage risk score. *Stroke* 2012;43(6):1524–1531.

52. Powers WJ, et al. Extracranial-intracranial bypass surgery for stroke prevention in hemodynamic cerebral ischemia: The Carotid Occlusion Surgery Study randomized trial. *JAMA* 2011;306(18):1983–1992.

53. Gonzalez NR, et al. Encephaloduroarteriosynangiosis for adult intracranial arterial steno-occlusive disease: Long-term single-center experience with 107 operations. *J Neurosurg* 2015;123(3):654–661.

54. Chaturvedi S, et al. Do patient characteristics explain the differences in outcome between medically treated patients in SAMMPRIS and WASID? *Stroke* 2015;46:2562–2567.

55. Kernan WN, et al. Guidelines for the prevention of stroke in patients with stroke and transient ischemic attack: A guideline for healthcare professionals from the American Heart Association/American Stroke Association. *Stroke* 2014;45(7):2160–2236.

53

Endovascular aneurysm repair

SAAD HUSSAIN SYED AND AAMER ABBAS

INTRODUCTION

An abdominal aortic aneurysm (AAA) is defined as an area of the aorta with an arterial diameter of more than 30 mm and is most commonly located in the infrarenal aorta. Another definition that has been postulated is an increase of more than 50% of the estimated normal infrarenal aortic diameter.[1-3] The normal adult human aortic diameter can differ due to age, gender, and body habitus, while the normal infrarenal aortic diameter is 2 cm and always less than 3 cm.[4]

The prevalence of AAAs in men with a diameter of 2.9–4.9 cm in two age groups of 45–54 and 75–84 are 1.3% and 12.5%, respectively. In women, it ranges from 0% in the youngest to 5.2% in the oldest age groups.[5] Typically, AAAs are found in older individuals. In 2013, the U.S. Centers for Disease Control and Prevention (CDC) reported AAAs being the 15th leading cause of death with 4.1 deaths per 100,000 people in the age range of 60–64 years; when stratified by gender, most of the deaths were found in men.[6] AAA is the cause of death for 0.13% of males, compared with 0.07% of females.[7] A meta-analysis of 18 studies reported a mean growth rate of 2.21 mm per year, independent of age and gender, with small AAAs having a diameter range of 3–5.4 cm. Subgroup analysis showed growth rate was higher in smokers than ex- or nonsmokers, and lower in patients with diabetes than nondiabetics. Furthermore, incidence of AAA rupture ranges from 0.71 to 11.03 per 1,000 person-years and is more frequent in smokers (pooled HR, 2.02; 95% CI, 1.33–3.06) and women (pooled HR, 3.76; 95% CI, 2.58–5.47).[8]

The reasons for the development of AAA are not clearly apparent. The postulated mechanism is migration of inflammatory cells into the aortic wall, which increases collagen degradation and leads to aneurysm formation. Transmural inflammation seen in AAA encompasses many different types of inflammatory cells, predominantly macrophages and lymphocytes, as compared to mast cells and neutrophils. Most of the lymphocytes are CD^{4+} T cells, T helper 1 (Th1) and Th17 cells, whereas infiltration by anti-inflammatory regulatory T cells (Treg) and Th2 cells is found at a lower rate. Proinflammatory M1 macrophages are more common as compared to anti-inflammatory M2 macrophages, and the levels of M1-associated proinflammatory cytokines, like interleukin (IL)-1b, IL-6, IL-8, interferon (IFN)-g, tumor necrosis factor (TNF)-a, and monocyte chemoattractant protein-1 (MCP-1), are elevated in both human aneurysmal tissue and serum.[9,10]

CLASSIFICATION AND RISK FACTORS

Several classifications are used to describe AAA. The following two are based on size and location:

1. AAA can be classified on the basis of size of the aortic aneurysm:

   - Small aneurysms—diameter <4 cm
   - Medium aneurysms—diameter between 4 and 5.5 cm
   - Large aneurysms—diameter >5.5 cm
   - Very large aneurysms—diameter ≥6 cm

2. The Crawford classification of aortic aneurysm is as follows (Figure 53.1):

- Extent I, from just distal to the left subclavian artery to above the renal arteries
- Extent II, from just distal to the left subclavian artery to below the renal arteries
- Extent III, from the sixth intercostal space to below the renal arteries
- Extent IV, from the 12th intercostal space to below the renal arteries (total AAA)
- Extent V, below the sixth intercostal space to just above the renal arteries[11]

Advanced age, male gender, and smoking are important risk factors for AAA. In addition, positive family history of AAA in a first-degree relative leads to increased risk for developing AAA. Studies have reported smoking being a strong individual risk factor, with odds ratio of >3 as compared to coronary artery disease or stroke. On the contrary, the incidence is lower among diabetics and ethnicities other than Caucasians.[15] Furthermore, certain factors have been associated with the development of AAA, such as greater height, hypertension, coronary artery disease, cerebrovascular disease, atherosclerosis, and high cholesterol; however, the data for some of these factors are not consistent to show a strong relationship with AAA.[12] Genetic studies showed an association of AAA with some variants of chromosome 9p21, and the occurrence of rs7025486[13] in the *DAB21P* gene increased the risk of AAA by 20%, with an odds ratio of 1.21 (95% CI 1.14–1.28).[14]

CLINICAL PRESENTATION AND DIAGNOSIS

Most patients are asymptomatic, and AAA is detected as an incidental finding on a routine imaging study performed for other medical reasons, or as part of the screening exam. Symptomatic AAA presents commonly with abdominal, back, or flank pain, and occasionally with thromboembolic phenomena causing symptoms of limb ischemia and systemic symptoms, such as fever and malaise. Severe pain, hypotension, and a pulsatile abdominal mass are considered symptoms of ruptured or rapidly expanding AAA in 50% of cases. Whereas, for other cases where presentation is atypical, delayed medical attention leads to complications.[12,16–19]

For diagnostic purposes, ultrasound is considered a safe, reliable, and inexpensive initial imaging test for confirming AAA in asymptomatic patients who are suspected of having AAA on physical exam. Sensitivity and specificity of ultrasound is 100% if AAA is more than 3 cm.[20] In addition, ultrasound is useful in following up asymptomatic small and medium-sized AAA patients. In contrast, physical exam has poor sensitivity specificity and is only helpful in large aneurysms. High-resolution computed tomography (CT) scans are routinely done for preoperative planning purposes and are considered the diagnostic test of choice in symptomatic AAA patients presenting with an impending rupture. Contrast is not usually required for diagnosis, but it can easily show extravasation of contrast in ruptured AAA.[21–22] In symptomatic AAA without rupture, CT can show signs, such as the crescent sign, breaks in wall calcification, or aortic blebs.[13,23–25]

SCREENING GUIDELINES

Three specific screening guidelines by various societies are outlined in Tables 53.1, 53.2, and 53.3.[12,26]

TREATMENT

The following are the main indications for treatment of AAA and are outlined in Tables 53.4, 53.5, and 53.6, as specified by the American College of Cardiology (ACC), American Heart Association (AHA) and European guidelines:[26,136]

1. Size >5.5 cm (as mortality increases significantly beyond this cutoff)
2. Aggressive nature of enlargement with >0.5 cm increase in size in last 6 months (regardless of the overall size)
3. Symptomatic regardless of the size

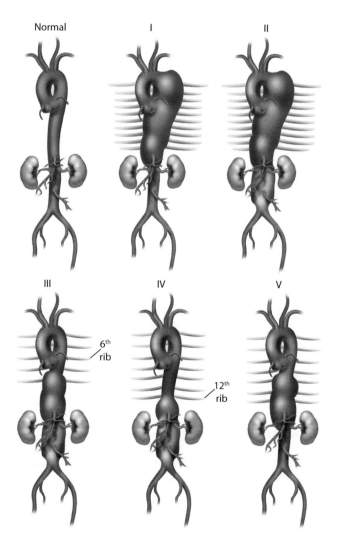

Figure 53.1 Modified Crawford Classification of Thoracoabdominal Aortic Aneurysm. (Courtesy of Warren Love.)

Randomized trials: open surgical versus endovascular aneurysm repair in nonruptured abdominal aortic aneurysm

The UK Endovascular Aneurysm Repair (EVAR) 1 trial[28] enrolled 1,252 patients in 37 UK hospitals with a maximum aortic aneurysm diameter of >5.5 cm; patients were randomized for open or endovascular repair. The 30-day immediate postoperative death rates were 1.8% for EVAR and 4.3% for open repair (P = 0.02), a remarkable advantage for EVAR. However, at the end of follow-up, both all-cause death rates (survival curve convergence at 2 years) and aneurysm-related death rates (survival curve convergence at 6 years) were equivalent between the two groups (Table 53.7).

The Dutch Randomized Endovascular Aneurysm Management (DREAM) Trial[29] enrolled 351 patients from 30 centers in the Netherlands and Belgium with a maximum AAA diameter of >5 cm; these patients were randomized to undergo either open or endovascular repair. The 30-day postoperative death rates were 1.2% after EVAR and 4.6% after open repair (risk ratio 3.9; 95% CI, 0.9–32.9). By the end of follow-up, all-cause death rates (survival curve convergence at 1 year) were equivalent between groups (Table 53.7).

The Open Versus Endovascular Repair (OVER) trial[30] enrolled 881 patients from 42 U.S. Veterans Affairs Medical Centers with an AAA maximum diameter of >5 cm, an iliac aneurysm of >3 cm, or an AAA of >4.5 cm and who had rapid AAA enlargement (>0.5 mm in 6 months) or saccular morphology. Patients were randomized to undergo either open or endovascular repair. The 30-day death rates were 0.5% after EVAR and 3% after open repair (P = 0.004). By the end of follow-up, all-cause death rates (survival curve convergence at 2 years) were equivalent between groups. Patients in the EVAR group had reduced procedure time, blood loss, transfusion requirement, duration of mechanical ventilation, length of hospital stay, and length of intensive care unit stay (Table 53.7).

Hence, short-term mortality and morbidity are significantly better with EVAR as compared to open repair; however, long-term outcomes are similar in both groups.

Table 53.1 American College of Cardiology/American Heart Association screening recommendations for abdominal aortic aneurysm (AAA)

Men 60 years of age or older who are either the siblings or offspring of patients with AAAs should undergo physical examination and ultrasound screening for detection of aortic aneurysms. (Level of Evidence: B)	Class I
Men who are 65 to 75 years of age who have ever smoked should undergo a physical examination and one-time ultrasound screening for detection of AAAs. (Level of Evidence: B)	Class IIa

Source: Adapted from Anderson, J.L., et al., Circulation, 127(13), 1425–1443, 2013.

Table 53.2 U.S. Preventive Services Task Force screening recommendations

One time screening for AAA in men between the ages of 65 and 75 who ever smoked	Grade B	Offer or provide service
Clinicians selectively offer screening of AAA in men with ages between 65 and 75 who never smoked, rather than screening all men in this group	Grade C	Offer or provide service for selected patients based on individual circumstance
Insufficient evidence for screening for AAA in women aged 65 to 75 years who have ever smoked.	Grade I	Insufficient evidence
Recommend against screening in women with AAA who never smoked	Grade D	Not recommended

Source: Adapted from LeFevre, M.L., Ann. Intern. Med., 161(4), 281–290, 2014.
Note: AAA, abdominal aortic aneurysm.

Table 53.3 Society of Vascular Surgery screening guidelines for abdominal aortic aneurysm (AAA)

Patient category	Level of recommendation	Quality of evidence
One-time ultrasound screening for AAA is recommended for all men at or older than 65 years. Screening men as early as 55 years is appropriate for those with a family history of AAA.	Strong	High
One-time ultrasound screening for AAA is recommended for all women at or older than 65 years with a family history of AAA or who have smoked.	Strong	Moderate
Re-screening patients for AAA is not recommended if an initial ultrasound scan performed on patients 65 years of age or older demonstrates an aortic diameter of <2.6 cm.	Strong	Moderate

Source: From Chaikof, E.L., et al., J. Vasc. Surg., 50(4 Suppl), S2–S49, 2009. With permission.

Table 53.4 Treatment guidelines: American College of Cardiology / American Heart Association recommendations for abdominal aortic aneurysm (AAA) repair on basis of size

Patients with infrarenal or juxtarenal AAAs measuring 5.5 cm or larger should undergo repair to eliminate the risk of rupture. *(Level of Evidence: B)*	Class I
Patients with infrarenal or juxtarenal AAAs measuring 4.0 to 5.4 cm in diameter should be monitored by ultrasound or computed tomographic scans every 6 to 12 months to detect expansion. *(Level of Evidence: A)*	Class I
Repair can be beneficial in patients with infrarenal or juxtarenal AAAs 5.0 to 5.4 cm in diameter. *(Level of Evidence: B)*	Class IIa
Repair is probably indicated in patients with suprarenal or type IV thoracoabdominal aortic aneurysms larger than 5.5 to 6.0 cm. *(Level of Evidence: B)*	Class IIa
In patients with AAAs smaller than 4.0 cm in diameter, monitoring by ultrasound examination every 2 to 3 years is reasonable. *(Level of Evidence: B)*	Class IIa
Intervention is not recommended for asymptomatic infrarenal or juxtarenal AAAs if they measure less than 5.0 cm in diameter in men or less than 4.5 cm in diameter in women. *(Level of Evidence: A)*	Class III

Source: Adapted from Anderson, J.L., et al., *Circulation*, 127(13), 1425–1443, 2013.

Table 53.5 American College of Cardiology / American Heart Association recommendations for abdominal aortic aneurysm repair on basis of symptoms

In patients with the clinical triad of abdominal and/or back pain, a pulsatile abdominal mass, and hypotension, immediate surgical evaluation is indicated. *(Level of Evidence: B)*	Class I
In patients with symptomatic aortic aneurysms, repair is indicated regardless of diameter. *(Level of Evidence: C)*	Class I

Source: Adapted from Anderson, J.L., et al., *Circulation*, 127(13), 1425–1443, 2013.

Table 53.6 Management of abdominal aortic aneurysms in clinical practice—Guidelines of the European Society for Vascular Surgery

Men should be considered for surgery when the maximum aortic diameter reaches 5.5 cm or more. Level 1b, Recommendation A.
Patients with a higher risk of rupture should be considered for surgery when the maximum aortic diameter reaches 5.0 cm. Level 3, Recommendation C.

Source: Adapted from Erbel R, Aboyans V, Boileau C, et al., *Eur Heart J* 2014;35(41):2873–2926.

Open repair versus endovascular aneurysm repair in ruptured abdominal aortic aneurysms

Similar mortality rates have been reported for open versus endovascular repair of ruptured AAAs. However, some evidence does favor better perioperative (30-day) outcomes for EVAR after ruptured AAA.[31–39] Therefore, for high-risk patients with multiple comorbidities and with suitable anatomy, an endovascular approach is recommended. Certain studies, including randomized controlled trials (RCTs) and registries, link endovascular repair of ruptured AAA to lower mortality rates when compared with open repair of ruptured AAA (EVAR, 16%–31%; open, 34%–44%).[33,38,40–50] However, selection bias was a concern as hemodynamically stable patients with ruptured AAA were treated with EVAR, whereas unstable patients with ruptured AAA were taken to the operating room for open approach.

In the setting of ruptured AAA, the IMPROVE trial is the largest with 613 patients. It was conducted in 30 centers in the United Kingdom and Canada and compared endovascular versus open repair. Thirty-day mortality was 35.4% (112/316) in the endovascular strategy group and 37.4% (111/297) in the open repair group; odds ratio 0.92 (95% CI 0.66–1.28; $P = 0.62$). At 1 year, all-cause mortality was 41.1% for the endovascular strategy group and 45.1% for the open repair group; odds ratio 0.85 (95% CI 0.62–1.17; $P = 0.325$), with similar re-intervention rates in each group (Table 53.7).[52]

In the multicenter Dutch AJAX trial, 116 patients were assigned to open repair or EVAR on the basis of anatomically suitability. The 30-day mortality was 21% (12 of 57) in patients who had EVAR versus 25% (15 of 59) in those who had open repair (ARR = 4.4%; 95% CI: −11% to +20%) (Table 53.7).[53]

The French ECAR (Endovasculaire ou Chirurgie dans les Anévrysmes aorto-iliaques Rompus) trial compared EVAR versus open repair in ruptured AAA patients who were hemodynamically stable at time of presentation and clinically and anatomically suitable for both EVAR or open repair. The ECAR trial was designed to avoid as many potential biases as possible. A total of 107 patients were enrolled, and 30-day mortality in EVAR versus open repair. was 19% versus 24%, and 1-year mortality was 33% versus 35%, respectively (Table 53.7).[54]

Perioperative morbidity has been considerably lower for EVAR as opposed to open repair in randomized trials of elective EVAR.[55–60] In looking at these results, it can be said that EVAR would be very favorable in patients with ruptured AAA who have unfavorable prognostic factors for open repair. The main benefit of EVAR in patients with ruptured AAA is likely due to its minimally invasive nature, which reduces physiologic stress of blood loss and ischemia and decreases the risk of subsequent cardiovascular,

Table 53.7 Summary of the results from the randomized controlled trials for both ruptured and non-ruptured abdominal aortic aneurysm (AAA) treated either with endovascular aneurysm repair (EVAR) or open repair

Trial	Short-term mortality	Long-term mortality
EVAR1 trial[28]		
EVAR (n=626)	1.8% at 30 days	23.1% at 4 years
Open AAA (n=626)	4.3% at 30 days	22.3% at 4 years
DREAM trial[29]		
EVAR (n=173)	1.2% at 30 days	31.1% at 6 years
Open AAA (n=178)	4.6% at 30 days	30.1% at 6 years
OVER trial[30]		
EVAR (n=444)	0.5% at 30 days	7.0% at 2 years
Open AAA (n=437)	3.0% at 30 days	9.8% at 2 years
AJAX trial[53]		
EVAR (n=116)	21% at 30 days	
Open AAA (n=116)	25% at 30 days	
ECAR trial[54]		
EVAR (n=107)	19% at 30 days	30%at 1 year
Open AAA (n=107)	24% at 30 days	35% at 1 year
IMPROVE trial[51,52]		
EVAR (n=275)	35.4% at 30 days	41.1% at 1 year
Open AAA (n=261)	37.4% at 30 days	45.1% at 1 year

Source: Courtesy of Saad Syed, M.D.

pulmonary, and renal morbidity. Even though efforts have been made to measure the risk of mortality with ruptured AAA, no variable or classification seems dependable for calculating mortality with certainty.[61] Summary data for both ruptured and nonruptured AAA treated with EVAR versus the open approach are outlined in Table 53.7.

TECHNICAL ASPECTS OF GRAFT DEPLOYMENT

Endovascular repair of ruptured AAA is restricted to facilities with a defined program for emergency endovascular surgery. Certain centers have taken upon an "EVAR first" approach to ruptured AAA, where EVAR is tried initially with an option to open conversion if needed.[21,43,55,62] The majority of EVAR procedures is performed in hemodynamically stable patients. However, in unstable patients with ruptured aorta, an aortic occlusion balloon is positioned through a long femoral sheath.[63–65] For infrarenal aortic rupture, the balloon needs to be repositioned just distal to the renal arteries to reserve renal blood flow while the device is deployed. Intermittent deflation of the balloon might be needed throughout the course of endograft placement. Preprocedure planning and anatomical assessment based on imaging studies are key for a successful outcome of an EVAR procedure. Anatomical characteristics for pre-procedure planning of EVAR are provided in Table 53.8.

Table 53.8 Anatomical characteristic for pre-procedure planning of endovascular aneurysm repair

Landing zone (Neck length)
Angle of neck
Diameter of healthy aortic segment
Diameter of iliac artery and common femoral artery
Tortuosity of aorta and access site vessels
Calcification and thrombosis of thrombus
Identify branch vessel inferior mesenteric, lumbar, and internal iliac arteries

Source: Courtesy of Saad Syed, M.D.

Preprocedure planning

EVAR in an elective setting entails a detailed preprocedure plan. High-resolution CT scans with three-dimensional (3D) reconstruction are usually required to assess the anatomy of the aorta and its branch vessels, the diameter of the access site vessel, neck angulation and length of neck, tortuosity of the aorta, and presence of calcification and thrombus. These are all important prerequisites of preprocedure planning. In addition, anticipation of coiling of branch vessels, which can become a potential source of a Type II endoleak, or preservation of branch vessels to avoid renal or pelvic ischemia, need to be considered as part of the planning (Table 53.8).

Access and imaging

The access site for the placement of a large delivery sheath for graft delivery plays a critical role in the successful outcome of EVAR. The choice of percutaneous femoral access or open femoral access is up to the discretion of the operator and based on the anatomic suitability of the access site. A list of U.S. Food and Drug Administration (FDA)–approved devices for infrarenal aneurysm repair is outlined in Tables 53.9 and 53.10. Percutaneous femoral access is closed with sutures based on the FDA's approved closure devices: Abbott Prostar XL and Abbott Perclose Proglide, which is deployed before sheath placement. As with open repair, vertical or oblique skin incisions may be used to expose the common femoral artery. However, reported wound complication rates with femoral access by an open surgical cutdown approach are 2%–2.8% in EVAR.[66,67] According to the study by Swinnen et al., less wound infections were noted with a vertical approach versus transverse approach (2.6% vs. 8.7%), with $P = 0.062$.[68]

Angiography is typically performed with low osmolar, nonionic agents, and is the standard method for obtaining landmarks for graft deployment and ensuring adequate aneurysm exclusion. Digital subtraction angiography, specifically, allows for optimal visualization of the contrast. Often, preoperative imaging can be used to guide wire, catheter, and graft placement, thereby limiting intravenous (IV) contrast exposure. The contrast may also be diluted to reduce the risk of contrast-induced nephropathy. Alternatively, carbon dioxide may be substituted as the contrast agent or intravascular ultrasound (IVUS) can help provide specific information and reduce or eliminate the use of contrast.[69] For aortic procedures, 8–15 MHz transducers are selected, with lower frequencies offering the ability to view the entire artery while sacrificing resolution.[70]

Deployment

Large femoral and iliac arteries are required to accommodate both the ipsilateral and contralateral limbs of the endograft. While a combination of angled catheters, angled wires, hydrophilic wires, and stiff wires may be used to track the sheaths proximally, three options are available when hypoplastic, stenotic, occluded, or tortuous vessels preclude traditional femoral access for device delivery. This includes direct puncture, use of a conduit, and controlled dilation or rupture of the artery.[71] There are a few large aortoiliac branches that must be addressed during endovascular repairs of infrarenal AAAs. These branches include lumbar arteries, the inferior mesenteric artery (IMA), internal iliac arteries, and renal and accessory renal arteries. Although most Type II endoleaks in the setting of stable aneurysms are currently treated expectantly, there is some controversy regarding preoperative and intraoperative branch occlusion.[72] Patent IMAs and large lumbar arteries, which are potential sources of Type II endoleaks, may be occluded; likewise, hypogastric arteries that must be covered for an adequate distal seal may be occluded. Typically, transarterial embolization is performed with a combination of coils placed at the origin of these branches to occlude the orifice, yet preserve collateral flow. In addition, the Amplatzer plug can be used and allows for controlled occlusion of both small and large branches.[69] Occasionally, special techniques are used during the graft deployment process to preserve flow in the renal and pelvic beds (Figures 53.2 and 53.3).[69,73]

Chimney and snorkel technique

Graft deployment steps vary based on the endograft selected; however, there are many common features and a few differences that are worth mentioning. First, determination of the side of main body and contralateral leg delivery is dependent on access vessel diameter, iliac artery tortuosity, main body length, and iliac artery diameter. Clearly, if an iliac artery stenosis is present, delivery of the large main body through the larger side would carry less risk of iliac artery injury. While placement of the main body through a tortuous iliac artery could potentially be difficult, tortuosity could also make wire and catheter management during access of the contralateral gate difficult, as stored energy leads to loss of torque and prevents extracorporeal wire manipulation. Additionally, as limited combinations of aortic diameters, iliac artery diameters, and endograft lengths exist, device delivery involves matching vessel size with endograft availability. Second, deployment close to the renal arteries is preferred, but the grafts should be placed within a neck of relatively uniform diameter. Currently, according to the manufacturer's instructions for use, the Medtronic Endurant 2 device is the only device approved for use with 10-mm-long infrarenal necks; the Ovation graft is approved for 13 mm neck length, and other devices require at least 15 mm for the proximal neck length. Mural thrombus, along the infrarenal neck and suprarenal portion of the aorta, may also guide endograft selection in order to avoid thromboembolic complications, graft migration, or endoleaks. Certainly, wire, catheter, sheath, and device manipulation should be limited in patients with tremendous mural thrombus burden. A patient with isolated suprarenal disease may be better suited for a device without a suprarenal stent in order to minimize embolization into the renal arteries or distally. Infrarenal thrombus located along the seal zone of the neck should be approached cautiously, as significant circumferential thrombus burden is a relative contraindication for endograft use. Deployment distal to the lowest renal is preferred, unless using a custom Fenestrated graft (Cook Medical) to gain seal zone in the visceral aorta. If the thrombus load is mild, suprarenal fixation to healthy aortic tissue should be considered. Third, aortic angulation, while usually not a problem, must be considered before graft selection and deployment. The majority of the endografts are contraindicated with necks of more than 60° of angulation.

Graft selection and deployment usually require consideration of aortic length, aortic diameter at the level of the contralateral gate, the narrowest aortic diameter, position

Table 53.9 FDA-approved devices for primary infrarenal aortic aneurysm repair

Company	Cook Medical	Endologix	Gore	Medtronic	TriVascular	Lombard	Cardinal Health
Product name	Zenith Flex	AFX	Excluder	Endurant II/EIIs	Ovation	Aorfix	Incraft
Stent material	Stainless steel, Nitinol[a]	Cobalt Chromium	Nitinol	Nitinol	Nitinol	Nitinol	Nitinol
Graft material	Polyester	DURAPLY ePTFE	ePTFE	Polyester	PTFE	Polyester	Polyester
Indications							
Neck length (seal zone)	≥15 mm	≥15 mm	≥15 mm	≥10 mm	@ 13 mm	≥15 mm	≥10 mm
Neck diameter	18–32 mm	18–32 mm	19–32 mm	19–32 mm	16–30 mm	19–34 mm	17–31 mm
Iliac length (seal zone)	≥10 mm	≥15 mm	≥10 mm	≥15 mm	≥10 mm	≥15 mm	≥10 mm
Iliac diameter	7.5–20 mm	10–23 mm	8–25 mm	8–25 mm	8–25 mm	9–19 mm	7–22 mm
Neck angle	≤60	≤60	≤60	≤60	≤45[g] or ≤60[h]	≤90	≤60
Graft Specs							
Main body diameter	22, 24, 26, 28, 30, 32, 36 mm	22, 25, 28 mm	23, 26, 28.5, 31, 35 mm	23, 25, 28, 32, 36 mm	20, 23, 26, 29, 34 mm	24, 26, 27, 28, 31, 36 mm	22, 26, 30, 34 mm
Main body length	112–179 mm	40–120 mm[c], 30–55 mm[d]	120–180 mm	124–166 mm; 103 mm[i]; 102 mm	80 mm	81–126 mm	96 mm
Ipsi limb diameter	12 mm	13, 16, 20 mm	12, 14.5 mm	13, 16, 20 mm; 14 mm[i/j]	14 mm	10, 12, 14, 16, 20 mm	11 mm
Main body profile (OD)	21, 23, 25 Fr	19.2 Fr	20.4 Fr	18, 20 Fr	14, 15 Fr	22 Fr	14, 16 Fr
Main body Profile (mm)	7.0, 7.7, 8.3 mm	6.5 mm	6.8 mm	6.0, 6.7 mm	4.7, 5.0 mm	7.3 mm	4.7, 5.3 mm
Method of fixation	Suprarenal, Active	Anatomical	Infrarenal, Active	Suprarenal, Active	Supraceliac, Active	Active	Suprarenal, Active
Method of seal	Radial force	Radial force	Radial force	Radial force	Polymer-filled O-rings	Radial force	Radial force
Iliac limb diameter	8–24 mm[b], 9–24 mm[a]	13–25 mm	10–27 mm	10–28 mm	10–28 mm	10–20 mm	10–24 mm
Iliac limb length	39–122 mm	55–88 mm	70–140 mm	82–199 mm	80–160 mm	54–106 mm	82–138 mm
Iliac limb profile (OD)	18, 20 Fr	19.2 Fr	15, 20.4 Fr	14, 16 Fr	12, 13, 14, 15 Fr	20 Fr	12, 13 Fr
Iliac limb profile (mm)	6.0, 6.7 mm	6.5 mm	5.0, 6.8 mm	4.7, 5.3 mm	4.0, 4.3, 4.7, 5.0 mm	6.7 mm	4.0, 4.3 mm
Aortic cuff diameter	22, 24, 26, 28, 30, 32, 36 mm	25, 28, 34 mm[f]	23, 26, 28.5, 32, 36 mm	23, 25, 28, 32, 36 mm	N/A	24, 26, 27, 28, 31 mm	N/A
Hydrophilic-coated	Yes	Yes	No	Yes	Yes	Yes	Yes
Sheath required	Integrated	Yes	Yes	No	Integrated	Integrated	Integrated

Source: Data courtesy of Endovascular Today 2017, Buyers Guide.
[a] Spiral-Z iliac limbs; [b] Flex limbs; [c] Main body length; [d] Main body limb length; [e] Ipsilateral limb diameter(s); [f] Infrarenal and Suprarenal cuffs available; [g] Neck length <10 mm; [h] Neck length ≥10 mm; [i] EIIs; [j] AUI.

Table 53.10 FDA-approved devices for primary infrarenal aortic aneurysm repair. (Continued from Table 53.9.)

Device	CT measurement method[a]	Delivery sheath required	Minimum access diameter for main body 1 French = 1/3 mm (or 1 mm = 3 Fr)	Minimum access diameter for contralateral limb	Treatable aortic neck diameter	Minimum aortic length to bifurcation	Minimum aortic neck length	Maximum aortic angulation[b]	Suprarenal Fixation	Treatable iliac diameter	Minimum iliac seal zone
Cook Zenith Flex	Outer diameter	No	22–26 mm graft = 7.1 mm 28–32 mm graft = 7.7 mm 36 mm graft	8–10 mm graft = 5.3 mm 12–24 mm graft = 6.0 mm	18–32 mm	22–32 mm graft = 82 mm 36 mm graft = 95 mm	15 mm	<60 degrees, <45 degrees[c]	Mandatory	7.5–20 mm	10 mm
Endologix Powerlink	Outer diameter	No	7 mm	3 mm	18–32 mm	25–28 mm graft = 80 mm 34 mm graft = 100 mm	15 mm	<60 degrees	Available	10–23 mm	15 mm
Gore Excluder	Inner diameter	Yes	23–8.5 mm graft = 6.8 31 graft = 7.6 mm	12–14.5 mm graft = 4.7 mm 16–20 mm graft = 6.8 mm	19–29 mm	70 mm	15 mm	<60 degrees	Not Available	10–18.5 mm	10 mm
Gore C3	Inner diameter	Yes	23–8.5 mm graft = 6.8 mm 31 mm graft = 7.6 mm	12–14.5 mm graft = 4.7 mm 16–20 mm graft = 6.8 mm	19–29 mm	70 mm	15 mm	<60 degrees	Not Available	10–18.5 mm	10 mm
Medtronic AneuRx	Outer diameter	No	7 mm	5 mm	16–26 mm	80 mm	15 mm	<45 degrees	Not Available	10–22 mm	25 mm
Medtronic Endurant	Inner diameter	No	23–25 mm graft = 5.7 mm 28–35 mm graft = 6.4mm	10–16 mm graft = 4.5 mm 20–28 mm graft = 5.1 mm	19–32 mm	124 mm length graft = 74 mm 145–166 mm length grafts = 84 mm	10 mm	≤60 degrees	Mandatory	8–25 mm	15 mm
Medtronic EII/EIIs	Inner diameter	No	23–28 mm graft = 18 Fr 32–36 mm graft = 20 Fr	10–16 mm = 14 Fr 20–28 mm = 16Fr All 156 mm and 199 mm limbs are 16 Fr	19–32 mm	124 mm length graft = 74 mm 145–166 mm length grafts = 84 mm EIIs = 103 mm length graft requires 84 mm	10 mm	≤ 60 degrees	Mandatory	8–25 mm	15 mm
Medtronic Talent	Outer diameter	No	22–28 mm graft = 7 mm 30–36 mm graft = 8 mm	6 mm	18–32 mm	80 mm	10 mm	<60 degrees	Available	8–22 mm	25 mm
Cook Renu Converter	Outer diameter	No	22–26 mm graft = 7.1 mm 28–32 mm graft = 7.7 mm 36 mm graft = 8.5 mm		18–32 mm[b]	22–32 mm graft = 82 mm 36 mm graft = 95 mm	15 mm[c]	<60 degrees, <45 degrees[d]	Mandatory	7.5–20 mm	10 mm

Source: Data courtesy of Endovascular Today 2017, Buyers Guide.

a Angulation of neck relative to long axis of aorta.

b New graft must be oversized 2 mm if placed within a pre-existing graft.

c Neck must be ≥10 mm if new graft is placed within pre-existing graft.

d Angulation of suprarenal stent relative to long axis of aorta.

Chimney technique

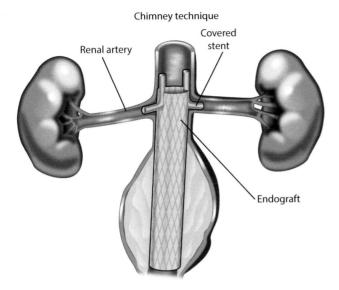

Figure 53.2 Chimney technique. The brachial or axillary approach is used to position and deploy the covered stent in the renal artery, with the stent extending into the aorta in a cranial direction. A standard endovascular aneurysm repair is then performed with care to simultaneously dilate the renal artery conduit and aortic graft to preserve renal perfusion and achieve an adequate proximal aortic seal. (Courtesy of Warren Love.)

of the iliac arteries, and iliac artery length. Currently, the Gore Excluder and Gore C3 have the shortest bodies, allowing the contralateral gate to be opened 70 mm below the top of the covered stents. Most often, however, long main bodies are preferred, as opening the contralateral gate in proximity to the common iliac artery orifice facilitates gate cannulation. Another factor in determining the main body length is the aortic diameter, both at the site of the contralateral gate and the narrowest point, as the diameter must be sufficient to prevent limb constriction. Circumferential calcification along narrow segments is particularly troublesome, as it often prevents graft expansion and seal. Additionally, depending on iliac artery position and length, the main body may be rotated up to 180° to facilitate contralateral gate cannulation or slightly shorten the iliac limbs. Conveniently, the Gore C3 is the only device that allows a portion of the graft to be recaptured to facilitate repositioning of the proximal graft and contralateral gate. Several programs, such as those of M2S and Tera Recon, are available to help with this planning by constructing 3D imaging and predicting center lines. Freestyle cannulation of the contralateral gate is most often performed with an angled catheter and wire. When this fails, a selective catheter placed from the ipsilateral limb or upper extremity can be used in combination with a snare to obtain wire access into the contralateral gate. If difficulty with contralateral gate cannulation is anticipated, the Endologix Powerlink graft may be used, as it employs a bifurcated unibody design that is deployed, pulled down onto the aortic bifurcation, and then modified with proximal and distal extensions, if needed.[69]

Snorkel-sandwich technique

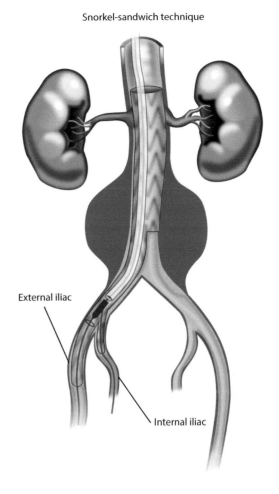

Figure 53.3 Snorkel—Sandwich technique. If the distal limbs must be extended into the external iliac arteries, the risk of pelvic ischemia and paralysis increases. Internal iliac arteries may be preserved with a "snorkel technique." The internal iliac artery can be accessed through a brachial, axillary, ipsilateral, or contralateral femoral approach, depending on the anatomy and angulation of the internal iliac artery with respect to the common and external iliac artery. Wire and catheter exchanges are performed as necessary to enable sheath advancement for covered stent placement. A standard iliac extension is then performed into the external iliac artery via ipsilateral femoral access. "Kissing balloons" are inflated in both the internal and external iliac limbs to fully expand the grafts. (Courtesy of Warren Love.)

In order to reduce contrast and radiation exposure, investigations are being performed on noninvasive remote aneurysm sac pressure measurements, primarily using the Cardio Mems Endosure Wireless AAA Pressure Sensor. This device, which is about the size of a paperclip, requires transcatheter placement through a 14-Fr delivery device into the aneurysm sac after main body deployment. The sensor is interrogated, the contralateral limb is deployed, the sensor pressures are measured again, and then the sensor is finally deployed. Despite the paucity of evidence demonstrating device durability and efficacy, preliminary studies have demonstrated promising short-term results.[74–76]

Management of early endoleaks and compressed limbs

After graft deployment and inflation of a molding balloon, digital subtraction angiography or IVUS is used to assess for endoleaks. Some Type I endoleaks can be managed with simple angioplasty or graft extensions. Additionally, bare stents can be used to juxtapose the endograft to the arterial wall. Most early Type II endoleaks are managed initially with observation, with prompt return for reintervention for those who are symptomatic or who have enlargement of the aneurysm sac. Mild external compression of the contralateral limb may be treated with angioplasty with selective stent placement. Alternatively, compressed limbs, inaccessible contralateral gates, and persistent endoleaks are sometimes treated with a hybrid conversion, combining an aorto-uni-iliac converter device with a femoro-femoral bypass.[69] During elective EVAR, a Type II endoleak (back bleeding into the aneurysm sac) may first be observed since the majority will correct over time. However, after endovascular repair for ruptured AAA, a Type II endoleak will not tamponade spontaneously; thus, when a Type II endoleak is seen, open surgical ligation of the back bleeding vessel is required. Finally, for those complications that cannot be managed via endovascular or hybrid approach, open conversion with explantation of the endoprosthesis and traditional open repair can be performed.[69]

Closure

The delivery devices and sheaths should be withdrawn while maintaining wire access. If a change in hemodynamics occurs or a segment of artery is withdrawn with the sheath, occlusive balloons can be inflated for hemostasis. If needed, arterial injuries can then be addressed under a more controlled situation. Arteriotomy closure depends on the initial approach for access. If femoral access was obtained via a traditional open approach, a standard arteriotomy repair should be performed with subsequent layered closure of the wound. Alternatively, if the "preclose" technique was utilized, manual pressure is maintained proximally while the wounds and sutures are rinsed free of thrombus and the tract is confirmed to be fully dilated. The sutures are then tied with the knots carefully pushed down to, but not into, the artery. The wire should be removed before tying the second suture and a brief period of manual compression may be required after successful closure. Several studies have reported a low incidence of short- and midterm complications using the "preclose" technique[77–80] and 95% success with percutaneous closure techniques. Emergent femoral artery repair should be performed if significant hemorrhage persists or extremity ischemia develops. As expected, extensive calcification, groin scarring, and operator inexperience increase the risk of complications. If a conduit is sutured to the aorta or iliac arteries, it may be ligated and transected proximally or preserved for an aortofemoral or iliofemoral bypass. Alternatively, the conduit can be conserved for later

reintervention by the subcutaneous placement of the ligated end. Last, a lower extremity pulse examination should be performed to exclude acute ischemic changes. Ankle-brachial indices and Doppler signals may be obtained on the operating table and compared to preoperative assessments as objective adjuncts to the clinical examination. Any significant issues can thereby be addressed immediately.[69]

In conclusion, EVAR requires extensive preoperative preparation, not only for graft selection, but also for optimal deployment. One must consider the method of access, device delivery, management of large branches, graft orientation, and contralateral limb deployment. Once deployed, the graft must be assessed for endoleaks and limb compression before arteriotomy and wound closure. Failure to understand these EVAR techniques and adequately plan for each step can result in endoleaks, visceral malperfusion, and extremity ischemia, precipitating the need for emergent complex open repair.[69] Video 53.1 depicts one case of an aneurysm.

COMPLICATIONS OF ENDOVASCULAR ANEURYSM REPAIR

Several peri- and postprocedural complications of EVAR are outlined in Table 53.11. Up to 20% of patients who receive EVAR need secondary intervention, usually to treat endoleaks.[58,81,82] Complications after EVAR can be life-threatening and may require prompt diagnosis and intervention. Overall complication percentages are as high as 30%, and the percentage of later complications needing intervention is 2%–3%,[83,84] which are mainly done via endovascular technique. According to one study, repetitive interventions are necessary in 12%–35% of cases.[86,87] Lifelong imaging follow-up is required as most of these complications are asymptomatic. Complications may arise instantly after endograft placement or can arise from hemodynamic stress incurred on the device over time. Cumulative radiation risk is a concern as techniques, devices, and longevity of patients improve after treatment.[85]

Endoleaks are found in 15%–25% of individuals within the initial 30 days after EVAR and are often asymptomatic.[89,90] Lifelong imaging surveillance is necessary for detection. Endoleaks are classified according to the origin

Table 53.11 Complications of endovascular aneurysm repair

Endoleak
Migration
Limb kinking or thrombosis
Infection
Renal complications
Bowel ischemia
Access site complications
Abdominal aortic aneurysm rupture

Source: Courtesy of Saad Syed, M.D.

Table 53.12 Endoleak classification

Type of endoleak	Source of blood flow
Type I	Stent-graft attachment sites
Type II	Inflow from collateral vessels
Type III	Structural stent-graft failure
Type IV	Endograft material porosity
Type V	Endotension

Source: Courtesy of Saad Syed, M.D.

of blood flow (Table 53.12). Although computed tomography angiography (CTA) is better for the identification of endoleaks, catheter angiography better shows the dynamics of blood flow critical for endoleak classification.[91]

A *Type I endoleak* results from a flow of blood into the aneurysm sac from an attachment site; this happens after approximately 10% of EVAR procedures[92] and an adequate proximal seal is needed to reduce the risk of a Type I endoleak. Stent grafts were formed with hooks and barbs to help reduce migration and proximal endoleak. Oversizing the endograft by 15%–20% also helps reach an adequate seal.[90] With a Type I endoleak, early intervention is necessary to reduce the risk of rupture. Treatment usually entails securing the attachment sites with angioplasty balloons, stents, or endograft extensions.[90,93] Treatment with coil embolization and glue has been effective in certain patients. If the neck has enlarged, placement of a fenestrated graft or chimney graft may avert surgical conversion.[94]

A *Type II endoleak* is most common, arising in 10%–25% of cases[92] due to retrograde flow into the aneurysm sac from collateral vasculature, usually the IMA or lumbar arteries. Pre-EVAR coil embolization of the IMA might decrease the incidence of Type II endoleaks and aneurysm sac enlargement.[95–98] Up to 40% of Type II endoleaks spontaneously thrombose, and immediate intervention is not always required.[90] Delayed Type II endoleaks arise more than 1 year after EVAR.[99] Treatment is usually started due to the potential for increased sac pressure and rupture.[100] Even though criteria are not evidence based, 5–10 mm of aneurysm sac expansion is usually the threshold for intervention. However, cases are present of rupture without sac expansion, suggesting that a more aggressive approach to Type II endoleak treatment might be needed.[101] Endovascular treatment entails embolization by a transarterial method or direct translumbar puncture. High-viscosity Onyx mixed with contrast agents has been used for postoperative embolization of clinically significant Type II endoleaks.[73]

A *Type III endoleak* arises from a structural stent-graft failure or disconnection between components, with an estimated incidence of 4% after 1 year.[90] CTA depicts contrast material next to the endograft, but often not within the aneurysm sac periphery, as is the case with a Type II endoleak. Arterial pulsation and sac shrinkage can alter the device or cause displacement and, therefore, result in a Type III endoleak.[102] Repair is needed due to the quick arterial pressurization of the aneurysm sac and the chance for

rupture. Endovascular repair typically involves the placement of a stent-graft extension or cuff in order to cover the site of leakage.

Type IV endoleaks are rare and arise from porosity in the graft material and can be viewed on the angiography instantly after placement. They typically resolve when coagulation is normalized. Type IV endoleaks were mostly noticed during placement of early generation devices and are usually of no clinical consequence.[89]

Type V endoleaks, also known as endotension, occur when there is amplification of the aneurysm sac without a noticeable leak on imaging.[89] This can be due to ultrafiltration of blood across the stent-graft with thrombus, providing an unsuccessful barrier to pressure transmission, infection, seroma, or unsuccessful attempt to catch the leak on imaging.[90,102] A Type V endoleak is a diagnosis of exclusion. Imaging with additional modalities, such as ultrasound and magnetic resonance angiography (MRA), need to be done in order to exclude an alternate type of endoleak that was not found on the initial surveillance study. Intervention, including conversion to open repair, might be needed in the presence of increasing aneurysm size (Table 53.8). Figure 53.4 summarizes the types of endoleaks and source of blood flow in the aneurysmal sac.

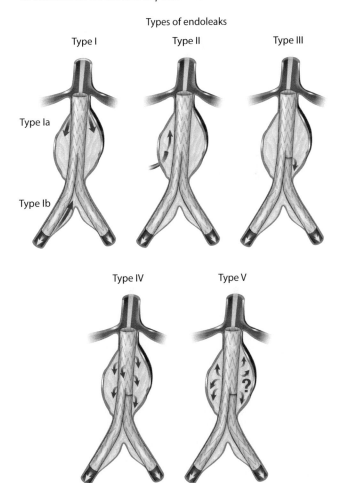

Figure 53.4 Types of endoleaks. (Courtesy of Warren Love.)

Graft migration of 5–10 mm is considered significant.[102] Landmarks, such as the superior mesenteric arteries (SMAs) and renal arteries, can be used to measure migration and provide a standard for comparison. The danger of migration is dependent on the type of device, neck diameter, configuration, and length of the landing zones.[103] Neck enlargement or other modifications in aneurysm morphologic structures over time can lead to migration, whereas suprarenal fixation is linked to a lower rate of migration.[104] Migration can result in endoleak, limb occlusion, and rupture. Extension cuffs are usually placed for treatment. Long-term results are predicted to yield lower rates of migration with new-generation devices.

Stent-graft kinking can arise from migration or decreasing aneurysm sac diameter and length. Kinking can cause migration, thrombosis, and a Type I or III endoleak. Excessive aortic neck angulation and a narrow distal aortic diameter are inclined to kink formation.[105] The reported incidence differs depending on the amount of kinking but is in the range of 1.7%–3.7%.[90,105] It is probable that new, low-profile devices will have higher rates of limb kinking and occlusion because of less radial force and columnar stent strength.[106] Additional high radial force uncovered stents may be placed in an effort to straighten kinks and avoid thrombosis. Limb occlusion is usually associated to kinking of the metallic skeleton, extension of the stent graft into tortuous or diminutive iliac arteries, or migration and dislocation of an endograft limb.[107]

Thrombosis of the graft can result due to excessive oversizing, causing folding of the graft material and twisting of the limbs during deployment.[108,109] The incidence of thrombosis is reported to be 0.5%–11%.[90] In scenarios of diminutive iliac arteries, it might be necessary to place an aorto-uni-iliac graft with a surgical bypass to avoid thrombosis. Thrombectomy and stent placement can be tried in order to salvage a thrombosed limb. Otherwise, a femoral-to-femoral artery bypass might be needed to revascularize the limb supplied by the thrombosed segment. In cases with an aneurysmal common iliac artery, snorkel stents or bifurcated iliac side-branch devices might be utilized to preserve flow to the internal iliac artery. Surveillance imaging needs to carefully analyze these devices for limb thrombosis, which can result in buttock claudication, especially when both internal iliac arteries are occluded.

Endograft infection is fairly rare, and occurs in less than 1% of cases.[110,111] Procedural contamination is the most probable cause of early infection. Although the stent-graft is secured by the intact aneurysm sac, remote sites of infection may lead to late colonization. Infection presents as leukocytosis, fever, and back pain. CT portrays mesenteric inflammation adjacent to the stent-graft, perigraft fluid collections, abnormal enhancement, or air bubbles. An aortoenteric fistula is an uncommon complication after EVAR that can cause massive hemorrhage, endograft infection, and hypovolemic shock.[112] Endoleaks resulting in aneurysm expansion may lead to erosion and aortoenteric fistula

formation.[113] Endograft infection and graft placement in inflammatory aneurysms are other frequently proposed causes for fistula formation.[112] Treatment can include *in situ* repair with resection of the infected graft and placement of an antibiotic-soaked polyester graft, autologous vein graft, or cryopreserved graft. Extra anatomic reconstruction is usually performed in high-risk cases. Patients will initially be given IV antibiotics, which will later be converted to an oral suppressive antibiotic regimen. The ideal duration of antibiotic therapy has not been determined and can be chronic in complicated cases.[111]

Renal failure incidence after EVAR is 6.7%;[114] a minimum of 50–100 mL of iodized IV contrast material is typically required during the case. The smallest possible dose of 50%/50% diluted iso-osmolar contrast material needs to be used in patients with renal insufficiency. A recent study proposes that patients who receive EVAR have a larger continuous decline in renal function over time as compared to those who undergo open aneurysm repair. This is probably due to the contrast agent given during the original procedure, secondary procedures to treat complications, and routine surveillance scans. Additional unenhanced surveillance protocols should lessen the long-term risk of renal function impairment.[115] Patients need to be well hydrated before and after the procedure. Pretreatment with sodium bicarbonate decreases contrast-induced nephrotoxicity, and acetylcysteine is also commonly given despite limited evidence of its efficacy. IVUS can be used to evaluate the anatomy prior to treatment and assess the endograft after placement.[116] Using IVUS can considerably reduce the amount of IV contrast material administered during stent-graft placement.[117]

Bowel ischemia is a serious but uncommon complication after EVAR. Thrombotic deposits and atheroma in the suprarenal aorta can be displaced during endograft placement and travel to the SMA, IMA, internal iliac arteries, and lower extremities. When involving the mesenteric circulation, microemboli might cause multifocal patchy bowel ischemia. Inadequate mesenteric collateral circulation is another proposed cause.[90,118] Colonic ischemia (CI) is a strong, independent predictor of postprocedural mortality. In one study, CI was more commonly associated with repair of ruptured aneurysms (8.9%, 756 patients) and elective open AAA repair (2.2%, 983 patients) than with EVAR (0.5%, 202 patients; $P < 0.001$).[112,119]

Structural endograft failure is now an uncommon complication and was more common with early generation devices.[120] It results from fatigue, corrosion, suture breakage, or graft fabric tear. Structural failures might happen in up to 5.5% of cases and result in unsuccessful attachment zone seal, migration, and endoleak.[108] Turbulent flow in the aneurysm sac because of an endoleak can contribute to early device fatigue and eventual failure.[102] It is probable that more device failures will be found as patients and devices age. A recent study showed that metallic ring failure and suture breakage can be detected on 3D CTA with the development of migration and Type I and Type III endoleaks, thus supporting the concept that fatigue degradation leads to delayed endoleaks.[121] Structural failures are often late occurrences, and vigilant long-term surveillance should be maintained for these complications.[120]

Access site complications arise in up to 3% of the percutaneous EVAR procedures,[112] which is conceivable in 76%–96% of patients, with success rates relying on patient selection.[122] Percutaneous EVAR reduces the rate of wound complications, operative time, and duration of hospital stay when looked at with traditional open femoral access.[122,123] Obesity, repeat groin access, larger sheath size, severe femoral artery calcification, access vessel size of less than 5 mm, and lack of operator capability are associated with percutaneous EVAR failure and conversion to open femoral access.[122,124,125] Research suggests that femoral artery calcification involving greater than 50% of the anterior vessel wall raises the risk of closure device failure.[123] Ultrasound guidance permits correct puncture in the common femoral artery and allows the operator to sidestep areas with large anterior calcifications. Several possible complications include arterial thrombosis, dissection, pseudoaneurysm formation, and local wound complications. Large delivery systems and sheath size can cause dissection and avulsion of the access arteries. Arterial dissection can be fixed with stenting if it is found during the procedure. Vessel rupture can happen when entering small or heavily calcified vessels and may not be obvious until the vascular sheath is removed at the end of the procedure.

Delayed AAA rupture after EVAR is uncommon and has been shown to occur in 0.5% of cases per year.[93] Treatment comprises endovascular revision or open surgical conversion. Ruptures can happen in patients without evidence of increasing aneurysm size on surveillance. This is probably due to sudden pressurization of the aneurysm sac from a Type I or III endoleak.[93] Mortality rates are significantly greater for secondary procedures performed after AAA rupture. Detailed imaging evaluation to narrow the cause of the endograft failure helps in surgical planning for either endovascular or open repair.[87] Endovascular therapy to treat the underlying failure usually involves graft extensions within the proximal or distal landing zones, or within the stent-graft components to adequately seal the rupture.

POST-ENDOVASCULAR ANEURYSM REPAIR SURVEILLANCE

CTA is the current reference standard for surveillance and is the primary imaging modality at most centers. CTA offers a sensitive evaluation for many imperative complications, and patients usually undergo numerous surveillance scans throughout their life. However, CT might not be the best modality for surveillance, mainly because of high accumulative radiation doses and the risk of contrast-induced nephropathy. Several studies portray the benefits of alternative ultrasound and magnetic resonance imaging (MRI) surveillance protocols. Each imaging modality comes with

its benefits and drawbacks, which should be carefully considered when developing a surveillance program.[85] CTA successfully detects migration, kinking, structural failure, endoleak, infection, and aneurysm growth.[126] Surveillance CTA typically includes unenhanced, arterial phase (30-second delay), and delayed phase (120- to 300-second delay) sequences. Unenhanced images are used to distinguish hyperdense calcifications from an endoleak, which may arise on the arterial or delayed phase. The delayed phase is critical to assess for a low-flow endoleak that may not be obvious on the earlier arterial phase images. A study utilizing a dynamic CT technique with multiple early scan phases[127] showed that the greatest rate of endoleak detection occurred 27 seconds after reaching the preset bolus tracking threshold. This study shows that the ideal timing for endoleak detection happens at a time point between standard arterial phase and venous phase images.[127] Contrast-induced nephropathy, cumulative radiation exposure, and cost are worries in lifelong CTA surveillance. Traditional surveillance protocols comprise a baseline CT at 1 month after repair, followed by 6-month interval scans with a transition to annual studies when complications are not present. Early aneurysm sac shrinkage might be linked with fewer late complications after EVAR.[128] Therefore, it may be appropriate to lengthen the interval to 1 year when the aneurysm sac is smaller than 5 cm or has reduced by 5 mm. When the sac size reduces to 4 cm, CT may then be obtained every 2–3 years.[129] Research also shows that the surveillance interval can be lengthened in the absence of complications on the 1-month post-treatment scan, and the 6-month follow-up scan may be excluded without negative outcomes.[130,131]

Limitations of ultrasound imaging are the presence of obesity and extensive arterial calcifications; but in the majority of cases, proximal and distal fixation sites and aneurysm sac size can be determined.[129]

MRA can identify luminal patency, device positioning, and residual sac flow. Nitinol stents are best suited for MRA, while stainless steel and cobalt-chromium-nickel alloy stents are ferromagnetic and might cause significant artifact.[89] Several reports show that MRA is more sensitive than CTA in endoleak identification.[102,132–135] With cases of endotension, the aneurysm sac increases in size without an appreciable endoleak on imaging. MRI should be considered in such cases as it is highly effective in detecting Type II endoleaks.

CONCLUSION

Based on available evidence, it appears that among AAA patients with suitable anatomy, EVAR is associated with a ~60% reduction in perioperative mortality, which comes at the cost of an increased reintervention rate. Despite the fact that the upfront mortality benefit is lost during follow-up, EVAR may be the preferred procedure in suitable patients. For all other AAA aneurysms that are not suitable for EVAR, open repair remains the standard of care.

VIDEO

- **Video 53.1 (https://youtu.be/qaz0wXFHQXg)**; Endovascular AAA Repair.

REFERENCES

1. Steinberg I, Stein HL. Arteriosclerotic abdominal aneurysms. Report of 200 consecutive cases diagnosed by intravenous aortography. *JAMA* 1966;195(12):1025–1029.
2. McGregor JC, Pollock JG, Anton HC. The value of ultrasonography in the diagnosis of abdominal aortic aneurysm. *Scott Med J* 1975;20(3):133–137.
3. Wanhainen A, Themudo R, Ahlström H, Lind L, Johansson L. Thoracic and abdominal aortic dimension in 70-year-old men and women—A population-based whole-body magnetic resonance imaging (MRI) study. *J Vasc Surg* 2008;47(3):504–512.
4. Johnston KW, Rutherford RB, Tilson MD, Shah DM, Hollier L, Stanley JC. Suggested standards for reporting on arterial aneurysms. Subcommittee on Reporting Standards for Arterial Aneurysms, Ad Hoc Committee on Reporting Standards, Society for Vascular Surgery and North American Chapter, International Society for Cardiovascular Surgery. *J Vasc Surg* 1991;13(3):452–458.
5. Witt BJ, Jacobsen SJ, Weston SA, et al. Cardiac rehabilitation after myocardial infarction in the community. *J Am Coll Cardiol* 2004;44(5):988–996.
6. *Deaths, percent of total deaths, and death rates for the 15 leading causes of death in 5-year age groups, by race, and sex.* www.cdc.gov/nchs/data/dvs/lcwk1_2013.pdf. (accessed June, 2016).
7. McPhee JT, Hill JS, Eslami MH. The impact of gender on presentation, therapy, and mortality of abdominal aortic aneurysm in the United States, 2001–2004. *J Vasc Surg* 2007;45(5):891–899.
8. Thompson SG, Brown LC, Sweeting MJ, et al. Systematic review and meta-analysis of the growth and rupture rates of small abdominal aortic aneurysms: Implications for surveillance intervals and their cost-effectiveness. *Health Technol Assess* 2013;17(41):1–118.
9. Dale MA, Ruhlman MK, Baxter BT. Inflammatory cell phenotypes in AAAs: Their role and potential as targets for therapy. *Arterioscler Thromb Vasc Biol* 2015;35(8):1746–1755.
10. Moxon JV, Parr A, Emeto TI, Walker P, Norman PE, Golledge J. Diagnosis and monitoring of abdominal aortic aneurysm: Current status and future prospects. *Curr Probl Cardiol* 2010;35(10):512–548.
11. Crawford ES, Crawford JL, Safi HJ, et al. Thoracoabdominal aortic aneurysms: Preoperative and intraoperative factors determining immediate and long-term results of operations in 605 patients. *J Vasc Surg* 1986;3(3):389–404.
12. Chaikof EL, Brewster DC, Dalman RL, et al. The care of patients with an abdominal aortic aneurysm: The Society for Vascular Surgery practice guidelines. *J Vasc Surg* 2009;50(4 Suppl):S2–S49.
13. Boules TN, Compton CN, Stanziale SF, et al. Can computed tomography scan findings predict "impending" aneurysm rupture? *Vasc Endovascular Surg* 2006;40(1):41–47.
14. Helgadottir A, Thorleifsson G, Magnusson KP, et al. The same sequence variant on 9p21 associates with myocardial infarction, abdominal aortic aneurysm and intracranial aneurysm. *Nat Genet* 2008;40(2):2172–2124.
15. Kent KC, Zwolak RM, Egorova NN, et al. Analysis of risk factors for abdominal aortic aneurysm in a cohort of more than 3 million individuals. *J Vasc Surg* 2010;52(3):539–548.
16. Rinckenbach S, Albertini JN, Thaveau F, et al. Prehospital treatment of infrarenal ruptured abdominal aortic aneurysms: A multicentric analysis. *Ann Vasc Surg* 2010;24(3):308–314.
17. Tsai YW, Blodgett JB, Wilson GS, Lucas RJ, Tumacder OC. Ruptured abdominal aortic aneurysm. Pathognomonic triad. *Vasc Surg* 1973;7(4):232–237.
18. Kiell CS, Ernst CB. Advances in management of abdominal aortic aneurysm. *Adv Surg* 1993;26:73–98.
19. Azhar B, Patel SR, Holt PJ, Hinchliffe RJ, Thompson MM, Karthikesalingam A. Misdiagnosis of ruptured abdominal aortic aneurysm: Systematic review and meta-analysis. *J Endovasc Ther* 2014;21(4):568–575.
20. LaRoy LL, Cormier PJ, Matalon TA, Patel SK, Turner DA, Silver B. Imaging of abdominal aortic aneurysms. *AJR Am J Roentgenol* 1989;152(4):785–792.
21. Mehta M, Taggert J, Darling RC, et al. Establishing a protocol for endovascular treatment of ruptured abdominal aortic aneurysms: Outcomes of a prospective analysis. *J Vasc Surg* 2006;44(1):1–8; discussion 8.
22. Chien DK, Chang WH, Yeh YH. Radiographic findings of a ruptured abdominal aortic aneurysm. *Circulation* 2010;122(18):1880–1881.
23. Siegel CL, Cohan RH, Korobkin M, Alpern MB, Courneya DL, Leder RA. Abdominal aortic aneurysm morphology: CT features in patients with ruptured and nonruptured aneurysms. *AJR Am J Roentgenol* 1994;163(5):1123–1129.
24. Arita T, Matsunaga N, Takano K, et al. Abdominal aortic aneurysm: Rupture associated with the high-attenuating crescent sign. *Radiology* 1997;204(3):765–768.
25. Mehard WB, Heiken JP, Sicard GA. High-attenuating crescent in abdominal aortic aneurysm wall at CT: A sign of acute or impending rupture. *Radiology* 1994;192(2):359–362.
26. Anderson JL, Halperin JL, Albert NM, et al. Management of patients with peripheral artery disease (compilation of 2005 and 2011 ACCF/AHA guideline recommendations): A report of the American College of Cardiology Foundation/American Heart Association Task Force on Practice Guidelines. *Circulation* 2013;127(13):1425–1443.
27. LeFevre ML, U.S Preventive Services Task Force. Screening for abdominal aortic aneurysm: U.S. Preventive Services Task Force recommendation statement. *Ann Intern Med* 2014;161(4):281–290.
28. Greenhalgh RM, Brown LC, Powell JT, et al. Endovascular versus open repair of abdominal aortic aneurysm. *N Engl J Med* 2010;362(20):1863–1871.
29. De Bruin JL, Baas AF, Buth J, et al. Long-term outcome of open or endovascular repair of abdominal aortic aneurysm. *N Engl J Med* 2010;362(20):1881–1889.
30. Lederle FA, Freischlag JA, Kyriakides TC, et al. Long-term comparison of endovascular and open repair of abdominal aortic aneurysm. *N Engl J Med* 2012;367(21):1988–1997.
31. Li Y, Li Z, Wang S, et al. Endovascular versus open surgery repair of ruptured abdominal aortic aneurysms in hemodynamically unstable patients: Literature review and meta-analysis. *Ann Vasc Surg* 2016;32:135–144.

32. van Beek SC, Conijn AP, Koelemay MJ, Balm R. Editor's choice—Endovascular aneurysm repair versus open repair for patients with a ruptured abdominal aortic aneurysm: A systematic review and meta-analysis of short-term survival. *Eur J Vasc Endovasc Surg* 2014;47(6):593–602.

33. Veith FJ, Lachat M, Mayer D, et al. Collected world and single center experience with endovascular treatment of ruptured abdominal aortic aneurysms. *Ann Surg* 2009;250(5):818–824.

34. Powell JT, Thompson SG, Thompson MM, et al. The immediate management of the patient with rupture: Open versus endovascular repair (IMPROVE) aneurysm trial—ISRCTN 48334791 IMPROVE trialists. *Acta Chir Belg* 2009;109(6):678–680.

35. Ten Bosch JA, Teijink JA, Willigendael EM, Prins MH. Endovascular aneurysm repair is superior to open surgery for ruptured abdominal aortic aneurysms in EVAR-suitable patients. *J Vasc Surg* 2010;52(1):13–18.

36. Ricotta JJ 2nd, Malgor RD, Oderich GS. Ruptured endovascular abdominal aortic aneurysm repair: Part II. *Ann Vasc Surg* 2010;24(2):269–277.

37. Coppi G, Gennai S, Saitta G, Silingardi R, Tasselli S. Treatment of ruptured abdominal aortic aneurysm after endovascular abdominal aortic repair: A comparison with patients without prior treatment. *J Vasc Surg* 2009;49(3):582–588.

38. Powell JT, Sweeting MJ, Thompson MM, et al. Endovascular or open repair strategy for ruptured abdominal aortic aneurysm: 30 day outcomes from IMPROVE randomised trial. *BMJ* 2014;348:f7661.

39. Mohan PP, Hamblin MH. Comparison of endovascular and open repair of ruptured abdominal aortic aneurysm in the United States in the past decade. *Cardiovasc Intervent Radiol* 2014;37(2):337–342.

40. Dillavou ED, Muluk SC, Makaroun MS. A decade of change in abdominal aortic aneurysm repair in the United States: Have we improved outcomes equally between men and women? *J Vasc Surg* 2006;43(2):230–238; discussion 238.

41. Thomas DM, Hulten EA, Ellis ST, et al. Open versus endovascular repair of abdominal aortic aneurysm in the elective and emergent setting in a pooled population of 37,781 patients: A systematic review and meta-analysis. *ISRN Cardiol* 2014;2014:149243.

42. Speicher PJ, Barbas AS, Mureebe L. Open versus endovascular repair of ruptured abdominal aortic aneurysms. *Ann Vasc Surg* 2014;28(5):1249–1257.

43. Starnes BW, Quiroga E, Hutter C, et al. Management of ruptured abdominal aortic aneurysm in the endovascular era. *J Vasc Surg* 2010;51(1):9–17; discussion 17–18.

44. McPhee J, Eslami MH, Arous EJ, Messina LM, Schanzer A. Endovascular treatment of ruptured abdominal aortic aneurysms in the United States (2001–2006): A significant survival benefit over open repair is independently associated with increased institutional volume. *J Vasc Surg* 2009;49(4):817–826.

45. Chagpar RB, Harris JR, Lawlor DK, DeRose G, Forbes TL. Early mortality following endovascular versus open repair of ruptured abdominal aortic aneurysms. *Vasc Endovascular Surg* 2010;44(8):645–649.

46. Lesperance K, Andersen C, Singh N, Starnes B, Martin MJ. Expanding use of emergency endovascular repair for ruptured abdominal aortic aneurysms: Disparities in outcomes from a nationwide perspective. *J Vasc Surg* 2008;47(6):1165–1170; discussion 1170–1171.

47. Mureebe L, Egorova N, Giacovelli JK, Gelijns A, Kent KC, McKinsey JF. National trends in the repair of ruptured abdominal aortic aneurysms. *J Vasc Surg* 2008;48(5):1101–1107.

48. Davenport DL, O'Keeffe SD, Minion DJ, Sorial EE, Endean ED, Xenos ES. Thirty-day NSQIP database outcomes of open versus endoluminal repair of ruptured abdominal aortic aneurysms. *J Vasc Surg* 2010;51(2):305–309.e1.

49. Ali MM, Flahive J, Schanzer A, et al. In patients stratified by preoperative risk, endovascular repair of ruptured abdominal aortic aneurysms has a lower in-hospital mortality and morbidity than open repair. *J Vasc Surg* 2015;61(6):1399–1407.

50. Mehta M, Byrne J, Darling RC, et al. Endovascular repair of ruptured infrarenal abdominal aortic aneurysm is associated with lower 30-day mortality and better 5-year survival rates than open surgical repair. *J Vasc Surg* 2013;57(2):368–375.

51. Powell JT, Hinchliffe RJ, Thompson MM, et al. Observations from the IMPROVE trial concerning the clinical care of patients with ruptured abdominal aortic aneurysm. *Br J Surg* 2014;101(3):216–224; discussion 224.

52. Improve Trial Investigators. Endovascular strategy or open repair for ruptured abdominal aortic aneurysm: One-year outcomes from the IMPROVE randomized trial. *Eur Heart J* 2015;36(31):2061–2069.

53. Reimerink JJ, Hoornweg LL, Vahl AC, et al. Endovascular repair versus open repair of ruptured abdominal aortic aneurysms: A multicenter randomized controlled trial. *Ann Surg* 2013;258(2):248–256.

54. Desgranges P, Kobeiter H, Katsahian S, et al. Editor's Choice—ECAR (Endovasculaire ou Chirurgie dans les Anévrysmes aorto-iliaques Rompus): A French randomized controlled trial of endovascular versus open surgical repair of ruptured aorto-iliac aneurysms. *Eur J Vasc Endovasc Surg* 2015;50(3):303–310.

55. Antoniou GA, Georgiadis GS, Antoniou SA, et al. Endovascular repair for ruptured abdominal aortic aneurysm confers an early survival benefit over open repair. *J Vasc Surg* 2013;58(4):1091–1105.

56. von Meijenfeldt GC, Ultee KH, Eefting D, et al. Differences in mortality, risk factors, and complications after open and endovascular repair of ruptured abdominal aortic aneurysms. *Eur J Vasc Endovasc Surg* 2014;47(5):479–486.

57. Prinssen M, Verhoeven EL, Buth J, et al. A randomized trial comparing conventional and endovascular repair of abdominal aortic aneurysms. *N Engl J Med* 2004;351(16):1607–1618.

58. EVAR trial participants. Endovascular aneurysm repair versus open repair in patients with abdominal aortic aneurysm (EVAR trial 1): Randomised controlled trial. *Lancet* 2005;365(9478):2179–2186.

59. Lederle FA, Freischlag JA, Kyriakides TC, et al. Outcomes following endovascular vs open repair of abdominal aortic aneurysm: A randomized trial. *JAMA* 2009;302(14):1535–1542.

60. Becquemin JP, Pillet JC, Lescalie F, et al. A randomized controlled trial of endovascular aneurysm repair versus open surgery for abdominal aortic aneurysms in low- to moderate-risk patients. *J Vasc Surg* 2011;53(5):1167–1173.e1.

61. Tambyraja AL, Murie JA, Chalmers RT. Prediction of outcome after abdominal aortic aneurysm rupture. *J Vasc Surg* 2008;47(1):222–230.

62. Setacci F, Sirignano P, De Donato G, et al. Endovascular approach for ruptured abdominal aortic aneurysms. *J Cardiovasc Surg (Torino)* 2010;51(3):313–317.

63. Philipsen TE, Hendriks JM, Lauwers P, et al. The use of rapid endovascular balloon occlusion in unstable patients with ruptured abdominal aortic aneurysm. *Innovations (Phila)* 2009;4(2):74–79.

64. Assar AN, Zarins CK. Endovascular proximal control of ruptured abdominal aortic aneurysms: The internal aortic clamp. *J Cardiovasc Surg (Torino)* 2009;50(3):381–385.

65. Arthurs ZM, Sohn VY, Starnes BW. Ruptured abdominal aortic aneurysms: Remote aortic occlusion for the general surgeon. *Surg Clin North Am* 2007;87(5):1035–1045, viii.

66. Rachel ES, Bergamini TM, Kinney EV, et al. Percutaneous endovascular abdominal aortic aneurysm repair. *Ann Vasc Surg* 2002;16(1):43–49.

67. Slappy AL, Hakaim AG, Oldenburg WA, Paz-Fumagalli R, McKinney JM. Femoral incision morbidity following endovascular aortic aneurysm repair. *Vasc Endovascular Surg* 2003;37(2):105–109.

68. Swinnen J, Chao A, Tiwari A, Crozier J, Vicaretti M, Fletcher J. Vertical or transverse incisions for access to the femoral artery: A randomized control study. *Ann Vasc Surg* 2010;24(3):336–341.

69. Phade SV, Garcia-Toca M, Kibbe MR. Techniques in endovascular aneurysm repair. *Int J Vasc Med* 2011;2011:964250.

70. Pearce BJ, Jordan WD. Using IVUS during EVAR and TEVAR: Improving patient outcomes. *Semin Vasc Surg* 2009;22(3):172–180.

71. Carpenter JP. Delivery of endovascular grafts by direct sheath placement into the aorta or iliac arteries. *Ann Vasc Surg* 2002;16(6):787–790.

72. Jonker FH, Aruny J, Muhs BE. Management of type II endoleaks: Preoperative versus postoperative versus expectant management. *Semin Vasc Surg* 2009;22(3):165–171.

73. Ohrlander T, Sonesson B, Ivancev K, Resch T, Dias N, Malina M. The chimney graft: A technique for preserving or rescuing aortic branch vessels in stent-graft sealing zones. *J Endovasc Ther* 2008;15(4):427–432.

74. Ellozy SH, Carroccio A, Lookstein RA, et al. First experience in human beings with a permanently implantable intrasac pressure transducer for monitoring endovascular repair of abdominal aortic aneurysms. *J Vasc Surg* 2004;40(3):405–412.

75. Hoppe H, Segall JA, Liem TK, Landry GJ, Kaufman JA. Aortic aneurysm sac pressure measurements after endovascular repair using an implantable remote sensor: Initial experience and short-term follow-up. *Eur Radiol* 2008;18(5):957–965.

76. Ohki T, Ouriel K, Silveira PG, et al. Initial results of wireless pressure sensing for endovascular aneurysm repair: The APEX trial—Acute Pressure Measurement to Confirm Aneurysm Sac EXclusion. *J Vasc Surg* 2007;45(2):236–242.

77. Eisenack M, Umscheid T, Tessarek J, Torsello GF, Torsello GB. Percutaneous endovascular aortic aneurysm repair: A prospective evaluation of safety, efficiency, and risk factors. *J Endovasc Ther* 2009;16(6):708–713.

78. Bent CL, Fotiadis N, Renfrew I, et al. Total percutaneous aortic repair: Midterm outcomes. *Cardiovasc Intervent Radiol* 2009;32(3):449–454.

79. Heyer KS, Resnick SA, Matsumura JS, Amaranto D, Eskandari MK. Percutaneous Zenith endografting for abdominal aortic aneurysms. *Ann Vasc Surg* 2009;23(2):167–171.

80. Lee WA, Brown MP, Nelson PR, Huber TS, Seeger JM. Midterm outcomes of femoral arteries after percutaneous endovascular aortic repair using the Preclose technique. *J Vasc Surg* 2008;47(5):919–923.

81. Schermerhorn ML, O'Malley AJ, Jhaveri A, et al. Endovascular vs. open repair of abdominal aortic aneurysms in the Medicare population. *N Engl J Med* 2008;358(5):464–474.

82. Brown LC, Brown EA, Greenhalgh RM, et al. Renal function and abdominal aortic aneurysm (AAA): The impact of different management strategies on long-term renal function in the UK EndoVascular Aneurysm Repair (EVAR) trials. *Ann Surg* 2010;251(5):966–975.

83. d'Audiffret A, Desgranges P, Kobeiter DH, Becquemin JP. Follow-up evaluation of endoluminally treated abdominal aortic aneurysms with duplex ultrasonography: Validation with computed tomography. *J Vasc Surg* 2001;33(1):42–50.

84. Kranokpiraksa P, Kaufman JA. Follow-up of endovascular aneurysm repair: Plain radiography, ultrasound, CT/CT angiography, MR imaging/MR angiography, or what? *J Vasc Interv Radiol* 2008;19(6 Suppl):S27–S36.

85. Picel AC, Kansal N. Essentials of endovascular abdominal aortic aneurysm repair imaging: Postprocedure surveillance and complications. *AJR Am J Roentgenol* 2014;203(4):W358–W372.

86. Becquemin JP, Kelley L, Zubilewicz T, Desgranges P, Lapeyre M, Kobeiter H. Outcomes of secondary interventions after abdominal aortic aneurysm endovascular repair. *J Vasc Surg* 2004;39(2):298–305.

87. Mehta M, Sternbach Y, Taggert JB, et al. Long-term outcomes of secondary procedures after endovascular aneurysm repair. *J Vasc Surg* 2010;52(6):1442–1449.

88. Elkouri S, Gloviczki P, McKusick MA, et al. Perioperative complications and early outcome after endovascular and open surgical repair of abdominal aortic aneurysms. *J Vasc Surg* 2004;39(3):497–505.

89. Shah A, Stavropoulos SW. Imaging surveillance following endovascular aneurysm repair. *Semin Intervent Radiol* 2009;26(1):10–16.

90. Liaw JV, Clark M, Gibbs R, Jenkins M, Cheshire N, Hamady M. Update: Complications and management of infrarenal EVAR. *Eur J Radiol* 2009;71(3):541–551.

91. Stavropoulos SW, Clark TW, Carpenter JP, et al. Use of CT angiography to classify endoleaks after endovascular repair of abdominal aortic aneurysms. *J Vasc Interv Radiol* 2005; 16(5):663–667.

92. Veith FJ, Baum RA, Ohki T, et al. Nature and significance of endoleaks and endotension: Summary of opinions expressed at an international conference. *J Vasc Surg* 2002;35(5):1029–1035.

93. Becquemin JP, Allaire E, Desgranges P, Kobeiter H. Delayed complications following EVAR. *Tech Vasc Interv Radiol* 2005;8(1):30–40.

94. Arko FR, Murphy EH, Boyes C, et al. Current status of endovascular aneurysm repair: 20 years of learning. *Semin Vasc Surg* 2012;25(3):131–135.

95. Ward TJ, Cohen S, Fischman AM, et al. Preoperative inferior mesenteric artery embolization before endovascular aneurysm repair: Decreased incidence of type II endoleak and aneurysm sac enlargement with 24-month follow-up. *J Vasc Interv Radiol* 2013;24(1):49–55.

96. Axelrod DJ, Lookstein RA, Guller J, et al. Inferior mesenteric artery embolization before endovascular aneurysm repair: Technique and initial results. *J Vasc Interv Radiol* 2004;15(11):1263–1267.

97. Alerci M, Giamboni A, Wyttenbach R, et al. Endovascular abdominal aneurysm repair and impact of systematic preoperative embolization of collateral arteries: Endoleak analysis and long-term follow-up. *J Endovasc Ther* 2013;20(5):663–671.

98. Burbelko M, Kalinowski M, Heverhagen JT, et al. Prevention of type II endoleak using the AMPLATZER vascular plug before endovascular aneurysm repair. *Eur J Vasc Endovasc Surg* 2014;47(1):28–36.

99. Nolz R, Teufelsbauer H, Asenbaum U, et al. Type II endoleaks after endovascular repair of abdominal aortic aneurysms: Fate of the aneurysm sac and neck changes during long-term follow-up. *J Endovasc Ther* 2012;19(2):193–199.

100. Zhou W, Blay E, Varu V, et al. Outcome and clinical significance of delayed endoleaks after endovascular aneurysm repair. *J Vasc Surg* 2014;59(4):915–920.

101. Sidloff DA, Stather PW, Choke E, Bown MJ, Sayers RD. Type II endoleak after endovascular aneurysm repair. *Br J Surg* 2013;100(10):1262–1270.

102. Stavropoulos SW, Charagundla SR. Imaging techniques for detection and management of endoleaks after endovascular aortic aneurysm repair. *Radiology* 2007;243(3):641–655.

103. Sampaio SM, Panneton JM, Mozes G, et al. AneuRx device migration: Incidence, risk factors, and consequences. *Ann Vasc Surg* 2005;19(2):178–185.

104. Resch T, Ivancev K, Brunkwall J, Nyman U, Malina M, Lindblad B. Distal migration of stent-grafts after endovascular repair of abdominal aortic aneurysms. *J Vasc Interv Radiol* 1999;10(3):257–264; discussion 265–266.

105. Fransen GA, Desgranges P, Laheij RJ, Harris PL, Becquemin JP, EUROSTAR Collaborators. Frequency, predictive factors, and consequences of stent-graft kink following endovascular AAA repair. *J Endovasc Ther* 2003;10(5):913–918.

106. Early H, Atkins M. Technical tips for managing difficult iliac access. *Semin Vasc Surg* 2012;25(3):138–143.

107. Maleux G, Koolen M, Heye S, Nevelsteen A. Limb occlusion after endovascular repair of abdominal aortic aneurysms with supported endografts. *J Vasc Interv Radiol* 2008;19(10):1409–1412.

108. Hellinger JC. Endovascular repair of thoracic and abdominal aortic aneurysms: Pre- and postprocedural imaging. *Tech Vasc Interv Radiol* 2005;8(1):2–15.

109. Lalka S, Dalsing M, Cikrit D, et al. Secondary interventions after endovascular abdominal aortic aneurysm repair. *Am J Surg* 2005;190(5):787–794.

110. Cernohorsky P, Reijnen MM, Tielliu IF, van Sterkenburg SM, van den Dungen JJ, Zeebregts CJ. The relevance of aortic endograft prosthetic infection. *J Vasc Surg* 2011;54(2):327–333.

111. Fatima J, Duncan AA, de Grandis E, et al. Treatment strategies and outcomes in patients with infected aortic endografts. *J Vasc Surg* 2013;58(2):371–379.

112. Maleux G, Koolen M, Heye S. Complications after endovascular aneurysm repair. *Semin Intervent Radiol* 2009;26(1):3–9.

113. Saratzis N, Saratzis A, Melas N, Ktenidis K, Kiskinis D. Aortoduodenal fistulas after endovascular stent-graft repair of abdominal aortic aneurysms: Single-center experience and review of the literature. *J Endovasc Ther* 2008;15(4):441–448.

114. Wald R, Waikar SS, Liangos O, Pereira BJ, Chertow GM, Jaber BL. Acute renal failure after endovascular vs open repair of abdominal aortic aneurysm. *J Vasc Surg* 2006;43(3):460–466; discussion 466.

115. Antonello M, Menegolo M, Piazza M, Bonfante L, Grego F, Frigatti P. Outcomes of endovascular aneurysm repair on renal function compared with open repair. *J Vasc Surg* 2013;58(4):886–893.

116. Murphy EH, Arko FR. Technical tips for abdominal aortic endografting. *Semin Vasc Surg* 2008;21(1):25–30.

117. Belenky A, Atar E, Orron DE, et al. Endovascular abdominal aortic aneurysm repair using transvenous intravascular US catheter guidance in patients with chronic renal failure. *J Vasc Interv Radiol* 2014;25(5):702–706.

118. Dadian N, Ohki T, Veith FJ, et al. Overt colon ischemia after endovascular aneurysm repair: The importance of microembolization as an etiology. *J Vasc Surg* 2001;34(6):986–996.

119. Perry RJ, Martin MJ, Eckert MJ, Sohn VY, Steele SR. Colonic ischemia complicating open vs endovascular abdominal aortic aneurysm repair. *J Vasc Surg* 2008;48(2):272–277.

120. Rutherford RB. Structural failures in abdominal aortic aneurysm stentgrafts: Threat to durability and challenge to technology. *Semin Vasc Surg* 2004;17(4):294–297.

121. Ueda T, Takaoka H, Petrovitch I, Rubin GD. Detection of broken sutures and metal-ring fractures in AneuRx stent-grafts by using three-dimensional CT angiography after endovascular abdominal aortic aneurysm repair: Association with late endoleak development and device migration. *Radiology* 2014;272(1):275–283.

122. Bensley RP, Hurks R, Huang Z, et al. Ultrasound-guided percutaneous endovascular aneurysm repair success is predicted by access vessel diameter. *J Vasc Surg* 2012;55(6):1554–1561.

123. Manunga JM, Gloviczki P, Oderich GS, et al. Femoral artery calcification as a determinant of success for percutaneous access for endovascular abdominal aortic aneurysm repair. *J Vasc Surg* 2013;58(5):1208–1212.

124. Mousa AY, Campbell JE, Broce M, et al. Predictors of percutaneous access failure requiring open femoral surgical conversion during endovascular aortic aneurysm repair. *J Vasc Surg* 2013;58(5):1213–1219.

125. Minion DJ, Davenport DL. Access techniques for EVAR: Percutaneous techniques and working with small arteries. *Semin Vasc Surg* 2012;25(4):208–216.

126. van der Vliet JA, Kool LJ, van Hoek F. Simplifying post-EVAR surveillance. *Eur J Vasc Endovasc Surg* 2011;42(2):193–194.

127. Lehmkuhl L, Andres C, Lücke C, et al. Dynamic CT angiography after abdominal aortic endovascular aneurysm repair: Influence of enhancement patterns and optimal bolus timing on endoleak detection. *Radiology* 2013;268(3):890–899.

128. Bastos Gonçalves F, Baderkhan H, Verhagen HJ, et al. Early sac shrinkage predicts a low risk of late complications after endovascular aortic aneurysm repair. *Br J Surg* 2014;101(7):802–810.

129. Back MR. Surveillance after endovascular abdominal aortic aneurysm repair. *Perspect Vasc Surg Endovasc Ther* 2007;19(4):395–400; discussion 401–402.

130. Go MR, Barbato JE, Rhee RY, Makaroun MS. What is the clinical utility of a 6-month computed tomography in the follow-up of endovascular aneurysm repair patients? *J Vasc Surg* 2008;47(6):1181–1186; discussion 1186–1187.

131. Kirkpatrick VE, Wilson SE, Williams RA, Gordon IL. Surveillance computed tomographic arteriogram does not change management before 3 years in patients who have a normal post-EVAR study. *Ann Vasc Surg* 2014;28(4):831–836.

132. Alerci M, Oberson M, Fogliata A, Gallino A, Vock P, Wyttenbach R. Prospective, intraindividual comparison of MRI versus MDCT for endoleak detection after endovascular repair of abdominal aortic aneurysms. *Eur Radiol* 2009;19(5):1223–1231.

133. Pitton MB, Schweitzer H, Herber S, et al. MRI versus helical CT for endoleak detection after endovascular aneurysm repair. *AJR Am J Roentgenol* 2005;185(5):1275–1281.

134. van der Laan MJ, Bartels LW, Viergever MA, Blankensteijn JD. Computed tomography versus magnetic resonance imaging of endoleaks after EVAR. *Eur J Vasc Endovasc Surg* 2006;32(4):361–365.

135. Habets J, Zandvoort HJ, Reitsma JB, et al. Magnetic resonance imaging is more sensitive than computed tomography angiography for the detection of endoleaks after endovascular abdominal aortic aneurysm repair: A systematic review. *Eur J Vasc Endovasc Surg* 2013;45(4):340–350.

136. Erbel R, Aboyans V, Boileau C, et al. 2014 ESC Guidelines on the diagnosis and treatment of aortic diseases: Document covering acute and chronic aortic diseases of the thoracic and abdominal aorta of the adult. The Task Force for the Diagnosis and Treatment of Aortic Diseases of the European Society of Cardiology (ESC). *Eur Heart J* 2014;35(41):2873–2926.

PART **10**

Credentialing and Documentation

54

Training program guidelines, case numbers, and maintenance of certification

MICHELE DOUGHTY VOELTZ

BACKGROUND

Percutaneous coronary intervention (PCI), pioneered by Andreas Gruentzig in the 1970s, is a relatively recent addition to cardiovascular medicine. The field has grown and expanded to include a number of different aspects of training, including coronary and peripheral intervention, and structural heart disease (SHD).

As interventional cardiology has expanded, the formalization of and requirements for training in this area have been updated and refined as well. The American College of Cardiology's (ACC's) Core Cardiology Training Symposium (COCATS) consensus statements[1] have worked to standardize training requirements across the field of invasive and interventional cardiology. This chapter reviews the most recent recommendations for training programs, case numbers, and maintenance of certification for interventional cardiology.

TRAINING PROGRAM REQUIREMENTS

Training program structure

Numerous organizations oversee the structure, content, and evaluation of medical training, the largest of these being the Accreditation Council for Graduate Medical Education (ACGME), a private, nonprofit organization whose role is to review and accredit graduate medical education (residency

and fellowship) programs, and the institutions through which they are sponsored.[2] The ACGME assesses training programs through its 27 Residency Review Committees (RRC), each consisting of 8–20 physicians. The RRC's purpose is to conduct on-site evaluations of each program and make recommendations regarding accreditation. Training programs must adhere to a standard set of program guidelines set forth by the ACGME. ACGME accreditation is required for program graduates to be eligible to sit for the American Board of Internal Medicine (ABIM) certifying examination in interventional cardiology, a critical element for developing a career in this specialty.

The role of the sponsoring institution is the assumption of responsibility for the education and well-being of its trainees.[2] The ACGME publishes Common Program Requirements, which detail its expectations of training programs and personnel. The goals of the Common Program Requirements are "assuring the provision of safe and effective care to the individual patient; assuring each resident's and fellow's development of the skills, knowledge, and attitudes required to enter the unsupervised practice of medicine; and establishing a foundation for continued professional growth."[3] The ACGME requires every interventional cardiology training program to have a single, dedicated program director. The program director must maintain ABIM certification in interventional cardiology and is expected to "possess the requisite specialty expertise," along with "documented educational and administrative abilities" at the primary teaching site. In addition to the program director, there must be a group of core faculty also possessing documented clinical experience, academic productivity, and procedural expertise within the program. The ratio of faculty to trainees must be at least 1.5:1.

The ACGME requires sufficient procedural volume by both the sponsoring institution (400 interventions annually) and the core faculty (75 interventions annually).[4] The availability of on-site cardiac surgical support, a cardiac surgical intensive care unit (ICU), and cardiac ICU are also required components of all interventional training programs.

The COCATS 4 Taskforce document, approved and published by the ACC and endorsed by the Society for Cardiovascular Angiography and Interventions (SCAI), drives training program content. Testing and certification of trainees are conducted by the ABIM, which is in turn affiliated with the American Board of Medical Specialties (ABMS).

Core Cardiology Training Symposium and Accreditation Council for Graduate Medical Education specifications

The goals and standards for interventional cardiology training are established by the ACGME and the COCATS training statements.[1] COCATS is a sequence of consensus documents, which address training requirements in all areas of cardiology, including invasive and interventional cardiology, developed by the ACC and SCAI and approved by the American Heart Association (AHA). COCATS 4[1] was published in 2015 and represents the most recent version of the principal documentation for interventional cardiology training program requirements.

The spirit of COCATS 4 is to guide training programs according to the six governing principles of the ACGME.[1,3] These principles are detailed in Table 54.1.[3] It is believed that these core competencies encourage development of professionalism, quality, and skills throughout a lifelong career.

Table 54.1 The six accreditation councils for Graduate Medical Education core competencies in medical education

1. Medical knowledge
2. Patient care
3. Practice-based learning and improvement in evidence-based medicine
   Quality improvement
4. Systems-based practice cost effectiveness
   Health care delivery and safety
5. Interpersonal and communications skills
6. Professionalism

Source: From Accreditation Council for Graduate Medical Education (ACGME), ACGME Common Program Requirements, July 2011, Available from: http://www.acgme.org/acWebsite/dutyHours/dh_duty-hoursCommonPR07012007.pdf.

CERTIFICATION AND CREDENTIALING

Training and procedural requirements for certification

The certification process, implemented by the ABIM, focuses on individual practice knowledge and quality through the maintenance of certification requirements and examination administration.[5] The ABIM addresses the needs of internal medicine, as well as its 20 subspecialties, and is the largest member of the ABMS, currently certifying one in every four physicians practicing in the United States.[5,6]

ABIM certification is designed to ensure that a physician has adequate training and knowledge in a particular medical specialty.[5] With regard to terminology, "board eligible" refers to a doctor who has completed all of the required training to qualify for examination in a subspecialty, but has not yet passed the certification test, either because he or she has not yet taken the exam or because of failure of the test. "Board certified," on the other hand, refers to a physician who has taken and passed the required initial and recertification examinations within the past 10 years. Any candidate may maintain "board eligible" status for up to 7 years; however, after that time, if the examination has not been successfully completed, "board eligible" status is lost. The pathway to certification in interventional cardiology involves a series of steps, including initial credentialing in internal medicine, followed by credentialing in cardiovascular diseases and, finally, in interventional cardiology.

Board certification is open to both graduates of accredited U.S. and Canadian medical schools, as well as international graduates with a standard certificate from the Educational Commission for Foreign Medical Graduates (ECFMG).[7] Thirty-six months of approved training in internal medicine must be completed prior to admission to the certification examination. Each candidate's demonstration of the six core competencies outlined in Table 54.1 must also be confirmed by the program director.[2] The breakdown of topics addressed by the ABIM examination is shown in Figure 54.1.[8] Once the aforementioned requirements are met and a passing score is achieved on the ABIM exam, certification is granted. The ABIM certification examinations may be repeated to secure a passing score, as long as the candidate meets other appropriate licensure and professional standing requirements.

Certification in cardiovascular disease requires preexisting certification in internal medicine followed by an additional 36 months of training, including at least 24 months of clinical patient care. Specific procedural and knowledge requirements include advanced cardiac life support, cardioversion, electrocardiography, exercise testing, echocardiography, arterial cannulation with catheter placement, right heart catheterization, temporary pacemaker insertion and management, and left heart catheterization. Documentation of procedural competence, satisfactory demonstration of the six core competencies, and passing scores on the ABIM examination in cardiovascular disease are required to finalize certification.

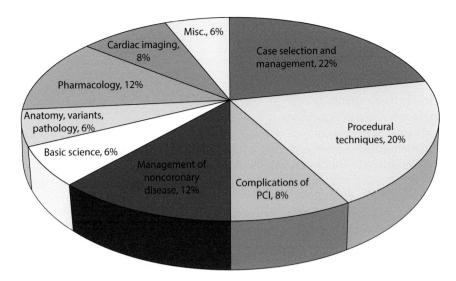

Figure 54.1 Breakdown of components of ABIM examination for interventional cardiology. Misc; miscellaneous; PCI, percutaneous coronary intervention. (Modified from American Board of Internal Medicine [ABIM], *Interventional Cardiology Certification Exam Blueprint*, January 2016, Retrieved from http://www.abim.org/~/media/ABIM%20Public/Files/pdf/exam-blueprints/certification/interventional-cardiology.pdf.)

ABIM endorsement in interventional cardiology requires prior certification in cardiovascular disease and an additional 12 *continuous* months of clinical training in coronary intervention at an ACGME-accredited institution. During this time, fellows must perform at least 250 therapeutic cardiac procedures. The ACGME requires demonstration of mastery of specific procedural and cognitive aspects of interventional practice (Tables 54.2 and 54.3).[1,4] Again, documentation of mastery of the core competencies and passing the ABIM certification are critical components of a successful interventional cardiology career.

MAINTENANCE OF CERTIFICATION

Overview

In an effort to encourage education on evolving techniques and technologies, ABIM certification is time limited.

The purpose of the Maintenance of Certification (MOC) is to ensure that an individual physician participates in certain continuous learning and education activities.[9] There are three components for eligibility for the maintenance of (re-) certification: holding a valid and unrestricted license to practice medicine, completing self-evaluation and education components, and achieving a passing score on the recertification examination. For candidates in the subspecialty of interventional cardiology, successful maintenance of certification in cardiovascular disease is also required, although it is not necessary to maintain certification in internal medicine. These certificates are valid for 10 years.

The MOC program requires physicians to accumulate MOC points every 2 years to be considered active. To be reported as certified, a physician must earn 100 points every 5 years (the points earned every 2 years count toward the 100 point total) and pass the MOC recertification examination every 10 years. There are multiple opportunities to earn MOC points in such categories as medical knowledge, patient assessment, patient voice, and patient safety.[10] These modules are available through the ABIM as web-based exercises. The practice performance self-evaluation is an opportunity for physicians to evaluate and reflect on the medical care they provide. Points can be earned through a variety of approved exercises, may be eligible for additional continuing medical education credit, and are valid for both cardiovascular disease and interventional cardiology MOC.

Among practicing physicians and professional organizations, the MOC requirements have caused controversy. In fact, in an ongoing lawsuit filed by the Association of American Physicians and Surgeons (AAPS), the ABMS is being criticized for the MOC program. The lawsuit states, "There is no justification for requiring the purchase of Defendant's product as a condition of practicing medicine or being on hospital medical staffs, yet ABMS has agreed with others to cause exclusion of physicians who do not purchase or comply with Defendant's program." The results of this lawsuit are still pending.[11]

The practice of interventional cardiology requires expertise in a number of technical, pharmacological, and conceptual arenas. The ABIM certification and recertification requirements are an effort to ensure that physicians attain and maintain mastery of these areas.

Institutional credentialing

Credentialing is the duty of the local hospital organization. According to Joint Commission mandates, medical staff are responsible for the development of appropriate practice and competency standards and the documentation of these

862 Training program guidelines, case numbers, and maintenance of certification

Table 54.2 Accreditation Council for Graduate Medical Education—Specific procedural and cognitive training requirements for Level 3 training in interventional cardiology

Fellows must demonstrate competence in the prevention, evaluation, and treatment of:

1. Acute ischemic syndromes
2. Antiarrhythmic medications
3. Bleeding disorders and complications
4. Chronic ischemic heart disease
5. Coronary arteriography, ventriculography, and hemodynamic measurement
6. Coronary intervention, including documented performance of at least 250 coronary interventions (each patient can count only once regardless of the number of procedures performed)
   a. Distal protection devices
   b. Intracoronary and Doppler pressure measurement
   c. Intravascular ultrasound
   d. Use of balloons, stents, and other commonly used interventional devices
7. Intra-aortic balloon counterpulsation and hemodynamic support
8. Intravascular ultrasound
9. Knowledge of:
   a. Advantages and disadvantages of PCI in varying anatomy
   b. Advantages and disadvantages of PCI vs. thrombolytic therapy in ST-elevation myocardial infarction
   c. Assessment of plaque composition
   d. Clinical importance of complete versus incomplete revascularization
   e. Detailed coronary anatomy
   f. Interpretation of randomized control trials in clinical medicine
   g. Pathophysiology and treatment of restenosis
   h. Physiology of coronary flow
   i. Platelets and clotting cascade
   j. Radiation physics
   k. Role of emergent CABG
   l. Strengths and limitations of invasive and non-invasive testing
   m. Treatment of valvular and structural heart disease
   n. Use of pharmacologic agents in PCI management
10. Management of PCI complications
11. Management of procedural complications:
    a. Cardiac tamponade
    b. Cardiogenic shock
    c. Coronary dissection
    d. No reflow
    e. Perforation
    f. Spasm
    g. Thrombosis
    h. Vascular complications
12. Patient care in outpatient, inpatient, ICU, and ED setting related to interventional procedures
13. Valvular and structural heart disease
14. Vasoactive medications

Source: From Accreditation Council for Graduate Medical Education (ACGME), ACGME Program Requirements for Graduate Medical Education in Interventional Cardiology (Internal Medicine), February 2011 [July 2016], Available from: http://www.acgme.org/Portals/0/PFAssets/ProgramRequirements/152_interventional_card_int_med_2016_1-YR.pdf?ver=2016-03-23-113035-420.

Note: CABG, coronary artery bypass grafting; ICU, intensive care unit; ED, emergency department; PCI, percutaneous coronary intervention.

principles in medical staff bylaws. These bylaws guide initial credentialing and periodic review (recredentialing), thereby assuring maintenance of standards and professional proficiency of all active hospital physician staff. Many hospitals require board eligibility or certification, at minimum,

for granting privileges as recent data have suggested an association between ABIM certification and improved health care delivery.[12–14] This stance is supported by research suggesting physician scores in the highest quartile on ABIM recertification have been linked to improved quality care

Table 54.3 Specific requirements for training in invasive cardiology as outlined by the COCATS-4 of the American College of Cardiology

Level 1

- Four months minimum participating in a minimum of 100 diagnostic procedures, including both hemodynamics and angiography
- Technical skills include vascular access, right heart catheterization, management of post-procedural complications, and coronary and left ventricular angiography
- Cognitive knowledge base including, but not limited to: coronary anatomy and physiology, hemodynamics, indications and contraindications for cardiac, biopsy, structural, and peripheral procedures, complications, treatment selection for coronary disease, pacing, radiation safety, adjunctive pharmacotherapy, hemodynamic assist devices, and vascular closure devices

Level 2

- An additional 4 months performing at least 300 total cardiac procedures (another 100 diagnostic peripheral procedures are required for those desiring Level II competency in peripheral vascular angiography)
- Technical skills include proficiency to an independent level in the following: hemodynamic catheterization, pericardiocentesis, endomyocardial biopsy, peripheral angiography (excluding carotid), intra-aortic balloon pump insertion
- All required skills for Level I training

Level 3

- Must be a fourth year of advanced training
- Technical skills include: PCI, peripheral, carotid, valvular, and structural heart interventions, including insertion and management of percutaneous left ventricular support devices
- All required skills for Level I and Level II training

Source: Modified from King, S.B. III, et al., *J. Am. Coll. Cardiol.*, 65(17), 1844–1853, 2015.
Note: COCATS, Core Cardiology Training Symposium; PCI, percutaneous coronary interventions.

measures among Medicare patients with diabetes after adjustment for patient and physician covariates (OR 1.17; 95% CI, 1.08–1.27).[12] Further suggestion of an association between certification exam performance and physician quality includes data reporting better ratings by program directors[14] and colleagues[15] for physicians who score higher on the initial certification exams. Early data suggest that exam performance may be linked to improvement in clinical care quality; however, further studies are necessary to evaluate the association between certification and achievement of quality outcomes in interventional cardiology.

In addition to board certification, hospitals require exposure to adequate teaching and experience in each individual procedure a physician wishes to perform. As a large number of novel techniques and procedures are introduced into the realm of interventional cardiology, many hospitals are introducing regulatory bodies, such as innovation committees, to assess credentialing requirements. Trainees planning a career in invasive cardiology should familiarize themselves with both programmatic and hospital-based requirements for credentialing at their chosen institution.

TRAINING IN EUROPE

Training standards in Europe are evolving rapidly. The European Society of Cardiology (ESC) Working Group 10 has recommended curriculum and syllabi for interventional cardiology subspecialty training in Europe.[16] Among other recommendations, the workgroup suggested that the trainee will have performed at least 200 coronary interventional procedures as first or only operator, from which one-third should have been emergency or acute coronary syndrome procedures. Additional recommendations were made for advanced structural and peripheral interventional training. The European Union of Medical Specialists (UEMS) has a list of core competencies, similar to those published by the ACGME, which must be achieved during the required 4-year training period.[17] Additionally, the ESC provides support for post-training physicians, much like the ACC in the United States. Formal training programs in interventional cardiology do not exist in most countries; however, concentrated experiences in interventions are provided. Board examinations similarly do not exist in many, if not most, other locations, including Canada, Europe, and Asia.

FUTURE DIRECTIONS

Interventional cardiology is one of the most rapidly growing fields in medicine as novel procedures and technologies are constantly being integrated into clinical practice. As such, training requirements must evolve to keep pace with these innovations. The training pathway must be continuously assessed to assure adequate exposure to critical components of modern intervention. Enhanced training pathways to assure proficiency in noncoronary cardiac and vascular interventions are in nascent stages of development. Continued trainee exposure to these disease entities will likely be followed by further educational initiatives, expectations of competency, and expansion of training and certification requirements to document mastery. Whether training standards for peripheral vascular disease and interventions should remain distinct from those established for cardiovascular interventional training remains a point of debate.

ENDOVASCULAR TRAINING

Since the development of the ABIM process for interventional cardiology training and curriculum,[18] endovascular procedures and techniques have rapidly evolved. Although training in vascular medicine, carotid and peripheral vascular intervention, and SHD is not required as part of the coronary interventional cardiology training program currently constructed,[4] many interventional cardiology trainees now desire certification in these areas as well. The most recent COCATS document addresses recommendations for vascular medicine fellowship training.[19] In addition to the ABIM examination in interventional cardiology, the American Board of Vascular Medicine (ABVM) offers both general vascular and endovascular board certification.[20]

Current interventional cardiology fellows are exposed to varying degrees of peripheral vascular intervention, image interpretation, and complex SHD procedures during training. Most fellowship programs ensure at least exposure to noncardiac intervention, though many do not reach the numbers required for Level III certification and board eligibility (Table 54.3). Many programs have added an additional year (total of 24 months) of fellowship training to ensure both coronary and noncoronary proficiency. There is some controversy about whether 12 months alone is adequate for both coronary and peripheral intervention, and this issue remains a source of great debate among training programs throughout the country. Fellows in 1-year programs often seek additional postgraduate training to achieve expertise in these areas.

The ABVM training requirements for general vascular medicine board eligibility include a cardiology fellowship that allows formal Level II vascular medicine training as detailed in COCATS-4 (Table 54.4),[18] or a vascular medicine fellowship training program of at least 12 months duration that meets society standards.[20] The practice pathway allows those with a general internal medicine or subspecialty of this discipline in the arena, if they demonstrate commitment to vascular patient care and clinical competency. For endovascular certification, those with a board certification in cardiology, cardiothoracic surgery, interventional radiology, vascular surgery, or vascular medicine may apply. The fellowship track requires completion of an ABIM-accredited fellowship including peripheral interventional procedures within 3 years of application. Also, performance of 100 diagnostic and 50 peripheral interventional procedures (at least half as primary operator) is required. For those already in practice, documentation of performance of 100 diagnostic peripheral angiograms (at least 50 as primary operator) and 50 peripheral interventional procedures (at least 25 as primary operator) within 24 months of application is required.

Noncoronary interventional training, like many aspects of cardiology, is a rapidly growing and evolving field involving a number of different disciplines and training backgrounds. Maintenance of balance between appropriate duration and scope of training remains a source of debate.

Structural heart disease training

In addition to endovascular procedures, the development of percutaneous approaches to the treatment of structural cardiac pathology is rapidly taking place. For years, SHD has been treated in pediatric catheterization laboratories by congenital interventionalists. In adult catheterization laboratories, SHD was traditionally limited to palliative and rescue procedures, such as balloon valvuloplasty and atrial septostomy. More recently, percutaneous closure of patent foramen ovale and atrial septal defects increased in frequency. Percutaneous implantation of bioprosthetic aortic valves, mitral valve annuloplasty and clipping, and left atrial appendage closure has catapulted SHD into the spotlight. Specialty SHD training has become increasingly popular as these techniques have developed. Currently, there are 24 SHD fellowship programs with 29 available positions in the United States.[21] All of these programs require completion of adult cardiology and interventional cardiology fellowship training prior to consideration. Further definition of the cognitive and procedural requirements and development of evaluative measures for certification will be required in the near future as this field grows.

Congenital heart disease training

As patients with congenital heart disease live longer with medical therapy, percutaneous intervention, and surgical treatment, the field of adult congenital heart disease (ACHD) has developed swiftly. In 2015, the first ABIM certifying examination in ACHD was administered, providing formal evaluation of knowledge and training in this subspecialty.[22] The examination was offered to candidates who have been previously certified in cardiovascular disease or pediatric cardiology. The formal training pathway requires 24 months of ACHD fellowship training, 18 of these clinical. The practice pathway grants board eligibility to those who have spent at least 40% of their clinical practice time, or 25% of their total post-training professional time, in the clinical practice of ACHD. There are currently eight programs in the United States offering formal ACHD training. Most of these require a pediatric

Table 54.4 Summary of COCATS-4 requirements for training in vascular medicine

Level	Months	Skills
1	2	Evaluation and management of arterial and venous disease, atherosclerotic risk factors, and hypercoaguable states.
		Knowledge of pathophysiology, causes, and clinical epidemiology of a variety of peripheral vascular conditions.
		Testing methods, including noninvasive vascular laboratory and vascular imaging (i.e., ultrasound, MRA, and CTA)
2	12	Outpatient vascular medicine clinic.
		Inpatient vascular medicine consultation service.
		Diagnostic testing procedures, equipment, indications, diagnostic criteria, technical limitations.
		Extensive mentoring and interpretation of at least 500 studies across vascular testing areas.
		Peripheral vascular catheterization and vascular surgery.
		All requirements outlined for Level I training.
3	12	Outpatient vascular medicine clinic.
		Inpatient medical consultation service.
		Vascular imaging as detailed above.
		Peripheral vascular catheterization and intervention.

Source: American Board of Internal Medicine (ABIM), Interventional Cardiology Policies, 2008, Available from: http://www.abim.org/certification/policies/imss/icard.aspx.

Note: COCATS, Core Cardiology Training Symposium; CTA, computed tomography angiogram; MRA, magnetic resonance angiogram.

cardiology background; however, it is expected that the number of training spots available to those with adult cardiology and interventional cardiology training will increase dramatically over the next several years.

Learning in practice

As stated above, interventional cardiology is an ever-changing and evolving subspecialty. As such, a career in this field requires a commitment to lifelong learning as new techniques, equipment, approaches, and procedures develop. Future training techniques are both progressive and regressive. In many ways, we are back to the days of Andreas Gruentzig, which was characterized by observation and proctorship. The progressive aspect includes medical simulation and other virtual training sources. As we approach a very exciting future in our chosen field, we must do so with a willingness to learn and progress, a desire to improve our own expertise, and, always, a focus on providing exceptional care to the patients whom we serve.

REFERENCES

1. King SB III, et al. COCATS 4 Task Force 10: Training in cardiac catheterization. *J Am Coll Cardiol* 2015;65(17):1844–1853.
2. Accreditation Council for Graduate Medical Education (ACGME). *ACGME Institutional Requirements*; June 2013 [September 2014]. Available from: http://www.acgme.org/acWebsite/irc/irc_IRCpr07012007.pdf (accessed July 2016).
3. Accreditation Council for Graduate Medical Education (ACGME). *ACGME Common Program Requirements*; July 2011. Available from: http://www.acgme.org/acWebsite/dutyHours/dh_duty-hoursCommonPR07012007.pdf.
4. Accreditation Council for Graduate Medical Education (ACGME). *ACGME Program Requirements for Graduate Medical Education in Interventional Cardiology (Internal Medicine)*; February 2011. Available from: http://www.acgme.org/ (accessed July 2016).
5. American Board of Internal Medicine (ABIM). *Policies and Procedures for Certification*; 2008. Available from: http://www.abim.org/about/.
6. American Board of Medical Specialties (ABMS). *About ABMS*. Available from: http://www.abms.org/about-abms/.
7. Educational Commission for Foreign Medical Graduates (ECFMG). *About ECFMG*. Available from: http://www.ecfmg.org/about/statement-of-values.html/.
8. American Board of Internal Medicine (ABIM). *Interventional Cardiology Certification Exam Blueprint*; January 2016. Available from: http://www.abim.org/~/media/ABIM%20Public/Files/pdf/exam-blueprints/certification/interventional-cardiology.pdf.
9. American Board of Internal Medicine (ABIM). *Maintenance of Certification*. Available from: http://www.abim.org/maintenance-of-certification/default.aspx.
10. American Board of Internal Medicine (ABIM). *How to Earn Maintenance of Certification Points*. Available from: http://www.abim.org/maintenance-of-certification/earning-points.aspx.
11. Association of American Physicians and Surgeons (AAPS). *AAPS takes MOC to court*; February 2016. Available from: http://www.aapsonline.org/index.php/site/article/aaps_takes_moc_to_court/.
12. Holmboe ES, et al. Association between maintenance of certification examination scores and quality of care for medicare beneficiaries. *Arch Intern Med* 2008;168(13):1396–1403.
13. Pham HH, et al. Delivery of preventive services to older adults by primary care physicians. *JAMA* 2005;294(4):473–481.

14. Shea JA, et al. Relationships of ratings of clinical competence and ABIM scores to certification status. *Acad Med* 1993;68(10 Suppl):S22–S24.

15. Ramsey PG, et al. Use of peer ratings to evaluate physician performance. *JAMA* 1993;269(13):1655–1660.

16. Di Mario C, et al. Curriculum and syllabus for Interventional Cardiology subspecialty training in Europe. *EuroIntervention* 2006;2(1):31–36.

17. Union Europeenne Des Medecins Specialistes (UEMS). *Training Requirements for the Specialty of Cardiology, European Standards of Postgraduate Medical Specialist Training*; 2013. Available from: http://www.uems. eu/—data/assets/pdf_file/0011/19577/UEMS-2013.24-SECTIONS-AND-BOARDS-Cardiology-European-Training-Requirements-2013.10.19.pdf.

18. American Board of Internal Medicine (ABIM). *Interventional Cardiology Policies*; 2008. Available from: http://www.abim.org/certification/policies/imss/icard.aspx.

19. Creager MA, et al. COCATS 4 Task force 9: Training in vascular endorsed by the society for vascular medicine. *Vasc Med* 2015;20(4):384–394.

20. American Board of Vascular Medicine (ABVM). *ABVM Requirements for Board Eligibility*; 2016. Available from: https://www.vascularboard.org/cert_reqs.cfm.

21. American College of Cardiology (ACC). *Structural Heart Disease and Congenital Interventional Fellowship Programs*; 2016. Available from: http://www.acc.org/membership/sections-and-councils/fellows-in-training-section/training-resources/structural-heart-disease-and-congenital-interventional-fellowship-programs.

22. American Board of Internal Medicine (ABIM). *Adult Congenital Heart Disease Certification Policies*; 2016. Available from: http://www.abim.org/certification/policies/internal-medicine-subspecialty-policies/adult-congenital-heart-disease.aspx.

55

Electronic catheterization records and data collection for quality improvement

PARTHA SARDAR, AMARTYA KUNDU, SAURAV CHATTERJEE, AND THEOPHILUS OWAN

INTRODUCTION

With recent advances in the field of cardiovascular medicine, cardiac catheterization has become one of the most common invasive procedures performed in the United States.[1,2] Although catheterization is generally considered to be a safe procedure, the large volume of interventions performed carry with them the risk of infrequent but potentially significant complications. Hence, the cardiac catheterization laboratory is a key environment where physicians strive to constantly improve quality outcomes.[1,2] For optimal quality management, there remains an obligation for detailed documentation, especially with the introduction of newer technologies to the field of interventional cardiology every year.[3–5] Moreover, there is a continuous increase in the volume of imaging and other data within invasive cardiology, thereby making the use of electronic databases in the cardiac catheterization laboratory of paramount importance. Not surprisingly, the Centers for Medicare and Medicaid Services (CMS) called electronic health records (EHR) "the next step in continued progress of health care." Additionally, the American Recovery and Reinvestment Act of 2009 required the adoption of EHR and allowed CMS to incentivize the implementation and "meaningful use" of EHR.[6,7] Electronic catheterization records (ECRs) and data collection as a part of EHR can lead to better cardiac procedural outcomes and improved quality. Although

achieving better patient outcomes remains at the top of the priority list, state and national regulatory requirements, public reporting, and payers' interests in both outcomes and cost, raise the importance of quality measurement and improvement in the cardiac catheterization laboratory.

THE CONCEPT OF ELECTRONIC CATHETERIZATION RECORDS

The use of health information technology (HIT) has revolutionized the way medicine is practiced. Both people within and outside the health care system see HIT as a key component in improving the efficacy, quality, and safety of health care delivery. A number of recent studies have shown measurable benefits emerging from the adoption of HIT in health care.[8] Among the many types of information technology that have been adopted in the health care system over the past decades, EHR is arguably the most important. EHR symbolizes a technological advancement that not only has profound effects on day-to-day work of physicians, but also has a long-standing impact on the quality of care individual patients receive, in addition to being a rich resource for learning and medical research. EHR offers the potential to increase the involvement of patients in the active management of their own health care plan.[9,10]

Our health care system has entered a new phase where the focus on quality improvement is universal. ECR as a part of EHR can improve the efficacy of cardiac interventions and represent an important quality metrics tool. The American College of Cardiology (ACC), the American Heart Association (AHA), and the Society for Cardiac Angiography and Interventions (SCAI) have been committed to improving quality outcomes and carefully reviewing the available evidence to synthesize guidelines to better guide patient care.[4,5,11] Adherence to these guidelines is the foundation of improving quality in the cardiac catheterization laboratory. HIT can enhance this adherence by integrating evidence-based medicine into our daily practice in the catheterization laboratory. It has the potential to improve our ability to treat patients in a more efficient and cost-effective manner.

ELECTRONIC CATHETERIZATION RECORDS: STRUCTURED REPORTING

The ACC/AHA/SCAI 2014 Health Policy Statement on Structured Reporting for the Cardiac Catheterization Laboratory published a detailed report on the standard of structured reporting of cardiovascular catheterization data.[1] According to this statement, the key characteristics of a proper structured report are as follows: (1) it must be inclusive of all information relevant to both clinical care and operational administration; (2) it should be clear, concise, organized, and reproducible, as well as straightforward to cognitively assimilate and comprehend, while being sufficiently flexible to accommodate evolutionary changes in procedures and documentation requirements; (3) it should contain all the required elements for documenting

procedure indications and assessing appropriateness per local coverage determination rules and/or published appropriate use criteria (AUC);[5] (4) a consistent minimum dataset should be included in the content of each report, anticipating clinical, operational, regulatory, and financial uses of the data therein; and (5) the report should be devoid of extraneous content and be brief yet thorough.

The process of structured reporting

The process of structured reporting emphasizes the importance of not only standard formats of reports, but also integration of data acquisition with workflow to maximize the accuracy, completeness, and efficiency of procedural report generation.[1,12] The first tenet of structured reporting is that the entire process mandates the capture of information as discrete, defined, computable, and reusable data elements instead of dictated or typed (free text) prose. The physician operator is primarily responsible for interpretation, description, and documentation of results and findings (i.e., the "meaning" of the data). The physician also validates (and assumes responsibility for) data that others have entered throughout the sequence of events related to the catheterization. The data flow diagram for cardiovascular catheterization procedures is presented in Figure 55.1.[1]

The prototype formatted, tabular, structured procedure report

The ACC/AHA/SCAI 2014 Health Policy Statement on Structured Reporting for the Cardiac Catheterization

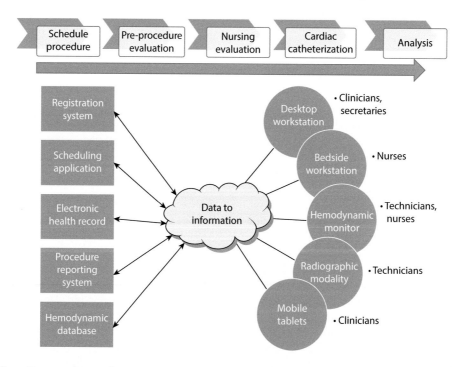

Figure 55.1 Data flow diagram for cardiovascular catheterization procedures. This diagram identifies sources, contributors, outputs, and users of data associated with cardiovascular catheterization procedures. (Reproduced from Sanborn, T.A., et al., *Circulation*, 129, 2578–2609, 2014. With permission.)

Laboratory provided a useful prototype for structured procedure reports.[1] The final catheterization procedure report is to be organized into three primary sections, with each section containing specific content (Table 55.1).[1] The first section should ideally consist of a single page of text in an easily understood layout that incorporates a focused summary of salient points of the case directed to the clinical community. All clinicians (spanning the spectrum from

Table 55.1 Organization of the structured catheterization procedure report

Header (top of summary page, top of details section)
- Facility information: health care entity, catheterization laboratory location
- Patient identifiers: name, medical record number, date of birth, age
- Procedure date
- Physician operator
- Referring provider(s)

Section 1: Summary page
1. Primary indication (*ICD* terminology)
2. History
   a. 1–3 sentences of prose describing circumstances of the presentation
3. Procedures (list of procedures, grouping individual procedures together by composite CPT code)
4. Procedure details
   a. Vascular access site(s)
      i. Sheath size, sheath status at end of procedure, vascular closure method
   b. Catheters *[diagnostic imaging/guide catheters]*
      i. Diagnostic
      ii. Intervention
   c. Diagnostic findings
      i. Findings, hemodynamics, calculations
   d. Interventions
      i. Target lesions: devices implanted, results
5. Adverse events
6. Medication and contrast totals
7. Impressions
   a. Prose listing of summary findings
8. Recommendations
   a. Prose listing of care recommendations

Section 2: Graphics and images
1. Diagram (graphical tree representation) of vascular anatomy, annotated
   a. Diagnostic findings
   b. Intervention results
2. Image capture
   a. Hemodynamic tracings
   b. Images ± annotations (embedded at a reduced resolution, with reference to DICOM image)

(Continued)

Table 55.1 (Continued) Organization of the structured catheterization procedure report

Section 3: Report body
1. Administrative information
   Patient
   - Patient full name, date of birth, age, gender
   - Race, ethnicity
   - Insurance
   - Medical record number
   - Case accession number (or other unique study ID)
2. Health care facility
   - Complete facility information: name of health care entity, catheterization location (laboratory), address, FAX number, phone number, laboratory accreditation
3. Operator, staff
   - Referring providers
   - Primary care provider
   - Cardiologist
   - Reason for request (ideally, replica of information received via EHR)
   - Procedure requested, date of request
   - Requestor
4. Encounter category
   - Elective, urgent, emergency, salvage (and subcategories)
5. History and physical
   - Symptom class
   - Medical history (risk factors-pertinent positives only, unless a negative finding is explicitly captured)
   - Family history (pertinent positives only)
   - Previous procedures and previous events, with pertinent results
   - Allergies and sensitivities
   - Physical examination (limited)
   - Laboratory values (limited: BMP, WBC, Hgb, Hct, platelet, PT, INR, PTT)
   - Procedure-indications (*ICD* terminology)
6. Procedure
   - Individual (component) procedures performed (as CPT codes, or using other standardized procedure terminology – these are not the aggregate procedures reported on the summary page)
   - Logistics (time in, time out, consent/sedation consents, timeout performed, final patient condition, and logistics)
   - Starting vital signs: BP, pulse
   - Access site (location(s), sheath(s) size and manufacturer, brand, other sheath information); sheath disposition at end of case, vascular hemostasis method
   - Anesthesia support (if applicable)

(Continued)

Table 55.1 (Continued) Organization of the structured catheterization procedure report

- Surgical support (if applicable)
- Hemodynamic support (if applicable)
  - Type of support: when initiated (e.g., elective at the start of the case, planned for the case, urgent in response to a complication), and disposition at end of case
7. Diagnostic findings
  - Diagnostic findings (organized by anatomic structure or physiologic function)
  - Equipment
  - Hemodynamic measurements, calculations (plus reference to DICOM Hemodynamics Report, if applicable)
  - Angiography findings, interpretations (plus reference to DICOM Quantitative Analysis Report, if applicable)
8. Intervention (grouped by anatomic target, if multiple lesions treated)
  - Equipment
  - Baseline anatomy
  - Devices deployed, device deployment parameters
  - Intervention results
9. Summaries
  - Medications in-lab (time-stamped)
  - Drips running at completion of case (if applicable)
  - Contrast type and total
  - Radiation exposure (fluoroscopy time, dose area product, cumulative air kerma, reference to DICOM Dose Report)
  - Estimated blood loss
  - Specimens removed
  - Final *ICD* diagnoses
  - Final procedure notes

Source: Reproduced from Sanborn, T.A., et al., *Circulation,* 129(24), 2578–2609, 2014. With permission.

Note: BMP, basic metabolic profile; BP, blood pressure; CPT, current procedural terminology; DICOM, digital imaging and communications in medicine; EHR electronic health records; Hct, hematocrit; Hgb, hemoglobin; ICD, International Classification of Diseases; INR, international normalized ratio; PT, prothrombin time; PTT, partial thromboplastin time; WBC, white blood cell.

the highly technical procedural cardiologists to nurses and other members of the clinical care team) should not have to look beyond this first page to understand the procedures performed, diagnostic findings, and management recommendations. The second section should focus on clinical images, including a computerized depiction of the observed anatomy, findings, and results. Optionally, captured images (with or without annotations) can be included in this section. Finally, the third section should contain more elaborate details of the procedure. This includes administrative data, the preprocedural history (particularly information captured as structured data), narrative description of the procedure itself, free-text descriptions of technical details, and other content relevant to the final procedure report.

Reporting of procedure and intervention details

All relevant events in the catheterization laboratory are to be captured in a time-stamped log, typically via the hemodynamic monitoring system of the laboratory. This includes the component parts of the diagnostic procedure as it is being performed, patient status and hemodynamics during the procedure, names and doses of medications administered, procedure-related observations and measurements, and other pertinent actions and events.

A dedicated section for interventions should explicitly separate diagnostic components from interventional procedures. The reporting in the intervention section is organized by the anatomic treatment target of the intervention. The standard layout paradigm of the intervention section is to describe the treatment target first, followed by the specific equipment used, parameters of that particular equipment, and the results of the intervention performed. The formats for the diagnostic procedures and intervention report's content are presented in Tables 55.2 and 55.3.

Extending the structured reporting use case

Professional societies in the field of cardiovascular medicine play a critical role in defining and establishing guidelines and performance metrics for various cardiovascular procedures. Comprising voluntary representatives, each society has the responsibility of establishing standards, norms, and expectations of professionalism for their members. The professional societies must lead the effort to establish standards in reporting of cardiovascular procedures. One critically important task is establishing a controlled vocabulary or terminology of relevant data elements for cardiovascular procedures. The individual terms selected for inclusion in this controlled vocabulary for the catheterization procedures must be clinically appropriate and relevant to both the patient and the procedure, and should have precise and mutually agreed upon definitions so that the elements have unambiguous shared meanings (i.e., semantic interoperability).

Closely linked with data element specification is determination of the data structure that combines individual elements into meaningful statements. Semantic interoperability is achieved by the combination of a controlled vocabulary as well as a data structure. Although these concepts may seem unfamiliar to clinicians, they are important for ensuring that data can be transmitted, received, and used as real information. In order to obtain compatibility with EHRs and operate across different computer networks, the standardized data elements and structures must meet technical language standards for interchange of data. The primary technical standard for procedural report structures

Table 55.2 Diagnostic procedures report content

For each procedure, the content listed under the header "Summary Page" corresponds to the content placed in Box 1 on the prototype report. Content listed under the header "Details Section" corresponds to the content placed in Box 3 on the prototype report.

Diagnostic: Right/left heart catheterization

- Summary page
  - Right heart catheterization
    - RA mean
    - RV systolic, diastolic, EDP
    - PA mean
    - PCW mean
    - AV O_2 diff
    - Cardiac output, cardiac index
    - Q_pQ_s [only if not 1.0]
    - PVR, SVR
- Details section
  - Right heart | right/left heart catheterization
  - Assessment conditions: baseline/rest; [challenge with vasoactive agent]
    - Patient height, weight, BSA
    - Patient blood pressure, heart rate
    - Inspired O_2
    - Vasoactive agent [intravenous vasodilator, inhaled vasodilator, vasopressor, inotrope]
  - Oxygen saturation (%)
    - Innominate
    - SVC
    - IVC
    - RA
    - RV
    - MPA
    - LPA
    - RPA
    - LA
    - Pulmonary vein
    - LV
    - Asc ao
    - Desc ao
  - Pressures (mmHg)
    - Hepatic wedge: mean
    - RA: a wave, v wave, mean
    - RV: systolic/diastolic, end diastolic
    - MPA: systolic/diastolic, mean
    - RPA: systolic/diastolic, mean
    - LPA: systolic/diastolic, mean
    - RPCW: a wave, v wave, mean
    - LPCW: a wave, v wave, mean
    - LV: systolic/diastolic, end diastolic
    - Asc ao: systolic/diastolic, mean
    - Desc ao: systolic/diastolic, mean

(Continued)

Table 55.2 (Continued) Diagnostic procedures report content

- Pressure gradients [specify mean/peak-peak/or both] (mmHg)
  - PCW-PA
  - RPA-MPA
  - LPA-MPA
  - MPA-RV
  - RV inflow-RV outflow
  - RV-RA
  - RA-hepatic wedge
  - LA-LV diastolic
  - LV inflow-LV outflow
  - LV-Asc ao
  - Asc ao-Desc ao
- Calculations
  - Hemoglobin: gm/dL
  - O_2 consumption: mL O_2/min
  - CO [method]: L/min
  - CI: L/min/m^2
  - AVO$_2$ diff: vol%
  - Q_p: L/min
  - Q_p index: L/min/m^2
  - Q_s: L/min
  - Q_s index: L/min/m^2
  - Q_p: Q_s
  - PVR: Wood units [or] dynes-sec/cm
  - SVR: Wood units [or] dynes-sec/cm
  - Valve area by [method]: cm^2

Diagnostic: Congenital disease angiography

- Summary page
  - Angiography of [structure]: summary findings
- Details section *(table)*
  - Structure, catheter, angles, findings
  - RA angiogram
  - Right ventriculogram
  - MPA angiogram
  - RPA angiogram
  - LPA angiogram
  - RPAW angiogram
  - LPAW angiogram
  - RUPV angiogram
  - Left ventriculogram
  - Ascending aortogram
  - Descending aortogram
  - Other angiogram [specify location, e.g., MAPCA, decompressing vein, collaterals]

Diagnostic: Left heart catheterization/left ventriculography/aortography

- Summary page
  - Pressures:
    - Aorta: systolic/diastolic, mean
    - Left ventricle: systolic/diastolic, LVEDP

(Continued)

Table 55.2 (Continued) Diagnostic procedures report content

- Left ventriculogram
  - Ejection fraction
  - LV segmental wall motion: [abnormal only; if none, then "normal"]
  - Mitral regurgitation: [grade]
  - Other findings: [describe]
- Details section
  - Pressures:
    - Aorta: systolic/diastolic, mean
    - Left ventricle: systolic/diastolic, LVEDP
  - Left ventriculogram
    - Ejection fraction
    - LV segmental wall motion: [table of all segments per the 5 segment model:
    - RAO includes anterior, apical, inferior; LAO includes septal, posterolateral segments]
    - Mitral regurgitation: [grade]
    - Other findings: [describe]
  - Aortogram
    - Findings: [describe]

Diagnostic: Coronary arteriography
- Summary page
  - Pressures:
    - Aorta: systolic/diastolic, mean
  - Coronary angiography (summary findings)
    - Dominance: [if not right dominant]
    - Left main: [normal, insignificant, or list of significant lesions]
    - Left anterior descending: [normal, insignificant, or list of significant lesions]
    - Left circumflex: [normal, insignificant, or list of significant lesions]
    - Right coronary: [normal, insignificant, or list of significant lesions]
    - Number of diseased vessels: [0, 1, 2, 3]
  - Graft angiography
    - Number of grafts (origins)
    - Number of distal anastomoses placed
    - Number of distal anastomoses patent
    - Significant graft lesions
- Details section
  - Coronary angiography(table)
    - Dominance
    - Artery-segment (size), % Stenosis descriptors, TIMI flow
  - Graft angiography (table)
    - Graft type-anastomosis, Segment, % Stenosis descriptors, TIMI flow
  - Adjunctive diagnostic assessment (table)
    - Modality Segment Findings
    - [FFR]
    - [IVUS]
    - [OCT]

Table 55.2 (Continued) Diagnostic procedures report content

Diagnostic: Peripheral arteriography
- Summary page
  - Peripheral vascular angiography (summary findings)
  - [Vessel/segment]: [normal, insignificant, or list of significant lesions]
  - Graft angiography: [normal, insignificant, or list of significant lesions]
  - Number of diseased leg vessel segments: [based on aorto-iliac, femoro-popliteal, and tibial-crural segmentation schema]
- Details section
  - Number of diseased leg vessel segments: [based on aorto-iliac, emoro-popliteal, and tibial-crural segmentation schema]
  - Peripheral vascular angiography (table)
    - Artery-segment, % stenosis, Lesion types
  - Graft angiography (table)
    - Graft type-anastomosis, Segment, % stenosis, Lestion type
  - Adjunctive imaging (table)
    - Modality, segment, findings
    - [IVUS]
    - [OCT]

Diagnostic: Cerebrovascular arteriography
- Summary page
  - Aortic arch type
  - Cerebrovascular angiography (summary of lesions in injected arteries): [normal, insignificant, or list of significant lesions]
- Details section
  - Aortic arch type (i.e., Types 1–3, bovine)
  - Hemispheric cross-filling
  - Cerebrovascular angiography (table)
    - Artery-segment, % stenosis, Lesion type

Source: Reproduced from Sanborn, T.A., et al., *Circulation*, 129(24), 2578–2609, 2014. With permission.
Note: ASC ao, ascending aorta; AV O2 diff, arteriovenous oxygen difference; BSA, body surface area; CI, cardiac index; CO, carbon monoxide; Desc ao, descending aorta; EDP, end diastolic pressure; FFR, fractional flow reserve; IVC, inferior vena cava; IVUS, intravascular ultrasound; LA, left atrium; LAO, left anterior oblique; LPA, left pulmonary artery; LPAW, left pulmonary artery wedge; LPCW, left pulmonary capillary wedge; LV, left ventricle; LVEDP, left ventricular end diastolic pressure; MAPCA, major aortopulmonary collateral artery; MPA, main pulmonary artery; OCT, optical coherence tomography; PA, pulmonary artery; PCW, pulmonary capillary wedge; PVR, pulmonary vascular resistance; Q$_P$; pulmonary blood flow; Q$_p$Q$_s$, pulmonary systemic flow ratio; Q$_S$, systemic blood flow; RA, right atrium; RAO, right anterior oblique; RPA, right pulmonary artery; RPAW, right pulmonary artery wedge; RPCW, right pulmonary capillary wedge; RUPV, right upper pulmonary vein; RV, right ventricle; SVC, superior vena cava; SVR, systemic vascular resistance.

(Continued)

Table 55.3 Intervention: Coronary artery disease

- Summary page
  - PCI of [coronary segment]
  - Devices: [type(s) of interventions—e.g., balloon angioplasty, atherectomy, stent implantation, aspiration thrombectomy, etc.]; stent—brand name, diameter × length, bare metal or drug-eluting, UDI; final balloon if no stent
  - Results: pre % stenosis to post % stenosis [pre TIMI flow to post TIMI flow, if either abnormal (i.e., not TIMI 3); no reflow]
- Details section
  - PCI of [coronary segment]
  - Intervention:
    - Guide catheters: manufacturer, Fr size, model
    - Guidewires: manufacturer, diameter, model
    - Devices: balloons—timing (pre vs. post stent implantation), diameter x length, max pressure × duration; other devices—with parameters; stent—manufacturer, brand name, diameter × length, max pressure × duration, bare metal or drug-eluting, UDI
  - Results: pre % stenosis to post % stenosis [pre TIMI flow to post TIMI flow, if either abnormal (i.e., not TIMI 3); no reflow]
  - Technical notes (analog text)

Intervention: Peripheral artery disease
- Summary page
  - PVI of [peripheral artery segment]
  - Devices: [type(s) of interventions—e.g., balloon angioplasty, atherectomy, stent implantation, etc.]; stent—brand name, diameter × length, bare metal or drug-eluting, UDI; final balloon if no stent
  - Results: pre % stenosis to post % stenosis [pre TIMI flow to post TIMI flow, if either abnormal (i.e., not TIMI 3)]
- Details section
- PVI of [peripheral artery segment]
  - Intervention:
    - Guide catheters: manufacturer, Fr size, model
    - Guidewires: manufacturer, diameter, model
    - Devices: balloons—timing (pre vs. post stent implantation), diameter x length, max pressure × duration; other devices—with parameters; stent—manufacturer, brand name, diameter × length, max pressure × duration, bare metal or drug-eluting, UDI
  - Results: pre % stenosis to post % stenosis [pre TIMI flow to post TIMI flow, if either abnormal (i.e., not TIMI 3)]
  - Technical notes (analog text)

Intervention: Cerebrovascular disease
- Summary page
  - PTA of [cerebrovascular artery segment]
  - Devices: [type(s) of interventions—e.g., balloon angioplasty, atherectomy, stent implantation]; embolism protection; stent—brand name, diameter × length, bare metal or drug-eluting, UDI
  - Results: pre % stenosis to post % stenosis
- Details section
- PTA of [cerebrovascular artery segment]
  - Intervention:
    - Guide catheters: manufacturer, Fr size, model
    - Guidewires: manufacturer, diameter, model
    - Devices: balloons—timing (pre versus post stent implantation), diameter x length, max pressure × duration; embolism protection—manufacturer, brand name, timing; other devices—with parameters; stent—manufacturer, brand name, diameter × length, max pressure × duration, bare metal or drug-eluting, UDI
  - Results: pre % stenosis to post % stenosis
  - Technical notes (analog text)

(Continued)

Table 55.3 (Continued) Intervention: Coronary artery disease

Intervention: Transcatheter aortic valve replacement (TAVR)
- Summary page
  - Intervention: valve—manufacturer, brand name, size; de novo or valve in valve
  - Results: mean gradient pre to mean gradient post; regurgitation post—grade and location (paravalvular, central)
- Details section
  - Angiography
    - Femoral artery angiogram: RFA/LFA, findings
    - Ascending aorta angiogram: findings
  - Aortic valve-baseline
    - Previous aortic valve bioprosthesis (make and size)
    - Dimensions by [CT/MR/echo]
      - Annulus (mm)
      - STJ (mm)
      - Sinus segment (mm)
    - Hemodynamic assessment
      - LV pressure
      - Asc aorta pressure
      - Peak-peak gradient, mean gradient
      - Valve area by [method]
      - Measurement condition: resting/inotrope and dose
  - Intervention
    - RV pacing
      - Rate
      - Timing: (when pacing used during procedure)
    - Balloon aortic valvuloplasty:
      - Guidewire: manufacturer, diameter, model
      - Balloon—manufacturer, brand name, diameter × length
      - Inflation duration (sec)
      - Inflation pressure (atm)
    - Transcatheter aortic valve replacement
      - Valve system—manufacturer, brand name, size
      - De novo or valve in valve
    - Maldeployment—present or absent; if present:
      - Valve embolization: LV or aortic
      - Management: open conversion, deployment in desc thoracic ao
  - Results:
    - Hemodynamic assessment
      - LV pressure
      - Asc aorta pressure
      - Peak-peak gradient, mean gradient
      - Valve area by [method]
      - Measurement condition: resting/inotrope and dose
    - Ascending aorta angiogram:
      - Paravalvular regurgitation: [none, 1+, 2+, 3+, 4+]
    - Iliac/femoral artery angiogram: findings
    - Transesophageal echocardiogram
      - Paravalvular regurgitation: [none, 1+, 2+, 3+, 4+]
      - Central regurgitation: [none, 1+, 2+, 3+, 4+]
- Access site closure
  - Closure method: open surgical, closure device—manufacturer, brand name
  - Angiogram: findings
  - Crossover technique
    - Sheath used—manufacturer, brand, size; balloon used—manufacturer, brand, size

(Continued)

Table 55.3 (Continued) Intervention: Coronary artery disease

Intervention: Congenital stenosis
- Summary page
  - Target: RPA, LPA, Coarcation, other stenosis [specify lesion]
  - Devices: [type(s) of interventions—e.g., balloon angioplasty, stent implantation]; stent—brand name, diameter × length, bare metal or covered, UDI
  - Results: gradient pre to gradient post; MLD pre to MLD post
- Details section
- Target: RPA, LPA, coarcation, other stenosis [specify lesion]
- Intervention:
  - Guide catheters: manufacturer, Fr size, model
  - Guidewires: manufacturer, diameter, model
  - Devices: balloons—timing (pre vs. post stent implantation), diameter × length, max pressure × duration; other devices—with parameters; stent—manufacturer, brand name, diameter × length, max pressure × duration, bare metal or covered, UDI
- Results: gradient pre to gradient post; MLD pre to MLD post; nominal (adjacent) diameter (PA stenosis); isthmus and descending ao @ diaphragm diameter (coarct)
- Technical notes (analog text)

Intervention: Valvuloplasty
- Summary page
  - Target: aortic valve, mitral valve, pulmonic valve, tricuspid valve
  - Devices: final balloon—diameter × length
  - Results: gradient pre to gradient post; MLD pre to MLD post
- Details section
  - Target: aortic valve, mitral valve, pulmonic valve, tricuspid valve; annulus diameter
  - Intervention:
    - Guide wires: manufacturer, diameter, model
    - Devices: balloons—diameter × length, max pressure × duration
  - Results: peak-peak gradient pre to post; mean gradient pre to post; valve area by [method] pre to post
    - Measurement condition, pre: resting/inotrope and dose
    - Measurement condition, post: resting/inotrope and dose
  - Technical notes (analog text)

Intervention: Defect closure
- Summary page
  - Target: ASD, PFO, PDA, VSD, fistula, other defect [specify defect]
  - Devices: closure device—brand name, size, UDI
  - Result: successful closure, unsuccessful closure
- Details section
  - Target: ASD, PDA, VSD, other defect [specify defect]
    - ASD characteristics:
      - ASD type
      - Size by echo (mm)
      - Size by balloon (mm)
      - Anterior rim, posterior rim, inferior rim, superior rim
    - PFO characteristics:
      - Size by echo (mm)
      - Size by balloon (mm)
    - PDA characteristics:
      - Size at pulmonic end (mm)
      - Length (mm)

(Continued)

Table 55.3 (Continued) Intervention: Coronary artery disease

- – VSD characteristics:
  - – VSD location
  - – VSD size (mm)
- – Aortopulmonary collateral:
  - – APC location
- – Coronary fistula
  - – Fistula location
- – Other abnormal conduit:
  - – Conduit location/description
- • Intervention:
  - – Guide catheters: manufacturer, Fr size, model
  - – Guidewires: manufacturer, diameter, model
  - – Devices: balloons—manufacturer, brand name, diameter × length; closure device—manufacturer, brand name, size, UDI
- • Results: successful closure, unsuccessful closure

Intervention: Cardiac biopsy
- • Summary page
  - • Biopsy: [location] × [# specimens]
- • Details section
  - • Biopsy: right ventricle [or other location]
    - – Guide catheter: manufacturer, Fr size, model
    - – Bioptome: manufacturer, model
    - – Number of specimens removed
    - – Pathology requisition number

Source: Reproduced from Sanborn, T.A., et al., *Circulation* 129(24), 2578–2609, 2014. With permission.
Note: Ao I, aorta; APC, aortopulmonary collateral; Asc, ascending; ASD, atrial septal defect; Atm, atmospheres; Desc, descending; Fr, French; LFA, left femoral artery; LPA, left pulmonary artery; L, left ventricle; MLD, minimum luminal diameter; PA, pulmonary artery; PCI, percutaneous coronary intervention; PDA, patent ductus arteriosus; PFO, patent foramen ovale; PTA, percutaneous transluminal angioplasty; PVI, peripheral vascular intervention; RFA, right femoral artery; RPA, right pulmonary artery; RV, right ventricle; Sec, seconds; STJ, sinotubular junction; TIMI, Thrombolysis in Myocardial Infarction; UDI, unique device identifier; VSD, ventricular septal defect.

is the HL7 Clinical Document Architecture (CDA) with terminology encoded using recognized vocabulary standards such as the SNOMED/CT, *International Classification of Diseases* (ICD)-9 , ICD-10, the Logical Observation Identifiers Names and Codes for laboratory values, and RxNorm for drugs and pharmacy systems. However, these systems are relatively incomplete for representing the complete depth and breadth of cardiovascular terminology, so stewardship of the controlled vocabulary of standardized data elements is required from professional cardiovascular societies. As primary performers and interpreters of different procedures, cardiologists must maintain close supervision of this specialized vocabulary. Other data element terminology coding systems will have to be mapped and cross-referenced with professional societies in order to ensure appropriate correspondences and reduce ambiguity. This entails collaboration to help establish and maintain the formal technical features required for vocabulary to be compatible with EHRs and have the ability to operate on multiple computer networks in the health care environment. An example of this is the International Society for Pediatric and Congenital Heart Disease—a multinational group founded in the year 2000, which is composed of cardiologists, cardiac surgeons, cardiac pathologists, and morphologists.

Since its inception, the group has been tasked with developing a common hierarchical coding structure of terms and definitions identified as the International Pediatric and Congenital Cardiac Code (IPCCC).[13,14] The IPCCC has been endorsed or adopted by a number of pediatric specialty societies in Europe and the United States. It requires constant interaction among all subgroups, with regular reviews and periodic revisions.

In the past, catheterization laboratory accreditation standards did not mandate structured reporting. However, in the 2012 Expert Consensus Document on Cardiac Catheterization Laboratory Standards, the recommendation was made that a structured report using standardized data elements should be finalized in a timely fashion following catheterization procedure completion.[3] The ACC- and SCAI-endorsed Accreditation for Cardiovascular Excellence program (http://www.cvexcel.org) requires the generation of structured reports as a criterion for accreditation. Similar criteria were established by the respective Intersocietal Commissions in echocardiography, nuclear cardiology, and cardiac magnetic resonance imaging (http://www.intersocietal.org). In conclusion, structured reporting must be considered an integral component of overall quality improvement, which is imperative for better cardiovascular care.

INTEGRATION OF ELECTRONIC CATHETERIZATION RECORDS TO REGISTRIES

Clinical registries are observational databases that provide detailed information about a patient population, a specific disease, or a clinical condition, therapy, or procedure. These can be utilized in estimating appropriateness of health care delivery and providing feedback to providers and health care organizations for gauging their performance at regional and national levels. The introduction of ECR has immensely helped the workflow and maintenance of clinical registries with their integrated software. Several larger health care organizations have integrated registries in their electronic medical record system. Computerized registries can also be used as a separate entity; however, they require manual entry of patient information into the system which can become labor intensive. Computerized procedure registries have made it easier for providers to graph outcomes in the catheterization laboratory, create reports, track their progress, and evaluate if they are meeting their guideline-directed goals. These also indirectly give feedback to providers regarding their adherence to guideline-recommended interventions.[15,16]

Cardiac catheterization–related registries

In an attempt to improve cardiovascular care by using clinical data from reliable institutions in the United States, the ACC developed the NCDR, the National Cardiovascular Data Registry, in the year 1997.[16,17] This has helped in gathering more data and assessing the utility of various management strategies at different institutional levels. The different registries that have been created for cardiovascular catheterizations are as follows:

1. The Cath PCI Registry: This registry collects data on both diagnostic catheterizations and percutaneous intervention (PCI) revascularization procedures. It also analyzes data on different characteristics of patients who receive PCI, appropriate adherence to established criteria and ACC/AHA guidelines, and the results of the procedures on patient outcomes.
2. The ICD Registry: CMS mandates all hospitals that perform implantable cardioverter defibrillator (ICD) implantation procedures to maintain an ICD Registry. This registry plays an important role in determining the association between evidence-based treatment strategies and clinical outcomes. This registry helps in creating a national standard for understanding different treatment patterns, clinical outcomes, device safety, and the overall quality of care provided to patients with ICDs.
3. The STS/ACC Transcatheter Valve Therapy (TVT) Registry: This registry was created for monitoring patient safety and outcomes related to transcatheter valve replacement and repair procedures for patients with valvular heart disease. The Society of Thoracic Surgeons (STS) and the ACC co-manage this registry with the same goal of achieving better clinical outcomes for transcatheter valvular procedures.

4. The Peripheral Vascular Intervention (PVI) Registry: This registry gathers information from the catheterization laboratory, radiology department, and outpatient vascular clinics on the prevalence, demographics, management, and outcomes of patients who have had carotid artery stenting, carotid endarterectomy, and peripheral lower extremity catheter interventions.
5. The LAAO Registry: This registry monitors the results of left atrial appendage occlusion (LAAO) with different closure devices. LAAO is a therapeutic option to prevent strokes in patients with nonvalvular atrial fibrillation who cannot be anticoagulated. The registry helps to maintain data on real-life clinical outcomes of this procedure, short and long-term safety, and cost-effectiveness.
6. The AFib Ablation Registry: This registry assesses the prevalence, demographics, outcomes, and acute management of patients with atrial fibrillation (AFib) ablation. Data gathered from this registry will help in the development of guidelines to improve clinical outcomes on ablation procedures for patients with Afib.

Role of registries and electronic catheterization records in quality care and reduction of health care costs

Rising health care costs have been a major concern for nations all over the world, and various strategies have been adopted by different countries to curb this. One of the major areas of interest for every health care managing body is to decrease health care costs, while achieving better patient outcomes. The primary objective, however, of all quality improvement endeavors, whether it be establishment of registries or ECR, is to practice evidence-based medicine that would lead to improved medical decision-making and better patient care. Registries provide an opportunity to institutions as well as researchers to monitor adherence to guideline-directed therapy. They have helped in reducing health care costs in many developed nations. Unfortunately, registries across the United States neither have a unique identifier number nor contain standard metrics even in the same specialty. This prevents researchers from integrating data, and as a result, there may be duplication of patient information. Recently, however, improved databases and registries have been developed under the guidance of medical societies. The Ontario Ministry of Health and Long-Term Care performed extensive analyses to derive a cost-effective model that accounted for a standardized pathway of care. They found that when left heart catheterization, PCI, and isolated coronary artery bypass graft (CABG) were compared, the maximum financial burden was for those patients who had a left ventricular ejection fraction of less than 50%, cardiogenic shock, intra-aortic balloon pump, or chronic obstructive pulmonary disease. It also showed that patient compliance had a direct impact on health care expenditure.[18] The Kaiser Permanente group developed the ICD and pacemaker, heart valve replacement, and endovascular stent graft registries. The implant registries, consisting of cardiac device implants, have been instrumental in improving quality, patient safety, and cost-effectiveness. These registries have helped to recall various devices and prevented serious complications. This has resulted in long-term patient safety and has ultimately reduced the cost burden from complications. These registries also guide in the purchase of implants in the future for improved patient outcomes.[19]

VETERANS AFFAIRS - CLINICAL ASSESSMENT REPORTING AND TRACKING: A POWERFUL EXAMPLE OF ELECTRONIC CATHETERIZATION RECORDS

A team of clinicians, health services researchers, and information technology developers designed the U.S. Department of Veterans Affairs (VA)-Clinical Assessment Reporting and Tracking (CART) program, which is a national clinical quality program for VA catheter laboratories.[20,21] The program began in 2005 and as of April 2014, contains data on 434,967 catheterization laboratory procedures, including 272,097 coronary angiograms and 86,481 PCIs performed by 801 clinicians on 246,967 patients. The foundation of the program is a clinical software application, which is integrated into the VA EHR. When any coronary procedure (i.e., diagnostic angiogram or PCI) in any VA catheterization laboratory is performed, patient and procedural data are recorded into the central database by clinicians. Data are automatically recorded in the EHR as a procedural note. In addition, this program is available for analysis to support quality-monitoring and research efforts, both locally and nationally. In order for the CART data to serve as a tool for future research and quality improvement, comprehensive and standardized data about both patients and procedures are needed. The CART software application enables standardized clinical data entry at the point of care using data elements and definitions from the ACC-NCDR. This synchronization of data elements permits direct comparisons between different VA sites, as well as comparisons between VA care and that of more than 1,500 non-VA medical centers that participate in the NCDR/CathPCI Registry. Regular communication between the CART program leadership, advisory committee of VA interventional cardiologists, NCDR, and "front-line" clinicians in the VA catheterization laboratories ensures that the system remains up to date. At the time of a catheterization procedure, clinicians record discrete data elements in the standardized data fields for both preprocedural and procedural clinical notes (Figure 55.2).[20] To maximize efficiency, information that is already available from the EHR, such as patient demographics, clinical history, medications, vital signs, and laboratory results, is automatically imported into the preprocedural note. After completion of the catheterization procedure, the clinician then enters procedural information and outcomes, again using the standardized data fields. Once completed, standardized and comprehensive preprocedural, cardiac catheterization, and/or PCI reports are immediately available in the EHR, thus providing "real-time" information to the primary care team.

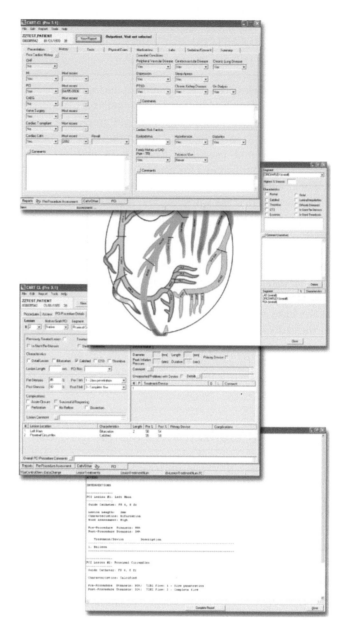

Figure 55.2 VA- CART user interface screen. (Reproduced from Maddox, T.M., et al., *Am. J. Cardiol.*, 114, 1750–1757, 2014. With permission.)

The CART program was implemented in 2004, and by the end of 2010, this program was used to record the procedural data on all coronary angiographies and interventions performed in all VA catheterization laboratories nationwide. By virtue of its design, the CART program establishes the foundation for high data quality in three important domains: data representativeness, completeness, and validity. As the CART program is embedded within the medical record for all VA patients receiving coronary procedures nationwide instead of a separate data registry, it captures complete data on the population it represents (i.e., of all veterans undergoing coronary procedures at any VA cardiac catheterization laboratory in the United States).

Data completeness in CART is facilitated by its user-friendly interface and the use of nationally established data standards for recording catheterization procedures.

Data validity in the CART system is optimized by the tight integration of CART and EHR into clinical workflow. CART's impact on data validity, completeness, and timeliness has resulted in significant improvements in data quality.[22] Initial quality-monitoring efforts using CART data focuses on mainly three areas: periodic feedback to individual catheterization laboratories for tracking and evaluation of procedures, peer review of major adverse events, and coronary device surveillance in association with the U.S. Food and Drug Administration (FDA). Using patient and procedural data, CART generates quality benchmark reports that are communicated to catheterization laboratory directors and leadership monthly for audit purposes. To monitor coronary devices, the CART application includes specific data fields to capture any unexpected device problems (UDPs) that occur during a catheterization procedure. If the investigation uncovers a potential quality or safety issue with the device, the CART coordination center then submits a formal report to the FDA's MedWatch reporting program.[23] As this program continues to develop, it can serve as a model for effective surveillance of medical device safety. The CART major adverse events program continually monitors VA catheterization laboratory procedures for any in-lab deaths, strokes, or need for emergency CABG surgeries that may occur. If a major adverse event occurs, a national committee of VA interventional cardiologists conducts a formal, protected peer review of the event. Reviewers are specifically directed to focus on system-level issues that may have led to the event and provide action items to correct any identified issues.

The VA-CART program is an innovative approach to EHR design that supports clinical care, quality, and safety in the catheterization laboratories. This novel approach holds promise in achieving the goals of a learning health care system.

Improvements on the horizon

Imitating the VA-CART program in other health care systems would require the commitment of EHR vendors, which have thus far focused more on market share than on making the programs work for clinicians. However, the ACC is now getting directly involved, and as a part of its strategic plan, the organization is working toward the development of a "digital platform" for education and decision-making, along with the creation of more standardized data fields that would be clinically meaningful to cardiologists.

CONTINUOUS QUALITY IMPROVEMENT MODEL

The continuous quality improvement (CQI) model is a proactive approach, which is designed to dynamically evaluate processes, procedural performance, outcomes, and most

importantly, to implement changes to improve them. The nascent concepts of the CQI model can be traced largely to techniques and ideas developed by pioneers within the industry.[24] Concepts central to this field focused on using data and statistics to reduce variation and focus, not merely on individuals, but also on processes. Examples of elements collected to track processes include door-to-balloon time, use of appropriate intervention strategy, or adherence to appropriate pharmacotherapy during PCI. The development of critical care pathways, collaborative efforts among emergency medical services, emergency department, and interventional cardiology personnel, and safety checklists and utilization of EHR are all examples of interventions that can be customized locally to profoundly impact patient care and process improvement.

APPROPRIATE USE OF CARDIAC CATHETERIZATION

Assessing the appropriateness of invasive catheterization techniques is challenging due to the complex nature of clinical case presentations and unique patient characteristics. Moreover, significant regional and operator-dependent variations in practice patterns exist.[5,25,26] Despite this, appropriate use criteria for coronary revascularization have been developed by professional organizations.[5] Adherence to these criteria should remain an area of focus for clinicians nationwide for demonstration of standardized quality in the catheterization laboratory. A standardized, transparent, and collaborative review of cases ensures that procedures are performed on patients who are likely to derive maximum benefit with least chances of adverse events. Data elements reflecting appropriate use criteria have been included in the most recent NCDR CathPCI Registry collection forms. Findings from this dataset suggest that there is room for improvement due to substantial variation across hospitals and a significant number of procedures classified as inappropriate. [5,25,26]

DISADVANTAGES OF ELECTRONIC CATHETERIZATION RECORDS

Despite the growing evidence on benefits of various ECR modalities, potential disadvantages associated with this technology have been identified.[1,27] These include high financial burden, changes in workflow, temporary loss of productivity associated with ECR adoption, privacy and security concerns, as well as several unintended consequences. Financial issues, such as adoption and implementation costs, ongoing maintenance costs, and loss of revenue associated with temporary loss of productivity, represent an impediment for hospitals and physicians to adopt and implement an ECR. ECR adoption and implementation costs include purchasing and installing hardware and software, converting paper charts to electronic ones, and training end-users. Costs for maintaining an ECR can also be significant. Hardware must be replaced and software needs to be upgraded on a regular basis. Institutions must provide ongoing training and support for end-users of an ECR. Another disadvantage of an ECR is disruption of workflow for medical staff and providers, which results in temporary losses in productivity.

CONCLUSION

EHR systems have the potential to transform health care from a mostly paper-based industry to one that utilizes intervention and related clinical and nonclinical data to assist providers in delivering a higher quality of care to their patients, in addition to being a powerful tool for medical research. In a primary health care setting, a computer-guided QI effort requiring minimal support improved cardiovascular disease risk measurement but did not increase prescription rates in the high-risk group.[28] ECR as a tool for data repository is intended to improve clinical care/communication, support local and national quality improvement, monitor patient safety, capture workload of cardiac catheterization lab procedures, and inform hospital systems to maximize operational efficiency and patient outcomes. The future of interventional cardiology in the United States is going to be centered around the use of ECR. Further integration of ECR with national registries is required, and nationwide implementation of ECRs is a necessary part in transforming the U.S. health care system. ECR adoption must be considered one of many approaches that diversify our focus on quality improvement and cost reduction. Overall, experts and policy-makers believe that significant benefits to patients and society can only be realized when ECRs are widely adopted and used in a meaningful way.

REFERENCES

1. Sanborn TA, et al. ACC/AHA/SCAI 2014 health policy statement on structured reporting for the cardiac catheterization laboratory: A report of the American College of Cardiology Clinical Quality Committee. *Circulation* 2014;129(24):2578–2609.
2. Klein LW, et al. Quality assessment and improvement in interventional cardiology: A position statement of the Society of Cardiovascular Angiography and Interventions, part 1: Standards for quality assessment and improvement in interventional cardiology. *Catheter Cardiovasc Interv* 2011;77(7):927–935.
3. Bashore TM, et al. 2012 American College of Cardiology Foundation/Society for Cardiovascular Angiography and Interventions expert consensus document on cardiac catheterization laboratory standards update. A report of the American College of Cardiology Foundation Task Force on Expert Consensus documents developed in collaboration with the Society of Thoracic Surgeons and Society for Vascular Medicine. *J Am Coll Cardiol* 2012;59(24):2221–2305.
4. Nallamothu BK, et al. ACC/AHA/SCAI/AMA-Convened PCPI/NCQA 2013 performance measures for adults undergoing percutaneous coronary intervention: A report of the American College of Cardiology/American Heart Association Task Force on Performance Measures, the Society for Cardiovascular Angiography and Interventions, the American Medical Association–Convened Physician Consortium for Performance Improvement, and the National Committee for Quality Assurance. *Circulation* 2014;129(8):926–949.
5. Patel MR, et al. ACCF/SCAI/STS/AATS/AHA/ASNC/HFSA/SCCT 2012 appropriate use criteria for coronary revascularization focused update: A report of the American College of Cardiology Foundation Appropriate Use Criteria Task Force, Society for Cardiovascular Angiography and Interventions, Society of Thoracic Surgeons, American Association for Thoracic Surgery, American Heart Association, American Society of Nuclear Cardiology, and the Society of Cardiovascular Computed Tomography. *J Thorac Cardiovasc Surg* 2012;143(4):780–803.
6. 111th United States Congress. *American Recovery and Reinvestment Act of 2009*. http://www.gpo.gov/fdsys/pkg/BILLS-111 hr1enr/pdf/BILLS-111hr1enr.pdf. Accessed March 16, 2016.
7. *An Introduction to the Medicare EHR Incentive Program for Eligible Professionals*. https://www.cms.gov/Regulations-and-Guidance/Legislation/EHRIncentivePrograms/downloads/beginners_guide.pdf. Accessed April 20, 2016.
8. Buntin MB, et al. The benefits of health information technology: A review of the recent literature shows predominantly positive results. *Health Aff (Millwood)* 2011;30(3):464–471.
9. Blumenthal D, Glaser JP. Information technology comes to medicine. *N Engl J Med* 2007;356(24):2527–2534.
10. Bates DW, et al. Effect of computerized physician order entry and a team intervention on prevention of serious medication errors. *JAMA* 1998;280(15):1311–1316.
11. Spertus JA, et al. American College of Cardiology and American Heart Association methodology for the selection and creation of performance measures for quantifying the quality of cardiovascular care. *Circulation* 2005;111(13):1703–1712.
12. Clunie D. *DICOM Structured Reporting*. PixelMed Publishing, Bangor, PA, 2000.
13. Bergersen L, et al. Report from The International Society for Nomenclature of Paediatric and Congenital Heart Disease: Cardiovascular catheterisation for congenital and paediatric cardiac disease (Part 1-Procedural nomenclature). *Cardiol Young* 2011;21(3):252–259.
14. Bergersen, et al. Report from The International Society for Nomenclature of Paediatric and Congenital Heart Disease: Cardiovascular catheterisation for congenital and paediatric cardiac disease (Part 2-Nomenclature of complications associated with interventional cardiology). *Cardiol Young* 2011;21(3):260–265.
15. Roumia M, Steinhubl S. Improving cardiovascular outcomes using electronic health records. *Curr Cardiol Rep* 2014;16(2):451.
16. ACC/NCDR Registries. http://cvquality.acc.org/en/NCDR-Home/Registries.aspx. Accessed May 27, 2016.
17. Brindis RG, et al. The American College of Cardiology-National Cardiovascular Data Registry (ACC-NCDR): Building a national clinical data repository. *J Am Coll Cardiol* 2001;37(8):2240–2245.

18. Cohen EA, et al. The cost drivers of care: A provincial cardiac registry-based costing analysis. *Can J Cardiol* 2014;30(10):s84–s85.

19. Paxton EW, et al. The Kaiser Permanente implant registries: Effect on patient safety, quality improvement, cost effectiveness, and research opportunities. *Perm J* 2012;16(2):36–44.

20. Maddox TM, et al. A national clinical quality program for Veterans Affairs catheterization laboratories (from the Veterans Affairs clinical assessment, reporting, and tracking program). *Am J Cardiol* 2014;114(11):1750–1757.

21. Box TL, et al. Strategies from a nationwide health information technology implementation: The VA CART story. *J Gen Intern Med* 2010;25 Suppl 1:72–76.

22. Byrd JB, et al. Data quality of an electronic health record tool to support VA cardiac catheterization laboratory quality improvement: The VA Clinical Assessment, Reporting, and Tracking System for Cath Labs (CART) program. *Am Heart J* 2013;165(3):434–440.

23. Kessler DA. Introducing MEDWatch. A new approach to reporting medication and device adverse effects and product problems. *JAMA* 1993;269(21):2765–2768.

24. Frey P, et al. Quality measurement and improvement in the cardiac catheterization laboratory. *Circulation* 2012;125(4):615–619.

25. Ko DT, et al. Regional variation in cardiac catheterization appropriateness and baseline risk after acute myocardial infarction. *J Am Coll Cardiol* 2008;51(7):716–723.

26. Chan PS, et al. Appropriateness of percutaneous coronary intervention. *JAMA* 2011;306(1):53–61.

27. Menachemi N, Collum TH. Benefits and drawbacks of electronic health record systems. *Risk Manag Healthc Policy* 2011;4:47–55.

28. Peiris D, et al. Effect of a computer-guided, quality improvement program for cardiovascular disease risk management in primary health care: The treatment of cardiovascular risk using electronic decision support cluster-randomized trial. *Circ Cardiovasc Qual Outcomes* 2015;8(1):87–95.

Index